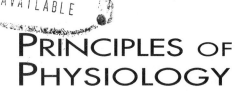

PRINCIPLES OF PHYSIOLOGY

This book is to be returned on or before
the last date stamped below.

PRINCIPLES OF PHYSIOLOGY

ROBERT M. BERNE, MD, DSC (HON)

Professor Emeritus
Department of Molecular Physiology and Biological Physics
University of Virginia Health Sciences Center
Charlottesville, Virginia

MATTHEW N. LEVY, MD

Senior Scientist, Rammelkamp Center;
Professor Emeritus of Physiology and Biomedical Engineering
Case Western Reserve University
Cleveland, Ohio

third edition

with 626 illustrations

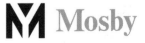

St. Louis Baltimore Boston Carlsbad Chicago Minneapolis New York Philadelphia Portland
London Milan Sydney Tokyo Toronto

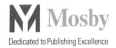

Project Manager: Carol Sullivan Weis
Project Specialist: Pat Joiner
Designer: Jen Marmarinos
Cover Photo: © PhotoDisc, Inc.

third edition

Mosby, Inc.
A Harcourt Health Sciences Company
11830 Westline Industrial Drive
St. Louis, Missouri 63146

Printed in the United States

Library of Congress Cataloging in Publication Data

Principles of physiology / editors, Robert M. Berne, Matthew N. Levy.
— 3rd ed.
        p.   cm.
    Includes bibliographical references and index.
    ISBN 0-323-00813-5
    1. Human physiology.   I. Berne, Robert M., 1918–   .   II. Levy,
Matthew N., 1922–   .
    [DNLM: 1. Physiology.   QT 104 P957 1999]
QP34.5.P744   1999
612—dc21
DNLM/DLC
for Library of Congress   99-19992
                                                            CIP

99 00 01 02 03 CL/KPT 9 8 7 6 5 4 3 2 1

Contributors

ROBERT M. BERNE, MD, DSc (HON)
Professor Emeritus
Department of Molecular Physiology and Biological
  Physics
University of Virginia Health Sciences Center
Charlottesville, Virginia
Part IV, Cardiovascular System

MARIO CASTRO, MD, MPH
Assistant Professor of Medicine
Pulmonary and Critical Care Medicine
Washington University School of Medicine;
Director, Pulmonary Function Lab
St. Louis, Missouri
Part V, Respiratory System

SAUL M. GENUTH, MD
Professor of Medicine
Division of Clinical and Molecular Endocrinology
Case Western Reserve University
Cleveland, Ohio
Part VIII, Endocrine System

BRUCE M. KOEPPEN, MD, PhD
Professor of Medicine and Physiology
Dean, Academic Affairs and Education
University of Connecticut Health Center
Farmington, Connecticut
Part VII, Renal System

HOWARD C. KUTCHAI, PhD
Professor
Department of Molecular Physiology and Biological
  Physics
University of Virginia School of Medicine
Charlottesville, Virginia
Part I, Cellular Physiology
Part VI, Gastrointestinal System

MATTHEW N. LEVY, MD
Senior Scientist, Rammelkamp Center;
Professor Emeritus of Physiology and Biomedical
  Engineering
Case Western Reserve University
Cleveland, Ohio
Part IV, Cardiovascular System

RICHARD A. MURPHY, PhD
Professor
Department of Molecular Physiology and Biological
  Physics
University of Virginia Health Sciences Center
Charlottesville, Virginia
Part III, Muscle

BRUCE A. STANTON, PhD
Professor
Department of Physiology
Dartmouth Medical School
Hanover, New Hampshire
Part VII, Renal System

WILLIAM D. WILLIS, JR., MD, PhD
Professor and Chairman
Department of Anatomy and Neurosciences
Cecil H. and Ida M. Green Chair and Director
Marine Biomedical Institute
University of Texas Medical Branch
Galveston, Texas
Part II, Nervous System

Reviewers

BEAU M. ANCES
Senior Medical Student
University of Pennsylvania
Philadelphia, Pennsylvania

SAMUEL C. BLACKMAN
MD/PhD Candidate
University of Illinois College of Medicine
Chicago, Illinois

TONY CHU
Medical Student
Yale University School of Medicine
New Haven, Connecticut

ELIZABETH M. GEGRUERS, MSc, PhD
Statutory Lecturer in Physiology
National University of Ireland–Cork
Cork, Ireland

LOREN W. KLINE, PhD
Professor
Department of Dentistry
Department of Physiology
University of Alberta
Edmonton, Alberta, Canada

EDWARD K. STAUFFER, PhD
Associate Professor
Department of Medical and Molecular Physiology
University of Minnesota
Duluth, Minnesota

To Alex, Ari, Chris, Daniel, Kyle, Madelyn, Maggie,
Molly, Nicholas, Sarah, Todd, and Tracy

Preface

The third edition of *Principles of Physiology* has been designed to clearly and concisely present the important features of mammalian physiology. General principles and underlying mechanisms are emphasized, and nonessential details are minimized. The first section of the text is devoted to cell physiology, which serves as the basis for body functions. Furthermore, the relevant cell physiology has been included in each of the succeeding sections. We have tried to show that these basic processes generally operate in the different cell types in the various organ systems.

The major emphasis in this book is on regulation. The mechanisms that regulate the individual organ systems are thoroughly described. These mechanisms are then applied to the complex interactions among the systems as they maintain the internal environment constant, a process that is so important for optimal function.

Each chapter begins with a list of objectives and a brief paragraph that denotes the relationship between that chapter and the chapters that immediately precede and follow it. Multicolored illustrations are used to depict concepts as simply as possible. When sequential mechanisms are involved, multipaneled diagrams have been designed to illustrate each step clearly. Block diagrams are used to depict the interrelationships among the various factors that may affect a specific function. Important data are accumulated in tables, and glossaries are included in sections in which many abbreviations and symbols are used.

The use of mathematics has been minimized, and succinct lucid descriptions have been substituted wherever feasible. Controversial issues have been omitted to allow ample room for the explanation of important, generally accepted physiological mechanisms. We have refrained from citing the sources of the statements or assertions that appear in the text to keep nonessential details to a minimum. Throughout the book, we have used small capital letters to emphasize important concepts, and we have used boldface to denote new terms and definitions. We have also emphasized many of the important physiological concepts by describing important clinical conditions in which such concepts are relevant. These clinical illustrations are framed in yellow rectangles.

Summaries are provided at the end of each chapter to highlight the key points in the chapter, and brief bibliographies are included to direct the student to more detailed information. The references listed in these bibliographies are mainly review articles or recent, relevant scientific papers. Also, at the end of each chapter, we have included a number of multiple-choice review questions based on illustrative clinical case studies. Answers with explanations are given at the end of the book. These questions and answers can help readers evaluate their comprehension of the material covered in the text and help in linking physiological concepts and mechanisms to clinical situations.

ROBERT M. BERNE
MATTHEW N. LEVY

Contents

Part II   Nervous System
William D. Willis, Jr.

Part III   Muscle
Richard A. Murphy

Part IV Cardiovascular System
Robert M. Berne
Matthew N. Levy

Part VIII   Endocrine System
Saul M. Genuth

PRINCIPLES OF PHYSIOLOGY

Introduction

As the reader embarks on the study of human physiology, it is instructive to briefly consider what physiology is and how it relates to other disciplines.

Physiology and anatomy originated in the western world with the ancient Greeks, and for centuries, they were the only recognized basic biomedical sciences. More recently, physiology and anatomy, together with biology, chemistry, physics, psychology, and other sciences, have given rise to other biomedical disciplines whose areas of inquiry overlap to a considerable degree. Among the newer biomedical sciences are biochemistry, genetics, pharmacology, biophysics, molecular biology, cell biology, neuroscience, and biomedical engineering. Because the overlap among the interests of the different biomedical sciences is so extensive, it is often difficult and sometimes not even useful to decide where one discipline begins and the other ends.

Physiology may be distinguished from the other basic biomedical sciences by its concern with the function of the intact organism and its emphasis on the processes that control and regulate important properties of living systems. In the healthy human, many variables are actively maintained within narrow physiological limits. The list of controlled variables is long; it includes body temperature, blood pressure, blood glucose levels, the oxygen and carbon dioxide contents of blood, and a host of other properties. The tendency to maintain the relative constancy of important variables, even in the face of significant environmental changes, is known as **homeostasis.** A central goal of physiological research is the elucidation of the mechanisms responsible for homeostasis.

In studying a homeostatic mechanism, physiologists attempt to characterize the components of the control system. What is the **sensor** that detects the difference between a physiological variable and its **set point?** How does the sensor operate? What is the **integrating center** that receives information from the sensor via **afferent pathways** and communicates with effectors by **efferent pathways?** The afferent and efferent pathways frequently involve nerves or hormones. What effectors function to bring the level of the controlled variable closer to its set point? The **steady-state value** of a controlled variable typically results from a dynamic balance among certain effectors that increase the value of the variable and other effectors that act to decrease it.

Mankind is in the midst of an explosion of knowledge of biological systems. This information expansion is characterized by greater understanding of the behavior of individual cells and of the molecules that make up those cells. The precise nucleotide sequences of many thousands of genes have been determined. The physiological regulation of the oxygen affinity of the blood is understood in terms of precise knowledge of conformational changes in the hemoglobin molecule. The structures of certain ion channels and the nature of the processes by which the channels open and close are being precisely determined. The mechanisms that control important variables in individual cells, such as the level of free Ca^{++} in cytosol, are being elucidated in great detail.

The methods of modern cellular and molecular biology, including the ability to manipulate the genomes of specific types of cells in the body, have enhanced the ability to characterize the cells and molecules involved in physiological processes. Partly because of the power of these methods for characterizing molecules and cells, many physiologists now study biological processes at the level of single cells or even of single molecules to explain their functions in vivo. Scientists in related disciplines also concentrate inquiries on the behavior of cells and biological molecules. What distinguishes physiology as a scientific discipline is its emphasis on homeostatic mechanisms at all levels of organization and its concern with synthesizing knowledge of the functions of tissues, cells, and molecules to achieve a more complete understanding of the behavior of the intact organism.

This textbook describes what is now known about the function of the major organ systems of mammals and the mechanisms that control and regulate their behavior. Physiological knowledge is being broadened continually and especially deepened. "The fabric of knowledge is being continually woven, and altered by the introduction of new threads, the texture and device even are mobile, yet it is the object of a comprehensive work to attempt to capture the fleeting pattern. That the design is of growing complexity, and less and less easy of discernment, may be matter for regret though not for surprise."* In an attempt to "capture the fleeting pattern," the authors have tried to describe important physiological processes and their mechanisms of control. They have also tried to integrate the descriptions of individual organ systems and homeostatic mechanisms to provide a broad appreciation of the physiological function of the whole organism. The authors hope that this text will stimulate its readers to actively pursue the study of physiology.

---

*Evans CL: Preface. In Evans CL, Hartridge H, eds: *Starling's principles of human physiology,* ed 7, Philadelphia, 1936, Lea & Febiger.

CELL PHYSIOLOGY

I

Howard C. Kutchai

CHAPTER 1

Cellular Membranes and Transmembrane Transport of Solutes and Water

OBJECTIVES

- Describe the "fluid mosaic model" of biological membranes.
- Estimate the rate of diffusion across a membrane using Fick's first law.
- State and apply van't Hoff's law to estimate the osmotic pressure of an electrolyte solution.
- Explain the ability of a solute to cause osmotic water flow across a membrane in relation to the permeability of the membrane for that solute.
- List the properties of facilitated and active transport.
- Define transcellular and paracellular transport across an epithelium.

The section on cellular physiology (see Chapters 1 to 5) discusses aspects of the functioning of individual cells that are later applied in the context of various organ systems. Each cell is surrounded by a plasma membrane that separates it from the extracellular milieu. Cellular organelles, such as the nucleus, mitochondria, Golgi apparatus, and endoplasmic reticulum, are bounded by membranes or contain multiple types of membranes. This chapter considers the basic structure and properties of biological membranes and some of the processes whereby molecules are transported across membranes. Chapters 2 and 3 present the basic properties of electrically excitable cells, such as neurons and muscle cells, and Chapter 4 discusses the means whereby electrical signals are communicated between cells. Chapter 5 explains the signal-transduction mechanisms whereby extracellular regulatory molecules, such as hormones, influence cellular processes.

Membranes

Membranes divide the cell into compartments with specific biochemical functions

The plasma membrane serves as a permeability barrier that allows the cell to maintain a cytoplasmic composition far different from the composition of the extracellular fluid. The plasma membrane contains enzymes, receptors, and antigens that play central roles in the interaction of the cell with other cells and with hormones and other regulatory agents in the extracellular fluid.

The membranes that enclose the various organelles divide the cell into discrete compartments and allow the localization of particular biochemical processes in specific organelles. Many vital cellular processes take place in or on the membranes of the organelles. Striking examples are the processes of electron transport and oxidative phosphorylation, which occur on, within, and across the mitochondrial inner membrane.

Most biological membranes have certain features in common. However, in keeping with the diversity of membrane functions, the composition and structure of the membranes differ from one cell to another and among the membranes of a single cell.

The lipid bilayer matrix of membranes is a barrier to the permeability of most substances

Proteins and phospholipids are the most abundant constituents of cellular membranes. A **phospholipid** molecule has a polar head group and two very nonpolar, hydrophobic fatty acyl chains (Figure 1-1, *A*). In an aqueous environment, phospholipids tend to form structures that allow the fatty acyl chains to be kept away from contact with water. One such structure is the **lipid bilayer** (Figure 1-1, *B*). Many phospholipids, when dispersed in water, spontaneously form lipid bilayers. Most of the phospholipid molecules in biological membranes have a lipid bilayer structure.

The phospholipid bilayer is responsible for certain passive permeability properties of biological membranes. Substances that are highly soluble in water typically permeate cellular membranes very slowly, whereas nonpolar compounds that are more soluble in nonpolar organic solvents cross cell membranes more rapidly. High concentrations of barium salts are administered by mouth or by enema to make the interior of the gastrointestinal tract opaque to x rays and improve the contrast of diagnostic x-ray films

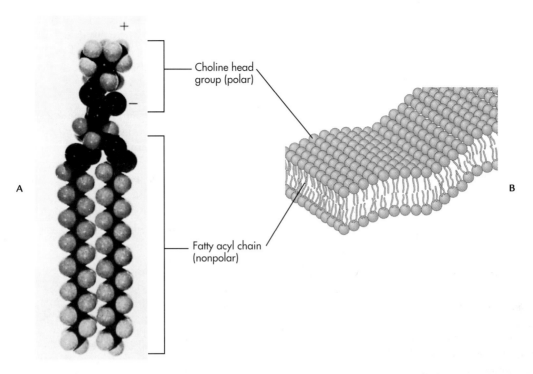

Figure 1-1 A, Structure of a membrane phospholipid molecule, in this case phosphatidylcholine. **B,** Structure of a phospholipid bilayer. The blue spheres represent the polar head groups of the phospholipid molecules. The wavy lines represent the fatty acyl chains of the phospholipids.

of the gastrointestinal tract. Barium ions in this concentration would be highly toxic, but because barium is highly water soluble and insoluble in the hydrophobic interior of membranes, it is barely absorbed from the gastrointestinal tract. Hence the concentration of barium in the blood rises very little after the administration of barium salts.

Most membranes are a "fluid mosaic" of phospholipids and proteins

Figure 1-2 depicts the **fluid mosaic model** of membrane structure. This model is consistent with many of the properties of biological membranes. Note the bilayer structure of most of the membrane phospholipids. There are two major classes of membrane proteins: (1) **integral** or **intrinsic membrane proteins** that are embedded in the phospholipid bilayer and (2) **peripheral** or **extrinsic membrane proteins** that are associated with the surface of the membrane. The peripheral membrane proteins interact with the membrane predominantly by charge interactions with integral membrane proteins. Thus peripheral proteins may often be removed from the membrane by altering the ionic composition of the medium. Integral membrane proteins have important hydrophobic interactions with the interior of the membrane.

These hydrophobic interactions can be disrupted only by detergents that make the integral proteins soluble by interacting hydrophobically with nonpolar amino acid side chains. Cellular membranes are fluid structures in which

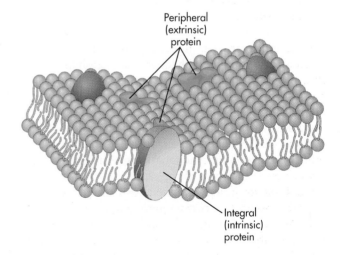

Figure 1-2 Fluid mosaic model of membrane structure. The integral proteins *(pink)* are embedded in the lipid bilayer matrix of the membrane, and the peripheral proteins *(green)* are associated with the external surfaces of integral membrane proteins.

many of the constituent molecules are free to diffuse in the plane of the membrane. Most lipids and proteins can move freely in the bilayer plane, but they "flip-flop" from one phospholipid monolayer to the other at much slower rates. A large hydrophilic moiety is unlikely to flip-flop if it must be dragged through the nonpolar interior of the lipid bilayer.

In some cases, membrane components are not free to diffuse in the plane of the membrane. Examples of this motional constraint are the sequestration of acetylcholine receptors (integral membrane proteins) at the motor endplate of skeletal muscle and the presence of different membrane proteins in the apical and basolateral plasma membranes of epithelial cells. The cytoskeleton appears to tether certain membrane proteins. The **anion exchanger,** a major protein of the human erythrocyte membrane, is bound to the **spectrin** network that undergirds the membrane via a protein called **ankyrin.**

If the motor nerve that innervates a skeletal muscle is accidentally severed, the acetylcholine receptors are no longer sequestered at the motor endplate; instead, they spread over the entire plasma membrane of the muscle cells. Then the entire surface of the cell becomes excitable by acetylcholine, a phenomenon known as **denervation supersensitivity.**

Membrane Composition

Phospholipids and cholesterol are the major lipid components of membranes

Choline-containing phospholipids and aminophospholipids are the most prevalent phospholipid classes

In animal cell membranes the most abundant phospholipids are often the choline-containing phospholipids: the lecithins (phosphatidylcholines) and the sphingomyelins. Often next in abundance are the amino phospholipids: phosphatidylserine and phosphatidylethanolamine. THE PHOSPHOLIPID BILAYER IS RESPONSIBLE PRIMARILY FOR THE PASSIVE PERMEABILITY PROPERTIES OF THE MEMBRANE. Other important phospholipids present in smaller amounts are phosphatidylglycerol, phosphatidylinositol, and cardiolipin.

Certain phospholipids present in tiny proportions in the plasma membrane play a vital role in cellular signal-transduction processes. **Phosphatidylinositol bisphosphate,** when cleaved by a receptor-activated phospholipase C, releases **inositol 1,4,5-trisphosphate (IP$_3$)** and **diacylglycerol.** IP$_3$ is released into the cytosol, where it acts on receptors in the endoplasmic reticulum to cause the release of stored Ca^{++}, an action that affects a wide variety of cellular processes (see Chapter 5). Diacylglycerol remains in the plasma membrane, where it participates, along with Ca^{++}, in activating **protein kinase C,** an important signal-transduction protein.

Cholesterol serves as a "fluidity buffer" in membranes

Cholesterol is a major constituent of plasma membranes, and its steroid nucleus lies parallel to the fatty acyl chains of membrane phospholipids. Cholesterol functions as a "fluidity buffer" in the plasma membrane

in that its presence tends to keep the fluidity of the acyl chain region of the phospholipid bilayer in an intermediate range in the presence of agents that tend to fluidize biological membranes, such as alcohols and general anesthetics.

Outward-facing carbohydrate moieties of glycolipids and glycoproteins serve as receptors and antigens

Glycolipids are not abundant but have important functions. They are found mostly in plasma membranes, where their carbohydrate moieties protrude from the external surface of the membrane. The carbohydrate parts of glycolipids frequently function as receptors or antigens.

The receptor for cholera toxin (see Chapter 34) is the carbohydrate moiety of a particular glycolipid, ganglioside (GM$_1$). The A and B blood group antigens (see Chapter 16) are the carbohydrate moieties of other gangliosides on the human erythrocyte membrane.

Phospholipids are distributed asymmetrically between the inner and outer lipid monolayers of the membrane

In many membranes the lipid components are not distributed uniformly across the bilayer. The glycolipids of the plasma membrane are located almost exclusively in the outer monolayer. Phospholipids are also distributed asymmetrically between the inner and outer monolayers of membranes. In the red blood cell membrane, for example, the outer (extracellular) monolayer contains most of the choline-containing phospholipids, whereas the inner monolayer contains most of the amino phospholipids.

Membrane proteins are enzymes, transporters, and receptors

The protein composition of membranes may be simple or complex. The functionally specialized membranes of the sarcoplasmic reticulum of skeletal muscle and the discs of the rod outer segment of the retina contain only a few different proteins. In contrast, plasma membranes, which perform many functions, may have more than 100 different protein constituents. Membrane proteins include enzymes, transport proteins, and receptors for hormones and neurotransmitters.

Membrane glycoproteins mediate interactions with the extracellular matrix

Some membrane proteins are glycoproteins with covalently bound carbohydrate side chains. As with glycolipids, the carbohydrate chains of glycoproteins are located almost exclusively on the extracellular surfaces of plasma membranes. The carbohydrate moieties of membrane glycoproteins and glycolipids have important functions. The negative surface charge of cells is caused by the negatively charged sialic acid of glycolipids and glycoproteins.

Fibronectin is a large fibrous glycoprotein that helps cells attach, via cell surface glycoproteins called **integrins,** to proteins of the extracellular matrix. This link mediates communication between the extracellular matrix and the cell's cytoskeleton.

> The major membrane proteins of enveloped viruses are glycoproteins. Their carbohydrate moieties stud the outer surface of the virus with "spikes" that are required for the virus to bind to a host cell.

Membrane proteins have a specific orientation in the membrane

The Na^+,K^+-ATPase of the plasma membrane and the Ca^{++} pump protein (Ca^{++}-ATPase) of the sarcoplasmic reticulum membrane are examples of the asymmetrical disposition of membrane proteins. In both cases, ATP is split on the cytoplasmic face of the membrane, and some of the energy liberated is used to pump ions in specific directions across the membrane. In the case of Na^+,K^+-ATPase, K^+ is pumped into the cell, and Na^+ is pumped out, whereas the Ca^{++}-ATPase actively pumps Ca^{++} into the sarcoplasmic reticulum. Both of these ion-transporting ATPases are disposed in the membrane so that the part of the protein responsible for binding ATP is on the cytosolic side of the membrane.

Membranes as Permeability Barriers

Membranes are impermeable to most water-soluble substances

Biological membranes serve as **permeability barriers.** Most of the molecules present in living systems are highly soluble in water and poorly soluble in nonpolar solvents. Such molecules are poorly soluble in the nonpolar environment in the interior of the lipid bilayer of biological membranes. Consequently, BIOLOGICAL MEMBRANES POSE A FORMIDABLE BARRIER TO THE DIFFUSION OF MOST WATER-SOLUBLE MOLECULES. The plasma membrane is a permeability barrier between the cytoplasm and the extracellular fluid. For many substances, this barrier allows the maintenance of large concentration differences between the cytoplasm and the extracellular fluid.

The localization of various cellular processes in certain organelles depends on the barrier properties of cellular membranes. For example, the inner mitochondrial membrane is impermeable to the enzymes and substrates of the tricarboxylic cycle; thus it allows the localization of this cycle in the mitochondrial matrix. The spatial organization of chemical and physical processes in the cell depends on the barrier functions of cellular membranes, much as the walls in a house separate rooms with different functions.

The passage of important molecules across membranes at controlled rates is central to the life of the cell. Examples are the uptake of nutrient molecules, the discharge of waste products, and the release of secreted molecules. As discussed in the next section, molecules may move from one side of a membrane to another without actually moving through the membrane itself. In other cases, molecules cross a particular membrane by passing through or between the molecules that make up the membrane.

Material may cross membranes without passing among the molecules that make up the membrane

Cells take up small samples of the extracellular medium via endocytosis

Endocytosis, a process that allows material to enter the cell without passing through the membrane (Figure 1-3), includes **phagocytosis** and **pinocytosis.** The uptake of particulate material is termed phagocytosis (Figure 1-3, *A*). The uptake of soluble molecules is called pi-

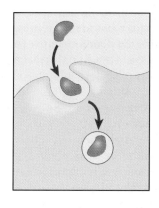 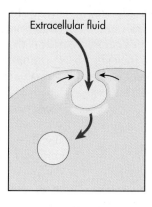 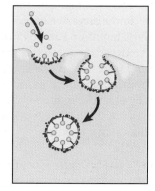

Extracellular fluid

A   B   C

Figure 1-3 Endocytotic processes. **A,** Phagocytosis of a solid particle. **B,** Pinocytosis of extracellular fluid. **C,** Receptor-mediated endocytosis by coated pits.

nocytosis (Figure 1-3, *B*). Sometimes, special regions of the plasma membrane are involved in endocytosis. In these regions the cytoplasmic surface of the plasma membrane is covered with bristles made primarily of a protein called **clathrin.** These clathrin-covered regions are called **coated pits,** and their endocytosis gives rise to coated vesicles. The coated pits are involved in receptor-mediated endocytosis (Figure 1-3, *C*). Proteins to be taken up are recognized and bound by specific membrane receptor proteins in the coated pits. The binding often leads to aggregation of receptor-ligand complexes, and the aggregation triggers endocytosis. Endocytosis is an active process that requires metabolic energy. Endocytosis can also occur in regions of the plasma membrane that do not contain coated pits.

Most cells cannot synthesize cholesterol, which is needed for the synthesis of new membranes (see Chapter 41). Cholesterol is carried in the blood, predominantly in low-density lipoproteins (LDLs). Many cells have LDL receptors in their plasma membranes. When LDL binds to these receptors, the receptor-LDL complexes migrate to coated pits, where they aggregate and are taken into the cell by receptor-mediated endocytosis. Individuals who lack LDL receptors have high levels of cholesterol-laden LDL in the blood. Consequently, such individuals tend to develop arterial disease **(atherosclerosis)** at an early age, which makes them more likely to experience heart attacks prematurely.

Certain substances are extruded from cells by exocytosis

Molecules can be ejected from cells by **exocytosis,** a process that resembles endocytosis in reverse. The release of neurotransmitters, which is considered in more detail in Chapter 4, takes place by exocytosis. Exocytosis is responsible for the release of secretory proteins by many cells; the release of pancreatic enzymes from the acinar cells of the pancreas is a well-studied example. The pancreatic enzymes play vital roles in the digestion of protein, carbohydrates, and lipids (see Chapters 33 and 34). In such cases the proteins to be secreted are stored in secretory vesicles in the cytoplasm. A stimulus to secrete causes the secretory vesicles to fuse with the plasma membrane and to release the vesicle contents by exocytosis.

Vesicle fusion allows the mixing of vesicular contents

The contents of one type of organelle can be transferred to another type by fusion of the membranes of the organelles. In some cells, secretory products are transferred from the endoplasmic reticulum to the Golgi apparatus by the fusion of the vesicles of the endoplasmic reticulum with the

membranous sacs of the Golgi apparatus. The fusion of phagocytic vesicles with lysosomes allows the phagocytosed material to be digested by proteolytic enzymes in the lysosomes. The turnover of many normal cellular constituents involves their destruction in lysosomes, followed by their resynthesis.

Influenza viruses have membrane proteins that undergo a dramatic conformational change to insert a "fusion peptide" into the host cell. The fusion peptide promotes the fusion of the viral membrane with the plasma membrane of the host cell, allowing entry of the viral genome into the host cell.

The Transport of Molecules through Membranes Occurs by Diffusion, Osmosis, and Protein-Mediated Processes

The traffic of molecules through biological membranes is vital for most cellular processes. Some molecules move through biological membranes simply by diffusing among the molecules that make up the membrane, whereas the passage of other molecules involves the mediation of specific transport proteins in the membrane.

O_2, for example, is a small molecule that is fairly soluble in nonpolar solvents. It crosses biological membranes by diffusing among membrane lipid molecules. Glucose, on the other hand, is a much larger molecule that is not very soluble in the membrane lipids. Glucose enters cells via specific glucose transport proteins in the plasma membrane.

Any substance tends to diffuse from where it is more concentrated to where it is less concentrated

Diffusion is the process whereby atoms or molecules intermingle because of their random thermal motion; it is also called **brownian motion.** Imagine a container divided into two compartments by a removable partition. A much larger number of molecules of a compound is placed on side A than on side B, and then the partition is removed. Every molecule is in random thermal motion. It is equally probable that a molecule that begins on side A will move to side B in a given time and that a molecule on side B will move to side A. Because many more molecules are present on side A, the total number of molecules moving from A to B will be greater than the number moving from B to A. In this way the number of molecules on side A decreases, whereas the number of molecules on side B increases. This process continues until the concentration of molecules on side A equals that on side B. Thereafter the rate of diffusion of molecules from A to B equals that from B to A, and no further net movement occurs; a dynamic equilibrium exists.

Diffusion occurs rapidly over microscopic distances but slowly over macroscopic distances

Diffusion is a rapid process when the distance over which it takes place is small. A rule of thumb is that a typical molecule takes 1 msec to diffuse 1 μm. However, the time required for diffusion increases with the square of the distance over which diffusion occurs. Thus A TEN-FOLD INCREASE IN THE DIFFUSION DISTANCE MEANS THAT THE DIFFUSION PROCESS WILL REQUIRE ABOUT 100 TIMES LONGER TO REACH A GIVEN DEGREE OF COMPLETION.

Table 1-1 shows the results of calculations for a typical small water-soluble solute. Diffusion is extremely rapid on a microscopic scale of distance. For macroscopic distances, diffusion is rather slow. A cell that is 100 μm away from the nearest capillary can receive nutrients from the blood by diffusion with a time lag of only 5 seconds or so. This is sufficiently fast to satisfy the metabolic demands of many cells. However, a skeletal muscle cell that is 1 cm long cannot rely on diffusion for the intracellular transport of vital metabolites because the 14 hours required for diffusion over the 1-cm distance is too long on the time scale of cellular metabolism. Some nerve fibers are longer than 1 m. Therefore it is no wonder that intracellular axonal transport systems are involved in transporting important molecules along nerve fibers. Because of the slowness of diffusion over macroscopic distances, it is not surprising that even small multicellular organisms have evolved circulatory systems to bring the individual cells of the organisms within a reasonable diffusion range of nutrients.

The diffusion coefficient depends on the diffusing molecule and the medium through which it is diffusing

The **diffusion coefficient (D)** is proportional to the speed with which the diffusing molecule can move in the surrounding medium. The larger the molecule and the more viscous the medium, the smaller D is. For small molecules, D is inversely proportional to $MW^{1/2}$ (*MW* refers to molecular weight.) For macromolecules, D is inversely proportional to $MW^{1/3}$. Thus a protein that has eight times the mass of another molecule has a D half that of the smaller molecule.

Table 1-1	Time Required for Diffusion to Occur over Various Diffusion Distances*
Diffusion Distance (μm)	**Time Required for Diffusion**
1	0.5 msec
10	50 msec
100	5 sec
1000 (1 mm)	8.3 min
10,000 (1 cm)	14 hr

*The time required for the "average" molecule (with diffusion coefficient taken to be 1×10^{-5} cm/sec) to diffuse the required distance was computed.

Diffusion of a substance across a membrane is described by Fick's first law of diffusion

Diffusion leads to a state in which the concentration of the diffusing species is constant in space and time. Diffusion across cellular membranes tends to equalize the concentrations on the two sides of the membrane. The diffusion rate across a membrane is proportional to the area of the membrane and to the difference in the concentration of the diffusing substance on the two sides of the membrane. **Fick's first law of diffusion** states the following:

$$J = -DA\frac{\Delta c}{\Delta x} \qquad \text{1-1}$$

where:

J   =   Net rate of diffusion in moles or grams per unit time

D   =   Diffusion coefficient of the diffusing solute in the membrane

A   =   Area of the membrane

Δc   =   Concentration difference across the membrane

Δx   =   Thickness of the membrane

Membranes are more permeable to lipid-soluble substances than to water-soluble substances

The permeability of membranes to lipid-soluble molecules is proportional to their solubility in the interior of the lipid bilayer

The plasma membrane serves as a diffusion barrier that enables the cell to maintain cytoplasmic concentrations of many substances that differ greatly from their extracellular concentrations. As early as a century ago, the relative impermeability of the plasma membrane to most water-soluble substances was attributed to its "lipoid nature."

The hypothesis that the plasma membrane has a lipoid character is supported by experiments showing a strong positive correlation between the permeability of biological membranes to various compounds and the solubility of those compounds in nonpolar solvents (e.g., benzene, olive oil). For compounds with similar solubilities in nonpolar solvents, permeability decreases with increasing MW. A good deal of experimental data support the idea that THE LIPID BILAYER IS THE PRINCIPAL BARRIER TO SUBSTANCES THAT PERMEATE THE MEMBRANE BY SIMPLE DIFFUSION.

Fat-soluble vitamins are absorbed by the epithelial cells of the small intestine by simply diffusing across their luminal plasma membranes. In contrast, water-soluble vitamins do not readily diffuse across biological membranes, so special membrane transport proteins are required for the absorption of most water-soluble vitamins (see Chapter 34).

Only rather small water-soluble molecules can diffuse rapidly across membranes

Very small uncharged, water-soluble molecules pass through cell membranes more rapidly than predicted by their lipid solubility. For example, water permeates cell membranes about 100 times more rapidly than predicted from its molecular radius and its olive oil/water partition coefficient. There are two reasons for the unusually high permeability to water. Water and certain very small water-soluble molecules can pass between adjacent phospholipid molecules without dissolving in the region occupied by the fatty acid side chains. Moreover, the plasma membranes of many cells contain membrane proteins called **aquaporins** that form channels permitting a high rate of water flow across the membrane (Figure 1-4). At least four isoforms of aquaporin are present in the kidney. Mutations in these water transport proteins result in defects in the ability of the kidney to produce urine that is more or less concentrated than body fluids (see Chapters 36 and 37).

The permeability of membranes to uncharged, water-soluble molecules decreases as the size of the molecules increases. Most membranes permit significant diffusion only of water-soluble molecules whose MWs are less than about 200. Because of their net charges, ions are relatively insoluble in membrane lipids, so membranes are not very permeable to most ions. Ionic diffusion across membranes occurs mainly through protein **ion channels** that span the membrane. Some ion channels are highly specific with respect to the ions allowed to pass, whereas others allow all ions below a certain size to pass. Some ion channels are controlled by the voltage difference across the membrane, and others are controlled by neurotransmitters or other regulatory molecules (see Chapters 3 and 4).

Although certain water-soluble molecules such as sugars and amino acids are essential for cellular survival, they do not cross plasma membranes appreciably by simple diffusion. Plasma membranes have specific proteins that allow the transfer of vital metabolites into or out of the cell. The characteristics of membrane **protein-mediated transport** are discussed later.

Water Flows by Osmosis When There Is a Solute Concentration Difference Across a Membrane

Osmosis is defined as the flow of water across a semipermeable membrane from a compartment in which the solute concentration is lower to one in which the solute concentration is greater. A SEMIPERMEABLE MEMBRANE IS A MEMBRANE PERMEABLE TO WATER BUT IMPERMEABLE TO SOLUTES. OSMOSIS TAKES PLACE BECAUSE THE PRESENCE OF SOLUTE DECREASES THE CHEMICAL POTENTIAL OF WATER. Water tends to flow from where its chemical potential is higher to where its chemical potential is lower. Other effects caused by the decrease in the chemical potential of water (because of the presence of solute) include reduced vapor pressure, lower freezing point, and higher boiling point of the solution compared with pure water. Because these properties, and osmotic pressure as well, depend primarily on the concentration of the solute present rather than on its chemical properties, they are called **colligative properties.**

The osmotic pressure of a solution is the pressure that must be applied to it to prevent water from entering the solution across a semipermeable membrane

In Figure 1-5 a semipermeable membrane separates a solution from pure water. Water flows from side B to side A by osmosis because the presence of solute on side A reduces the chemical potential of water in the solution. Pushing on the piston increases the chemical potential of the water in

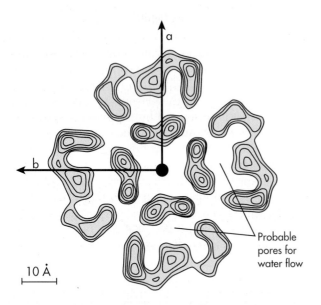

Figure 1-4 Structure of a water channel protein. Electron crystallography was used to determine the structure of aquaporin-1, a water channel protein in erythrocyte membranes and in cells of the renal proximal tubules. Section through the three-dimensional electron density map of aquaporin-1 is viewed perpendicular to the plane of the membrane. Aquaporin-1 exists in the membrane as a tetramer. Each monomer can conduct water through the membrane. *(Redrawn from Cheng A et al: Nature 387:627, 1997.)*

Probable pores for water flow

10 Å

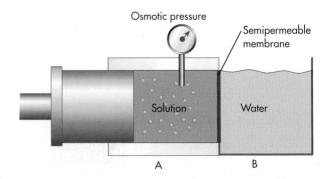

Figure 1-5 Osmotic pressure. When the hydrostatic pressure applied to the solution in chamber A is equal to the osmotic pressure of that solution, there is no net water flow across the membrane.

the solution of side A and slows the net rate of osmotic water flow. If the force on the piston is increased gradually, a pressure is eventually reached at which net water flow stops. The application of still more pressure causes water to flow in the opposite direction. The pressure on side A that is just sufficient to keep pure water from entering is called the **osmotic pressure** of the solution on side A.

THE OSMOTIC PRESSURE OF A SOLUTION DEPENDS ON THE CONCENTRATION OF PARTICLES IN SOLUTION. Thus the degree of ionization of the solute must be taken into account. A 1 M solution of glucose, a 0.5 M solution of NaCl, and a 0.333 M solution of $CaCl_2$ have approximately the same osmotic pressure. (Actually, their osmotic pressures differ somewhat because of the deviations of real solutions from ideal behavior.) One form of **van't Hoff's law** or the calculation of osmotic pressure is:

$$\pi = RT(\Phi ic) \qquad \textbf{1-2}$$

where:

π = Osmotic pressure
R = Ideal gas constant
T = Absolute temperature
Φ = Osmotic coefficient
i = Number of ions formed by the dissociation of a solute molecule
c = Molar concentration of the solute (moles of solute per liter of solution)

The osmotic coefficient (Φ) accounts for the deviation of the solution from the ideal. It depends on the particular compound, its concentration, and the temperature. The value of Φ is less than 1 for electrolytes of physiological importance, and for all solutes it approaches 1 as the solution becomes more and more dilute. The term **Φic** can be regarded as the **osmotically effective concentration,** and Φic, called the **osmolarity** of the solution, is expressed in osmoles per liter. Sometimes, a less precise estimate of osmotic pressure is computed by assuming that Φ is equal to 1.

Values of Φ for different substances can be obtained from handbooks that list such values as functions of concentration. Solutions of proteins deviate greatly from ideal behavior, and different proteins may deviate to different extents. Values of Φ depend on the concentration of the solute and on its chemical properties.

The osmotic pressure of a solution can be estimated from its freezing point

The osmotic pressure of a solution can be obtained by determining the pressure required to prevent water from entering the solution across a semipermeable membrane (Figure 1-5). More often, however, the osmotic pressure is estimated from another colligative property, such as depression of the freezing point. The relationship that describes the osmolarity (Φic) of a solution in terms of the depression of the freezing point of water by the solute is:

$$\Phi ic = \Delta T_f / 1.86 \qquad \textbf{1-3}$$

where ΔT_f is the freezing point depression in degrees centigrade. When the freezing point depression of a multicomponent solution is determined, the effective osmolarity (in osmoles per liter) of the solution as a whole can be obtained.

If the total osmotic pressures of two solutions (as measured by freezing point depression or by the osmotic pressure developed across a semipermeable membrane) are equal, the solutions are said to be **isoosmotic** (or **isosmotic**). If solution A has greater osmotic pressure than solution B, A is said to be **hyperosmotic** with respect to B. If solution A has less total osmotic pressure than solution B, A is said to be **hypoosmotic** to B.

Cells swell or shrink in response to changes in the solute content of extracellular fluid

The plasma membranes of most of the body's cells are relatively impermeable to many of the solutes of the extracellular fluid but are highly permeable to water. Therefore when the osmotic pressure of the extracellular fluid is increased, water leaves the cells by osmosis, and the cells shrink. Thus the cellular solutes become more concentrated until the effective osmotic pressure of the cytoplasm is again equal to that of the extracellular fluid. Conversely, if the osmotic pressure of the extracellular fluid is decreased, water enters the cells. The cells continue to swell until the intracellular and extracellular osmotic pressures are equal.

Red blood cells are often used to illustrate the osmotic properties of cells because they are readily obtained and are easily studied. Within a certain range of external solute concentrations, the red cell behaves as an osmometer because its volume is inversely related to the solute concentration in the extracellular medium. In Figure 1-6 the red cell volume, as a fraction of its normal volume in plasma, is shown as a function of the concentration of NaCl solution in which the red cells are suspended. At an NaCl concentration of 154 mM (308 mM osmotically active particles), the volume of the cells is the same as their volume in plasma; this concentration of NaCl is said to be **isotonic** to the red cell.

Isotonic NaCl solution (also known as **isotonic saline**) is used for intravenous rehydration or for the administration of medications. Almost every patient undergoing surgery has an intravenous drip of isotonic saline.

A concentration of NaCl greater than 154 mM is called **hypertonic** (greater strength, causes cells to shrink), and a solution less concentrated than 154 mM is termed **hypotonic** (cells swell). When red cells have swollen to about 1.4 times their original volume, some cells lyse (burst). At this volume the properties of the red cell membrane abruptly change; hemoglobin leaks out of the cell, and the membrane becomes transiently permeable to other large molecules as well.

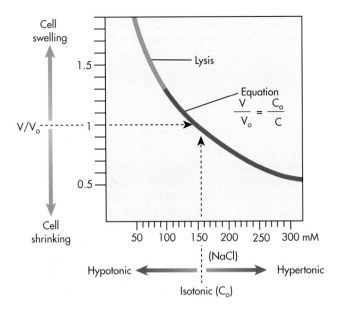

Figure 1-6 Osmotic behavior of human red blood cells in NaCl solutions. At 154 mM NaCl (isotonic), the red cell has a normal volume. It shrinks in more concentrated (hypertonic) solutions and swells in more dilute (hypotonic) solutions. V_o and C_o are the red cell volume and intracellular solute concentration, respectively, for the red cell in blood or in an isotonic solution. V and C are, respectively, the cell volume and intracellular solute concentration in a solution that is not isotonic.

The erythrocyte's intracellular substances producing an osmotic pressure that just balances the osmotic pressure of the extracellular fluid include hemoglobin, K^+, organic phosphates (e.g., ATP; 2,3-diphosphoglycerate), and glycolytic intermediates. Regardless of the chemical nature of its contents, the red cell behaves as though it is filled with a solution of impermeant molecules with an osmotically effective concentration of 286 milliosmolar, which is the same as the osmolarity of isotonic saline, as follows:

$$\Phi_{NaCl} i_{NaCl} C_{NaCl} = 0.93 \times 2 \times 0.154\ M = \qquad \textbf{1-4}$$
$$0.286\ osmolar = 286\ milliosmolar$$

Permeant solutes have only a transient effect on cell volume

Permeating solutes eventually equilibrate across the plasma membrane. For this reason, permeating solutes exert only a transient effect on cell volume. Consider a red blood cell placed in a large volume of 0.154 M NaCl that contains 0.050 M glycerol. Because of the extracellular NaCl and glycerol, the osmotic pressure of the extracellular fluid initially exceeds that of the cell interior, so the cell shrinks. With time, however, glycerol equilibrates across the plasma membrane of the red cell, and the cell swells back toward its original volume. THE STEADY-STATE VOLUME OF THE CELL IS DETERMINED ONLY BY THE IMPERMEANT SOLUTES IN THE EXTRACELLULAR FLUID. In this case the impermeant solutes (NaCl) have a total concentration that is isotonic, so the final volume of the cell is equal to the normal red cell volume. Because the red cell ultimately returns to its normal volume, the solution

(0.050 M glycerol in 0.154 M NaCl) is isotonic. Because the red cell initially shrinks when put in this solution, the solution is hyperosmotic with respect to the normal red cell. The transient changes in cell volume depend on the equilibration of glycerol across the membrane. If urea (a more rapidly permeating substance) had been used, the cell would have reached steady-state volume sooner. The following rules help predict the volume changes a cell undergoes when suspended in solutions of permeant and impermeant solutes:

1. THE STEADY-STATE VOLUME OF THE CELL IS DETERMINED ONLY BY THE CONCENTRATION OF IMPERMEANT SOLUTES IN THE EXTRACELLULAR FLUID.
2. PERMEANT SOLUTES CAUSE ONLY TRANSIENT CHANGES IN CELL VOLUME.
3. THE GREATER THE PERMEABILITY OF THE MEMBRANE TO THE PERMEANT SOLUTE, THE MORE RAPID THE TRANSIENT CHANGES.

The more permeable a membrane is to a particular solute, the smaller the osmotic flow that can be caused by that solute

In the preceding example, it was explained that permeants such as glycerol exert only a transient osmotic effect. It is sometimes important to determine the rate of the osmotic flow caused by a particular permeant.

When a difference in hydrostatic pressure (ΔP) causes water flow across a membrane, the rate of water flow ($\dot{V}_w$) is as follows:

$$\dot{V}_w = L\Delta P \qquad \textbf{1-5}$$

where L is a constant of proportionality called the **hydraulic conductivity**.

THE OSMOTIC FLOW OF WATER ACROSS A MEMBRANE IS DIRECTLY PROPORTIONAL TO THE OSMOTIC PRESSURE DIFFERENCE ($\Delta\Pi$) BETWEEN THE SOLUTIONS ON THE TWO SIDES OF THE MEMBRANE, then:

$$\dot{V}_w = L\Delta\pi \qquad \textbf{1-6}$$

Equation 1-6 holds only for osmosis caused by impermeant solutes. Permeant solutes cause less osmotic flow. THE GREATER THE PERMEABILITY OF A SOLUTE, THE SMALLER THE OSMOTIC FLOW IT CAUSES. Table 1-2 shows the osmotic water flows induced across a porous membrane by solutes of different molecular sizes. The solutions have identical freezing points, so the total osmotic pressures are the same. The larger the solute molecule, the more impermeable the membrane to the solute, and the greater the osmotic water flow it causes.

The σ of a solute allows the prediction of how much osmotic flow it can cause across a particular membrane

Equation 1-6 can be rewritten to take solute permeability into account by including the **reflection coefficient (σ),** as follows:

$$\dot{V}_w = \sigma L\Delta\pi \qquad \textbf{1-7}$$

Table 1-2   Osmotic Water Flow across a Porous Dialysis Membrane Caused by Various Solutes

Gradient Producing the Water Flow	Net Volume Flow (μl/min)*	Solute Radius (Å)	Reflection Coefficient (σ)
D_2O	0.06	1.9	0.0024
Urea	0.6	2.7	0.024
Glucose	5.1	4.4	0.205
Sucrose	9.2	5.3	0.368
Raffinose	11	6.1	0.440
Inulin	19	12	0.760
Bovine serum albumin	25.5	37	1.02
Hydrostatic pressure	25		

Data from Durbin RP: *J Gen Physiol* 44:315, 1960.
*Flow is expressed as microliters per minute caused by a 1 M concentration difference of solute across the membrane. The flows are compared with the flow caused by a theoretically equivalent hydrostatic pressure.

σ is a dimensionless number that ranges from one for completely impermeant solutes to zero for extremely permeant solutes. σ is a property of a particular solute and a particular membrane and represents the osmotic flow induced by the solute as a fraction of the theoretical maximum osmotic flow (Table 1-2). The more permeant a substance across a particular membrane, the smaller the σ of the membrane for that substance, and the smaller the osmotic water flow the substance can cause.

> The mechanism by which the kidney produces urine more concentrated than extracellular fluid (see Chapter 36) involves various parts of the nephron that have a different σ for each important solute, such as NaCl and urea. The osmotic water flows induced by NaCl and urea in a particular segment of the nephron depend on the values of σ for the epithelium in that segment to these solutes.

Transport Proteins Are Responsible for Moving Important Substances Across Membranes

Certain substances enter or leave cells by way of specific carriers or channels that are intrinsic proteins of the plasma membrane. Transport via such protein carriers or channels is called **protein-mediated transport** or simply **mediated transport.** Specific ions or molecules may cross the membranes of the mitochondrion, the endoplasmic reticulum, and other organelles by mediated transport. Mediated transport systems include **active transport** and **facilitated transport,** which have several properties in common. The principal distinction between these two processes is that ACTIVE TRANSPORT IS CAPABLE OF "PUMPING" A SUBSTANCE AGAINST A GRADIENT OF CONCENTRATION (OR ELECTROCHEMICAL POTENTIAL), WHEREAS FACILITATED TRANSPORT TENDS TO EQUILIBRATE THE SUBSTANCE ACROSS THE MEMBRANE.

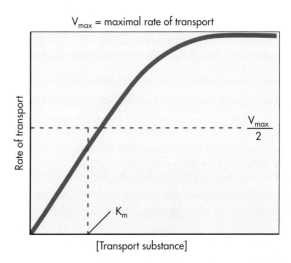

Figure 1-7 Movement via a transport protein shows saturation kinetics. As the concentration of the transported substance increases, the rate of its transport approaches a maximum value, the V_{max} for the transporter. The concentration of the transported substance required for the transport rate to be half-maximal is termed the K_m of the transporter.

Protein-mediated transport has some of the properties of enzyme catalysis

1. A substance moved by mediated transport is moved more rapidly than molecules that have a similar MW and lipid solubility but that cross the membrane by simple diffusion.
2. The transport rate shows **saturation kinetics:** as the concentration of the transported compound is increased, the rate of transport at first increases, but eventually a concentration is reached after which the transport rate increases no further (Figure 1-7). At this point the transport system is said to be SATURATED WITH THE TRANSPORTED COMPOUND.
3. The mediating protein has **chemical specificity:** only molecules with the requisite chemical structure are transported. The specificity of most trans-

port systems is not absolute, and in general, it is broader than the specificity of most enzymes. The lock-and-key relationship between an enzyme and its substrate applies to transport proteins as well.

4. Structurally related molecules may compete for transport. Typically, one transport substrate decreases the transport rate of a second substrate by competing for the transport protein. The competition is analogous to competitive inhibition of an enzyme.

5. Transport may be inhibited by compounds not structurally related to transport substrates. An inhibitor may bind to the transport protein in a way that decreases the affinity of the protein for the normal transport substrate. The compound **phloretin** does not resemble a sugar molecule; yet it strongly inhibits red cell sugar transport. Active transport systems, which require some link to metabolism, may be inhibited by metabolic inhibitors. The rate of Na^+ transport out of cells by Na^+,K^+-ATPase is decreased by substances that interfere with ATP generation.

A facilitated transport enhances the rate a substance can flow down its concentration gradient

SOMETIMES CALLED **FACILITATED DIFFUSION,** FACILITATED TRANSPORT OCCURS VIA A TRANSPORT PROTEIN THAT IS NOT LINKED TO METABOLIC ENERGY. Facilitated transport has the properties discussed previously, except that it is not generally depressed by metabolic inhibitors. Because facilitated transport processes are not linked to energy metabolism, they cannot move substances against concentration gradients. Facilitated transport systems act to equalize concentrations of the transported substances on the two sides of the membrane.

Monosaccharides enter muscle cells by facilitated transport. Glucose, galactose, arabinose, and 3-0-methylglucose compete for the same carrier. The rate of transport shows saturation kinetics. The nonphysiological stereoisomer L-glucose enters the cells very slowly, and nontransported sugars, such as mannitol or sorbose, enter muscle cells very slowly, if at all. Phloretin inhibits sugar uptake, and insulin stimulates it.

A major action of the hormone **insulin** is to stimulate the transport of glucose across the plasma membranes of muscle and fat cells. People with **type 1 diabetes** secrete insulin at markedly subnormal rates (see Chapter 42). In this disease the rate of glucose uptake by muscle and adipose cells is so slow that the ability of these tissues to use glucose as a metabolic fuel is markedly impaired. Some of the pathological consequences of type 1 diabetes are caused by the inability to metabolize glucose at normal rates.

An active transport protein can transport a substance from where its concentration is lower to where it is higher: this requires energy

Active transport processes have most of the properties of facilitated transport. In addition, active transport systems can concentrate their substrates against concentration or electrochemical potential gradients. This requires energy; hence ACTIVE TRANSPORT PROCESSES MUST BE LINKED TO ENERGY METABOLISM IN SOME WAY. Active transport systems may use ATP directly, or they may be linked more indirectly to metabolism. Because of their dependence on metabolism, active transport processes may be inhibited by any substance that interferes with energy metabolism.

A *primary active transport process has a direct link to metabolic energy*

An active transport process linked directly to cellular metabolism (i.e., by using ATP to power the transport) is called **primary active transport.** In the cytoplasm of most animal cells the concentration of Na^+ is much less and the concentration of K^+ is much greater than their extracellular concentrations. These concentration gradients are brought about by the action of Na^+,K^+-ATPase, an integral protein in the plasma membrane. Na^+,K^+-ATPase uses the energy of ATP to pump Na^+ out of the cell and K^+ into the cell. Na^+,K^+-ATPase transports three sodium ions out of the cell and transports two potassium ions into the cell for each molecule of ATP hydrolyzed. The cyclic phosphorylation and dephosphorylation of the protein causes the protein to alternate between two conformations, E1 and E2. In the E1 conformation the ion-binding sites of the protein have a high affinity for Na^+ and a low affinity for K^+, and the binding sites face the cytoplasm. In the E2 conformation the ion-binding sites face the extracellular fluid, and their affinities favor the binding of K^+ and the dissociation of Na^+. In this way, Na^+,K^+-ATPase alternates between the E1 and the E2 conformations and transports K^+ into the cell and Na^+ out of the cell by a process resembling "molecular peristalsis."

Because Na^+,K^+-ATPase uses the energy in the terminal phosphate bond of ATP to power the transport cycle, it is said to be a primary active transport system. A transport process powered by some other high-energy metabolic intermediate or linked directly to a primary metabolic reaction would also be classified as primary active transport.

A *secondary active transport protein derives energy from the concentration gradient of another substance that is actively transported*

The previous section emphasized that energy is required to create a concentration gradient for a transported substance. ONCE CREATED, A CONCENTRATION GRADIENT REPRESENTS A STORE OF CHEMICAL POTENTIAL ENERGY THAT CAN BE HARNESSED TO DO WORK (see Chapter 2). In many cell types the

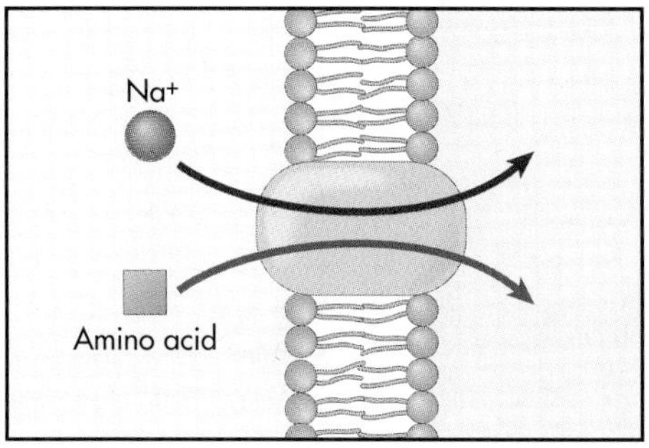

Figure 1-8 Many cells take up neutral amino acids via secondary active transport. The transport protein binds both Na^+ and the amino acid. Na^+ is transported down its electrochemical gradient, and the transport protein uses the energy released by Na^+ flux to transport the amino acid against a concentration gradient.

concentration gradient of Na^+ created by Na^+,K^+-ATPase is used to actively transport other solutes into the cell. Many cells take up neutral, hydrophilic amino acids by membrane transport proteins that link the inward transport of Na^+ down its electrochemical potential gradient to the inward transport of amino acids against their gradients of concentration (Figure 1-8). The energy for the transport of the amino acid is provided, not directly by ATP or another high-energy metabolite, but indirectly from the gradient of Na^+ that is itself actively transported. Hence the amino acid is said to be transported by **secondary active transport.** In the secondary active transport of amino acids, both the rate of amino acid transport and the extent to which the amino acid is accumulated depend on the electrochemical potential gradient of Na^+. Certain other secondary active transport processes, such as the absorption of small peptides from the small intestine (see Chapter 34), are powered by an electrochemical potential gradient of H^+.

Cells depend on a number of membrane transport processes

Ca++ is transported across membranes by Ca++-ATPases and by Na+/Ca++ exchange proteins

Under most circumstances the concentration of Ca^{++} in the cytosol of cells is maintained at low levels, below 10^{-7} M, whereas the concentration of Ca^{++} in extracellular fluids is on the order of 10^{-3} M. Plasma membranes contain Ca^{++}-ATPase that helps maintain the large gradient of Ca^{++} across the plasma membrane. The plasma membrane Ca^{++}-ATPase is a close relative of the Ca^{++}-ATPase responsible for sequestering Ca^{++} in the sarcoplasmic reticulum of muscle (see Chapter 13). The plasma membrane Ca^{++}-ATPase shares important properties with the Ca^{++}-ATPase of the sarcoplasmic reticulum and the Na^+,K^+-ATPase of plasma membranes. These proteins carry out the primary active transport of ions across membranes, and they use the

energy of the terminal phosphate bond of ATP to accomplish this task.

In addition, most cells store Ca^{++} in the endoplasmic reticulum or other intracellular storage vesicles. Ca^{++} is concentrated in these vesicles by a Ca^{++}-ATPase closely related to the Ca^{++}-ATPase of the sarcoplasmic reticulum of muscle cells. Because Ca^{++} is a key second messenger (see Chapter 5), many hormones or agonists elevate the intracellular level of Ca^{++} by opening Ca^{++} channels in the plasma membrane, the membranes of Ca^{++}-storage vesicles, or both sites.

Certain electrically excitable cells, such as those of the heart, have an additional mechanism for controlling the level of intracellular Ca^{++}. A Na^+/Ca^{++} exchange protein in the plasma membrane uses the energy in the Na^+ gradient to extrude Ca^{++} from the cell. In heart cells the rapid, transient changes in intracellular Ca^{++} appear to be mediated by the Na^+/Ca^{++} exchange protein, whereas the resting level of intracellular Ca^{++} is set mainly by the Ca^{++}-ATPases of the plasma membrane and sarcoplasmic reticulum (see Chapters 14 and 18).

Glucose is transported into muscle and fat cells by facilitated transporters

Glucose is a primary fuel for most of the cells of the body, but glucose diffuses across plasma membranes very slowly. The plasma membranes of many cell types contain sugar transport proteins that mediate the facilitated transport of glucose and related monosaccharides. Red blood cells, hepatocytes, adipocytes, and muscle cells (skeletal, cardiac, smooth) all possess glucose transporters. The uptake of glucose in these cell types depends neither on the electrochemical potential difference of Na^+ across the plasma membrane nor on cellular metabolism in any direct way. In adipocytes and muscle cells, the transport of glucose across the plasma membrane is increased by insulin (see Chapter 42), which causes more glucose transport proteins to be inserted into the plasma membrane. The source of the newly inserted protein is a preformed pool of transporters in the membranes of the endoplasmic reticulum within the cell.

Amino acids are taken up into cells via several different types of amino acid transport proteins

Most of the cells in the body synthesize proteins and therefore require amino acids. The synthesis of proteins is required for the turnover of cells and tissues and in processes such as wound healing. Several different amino acid transport proteins are present in plasma membranes. The amino acid transport systems include three distinct classes of transporters: neutral, basic, and acidic amino acids (see Chapter 34). Amino acid transport proteins overlap significantly in specificities, and the distribution of the different transport proteins varies from one cell type to another. Some of these transport proteins are secondary active transporters powered

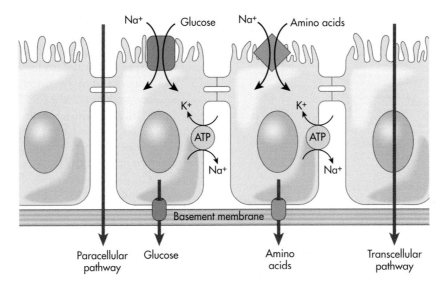

Figure 1-9 Epithelial transport processes that occur in the small intestine and renal tubules. Epithelia are polarized such that the transport processes on one side of the cell differ from those on the other side. Glucose and neutral amino acids enter the epithelial cell at the brush border via Na$^+$-powered secondary active transport but leave the cell across the basolateral membrane by facilitated transport.

by the concentration gradient of Na$^+$. Others are facilitated transport proteins.

Epithelial cells are polarized: the apical and basolateral plasma membranes contain different transport proteins

Epithelial cells are polarized with respect to their transport properties. That is, the transport properties of the plasma membrane facing one side of the epithelial cell layer are different from those of the membrane facing the other side.

The epithelial cells of the small intestine (see Chapter 34) and the proximal tubule of the kidney (see Chapter 36) are good examples of this polarity. The complement of membrane transport proteins in the brush border that faces the lumen of the small bowel or the renal tubule differs from that of the basolateral plasma membrane of the cell. The tight junctions that join the epithelial cells side to side prevent mixing of the transport proteins of the luminal and basolateral plasma membranes. The brush border plasma membranes of these epithelia contain very few Na$^+$,K$^+$-ATPase molecules, which reside mainly in the basolateral plasma membrane. Glucose (and galactose) and neutral amino acids enter these epithelial cells at the brush border by secondary active transporters driven by the Na$^+$ gradient. However, these substances leave the cells at the basolateral membrane primarily by facilitated transporters (Figure 1-9).

The tight junctions that join the cells are leaky to water and small water-soluble molecules and ions. The tightness of the tight junctions varies among epithelia. There are thus two types of pathways for transport across the epithelia: (1) **transcellular pathways** (through the cells) and (2) **paracellular pathways** (in between the cells) (Figure 1-9).

SUMMARY

- Biological membranes are phospholipid bilayers with integral membrane proteins imbedded in the bilayer and peripheral membrane proteins adherent to the surfaces of the membrane.

- Membranes serve as permeability barriers that separate the cell from the extracellular milieu and divide the cell into biochemically specialized compartments.

- Endocytosis and exocytosis permit material to enter or leave the cell without passing through the membrane.

- Diffusion is an effective biological transport process on the microscopic scale of distances.

- Only very small water-soluble molecules and lipid-soluble molecules can diffuse across biological membranes at appreciable rates.

- Gradients of solutes across membranes power the flow of water by osmosis. Impermeant solutes determine the steady-state volumes of cells, but permeant solutes have only transient effects.

- The osmotic water flow caused by a particular solute depends on the permeability of the membrane to that species: the greater the permeability, the smaller the osmotic water flow.

- Biological membranes contain transport proteins (transporters) to promote the permeation of various classes of molecules. Facilitated transporters allow the transported substance to equilibrate across the membrane. Active transporters can pump the transported species against a concentration or energy gradient. This requires a link to metabolism.

- Primary active transport proteins have a direct link to metabolism, frequently by consuming ATP.

■ Secondary active transport proteins use the gradient of another substance, frequently Na$^+$, to power the transport of substances such as sugars and amino acids.

BIBLIOGRAPHY

Carruthers A: Facilitated diffusion of glucose, *Physiol Rev* 70:1135, 1990.

Christensen HN: Role of amino acid transport and countertransport in nutrition and metabolism, *Physiol Rev* 70:43, 1990.

Griffith JK: Membrane transport proteins: implications of sequence comparisons, *Curr Opin Cell Biol* 4:684, 1992.

Henderson PJF: The 12-transmembrane helix transporters, *Curr Opin Cell Biol* 5:708, 1993.

Kaplan JH, De Weer P, eds: *The sodium pump: structure, mechanism, and regulation—Symposium of the Society of General Physiologists,* New York, 1990, Rockefeller Press.

Lauger P: *Electrogenic ion pumps,* Sunderland, Mass, 1991, Sinauer Associates.

Mercer RW: Structure of the Na,K-ATPase, *Int Rev Cytol* 137C:139, 1993.

Sachs G, Munson K: Mammalian phosphorylating ion-motive ATPases, *Curr Opin Cell Biol* 3:685, 1991.

Schultz SG et al, eds: *Molecular biology of membrane disorders,* New York, 1996, Plenum.

Stein WH: *Channels, carriers, and pumps: an introduction to membrane transport,* San Diego, 1990, Academic.

Wright EM, Hager KM, Turk E: Sodium co-transport proteins, *Curr Opin Cell Biol* 4:696, 1992.

▷ CASE STUDIES

Case 1-1

A 38-year-old man visits his physician complaining of occasional chest pain. The patient has xanthomas (fatty tumors) on both Achilles tendons and some of the tendons of the dorsum of the hand, xanthelasma (fatty tumors on the eyelids), and arcus corneae (opaque rings near the corneal margins). The patient reveals that routine cholesterol screening at his place of employment found an elevated total serum cholesterol level (425 mg/dl compared with an average of about 200 mg/dl for white men of this age). The physician orders additional laboratory analyses, which determine that the elevation of serum cholesterol is due primarily to an elevation of low-density lipoprotein (LDL) cholesterol (380 mg/dl compared with an average of 132 mg/dl for white men of this age). The provisional diagnosis is the **heterozygous form of familial hypercholesterolemia.** This disorder is caused by a mutation in the LDL receptor that prevents cells from taking up LDL from the extracellular fluid via receptor-mediated endocytosis.

1. Which of the following statements is true?

A. The patient's elevated serum LDL level is caused only by the inability of cells to take up and metabolize cholesterol.

B. Increased cholesterol synthesis by hepatocytes contributes to the patient's elevated level of serum LDL.

C. The patient's xanthomas are due primarily to the increased serum triglyceride levels.

D. The patient's disorder is quite rare.

E. The patient is not very likely to have atherosclerosis.

2. If skin fibroblasts from this patient were grown in culture and then deprived of serum for 24 hours, what would occur?

A. The high-affinity binding of LDL to the plasma membranes of the patient's fibroblasts might be about 50% that of binding to normal fibroblasts.

B. The high-affinity binding of LDL to the plasma membranes of the patient's fibroblasts might be much greater than that to the fibroblasts of a person with homozygous familial hypercholesterolemia.

C. The high-affinity binding of LDL to the plasma membrane of the patient's fibroblasts might be about the same as the binding of LDL to normal fibroblasts.

D. The rate of catabolism of LDL by the patient's fibroblasts would be less than that of normal fibroblasts.

E. All of the above.

3. Which of the following statements is true?

A. If the patient follows a diet extremely low in fat, his plasma LDL level may approach normal.

B. A diet very low in fat will allow the patient's risk for heart attack to approach that of the overall population in his age group.

C. A medication that suppresses cholesterol synthesis by hepatocytes is not likely to be useful in treating this condition.

D. A liver transplant would normalize the patient's LDL levels.

E. The combination of a low-fat diet and treatment with a medication that suppresses cholesterol synthesis is advisable for this patient.

Case 1-2

A 3-week-old infant is admitted to the hospital with dehydration, acidosis, and hypokalemia, all apparently caused by persistent diarrhea. Intravenous fluids are used to correct the baby's hydration and electrolyte problems. Then the baby is fed formulas containing different sugars. When she was fed formulas with lactose, sucrose, or glucose, diarrhea resulted. When she was fed formula whose only sugar was fructose, the diarrhea abated. (Disaccharides and larger oligosaccharides cannot be absorbed in the small intestine; only monosaccharides can be absorbed there. The only monosaccharides that can be absorbed are glucose, galactose, and fructose. Glucose and galactose are absorbed by a common Na^+-powered facilitated transport protein called *SGLT1;* fructose is absorbed by a different facilitated transport protein [see Chapter 34].) (Assume that there is only one defective process.)

1. Which of the following statements is true?

   A. If the patient were fed maltose, the diarrhea would abate.

   B. If the patient were fed plant starch, the diarrhea would abate.

   C. The cause of the patient's disorder might be a congenital deficiency of lactase, the enzyme in the intestinal brush border that hydrolyzes lactose into glucose and galactose.

   D. The patient's disorder might result from a deficiency of glucoamylase, the brush border enzyme that hydrolyzes linear polymers of glucose.

   E. None of the above.

2. Which of the following statements is true?

   A. The baby's only deficit may be the intestine's inability to absorb only glucose.

   B. The problem may be a lack of the brush border α-dextrinase (also called *isomaltase*) that debranches branched starch molecules.

   C. The baby's intestines may be unable to absorb any monosaccharides.

   D. The baby's intestines may be unable to absorb glucose and galactose.

   E. None of the above.

3. Which of the following statements is true?

   A. The failure to absorb glucose and galactose would probably be rectified by placing NaCl in the baby's formula to enhance the gradient for Na^+ influx to power monosaccharide absorption.

   B. If the baby's formula contained NaCl at three times the concentration of NaCl in plasma, no untoward consequences would occur.

   C. If the baby were fed a formula containing galactose, diarrhea would abate.

   D. If an intestinal biopsy were probed with antibodies against the Na^+-powered glucose/galactose transporter (SGLT1), this protein would probably be deficient.

   E. None of the above.

CHAPTER 2

Ionic Equilibria and Resting Membrane Potentials

OBJECTIVES

- Define the electrochemical potential of an ion and write the equation for the electrochemical potential difference of an ion on the two sides of a membrane.
- Identify the Nernst equation and use it to determine whether an ion is in equilibrium across a membrane. If the ion is not in equilibrium, decide in which direction the ion will tend to flow.
- Identify the Gibbs-Donnan equation and explain the circumstances under which it applies.
- Compute the equilibrium transmembrane electrical potential difference across a membrane that is permeable to only one ionic species.
- Estimate a cell's resting membrane potential using the chord conductance equation.

Cells have an electrical potential difference (voltage difference), called the **resting membrane potential,** across their plasma membranes. THE CYTOPLASM IS USUALLY ELECTRICALLY NEGATIVE RELATIVE TO THE EXTRACELLULAR FLUID. The resting membrane potential is necessary for the electrical excitability of neurons (see Chapters 2 to 4 and 6 to 11), skeletal muscle (see Chapter 13), smooth muscle (see Chapter 14), and the heart (see Chapter 17). This chapter discusses the basic physical chemical principles of ionic equilibria and the processes that generate the resting membrane potential in all the cells of the body.

Ionic Equilibria

The difference in potential energy of an ion across a membrane depends on the concentration difference and the electrical potential difference across the membrane

A membrane separates aqueous solutions in two chambers (A and B). The ion X^+ is at a higher concentration on side A than on side B (Figure 2-1). If no electrical potential difference exists between A and B, X^+ tends to diffuse from A to B, just as if it were an uncharged molecule. If, however, A is electrically negative with respect to B, the situation is more complex. The tendency of X^+ to diffuse

from A to B because of the concentration difference remains, but now X^+ also tends to move in the opposite direction (from B to A) because of the electrical potential difference across the membrane. The direction of net X^+ movement depends on whether the effect of the concentration difference or the effect of the electrical potential difference is larger. By comparing the two tendencies—concentration and electrical—one can predict the direction of net X^+ movement.

The quantity that allows a comparison of the relative contributions of ionic concentration and electrical potential is called the **electrochemical potential (μ)** of an ion. The electrochemical potential difference of X^+ across the membrane is defined as follows:

$$\Delta\mu(X) = \mu_A(X) - \mu_B(X) = RT \ln\frac{[X]_A}{[X]_B} + zF(E_A - E_B) \qquad \textbf{2-1}$$

where:

$$\Delta\mu = \text{Electrochemical potential difference of the ion between sides A and B of the membrane}$$

$$R = \text{Ideal gas constant}$$

$$T = \text{Absolute temperature}$$

$$\ln\frac{[X]_A}{[X]_B} = \text{Natural logarithm of concentration ratio of } X^+ \text{ on the two sides of the membrane}$$

$$z = \text{Charge number of the ion } (+2 \text{ for } Ca^{++}, -1 \text{ for } Cl^-, \text{ etc.})$$

$$F = \text{Faraday's number}$$

$$E_A - E_B = \text{Electrical potential difference across the membrane}$$

THE FIRST TERM ON THE RIGHT-HAND SIDE OF EQUATION 2-1 (THE LOGARITHM) EXPRESSES THE TENDENCY FOR X^+ IONS TO MOVE FROM A TO B BECAUSE OF THE CONCENTRATION DIFFERENCE, AND THE SECOND TERM, $zF(E_A - E_B)$, EXPRESSES THE TENDENCY FOR THE IONS TO MOVE FROM A TO B BECAUSE OF THE ELECTRICAL POTENTIAL DIFFERENCE. The first term represents the potential energy difference between a mole of X^+ ions on side A and a mole of X^+ ions on side B as a result of the concentration difference. The second term represents the potential energy difference between a mole of X^+ ions on side A and a mole of X^+ ions on side B caused by the electrical potential difference between A and B. Thus

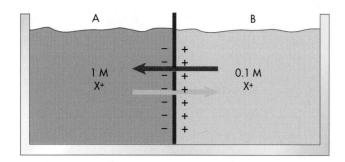

Figure 2-1 X^+ is present at 1 M in chamber A and at 0.1 M in chamber B. A concentration force for X^+ tends to cause X^+ to flow from A to B. However, chamber A is electrically negative with respect to chamber B, so an electrical force tends to cause X^+ to flow from B to A. The red arrow indicates the electrical gradient; the yellow arrow indicates the concentration gradient.

$\Delta\mu(X)$ describes the difference that exists in potential energy between a mole of X^+ ions on side A and a mole of X^+ ions on side B and that results from both concentration and electrical potential differences, hence the name **electrochemical potential difference.** The unit of electrochemical potential, and of both terms on the righthand side of Equation 2-1, is energy per mole.

The X^+ ions tend to move spontaneously from higher to lower electrochemical potential. The term $\Delta\mu$ has been defined as the electrochemical potential of the ion on side A minus that on side B. If $\Delta\mu$ is positive, the ions tend to move from A to B; if $\Delta\mu$ is zero, there is no net tendency for the ions to move at all; and if $\Delta\mu$ is negative, the ions tend to move from B to A.

If μ_A is greater than μ_B, ions tend to flow spontaneously from A to B. For ions to flow from B to A, work must be done. Specifically, $\mu_A - \mu_B$ is the minimal amount of work that must be done to cause 1 mole of ions to flow from B to A. When ions flow from A to B, on the other hand, energy is released. In fact, this energy can be harnessed to perform work. The maximal amount of work that can be done by 1 mole of ions flowing from A to B is $\mu_A - \mu_B$. THE ELECTROCHEMICAL POTENTIAL DIFFERENCE OF AN ION ACROSS A MEMBRANE THUS REPRESENTS POTENTIAL ENERGY THAT CAN BE USED TO PERFORM WORK.

What sort of work can be done by the electrochemical potential energy stored in an ion gradient? Chapter 1 mentioned that the electrochemical potential of the Na^+ gradient is used to power the secondary active transport of sugars and amino acids. In mitochondria, the action of the electron transport enzymes creates an electrochemical potential difference of H^+ across the mitochondrial inner membrane. The H^+ ions flow back into the mitochondrial matrix via the ATP synthase enzyme complex in the mitochondrial inner membrane. The ATP synthase uses the energy released by the H^+ ions to drive the synthesis of ATP. Drugs that increase the permeability of the mitochondrial inner membrane to H^+, such as the poison dinitrophenol, collapse the H^+ gradient and prevent the synthesis of ATP.

An ion in equilibrium across a membrane satisfies the Nernst equation

In Equation 2-1, $\Delta\mu$ may be thought of as the net force on the ion, whereas the logarithm is the force caused by the concentration difference, and $zF(E_A - E_B)$ is the force caused by the electrical potential difference. When the two forces are equal and opposite, $\Delta\mu$ equals zero, and there is no net force on the ion. When there is no net force on the ion, no net movement of the ion occurs, and the ion is said to be in **electrochemical equilibrium** across the membrane. At equilibrium, $\Delta\mu$ equals zero. From Equation 2-1 therefore, at equilibrium:

$$RT \ln \frac{[X]_A}{[X]_B} + zF(E_A - E_B) = 0 \qquad \textbf{2-2}$$

Solving for $E_A - E_B$, one obtains:

$$E_A - E_B = -\frac{RT}{zF} \ln \frac{[X]_A}{[X]_B} = \frac{RT}{zF} \ln \frac{[X]_B}{[X]_A} \qquad \textbf{2-3}$$

Equation 2-3 is called the **Nernst equation.** The condition of equilibrium was assumed in its derivation, and THE NERNST EQUATION IS SATISFIED ONLY FOR IONS IN EQUILIBRIUM. It allows the computation of the electrical potential difference, $E_A - E_B$, required to produce an electrical force, $zF(E_A - E_B)$, equal and opposite to the concentration force, which equals:

$$-\frac{RT}{zF} \ln \frac{[X]_A}{[X]_B}$$

The Nernst equation can be used to determine whether an ion is in equilibrium across a membrane

It is often convenient to convert the Nernst equation to a form involving the logarithm to the base 10 (log) rather than natural logarithms (ln). The formula for this conversion is $\ln(x) = 2.303 \log(x)$. Because biological potentials are usually expressed in millivolts (mV), the units of R may be selected so that RT/F comes out in millivolts. At 29.2° C the quantity 2.303 RT/F is equal to 60 mV. Because this quantity is proportional to the absolute temperature, it changes by approximately 1/300 (0.33%) for each centigrade degree. Thus the value of 60 mV for 2.303 RT/F holds approximately for most experimental conditions in biology, and a useful form of the Nernst equation follows:

$$E_A - E_B = \frac{-60 \text{ mV}}{z} \log \frac{[X]_A}{[X]_B} = \frac{60 \text{ mV}}{z} \log \frac{[X]_B}{[X]_A} \qquad \textbf{2-4}$$

Examples of uses of the Nernst equation

EXAMPLE 1.   In Figure 2-2, K^+ is 10 times more concentrated on side A than on side B. The following is a calculation of the electrical potential difference that

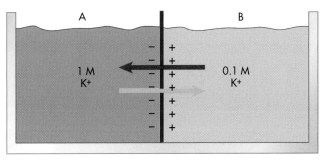

$$E_A - E_B = -60 \text{ mV}$$

Figure 2-2 A membrane separates chambers containing K^+ at different concentrations. At an electrical potential difference ($E_A - E_B$) of -60 mV, K^+ is in electrochemical equilibrium across the membrane. The red arrow indicates the electrical gradient; the yellow arrow indicates the concentration gradient.

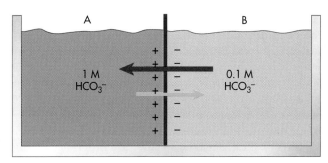

$$E_A - E_B = +100 \text{ mV}$$

Figure 2-3 A membrane separates chambers containing different HCO_3^- concentrations. $E_A - E_B = +100$ mV. HCO_3^- is not in electrochemical equilibrium. If $E_A - E_B$ were $+60$ mV, HCO_3^- would be in equilibrium. $E_A - E_B$ ($+100$ mV) is stronger than it needs to be ($+60$ mV) to just balance the tendency for HCO_3^- to move from A to B because of its concentration difference. Thus a net movement of HCO_3^- from B to A occurs. The red arrow indicates the electrical gradient; the yellow arrow indicates the concentration gradient.

must exist between the chambers for K^+ to be in equilibrium across the membrane. Because K^+ should be in equilibrium, the Nernst equation holds:

$$E_A - E_B = \frac{-60 \text{ mV}}{1} \log \frac{[K^+]_A}{[K^+]_B} = -(60 \text{ mV}) \log \frac{0.1}{0.01} = \qquad \textbf{2-5}$$
$$-60 \text{ mV} \log(10) = -60 \text{ mV}$$

The Nernst equation reveals that at equilibrium, A must be -60 mV relative to B. This polarity is correct because K^+ tends to move from B to A driven by this electrical force, which counteracts the tendency for it to move from A to B as a result of the concentration difference.

This example shows that AN ELECTRICAL POTENTIAL DIFFERENCE OF ABOUT **60 MV** IS REQUIRED TO BALANCE A TENFOLD CONCENTRATION DIFFERENCE OF A UNIVALENT ION. This is a useful rule of thumb.

EXAMPLE 2. In Figure 2-3 the Nernst equation can aid in the determination of whether HCO_3^- is in equilibrium. If HCO_3^- is not in equilibrium, the equation allows a prediction regarding the direction of net flow of HCO_3^-.

The Nernst equation reveals that the electrical potential difference, $E_A - E_B$, just balances the concentration difference of HCO_3^- across the membrane, as follows:

$$E_A - E_B = \frac{-60 \text{ mV}}{-1} \log \frac{[HCO_3^-]_A}{[HCO_3^-]_B} = +(60 \text{ mV}) \log \frac{1}{0.1} = \qquad \textbf{2-6}$$
$$+60 \text{ mV} \log(10) = +60 \text{ mV}$$

Thus a potential difference of $+60$ mV between A and B would just balance the tendency of HCO_3^- to move from A to B because of its concentration difference. However, $E_A - E_B$ is actually $+100$ mV. Therefore the electrical force is in the right direction to balance the concentration force, but it is 40 mV larger than it needs to be to just balance the concentration force. Because

the electrical force on HCO_3^- is larger than the concentration force, the electrical force determines the direction of net HCO_3^- movement. Net HCO_3^- flow occurs from B to A.

In summary, the Nernst equation can be used to predict the direction that ions tend to flow, as follows:

1. If the potential difference measured across a membrane is equal to the potential difference calculated from the Nernst equation for a particular ion, then that ion is **in electrochemical equilibrium** across the membrane, and no net flow of that ion will occur across the membrane.

2. If the measured electrical potential is of the same sign as that calculated from the Nernst equation for a particular ion but is larger in magnitude than the calculated value, then the electrical force is larger than the concentration force, and net movement of that particular ion tends to occur in the direction determined by the electrical force.

3. When the electrical potential difference is of the same sign but is numerically less than that calculated from the Nernst equation for a particular ion, then the concentration force is larger than the electrical force, and net movement of that ion tends to occur in the direction determined by the concentration difference.

4. If the electrical potential difference measured across the membrane is of the opposite sign to that predicted by the Nernst equation for a particular ion, then the electrical and concentration forces are in the same direction. Thus that ion cannot be in equilibrium, and it tends to flow in the direction determined by both electrical and concentration forces.

Gibbs-Donnan equilibrium: certain properties of cells are due to the presence of impermeant anions in the cytosol

Cytoplasm typically contains proteins, organic polyphosphates, nucleic acids, and other ionized substances that cannot permeate the plasma membrane. The majority of these impermeant intracellular ions are negatively charged at physiological pH. The steady-state properties of this mixture of permeant and impermeant ions are described by the **Gibbs-Donnan equilibrium.**

As a model of a cell with impermeant anions, consider a membrane separating a solution of KCl from a solution of KY, where Y^- is an anion to which the membrane is completely impermeable (Figure 2-4, *top*). The membrane is permeable to water, K^+, and Cl^{-4}. Suppose that initially chamber A contains a 0.1 M solution of KY and that chamber B contains an equal volume of 0.1 M KCl. Because $[Cl^-]_B$ exceeds $[Cl^-]_A$, there is a net flow of Cl^- from B to A. Negatively charged Cl^- ions flowing from B to A create an electrical potential difference (chamber A negative) that causes K^+ to also flow from B to A. Given enough time, K^+ and Cl^- come to equilibrium. At equilibrium, both $\Delta\mu(K^+)$ and $\Delta\mu(Cl^-)$ must equal zero. When both K^+ and Cl^- are at equilibrium:

$$[K^+]_A[Cl^-]_A = [K^+]_B[Cl^-]_B \qquad \textbf{2-7}$$

Equation 2-7 is called the **Donnan relation** or the **Gibbs-Donnan equation,** and it holds for any pair of univalent cation and anion in equilibrium between the two chambers. If other univalent ions that could attain an equilibrium distribution were present, the same reasoning and an equation similar to Equation 2-7 would apply to each cation-anion pair among them as well.

For this model situation, application of the Gibbs-Donnan equation results in the final concentrations shown in Figure 2-4, *bottom*. In this Gibbs-Donnan equilibrium, K^+ and Cl^- (but not Y^-) are in electrochemical equilibrium. This means that both K^+ and Cl^- must satisfy the Nernst equation, so the equilibrium transmembrane electrical potential difference can be computed from the Nernst equation for either K^+ or Cl^-. Applying the Nernst equation to either K^+ or Cl^- results in:

$$E_A - E_B = -60 \text{ mV} \log(2) = -18 \text{ mV}$$

The presence of the impermeant Y^- anions results in a negative electrical potential in the chamber that contains them. In this way the impermeant anions in the cytoplasm of a typical cell contribute on the order of -10 mV to the resting membrane potential of the cytoplasm relative to the extracellular fluid.

Only the permeant ions (K^+ and Cl^- in this example) attain equilibrium. The impermeant anion, Y^-, cannot reach an equilibrium distribution. It may not be evident

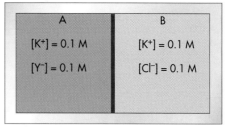

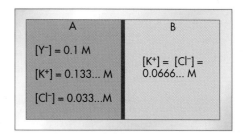

Membrane permeable to HCO_3^- and Cl^- but impermeable to Y^-

Figure 2-4 *Top,* Initial concentrations. Before a Gibbs-Donnan equilibrium is established, a membrane separates two aqueous compartments. The membrane is permeable to water, K^+, and Cl^- but is impermeable to Y^-. *Bottom,* Equilibrium concentrations. Ion concentrations after a Gibbs-Donnan equilibrium has been attained.

that water also does not achieve equilibrium, unless provision is made for that to occur. The sum of the concentrations of K^+ and Cl^- ions in chamber A in the preceding example exceeds that in chamber B. This is a general property of Gibbs-Donnan equilibria. When the impermeant Y^- is also taken into account, the total concentration of osmotically active ions is considerably greater in A than in B. Water tends to flow by osmosis from B to A until the total osmotic pressure of the two solutions is equal. However, ions then flow to set up a new Gibbs-Donnan equilibrium, and this requires that there be more osmotically active ions on the side with Y^-. All the water from B ends up in A unless water is restrained from moving.

This can be done by enclosing the solution in chamber A in a rigid container (Figure 2-5). Then as fluid flows from B to A, pressure builds up in A, and this pressure opposes further osmotic water flow. The pressure in A at equilibrium is equal to the difference between the total osmotic pressures of the solutions in A and B. The rigid cell wall of plant cells allows turgor pressure to build up in the cell and to partly compensate for the osmotic effects of the Gibbs-Donnan equilibrium. Left to its own devices, the Gibbs-Donnan equilibrium results in an osmotic pressure in the cytoplasm that is in excess of that in the extracellular fluid. This poses a threat to the maintenance of the normal cellular volume. Animal cells do not have rigid cell walls and have thus evolved other ways that involve ion transport processes to deal with the osmotic consequences of the Gibbs-Donnan equilibrium.

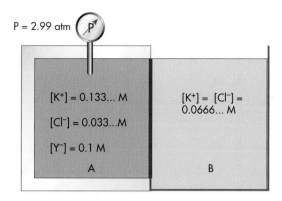

Figure 2-5 A hydrostatic pressure *(P)* of 2.99 atm is required to prevent water from flowing from B to A in the Gibbs-Donnan equilibrium in Figure 2-4. This 2.99 atm is equal to the osmotic pressure in chamber A minus that in chamber B.

Ion transport processes are required for the regulation of cell volume

Both K^+ and Cl^- are nearly in equilibrium across many plasma membranes, and their distribution is influenced by the predominantly negatively charged impermeant ions, such as proteins and nucleotides, in the cytoplasm. This being the case, why does the osmotic imbalance previously discussed not cause the cells to swell and finally burst? One reason is that CELLS ACTIVELY PUMP Na^+ OUT OF THE CYTOPLASM TO THE EXTRACELLULAR FLUID. The extrusion of Na^+ decreases the osmotic pressure of the cytoplasm and increases that of the extracellular fluid. The pumping of Na^+ is done by the Na^+ pump (i.e., Na^+,K^+-ATPase) in the plasma membrane. The Na^+,K^+-ATPase splits an ATP and uses some of the energy released to extrude three sodium ions from the cytoplasm and to pump two potassium ions into the cell. Whereas K^+ is only slightly removed from an equilibrium distribution, Na^+ is pumped out against a large electrochemical potential difference.

When the ATP production of a cell is compromised (e.g., in the presence of metabolic inhibitors or low O_2 levels) or when the Na^+,K^+-ATPase is specifically inhibited, Na^+ enters the cell more rapidly than it can be pumped out. As a result, the cell swells.

The plasma membranes of red blood cells from patients with **hereditary spherocytosis (HS)** are about three times more permeable to Na^+ than red blood cells from normal individuals. The level of Na^+,K^+-ATPase in the erythrocyte membranes of such patients is also substantially elevated. When these red cells have sufficient glucose to maintain normal ATP levels, they extrude Na^+ as rapidly as it diffuses into the cell cytosol, and the red cell volume is maintained. However, when such erythrocytes are delayed in the venous sinuses of the spleen, where glucose and ATP are present at low levels, the intracellular ATP concentrations fall; Na^+ cannot be pumped out by Na^+,K^+-

ATPase as rapidly as it enters; and the red cells swell. The swollen erythrocytes are prone to destruction by the spleen; consequently, patients with HS become anemic.

Resting Membrane Potentials

The cytosol of a cell at rest is electronegative relative to the extracellular fluid

Communication between nerve cells depends on an electrical disturbance called an **action potential** that is propagated in the plasma membrane of the nerve cell. In striated muscle an action potential propagates rapidly over the entire cell surface and allows the cell to contract synchronously (see Chapter 13). The action potential in nerve and muscle cells and the ionic mechanisms that account for its properties are discussed in Chapter 3. All cells that can produce action potentials have sizable resting membrane potentials (cytoplasm negative) across their plasma membranes. Inexcitable cells also have negative resting membrane potentials.

The resting membrane potential of a skeletal muscle cell is about −90 mV. By convention, membrane potential differences are expressed as the voltage in the cytoplasm minus the voltage in the extracellular fluid. A negative value denotes that the cytoplasm is electrically negative relative to the extracellular fluid. The resting membrane potential is necessary for the cell to fire an action potential.

Actively transported ions are not in electrochemical equilibrium across the plasma membrane. It is shown later that the flow of ions across the plasma membrane, down their electrochemical potential gradients, is directly responsible for generating much of the resting membrane potential. An understanding of how an ion's electrochemical potential gradient can give rise to a transmembrane difference in electrical potential can be gained by first considering a model system known as a **concentration cell.**

Concentration cells: a concentration gradient of a permeant ionic species across a membrane produces an electrical potential difference across the membrane

In Figure 2-6 the membrane that separates chambers A and B is permeable to cations but not to anions. Initially, no electrical potential difference exists across the membrane. K^+ flows from A to B because of the concentration force acting on it. Cl^- has the same force on it but cannot flow because the membrane is impermeable to anions. The flow of K^+ from A to B transfers a net positive charge to B and leaves a very slight excess of negative charges behind on A. A thus becomes electrically negative to B (Figure 2-6). This electrical force is oppositely directed to the concentration force on K^+. The more K^+ that flows, the larger the opposing electrical force. Net K^+ flow stops when the electrical force just balances the concentration force, which occurs

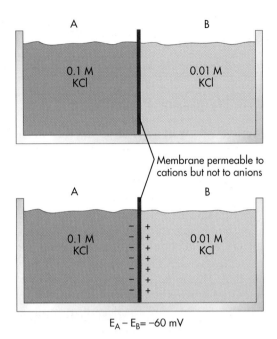

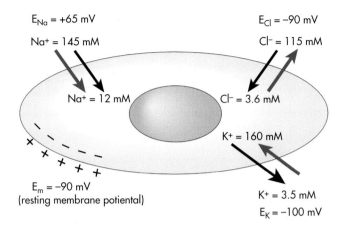

$E_A - E_B = -60$ mV

Figure 2-6 *Top,* Initial concentrations. A membrane that is permeable to cations but not to anions separates KCl solutions of different concentrations. *Bottom,* Equilibrium concentrations. Electrochemical equilibrium has been established. The flow of an infinitesimal amount of K$^+$ generated an electrical potential difference across the membrane that is equal to the equilibrium potential for K$^+$.

Figure 2-7 Approximate concentrations of Na$^+$, K$^+$, and Cl$^-$ in the cytoplasm of a human skeletal muscle cell and in the surrounding extracellular fluid. The equilibrium potentials of the ions are indicated. The concentration forces on the ions are indicated by black arrows and the electrical forces by green arrows.

when the electrical potential difference is equal to the equilibrium (Nernst) potential for K$^+$:

$$E_A - E_B = \frac{-60 \text{ mV}}{+1} \log \frac{[\text{K}^+]_A}{[\text{K}^+]_B} = -(60 \text{ mV}) \log \frac{0.1}{0.01} = -60 \text{ mV}$$

Only a very small amount of K$^+$ flows from A to B before equilibrium is reached. This is because the separation of positive and negative charges requires a large amount of work. The electrical potential difference that builds up to oppose further K$^+$ movement is a manifestation of that work.

THE K$^+$ CONCENTRATION DIFFERENCE IN THIS EXAMPLE ACTS LIKE A BATTERY. The natural tendency for any ion that can flow is to seek equilibrium; thus K$^+$ tends to flow until its equilibrium potential difference is established. As explained later, when more than one type of ion can permeate a membrane, each ion "strives" to make the transmembrane potential difference equal to its equilibrium potential. The more permeant an ion, the greater its ability to force the electrical potential difference toward its equilibrium potential.

Gradients of ion concentrations across the plasma membrane help generate the resting membrane potential

In most tissues a number of ions are not in equilibrium between the extracellular fluid and the cytoplasm. Figure 2-7 gives approximate concentrations of Na$^+$, K$^+$, and Cl$^-$ in the extracellular fluid and in the cytoplasmic water of hu-

man skeletal muscle. The resting membrane potential of a typical skeletal muscle cell is about -90 mV. Cl$^-$ is very close to being in equilibrium across the plasma membrane of skeletal muscle cells. This is known because chloride's equilibrium potential (E_{Cl}), as calculated from the Nernst equation, is about equal to the measured transmembrane potential difference (Figure 2-7). K$^+$ has a concentration force that tends to make it flow out of the cell. The electrical force on K$^+$ is oppositely directed to the concentration force. If the $E_{in} - E_{out}$ in skeletal muscle were -100 mV, the value of E_K, electrical and concentration forces on K$^+$ would exactly balance. Because $E_{in} - E_{out}$ is only -90 mV, the concentration force on K$^+$ is greater than the electrical force. Therefore K$^+$ has a net tendency to flow out of the cell. Both the concentration and the electrical forces on Na$^+$ tend to cause it to flow into the cell. Na$^+$ is the ion farthest from an equilibrium distribution. The larger the difference between the measured membrane potential and the equilibrium potential for an ion, the larger the net force tending to make that ion flow.

By extruding more Na$^+$ than the K$^+$ taken up, Na$^+$, K$^+$-ATPase contributes directly to generation of the resting membrane potential

The Na$^+$,K$^+$-ATPase located in the plasma membrane uses the energy of the terminal phosphate ester bond of ATP to extrude Na$^+$ actively from the cell and to take K$^+$ actively into the cell. The Na$^+$-K$^+$ pump is responsible for the high intracellular K$^+$ concentration and the low intracellular Na$^+$ concentration. Because the pump moves a larger number of Na$^+$ ions out than K$^+$ ions in (three Na$^+$ to two K$^+$), it causes a net transfer of positive charge out of the cell and thus contributes to the resting membrane potential. Because it brings about net movement of charge across the membrane, the pump is termed **electrogenic.**

The size of the pump's electrogenic contribution to the resting potential can be estimated by completely inhibiting the pump with a cardiac glycoside such as **ouabain.** Such studies show that in some cells the electrogenic Na^+-K^+ pump is responsible for a large fraction of the resting potential. In many vertebrate nerve and skeletal muscle cells, however, the direct contribution of the pump to the resting potential is small: less than 5 mV. The resting membrane potential in nerve and skeletal muscle results mainly from the diffusion of ions down their electrochemical potential gradients. The ionic gradients are maintained by active ion pumping. In other types of excitable cells, electrogenic pumping of ions may contribute more to the resting membrane potential. In certain smooth muscle cells, for example, the electrogenic effect of the Na^+-K^+ pump is responsible for at least 20 mV of the resting membrane potential.

Cardiac glycosides, such as **digitalis** and related medications, can increase the heart's strength of contraction (see Chapter 18). These compounds inhibit the Na^+-K^+ pump. Consequently, the intracellular level of Na^+ in cardiac cells is elevated. Each contraction of the heart is initiated by an increase in the cytosolic concentration of Ca^{++} (see Chapter 17). For cardiac muscle to relax, Ca^{++} must be removed from the cytosol, which is accomplished by its being pumped into the sarcoplasmic reticulum (SR) by a Ca^{++}-ATPase in the SR membrane and out across the plasma membrane by plasma membrane Ca^{++}-ATPase and by Na^+/Ca^{++} exchangers in the plasma membrane (see Chapter 1). In the presence of cardiac glycosides, because of the elevated cytosolic Na^+ concentration, the Na^+/Ca^{++} exchanger is not as effective in extruding Ca^{++} from the cell. Consequently, Ca^{++}-ATPase can accumulate more Ca^{++} in the SR, so more Ca^{++} is released from the SR to power the next cardiac contraction, which is stronger than normal because of the higher peak level of Ca^{++} in the cytosol.

The diffusion of ions down their electrochemical potential gradients contributes to generation of the resting membrane potential

The earlier discussion of concentration cells shows how an ion gradient can act as a battery. WHEN A NUMBER OF IONS ARE DISTRIBUTED ACROSS A MEMBRANE, ALL BEING REMOVED FROM ELECTROCHEMICAL EQUILIBRIUM, EACH ION TENDS TO FORCE THE TRANSMEMBRANE POTENTIAL TOWARD ITS OWN EQUILIBRIUM POTENTIAL AS CALCULATED FROM THE NERNST EQUATION. THE MORE PERMEABLE THE MEMBRANE TO A PARTICULAR ION, THE GREATER STRENGTH THAT ION WILL HAVE IN FORCING THE MEMBRANE POTENTIAL TOWARD ITS EQUILIBRIUM POTENTIAL. In skeletal muscle (Figure 2-7) the Na^+ concentration difference can be regarded as a battery that tries to make E_{in} − E_{out} equal to +65 mV. The K^+ concentration difference resembles a battery that attempts to make E_{in} − E_{out}

equal to −100 mV. The Cl^- concentration difference resembles a battery trying to make E_{in} − E_{out} equal to −90 mV.

THE CHORD CONDUCTANCE EQUATION DESCRIBES THE CONTRIBUTIONS OF PERMEANT IONS TO THE RESTING MEMBRANE POTENTIAL.   The way in which the interplay of ion gradients creates the resting membrane potential (E_m) is illustrated by a simple mathematical model. For the distribution of K^+, Na^+, and Cl^- across the plasma membrane of a cell, the following equation predicts the transmembrane potential difference across the membrane:

$$E_m = \frac{g_K}{\Sigma g} E_K + \frac{g_{Na}}{\Sigma g} E_{Na} + \frac{G_{Cl}}{\Sigma g} E_{Cl} \qquad \textbf{2-8}$$

where:

g = the conductance of the membrane to the ion indicated by the subscript
Σg = $(g_K + g_{Na} + g_{Cl})$
E = the equilibrium potentials of the ion denoted by the subscript

Conductance is the reciprocal of resistance ($g = 1/R$). The more permeable the membrane to a particular ion, the greater the conductance of the membrane to that ion.

Equation 2-8 is called the **chord conductance equation.** It states that the membrane potential is a weighted average of the equilibrium potentials of all the ions to which the membrane is permeable, in this case K^+, Na^+, and Cl^-. The weighting factor for each ion is the fraction of the total ionic conductance of the membrane (the sum of the individual ionic conductances) that results from the conductance of the ion in question. The sum of the weighting factors for the ions must equal one, so if one weighting factor grows larger, the others must become smaller. The chord conductance equation shows that THE GREATER THE CONDUCTANCE OF THE MEMBRANE TO A PARTICULAR ION, THE GREATER THE ABILITY OF THAT ION TO BRING THE MEMBRANE POTENTIAL TOWARD THE EQUILIBRIUM POTENTIAL OF THAT ION.

For the skeletal muscle fiber discussed earlier, E_{in} − E_{out} = −90 mV. The membrane potential is much closer to E_K (−100 mV) than to E_{Na} (+65 mV) because in the resting cell, g_K is larger than g_{Na} The chord conductance equation predicts that in resting muscle, g_K is about 10 times larger than g_{Na}. This has been confirmed by ion flux measurements with radioactive tracers. In other types of excitable cells the relationship between g_K and g_{Na} may be somewhat different. Other ions also may play a role in generating the resting membrane potential. Resting membrane potentials vary from approximately −10 mV in human erythrocytes to around −40 mV in some types of smooth muscle and up to −90 mV or more in vertebrate skeletal muscle and cardiac ventricular cells.

K+ has the largest resting conductance and thus has the largest influence on the resting membrane potential. For this reason, changes that occur in the concentration of K+ in a patient's extracellular fluid affect the resting membrane potentials of all cells. An increase in extracellular K+ partially depolarizes cells (decreases the magnitude of the resting membrane potential), whereas a decrease in the level of extracellular K+ hyperpolarizes cells (increases the magnitude of the resting membrane potential). Either a depolarization or a hyperpolarization of cardiac cells (see Chapter 17) may lead to cardiac arrhythmias, some of which are life threatening. **Hypokalemia** (low serum K+ levels) may result from long-term use of diuretics. **Hyperkalemia** (elevated serum K+ level) occurs in acute renal failure and in a disorder called **primary hyperkalemic periodic paralysis,** which is characterized by episodes of muscle weakness and flaccid paralysis.

Na+,K+-ATPase contributes directly and indirectly to the establishment of the resting membrane potential

The Na+-K+ pump establishes gradients of Na+ and K+ across the plasma membranes of cells. Because the amount of Na+ pumped out is larger than the amount of K+ pumped in, THE PUMP TRANSFERS NET CHARGE ACROSS THE MEMBRANE AND IN THIS WAY CONTRIBUTES DIRECTLY TO THE RESTING MEMBRANE POTENTIAL. In vertebrate skeletal and cardiac muscles and in nerves, the electrogenic activity of the pump is directly responsible for only a small fraction of the resting membrane potential. The major portion of the resting membrane potential in these tissues results from the diffusion of Na+ and K+ down their electrochemical potential gradients, with each ion tending to bring the transmembrane potential toward its own equilibrium potential. THIS CONTRIBUTION TO THE RESTING MEMBRANE POTENTIAL IS INDIRECTLY CAUSED BY Na+,K+-ATPASE. The relative magnitude of the direct and indirect contributions of Na+,K+-ATPase to the resting membrane potential varies from one cell type to another.

SUMMARY

- An ion tends to flow across a membrane if there is a concentration difference of that ion or an electrical potential difference across the membrane.
- The electrochemical potential difference ($\Delta\mu$) of an ion across a membrane includes the contributions of both the concentration difference and the electrical potential difference to the tendency of the ion to flow across the membrane.
- The electrochemical potential difference of an ion across a membrane represents a difference of chemical potential energy. This potential energy difference can be harnessed to do work.

- An ion that is distributed in equilibrium across a membrane satisfies the Nernst equation, which can be used to tell whether an ion is in equilibrium or to compute what the electrical potential difference across the membrane would have to be for a particular ion to be in equilibrium.
- Cytoplasm contains an excess of negative ions that are impermeant to the plasma membrane. A permeant univalent ion pair that can attain equilibrium across the membrane, X^+ and Z^-, satisfies the Gibbs-Donnan equilibrium, which is represented by the relationship: $[X]_{in}[Z]_{in} = [X]_{out}[Z]_{out}$, where *in* and *out* refer to cytoplasm and extracellular fluid, respectively.
- All cells have a negative resting membrane potential; that is, the cytoplasm is electrically negative relative to the extracellular fluid.
- The diffusion of ions across the plasma membrane and down their electrochemical potential gradients contributes to the resting membrane potential.
- The flow of each ion across the plasma membrane tends to bring the resting membrane potential toward the equilibrium potential for that ion. The more conductive the membrane to a particular ion, the greater the ability of that ion to bring the membrane potential toward its equilibrium potential. This is described by the chord conductance equation.
- Three processes contribute to generation of the resting membrane potential: ionic diffusion as just described (major), the electrogenic effect of Na+,K+-ATPase (variable in importance), and the Gibbs-Donnan equilibrium (minor in excitable cells).

BIBLIOGRAPHY

Aidley DJ: *The physiology of excitable cells,* ed 3, Cambridge, 1990, Cambridge University Press.

Hille B: *Ion channels of excitable membranes,* ed 2, Sunderland, Mass, 1992, Sinauer Associates.

Hodgkin AL: *The conduction of the nervous impulse,* Springfield, Ill, 1964, Charles C Thomas.

Kandel ER, Schwartz JH, Jessell TM: *Principles of neural science,* ed 3, New York, 1992, Elsevier Science.

Katz B: *Nerve, muscle, and synapse,* New York, 1966, McGraw-Hill.

Keynes RD, Aidley DJ: *Nerve and muscle,* ed 2, New York, 1991, Cambridge University Press.

Laüger P: *Electrogenic ion pumps,* Sunderland, Mass, 1991, Sinauer Associates.

Levitan IB, Kaczmarek LK: *The neuron: cell and molecular biology,* ed 2, New York, 1997, Oxford University Press.

Nicholls JG, Martin AR, Wallace BG: *From neuron to brain,* ed 3, Sunderland, Mass, 1992, Sinauer Associates.

Shepherd GM: *Neurobiology,* ed 3, New York, 1994, Oxford University Press.

▷ CASE STUDIES

Case 2-1

A 20-year-old woman suffers from anemia and occasional bouts of jaundice. Her medical records reveal that over the last 10 years, she has had episodes of moderate to severe anemia, usually after a febrile illness. Her spleen is markedly enlarged. A blood smear shows a large number of microspherocytes (erythrocytes that are round and somewhat smaller than normal). The osmotic fragility of the patient's erythrocytes (measured by putting the erythrocytes in hypotonic solutions) is much greater than that of erythrocytes from normal individuals. Her erythrocytes had normal content of Na^+ and K^+. Membrane permeabilities to Na^+ and K^+ and the level of Na^+,K^+-ATPase in the red cell membrane were about three times normal. The average life span of the patient's erythrocytes is well below normal. When an aliquot of the patient's erythrocytes was labeled and injected intravenously into a normal individual, the patient's erythrocytes had a markedly reduced survival time compared with that of normal erythrocytes. When labeled erythrocytes from a normal individual were infused into the patient, their survival time was comparable to that in the normal donor. After a splenectomy, the patient's anemia was mostly reversed. The patient's disorder was diagnosed as **hereditary spherocytosis.**

1. For which reason does the patient's erythrocytes have a higher osmotic fragility?
   A. The erythrocytes are smaller than normal.
   B. They are round.
   C. Their Na^+ permeability is elevated.
   D. Their Na^+,K^+-ATPase level is higher than normal.
   E. Their ability to use ATP for ion pumping is compromised.

2. Which statement is true about the patient's anemia?
   A. It is due partly to a decreased rate of erythropoiesis.
   B. It is due to an abnormality in the patient's spleen.
   C. It is due partly to the elevated Na^+,K^+-ATPase level in the patient's erythrocytes.
   D. It is due partly to the increased permeability of the erythrocytes to Na^+.
   E. It is increased after febrile illness because fever increases the rate that the spleen destroys erythrocytes.

3. Which of the following statements is true?
   A. Even in the presence of adequate ATP levels the Na^+,K^+-ATPase activity of the patient's erythrocytes cannot compensate for the increased permeabilities to Na^+ and K^+.
   B. Diminished deformability of the patient's erythrocytes contributes to their destruction in the spleen.
   C. If the patient's erythrocytes were infused into a normal individual, their life span would be the same as those of the normal individual.
   D. Removal of the patient's spleen contributes to an increased rate of hematopoiesis.

E. The increased permeability to K^+ contributes to the increased hemolysis in the absence of glucose and ATP.

Case 2-2
A 10-year-old boy experiences sporadic attacks of muscle paralysis. The onset of these attacks is characterized by pain associated with contractures of the affected muscles. Later in the attack, these muscles may become paralyzed and more flaccid. Episodes of pain and contracture frequently occur without subsequent paralysis. Analysis of blood samples taken during an attack indicate that the patient is hyperkalemic. Plasma K^+ levels are in the normal range when the patient is not having an attack. Biopsies of the patient's muscle show a significantly diminished level of intracellular K^+ compared to control muscle. The basal tissue activity of Na^+,K^+-ATPase is within the normal range. Paralytic attacks are accompanied by diuresis with increased K^+ excretion. Microelectrode studies found that during an attack, the magnitude of the resting membrane potential of skeletal muscle cells is diminished compared to control muscle fibers. Electromyography shows that early in an attack, the muscle contractures are associated with spontaneous action potentials in the affected muscle fibers. Later, during the paralytic phase of an attack, muscle cells become electrically inexcitable. A paralytic attack can be relieved by an insulin injection. Long-term administration of the β_2-agonist albuterol dramatically diminishes the occurrence of episodes of both contractures and subsequent paralytic attacks. The diagnosis is **primary hyperkalemic periodic paralysis.**

1. Which of the following statements is correct?
   A. The disorder is likely to involve increased membrane Cl^- conductance.
   B. Because the resting membrane potential of muscle cells is smaller (less negative), the intracellular $[Cl^-]$ is expected to be decreased.
   C. A decrease in intracellular $[Na^+]$ has occurred in the patient's skeletal muscle cells.
   D. An increasing resting conductance to Na^+ might contribute to this disorder.
   E. The decreased intracellular $[K^+]$ would be expected to lead to hyperpolarization (more negative resting membrane potential).

2. Which of the following statements is correct?
   A. Because the muscle does not contract during an attack when its motor nerve is stimulated, a defect in the neuromuscular junction is probably involved.
   B. Insulin improves the patient's condition by enhancing glucose metabolism.
   C. Albuterol improves the patient's condition by promoting the production of ATP from fatty acids in the muscle.

D. Diminished resting K^+ conductance could be responsible for the diminished (depolarized) resting membrane potential.

E. None of the above.

3. **Some cases of primary hyperkalemic periodic paralysis are associated with a mutation in the voltage-gated Na^+ channel. The mutation decreases the rate and extent of inactivation of the Na^+ channel that occurs when the membrane is depolarized (see Chapter 3). Which of the following statements is correct?**

   A. The mutated channel might lead to persistently elevated Na^+ influx into the muscle cells after muscle activity.

   B. If A were true, the patient's muscles should have decreased levels of intracellular $[Na^+]$.

   C. If A were true, the activity of Na^+,K^+-ATPase in the patient's muscle cells would be lower than normal.

   D. The described mutation is not consistent with the decreased resting membrane potential during an attack.

   E. Paralysis should be associated with hyperpolarization (larger, more negative resting potential) rather than with depolarization.

CHAPTER 3

Generation and Conduction of Action Potentials

- Describe in terms of the chord conductance equation how the changes in the conductances to Na^+ and K^+ account for the form of the action potential.
- Define the absolute and relative refractory periods and accommodation and explain these phenomena in terms of the voltage-dependent properties of Na^+ and K^+ channels.
- Explain electrotonic conduction in terms of local circuit currents.
- Describe the local response and define the length constant and explain its determinants.
- Explain why an axon with large diameter conducts faster than a smaller axon.
- Explain how myelination of an axon greatly increases its conduction velocity.

An action potential is a rapid change in the membrane potential that is propagated along the length of the cell. Action potentials are the basis for most communication between neurons (see Chapters 4 and 6 to 11). Action potentials elicit the contraction of skeletal muscle cells and permit contraction to occur nearly synchronously along the length of the cell (see Chapters 4 and 13). Action potentials in cardiac muscle cells spread from one cell to another via gap junctions, causing contractions of the ventricle to occur in a coordinated manner that permits the effective pumping of blood (see Chapters 17 and 18).

Action Potentials Have Different Forms in Different Tissues

An **action potential** is a rapid change in the membrane potential followed by a return to the resting membrane potential (Figure 3-1). The size and shape of action potentials differ considerably from one excitable tissue to another. An action potential is propagated with the same shape and size along the whole length of a nerve or muscle cell. Voltage-dependent ion channel proteins in the plasma membrane are responsible for action potentials. Different action potentials in the cell types shown in Figure 3-1 occur because these cells have different populations of voltage-dependent ion channels.

Membrane Potentials

The membrane potential of a cell can be measured by penetrating its plasma membrane with a microelectrode

Knowledge of the ionic mechanisms of action potentials was first obtained from experiments on the squid giant axon. The large diameter (≤ 0.5 mm) of the squid giant axon makes it a convenient model for electrophysiological research with intracellular electrodes. The information learned from the squid axon applies in large part to mammalian neurons. The frog sartorius muscle is another useful preparation.

If the plasma membrane of a single muscle cell of a frog sartorius muscle is penetrated by a microelectrode (tip diameter < 0.5 μm), a potential difference is observed between the microelectrode whose tip is inside the cell and an extracellular electrode. The internal electrode is about −90 mV with respect to the external electrode. This 90-mV potential difference is the resting membrane potential of the muscle fiber. In the absence of perturbing influences, the resting membrane potential remains at 90 mV.

Subthreshold changes in membrane potential are conducted with decrement

If a pulse of current flows across a cell's plasma membrane, the membrane potential changes. Current pulses are **depolarizing** or **hyperpolarizing** depending on the direction of current flow. The terms depolarizing and hyperpolarizing may be confusing. A change in the membrane potential from −90 to −70 mV is a depolarization because it is a decrease in the potential difference, or polarization, across the cell membrane. If the membrane potential changes from −90 to −100 mV, the polarization of the membrane has increased; this is hyperpolarization. The

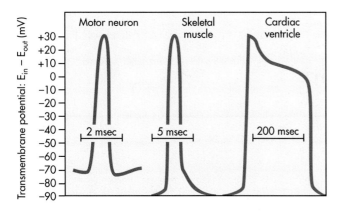

Figure 3-1 Action potentials from three vertebrate cell types. Note the different time scales. *(Redrawn from Flickinger CJ et al: Medical cell biology, Philadelphia, 1979, WB Saunders.)*

larger the current passed, the larger the perturbation of the membrane potential.

When subthreshold current pulses are passed, the size of the potential change observed depends on the distance of the recording electrode from the point of current passage (Figure 3-2, *A*). THE CLOSER THE RECORDING ELECTRODE TO THE SITE OF CURRENT PASSAGE, THE LARGER THE POTENTIAL CHANGE OBSERVED. The size of the potential change decreases exponentially with distance from the site of current passage (Figure 3-2, *B*). The response is said to be **conducted with decrement.** The distance over which the potential change decreases to 1/e (37%) of its maximum value is called the **length constant** or space constant. (*e* is the base of natural logarithms and is equal to 2.7182.) A LENGTH CONSTANT OF 1 TO 2 MM IS TYPICAL FOR MAMMALIAN NERVE OR MUSCLE CELLS. Because these potential changes are observed primarily near the site of current passage and the changes are not propagated along the length of the cell (as are action potentials), they are called **local responses.**

An action potential remains the same size and shape as it spreads across the membrane

If progressively larger depolarizing current pulses are applied, a condition is reached at which a different sort of response, the action potential, occurs (Figure 3-3). AN ACTION POTENTIAL IS TRIGGERED WHEN THE DEPOLARIZATION IS SUFFICIENT FOR THE MEMBRANE POTENTIAL TO REACH A THRESHOLD VALUE. The action potential differs from the local response in two important ways: (1) it is a much larger response, with the polarity of the membrane potential reversing (i.e., the cell interior becoming positive with respect to the exterior), and (2) the action potential is propagated without decrement down the entire length of the nerve or muscle fiber. THE SIZE AND SHAPE OF AN ACTION POTENTIAL REMAIN THE SAME AS THE POTENTIAL TRAVELS ALONG THE CELL. Unlike the local response, the potential does not decrease in size with distance. When a stimulus larger than the threshold stimulus is applied, the size

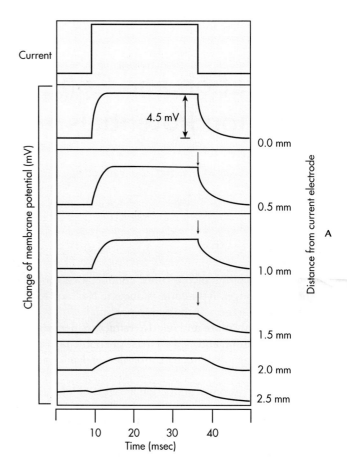

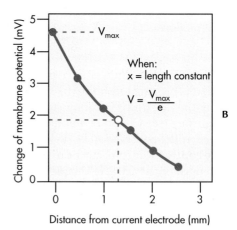

Figure 3-2 A, Responses of an axon of a shore crab to a subthreshold rectangular pulse of current recorded extracellularly by an electrode located different distances from the current-passing electrode. As the recording electrode is moved farther from the point of stimulation, the response of the membrane potential is slower and smaller. **B,** The maximum change in membrane potential from **A** is plotted versus distance from the point of current passage. The distance over which the response falls to 1/e (37%) of the maximal response *(Vmax)* is the length constant. *(A redrawn from Hodgkin AL, Rushton WAH: Proc R Soc B133:97, 1946.)*

and shape of the action potential do not change. Either a stimulus fails to elicit an action potential (a subthreshold stimulus), or it produces a full-sized action potential. For this reason the action potential is an **all-or-none response.**

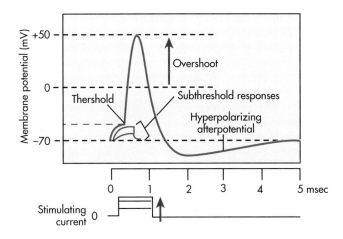

Figure 3-3 Responses of the membrane potential of a squid giant axon to increasing pulses of depolarizing current. When the cell is depolarized to threshold, it fires an action potential.

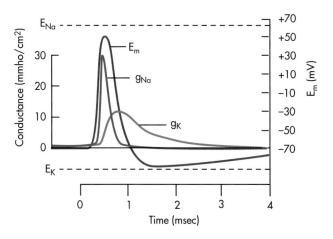

Figure 3-4 The action potential E_m of a squid giant axon is shown on the same time scale as the associated changes in g_{Na} and g_K. *(Redrawn from Hodgkin AL, Huxley AF: J Physiol 117:500, 1952.)*

Ionic Mechanisms of Action Potentials

Action potentials in neurons have a characteristic form

The form of an action potential of a squid giant axon is shown in Figure 3-3. Action potentials in many mammalian neurons have a similar shape. Once the membrane is depolarized to the threshold, an explosive depolarization occurs and completely depolarizes the membrane and even overshoots so that the membrane becomes polarized in the reverse direction. The peak of the action potential reaches about +50 mV. The membrane potential then returns toward the resting membrane potential almost as rapidly as it was depolarized. After repolarization, a transient hyperpolarization occurs that is known as the **hyperpolarizing afterpotential.** It persists for about 4 msec.

The neuronal action potential is caused by changes in the conductance of the membrane to Na+ and K+

In Chapter 2 the resting membrane potential was seen to be a weighted sum of the equilibrium potentials for ions such as Na+, K+, and Cl−. The weighting factor for each ion is the fraction that its conductance contributes to the total ionic conductance of the membrane (the chord conductance equation, Equation 2-8). In squid giant axon the resting membrane potential (E_m) is about −70 mV. E_K is about −100 mV in squid axon; hence an increase in the conductance to K+ (g_K) would hyperpolarize the membrane, and a decrease in g_K would tend to depolarize the membrane. E_{Cl} is about −70 mV, so an increase in the conductance to Cl− (g_{Cl}) would stabilize E_m at −70 mV. An increase in the conductance to Na+ (g_{Na}) of sufficient magnitude would cause depolarization and reversal of the membrane polarity because E_{Na} is about +65 mV in squid giant axon.

In the 1950s, Hodgkin and Huxley showed that the action potential of squid giant axon is caused by successive increases in conductance to Na+ and K+. They found that g_{Na} increases very rapidly during the early part of the action potential (Figure 3-4). g_{Na} reaches a peak about the same time as the peak of the action potential; then it decreases rapidly. g_K increases more slowly, reaches a peak at about the middle of the repolarization phase, and then returns more slowly to resting levels.

As described in Chapter 2, the chord conductance equation shows that the membrane potential is a result of the opposing tendencies of the K+ gradient to bring E_m toward the equilibrium potential for K+ and the Na+ gradient to bring E_m toward the equilibrium potential for Na+. Increasing the conductance of either ion increases its ability to pull E_m toward its equilibrium potential. The rapid increase in g_{Na} during the early part of the action potential causes the membrane potential to move toward the equilibrium potential for Na+ (+65 mV). The peak of the action potential reaches only about +50 mV because g_{Na} quickly decreases toward resting levels and because g_K increases to provide an opposing tendency to the depolarization. The rapid return of the membrane potential toward the resting potential is caused by the rapid decrease in g_{Na} and the continued increase in g_K. These conductance changes decrease the size of the Na+ term in the chord conductance equation and increase the size of the K+ term. During the hyperpolarizing afterpotential, when the membrane potential is actually more negative (more polarized) than the resting potential, g_{Na} returns to baseline levels, but g_K remains elevated above resting levels. Thus E_m is pulled closer to the K+ equilibrium potential (−100 mV) as long as g_K remains elevated.

Na+ and K+ channels open and close in response to changes in the membrane potential

Hodgkin and Huxley proposed that the ion currents pass through separate Na+ and K+ channels, each with distinct characteristics, in the plasma membrane. Subsequent re-

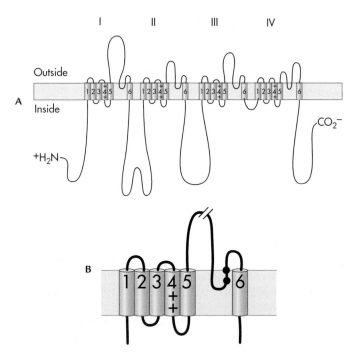

Figure 3-5 Model of the voltage-dependent Na$^+$ channel protein. **A,** Two-dimensional model. The cylinders represent transmembrane α-helices. There are four repeats of six-cylinder domains of homologous α-helices. The S4 helices, marked with plus signs, function as voltage sensors, and movements of these helices are responsible for activation (opening) of the channel. The intracellular loop connecting domains III and IV functions as the inactivation gate: after depolarization, with a slight delay, this loop apparently swings up into the mouth of the channel to block ion conduction. **B,** Domain IV. The part of the extracellular loop that connects helices 5 and 6 and that dips into the membrane helps form the selectivity filter of the channel. The residues indicated by solid circles are key determinants of the ionic selectivity of the channel. *(**B** redrawn from Catterall W: J Bioenergetics Biomemb 28:219, 1996.)*

Tetrodotoxin (TTX), one of the most potent poisons known, is a specific blocker of the Na$^+$ channel. It binds to the extracellular side of this channel. **Tetraethylammonium** (TEA$^+$) blocks the K$^+$ channel. It enters the K$^+$ channel from the cytoplasmic side and blocks the channel because it cannot pass through it.

> The ovaries of certain species of puffer fish, also known as **blowfish,** contain TTX. Raw puffer fish is a highly prized dish in Japan. Connoisseurs of puffer fish enjoy the tingling numbness of the lips that is caused by minuscule quantities of TTX present in the flesh. Sushi chefs who are trained to remove the ovaries safely are licensed by the government to prepare this dish. Nevertheless, several people die each year from eating improperly prepared puffer fish.

Saxitoxin is another blocker of Na$^+$ channels. Saxitoxin is produced by reddish dinoflagellates that are responsible for the so-called red tide. Shellfish eat the dinoflagellates, and saxitoxin becomes concentrated in their tissues. A person who eats these shellfish may experience life-threatening paralysis about 30 minutes after the meal.

An ion channel has an open state and a closed state

It is possible to study the behavior of individual ion channels. One way to do this is to incorporate either purified ion channel proteins or bits of membrane into planar lipid bilayers that separate two aqueous compartments. Then electrodes placed in the aqueous compartments can be used to monitor or impose currents and voltages across the membrane. Under some conditions, only one or a few ion channels of a particular type may be present in the planar membrane. The ion channels spontaneously oscillate between an open state and a closed state.

Another way to study individual ion channels involves the use of so-called **patch electrodes.** A fire-polished microelectrode is placed against the surface of a cell, and suction is applied to the electrode to form a high-resistance seal around the tip of the electrode (Figure 3-6, *A*). The sealed patch electrode can then be used to monitor the activity of whatever channels happen to be trapped inside the seal. Sometimes, the patch trapped inside the electrode contains more than one functional ion channel (Figure 3-6, *B*).

During an action potential, there is a rapid influx of Na$^+$. The time course of this inward Na$^+$ current resembles that of the change in the Na$^+$ conductance shown in Figure 3-4. In contrast, the behavior of each Na$^+$ channel is random, like the behavior of the channels shown in Figure 3-6, *B*. The probability of each Na$^+$ channel being in the open state is increased when the membrane is depolar-

search has supported this interpretation and has determined some of the properties of proteins that form the channels. The amino acid sequences of several K$^+$ and Na$^+$ channels have been determined, and knowledge of the structure of ion channels is rapidly expanding (Figure 3-5). Although the three-dimensional structure of the Na$^+$ channel remains to be determined, its intramembrane domain is known to consist of a number of α-helices that span the membrane and probably surround the ion channel. The Na$^+$ channel has both an **activation gate** and an **inactivation gate** that account for the changes in g_{Na} during an action potential (Figure 3-4). Groups of charged amino acid residues that form these gates have been tentatively identified. To enter the channel's narrowest part, known as the **selectivity filter,** K$^+$ and Na$^+$, it is believed, must shed most of their waters of hydration. To strip K$^+$ or Na$^+$ of its associated water molecules, negative amino acid residues that line the pore of the channel must have a particular geometric shape, the precise geometry being different for K$^+$ than for Na$^+$. This requirement is believed to confer the specificity of ion channels.

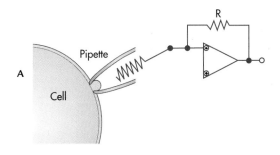

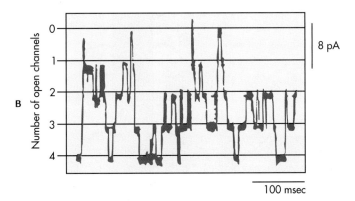

Figure 3-6 A, Patch electrode and circuitry required to record the ionic currents that flow through the small number of ion channels isolated in the electrode patch. **B,** Current recording from a patch electrode on the plasma membrane of a skeletal muscle cell. The five current levels show that this particular patch contains four different ion channels, each opening and closing independently of the others. *(A redrawn from Sigworth FJ, Neher E:* Nature *287:447, 1980.* **B** *redrawn from Hammill OP et al:* Pflügers Arch *391:85, 1981.)*

ized to threshold, and then the probability of being open decreases (channel inactivation). The macroscopic Na^+ current is the average current through thousands of Na^+ channels. The "average channel" opens (activates) promptly in response to depolarization; then after a short delay, the channel closes (inactivates) even though the applied depolarization is maintained.

Action potentials in cardiac muscle cells have a different shape than nerve and muscle action potentials because different voltage-gated ion channels are present in cardiac cells

An action potential in a cardiac ventricular cell is shown in Figure 3-1. The initial rapid depolarization and overshoot are caused by the rapid entry of Na^+ through channels that are very similar to the Na^+ channels of nerve and skeletal muscle. After the initial depolarization and overshoot, the cardiac ventricular action potential has a plateau phase. The plateau is caused by another set of channels that are distinct from the fast Na^+ channels, open and close more slowly than the fast Na^+ channels, and are sometimes called **slow channels.** The slow channels belong to a particular class of Ca^{++} channels called **L-type Ca^{++} channels** (for long lasting). The Ca^{++} that enters the cell via the

L-type Ca^{++} channels during the plateau phase helps initiate contraction of the ventricular cell and stimulates release of more Ca^{++} from the sarcoplasmic reticulum of the heart cell. The repolarization of the ventricular cell is brought about by the closing of the L-type Ca^{++} channels and by a much delayed opening of the K^+ channels. The ionic mechanisms of cardiac action potentials are discussed in more detail in Chapter 17.

Properties of Action Potentials

The voltage inactivation of Na^+ channels is responsible for refractory periods and accommodation

If a neuron or skeletal muscle cell is partially depolarized (e.g., by increasing the concentration of K^+ in the extracellular fluid), its action potential has a slower rate of rise and a smaller overshoot than the action potential of the normally polarized cell. This is a result of a smaller electrical force driving Na^+ into the depolarized cell and voltage inactivation of some of the Na^+ channels. The increase in g_{Na} in response to a depolarization is self-inactivating; that is, the inactivation gates close soon after the activation gates open. Once the Na^+ channels are inactivated, the membrane must be repolarized toward the normal resting membrane potential before the channels can be reopened. As the membrane potential is restored toward normal resting levels, more and more of the Na^+ channels again become capable of being activated.

The explosive depolarizing phase of the action potential may be compared to a chemical explosion. A chemical explosion requires a critical mass of material; the spike of the action potential can be generated only if a critical number of Na^+ channels are recruited. WHEN A CELL IS PARTLY DEPOLARIZED, THE POOL OF ACTIVABLE Na^+ CHANNELS IS REDUCED; consequently a stimulus may not be able to recruit a sufficient number of Na^+ channels to generate an action potential. Voltage inactivation of Na^+ channels partially accounts for important properties of excitable cells, such as refractory periods and accommodation.

During the first part of an action potential, it is impossible to elicit another action potential

During much of the action potential, the membrane is completely refractory to further stimulation. This means that no matter how strongly the cell is stimulated, it is unable to fire a second action potential. This unresponsive state is called the **absolute refractory period** (Figure 3-7). The cell is refractory because a large number of its Na^+ channels are voltage inactivated and cannot be reopened until the membrane is repolarized.

During the latter part of the action potential, the cell is able to fire a second action potential, but a stronger-than-normal stimulus is required. This is the **relative refractory period.** Early in the relative refractory period, before

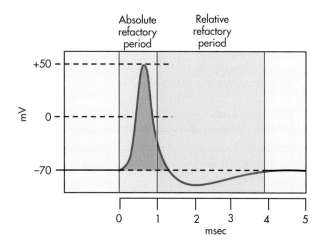

Figure 3-7 Action potential of a nerve, illustrating the associated absolute and relative refractory periods.

the membrane potential has returned to the resting potential level, some Na$^+$ channels are voltage inactivated; hence a stronger-than-normal stimulus is required to open the critical number of Na$^+$ channels needed to trigger an action potential. Throughout the relative refractory period, the conductance to K$^+$ is elevated, which opposes depolarization of the membrane. This also contributes to the refractoriness.

A cell that is depolarized too slowly may fail to fire an action potential

When a nerve or muscle cell is depolarized slowly, the normal threshold may be passed without an action potential being fired; this is called **accommodation.** Na$^+$ and K$^+$ channels are both involved in accommodation. During slow depolarization, some of the Na$^+$ channels that are opened by depolarization have enough time to become voltage inactivated before the threshold potential is attained. If depolarization is slow enough, the critical number of open Na$^+$ channels required to trigger the action potential may never be attained. In addition, K$^+$ channels open in response to the depolarization. The increased g_K tends to repolarize the membrane, making it still more refractory to depolarization.

In an inherited disorder called **primary hyperkalemic periodic paralysis,** patients suffer episodes of painful spontaneous contractures of muscles followed by periods of paralysis of the affected muscles. These symptoms are accompanied by elevated levels of K$^+$ in the plasma and extracellular fluid. The elevation of extracellular K$^+$ contributes to depolarization of skeletal muscle cells. Initially the depolarization brings muscle cells closer to threshold, so spontaneous action potentials and contractions are more likely. As depolarization of the cells becomes more marked, the cells accommodate because of

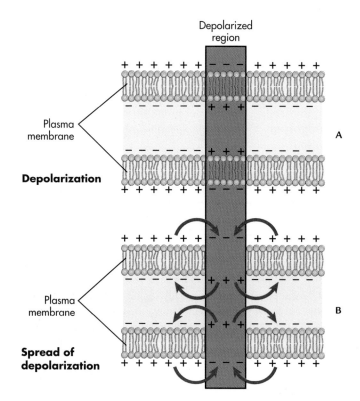

Figure 3-8 Mechanism of electrotonic spread of depolarization. **A,** Reversal of membrane polarity that occurs with local depolarization. **B,** Local currents that flow to depolarize adjacent areas of the membrane and allow conduction of the depolarization.

voltage-inactivated Na$^+$ channels. Thus they become unable to fire action potentials and are unable to contract in response to action potentials in their motor axons.

Conduction of Action Potentials

Local circuit currents are responsible for the conduction of action potentials and subthreshold responses

Action potentials and subthreshold responses are conducted along a nerve or muscle fiber by local current flows (Figure 3-8). The same factors that govern the velocity of electrotonic conduction also determine the speed of action potential propagation. Figure 3-8, *A*, shows the membrane of an axon or muscle fiber that has been depolarized in a small region. In this region the external surface of the membrane is negative relative to the adjacent membrane, and the internal face of the depolarized membrane is positively charged relative to neighboring internal areas. The potential differences cause **local circuit currents** to flow (Figure 3-8, *B*), which depolarize the membrane adjacent to the initial site of depolarization. These newly depolarized areas then cause current flows that depolarize other segments of the membrane still farther removed from the initial site of depolarization. This mechanism of conduction is known as **electrotonic conduction.**

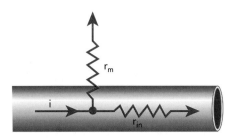

Figure 3-9 An axon or a muscle fiber resembles an electrical cable. Currents *(i)* that flow across the membrane resistance (r_m) are lost from the cable. Currents that flow through the longitudinal resistance (r_{in}) carry the electrical signal along the cable. The larger the ratio r_m/r_{in}, the more efficient the signal transmission along the fiber.

The length constant is determined by resistance properties of the cell

A subthreshold depolarization is conducted electrotonically, and it diminishes in strength as it moves along the cell. Thus it is conducted with decrement. As shown in Figure 3-2, *B*, an electrotonically conducted signal dies away to 37% of its maximal strength over a distance of one length constant (about 1 to 2 mm) and decreases to almost nothing over about 5 mm.

A nerve or muscle fiber has some of the properties of an electrical cable. In a perfect cable the insulation surrounding the core conductor prevents all loss of current to the surrounding medium, so a signal is transmitted along the cable with undiminished strength (Figure 3-9). The plasma membrane of an unmyelinated nerve or muscle fiber serves as the insulation, the cytoplasm being the core conductor. The membrane has a resistance (r_m) much higher than the resistance of the cytoplasm (r_{in}), but (partly because of its thinness) the plasma membrane is not a perfect insulator. The higher the ratio of r_m to r_{in}, the less current lost across the plasma membrane, the better the cell can function as a cable, and the longer the distance that a signal can be transmitted electrotonically without significant decrement. r_m/r_{in} determines the **length constant** of a cell: the length constant is equal to $(r_m/r_{in})^{1/2}$.

An action potential does not diminish in size because it is self-reinforcing

Many nerve and muscle fibers are much longer than their length constants (1 to 2 mm). Skeletal muscle cells can be as long as 1 to 2 cm. Nerve axons can be around 1 m in length. Conduction with decrement will not work for such long cells. The action potential conducts an electrical impulse with undiminished strength along the full length of these cells. To do this, the action potential reinforces itself as it is conducted along the fiber. Thus the action potential may be said to be **propagated** as well as conducted. The conduction of the action potential occurs via local circuit currents by the electrotonic mechanism depicted in Figure 3-8. When the areas on either side of the depolarized region reach threshold, these areas also fire action potentials,

which locally reverses the polarity of the membrane potential. By local current flow, the areas of the fiber adjacent to these areas are next brought to threshold, and these areas in turn fire action potentials. A cycle of depolarization occurs by local current flow followed by generation of an action potential in a restricted region that then is conducted along the length of the fiber, with "new" action potentials being generated as they spread. In this way the action potentials are regenerated as they spread, and the action potential propagates over long distances, keeping the same size and shape.

BECAUSE THE SHAPE AND SIZE OF THE ACTION POTENTIAL ARE USUALLY INVARIANT, ONLY VARIATIONS IN THE FREQUENCY OF THE ACTION POTENTIALS CAN BE USED IN THE CODE FOR INFORMATION TRANSMISSION ALONG AXONS. The maximum frequency is limited by the duration of the absolute refractory period (≈ 1 msec) to about 1000 impulses/sec in large mammalian nerves.

The conduction velocity is determined by the resistance and capacitance of the cell

The speed of electrotonic conduction of an action potential or a local response along a nerve or muscle fiber is determined by the electrical properties of the cytoplasm and of the plasma membrane that surrounds the fiber. The following discussion focuses on the mechanism of electrotonic conduction, but it applies equally well to the mechanism of propagation of the action potential.

FIBERS THAT ARE LARGER IN DIAMETER HAVE A GREATER CONDUCTION VELOCITY. This is caused principally by the decrease in resistance to conduction in the cytoplasm along the length of the fiber as the radius (and hence the cross-sectional area) of the fiber increases.

Myelination results in a dramatic increase in conduction velocity

In vertebrates, certain nerve fibers are coated with **myelin;** such fibers are said to be **myelinated.** Myelin is formed from multiple wrappings of the plasma membranes of **Schwann cells** that wind themselves around the nerve fiber (Figure 3-10). The myelin sheath consists of several to more than 100 layers of plasma membrane. Gaps that occur in the sheath every 1 to 2 mm are known as **nodes of Ranvier.** These nodes are about 1 µm wide and are the lateral spaces between adjacent Schwann cells along the axon. MYELIN ALTERS THE ELECTRICAL PROPERTIES OF THE NERVE FIBER AND RESULTS IN A GREAT INCREASE IN THE CONDUCTION VELOCITY OF THE FIBER.

A squid giant axon with a 500-µm diameter has a conduction velocity of 25 m/sec and is unmyelinated. If conduction velocity were directly proportional to fiber radius, a human nerve fiber with a 10-µm diameter would conduct at 0.5 m/sec. With this conduction velocity a reflex withdrawal of the foot from a hot coal would take about 4 seconds. Even though human nerve fibers are much smaller in diameter than squid giant ax-

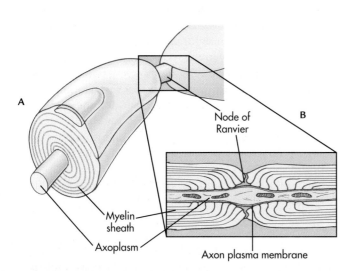

Figure 3-10 Myelin sheath. **A,** Drawing of Schwann cells wrapping around an axon to form a myelin sheath. **B,** Drawing of a cross section through a myelinated axon near a node of Ranvier.

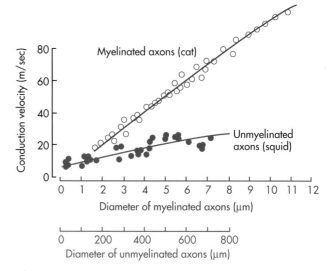

Figure 3-11 Conduction velocities of myelinated and unmyelinated axons as functions of axon diameter. Myelinated axons are from cat saphenous nerve at 38° C. Unmyelinated axons are from squid at 20° to 22° C. Note that myelinated axons have greater conduction velocities than unmyelinated axons 100 times greater in diameter. *(Data for myelinated axons from Gasser HS, Grundfest H: Am J Physiol 127:393, 1939. Data for unmyelinated axons from Pumphrey RJ, Young JZ: J Exp Biol 15:453, 1938.)*

ons, human reflexes are much faster than this. The myelin sheath that surrounds certain vertebrate nerve fibers results in a much greater conduction velocity than that of unmyelinated fibers of similar diameters. A 10-μm myelinated fiber has a conduction velocity of about 50 m/sec, which is twice that of the 500-μm squid giant axon. The high conduction velocity permits reflexes that are fast enough to allow humans to avoid dangerous stimuli. A myelinated axon has a greater conduction velocity than an unmyelinated fiber that is 100 times larger in diameter (Figure 3-11). As discussed next, the myelin sheath increases the velocity of action potential conduction by increasing the length constant of the axon, decreasing the capacitance of the axon, and restricting the generation of action potentials to the nodes of Ranvier.

Myelination greatly alters the electrical properties of the axon. The many wrappings of membrane around the axon increase the effective membrane resistance so that r_m/r_{in} (Figure 3-9), and thus the length constant is much greater. Less of the conducted signal is lost through the electrical insulation of the myelin sheath; hence the amplitude of a conducted signal declines less with distance along the axon. The myelin-wrapped membrane has a much smaller electrical capacitance than the naked axonal membrane. Therefore the local currents can more rapidly depolarize the membrane as a signal is conducted. For this reason the conduction velocity is greatly increased by myelination. BECAUSE OF THE INCREASE IN LENGTH CONSTANT AND CONDUCTION VELOCITY, AN ACTION POTENTIAL IS CONDUCTED WITH LITTLE DECREMENT AND AT GREAT SPEED FROM ONE NODE OF RANVIER TO THE NEXT.

The resistance to the flow of ions across the many layers of Schwann cell membrane that make up the myelin sheath is so high that the ionic currents are effectively localized to the short stretches of naked plasma membrane that occur at the nodes of Ranvier. Also the ion channels that participate in the action potential are especially concentrated at the nodes of Ranvier. For these reasons, the action potential is regenerated only at the nodes of Ranvier (1 to 2 mm apart) rather than at each place along the fiber, as is the case in an unmyelinated fiber. The action potential is rapidly conducted from one node to the next (in about 20 μsec) and "pauses" to be regenerated at each node. The action potential appears to "jump" from one node of Ranvier to the next, a process called **saltatory conduction.**

Myelinated axons are also more efficient metabolically than unmyelinated axons. The Na^+-K^+ pump extrudes the Na^+ that enters and reaccumulates the K^+ that leaves the cell during action potentials. In myelinated axons, ionic currents are restricted to the small fraction of the membrane surface at the nodes of Ranvier. For this reason, far fewer sodium and potassium ions traverse a unit area of fiber membrane, and much less ion pumping is required to maintain Na^+ and K^+ gradients.

In some diseases known as **demyelinating disorders,** the myelin sheath deteriorates. In **multiple sclerosis,** scattered progressive demyelination of axons in the central nervous system results in loss of motor control. The neuropathy common in severe cases of **diabetes mellitus** is due to demyelination of peripheral axons. When myelin is lost, the length constant, which is dramatically increased by myelination, becomes much shorter. Hence when the action potential is electrotonically conducted from one node of Ranvier to the next, it loses amplitude. If demyelination is sufficiently severe, the action potential may arrive at the next node of Ranvier with insufficient strength to fire an action potential. The axon then fails to propagate action potentials.

SUMMARY

■ Different cell types have differently shaped action potentials because their populations of voltage-dependent ion channels differ.

■ The action potential in a squid giant axon is generated by the rapid activation and subsequent voltage inactivation of voltage-dependent Na^+ channels and the delayed opening and closing of voltage-dependent K^+ channels.

■ Ion channels are integral membrane proteins that have ion-selective pores. Charged polypeptide regions of an ion channel protein act as gates that are responsible for the activation and inactivation of the channel.

■ An ion channel typically has two states: high conductance (open) and low conductance (closed). The channel oscillates randomly between the open and closed states. For a voltage-dependent channel the fraction of time the channel spends in the open state is a function of the transmembrane potential difference.

■ Cardiac muscle cells have L-type Ca^{++} channels that open and close slowly and are responsible for the long duration of the action potential in these cell types.

■ The voltage inactivation of Na^+ channels is an important factor in the absolute and relative refractory periods and in the accommodation of an excitable cell to a slowly rising stimulus.

■ Local circuit currents produce electrotonic conduction. This is the mechanism by which both subthreshold signals and action potentials are conducted along the length of a cell.

■ A subthreshold signal is conducted with decrement. It dies away to 37% of its maximal strength over a distance of 1 length constant. The length constant is equal to $(r_m/r_{in})^{1/2}$. A typical value for the length constant is 1 to 2 mm.

■ The action potential is propagated, rather than merely conducted: it is regenerated as it moves along the cell. In this way an action potential remains the same size and shape as it is conducted.

■ The velocity of conduction is determined by the electrical properties of the cell. A large-diameter cell has a faster conduction velocity.

■ Myelination dramatically increases the conduction velocity of a nerve axon. Because of myelination, an action potential is conducted very rapidly and with little decrement from one node of Ranvier to the next.

■ Action potentials are regenerated only at the nodes of Ranvier; the internodal membrane cannot fire an action potential. Because it takes much longer to generate an action potential at each node than it does for the action potential to be conducted between nodes, the action potential appears to jump from node to node; this is saltatory conduction.

BIBLIOGRAPHY

Aidley DJ: *The physiology of excitable cells,* ed 3, Cambridge, 1990, Cambridge University Press.

Armstrong C, Hille B: Voltage-gated ion channels and electrical excitability, *Neuron* 20:371, 1998.

Catterall WA: Structure and function of voltage-gated ion channels, *Annu Rev Biochem* 64:493, 1995.

Hille B: *Ionic channels of excitable membranes,* ed 2, Sunderland, Mass, 1992, Sinauer Associates.

Hodgkin AL: *The conduction of the nervous impulse,* Springfield, Ill, 1964, Charles C Thomas.

Hoffman F, Biel M, Flockerzi V: Molecular basis for Ca^{2+} channel diversity, *Annu Rev Neurosci* 17:399, 1994.

Jan LY, Jan YN: Structural elements involved in specific K^+ channel functions, *Annu Rev Physiol* 54:537, 1992.

Katz B: *Nerve, muscle, and synapse,* New York, 1966, McGraw-Hill.

Levitan IB, Kaczmarek LK: *The neuron: cell and molecular biology,* ed 2, New York, 1997, Oxford University Press.

Neher E, Sakmann B: The patch clamp technique, *Sci Am* 266(3):28, 1992.

CASE STUDIES

Case 3-1

A 30-year-old woman is brought into the emergency room. Shortly after eating supper in a local restaurant, the woman experienced the following symptoms. First, there was a tingling sensation that affected the mouth and lips but then spread to the face and neck. Then the tingling spread down the arms and legs to the fingers and toes. At presentation the patient reports numbness of the areas that previously tingled and difficulty walking in a coordinated fashion. The patient says that she had shrimp cocktail as an appetizer, followed by salad, steak with baked potatoes and green beans, and apple pie and coffee for dessert. The patient says she has no history of allergic response to shellfish. The patient's superficial reflexes are almost absent, and her deep reflexes are markedly hypoactive. An extracellular electrode is placed in the patient's ulnar nerve. Then the palmar surface of the patient's little finger is scraped with the physician's fingernail in a way that should be painful to the patient. The patient cannot feel this stimulus, and no action potentials in the ulnar nerve are detected in response to the stimulus. When an intracellular microelectrode is placed in a sensory nerve fiber in the ulnar nerve, the resting membrane potential is found to be near −70 mV (normal). When an action potential is evoked by repeated vigorous scraping of the skin of the little finger as previously described, the action potential is slower to rise and of shorter height than expected from measurements in normal individuals. The diagnosis is **paralytic shellfish poisoning.**

1. **Paralytic shellfish poisoning is due to a compound called *saxitoxin* that is produced by dinoflagellates that are eaten by shellfish, which concentrate the toxin in their tissues. Which of the following is likely to be caused by the toxin?**

   A. Reducing the resting K^+ conductance in nerve and muscle cells

   B. Preventing K^+ channels from opening in response to a depolarization

   C. Preventing Na^+ channels from opening

   D. Slowing the voltage inactivation of Na^+ channels

   E. Slowing the normal closing of K^+ channels during an action potential

2. **The patient's symptoms are consistent with which of the following?**

   A. A malfunction of the cutaneous sensory system only

   B. A malfunction of the motor system only

   C. Malfunctions in both the cutaneous sensory system and the motor system

   D. Malfunction of neurons but not of muscle cells

   E. None of the above

3. **Which of the following is true?**

   A. This woman appears to have an unusual sensitivity to saxitoxin.

   B. There was no good reason to keep this patient in the hospital.

   C. The patient's recovery is due to the excretion of saxitoxin in the urine, limited by the slow dissociation of saxitoxin from Na^+ channels.

   D. This patient should be advised to never eat shellfish again.

   E. The patient is likely to have episodes of tingling sensation of mouth and lips for about 1 week.

Case 3-2

A 14-year-old boy complains of muscle stiffness that is not associated with pain. After shaking hands with the physician, the patient requires a few seconds to relax his grip. The patient's musculature is well developed with no signs of muscle atrophy. When a muscle is tapped, a dimpling of the belly of the muscle can be seen for several seconds. Electromyography shows spontaneous repetitive action potentials in response to placement of the needle electrode and repetitive action potentials elicited by tapping of the muscle. After a voluntary contraction, a series of spontaneous action potentials lasting several seconds is observed. A biopsy of an external intercostal muscle is performed. Analysis of the biopsy shows that the muscle levels of Na^+, K^+, and Cl^- are not signifi-

cantly different from normal. The resting membrane potential is not significantly different from the normal value, but the electrical resistance of the membrane is about two times normal. The diagnosis is **myotonia congenita.**

1. **The increase in membrane resistance implies a reduction in the conductance of the membrane to one or more ionic species. Which of the following is true?**

   A. The conductance of the plasma membrane to Na^+ is reduced.

   B. The conductance of the plasma membrane to K^+ is reduced.

   C. The conductance of the plasma membrane to Cl^- is reduced.

   D. The conductance of the plasma membrane to Ca^{++} is reduced.

   E. None of the above.

2. **Further studies have revealed that the cause of myotonia congenita is a mutation in the Cl^- channel that results in markedly lower Cl^- conductance. Which of the following is true?**

   A. There should be no change in the duration of the action potential.

   B. When the muscle is stimulated electrically, the threshold current should be larger.

   C. The repetitive action potentials cannot be explained on the basis of the lower Cl^- conductance.

   D. There is no reason that decreased Cl^- conductance should cause the increased mechanical excitability of the muscle.

   E. None of the above.

3. **The Cl^- channel is known to be a homotetramer. Dominant and recessive forms of myotonia congenita have been described, and both forms are associated with mutations of Cl^- channels. In both cases, muscle Cl^- conductance is reduced to about 10% of the normal value. Which of the following statements is true?**

   A. In the dominant form of the disease, it is likely that one mutant polypeptide in a tetramer is sufficient to greatly diminish the Cl^- conductance of the tetramer.

   B. In the recessive form of the disease, it is likely that one mutant polypeptide in a tetramer is sufficient to greatly diminish the Cl^- conductance of the tetramer.

   C. In the dominant form of the disease, it is likely that three or more mutant polypeptides in a tetramer are required to greatly diminish the Cl^- conductance of the tetramer.

   D. In the recessive form of the disease, it is likely that three or more mutant polypeptides in a tetramer are required to greatly diminish the Cl^- conductance of the tetramer.

   E. None of the above.

CHAPTER 4

Synaptic Transmission

OBJECTIVES

- Explain how gap junctions mediate electrical conduction between cells.
- Describe the sequence of events at a generalized chemical synapse.
- Contrast the synthesis, secretion, and recycling of small-molecule neurotransmitters with neuropeptides.
- Discuss the sequence of events at a neuromuscular junction.
- Explain how miniature endplate potentials reveal information about the quantal nature of transmitter release.
- Explain how integration can occur at a postsynaptic neuron.
- Contrast facilitation, posttetanic potentiation, synaptic fatigue, and long-term potentiation.
- Explain the criteria for establishing that a particular substance is a neurotransmitter at a particular synapse.

This chapter and the next deal with communication among cells. This chapter discusses communication among electrically excitable cells. Chapter 5 presents, in a more general context, the mechanisms whereby a regulatory molecule released by one cell can influence the activities of a target cell. A **synapse** is a site at which an electrical response is transmitted from one cell to another. At an **electrical synapse,** two excitable cells communicate directly by the passage of current between them via **gap junctions.** At a **chemical synapse** an action potential in the presynaptic cell causes an electrical response in the postsynaptic cell via the action of a **neurotransmitter** substance released by the presynaptic cell.

At Electrical Synapses, Gap Junctions Permit Ions to Flow from One Cell to Another

AT AN ELECTRICAL SYNAPSE A CHANGE IN THE MEMBRANE POTENTIAL OF ONE CELL IS TRANSMITTED TO ANOTHER CELL BY THE DIRECT FLOW OF CURRENT. Because current flows directly between two cells that make an electrical synapse, there is essentially no synaptic delay. Usually, electrical synapses allow conduction in both directions. In this respect, electrical synapses differ from chemical synapses, which are unidirectional (see later discussion). Certain electrical

synapses conduct more readily in one direction than in another; this property is called **rectification.**

Cells that form electrical synapses are joined by **gap junctions.** Gap junctions are plaquelike structures in which the plasma membranes of the coupled cells are very close (<3 nm). Freeze-fracture electron micrographs of gap junctions show regular arrays of intramembrane protein particles. The intramembrane particles consist of six subunits surrounding a central channel that is accessible to water, ions, and molecules as large as 1500 MW (Figure 4-1, *A*). The hexagonal array is called a **connexon.** Each of the six subunits is a single protein (one polypeptide chain) called **connexin** ($\approx$25,000 MW). At the gap junction the connexons of the coupled cells are aligned to form **connexon channels,** which allow the passage of ions and water-soluble molecules from one cell to another.

Connexon channels are not open continuously; they open and close (Figure 4-1, *B*) stochastically as do the voltage-gated ion channels discussed in Chapter 3. The probability of connexon channels being open may be changed by elevated intracellular Ca^{++} or H^+ in one of the cells or in response to depolarization of one or both of the cells.

Electrical synapses are widespread in the peripheral nervous system and the central nervous system (CNS) of invertebrates and vertebrates. Some neurons in the brain receive input by both electrical and chemical synapses. Electrical synapses are particularly useful in reflex pathways in which rapid transmission between cells (little synaptic delay) is necessary or when the synchronous response of a number of cells is required. AMONG THE MANY NONNEURONAL CELLS COUPLED BY GAP JUNCTIONS ARE HEPATOCYTES, MYOCARDIAL CELLS, INTESTINAL SMOOTH MUSCLE CELLS, AND EPITHELIAL CELLS OF THE LENS.

At a Chemical Synapse, a Neurotransmitter Substance Released by the Presynaptic Cell Evokes an Electrical Response in the Postsynaptic Cell

There are several types of chemical synapses. Most share the following properties:

1. The nerve ending of the presynaptic cell contains vesicles with neurotransmitter or neuromodulator substances (Figure 4-2). Vesicles that contain

"classic" small-molecule neurotransmitters, such as acetylcholine or norepinephrine, are small (≈ 50 nm in diameter), and many of the vesicles are docked near specialized release sites called **active zones** on the intracellular aspect of the presynaptic membrane. Vesicles that contain **neuropeptides** are larger and are distributed throughout the nerve terminal. Many nerve terminals contain both small vesicles with small-molecule transmitters and larger vesicles with neuropeptides.

2. An action potential in the presynaptic neuron opens voltage-gated Ca^{++} channels that are concentrated near the active zones in the nerve ter-

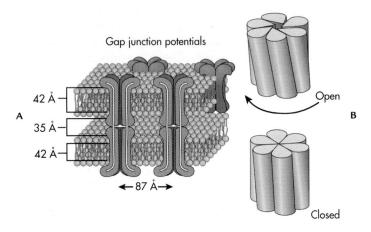

Gap junction potentials

42 Å

35 Å

42 Å

← 87 Å →

A

B

Open

Closed

Figure 4-1 A, Structure of gap junction channels. **B,** Opening and closing of a gap junction channel. *(A redrawn from Makowski L et al:* J Cell Biol *74:629, 1977.* **B** *redrawn from Unwin PNT, Zampighi G:* Nature *283:45, 1980.)*

minal. The influx of Ca^{++} into the nerve terminal raises the intracellular $[Ca^{++}]$; this is the trigger for the release of neurotransmitter via exocytosis into the **synaptic cleft,** the narrow (20 to 40 nm in width) space that separates the presynaptic and postsynaptic cells.

3. The neurotransmitter substance diffuses across the synaptic cleft to bind to specific **neurotransmitter receptor** proteins in the postsynaptic membrane. THE BINDING OF THE NEUROTRANSMITTER TO ITS RECEPTOR RESULTS IN A TRANSIENT CHANGE IN THE CONDUCTANCE OF THE POSTSYNAPTIC MEMBRANE TO ONE OR MORE IONS AND THEREBY CAUSES A TRANSIENT CHANGE IN THE MEMBRANE POTENTIAL OF THE POSTSYNAPTIC CELL. A transient depolarization of the postsynaptic cell is an **excitatory postsynaptic potential (EPSP);** a transient hyperpolarization of the postsynaptic cell is an **inhibitory postsynaptic potential (IPSP).**

4. THE RECEPTOR PROTEINS FOR MANY NEUROTRANSMITTERS ARE LIGAND-GATED ION CHANNELS. Binding of the neurotransmitter to its receptor alters the probability of the ion channel being open. In other cases the neurotransmitter receptor is the first protein in a signal-transduction cascade that alters the probability of an ion channel being open.

5. In some instances the neuroeffector substances, both nonpeptides and neuropeptides, function as **neuromodulators,** rather than as neurotransmitters. A neuromodulator usually binds to a receptor protein in the plasma membrane of the postsynaptic cell or the presynaptic nerve

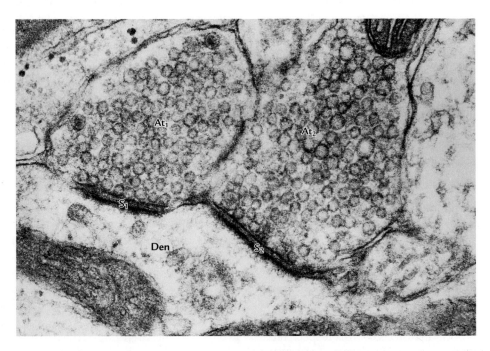

Figure 4-2 Synapses (S_1 and S_2) in the cerebral cortex. Two axon terminals (At_1 and At_2) synapse with a dendrite *(Den)* of a stellate cell. The axon terminals are packed with synaptic vesicles. *(From Peters A, Palay SL, Webster H deF:* The fine structure of the nervous system, *Philadelphia, 1976, WB Saunders.)*

terminal to initiate a signal-transduction cascade that influences the response of the postsynaptic cell to a neurotransmitter or alters the amount of neurotransmitter released by the presynaptic cell.

6. The action of most nonpeptide neurotransmitters is terminated when they are actively transported back into the presynaptic nerve ending by Na^+-powered secondary active transport. The action of neuropeptides is terminated by proteolysis or by diffusion away from the postsynaptic membrane.

7. Transmission at chemical synapses is one way. An action potential in the postsynaptic cell does not cause an electrical response of the presynaptic cell. The time that elapses between an action potential in the presynaptic nerve terminal and the postsynaptic potential it evokes, typically about 0.5 msec, is called a **synaptic delay.**

8. The presynaptic nerve terminal contains the enzymes for synthesizing small-molecule transmitters from simple precursors. The nerve terminal is the site of synthesis of nonpeptide neurotransmitters. In contrast, neuropeptides are synthesized in the rough endoplasmic reticulum of the cell body **(soma)** of the presynaptic neuron, and the peptide-loaded vesicles reach the nerve terminal via axonal transport.

9. After a vesicle containing a nonpeptide neurotransmitter fuses with the plasma membrane, its components are recycled as coated vesicles via endocytosis. The coated vesicles fuse with early endosomes, from which new synaptic vesicles bud. The nascent neurotransmitter vesicle membrane contains an ATPase that pumps H^+ ions into the vesicle interior and a neurotransmitter transporter that couples the downhill efflux of H^+ from the vesicles to the active accumulation of neurotransmitter into the vesicle. In contrast, neuropeptide-containing vesicles are not recycled; the membrane containing the components of these vesicles is degraded.

The Neuromuscular Junction Is a Chemical Synapse

The synapses between the axons of motor neurons and skeletal muscle fibers are called **neuromuscular junctions, myoneural junctions,** or **motor endplates.** Neuromuscular junctions were the first vertebrate synapses to be well characterized, and knowledge of them aids in the comprehension of other chemical synapses.

Near the neuromuscular junction the motor nerve loses its myelin sheath and divides into fine terminal branches, which lie in **synaptic troughs** on the surfaces of the muscle cells (Figures 4-3). The plasma membrane of the muscle cell lining the synaptic trough is thrown into numerous **junctional folds.** The axon terminals contain many 40-nm-diameter **synaptic vesicles** that contain **acetylcholine,** the neurotransmitter employed at this synapse. Many of the synaptic vesicles in the nerve terminals are docked at active zones on the prejunctional membrane; active zones are concentrated opposite the mouths of the junctional folds. **Acetylcholine receptor protein** molecules are concentrated near the crests of the junctional folds. The axon terminal and the muscle cell are separated by the **junctional cleft,** which contains a carbohydrate-rich amorphous material. When acetylcholine is released, it diffuses across the cleft to bind to acetylcholine receptors on the postjunctional membrane.

The enzyme **choline-O-acetyltransferase** in the motor nerve terminal catalyzes the condensation of acetyl coenzyme A (acetyl CoA) and choline. Acetyl CoA is produced by the neuron, as it is by most cells. CHOLINE CANNOT BE SYNTHESIZED BY THE MOTOR NEURON IN ADEQUATE AMOUNTS; IT IS OBTAINED BY ACTIVE UPTAKE FROM THE EXTRACELLULAR FLUID by a Na^+-coupled secondary active transporter in the nerve terminal membrane that can accumulate choline against a large electrochemical potential gradient.

Acetylcholine receptors are ligand-gated channels that conduct both Na^+ and K^+

The binding of acetylcholine to an acetylcholine receptor causes a transient opening of the ion channel that increases the conductance of the postjunctional membrane to Na^+ and K^+. Because the driving force on Na^+ is much greater than that on K^+ (see Chapters 2 and 3), the inward current of Na^+ predominates, causing a transient depolarization of the endplate region. The transient depolarization is called the **endplate potential (EPP)** (Figure 4-4).

THE EPP IS TRANSIENT BECAUSE THE ACTION OF ACETYLCHOLINE IS ENDED BY THE HYDROLYSIS OF ACETYLCHOLINE TO FORM CHOLINE AND ACETATE. The hydrolysis of acetylcholine is catalyzed by the enzyme **acetylcholinesterase,** which is present in high

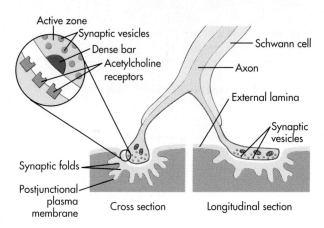

Figure 4-3 Structure of the neuromuscular junction in skeletal muscle. Docked vesicles are concentrated at active zones.

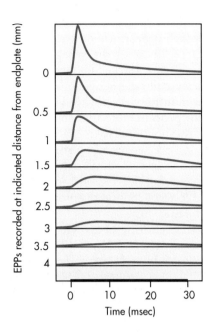

Figure 4-4 EPPs in a frog sartorius muscle. The preparation was treated with curare to bring the EPP just below threshold for eliciting an action potential. The EPP, recorded at increasing distances from the neuromuscular junction, decreases in amplitude and rate of rise. *(Redrawn from Fatt P, Katz B: J Physiol 115:320, 1951.)*

concentration on the postjunctional membrane. Choline liberated in the synaptic cleft is taken back up into the motor nerve terminal by a Na^+-powered secondary active transporter in the prejunctional plasma membrane.

> Drugs that inhibit acetylcholinesterase are called **anticholinesterases.** In the presence of an anticholinesterase, the EPP is both larger in magnitude and longer in duration. Anticholinesterases are useful in treating disorders in which the function of neuromuscular junctions is impaired, such as **myasthenia gravis** (see Case 4-2). **Hemicholiniums** are medications that block the plasma membrane choline transport system and inhibit choline uptake. Prolonged treatment with hemicholiniums depletes the store of transmitter and ultimately decreases the acetylcholine content of the vesicles.

The endplate potential elicits an action potential in the muscle cell plasma membrane

The EPP depolarizes the postjunctional membrane by 15 to 20 mV. BECAUSE THE POSTJUNCTIONAL MEMBRANE LACKS ADEQUATE NUMBERS OF VOLTAGE-GATED Na^+ AND K^+ CHANNELS, IT DOES NOT FIRE AN ACTION POTENTIAL. Local circuit currents (see Chapter 3) depolarize the muscle cell plasma membrane on either side of the neuromuscular junction to threshold, and action potentials are generated that propagate from near the neuromuscular junction to both ends of the muscle cell to cause the muscle cell to contract (see

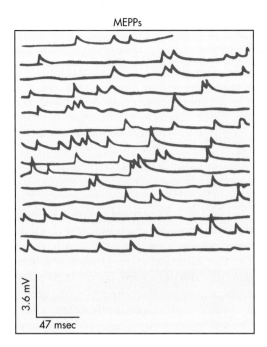

Figure 4-5 Spontaneous MEPPs recorded at a neuromuscular junction in a fiber of frog extensor digitorum longus muscle. *(Redrawn from Fatt P, Katz B: Nature 166:597, 1950.)*

Chapter 13). Under normal circumstances, a single action potential in the motor neuron causes a single action potential and a single twitch in each of the muscle cells innervated by that motor neuron (see Chapter 13).

Acetylcholine is released in small packets called quanta

The amount of acetylcholine released by the prejunctional nerve ending does not vary continuously; rather the amount varies in steps, with each step corresponding to the release of one synaptic vesicle. THE AMOUNT OF ACETYLCHOLINE CONTAINED IN ONE VESICLE CORRESPONDS TO A **QUANTUM** OF ACETYLCHOLINE.

Even if the motor neuron is not stimulated, small depolarizations of the postjunctional muscle cell occur spontaneously. These small spontaneous depolarizations are known as **miniature endplate potentials (MEPPs)** (Figure 4-5). They occur at random times with a frequency that averages about one per second. Each MEPP depolarizes the postjunctional membrane by only about 0.4 mV on average, not nearly enough to trigger an action potential in the adjacent muscle plasma membrane. The MEPP has the same time course as an EPP that is evoked by an action potential in the nerve terminal. The MEPP is similar to the EPP in its responses to most medications. The EPP and MEPP are both prolonged by medications that inhibit acetylcholinesterase, and both are similarly depressed by compounds that compete with acetylcholine for binding to the receptor protein. The frequency of MEPPs may vary, but their amplitudes are within a relatively narrow range (Figure 4-5). AN **MEPP** IS CAUSED BY THE SPONTANEOUS RELEASE OF ONE QUANTUM OF ACETYLCHOLINE INTO THE JUNCTIONAL CLEFT.

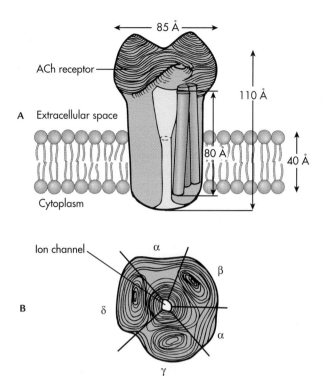

Figure 4-6 Structure of a nicotinic acetylcholine *(ACh)* receptor protein from *Torpedo,* an electric fish. **A,** Viewed from the side. **B,** Viewed looking down on the acetylcholine receptor from the extracellular surface. *(Redrawn from Kistler J et al: Biophys J 37:371, 1982).*

Acetylcholine receptor proteins are concentrated on the crests of the junctional folds

There are 10^7 to 10^8 acetylcholine receptor proteins per motor endplate. The acetylcholine receptor protein is an integral membrane protein that spans the hydrophobic lipid matrix of the postjunctional membrane. The acetylcholine receptor of the neuromuscular junction consists of five subunits (Figure 4-6), two of which (α subunits) are identical, so there are four different polypeptide chains (i.e., α, β, δ, γ). Each α subunit contains a binding site for acetylcholine; both α subunits must bind acetylcholine to open the ion channel.

So called α-**toxins** in cobra venoms are responsible for paralyzing the snakes' prey. (α-Toxins bind to the acetylcholine binding site on the α subunits of the **acetylcholine** receptor protein and prevent acetylcholine from acting. Poison arrows whose tips are dipped in **curare,** an α-toxin extracted from certain plants, are used by some South American Indians to paralyze their prey. **Succinylcholine,** which binds to the α subunit but cannot open the ion channel, is used an a paralytic agent in some surgical and medical procedures.

Acetylcholine receptor proteins are highly concentrated in the postjunctional membrane, and very few acetylcholine receptors are located elsewhere on the muscle plasma membrane. The mechanisms responsible for localizing the acetylcholine receptors in the postjunctional membrane are not completely understood, but it is clear that the motor neuron plays a role.

Chemical Synapses Between Neurons Share Many of the Properties of Neuromuscular Junctions

A presynaptic cell may make synapses with the dendrites, the soma, or the axon of a postsynaptic neuron. Synapses of a presynaptic axon with a dendrite of another cell, **axodendritic synapses,** are the most numerous synapses in the CNS. Synapses are particularly common on **dendritic spines,** protuberances on the dendrites that have a highly specialized structure. However, **axosomatic synapses,** synapses of axons with the cell body, or soma, of a postsynaptic neuron, and **axoaxonal synapses,** synapses of an axon with the axon of a postsynaptic neuron, also occur.

A postsynaptic cell may receive one or many presynaptic inputs

Each skeletal muscle cell has only one neuromuscular junction. A single action potential in the motor neuron elicits a single action potential in the muscle cell. The neuromuscular junction is a **one-to-one synapse.**

Certain neurons receive a single synaptic input; in some cases a single action potential in the presynaptic neuron evokes a burst of action potentials in the postsynaptic cell. This is a **one-to-many synapse.**

The most common situation is for a postsynaptic cell to receive many inputs; a **many-to-one** synaptic arrangement. In such cases, one action potential in a presynaptic cell is not typically sufficient to make the postsynaptic cell fire an action potential. The nearly simultaneous arrival of presynaptic action potentials in several input neurons that synapse on the postsynaptic cell is necessary to depolarize the postsynaptic cell to threshold.

Integration occurs at postsynaptic cells with multiple synaptic inputs

The spinal motor neuron has a many-to-one synaptic organization. About 10,000 presynaptic axons synapse on each spinal motor neuron (Figure 4-7): about 8000 on dendrites and about 2000 on the soma of the motor neuron. Some of these are excitatory inputs that cause a transient depolarization, an **EPSP,** of the postsynaptic cell (Figure 4-8). Other inputs cause a transient hyperpolarization, an IPSP. An EPSP brings the membrane potential of the postsynaptic cell closer to its threshold; an IPSP moves the membrane potential farther away from threshold. An EPSP depolarizes the postsynaptic cell by 1 to 2 mV; an IPSP hyperpolarizes it by about the same amount. The postsynaptic cell **integrates** its many synaptic inputs. IF THE MOMENTARY SUM OF THE INPUTS DEPOLARIZES THE POSTSYNAPTIC CELL TO ITS THRESHOLD, IT FIRES

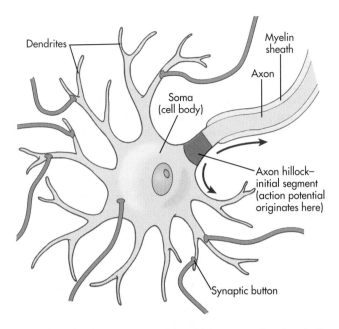

Figure 4-7 Spinal motor neuron with multiple synapses *(green)* on both soma and dendrites. There are about 10,000 synapses on a typical spinal motor neuron: 2000 on the soma and 8000 on the dendrites. The axon hillock–initial segment has the lowest threshold; as a result, action potentials tend to originate there.

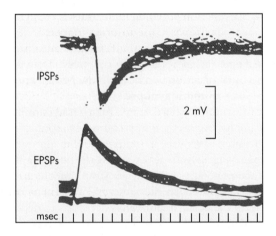

Figure 4-8 IPSPs and EPSPs recorded with a microelectrode in a cat spinal motor neuron in response to stimulation of appropriate peripheral afferent fibers. A total of 40 traces are superimposed. *(Redrawn from Curtis DR, Eccles JC: J Physiol 145:529, 1959.)*

AN ACTION POTENTIAL. THIS IS INTEGRATION AT THE LEVEL OF A SINGLE POSTSYNAPTIC NEURON.

Postsynaptic potentials in spinal motor neurons are caused by the opening of specific transmitter-gated ion channels

An EPSP (Figure 4-8) in a spinal motor neuron is caused by a transient increase of the conductance of the postsynaptic membrane to both Na^+ and K^+ in response to the neurotransmitter. At the cell's resting potential, the driving force

for Na^+ to enter the cell is much greater than the force for K^+ to leave. Hence in response to the neurotransmitter, a net inward flow of Na^+ ions predominates, and this depolarizes the postsynaptic cell.

An IPSP (Figure 4-8) in a cat spinal motor neuron is caused by a transient increase in the Cl^- conductance of the postsynaptic membrane in response to the binding of the inhibitory transmitter. At rest the net tendency is for Cl^- to enter the cell. The transmitter-induced increase in Cl^- conductance allows this ion to enter the postsynaptic cell and hyperpolarize it.

The part of the membrane of the postsynaptic neuron that forms the synapse is specialized for chemical rather than electrical sensitivity. ACTION POTENTIALS ARE NOT PRODUCED AT THE SYNAPSE. The change in membrane potential that occurs at the synapse, whether depolarization or hyperpolarization, is conducted electrotonically over the membrane of the postsynaptic neuron. The part of the neuron where its axon originates is called the **axon hillock;** the part of the axon very near to the neuronal cell body is called the **initial segment.** In many neurons the **axon hillock–initial segment** region of the cell has a lower threshold than the rest of the plasma membrane of the postsynaptic cell (Figure 4-7). An action potential is generated at this site if the sum of all the inputs to the cell exceeds threshold. Once the action potential has been generated, it is conducted back over the surface of the soma and dendrites of the postsynaptic cell and is propagated along its axon.

Summation of synaptic inputs occurs by spatial and temporal summation

Spatial summation occurs when two separate inputs arrive almost simultaneously (Figure 4-9, *A* and *B*). The two postsynaptic potentials are added so that two simultaneous excitatory inputs depolarize the postsynaptic cell about twice as much as either input alone. However, if an EPSP and an IPSP occur simultaneously, they tend to cancel each other. Even postsynaptic potentials from synapses at opposite ends of the postsynaptic cell body sum in this way. The postsynaptic potentials (EPSPs and IPSPs) sum with very little decrement because cellular dimensions ($<100\ \mu m$) are much smaller than the length constant (≈ 1 to $2mm$) for electronic conduction. In contrast, synaptic potentials that originate in fine dendritic branches decrease in magnitude as they are conducted to the cell body; the finer the dendrite, the greater the decrement.

Temporal summation occurs when two or more action potentials in a single presynaptic neuron occur in rapid succession so that the resulting postsynaptic potentials overlap in time (Figure 4-9, *A* and *C*). A train of impulses in a single presynaptic neuron can change the potential of the postsynaptic cell in a stepwise manner, each step caused by one of the presynaptic impulses.

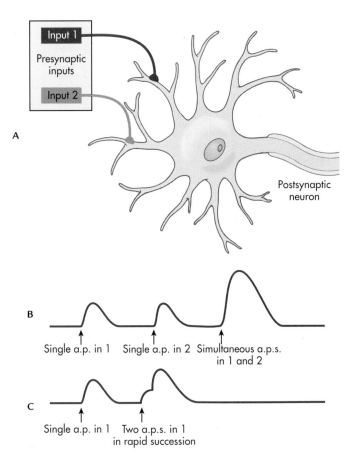

Figure 4-9 **A,** Spatial and temporal summation at a postsynaptic neuron with two synaptic inputs (*1* and *2*). **B,** Spatial summation. The postsynaptic potentials in response to single action potentials (*a.p.*) in inputs 1 and 2 occurring separately and simultaneously. **C,** Temporal summation. The postsynaptic response to two impulses in rapid succession in the same input.

Synaptic inputs to a presynaptic axon can influence the amount of transmitter it releases

The strength of individual synaptic inputs to a particular postsynaptic cell may be modulated by stimulatory or inhibitory effects on particular presynaptic axons that modulate the amount of transmitter released. **Presynaptic inhibition** and **presynaptic facilitation** are effected by means of axoaxonal synapses between modulatory neurons and presynaptic axons. Presynaptic inhibition may occur when the transmitter released at the axoaxonal synapse results in increased Cl^- conductance in the nerve terminal of the axon being modulated. The increased Cl^- conductance results in a shorter and smaller action potential, so less Ca^{++} enters the nerve terminal, and less transmitter is released. Presynaptic facilitation may result when the transmitter released by the modulatory neuron onto the axon being modulated results in diminished voltage-gated K^+ conductance. Thus the action potential is prolonged, which allows a greater influx of Ca^{++} and the release of more transmitter.

Repetitive stimulation can modulate the amount of transmitter released by a presynaptic neuron

When a presynaptic axon is stimulated repeatedly, the postsynaptic response may grow with each stimulation. This phenomenon is called **facilitation** (Figure 4-10, *A*). As shown in Figure 4-10, *B*, the extent of facilitation depends on the frequency of presynaptic impulses. Facilitation dies away rapidly, within tens to hundreds of milliseconds after stimulation stops.

When a presynaptic neuron is stimulated **tetanically** (many stimuli at high frequency) for several seconds, a longer enhancement of postsynaptic response **(posttetanic potentiation)** occurs (Figure 4-10, *C*). Posttetanic potentiation persists much longer than facilitation; it lasts for tens of seconds to several minutes after the cessation of tetanic stimulation.

Facilitation and posttetanic potentiation result from the effects of repeated stimulation on the presynaptic neuron. These phenomena do not involve a change in the sensitivity of the postsynaptic cell to transmitter. With repeated stimulation, an increased number of quanta of transmitter is released, partly because repetitive stimulation leads to increased levels of intracellular calcium.

When a synapse is repetitively stimulated for a long time, a point is reached at which each successive presynaptic stimulation elicits smaller postsynaptic responses. This phenomenon is called **synaptic fatigue** (neuromuscular depression at the neuromuscular junction). The postsynaptic cell at a fatigued synapse responds normally to transmitter applied from a micropipette; thus the defect is presynaptic. In some cases a decrease in **quantal content** (the amount of transmitter per synaptic vesicle) contributes to synaptic fatigue. A fatigued synapse typically recovers in a few seconds.

Long-term potentiation and long-term depression involve changes in postsynaptic neurons

Repetitive high-frequency stimulation of certain synapses in the brain increases the efficacy of transmission at those synapses, a reaction that can persist for days to weeks. This phenomenon is called **long-term potentiation,** and it is probably involved in learning and memory. Repetitive low-frequency stimulation of the same synapse may lead to **long-term depression,** a persistent decrease in synaptic efficacy. In contrast with the modulatory mechanisms that result from changes in the presynaptic nerve terminal (discussed in the previous section), LONG-TERM POTENTIATION AND INHIBITION APPEAR TO BE INITIATED IN THE POSTSYNAPTIC NEURON.

Ca^{++} entry into the postsynaptic region is an early required step in initiating the changes that result in long-term enhancement of the response of the postsynaptic cell to neurotransmitter. Ca^{++} entry occurs through *N*-methyl-D-aspartate (NMDA) receptors (see later discussion), a class of glutamate receptors that per-

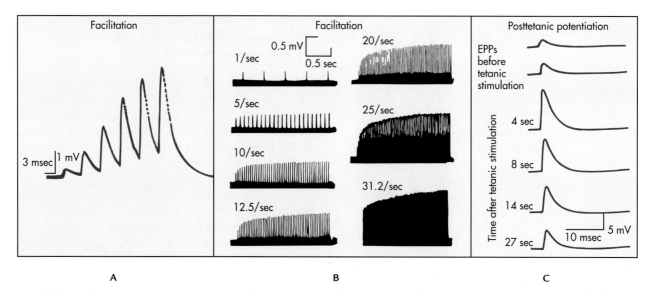

Figure 4-10 A, Facilitation at a neuromuscular junction. EPPs at a neuromuscular junction in toad sartorius muscle were elicited by successive action potentials in the motor axon. **B,** EPPs at a frog neuromuscular junction elicited by repeatedly stimulating the motor axon at different frequencies. Note that the degree of facilitation increases with the increasing frequency of stimulation. **C,** Posttetanic potentiation at a frog neuromuscular junction. The top two traces indicate control EPPs in response to single action potentials in the motor axon. Subsequent traces indicate EPPs in response to single action potentials after tetanic stimulation of the motor neuron. The time interval between the end of tetanic stimulation and the single action potential is shown on each trace. *(**A** redrawn from Belnave RJ, Gage PW: J Physiol 266:435, 1977. **B** redrawn from Magelby KL: J Physiol 234:327, 1973. **C** redrawn from Weinrich D: J Physiol 212:431, 1971.)*

mits Ca^{++} influx. The entry of Ca^{++} is believed to activate Ca^{++}–calmodulin kinase II, a multifunctional protein kinase (see Chapter 5) that is present in very high concentrations in postsynaptic densities. In the presence of high Ca^{++} concentrations, this kinase can phosphorylate itself and thereby become active whether or not Ca^{++} is present. Ca^{++}–calmodulin kinase II is believed to phosphorylate proteins that are essential for the induction of long-term potentiation.

Long-term potentiation may also have an anatomical component. After appropriate stimulation of a presynaptic pathway, the number of dendritic spines and the number of synapses on the dendrites of the postsynaptic neurons may rapidly increase.

Whether changes in the presynaptic nerve terminal also contribute to long-term potentiation remains unresolved. The postsynaptic neuron may release a signal (nitric oxide [NO] has been suggested) that enhances transmitter release by the presynaptic nerve terminal.

Many Compounds Serve as Neurotransmitters and Neuromodulators

Table 4-1 lists some of the substances that serve as neurotransmitters and neuromodulators. It is often difficult to prove that a substance is a neurotransmitter at a particular synapse. The candidate compound must satisfy the following criteria before it is accepted as a mediator of transmission at a particular synapse:

1. The presynaptic neurons must contain the compound and must be able to synthesize it.
2. The compound must be released by the presyn-

aptic neurons in response to appropriate stimulation.
3. The microapplication of the compound to the postsynaptic membrane must mimic the effects of stimulation of the presynaptic neuron.
4. The effects of presynaptic stimulation and of microapplication of the compound should be altered in the same way by drugs.

Some neurotransmitters and neuromodulators have rapid and transient effects on the postsynaptic cell; others have effects that are much slower in onset and may last for minutes or even hours. Most, but not all, known neurotransmitters and neuromodulators fall into the following major chemical classes: amines, amino acids, and oligopeptides.

Acetylcholine mediates transmission between motor neurons and skeletal muscle cells and in the autonomic nervous system and the central nervous system

As discussed previously, acetylcholine is the transmitter used by all motor axons that arise from the spinal cord. Acetylcholine also plays a central role in the autonomic nervous system; it is the transmitter for all autonomic preganglionic neurons and also for postganglionic parasympathetic fibers. Betz cells of the motor cortex use acetylcholine as their transmitter. Acetylcholine is apparently an important neurotransmitter in the basal ganglia, which are involved in the control of movement. In addition, acetylcholine may be the transmitter in many other central neural pathways.

Table 4-1   Selected Neurotransmitters and Neuromodulators

Compound	Site of Action of Neurons
Acetylcholine	Neuromuscular junction, autonomic endings, autonomic ganglia, sweat glands, brain, retina, GI tract
Biogenic amines	
Epinephrine	Brain, spinal cord
Norephinephrine	Sympathetic endings, brain, spinal cord, GI tract
Dopamine	Brain, sympathetic ganglia, retina
Serotonin	Brain, spinal cord, retina, GI tract
Histamine	Brain, GI tract
Amino acids	
GABA	Brain, retina
Glutamate	Brain
Aspartate	Spinal cord, brain?
Glycine	Spinal cord, brain, retina
Purines/purine nucleotides	
Adenosine	Brain
ATP	Autonomic ganglia, brain
Gas	
Nitric oxide	Brain, spinal cord, GI tract
Peptides	
Activins	Brain
Angiotensin II	Brain, spinal cord
Atrial natriuretic peptide	Brain
Calcitonin gene–related peptide	Spinal cord, brain
Cholecystokinin	Brain, retina
Corticotropin-releasing hormone	
β-Endorphins	Brain, retina, GI tract
Enkephalins	Brain, retina, GI tract
Endothelins	Brain, pituitary gland
FMRF amide	Brain
Galanin	Brain, spinal cord
Gastrin	Brain
Gastrin-releasing peptide	Brain
Gonadotropin-releasing hormone	Brain, autonomic ganglia, retina
Inhibins	Brain
Motilin	Brain, pituitary gland
Neuropeptide Y	Brain, autonomic nervous system
Neurotensin	Brain, retina
Oxytocin	Pituitary gland, brain, spinal cord
Secretin	Brain
Somatostatin	Brain, retina, GI tract
Vasoactive intestinal polypeptide	Autonomic nervous system, spinal cord, brain, retina, GI tract

GI, Gastrointestinal.

Deficits in pathways involving acetylcholine (**cholinergic pathways**) in the brain have been implicated in some forms of **senile dementia** (such as **Alzheimer's disease**). Treatment with long-lasting anticholinesterases that penetrate the blood-brain barrier may improve cognitive function in some individuals suffering from senile dementia.

Several amines serve as neurotransmitters

Dopamine, norepinephrine, and epinephrine are **catecholamines,** and they share a common biosynthetic pathway that starts with the amino acid tyrosine. Tyrosine is converted to L-dopa by tyrosine hydroxylase. L-Dopa is converted to dopamine by a specific decarboxylase. In dopaminergic neurons the pathway stops here.

Noradrenergic neurons have another enzyme, dopamine β-hydroxylase, that converts dopamine to norepinephrine. Norepinephrine is the primary transmitter for postganglionic sympathetic neurons. Chromaffin cells in the adrenal medulla add a methyl group to norepinephrine to produce the hormone epinephrine.

Neurons that contain high levels of dopamine are prominent in the midbrain regions known as the **substantia nigra** and the **ventral tegmentum.** Some of the axons of these neurons terminate in the **corpus striatum,** where they participate in controlling complex movements. Degeneration of dopaminergic synapses in the corpus striatum occurs in **Parkinson's disease** and may be a major cause of the muscular tremors and rigidity that characterize this condition. Treatment with **L-dopa,** the precursor of dopamine, may improve motor control but only temporarily.

In contrast, hyperactivity of dopaminergic synapses may be involved in some forms of **psychosis. Chlorpromazine** and related antipsychotic drugs inhibit the dopamine receptors on postsynaptic membranes and thus diminish the effects of dopamine released from presynaptic nerve terminals.

Neurons that contain **serotonin (5-hydroxytryptamine)** are present in high concentrations in certain nuclei in the brainstem. Serotonergic neurons may be involved in temperature regulation, sensory perception, onset of sleep, and control of mood. Serotonergic neurons have been implicated in aggressive behavior in certain animal species. About 13 different subtypes of serotonin receptors have been discovered, suggesting that many functions are regulated by this compound. About 12 distinct isoforms of the serotonin receptor are G protein–coupled receptors (see Chapter 5), and another type of serotonin receptor is a ligand-gated ion channel.

Amino acid transmitters are the most common inhibitory and excitatory neurotransmitters in the central nervous system

Glycine, the simplest amino acid, is an inhibitory neurotransmitter released by certain interneurons in the spinal cord and brainstem. **γ-Aminobutyric acid (GABA)** is not incorporated into proteins, nor is it present in all cells, as are the other naturally occurring amino acids. GABA IS PRODUCED FROM GLUTAMATE BY A SPECIFIC DECARBOXYLASE PRESENT ONLY IN CERTAIN NEURONS IN THE CNS. Among the cells that contain GABA are some neurons in the basal ganglia, cerebellar Purkinje cells, and certain spinal interneurons. In all known cases, GABA functions as an inhibitory transmitter. GABA may be the neurotransmitter at as many as one fourth of the synapses in the brain.

Glutamate and **aspartate,** dicarboxylic amino acids, strongly excite many neurons in the brain. GLUTAMATE IS THE MOST COMMON EXCITATORY NEUROTRANSMITTER IN THE BRAIN. There are five classes of **excitatory amino acid (EAA) receptors** (see later discussion).

Nitric oxide is an important neurotransmitter neuromodulator

NO mediates transmission between inhibitory motor neurons of the enteric nervous system and gastrointestinal smooth muscle cells (see Chapter 32). It also functions as a neurotransmitter and neuromodulator in the CNS. NO differs from other neuroactive compounds because it is a gas and because it is neither packaged into synaptic vesicles nor released by exocytosis. NO is highly permeant and simply diffuses from its site of production to neighboring cells. **NO synthase,** the enzyme that catalyzes the production of NO, is stimulated by an increase in cytosolic Ca^{++}.

The receptor for NO is soluble guanylyl cyclase in the target cell (see Chapter 5). NO potently stimulates this enzyme and thereby leads to an elevation of cyclic GMP in the target cell. The elevated levels of cyclic GMP can then influence multiple cellular processes, including certain ion channels.

Purine nucleotides and nucleosides are neurotransmitters and neuromodulators

ATP and adenosine function as neurotransmitters and neuromodulators in the central, autonomic, and peripheral nervous systems.

Many neuropeptides are neurotransmitters and neuromodulators

Certain cells release peptides that act at very low concentrations to excite or inhibit neurons. Many of these so-called **neuroactive peptides,** or **neuropeptides,** ranging from 2 to 40 amino acids long, have been identified (Table 4-1).

Although there are some exceptions, neuropeptides typically affect their target neurons at lower concentrations than the classic neurotransmitters discussed previously, and the effects of neuropeptides frequently are slower to occur and are more persistent. A number of neuropeptides are more familiar as hormones. A hormone is a substance that is released into the blood and that reaches its target cells via the circulation. A number of neuropeptides act as true transmitters at particular synapses and as neuromodulators at other synapses. Table 4-2 lists some of the differences between nonpeptide neurotransmitters and peptide neurotransmitters.

In many instances, neuropeptides coexist with classic transmitters in the same nerve terminals. The classic transmitters are present in the presynaptic nerve terminal in small vesicles clustered near active zones; the neuropeptides are present in larger vesicles distributed throughout

Table 4-2 Distinction Between Nonpeptide and Peptide Neurotransmitters

Nonpeptide Neurotransmitters	Peptide Neurotransmitters
Synthesized and packaged in presynaptic nerve terminal	Synthesized and packaged in soma of presynaptic neuron; transported to nerve terminal by axonal transport
Nonpeptide synthesized in active form	Active peptide formed by cleavage from much larger peptide that contains multiple neuropeptides or hormones
Present in small synaptic vesicles clustered near active zones	Present in large, clear synaptic vesicles distributed throughout nerve terminal
Action terminated by active reuptake into presynaptic nerve terminal	Action terminated by proteolysis or peptide diffusing away
Neurotransmitters and vesicle constituents recycled	Neuropeptide and vesicle constituents degraded
Released into synaptic cleft	May be released some distance from target neuron
Typically, action has short latency and short duration (milliseconds)	Action may have long latency and may persist for many seconds

the nerve terminal. It appears that low-frequency stimulation of the presynaptic neuron preferentially releases the nonpeptide transmitter, whereas the neuropeptide is released in response to high-frequency stimulation.

Neuropeptides are synthesized in the neuronal cell body. Secretory vesicles containing the neuropeptide are released from the mature face of the Golgi complex and are then transported by **fast axonal transport** to the axon terminal.

Some neuropeptides are synthesized as preprohormones (see also Chapter 40). Cleavage of a signal sequence converts a preprohormone to a prohormone. Proteolytic cleavage of the prohormone may then release one or more active peptides. In some cases, one prohormone may contain several active peptide sequences.

Opioid peptides modulate pain pathways and are important neuromodulators in the central nervous system and gastrointestinal tract

Opiates are drugs derived from the juice of the opium poppy. Compounds that are not derived from the opium poppy but that exert direct effects by binding to opiate receptors are called **opioids.** Operationally, opioids are defined as direct-acting compounds whose effects are stereospecifically antagonized by **naloxone,** a morphine derivative. Opiates are useful therapeutically as powerful **analgesics** (pain relievers). They exert this effect by binding to specific opiate receptors.

The three major classes of endogenous opioid peptides in mammals are **enkephalins, endorphins,** and **dynorphins.** Enkephalins are the simplest opioids; they are pentapeptides. (Met-enkephalin is Tyr-Gly-Gly-Phe-Met, and leu-enkephalin is Tyr-Gly-Gly-Phe-Leu.) Dynorphin and the endorphins are somewhat longer peptides that contain one or the other of the enkephalin sequences at their N-termini.

Opioid peptides are widely distributed in neurons of the CNS and intrinsic neurons of the gastrointestinal

tract. The endorphins are discretely localized in particular structures of the CNS, whereas the enkephalins and dynorphins are more widely distributed. Opioids also inhibit cerebral neurons that are involved in the perception of pain.

Substance P is a transmitter in the pain pathways and gastrointestinal tract

Most of the known neuropeptides are not opioids. **Substance P,** a peptide of 11 amino acids, is present in specific neurons in the brain, primary sensory neurons, and plexus neurons in the wall of the gastrointestinal tract. Substance P was the first so-called **gut-brain peptide** to be discovered. Enteric neurons contain many of the neuropeptides, including substance P, that are found in the brain and spinal column.

Substance P is the transmitter at synapses that primary sensory neurons (their cell bodies are in the dorsal root ganglia) make with spinal interneurons in the dorsal horn of the spinal column. Enkephalins decrease the release of substance P at these synapses and thereby inhibit the pathway for pain sensation at the first synapse in the pathway.

Vasoactive intestinal polypeptide, secretin, glucagon, and gastric inhibitory peptide are members of a family of neuropeptides

Vasoactive intestinal polypeptide (VIP) was first discovered as a gastrointestinal hormone, but it is now known to be a neuropeptide as well. VIP is widely distributed in the CNS and the intrinsic neurons of the gastrointestinal tract. In neurons in the brain, VIP has been localized in synaptic vesicles. VIP may function as an inhibitory transmitter to vascular and nonvascular smooth muscle and as an excitatory transmitter to glandular epithelial cells.

Secretin, glucagon, and **gastric inhibitory polypeptide (GIP)** are peptides whose functions as gastrointestinal hormones have been well characterized. These peptides have also been found in particular neurons in the CNS, but their functions in neurons remain undetermined.

Cholecystokinin is a member of a group of neuropeptides that includes gastrin and cerulein

The group of peptides that includes gastrin and cerulein have similar C-terminal sequences. Cholecystokinin (CCK) is a well-known gastrointestinal hormone that elicits contraction of the gallbladder and has other roles in the gastrointestinal tract (see Chapters 33 and 34). One form of CCK is present in particular neurons of the CNS.

Neurotransmitter Receptors Are Ligand-Gated Ion Channels or Signal-Transduction Proteins

As previously mentioned, some neurotransmitter receptors, such as the acetylcholine receptor of the neuromuscular junction, are ligand-gated ion channels. Other neurotransmitters influence the function of ion channels more indirectly.

Two major classes of acetylcholine receptors are nicotinic and muscarinic acetylcholine receptors

The acetylcholine receptor at the neuromuscular junction (Figure 4-6) is a **nicotinic acetylcholine receptor;** it can be stimulated by **nicotine.** Other receptors for acetylcholine, such as those on heart cells, smooth muscle cells, and many brain neurons, are stimulated not by nicotine but by **muscarine.** They are called **muscarinic acetylcholine receptors.** Subtypes of nicotinic and muscarinic receptors are classified by their sensitivities to agonist and antagonist drugs.

MUSCARINIC ACETYLCHOLINE RECEPTORS ARE NOT ION CHANNELS. Muscarinic receptors are seven-transmembrane helix receptor proteins that are linked to heterotrimeric guanine triphosphate–binding proteins. Binding of acetylcholine to M_2-muscarinic receptors in the heart's sinoatrial node activates G_i protein, which increases the probability of opening of K^+ channels (see Chapter 5). This tends to hyperpolarize the pacemaker cells of the sinoatrial node and thereby decreases the heart rate (see Chapter 19). There are five major subtypes of muscarinic receptors.

γ-Aminobutyric acid and glycine receptors mediate neurotransmission at most inhibitory synapses in the central nervous system

Glycine-mediated inhibitory synapses predominate in the spinal cord, and GABA-ergic synapses are the most numerous synapses in the brain. Most GABA and glycine receptors, and most other neurotransmitter receptors, belong to the superfamily of ligand-gated ion channels. They are heteropentamers, like acetylcholine

receptors, and their subunits have significant sequence homology and structural similarities with the subunits of nicotinic acetylcholine receptors. Even though there may be five distinct subunits, only one or two subunit isoforms are typically required to form a functional ion channel. Different cell types in the CNS may have different receptor subtypes that consist of different combinations of subunit isoforms.

Most GABA and glycine receptors are ligand-gated Cl^- channels that mediate Cl^- influx into neurons. The Cl^- current hyperpolarizes and thus inhibits the neurons. The following types of GABA receptors have been identified: $GABA_A$ and $GABA_B$. The $GABA_A$ receptor is a GABA-mediated Cl^- channel. The $GABA_B$ receptor is not an ion channel itself, but it acts via protein kinase C to increase the K^+ conductance and to decrease the Ca^{++} conductance of the postsynaptic cell.

General **anesthetics** prolong the open time of $GABA_A$ receptor chloride channels and thus prolong the inhibition of the postsynaptic neurons at GABA-ergic synapses. $GABA_A$ receptors may be a principal target of general anesthetics. $GABA_A$ receptors are also the targets of two major classes of medications: **benzodiazepines** and **barbiturates.** Benzodiazepines (such as **diazepam**) are widely used antianxiety and relaxant drugs. Barbiturates are used as sedatives and anticonvulsants. Both of these classes of drugs bind to distinct sites on $GABA_A$ receptors and enhance the opening of the receptors' Cl^- channels in response to GABA.

Excitatory amino acid receptors have glutamate as their most important ligand

Glutamate is the major neurotransmitter that mediates synaptic excitation in the CNS. Glutamate receptors are also known as **excitatory amino acid (EAA) receptors.** At present, five subtypes of EAA receptors are recognized (Table 4-3). The subtypes are classified principally on the synthetic amino acid analogues that bind tightly and specifically to them. Four of the subtypes are ligand-gated ion channels, and the fifth is a receptor (called the **metabotropic EAA receptor**) that is indirectly linked to an ion channel.

AMPA and **NMDA** receptors are widely distributed in the CNS. Stimulation of AMPA receptors by glutamate or another agonist elicits an EPSP caused by the flow of Na^+ and K^+. Stimulated NMDA receptors permit the flow of Ca^{++} as well as Na^+ and K^+. NMDA receptors are blocked by extracellular Mg^{++} at physiological levels. The Mg^{++} block is relieved when the cell is depolarized. Thus the first physiological response to glutamate is depolarization of the postsynaptic cell by glutamate acting on AMPA receptors. This depolarization relieves the Mg^{++} block of NMDA receptors, which then respond by permitting a Ca^{++} influx and further

Table 4-3   Different Classes of Excitatory Amino Acid Receptors

Receptor Class	Properties
AMPA	Is widely distributed in CNS; is channel selective for Na^+ and K^+; was known as *quisqualate receptor*
N-methyl-D-aspartate (NMDA)	Is widely distributed in CNS; is channel selective for Ca^{++}, Na^+, and K^+; is blocked by Mg^{++} (block relieved by depolarization)
Kainate	Is present in specific areas of CNS
L-2-Amino-4-phosphonobutyrate	Is not widely distributed; may function as presynaptic glutamate receptor that inhibits glutamate release
Metabotropic	Is not an ion channel; mobilizes inositol 1,4,5-trisphosphate; increases intracellular Ca^{++} levels

depolarization of the postsynaptic cell. NMDA receptors are also regulated by glycine, which binds to the receptor to enhance current flow in response to glutamate. The role of NMDA receptors in long-term potentiation was discussed previously.

SUMMARY

- Direct electrical transmission between neighboring cells is mediated by gap junctions.
- At a chemical synapse, an action potential in the presynaptic nerve terminal causes a Ca^{++} influx, which initiates the chain of events culminating in the release of neurotransmitter.
- Neurotransmitter diffuses across the synaptic cleft to bind to neurotransmitter receptor proteins on the postsynaptic membrane, which results in a transient change in the conductance of the postsynaptic membrane to one or more ions.
- At the neuromuscular junction, acetylcholine released by the prejunctional nerve terminal binds to acetylcholine receptors in the postjunctional membrane to open ion channels conductive to Na^+ and K^+. The resulting ion flow across the postjunctional membrane causes a depolarization, called an endplate potential (EPP).
- The EPP is terminated by the hydrolysis of acetylcholine by the enzyme acetylcholinesterase. When acetylcholine is hydrolyzed, the choline liberated in the synaptic cleft is actively transported back into the nerve terminal.

- The release of acetylcholine is quantal. A quantum corresponds to the amount of acetylcholine in a single presynaptic vesicle.
- An action potential in an excitatory input to a spinal motor neuron causes an EPSP that depolarizes the motor neuron and brings it closer to threshold.
- An action potential in an inhibitory input causes an IPSP that hyperpolarizes the motor neuron.
- The efficacy of synaptic transmission depends on the timing and frequency of action potentials in the presynaptic neuron.
- Facilitation, posttetanic potentiation, and long-term potentiation are examples of the results of an increased release of neurotransmitter in response to previous multiple stimulations of a synapse.
- Long-term potentiation involves biochemical changes that enhance the responsiveness of the postsynaptic neuron to neurotransmitter.
- Acetylcholine, biogenic amines, glutamate, glycine, and GABA are important neurotransmitters in the CNS.
- Glycine and GABA are the major transmitters at inhibitory synapses in the CNS.
- Glutamate is the major excitatory neurotransmitter in the CNS. There are five classes of EAA receptors.
- Many neuroactive peptides function as neuromodulators or neurotransmitters in the CNS.

BIBLIOGRAPHY

Amara SG, Kuhar MJ: Neurotransmitter transporters: recent progress, *Annu Rev Neurosci* 16:73, 1993.

Barnard EA: Receptor classes and the transmitter-gated ion channels, *Trends Biochem Sci* 17:368, 1992.

Bennett MK, Scheller RH: A molecular description of synaptic vesicle membrane trafficking, *Annu Rev Biochem* 63:63, 1994.

Bredt DS, Snyder SH: Nitric oxide: a physiologic messenger molecule, *Annu Rev Biochem* 63:175, 1994.

Froehner SC: Regulation of ion channel distribution at synapses, *Annu Rev Neurosci* 16:347, 1993.

Gingrich JA, Caron MG: Recent advances in the molecular biology of dopamine receptors, *Annu Rev Neurosci* 16:299, 1993.

Hökfelt T: Neuropeptides in perspective: the last ten years, *Neuron* 7:867, 1991.

Jahn R, Sudhof TC: Synaptic vesicles and exocytosis, *Annu Rev Neurosci* 17:219, 1994.

Jessel TM, Kandel ER: Synaptic transmission: a bi-directional and self-modifiable form of cell-cell communication, *Cell* 72(suppl):1, 1993.

Levitan IB, Kaczmarek LK: *The neuron: cell and molecular biology,* ed 2, New York, 1997, Oxford University Press.

Nakanishi S, Masu M: Molecular diversity and functions of glutamate receptors, *Annu Rev Biophys Biomolec Struct* 23:319, 1994.

Sakmann B: Elementary steps in synaptic transmission revealed by currents through single ion channels, *Science* 256:28, 1992.

Schuman EM, Madison DV: Nitric oxide and synaptic function, *Annu Rev Neurosci* 17:153, 1994.

Stevens CF: Quantal release of neurotransmitter and long-term potentiation, *Cell* 72(suppl):55, 1993.

CASE STUDIES

Case 4-1

A 43-year-old man experiences weakness of the lower limbs. He reports difficulty climbing stairs and complains of persistent dry mouth. The patient has diminished muscle stretch reflexes. There is a transient increase in muscle power after maximal exercise. Electromyographic (EMG) studies reveal a diminished amplitude of compound muscle action potentials. Nerve conduction velocities are normal. The compound muscle action potential is markedly (>200%) increased in amplitude after vigorous exercise of the muscle studied. Single-fiber muscle action potentials show significant blocking (instances in which an action potential in the motor neuron fails to elicit an action potential in the muscle). After purified immunoglobulin G from this patient is intravenously injected into a mouse, the mouse displays symptoms similar to the patient. The diagnosis is **Eaton-Lambert syndrome,** a disorder cause by circulating antibodies against voltage-gated Ca^{++} channels.

1. Which of the following statements is correct?

A. The patient's dry mouth is not consistent with his other symptoms.

B. The increase in muscle power after maximal exercise is likely due to facilitation at the neuromuscular junction.

C. Diminished magnitude of the compound action potential suggests a problem with the conduction of action potentials in motor axons.

D. The blocking of single muscle fiber action potentials is consistent with the presence of smaller EPPs.

E. None of the above.

2. If the patient does have Eaton-Lambert syndrome, which of the following statements is correct?

A. The patient should have diminished frequency of MEPPs.

B. Treating a biopsy of the patient's muscle with a calcium ionophore should not alter the frequency of MEPPs.

C. The patient should have decreased EPP amplitudes.

D. Increased extracellular K^+ levels should increase the frequency of MEPPs to the same extent in the patient as in a healthy individual.

E. None of the above.

3. Which of the following statements is not correct?

A. Immunosuppressive therapy might improve the patient's condition.

B. Treatment with 4-aminopyridine, which blocks voltage-gated K^+ channels, might improve the patient's condition.

C. Plasmapheresis might improve the patient's condition.

D. Treatment with a medication that diminishes voltage-inactivation of Na^+ channels might improve the patient's condition.

E. All of the above.

Case 4-2

A 28-year-old man complains of weakness. On examination the patient exhibits **ptosis** (drooping of the upper eyelid). The patient can lift a 20-pound weight by flexing his forearm but is unable to maintain the contraction for more than a few seconds. **Edrophonium** (Tensilon), a fast-acting but short-lived anticholinesterase, is administered. One minute after injection of the medication, the ptosis subsides, and the patient can lift the 20-pound weight by flexing his forearm and can maintain this contraction for 20 seconds. The diagnosis is **myasthenia gravis,** a disease characterized by circulating antibodies against nicotinic acetylcholine receptors (AChR).

1. Which of the following statements is correct?

A. The patient's anti-AChR antibody is unlikely to cross-react with AChR from *Torpedo,* an electric fish.

B. The patient's anti-AChR antibody is likely to be directed against the same epitope as the antibodies of other patients with myasthenia gravis.

C. The titer of anti-AChR antibody in the patient's serum is likely to be a good predictor of the severity of his disease.

D. The absence of anti-AChR rules out the diagnosis of myasthenia gravis.

E. None of the above.

2. Which of the following statements is correct?

A. Electromyography would likely show a decreased amplitude of the compound muscle action potential that does not change during sustained effort.

B. There is likely to be a slight increase in nerve conduction time in this patient.

C. A biopsy of external intercostal muscle from this patient would show a normal level of AChR protein.

D. Electromyography would likely show that the amplitude of the compound muscle action potential decreases during sustained effort.

E. None of the above.

3. Which of the following statements in incorrect?

A. The patient is unlikely to have an enlarged thymus.

B. Thymectomy is unlikely to improve this patient's condition.

C. Treatment with prednisone is unlikely to improve the patient's condition.

D. Treatment with azathioprine, a long-lasting anticholinesterase, is likely to improve the patient's condition.

E. None of the above.

CHAPTER 5

Membrane Receptors, Second Messengers, and Signal-Transduction Pathways

OBJECTIVES

- List the components of a generalized G protein–mediated signal-transduction pathway.
- Describe the roles of protein kinases and protein phosphatases in signal transduction.
- Identify the major classes of second messenger–dependent protein kinases.
- Describe the general functions of receptor tyrosine kinases.
- List the major classes of protein phosphatases.

This chapter discusses the signal-transduction pathways whereby extracellular regulatory molecules influence intracellular processes. Basic cellular processes are regulated by a host of substances. Some regulatory substances, such as steroid hormones (see Chapters 40 and 46), enter the cell and influence the transcription of certain genes. Other regulatory substances exert their influences from outside the cell.

A Signal-Transduction Pathway Links the Binding of a Regulatory Substance to Its Membrane Receptor with Its Intracellular Effect

An extracellular regulatory substance's first action is to bind to the extracellular domain of the specific protein **receptors** in the plasma membrane of the target cells. The neurotransmitters discussed in Chapter 4 and their receptors are examples of extracellular regulatory compounds. For the neurotransmitters discussed so far, the receptor is a ligand-gated ion channel, and the response of the cell is a ligand-induced ionic current. In such cases the ligand-gated ion channel is both the receptor and the **effector** for the action of the neurotransmitter.

For most regulatory molecules or **agonists,** however, a more complex series of events links the binding of the agonist and its specific membrane receptor with its final effects on cellular function. Extracellular agonists exert their effects on cells via **signal-transduction pathways,** whereby the binding of an agonist to its plasma membrane receptor elicits an intracellular response by altering the activities of particular cellular proteins. A comprehensive discussion of this subject is beyond the scope of this book. Therefore only certain signal-transduction pathways, especially those relevant to topics discussed in subsequent chapters, are described.

The extracellular agonists considered may be classified as **endocrine, neurocrine,** or **paracrine.** Endocrine regulatory substances **(hormones)** are released by endocrine cells, and they reach their target cells, which may be far from the endocrine cells, via the bloodstream. Neurocrine regulators are released by neurons in the immediate vicinity of the target cells. Neurotransmitters are neurocrine substances, as are most of the neuromodulators discussed in Chapter 4. Paracrine substances are released by cells that are not immediately adjacent to the target cells but are sufficiently close that the paracrine substance can reach the target cells by diffusion.

Paracrine regulators are secreted by one cell type and act on cells of a different type. However, some cells release regulators that act on that cell itself or on its neighbors of the same cell type. This is called **autocrine regulation.**

Protein kinases and protein phosphatases: phosphorylation of proteins is a common means of transferring information in signal-transduction pathways

Frequently, one or more steps in a signal-transduction pathway involves the phosphorylation of particular proteins that play central roles in eliciting cellular responses. When these proteins are phosphorylated, their activities may be enhanced or suppressed. **Protein kinases** in the

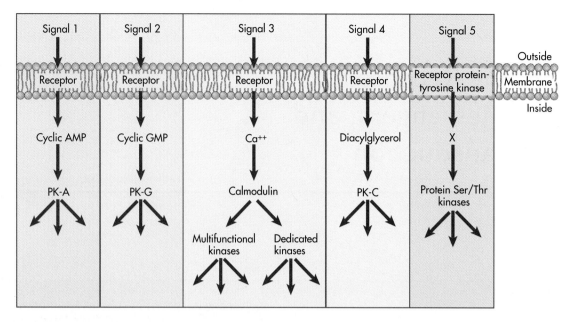

Figure 5-1 Signal-transduction pathways of mammalian cells involving protein kinases. *PK-A,* Cyclic AMP–dependent protein kinase; *PK-C,* protein kinase C; *PK-G,* cyclic GMP–dependent protein kinase; *X,* signaling pathways described later. *(Adapted from Cohen P:* Trends Biochem Sci *17:408, 1992.)*

cell are responsible for phosphorylating particular proteins, and **protein phosphatases** catalyze the removal of phosphates from proteins. THE STATE OF PHOSPHORYLATION OF AN EFFECTOR PROTEIN DEPENDS ON THE BALANCE OF THE ACTIVITIES OF THE KINASE THAT PHOSPHORYLATES IT AND THE PHOSPHATASE THAT DEPHOSPHORYLATES IT.

A signal-transduction pathway may alter the activity of a protein kinase in response to the binding of an agonist to an extracellular site on its membrane receptor. The major classes of agonist-activated protein kinases are shown in Figure 5-1.

The binding of an agonist to its receptor on the cell surface frequently begins a sequence of events that leads to a change in the intracellular concentration of a **second messenger** substance, which may act to increase the activity of a protein kinase. Second messengers that regulate the activities of protein kinases include **cyclic AMP, cyclic GMP, Ca^{++}, inositol 1,4,5-trisphosphate (IP$_3$),** and **diacylglycerol.**

Cells contain protein kinases whose activities are enhanced by cyclic AMP and cyclic GMP. These kinases are called **cyclic AMP–dependent protein kinases** and **cyclic GMP–dependent protein kinases,** respectively.

The activities of **calmodulin-dependent protein kinases** are enhanced when they bind the complex of Ca^{++} with a protein called **calmodulin.** Calmodulin is a protein (molecular weight [MW], 16,700 d) that is present in all cells. Calmodulin binds four Ca^{++} ions; the complex of Ca^{++} and calmodulin then regulates a host of other intracellular proteins, many of which are not kinases.

Protein kinases of the **protein kinase C** family are activated by Ca^{++}, diacylglycerol, certain membrane phospholipids, and some breakdown products of membrane phospholipids.

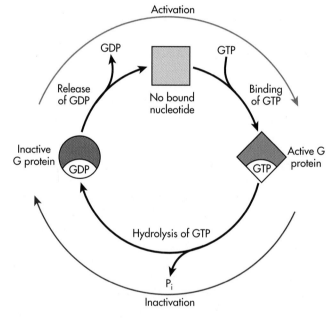

Figure 5-2 Activity cycle of a GTP-binding protein (G protein). The inactive form of the G protein *(blue circle)* binds GDP. The release of GDP and the binding of GTP causes the G protein to become activated *(green diamond).* The hydrolysis of bound GTP causes the G protein to become inactivated *(blue circle).* P$_i$, Inorganic phosphate.

Insulin and certain **growth factors** bind to membrane receptors that are themselves protein kinases that phosphorylate protein substrates on tyrosine residues. (The other protein kinases described phosphorylate proteins on serine or threonine residues.) The binding of a growth factor stimulates the **protein-tyrosine kinase** activity of the receptor.

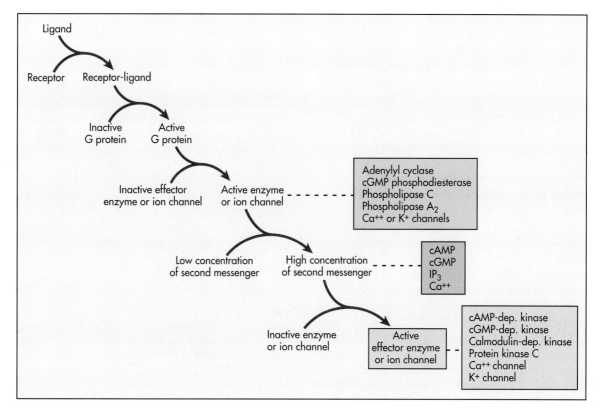

Figure 5-3 Signal-transduction cascade by which an extracellular ligand such as a peptide hormone can bind to its receptor to activate a G protein and via the cascade, to lead to the activation or inactivation of an ion channel, a protein kinase, or a phospholipase. *cAMP,* Cyclic AMP; *cGMP,* cyclic GMP; *dep.,* dependent.

G proteins are molecular switches in signal-transduction pathways

Many hormones, neuromodulators, and other regulatory molecules that alter cellular processes do so by signal-transduction pathways involving **heterotrimeric GTP-binding proteins,** also called simply **G proteins.** (Another class of GTP-binding proteins, monomeric GTP-binding protein, is discussed later.) A G protein is a molecular switch (Figure 5-2) that can exist in two states. In its activated ("on") state, a G protein has a higher affinity for GTP. The inactivated ("off") G protein preferentially binds GDP. When certain membrane receptors have agonist molecules bound to them, they interact with specific G proteins to promote the conversion of proteins to their activated state by binding GTP. An activated G protein can then interact with many effector proteins, most notably enzymes or ion channels, to alter their activities. The activated G protein has GTPase activity, so eventually the bound GTP is hydrolyzed to GDP, and the G protein reverts to its inactive state (Figure 5-2).

Among the most important targets of activated G proteins are molecules that change the cellular concentrations of the second messengers cyclic AMP, cyclic GMP, Ca^{++}, IP_3, and diacylglycerol (Figure 5-3). **Adenylyl cyclase** and **cyclic GMP phosphodiesterase,** the enzymes responsible for the synthesis of cyclic AMP and the breakdown of

cyclic GMP, respectively, are powerfully modulated by G protein–mediated mechanisms. Ca^{++} channels may be modulated directly by G proteins or indirectly by second messenger–dependent protein kinases. Other effectors that are modulated by G proteins include certain K^+ channels and phospholipases C, A_2, and D.

In general, a G protein–protein kinase—mediated signal-transduction pathway involves the following events (Figure 5-3):

1. A hormone or other agonist binds to its plasma membrane receptor.
2. The ligand-bearing receptor interacts with a G protein and activates it; the activated G protein binds GTP.
3. The activated G protein interacts with one or more of the following effectors to activate or inhibit them: adenylyl cyclase, cyclic GMP phosphodiesterase, Ca^{++} or K^+ channels, or phospholipases C, A_2, or D.
4. The cellular level of one or more of the following second messengers increases or decreases: cyclic AMP, cyclic GMP, Ca^{++}, IP_3, or diacylglycerol.
5. The increase or decrease of the concentration of a second messenger changes the activity of one or more of the second messenger–dependent protein kinases: cyclic AMP–dependent protein kinase, cyclic GMP–dependent protein kinase,

calmodulin-dependent protein kinase, or protein kinase C. It can also activate an ion channel.

6. The level of phosphorylation of an enzyme or an ion channel is altered, or an ion channel activity changes because of interaction with an activated G protein and causes the final cellular response.

AT EACH LEVEL OF THE SIGNAL-TRANSDUCTION CASCADE, AMPLIFI-CATION CAN OCCUR, SO ONE AGONIST-BEARING RECEPTOR CAN RESULT IN THE ACTIVATION OF HUNDREDS OF EFFECTORS.

Membrane inositol phospholipids are intermediates in certain signal-transduction pathways

Another class of extracellular agonists binds to receptors that activate via a G protein called G_q, the β isoform of **phospholipase C.** This isoform cleaves phosphatidylinositol 4,5-bisphosphate (a phospholipid present in minute quantities in the plasma membrane) into **IP₃** and **diacylglycerol** (Figure 5-4), both of which are second messengers. IP₃ binds to specific ligand-gated Ca^{++} channels in the endoplasmic reticulum and releases Ca^{++}, thereby increasing its cytosolic level. Diacylglycerol, together with Ca^{++}, activates protein kinase C. Among the substrates of protein kinase C are certain proteins involved in the control of gene transcription and cellular proliferation.

The enzymes **phospholipase A₂** and **phospholipase D** are also activated by some agonists via G protein–dependent pathways. Certain products of these enzymes' action on membrane phospholipids also activate protein kinase C. Phospholipase A₂ cleaves the second fatty acid from membrane phospholipids. Because some of the phospholipids are species with **arachidonic acid** esterified to the second carbon of the glycerol backbone, phospholipase A₂ releases significant amounts of arachidonic acid. Arachidonic acid is a regulatory molecule in its own right, and arachidonic acid is also the precursor for the cellular synthesis of **prostaglandins, prostacyclins, thromboxanes,** and **leukotrienes,** which are important classes of potent regulatory molecules.

One of the antiinflammatory actions of corticosteroids (see Chapter 46) is inhibition of the phospholipase A₂ that releases arachidonic acid from phospholipids. Aspirin and other nonsteroidal antiinflammatory agents inhibit the conversion of arachidonic acid to inflammatory prostaglandins, prostacyclins, and thromboxanes.

Signal-transduction cascades initiated by growth factors involve protein-tyrosine kinases

Proteins with intrinsic **protein-tyrosine kinase** activity make up another family of membrane receptors not linked to G proteins. When these receptors bind agonist, their tyrosine kinase activity is stimulated, and they phosphory-

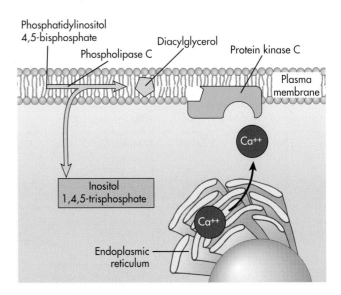

Figure 5-4 Signal-transduction pathway activated by the hydrolysis of inositol phospholipids of the plasma membrane. Activation of G_q by an agonist stimulates the hydrolysis of phosphatidylinositol 4,5-bisphosphate to inositol 1,4,5-trisphosphate (IP₃) and diacylglycerol. IP₃ releases Ca^{++} from the endoplasmic reticulum. Diacylglycerol, together with Ca^{++}, activates protein kinase C.

late specific effector proteins on particular tyrosine residues. The receptor for the hormone insulin and receptors for many growth factors are tyrosine kinases.

G protein–linked membrane receptors constitute a large family

Membrane receptors that mediate agonist-dependent activation of G proteins constitute a protein family with more than 500 members. This family includes α- and β-adrenergic receptors, muscarinic acetylcholine receptors, serotonin receptors, adenosine receptors, olfactory receptors, rhodopsin, and receptors for most peptide hormones. The members of the G protein–coupled receptor family have seven transmembrane α-helices, each made up of 22 to 28 predominantly hydrophobic amino acids. After a receptor binds an agonist, the receptor undergoes a conformational change that enables the receptor to interact with and activate a specific type of G protein.

Two Classes of G Proteins: Heterotrimeric and Monomeric

Heterotrimeric G proteins have three different subunits

A heterotrimeric G protein has three subunits: α (40,000 to 45,000 d), β (≈37,000 d), and γ (8000 to 10,000 d). Currently, about 20 different genes that encode α subunits, at least 4 genes that encode β subunits, and about 7 genes that encode γ subunits in mammals are known. In most

Table 5-1   Selected Mammalian Heterotrimeric G Proteins Classified on the Basis of Their α Subunits*

G Protein	Activated by Receptors for	Effectors	Signaling Pathways
G_s	Epinephrine, norepinephrine, histamine, glucagon, ACTH, luteinizing hormone, follicle-stimulating hormone, thyroid-stimulating hormone, others	Adenylyl cyclase Ca^{++} channels	↑ Cyclic AMP ↑ Ca^{++} influx
G_{olf}	Odorants	Adenylyl cyclase	↑ AMP (olfaction)
G_{t1} (rods)	Photons	Cyclic GMP phosphodiesterase	↓ Cyclic GMP (vision)
G_{t2} (cones)	Photons	Cyclic GMP phosphodiesterase	↓ Cyclic GMP (color vision)
G_{i1}, G_{i2}, G_{i3}	Norepinephrine, prostaglandins, opiates, angiotensin, many peptides	Adenylyl cyclase Phospholipase C Phospholipase A_2 K^+ channels	↓ Cyclic AMP ↑ Inositol 1,4,5-trisphosphate, diacylglycerol, Ca^{++}
G_q	Acetylcholine, epinephrine	Phospholipase Cβ	Membrane polarization ↑ Inositol 1,4,5-trisphosphate, diacylglycerol, Ca^{++}

Adapted from Bourne HR, Sanders DA, McCormick F: *Nature* 348:125, 1990.
ACTH, Adrenocorticotropic hormone.
*There is more than one isoform of each class of α subunit; more than 20 distinct α subunits have been identified.

cases the β and γ subunits are tightly associated with each other. Some heterotrimeric G proteins and the signal-transduction pathways they mediate are listed in Table 5-1.

Frequently the α subunit is the "business end" of the heterotrimeric G protein (Figure 5-5). The inactive G protein exists primarily as the αβγ heterotrimer, with GDP in its nucleotide binding site. The interaction of the heterotrimeric G protein with a ligand-bearing receptor causes a conformational change in the α subunit to the active form, which has a higher affinity for GTP and a lower affinity for the βγ pair. Therefore the activated α subunit releases GDP, binds GTP, and then dissociates from βγ. The dissociated α subunit then interacts with the next protein in the signal-transduction pathway. In some cases, however, the βγ dimer appears to be responsible for all or some of the receptor-mediated response.

Regulation of adenylyl cyclase was the first G protein–mediated regulatory pathway to be discovered

Cyclic AMP was the first of the second messengers to be discovered, and the regulation of adenylyl cyclase, the enzyme that produces cyclic AMP, is the prototype for G protein–mediated signal-transduction pathways. Adenylyl cyclase is subject to both positive and negative control by G protein–mediated pathways (Figure 5-5). The binding of a stimulatory ligand, such as epinephrine acting through β-adrenergic receptors, results in the activation of heterotrimeric G proteins with α subunits of the type called $α_s$ (*s* for stimulatory). Activation of the G_s-type G protein by the agonist-bearing receptor causes its $α_s$ subunit to bind GTP and then to dissociate from βγ. The $α_s$ subunit then interacts with adenylyl cyclase to activate it.

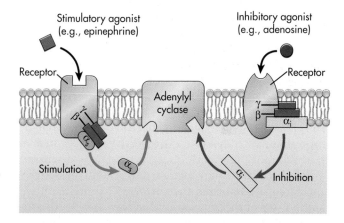

Figure 5-5 Receptors for agonists that stimulate adenylyl cyclase activate G_s, whose $α_s$ *(green)* subunit dissociates from βγ and then interacts with adenylyl cyclase to stimulate it. Receptors for agonists that inhibit adenylyl cyclase activate G_i, whose $α_i$ subunit *(yellow)* inhibits adenylyl cyclase.

Patients suffering from **cholera** experience profound diarrhea. A patient with cholera may produce up to 20 L/day of watery stool. Such patients are likely to die unless their bodies are promptly and adequately rehydrated. Cholera is caused by **cholera toxin** that is produced by the bacterium *Vibrio cholerae*. Cholera toxin catalyzes the transfer of ADP-ribose to $α_s$, thereby locking $α_s$ in the activated state. Consequently, adenylyl cyclase is persistently stimulated and thereby elevates the level of cyclic AMP in intestinal epithelial cells. The elevated cyclic AMP levels cause the secretion of Cl^-, Na^+, and water into the intestinal lumen by the cells in the crypts of Lieberkühn and

Table 5-2   Subfamilies of Monomeric GTP-Binding Proteins and Some of the Intracellular Processes They Regulate

Subfamily	Cellular Effects
Ras-like proteins	Control growth and differentiation
Rho-like proteins (including Rac)	Control polymerization of actin filaments and their assembly into particular structures such as focal adhesions
Rab-like proteins	Control vesicle trafficking by helping target vesicles to particular membranes
ARF-like proteins	Regulate the assembly and disassembly of vesicle coat proteins and thereby control vesicle traffic

diminished absorption of salts and water by intestinal epithelial cells near the tips of the intestinal villi. These responses cause the massive diarrhea associated with cholera.

Other regulatory substances, such as epinephrine acting at α_2-receptors and adenosine acting on A_1 receptors, inhibit adenylyl cyclase by activating G_i-type G proteins, which have α subunits of a different type, called α_i (*i* for inhibitory). Binding of the inhibitory ligand to its receptor activates the G_i-type G protein and causes its α_i subunit to dissociate from the $\beta\gamma$ dimers. The activated α_i binds to and inhibits adenylyl cyclase. In addition, the $\beta\gamma$ dimers may bind to free α_s subunits and thus diminish the stimulation of adenylyl cyclase by stimulatory agonists.

Certain ion channels are directly modulated by G proteins
In Chapter 4, several ligand-gated ion channels that are modulated directly by an extracellular agonist, such as acetylcholine or γ-aminobutyric acid, are discussed. Other ion channels are regulated by second messenger–mediated mechanisms that involve G proteins in the second step of the signal-transduction cascade. SOME ION CHANNELS, HOWEVER, ARE DIRECTLY MODULATED BY G PROTEINS WITHOUT THE INVOLVEMENT OF A SECOND MESSENGER. The binding of acetylcholine to M_2-muscarinic receptors in the heart and in certain neurons leads to the activation of a specific class of K^+ channels. Acetylcholine binding to the muscarinic receptor leads to the activation of a G protein of the G_i subclass. The activated α_i subunit then dissociates from the $\beta\gamma$ dimer. The $\beta\gamma$ dimer directly interacts with a particular class of K^+ channels to increase their probability of opening. The action of acetylcholine on muscarinic receptors to increase K^+ conductance of the pacemaker cells in the sinoatrial node of the heart is a major mechanism whereby parasympathetic nerves slow the heart rate (see Chapter 19).

Certain ion channels are directly modulated by a second messenger
IN SOME CASES A SECOND MESSENGER ACTS DIRECTLY ON AN ION CHANNEL TO PRODUCE A RESPONSE. Some cells have K^+ channels that are directly activated by Ca^{++}. When intracel-lular Ca^{++} levels rise, Ca^{++}-**activated K^+ channels** are stimulated, which leads to repolarization or hyperpolarization of the cell.

Vision (see Chapter 8) depends on cyclic GMP–gated ion channels. When a person is in the dark, the level of cyclic GMP in rod photoreceptors is high. Consequently, the **cyclic GMP–activated Na^+ channels** in the rod plasma membrane are open, and Na^+ entry maintains the rod cells in a depolarized state. **Rhodopsin** is a member of the family of G protein–coupled receptors. When rhodopsin is activated by light, it interacts with and activates a heterotrimeric G protein called **transducin (G_t).** Activated G_t interacts with cyclic GMP phosphodiesterase to greatly increase its activity, causing a rapid decrease in the intracellular cyclic GMP concentration. Hence the cyclic GMP–activated Na^+ channels close, and the photoreceptor cell becomes hyperpolarized.

Olfaction (see Chapter 8) involves cyclic AMP–gated ion channels. Humans can distinguish a large number of different odorants. Many of the odorants interact with G protein–coupled receptors in the plasma membrane of olfactory receptor cells. The odorant-bearing receptor activates **G_{olf},** a heterotrimeric G protein. Activated G_{olf} in turn stimulates adenylyl cyclase to produce cyclic AMP. Elevated cyclic AMP levels activate **cyclic AMP–gated Na^+ channels** in the plasma membrane of the olfactory receptor cell. Na^+ inflow leads to depolarization of the receptor, which may trigger an action potential in the axon of the olfactory receptor.

Monomeric GTP-binding proteins regulate several cellular processes

Cells contain another family of GTP-binding proteins called **monomeric GTP-binding proteins;** they are also known as **low-molecular-weight G proteins** or **small G proteins** (MW, 20,000 to 35,000). Table 5-2 lists the major subfamilies of monomeric GTP-binding proteins and some of their properties. The Ras-like and Rho-like monomeric GTP-binding proteins are involved in the signal-transduction pathways that link growth factor receptor tyrosine kinases to their intracellular effects. Among the processes regulated by pathways involving monomeric GTP-binding proteins are polypeptide chain elongation in

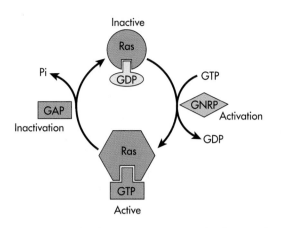

Figure 5-6 Activity cycle of Ras, a monomeric GTP-binding protein. The activation of Ras is enhanced by guanine nucleotide–releasing protein (*GNRP*). The inactivation of Ras is promoted by GTPase-activating protein (*GAP*). *P_i,* Inorganic phosphate.

protein synthesis, proliferation and differentiation of cells, neoplastic transformation of cells, control of the actin cytoskeleton and links between the cytoskeleton and the extracellular matrix, transport of vesicles among different organelles, and exocytotic secretion. Like their heterotrimeric cousins, monomeric GTP-binding proteins operate via the cycle of activation and inactivation shown in Figure 5-2. However, the activation and inactivation of the monomolecular GTP-binding proteins involves additional regulatory proteins that do not operate on the heterotrimeric G proteins (Figure 5-6). The activation of monomeric GTP-binding proteins is enhanced by **guanine nucleotide–releasing proteins (GNRPs),** and inactivation is promoted by **GTPase-activating proteins (GAPs).** The activation and inactivation of monomeric GTP-binding proteins can occur via upstream signals that influence the activity of GNRPs or GAPs, rather than via direct effects on the monomeric G protein.

A Second Messenger–Dependent Protein Kinase Is Modulated by the Cellular Level of a Second Messenger

Cyclic AMP–dependent protein kinase participates in regulating important metabolic pathways

Cyclic AMP was first identified as a second messenger in investigations of the mechanisms involved in the hormonal control of glycogen synthesis and breakdown (see Chapters 41 and 42). The phosphorylation of rate-determining enzymes in these metabolic pathways by cyclic AMP–dependent protein kinases is responsible for the hormonal regulation of glycogen metabolism.

In the absence of cyclic AMP, cyclic AMP–dependent protein kinase is composed of four subunits: two regulatory subunits and two catalytic subunits. The presence of the regulatory subunits greatly inhibits the enzymatic ac-

tivity of the complex. In the presence of micromolar levels of cyclic AMP, each regulatory subunit binds two molecules of cyclic AMP. The binding of cyclic AMP causes a conformational change in the regulatory subunits and diminishes their affinity for binding the catalytic subunits. Hence the regulatory subunits dissociate from the catalytic subunits, and in this way the catalytic subunits become activated. The active catalytic subunit phosphorylates target proteins on particular serine and threonine residues.

Comparison of the amino acid sequence of cyclic AMP–dependent protein kinase with representatives of the other classes of protein kinases shows that in spite of vast differences in their regulatory properties, the different classes of protein kinases share a common core with high amino acid homology (Figure 5-7). The core structure includes the ATP-binding domain and the enzyme's active center, where phosphate from ATP is transferred to the acceptor protein. Regions of the kinases outside the catalytic core are involved in the regulation of kinase activity.

Calmodulin-dependent protein kinases are activated by the complex of Ca^{++} with calmodulin

A host of vital cellular processes, including the release of neurotransmitters, the secretion of hormones, and muscle contraction, are regulated by the cytosolic level of Ca^{++}. One way that Ca^{++} exerts control is by binding to calmodulin. The complex of Ca^{++} and calmodulin can then influence the activity of many different proteins, among them a group of protein kinases known as **calmodulin-dependent protein kinases** (Figure 5-8). Dedicated calmodulin-dependent protein kinases, such as myosin light-chain kinase and phosphorylase kinase, have only one cellular substrate. Multifunctional calmodulin-dependent protein kinases phosphorylate more than one substrate protein.

Myosin light-chain kinase plays a central role in regulating the contraction of smooth muscle (see Chapter 14). Elevation of the cytosolic Ca^{++} concentration in a smooth muscle cell stimulates the activity of myosin light-chain kinase; the resulting phosphorylation of the regulatory light chains of myosin allows the contraction of smooth muscle cells to proceed.

Calmodulin-dependent protein kinase II is among the most abundant proteins in the nervous system. This kinase participates in the mechanism by which an increase in Ca^{++} in a nerve terminal causes the exocytotic release of neurotransmitter (see Chapter 4).

Protein kinase C is activated by Ca^{++} and membrane lipids

The primary action of certain lipophilic tumor-promoting substances, most notably the phorbol esters, is direct activation of protein kinase C. This powerfully stimulates cell division in many cell types and converts normal cells with

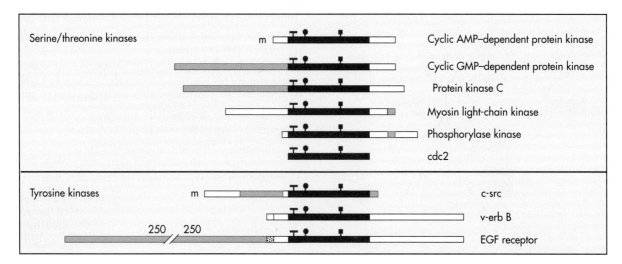

Figure 5-7 Protein kinase family. All known protein kinases share a common catalytic core *(blue)* that contains ATP- and peptide-binding domains and an active site where phosphoryl transfer occurs. Conserved residues are aligned with lysine 72 *(blue circles)*, aspartate 184 *(blue squares)*, and the glycine-rich loop *(blue rectangles)* of the catalytic subunit of cyclic AMP–dependent protein kinase. Regions important for regulation are orange. The membrane-spanning segment of the epidermal growth factor *(EGF)* receptor is stippled. Sites of myristoylation are indicated by *m*. A covalently attached myristic acid residue helps anchor the protein kinase in the plasma membrane. *(Adapted from Taylor S et al:* Annu Rev Cell Biol *8:429, 1992.)*

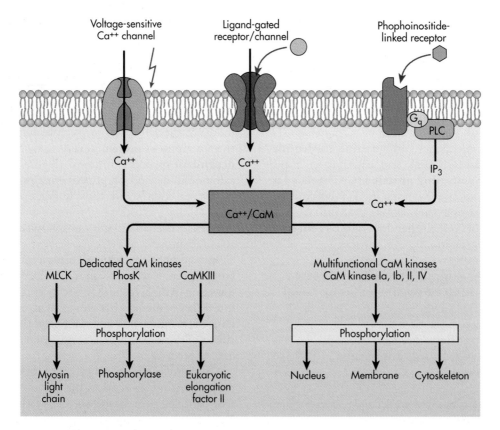

Figure 5-8 Dedicated calmodulin-dependent protein kinases phosphorylate specific effector proteins. Multifunctional calmodulin-dependent protein kinases phosphorylate multiple proteins of the nucleus or cytoskeleton or membrane proteins. *CaM,* Calmodulin; *CaMKIII,* calmodulin-dependent kinase III; *IP3,* inositol 1,4,5-trisphosphate; *MLCK,* myosin light-chain kinase; *PhosK,* phosphorylase kinase; *PLC,* phospholipase C. *(Adapted from Schulman H:* Curr Opin Cell Biol *5:247, 1993.)*

Table 5-3   Properties of Mammalian Isozymes of PKC

Group	Subspecies	Apparent Molecular Mass (d)	Activators	Tissue Expression
cPKC	α	76,799	Ca^{++}, DAG, PS, FFA, LysoPC	Universal
	βI	76,790	Ca^{++}, DAG, PS, FFA, LysoPC	Some tissues
	βII	76,933	Ca^{++}, DAG, PS, FFA, LysoPC	Many tissues
	γ	78,366	Ca^{++}, DAG, PS, FFA, LysoPC	Brain only
nPKC	δ	77,517	DAG, PS	Universal
	ϵ	83,474	DAG, PS, FFA	Brain, others
	η (L)	77,972	?	Lung, skin, heart
	θ	81,571	?	Skeletal muscle (mainly)
aPKC	ζ	67,740	PS, FFA	Universal
	λ	67,200	?	Ovary, testis, others

Adapted from Asaoka Y et al: *Trends Biochem Sci* 17:414, 1992.
PKC, Protein kinase C; *DAG*, diacylglycerol; *PS*, phosphatidylserine; *FFA*, *cis*-unsaturated fatty acids; *LysoPC*, lysophosphatidylcholine.

controlled growth properties into transformed cells (tumor cells) that grow uncontrollably.

In an unstimulated cell, much of the protein kinase C is present in the cytosol and is inactive. When cytosolic levels of Ca^{++} rise, Ca^{++} binds to protein kinase C. The binding of Ca^{++} causes protein kinase C to bind to the inner surface of the plasma membrane, where it can be activated by the diacylglycerol produced by the hydrolysis of phosphatidylinositol 4,5-bisphosphate. About 10 different isoforms of protein kinase C have been discovered (Table 5-3).

Tyrosine Kinases Play Key Roles in the Control of Cellular Proliferation

Receptors for certain growth factors are tyrosine kinases

The receptors for certain peptide hormones and growth factors are proteins with a glycosylated extracellular domain, a single transmembrane sequence, and an intracellular domain with protein-tyrosine kinase activity. Members of this superfamily of peptide receptors include the receptors for insulin and related growth factors, epidermal growth factor, nerve growth factor, platelet-derived growth factor, colony-stimulating factor, fibroblast growth factor, and hepatocyte growth factor. The binding of hormone or growth factor to its receptor triggers multiple cellular responses, including Ca^{++} influx, increased Na^+-H^+ exchange, stimulation of the uptake of sugars and amino acids, and stimulation of phospholipase Cβ to hydrolyze phosphatidylinositol 4,5-bisphosphate.

The known protein-tyrosine kinase receptors fall into eight subfamilies. The binding of ligand to the receptor results in dimerization of the receptor-ligand complexes. The dimerization enhances binding affinity and activates the protein-tyrosine kinase activity. Each monomer in a dimer phosphorylates the other monomer on multiple tyrosine residues. In subclass II receptors, the insulin receptor family, the unliganded receptor exists as a disulfide-

linked dimer, and binding of insulin results in a conformational change of both "monomers." This conformational change enhances insulin binding and activates the receptor's tyrosine kinase activity, which leads to enhanced autophosphorylation of the receptor.

> Protein-tyrosine kinases that are "out of control" play a central role in cell transformation and cancer. In some cell types, a mutation of a growth factor receptor renders the receptor active in phosphorylating tyrosines regardless of the presence or absence of the growth factor. Other tumor cells secrete a growth factor and overexpress its receptor. This leads to abnormally high rates of protein-tyrosine kinase activity and to uncontrolled cell division.

Monomeric GTP-binding proteins of the Ras family (Table 5-2) are involved in coupling the binding of mitogenic ligands and their protein-tyrosine kinase receptors to the resulting intracellular effects during cell proliferation. When Ras is inactive, cells cannot respond to the growth factors that operate via receptor tyrosine kinases.

> Mutations in Ras may produce overactive forms of Ras that constitutively activate the downstream effectors that normally are active only in the presence of growth factors. In such cases, cell growth may be uncontrolled, even in the absence of growth factors. Approximately 30% of human cancers involve mutated Ras proteins.

The activation of Ras by an activated receptor tyrosine kinase in turn activates a signal-transduction pathway that ultimately turns on the transcription of certain key genes that promote cell growth. The **mitogen-activated protein (MAP) kinase cascade** (Figure 5-9)

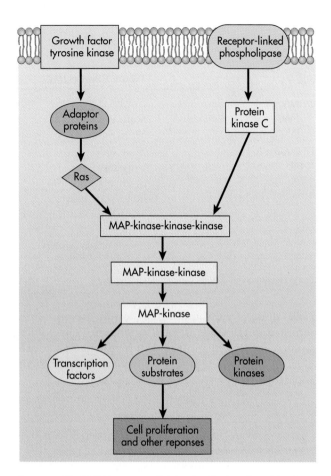

Figure 5-9 The MAP kinase cascade is involved in the cell-proliferation responses elicited by agonists that stimulate protein kinase C and by growth factors that act on membrane protein-tyrosine kinase receptors. MAP-kinase-kinase-kinase can be activated either by activated Ras or by protein kinase C. The cascade results in the phosphorylation and activation of MAP kinase, which in turn phosphorylates transcription factors, protein substrates, and other protein kinases important in eliciting proliferation and other cellular responses.

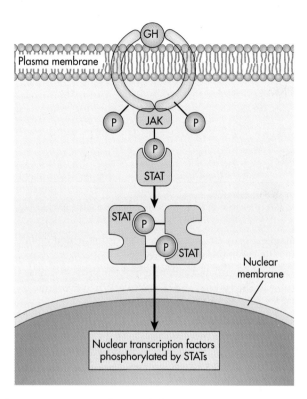

Figure 5-10 Receptors for growth hormone *(GH)* have no intrinsic tyrosine kinase activity. The receptor dimerizes in response to GH binding. The dimeric receptor binds one or more JAK tyrosine kinases, which phosphorylate themselves and the receptor. STAT tyrosine kinases bind to the complex and are phosphorylated. The phosphorylated STATs dissociate as dimers that are translocated to the nucleus, where they phosphorylate key transcription factors. *P,* Phosphate.

is involved in the responses to activated Ras. Protein kinase C also activates the MAP kinase cascade. The MAP kinase cascade is an important point of convergence for multiple effectors that promote cellular proliferation.

Certain other growth factor receptors form complexes with intracellular tyrosine kinases

The receptors for **growth hormone, prolactin,** and **erythropoietin** (as well as receptors for interferon and many cytokines) are not themselves protein kinases. However, on activation, these receptors form signaling complexes with intracellular tyrosine kinases that bring about their intracellular effects (Figure 5-10). The binding of hormone induces dimerization of the hormone receptor. The receptor dimer binds one or more members of the **Janus family, JAK** for short, of tyrosine kinases. Then the JAKs cross-phosphorylate one another and also phosphorylate the receptor. Members of the **signal transducers and acti-**

vators of transcription (STAT) family bind to phosphotyrosine domains on the complex of receptor and JAK proteins. The STAT proteins are phosphorylated by the JAKs and then dissociate from the signaling complex. The phosphorylated STAT proteins form dimers that move to the nucleus to activate the transcription of certain genes.

Protein Phosphatases Undo the Work of Protein Kinases

The extent of phosphorylation of a regulated protein depends on the activities of the protein kinase that phosphorylates the protein and the protein phosphatase that dephosphorylates it. In addition to the different types of protein kinases discussed, all cells also contain protein phosphatases whose task is to reverse the effects of protein phosphorylation. Protein phosphatases are classified as **serine-threonine protein phosphatases** or **protein-tyrosine-phosphatases.**

Table 5-4   Properties of Subtypes of Serine-Threonine Protein Phosphatases

Subtype	PP-1	PP-2A	PP-2B	PP-2C
Preference for the α or β subunit of phosphorylase kinase	β Subunit	α Subunit	α Subunit	α Subunit
Inhibition by interleukin-1 and interleukin-2	Yes	No	No	No
Absolute requirement for divalent cations	No	No	Yes (Ca^{++})	Yes (Mg^{++})
Stimulation by calmodulin	No	No	Yes	No
Inhibition by okadaic acid	Yes (20 nM)	Yes (0.2 nM)	Yes (5 μM)	No
Phosphorylase phosphatase activity	High	High	Very low	Very low

Adapted from Cohen P: *Annu Rev Biochem* 58:453, 1989.

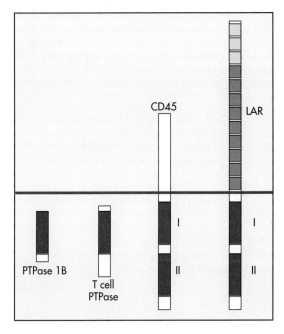

Figure 5-11 Four of more than sixty-five known protein-tyrosine-phosphatases *(PTPases)*. PTPase 1B from human placenta and PTPase from human T cells are small cytosolic PTPases. CD45 (leukocyte common antigen) and LAR (leukocyte common antigen–related protein) are transmembrane PTPases. The orange cytosolic segments of each protein are their PTPase catalytic domains. *(Adapted from Tonks NK, Charbonneau H: Trends Biochem Sci 14:497, 1989.)*

Serine-threonine protein phosphatases are subject to complex regulation

The serine-threonine protein phosphatases are a large family of structurally related molecules. They are classified as type 1 **(PP-1)** or type 2 **(PP-2).** The type is based on which subunit of phosphorylase kinase they prefer to dephosphorylate (Table 5-4). PP-2 is further classified into PP-2A, PP-2B, and PP-2C based on regulation by Ca^{++} and Mg^{++} and on susceptibility to being inhibited by okadaic acid, a complex fatty acid produced by marine dinoflagellates. PP-2B is also called **calcineurin,** and it is especially abundant in certain regions of the brain.

There are a large number of different protein-tyrosine-phosphatases

Protein-tyrosine-phosphatases are not structurally homologous to serine-threonine protein phosphatases. Figure 5-11 depicts 4 of the more than 65 known protein-tyrosine-phosphatases. Whereas two are small cytosolic proteins, two others are larger transmembrane proteins. Based on their structures, the transmembrane protein-tyrosine-phosphatases are probably receptors whose activity is modulated by extracellular ligands.

Atrial Natriuretic Peptide Receptors Have Guanylyl Cyclase Activity

Atrial natriuretic peptide (ANP) is released by cells in the atrium of the heart in response to an elevation of atrial pressure. This hormone increases the excretion of NaCl and water by the kidney (see Chapters 37 and 46) and diminishes the constriction of certain blood vessels. The membrane receptors for ANP themselves possess guanylyl cyclase activity that is stimulated when ANP is bound to the receptor. No second messenger is required to activate guanylyl cyclase.

ANP receptors have an extracellular ANP binding domain, a single transmembrane helix, and an intracellular guanylyl cyclase domain. The binding of ANP stimulates the guanylyl cyclase activity and elevates intracellular levels of the second messenger cyclic GMP.

Nitric Oxide Is a Short-Lived Paracrine Mediator

Nitric oxide (NO) is a paracrine mediator that is released by endothelial cells and certain neurons. NO is rapidly oxidized, so its biological lifetime is only several seconds. For this reason, NO affects only cells in the immediate vicinity of the cell that produces it. NO stimulates a soluble guanylyl cyclase in the target cell and thereby elevates the intracellular concentration of cyclic GMP in the target cell, thus stimulating cyclic GMP–dependent protein kinase.

The production of NO is catalyzed by **NO synthase,** a Ca^{++}-calmodulin–dependent enzyme that accelerates the conversion of arginine to citrulline plus NO. An increase in cytosolic Ca^{++} levels is often the stimulus for the enhanced formation and release of NO. NO is a neurotransmitter that is released by nerve terminals of certain neurons in the central nervous system (see Chapter 4) and by some neurons of the enteric nervous system (see Chapter 32). NO is released by endothelial cells in response to agonists such as acetylcholine. NO released by endothelial cells acts on nearby vascular smooth muscle cells to cause vasodilation (see Chapter 23).

SUMMARY

- Heterotrimeric GTP-binding proteins serve as intermediaries between a receptor that has been activated by binding an agonist and enzymes and ion channels whose activity is modulated in response to agonist binding.
- A GTP-binding protein is activated by interacting with an agonist-bearing receptor. It then changes the activity of an enzyme or an ion channel and thereby alters the intracellular concentration of a second messenger, such as cyclic AMP, cyclic GMP, Ca^{++}, IP_3, or diacylglycerol.
- An increased level of a second messenger may increase the activity of a second messenger–dependent protein kinase: cyclic AMP–dependent protein kinase, cyclic GMP–dependent protein kinase, calmodulin-dependent protein kinase, or protein kinase C.
- Myriad cellular processes are regulated via the phosphorylation of enzymes and ion channels.
- Certain membrane receptors for hormones and growth factors are protein-tyrosine kinases or are associated with tyrosine kinases activated by binding of the agonist.
- Monomeric GTP-binding proteins are intermediaries between the binding of growth factors to their protein-tyrosine kinase receptors and the downstream effects on cellular proliferation.
- The small G proteins also regulate the function of the actin cytoskeleton and intracellular vesicular trafficking.
- Protein phosphatases, themselves subject to complex regulation by agonists and second messengers, reverse the effects of protein phosphorylation.

BIBLIOGRAPHY

Berridge MJ: Elementary and global aspects of calcium signalling, *J Physiol (London)* 449(Pt 2):290, 1997.

Bourne HR: How receptors talk to trimeric G proteins, *Curr Opinion Cell Biol* 9:134, 1997.

Braun AP, Shulman H: The multifunctional calcium/calmodulin-dependent protein kinase: from form to function, *Annu Rev Physiol* 57:417, 1995.

Duhe RJ, Farrar WL: Structural and mechanistic aspects of Janus kinases: how the two-faced god wields a double-edged sword, *J Interferon Cytokine Res* 18:1, 1998.

Gilman AG: Nobel lecture: G proteins and regulation of adenylyl cyclase, *Biosci Reports* 15:65, 1995.

Gutkind JS: The pathways connecting G protein–coupled receptors to the nucleus through divergent mitogen-activated protein kinase cascades, *J Biol Chem* 273:1839, 1998.

Hall A: Rho GTPases and the actin cytoskeleton, *Science* 279:509, 1998.

Hamm HE: The many faces of G protein signaling, *J Biol Chem* 273:669, 1998.

Hancock JT: *Cell signalling,* Harlow, England, 1997, Longman.

McCormick F, Wittinghofer A: Interactions between Ras proteins and their effectors, *Curr Opinion Biotech* 7:449, 1996.

Michell RH: The multiplying roles of inositol lipids and phosphates in cell control processes, *Essays Biochem* 32:31, 1997.

Schulman H: Nitric oxide: a spatial second messenger, *Mol Psychiatry* 2:296, 1997.

Spiegel AM, ed: *G proteins, receptors, and disease,* Towata, NJ, 1998, Humana.

Tonks NK: Protein tyrosine phosphatases and the control of cellular signaling responses, *Adv Pharmacol* 36:91, 1996.

Vaughan M: Signaling by heterotrimeric G proteins, *J Biol Chem* 273:667, 1998.

CASE STUDIES

Case 5-1

An American archeologist studying Mayan ruins in Belize drinks water from a brook downstream from an Indian village. She is stricken with a violent diarrheal illness that does not respond to over-the-counter medications. She becomes very weak and is flown to a clinic in Belize City, where her illness is diagnosed as **cholera.** Several liters of isotonic saline intravenously are administered, and then oral rehydration therapy with a solution of NaCl, glucose, KCl, and $NaHCO_3$ is initiated. Stool cultures confirm the presence of *Vibrio cholerae,* the organism responsible for cholera. After 3 days of oral rehydration therapy, the woman's diarrhea abates, and she feels strong enough to leave the clinic.

1. **Which of the following statements is correct?**
    A. The toxin responsible for cholera is produced by certain strains of *Salmonella typhimurium.*
    B. Cholera toxin activates adenylyl cyclase by transferring ADP-ribose to it.
    C. The increased level of cyclic AMP stimulates the secretion of salts and water by cells in the crypts of Lieberkühn.
    D. The increased level of cyclic AMP causes a net secretion of salts and water by intestinal epithelial cells near the villous tips.
    E. The activity of G_i, the inhibitory G protein, is decreased by cholera toxin.

2. Which of the following statements is correct?

A. The patient's weakness was caused primarily by the bacterial infection.

B. Antibiotics administered at the clinic could have markedly shortened the duration of the diarrhea.

C. Dehydration was the primary cause of the patient's weakness.

D. Oral rehydration therapy alone could not have cured the patient.

E. Electrolyte imbalance is not likely to have been present in this patient.

3. Which of the following statements is correct?

A. Oral rehydration therapy stimulates the absorption of salts and water by intestinal epithelial cells.

B. If the patient is adequately hydrated, diarrhea should abate in about 1 week.

C. The administration of G_i by mouth might be a useful therapy for inhibiting adenylyl cyclase.

D. Treatment with antibiotics after the diarrhea has abated is necessary to prevent relapse of the disease.

E. Drugs that diminish intestinal motility are particularly useful in treating cholera.

Case 5-2

A 5-year-old boy enters the hospital with weakness, lethargy, and patches of pigmented skin, particularly on his trunk. He is at the 5th percentile in body weight for his age. Laboratory tests reveal low levels of blood glucose, very low serum levels of the hormone cortisol (see Chapter 46), and high levels of adrenocorticotrophic hormone (ACTH). ACTH is released from the anterior pituitary gland and is the major stimulus for the release of cortisol from the adrenal cortex (see Chapter 46). The administration of cortisol results in a decrease in serum levels of ACTH. The administration of ACTH does not result in increased serum levels of cortisol. The patient is diagnosed with an **ACTH resistance syndrome.** Over several years of regular administration of cortisol, he gains weight, which becomes normal for his age; his strength and energy improve substantially; and his pigmented skin patches disappear.

1. Which of the following statements is true?

A. The elevated level of ACTH is primarily responsible for the weakness and lethargy.

B. The patient's hypothalamus may be releasing inadequate amounts of corticotropin-releasing hormone.

C. The administration of cortisol will not diminish the elevated levels of ACTH.

D. Administration of corticotropin-releasing hormone might help alleviate the patient's symptoms.

E. The patient's weakness, lethargy, and low growth rate are due to low levels of cortisol.

2. Which of the following statements is true?

A. The disorder could not result from a decreased number of ACTH receptors in the plasma membrane of the adrenal gland cells (in the zona fasciculata) that synthesize and secrete cortisol.

B. This disorder could result from a greatly decreased affinity of the ACTH receptors for ACTH.

C. The disorder could not result from a diminished ability of the liganded ACTH receptor to activate adenylyl cyclase in the cells of the zona fasciculata.

D. The disorder could not result from a defect in one of the enzymes involved in the biosynthesis of cortisol.

E. If the cause of the disorder is decreased affinity of the ACTH receptor for ACTH, the administration of high levels of ACTH should result in increased plasma levels of cortisol.

3. Polymerase chain reaction was used to amplify the coding region of the genes for the ACTH receptor in DNA from white blood cells taken from this patient. Which of the following statements is true?

A. If the patient has one normal and one mutant form of the ACTH receptor gene, this would be consistent with the clinical findings presented.

B. Even if the patient has two normal copies of the ACTH receptor gene, a defect involving the ACTH receptor is still the most likely cause of the disorder.

C. If the patient has two mutant forms of the ACTH receptor, this could explain the clinical findings.

D. If the patient has two mutant forms of the ACTH receptor, then one of the patient's parents suffers from the same disorder.

E. An individual with one normal and one mutant form of the ACTH receptor could have no symptoms in common with the patient.

NERVOUS SYSTEM II

William D. Willis, Jr.

CHAPTER 6

Cellular Organization

- Introduce the cellular composition of the nervous system.
- Describe the organization of the peripheral and central nervous system, the environment of neurons, and the structure of neurons.
- Discuss the functional properties of neurons and the ways that information is distributed and chemical substances are transported in nervous tissue.
- Discuss the pathological responses of nervous tissue and some representative diseases that result from disorders of neural function.

The nervous system is responsible for most of the functions that characterize higher organisms. In humans, it is the source of conscious awareness, sensation, voluntary movement, thought, memory and learning, prediction, emotion, and other forms of cognitive behavior. On a simpler level, the nervous system mediates reflex activity and controls autonomic and endocrine responses. Elements of the nervous system are distributed throughout the body and influence all other systems.

The nervous system is a communications network that allows an organism to interact in appropriate ways with the environment. This system has **sensory components** that detect environmental events, **integrative components** that process sensory data and information that is stored in memory, and **motor components** that generate movements and other activity. The nervous system can be divided into peripheral and central parts, each with a number of further subdivisions.

Cellular Composition

The nervous system consists of a highly complex aggregation of cells, part of which is a communication network and another part a supportive matrix. The communication network is formed by **neurons,** which are the functional cellular units of the nervous system. The human brain contains approximately 10^{12} neurons. Neurons are specialized for receiving information, making decisions, and transmitting signals to other neurons or to effector cells such as muscle or gland cells. This specialization depends on different types of extensions of the cell body, or **soma,** of a neuron. Most neurons have several **dendrites** and an **axon.** Different types of neurons have consistent forms that relate to their functional properties (Figure 6-1). The dendrites receive contacts called **synapses** from other neurons, and the axon forms synapses with other neurons or effector cells. Information is transmitted in a neuron by conduction of an electrical signal, the nerve impulse or **action potential** from the soma and dendritic region, along the axon to the synaptic ending. A chemical **neurotransmitter** is then released and signals information to the next cell. **Synaptic transmission** can have an excitatory or an inhibitory effect.

The supportive cells of the nervous system include the **neuroglia** ("nerve glue"). The human brain has 10 times as many neuroglia as neurons. Different types of neuroglia are shown in Figure 6-2. Some neuroglia, called **astrocytes** because of their star-shaped appearance in stained histological sections, help maintain an appropriate local environment for neurons. Others, named **oligodendroglia** because they have a limited number of processes, ensheathe axons to increase the speed of propagation of nerve impulses (see Chapter 3). **Microglia** are phagocytes that remove the products of cellular damage from the central nervous system. They are probably derived from the circulation. **Ependymal cells** form an epithelium that separates the CNS from the ventricles, a series of cavities within the brain; these cavities contain cerebrospinal fluid (CSF).

The nervous system is also richly supplied with blood vessels.

Organization of the Nervous System

The nervous system can be divided into a **peripheral nervous system (PNS)** and a **central nervous system (CNS).**

The peripheral nervous system is an interface between the central nervous system and the environment

The PNS provides an interface between the CNS and the environment, including both the external world and the body apart from the nervous system. The PNS includes sensory and motor components. The sensory component detects environmental signals and is formed by **sensory receptor organs** and **primary afferent neurons.** Motor

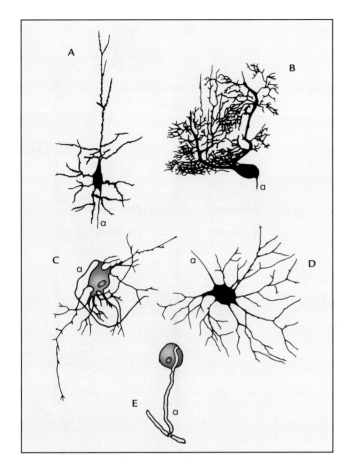

Figure 6-1 Various forms of neurons. **A,** Pyramidal cell from the cerebral cortex. **B,** Cerebellar Purkinje cell. **C,** Sympathetic postganglionic neuron. **D,** Spinal cord motor neuron. **E,** Dorsal root ganglion cell. *a,* Axon. *(Redrawn from Willis WD Jr, Grossman RG: Medical neurobiology: neuroanatomical and neurophysiological principles basic to clinical neuroscience, ed 3, St Louis, 1981, Mosby.)*

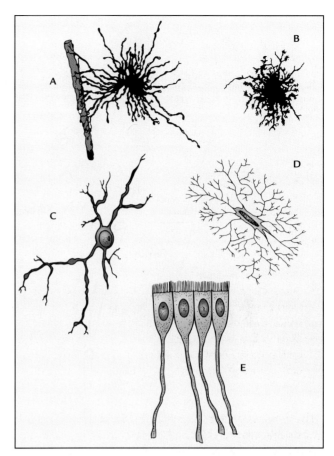

Figure 6-2 Different types of neuroglial cells of the central nervous system. **A,** Fibrous astrocyte; note the glial foot processes in association with a capillary. **B,** Protoplasmic astrocyte. **C,** Oligodendrocyte; each of the processes is responsible for the production of one or more myelin sheath internodes around central axons. **D,** Microglial cell. **E,** Ependymal cells. *(Redrawn from Willis WD Jr, Grossman RG: Medical neurobiology: neuroanatomical and neurophysiological principles basic to clinical neuroscience, ed 3, St Louis, 1981, Mosby.)*

components command effector organs to perform muscular or glandular activity and include the axons of **somatic motor neurons** as well as **autonomic preganglionic and postganglionic neurons** and their axons. Autonomic neurons can be further subdivided into **sympathetic, parasympathetic,** and **enteric neurons.** Somatic motor axons cause contractions of skeletal muscle fibers. Autonomic motor axons excite or inhibit cardiac muscle, smooth muscle, or glands. The sympathetic nervous system prepares the organism for emergency action, whereas the parasympathetic nervous system promotes more routine activities such as digestion. Ordinarily the sympathetic and parasympathetic nervous systems work together in regulating visceral function.

The central nervous system includes the spinal cord and brain

The CNS includes the **spinal cord** and **brain** (Figure 6-3). The brain can be subdivided into the following regions based on embryological development: **myelencephalon, metencephalon, mesencephalon, diencephalon,** and

telencephalon. In the adult brain the myelencephalon becomes the **medulla;** the metencephalon, the **pons** and **cerebellum;** the mesencephalon, the **midbrain;** the diencephalon, the **thalamus** and **hypothalamus;** and the telencephalon, the **basal ganglia** and various lobes of the **cerebral cortex.** The thalamus and basal ganglia are hidden from view in Figure 6-3.

Environment of the Neuron

The local environment of most neurons is controlled so that neurons are normally protected from extreme variations in the composition of the extracellular fluid that bathes them. This control is provided by regulation of the circulation of the CNS (see Chapter 25), the presence of a blood-brain barrier, the buffering function of astrocytes, and the exchange of substances with CSF. Substances are exchanged freely between the extracellular fluid of the CNS and the CSF. However, the entry of substances from the blood into the CNS is

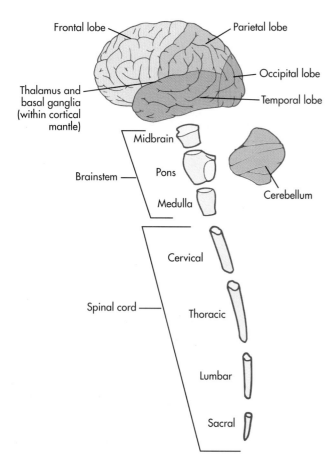

Figure 6-3 Exploded view showing the major components of the central nervous system. Also shown are four of the major divisions of the cerebral cortex: the frontal, parietal, occipital, and temporal lobes.

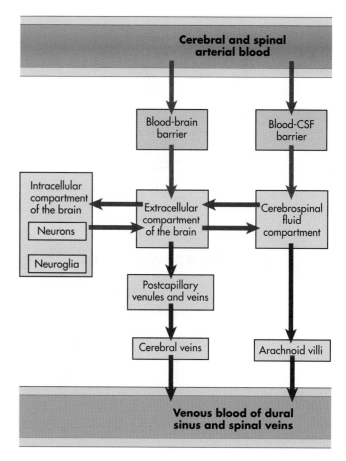

Figure 6-4 Structural and functional relationships involved in the blood-brain and blood-CSF barriers. Substances entering the neurons and neuroglial cells (i.e., intracellular compartment) must pass through the cell membrane. Arrows indicate the direction of fluid flow under normal conditions.

controlled by secretory processes in the choroid plexuses, which form CSF, and by the blood-brain barrier (Figure 6-4).

The fluid compartments of the cranium are the brain, blood, and cerebrospinal fluid

The cranial cavity contains the brain, blood, and CSF. The human brain weighs about 1350 g, of which approximately 15%, or 200 ml, is extracellular fluid. The intracranial blood volume is about 100 ml, half of it extracellular fluid, and the cranial CSF volume another 100 ml. Thus the extracellular fluid space in the cranial cavity totals approximately 350 ml.

The blood-brain barrier restricts the movement of substances into the brain

The movement of large molecules and highly charged ions from the blood into the brain and spinal cord is severely restricted by the **blood-brain barrier** (Figure 6-4). The restriction is at least partly caused by the presence of tight junctions between the capillary endothelial cells of the

CNS. Astrocytes may also help limit the movement of certain substances. For example, astrocytes can take up K^+ and thus regulate the K^+ concentration in the extracellular space. Some substances are removed from the CNS by transport mechanisms. For example, penicillin is transported from CSF across the epithelium of the choroid plexuses and into the blood.

Cerebrospinal fluid influences the environment of neurons of the central nervous system

The extracellular fluid within the CNS communicates directly with the CSF. Thus the composition of CSF indicates the composition of the extracellular environment of neurons in the brain and spinal cord. The main constituents of CSF in the lumbar cistern (from which CSF can readily be removed by lumbar puncture) are shown in Table 6-1. For comparison, the concentrations of the same constituents in the blood are also given. CSF has lower concentrations of K^+, glucose, and protein but greater concentrations of Na^+ and Cl^- than blood. Furthermore,

Table 6-1	Constituents of CSF and Blood	
Constituent	Lumbar CSF	Blood
Na^+ (mEq/L)	148	136-145
K^+ (mEq/L)	2.9	3.5-5
Cl^- (mEq/L)	120-130	100-106
Glucose (mg/dl)	50-75	70-100
Protein (mg/dl)	15-45	$6-8 \times 10^3$
pH	7.3	7.4

CSF, Cerebrospinal fluid.

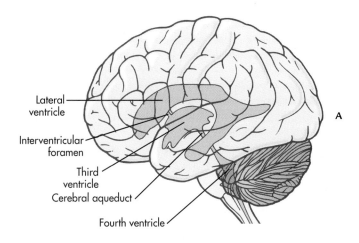

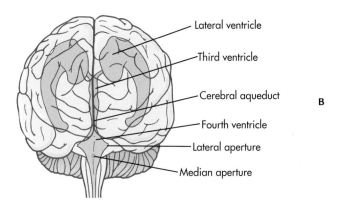

Figure 6-5 Ventricular system in situ as seen from the side **(A)** and front **(B).**

CSF contains practically no blood cells. The increased concentrations of Na^+ and Cl^- allow CSF to be isotonic to blood, despite the much lower concentration of protein in the former.

CSF is formed largely by the **choroid plexuses,** which are capillary loops covered by specialized ependymal cells and are located in the ventricular system of the brain. The **ventricular system** includes the two **lateral ventricles** in the telencephalon, the **third ventricle** of the diencephalon, and the **fourth ventricle** of the metencephalon and myelencephalon. Each lateral ventricle connects to the third ventricle via an **interventricular foramen,** and the third ventricle connects with the fourth through the **cerebral aqueduct.** Choroid plexuses are found in the lateral ventricles, third ventricle, and fourth ventricle (Figure 6-5).

CSF escapes from the fourth ventricle through openings in its connective tissue roof (Figure 6-5). These openings are the unpaired **median aperture** and the paired **lateral apertures.** After leaving the ventricular system, CSF circulates through the subarachnoid spaces surrounding the brain and spinal cord. Much of the CSF is removed by bulk flow through the valvular **arachnoid villi** into the dural venous sinuses.

The volume of CSF within the cerebral ventricles is approximately 35 ml, and that in the subarachnoid spaces of the brain and spinal cord is about 100 ml. CSF is produced at a rate of about 0.35 ml/min, which allows the CSF to be turned over approximately four times daily.

The pressure in the CSF column of adults is about 12.0 to 18.0 cm H_2O when a person is recumbent. The rate at which CSF is formed is relatively independent of the pressure in the ventricles and subarachnoid space and of the systemic blood pressure. However, the absorption rate of CSF is a direct function of CSF pressure.

Obstruction of the circulation of CSF leads to increased CSF pressure and hydrocephalus. In **hydrocephalus** the ventricles become distended. In young children the intracranial volume may be increased because the cranial sutures are not closed, so the head can enlarge. However, if the increase continues, brain substance may be lost. In adults, an increase in the ventricular size compromises the flow of blood and causes the loss of brain tissue. When the obstruction is within the ventricular system or in the roof of the fourth ventricle, the condition is called a **noncommunicating hydrocephalus.** If the obstruction is in the subarachnoid space or arachnoid villi, it is known as a **communicating hydrocephalus.**

Microscopic Anatomy of the Neuron

Most neurons have the following parts: a cell body or soma; one or more dendrites; and an axon. The **cell body** (Figure 6-6) contains the nucleus and nucleolus of the neuron. It possesses a well-developed biosynthetic apparatus for the manufacture of membrane constituents, synthetic enzymes, and other chemical substances needed for the specialized functions of the nerve cell. The neuronal biosynthetic apparatus includes **Nissl bodies,** which are stacks of **rough endoplasmic reticulum,** the organelle that is responsible for protein synthesis. The soma also contains a prominent **Golgi ap-**

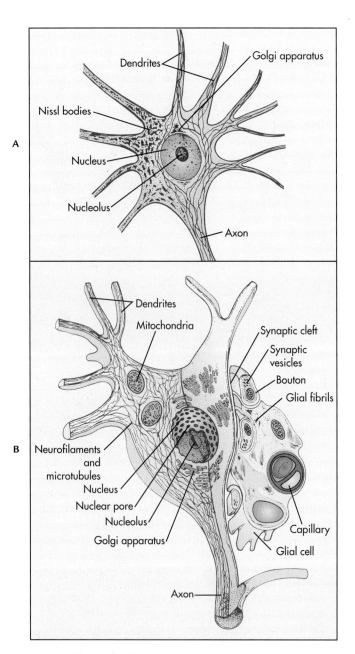

Figure 6-6 Organelles of the neurons. **A,** Organelles typical of a neuron shown as they are seen with the light microscope. The left side of the neuron includes structures seen with a Nissl's stain, whereas the right side includes structures seen with a heavy metal stain. **B,** Structures visible with an electron microscope. *(Redrawn from Willis WD Jr, Grossman RG: Medical neurobiology: neuroanatomical and neurophysiological principles basic to clinical neuroscience, ed 3, St Louis, 1981, Mosby.)*

paratus, which packages materials into vesicles for transport to other parts of the cell, and numerous mitochondria and cytoskeletal elements, including neurofilaments and microtubules. **Neurofilaments** are thin, rodlike structures, whereas **microtubules** are larger, cylinder-like structures. **Lipofuscin** is a pigment formed from incompletely degraded membrane components, and it accumulates in some neurons. A few groups of neurons in the brainstem contain melanin pigment.

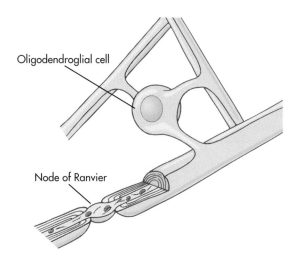

Figure 6-7 Myelin sheath in the CNS. Each oligodendroglial process forms the internode for one axon.

The **dendrites** (Figure 6-6) are extensions of the cell body. In some neurons, dendrites may be as long as 1 mm, and they account for more than 90% of the surface area of many neurons. The proximal dendrites (near the cell body) contain Nissl bodies and parts of the Golgi apparatus. However, the main cytoplasmic organelles in dendrites are microtubules and neurofilaments.

The **axon** (Figure 6-6) arises from the soma (or sometimes from a dendrite) in a specialized region called the **axon hillock.** The axon hillock and axon differ from the soma and proximal dendrites because they lack rough endoplasmic reticulum, **free ribosomes,** and the Golgi apparatus. The axon contains smooth endoplasmic reticulum and a prominent cytoskeleton. Axons may be short, and like dendrites, they terminate near the soma **(Golgi type 1 neurons),** or they may be long **(Golgi type 2 neurons)** and extend as far as a meter or more.

Axons may be ensheathed or bare. In the PNS, axons are always surrounded by **Schwann cells.** Many axons are surrounded by a spiral, multilayered wrapping of a Schwann cell membrane called a **myelin sheath.** A series of Schwann cells forms a series of internodes along the axon. Gaps between adjacent internodes are called the **nodes of Ranvier,** which are the sites of nerve impulse generation (see Chapter 3). In the CNS, myelinated axons are ensheathed by oligodendroglia (Figure 6-7). One oligodendroglia cell forms myelin internodes on many CNS axons. The presence of myelin allows nerve impulses to be conducted more rapidly. Other axons are unmyelinated. In the PNS, unmyelinated axons are embedded in Schwann cells but are not wrapped in myelin (Figure 6-8). A group of such axons and the accompanying Schwann cells are called a **bundle of Remak.** In the CNS, unmyelinated axons are bare. Unmyelinated axons conduct action potentials slowly.

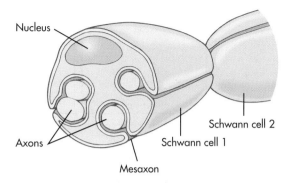

Figure 6-8 Three-dimensional view of a bundle of Remak. The cut face of the bundle is shown to the left. One of three unmyelinated axons is represented as protruding from the bundle. The mesaxon is a membrane indentation of the Schwann cell. To the right, the junction of adjacent Schwann cells is depicted.

In some diseases of the nervous system, myelin may be lost over one or more internodes of many axons without interruption of the axons. In such cases, conduction of nerve impulses may be slowed or blocked, and the function of the affected axons is therefore abnormal. Such demyelination occurs in the PNS in the **Guillain-Barré syndrome** and diphtheria. An important demyelinating disease of the CNS is **multiple sclerosis.**

General Functions of the Nervous System

Function of the nervous system include SENSORY DETECTION, INFORMATION PROCESSING, LEARNING AND MEMORY, AND BEHAVIOR. Learning and memory permit behavior to change appropriately in response to environmental challenges based on past experience. Other systems, such as the endocrine and immune systems, share these functions, but the nervous system is specialized for them.

Excitability is a cellular property that enables neurons to perform their functions. It is manifested by electrical events such as **nerve impulses** (or **action potentials**), **receptor potentials,** and **synaptic potentials** (see Chapters 3 and 4). Chemical events often accompany these electrical ones.

Sensory detection is accomplished by special nerve cells called **sensory receptors.** Various forms of energy, including mechanical events that impinge on the body wall, chemicals, temperature gradients, light, sound, and in some animals, electrical fields, are sensed.

Information processing in neural circuits depends on intercellular communication, which is accomplished by nerve cells as they respond to and generate chemical signals. The mechanisms involved require both electrical and chemical changes. Learning and memory require special forms of information processing and mechanisms for the storage and retrieval of the information.

Behavior may be covert, as in cognition or memory, but it is often readily observable as a motor act, such as a movement or an autonomic response. In humans a particularly important set of behaviors are those involved in language.

Transmission of Information

A major role of axons is to transmit information from the region of the cell body and dendrites of a neuron to the synapses on other neurons or effector cells. The information is generally transmitted as a series of **nerve impulses.**

The speed of transmission of information depends partly on the conduction velocity of the axon. Conduction velocity in turn depends on how wide the axon is and whether the axon is unmyelinated or myelinated. Unmyelinated axons are generally less than 1 μm in diameter and conduct at speeds less than 2.5 m/sec. About 1 second would be required for a signal in an unmyelinated axon that supplies a sensory receptor in a person's foot to reach the spinal cord if the axonal conduction velocity were 1 m/sec. Myelinated axons have diameters of 1 to 20 μm and conduct at speeds of 3 to 120 m/sec. A spinal motor neuron with an axon that conducts at 100 m/sec would be able to trigger the contraction of a toe muscle in about 10 msec.

In the CNS, certain neurons that lack axons (e.g., **amacrine cells** of the retina) signal information by electrical current flow rather than by the generation of action potentials. This current flow produces a **local potential,** which decays over a short distance (millimeters to hundreds of micrometers, depending on the length constant of the neuron involved). Local potentials differ from action potentials in that they do not propagate and therefore cannot spread over long distances. In contrast, action potentials can propagate over long distances along axons (see also Chapter 3).

Signaling by local potentials is also characteristic of sensory receptors, which produce **receptor potentials** (see Chapter 7), and of communication between nerve cells by **synaptic potentials** (see Chapter 4).

Neurons encode information

Information conveyed by axons may be coded in several ways. Sets of neurons may be dedicated to a general function, such as a particular sensory modality. For example, the visual pathway includes the retina, optic nerve and tract, lateral geniculate nucleus of the thalamus, and visual parts of the cerebral cortex (see Chapter 8). The normal means of activating the visual system is by light striking the retina, leading to axonal and synaptic transmission of visual information to higher levels in the visual pathway. However, mechanical or electrical stimulation of the visual system also produces a visual response, although a distorted one. Thus neurons of the visual system can be regarded as a **labeled line,** which when activated, causes a visual sensation. A labeled line consists of a set of neurons, including sensory receptors and CNS processing circuits, that together are responsible for signaling a particular type of sensation. A labeled line is usually activated by sensory stimulation. However, it may also be activated artificially: for example, one can cause a person to see flashes of light by pressing on the eye or by stimulating the cerebral cortex with electric shocks. Other sensory systems provide further examples of labeled lines.

Information is also coded by the nervous system through **spatial maps.** The body surface may be mapped by an array of neurons in a sensory or motor system. This type of map is termed a **somatotopic map** (or in humans, a **homunculus** [see Chapters 7 and 9]). In the visual system, there are **retinotopic maps**. In the auditory system the frequency of sounds is represented in **tonotopic maps** (see Chapter 8).

A third method for coding information is by **patterns of nerve impulses.** Axons transmit a sequence of nerve impulses that results in synaptic transmission of information to a new set of neurons. The information communicated is coded in terms of the structure of the nerve impulse trains. Several different types of nerve impulse codes have been proposed. A common code is likely to depend on the mean discharge frequency. Other candidate codes depend on the time of firing, temporal pattern, and duration of bursts.

Synaptic transmission allows neurons to communicate

Neurons communicate with one another at specialized junctions called **synapses** (see Chapter 4). Typically, synapses are formed between the terminals of the axon of one neuron and the dendrites of another (Figure 6-9); these are called **axodendritic synapses.** However, several other types of synapses, including **axosomatic, axoaxonal,** and **dendrodendritic** (Figure 6-9), occur. The synapse between a motor neuron and a skeletal muscle fiber is called an **end-plate** or **neuromuscular junction.**

Axonal transport is used to move substances within neurons

Many axons are too long to allow the effective movement of substances from the soma to the synaptic endings simply by diffusion. Certain membrane and cytoplasmic components that originate in the biosynthetic apparatus of the soma and proximal dendrites must be distributed along the processes, especially to the presynaptic elements of synapses, to replenish secreted or inactivated materials. A special transport mechanism, called **axonal transport,** accomplishes this distribution.

There are several types of axonal transport. Certain membrane-bound organelles and mitochondria are transported relatively rapidly by **fast axonal transport.** Sub-

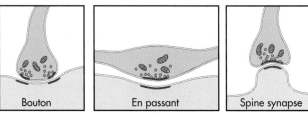

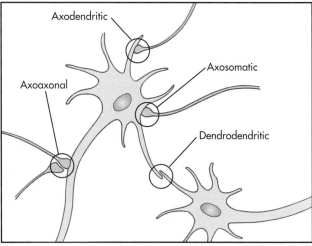

Figure 6-9 The drawings of electron micrographs at the top left show a synaptic bouton at the termination of an axon, an en passant synapse made by an axon that continues past the synapse, and a spine synapse on a dendritic spine. The drawing at the bottom illustrates axodendritic axosomatic, axoaxonal, and dendrodendritic synapses.

stances (e.g., proteins) that are dissolved in cytoplasm are moved by **slow axonal transport.** Fast axonal transport proceeds as rapidly as 400 mm/day, whereas slow axonal transport occurs at about 1 mm/day. This means that synaptic vesicles can travel from a motor neuron in the spinal cord to a neuromuscular junction in a person's foot in about 2½ days, whereas the transport of many soluble proteins over the same distance would take nearly 3 years.

Axonal transport requires metabolic energy and involves Ca^{++} ions. Microtubules in the cytoskeleton provide a system of guidewires along which membrane-bound organelles move during fast axonal transport. These organelles attach to transport filaments, which are moved along the microtubules through a link similar to that between the thick and thin filaments of skeletal muscle fibers. Ca^{++} triggers the movement of the organelles along the microtubules.

Axonal transport occurs in both directions. Transport from the soma toward the axonal terminals is called **anterograde axonal transport.** This process allows the replenishment of synaptic vesicles and enzymes responsible for neurotransmitter synthesis in synaptic terminals. Transport in the opposite direction is **retrograde axonal transport** (Figure 6-10). Retrograde axonal transport is rapid, although the speed is only about half that of fast anterograde transport. This process returns synaptic vesicle membrane to the soma for lysosomal degradation. Marker

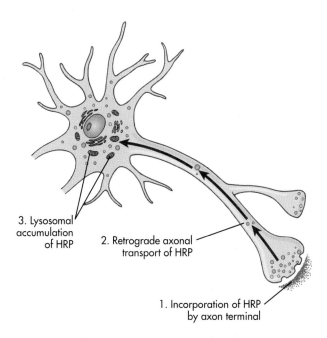

3. Lysosomal
accumulation
of HRP

2. Retrograde axonal
transport of HRP

1. Incorporation of HRP
by axon terminal

Figure 6-10 Incorporation *(1)*, retrograde axonal transport *(2)*, and lysosomal accumulation (3) of horseradish peroxidase *(HRP)* in a neuron.

substances, such as the enzyme horseradish peroxidase, can be transported anterogradely or retrogradely and can be used in experiments to trace neural pathways.

> Axonal transport is important in pathological processes. Primary afferent neurons and motor neurons link the CNS with the periphery and thus form a protoplasmic bridge that crosses the blood-brain barrier. Certain viruses, such as the rabies virus and the polio virus, and toxins, such as tetanus toxin, can enter the CNS from the periphery if they are taken up and transported in the axons of these neurons.

Reactions to Injury

Injury to nervous tissue elicits responses by neurons and neuroglia. Severe injury causes cell death. Once a neuron is lost, it cannot be replaced because neurons are postmitotic cells; that is, they are fully differentiated and no longer undergo cell division. Most neurons complete their differentiation before birth, although neuroglial cells continue to divide even in adulthood. Thus most tumors of the CNS originate from neuroglial precursor cells rather than from neurons.

The axonal reaction is a pathological response of a neuronal soma to axonal injury

When an axon is transected, the soma of the neuron may show the **axonal reaction.** Normally, Nissl bodies stain well with basic aniline dyes, which attach to the ribonucleic acid of the ribosomes (Figure 6-11, *A*). During the axonal

reaction, the cisterns of the rough endoplasmic reticulum become distended with the products of protein synthesis. The ribosomes become disorganized; thus the Nissl bodies are stained weakly by basic aniline dyes. This alteration in staining is termed **chromatolysis** (Figure 6-11, *C* and *D*). The soma may also become swollen and rounded, and the nucleus may assume an eccentric position in the cytoplasm. These morphological changes reflect the cytological processes that accompany protein synthesis. The damaged neuron is repairing itself.

Wallerian degeneration is the response of an axon to its interruption

If a nerve fiber is cut, the axon distal to the transection dies (Figure 6-11, *B* and C). Within a few days the axon and all of the synaptic endings formed by the axon disintegrate. If the axon was myelinated, the myelin sheath becomes fragmented and is eventually phagocytized and removed. However, the Schwann cells that formed the myelin sheath remain viable. This sequence of events was originally described by Waller and is thus called **wallerian degeneration.**

If the axons that provide the sole or predominant synaptic input to a neuron or an effector cell are interrupted, the postsynaptic cell may undergo degeneration and even death. The best known example of this is the atrophy of skeletal muscle fibers after their innervation by motor neurons is interrupted.

In neuroanatomical investigations, these pathological changes have been useful for tracing neural pathways. For example, retrograde chromatolysis has been used to reveal groups of neurons whose axons have been deliberately interrupted. The projection target of axons can be determined by following the course of interrupted axons undergoing wallerian degeneration. Synaptic targets can also be mapped if neurons undergo **transneuronal degeneration** after an axon bundle is transected.

Regeneration can occur in the peripheral nervous system but is unsatisfactory in the central nervous system

Many neurons can regenerate a new axon if the axon is lost through injury. The proximal stump of the damaged axon develops sprouts (Figure 6-11, *C*). In the PNS, these sprouts elongate and grow along the path of the original nerve if this route is available. The Schwann cells in the distal stump of the nerve not only survive the wallerian degeneration but also proliferate and form rows along the course previously taken by the axons. Growth cones of the sprouting axons find their way along the rows of Schwann cells and may eventually reinnervate the original peripheral target structures (Figure 6-11, *D* and *E*). The Schwann cells then remyelinate the axons. The rate of regeneration is limited by the rate of slow axonal transport to about 1 mm/day.

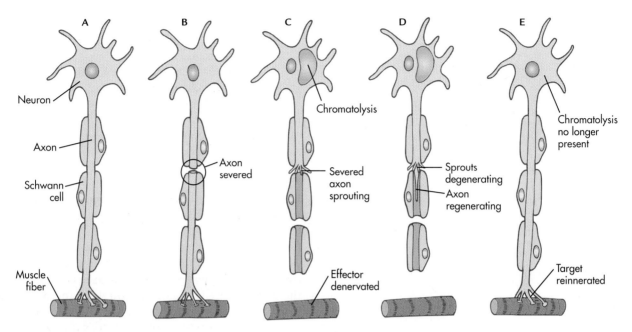

Figure 6-11 A, Normal motor neuron innervating a skeletal muscle fiber. **B,** The motor axon has been severed, and the motor neuron is beginning to undergo chromatolysis. **C,** The chromatolysis is associated eventually with sprouting. **D,** It is also associated with regeneration of the axon. The excess sprouts degenerate. **E,** When the target cell is reinnervated, chromatolysis is no longer present. *(Redrawn from Willis WD Jr, Grossman RG: Medical neurobiology: neuroanatomical and neurophysiological principles basic to clinical neuroscience, ed 3, St Louis, 1981, Mosby.)*

Nerve growth factor and other growth factors play an important role in the growth of sensory and autonomic axons in peripheral nerves during development, in their maintenance, and in their regeneration after injury.

Transection of axons in the CNS also results in wallerian degeneration followed by sprouting. Proper guidance for the sprouts is generally lacking, however, because the oligodendroglia do not form a path along which the sprouts can grow. Oligodendroglia do not form this path because a single oligodendroglial cell myelinates many central axons, whereas a given Schwann cell provides myelin for only a single axon in the PNS. Alternatively, different chemical signals, such as different growth factors or growth-inhibiting factors, may affect the peripheral and central attempts at regeneration differently. Another obstacle is the formation of glial scars by astrocytes.

SUMMARY

- The general functions of the nervous system include sensory detection, information processing, and behavior.
- The functional cellular unit of the nervous system is the neuron.
- Nervous tissue contains not only neurons but also supporting cells or neuroglia (Schwann cells in the PNS; astrocytes, oligodendroglia, microglia, and ependymal cells in the CNS) and blood vessels.
- The nervous system is subdivided into the PNS (sensory, somatic motor, and autonomic neurons) and the CNS (spinal cord and brain).

- The extracellular environment of neurons in the CNS is highly regulated. CSF is secreted by the choroid plexuses. The blood-brain barrier restricts the entry of substances into the brain.
- The parts of neurons include the cell body, dendrites, and axon. Axons may be myelinated or unmyelinated.
- Information is conducted along axons by nerve impulses, whose conduction velocity depends on the presence or absence of myelin and the diameter of the axon. The largest myelinated axons have the fastest conduction velocities.
- Several coding mechanisms are used by neurons to convey information in neural networks. These include labeled lines, spatial maps, and patterns of nerve impulses.
- Information is transmitted from neuron to neuron or from neuron to effector organ by means of synaptic transmission.
- Materials are moved along axons by axonal transport. The movements can be rapid or slow and away from or toward the cell body.
- Neurons respond to damage either by cell death or by less drastic changes, such as the axonal reaction (chromatolysis) and wallerian degeneration. Viable axons may subsequently regenerate.

BIBLIOGRAPHY

Brodal P: *The central nervous system: structure and function,* New York, 1992, Oxford University Press.

Cajal SR: *Degeneration and regeneration of the nervous system,* New York, 1959, Hafner.

Cajal SR: *Histology of the nervous system,* New York, 1995, Oxford University Press.

Gehrmann J, Matsumoto Y, Kreutzberg GW: Microglia: intrinsic immuneffector cell of the brain, *Brain Res Rev* 20:269, 1995.

Graham DI, Lantos PL, eds: *Greenfield's neuropathology,* London, 1997, Arnold.

Ip NY, Yancopoulos GD: The neurotrophins and CNTF: two families of collaborative neurotrophic factors, *Annu Rev Neurosci* 19:491, 1996.

Kettenmann H, Ranson BR, eds: *Neuroglia,* New York, 1995, Oxford University Press.

Nicholls JG, Martin AR, Wallace BG: *From neuron to brain,* ed 3, Sunderland, Mass, 1992, Sinauer Associates.

Peters A, Palay SL, Webster H deF: *The fine structure of the nervous system,* ed 3, New York, 1991, Oxford University Press.

Willis WD Jr, Grossman RG, *Medical neurobiology: neuroanatomical and neurophysiological principles basic to clinical neuroscience,* ed 3, St Louis, 1981, Mosby.

▷ **CASE STUDIES**

Case 6-1

A 59-year-old man became depressed over several years after a business failure. He became confused and had memory lapses. His family was concerned that he might be developing Alzheimer's disease. He experienced progressively greater difficulty in walking. On examination, he did not know the date and had difficulty with mental arithmetic. His gait was unsteady, and he tended to fall. He had signs of interruption of the voluntary motor pathways. The results of blood chemical analysis were normal. However, in the CSF the protein level was elevated, and the white blood cell count was high, but the glucose level was low. A magnetic resonance scan showed a massively dilated ventricular system. A microbe screening demonstrated the presence of cryptococci in the CSF.

1. **What is the most likely reason for the patient's changed mental state and motor difficulties?**
   A. Alzheimer's disease
   B. Brain tumor
   C. Encephalitis
   D. Hydrocephalus
   E. Hypoglycemia

2. **If all of the ventricles are dilated, where is the most likely site of the obstruction?**
   A. Arachnoid villi
   B. Cerebral aqueduct
   C. Interventricular foramen
   D. Roof of the fourth ventricle
   E. Third ventricle

Case 6-2

An 18-year-old woman was well until 3 years ago, when she suddenly lost sight in her right eye. Her vision then gradually improved. Then 2 years ago, she developed a hearing loss in her right ear lasting 3 weeks. A month later, she experienced numbness and tingling in her right leg, which improved over 2 weeks. A neurological examination revealed no significant abnormalities. However, 2 months later, she developed blurred vision and on examination, had weakness of adduction of the left eye and nystagmus. Some 6 months ago she became weak in the left leg. Currently, she is experiencing normal eye movements but a left-sided weakness, a left-sided facial weakness, and hyperactive phasic stretch reflexes in the left arm and leg; Babinski's sign was elicited on the left. The results of blood and spinal fluid chemical analysis were normal.

1. **Which nervous system cell type is most likely to be affected in this patient?**
   A. Astrocyte
   B. Motor neuron
   C. Oligodendroglial cell
   D. Pyramidal cell
   E. Schwann cell

2. **What is the basic defect caused by disrupted function of this cell type?**
   A. Abnormal axonal transport
   B. Blockade or slowed conduction velocity of axons
   C. Chromatolysis
   D. Failure of synaptic transmission
   E. Wallerian degeneration

CHAPTER 7

General Sensory System

OBJECTIVES

- Describe the basic principles of sensory physiology.
- Discuss the organization of the somatovisceral sensory system.
- Describe how pathways that descend from the brain can modulate sensory transmission.

The nervous system can be regarded as a complex of several subsystems with different functional roles. These subsystems interact, however, and their activity leads to unified behavior. Some neural subsystems are concerned with sensory function. This chapter considers the general sensory system, or **somatovisceral sensory system,** which analyzes sensory events relating to the mechanical, thermal, or chemical stimulation of the body and face. Chapter 8 describes the special sensory systems.

The somatovisceral sensory system involves **sensory receptors,** which respond to various stimuli via a process of **sensory transduction.** The sensory receptors then provide sensory information about these stimuli to the central nervous system (CNS). Sensory information is encoded in various ways, and this encoded information is then transmitted through sensory pathways that ascend in the spinal cord white matter to brain areas that process the information in ways that eventually lead to sensory perception. One of these ascending pathways is known as the **dorsal column–medial lemniscus** pathway. This pathway is largely responsible for the sensations of flutter-vibration and touch-pressure, as well as for proprioception. Another pathway is the **spinothalamic tract,** which is largely responsible for pain and temperature sensations. Components of the **trigeminothalamic tract** have similar roles in mediating sensations arising from the face and oral, nasal, and cranial cavities. Neural pathways also descend from the brain to control transmission in the ascending somatosensory pathways. The **endogenous analgesia system** is an example of this type of pathway.

Principles of Sensory Physiology

Transduction allows sensory receptors to respond to stimuli

Useful features of environmental events are detected by **sensory receptors,** which then provide information about the events to the CNS. The interaction of an environmental event with a sensory receptor is called a **stimulus.** The effect of the stimulus on the sensory receptor may lead to neural activity, a **response.** The process that enables a sensory receptor to respond usefully to a stimulus is called **sensory transduction.**

ENVIRONMENTAL EVENTS THAT LEAD TO SENSORY TRANSDUCTION CAN INVOLVE MECHANICAL, THERMAL, CHEMICAL, AND OTHER FORMS OF ENERGY, DEPENDING ON THE SENSORY APPARATUS. Although humans cannot sense electrical or magnetic fields, other animals, such as fish, can respond to such stimuli.

The manner in which sensory transduction is accomplished varies with the receptor type. For example, a **chemoreceptor** may respond when a molecule of a chemical stimulant reacts with a receptor molecule in the surface membrane of the chemoreceptor. The reaction may open an ion channel and induce the influx of ionic current. On the other hand, mechanically sensitive ion channels in the surface membrane of a **mechanoreceptor** are opened in response to the application of a mechanical force along the membrane. Ion channels in the outer segment of a **photoreceptor** are open in the dark but closed when photons are absorbed by pigment on the disc membrane. The signal for closure of the ion channels in photoreceptors is transmitted by second messenger molecules. Thus the details of sensory transduction vary with receptor type, but often, transduction depends on changes in ionic current through ion channels in response to the activation of receptor molecules. Receptor molecules and ion channels are sometimes directly coupled, but in other cases, they are coupled indirectly through second messenger cascades.

Sensory transduction generally induces a **receptor potential** in the peripheral terminal of a primary afferent sensory neuron. A receptor potential is usually a depolarizing event that results from inward current flow, and it brings the membrane potential of the sensory receptor toward or past the threshold needed to trigger a nerve impulse. For example, in Figure 7-1, *A,* a mechanical stimulus distorts

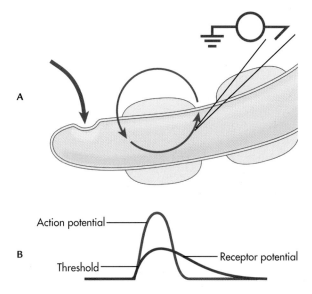

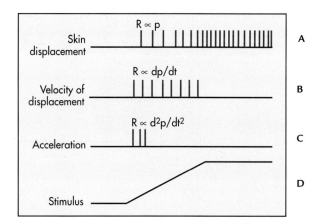

Figure 7-1 A, The terminal region of a myelinated mechanoreceptor afferent fiber is shown as if cut in longitudinal section. The surface membrane is indicated by a light yellow line, the axoplasm by the orange area, and the myelin internodes by the light blue areas. The current flow produced by stimulation of the mechanoreceptor at the site indicated by the large arrow is shown by the smaller arrows. The tip of an intracellular microelectrode has been placed in the axon, as indicated. **B,** The receptor potential produced by the current *(red line)* and an action potential that may be triggered by the receptor potential if the latter exceeds threshold *(blue line)* are shown.

Figure 7-2 Responses of slowly and rapidly adapting mechanoreceptors to displacement of the skin. The discharges of the primary afferent fibers supplying the receptors in response to the ramp and hold stimulus **(D)** are termed the responses *(R)*. **A,** *R* is proportional to skin position *(p)*. The receptor is slowly adapting and signals skin displacement. **B,** *R* is a function of the velocity of displacement *(dp/dt)*. **C,** *R* is a function of acceleration *(d²p/dt²)*. The receptors in **B** and **C** are rapidly adapting, but they signal different dynamic features of the stimulus.

the ending of a mechanoreceptor and causes inward current flow at the terminal and longitudinal and outward current flow along the axon. The outward current produces a depolarization, the receptor potential, which may exceed threshold for an action potential. In this case the action potential is generated at a trigger zone in the first node of Ranvier of the afferent fiber. However, in photoreceptors the cessation of inward current flow during phototransduction leads to a hyperpolarization of the receptor.

In some sensory receptor organs, the peripheral terminal of a primary afferent fiber contacts a separate, peripherally located sensory cell. For example, in the cochlea, primary afferent fibers contact hair cells. Sensory transduction in such sense organs is made more complex by this arrangement. In the cochlea a receptor potential is produced in the hair cells in response to sound. The receptor potential is a depolarization of the hair cell's membrane, and the depolarization liberates an excitatory neurotransmitter onto the primary afferent terminal. The resulting inward current depolarizes the primary afferent fiber terminal and produces a **generator potential.** This depolarization brings the membrane potential of the primary afferent fiber toward or beyond threshold for firing nerve impulses.

Sensory receptors have the property of **adaptation** to maintained stimuli. A long-lasting stimulus may produce a prolonged repetitive discharge, or it may result in a short response (one or a few discharges) depending on whether the sensory receptor is slowly or rapidly adapting. The ad-

aptation rates differ because a prolonged stimulus may produce either a maintained or a transient receptor potential in the sensory receptor. The functional implication of the adaptation rate is that different temporal features of a stimulus can be analyzed by receptors that have different adaptation rates. For example, during an indentation of the skin, a slowly adapting receptor may respond repetitively at a rate proportional to the amount of indentation (Figure 7-2, *A*). Such a response can signal skin position. On the other hand, rapidly adapting receptors in the skin respond best to transient mechanical stimuli. The information signaled may reflect stimulus velocity (Figure 7-2, *B*) or acceleration (Figure 7-2, *C*) rather than the amount of skin indentation.

The stimulation of receptive fields affects the discharges of sensory neurons

The relationship between the location of a stimulus and the activation of particular sensory neurons is a major theme in sensory physiology. The **receptive field** of a sensory neuron is the region that when stimulated, affects the discharge of the neuron. For example, a sensory receptor might be activated by the indentation of only a small area of skin. That area is the **excitatory receptive field** of the sensory receptor. A sensory neuron in the CNS might be excited by the stimulation of a receptive field several times as large as that of a primary afferent neuron. The receptive fields of sensory neurons in the CNS are typically larger than the receptive fields of sensory receptors because the central neurons receive information from many

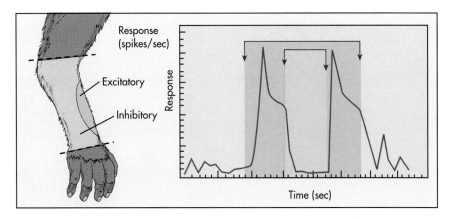

Figure 7-3 Excitatory and inhibitory receptive fields of a central somatosensory neuron located in the primary somatosensory cerebral cortex. The excitatory receptive field is on the forearm and is surrounded by an inhibitory receptive field. The graph shows the response to an excitatory stimulus and the inhibition of that response by a stimulus applied in the inhibitory field.

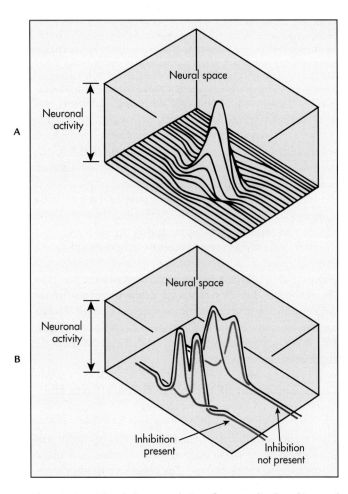

Figure 7-4 Activity of a large population of neurons distributed in neural space (e.g., in the cerebral cortex). **A,** The activity of the neurons in response to a stimulus applied to a single point on the skin is plotted on the vertical axis. Note that an excitatory peak is surrounded by an inhibitory trough; these are determined by the excitatory and inhibitory receptive fields of sensory neurons in the central somatosensory pathways. **B,** Neural activity in response to the stimulation of two adjacent points on the skin. Note that the sum of the activity *(black line)* is separated better into two peaks when inhibition is present than when it is not.

sensory receptors, each with a slightly different receptive field. The location of the receptive field is determined by the location of the sensory-transduction apparatus responsible for signaling information about the stimulus to the sensory neurons.

Generally, the receptive fields of sensory receptors are excitatory. However, a sensory neuron in the CNS can have either an excitatory or an **inhibitory receptive field** (Figure 7-3). Inhibition results from data processing in sensory neural circuits and is mediated by inhibitory interneurons.

Sensory coding depends on nerve impulses in sensory neurons

Sensory neurons encode stimuli. In the process of sensory transduction, one or more aspects of the stimulus must be encoded in a way that can be interpreted by the CNS. The **encoded information** is an abstraction based on the responses of sensory receptors to the stimulus and on information processing within the sensory pathway. SOME OF THE ASPECTS OF STIMULI THAT ARE ENCODED INCLUDE MODALITY, SPATIAL LOCATION, THRESHOLD, INTENSITY, FREQUENCY, AND DURATION. Other aspects encoded are presented in reference to particular sensory systems (see Chapter 8).

A **sensory modality** is a readily identified class of sensation. For example, maintained mechanical stimuli applied to the skin result in a sensation of **touch-pressure,** and transient mechanical stimuli may evoke a sensation of **flutter-vibration.** Other cutaneous modalities include **cold, warm,** and **pain. Vision, audition, position sense, taste,** and **smell** are examples of noncutaneous modalities. In most sensory systems the encoding of sensory modality is by labeled-line sensory channels (see Chapter 6). A **labeled-line sensory channel** consists of a set of neurons devoted to a particular sensory modality.

Stimulus location is often signaled by the activation of the particular population of sensory neurons whose receptive fields are affected by the stimulus (Figure 7-4, *A*). In some cases an inhibitory receptive field or a contrasting

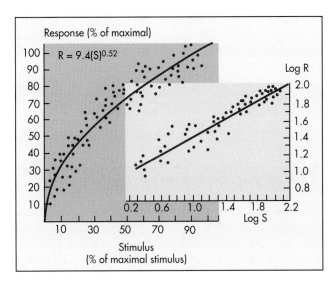

Figure 7-5 Stimulus-response function for a slowly adapting mechanoreceptor. The rate of discharge is plotted against stimulus strength (normalized to maximal). The plots are on linear and on log-log scales. The stimulus-response function is response $(R) = 9.4(S)^{0.52}$.

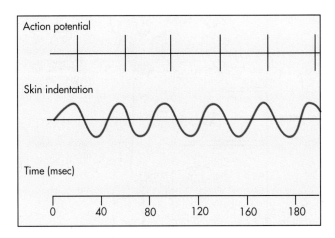

Figure 7-6 Coding for the frequency of stimulation: discharge of a rapidly adapting cutaneous mechanoreceptor in phase with a sinusoidal stimulus. *Top,* Action potential. *Center,* Stimulus. *Bottom,* Time in milliseconds.

border between an excitatory and an inhibitory receptive field can have localizing value. The resolution of two different adjacent stimuli may depend on the excitation of partially separated populations of neurons and also on inhibitory interactions (Figure 7-4, *B*).

A **threshold stimulus** is the weakest that can be detected. To be detected, a stimulus must produce receptor potentials large enough to activate one or more primary afferent fibers. Weaker intensities of stimulation can produce subthreshold receptor potentials; however, such stimuli would not excite central sensory neurons. Furthermore, the number of primary afferent fibers that need to be excited for sensory detection depends on the requirements for spatial and temporal summation in the sensory pathway (see Chapter 4). Thus a stimulus at threshold for detection may be much greater than threshold for activation of the most responsive primary afferent fibers. Conversely, a stimulus that excites some primary afferent fibers may not lead to perception of that stimulus.

Stimulus intensity may be encoded by the mean frequency of the discharge of sensory neurons. The relationship between stimulus intensity and response can be plotted as a stimulus-response function. For many sensory neurons, the stimulus-response function approximates an exponential curve (Figure 7-5). The general equation for such a curve follows:

$$\text{Response} = \text{Stimulus}^n \times \text{Constant}$$

The exponent, *n*, can be less than, equal to, or greater than 1. Many mechanoreceptors have stimulus-response functions with fractional exponents (Figure 7-5). Thermoreceptors have linear stimulus-response curves. Nociceptors may have linear or positively accelerating stimulus-response functions; that is, the exponent for these curves is 1 or more.

Another way in which stimulus intensity is encoded is by the number of sensory receptors activated. A stimulus that is threshold for perception may activate just one or a few primary afferent fibers, whereas a strong stimulus may excite many similar receptors. Central neurons that receive input from a particular class of sensory receptors would be more powerfully activated as more primary afferents are caused to discharge, and a greater activity in central sensory neurons will result in the perception of a stronger stimulus.

Stimuli of different intensities may activate different sets of receptors. For example, a weak mechanical stimulus applied to the skin might activate only mechanoreceptors, whereas a strong mechanical stimulus might activate both mechanoreceptors and nociceptors. In this case the sensation evoked by the stronger stimulus would be more intense, and the quality would be different.

Stimulus frequency can be encoded by the intervals between the discharges of sensory neurons. Sometimes the interspike intervals correspond exactly to the intervals between stimuli (Figure 7-6), but in other cases a given neuron may discharge at intervals that are multiples of the interstimulus interval.

Stimulus duration may be encoded in slowly adapting sensory neurons by the duration of the enhanced firing. In rapidly adapting neurons, the beginning and end of a stimulus may be signaled by transient discharges.

Sensory pathways conduct sensory information to sensory-processing areas of the brain

A **sensory pathway** can be viewed as a set of neurons arranged in series (Figure 7-7). First-, second-, third-, and higher-order neurons serve as sequential elements in a par-

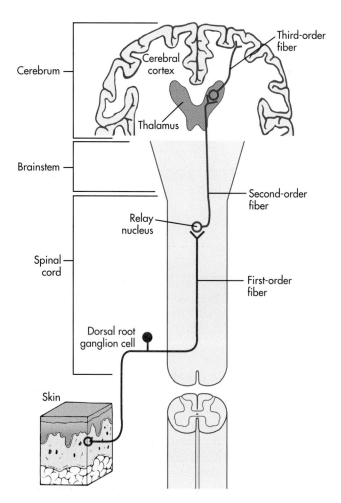

Figure 7-7 General arrangement of sensory pathways showing first-, second-, and third-order neurons. Note that the axon of the second-order neuron crosses the midline, so sensory information from one side of the body is transmitted to the opposite side of the brain.

ticular sensory pathway. However, several parallel sensory pathways often transmit similar sensory information.

The **first-order neuron** in a sensory pathway is the primary afferent neuron. The peripheral endings of this neuron form a sensory receptor (or receive input from an accessory sensory cell, such as a hair cell), and thus the neuron responds to a stimulus and transmits encoded information to the CNS. The primary afferent neuron often has its soma in a dorsal root or cranial nerve ganglion.

The **second-order neuron** is likely to be located in the spinal cord or brainstem. It receives information from first-order neurons and transmits information to the thalamus. The information may be transformed at the level of the second-order neuron by local neural processing circuits. The ascending axons of second-order neurons typically cross the midline; thus sensory information that originates on one side of the body reaches the contralateral thalamus.

The **third-order neuron** is generally located in a sensory nucleus of the thalamus. Again, local circuits may transform information from second-order neurons before the signals are transmitted to the cerebral cortex.

Fourth-order neurons in the appropriate sensory-receiving areas of the cerebral cortex and **higher-order neurons** in the same and in other cerebral cortical areas process the information further. There may also be interactions between the cerebral cortex and subcortical structures, such as the basal ganglia and cerebellum. At some undetermined site the sensory information results in sensory perception, which is a conscious awareness of the stimulus.

Somatovisceral Sensory System

The somatovisceral sensory system includes primary afferent neurons that form sensory receptor organs in the skin, muscle, joints, and viscera. Information arising from these sensory receptors reaches the CNS by way of the axons of the first-order sensory neurons. The cell bodies of the primary afferent neurons are generally in dorsal root or cranial nerve ganglia. Each ganglion cell gives off a branch or **neurite** that bifurcates into a peripheral process and a central process. The peripheral process has the structure of an axon and terminates peripherally as a sensory receptor. The central process is also an axon and enters the spinal cord through a dorsal root or the brainstem through a cranial nerve. The central process typically gives rise to numerous collateral branches that end synaptically on several second-order neurons.

The processing of somatovisceral sensory information involves a number of CNS structures, including the spinal cord, brainstem, thalamus, and cerebral cortex. The ascending pathways arise from second-order sensory neurons that are located in the spinal cord and brainstem and that generally project to the contralateral thalamus. The most important ascending somatovisceral pathways that carry information from the body are the **dorsal column–medial lemniscus pathway** and the **spinothalamic tract.** The main somatovisceral projection that represents the face is the trigeminothalamic tract. The organization of these pathways is described in the following sections. Ancillary somatovisceral pathways include the spinocervicothalamic pathway, the postsynaptic dorsal column pathway, the dorsal spinocerebellar tract, the spinoreticular tract, and the spinomesencephalic tract.

The somatovisceral sensory system can be regarded as a general sensory system. The sensory modalities mediated by the somatovisceral sensory system include touch-pressure, flutter-vibration, position sense, joint movement, thermal sense, pain, and visceral distention.

Sensory receptors detect stimuli

The somatovisceral sensory system includes various types of sensory receptors in the skin, muscles, joints, and viscera. **Cutaneous receptors** can be subdivided according to the type of stimulus to which they respond. The major

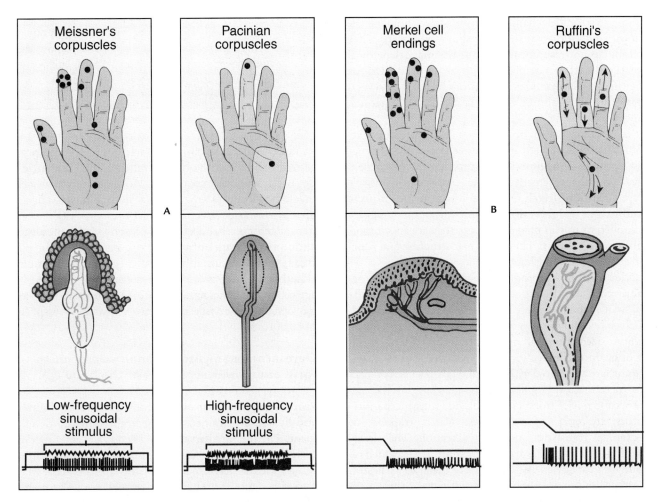

Figure 7-8 The receptive fields of several types of cutaneous mechanoreceptors are shown in the top row. Many more receptors are present than are indicated. Their density is greater on the more distal parts of the fingers. Red dots indicate the centers of the receptive fields, and yellow shading indicates the extent of the receptive fields. **A,** Rapidly adapting mechanoreceptors: Meissner's corpuscles and pacinian corpuscles. **B,** Slowly adapting mechanoreceptors: Merkel cell endings and Ruffini's corpuscles. The red arrows on the receptive fields of Ruffini's corpuscles show the directions of skin stretch that activated the afferent fibers. The second row of drawings shows the morphological structures of the receptors; the third row shows the responses to sinusoidal stimuli **(A)** or to step indentations of the skin **(B).**

types of cutaneous receptors include mechanoreceptors, thermoreceptors, and nociceptors. **Mechanoreceptors** respond to mechanical stimuli such as stroking or indenting the skin and can be rapidly or slowly adapting. Rapidly adapting cutaneous mechanoreceptors include **hair follicle receptors** in the hairy skin, **Meissner's corpuscles** in the nonhairy (glabrous) skin, and **pacinian corpuscles** in subcutaneous tissue (Figure 7-8, *A*). Hair follicle receptors and Meissner's corpuscles respond best to stimuli repeated at rates of about 30 to 40 Hz, and they contribute to the sensation of flutter. In contrast, pacinian corpuscles prefer stimuli repeated at approximately 250 Hz. They are responsible for vibratory sensation. Slowly adapting cutaneous mechanoreceptors include **Merkel cell endings** and **Ruffini's corpuscles** (Figure 7-8, *B*). Merkel cell endings have punctate receptive fields, whereas Ruffini's corpuscles have large receptive fields and can be activated by stretching or indenting the skin. Merkel cell endings contribute to touch-pressure sensation. Ruffini's corpuscles probably contribute both to touch-pressure sensation and to posi-

tion sense, at least with respect to distal joints such as those in the fingers. The axons of all of these receptor types are myelinated, so they conduct relatively rapidly, which permits signals transmitted from these receptors to be perceived soon after the stimulus occurs.

The two types of **thermoreceptors** in the skin are **cold receptors** and **warm receptors.** Both are slowly adapting, although they also discharge phasically when skin temperature rapidly changes. These are among the few receptor types that discharge spontaneously under normal circumstances. Cold receptors are supplied by small myelinated axons, whereas warm receptors are supplied by unmyelinated axons.

Nociceptors respond to stimuli that threaten to produce damage or actually do so. There are two major classes of cutaneous nociceptors: the **A-δ mechanical nociceptors** and **the C polymodal nociceptors.** A-δ mechanical nociceptors are supplied by finely myelinated (or A-δ) axons, whereas C polymodal nociceptors are supplied by unmyelinated (or C) fibers. The A-δ mechanical nociceptors respond to strong mechanical stimuli, such as pricking the skin with a needle or crushing the skin with forceps. They typically do not respond to noxious thermal or chemical stimuli unless they have previously been sensitized. On the other hand, C polymodal nociceptors respond to several types of noxious stimuli, including mechanical, thermal, and chemical.

Skeletal muscle also contains several types of sensory receptors. These are chiefly mechanoreceptors and nociceptors, although some muscle receptors possess thermosensitivity or chemosensitivity. The best-studied muscle receptors are the stretch receptors, which include **muscle spindles** and **Golgi tendon organs.** Although these play an important role in proprioception, they are also important in motor control. Therefore their structure and function are discussed in Chapter 9.

Other sensory receptors in muscle include nociceptors that respond to pressure applied to the muscle and to the release of metabolites, especially during **ischemia** (inadequate blood flow). Muscle nociceptors are supplied by medium-sized and small myelinated (group II and III) axons or by unmyelinated (group IV) afferent fibers.

Joints are associated with several types of sensory receptors, including rapidly and slowly adapting mechanoreceptors and nociceptors. The rapidly adapting mechanoreceptors are pacinian corpuscles, which respond to mechanical transients, including vibration. The slowly adapting joint receptors are Ruffini's corpuscles, which respond best to movements of a joint to extremes of flexion or extension; these endings signal pressure or torque applied to the joint. Joint mechanoreceptors are innervated by medium-sized (group II) afferent fibers. Joint nociceptors are activated by probing of a joint capsule or by hyperextension or hyperflexion, although many articular nociceptors fail to respond to joint movements under normal conditions. If sensitized by inflammation, however, they can respond to innocuous stimuli, such as movements or weak pressure. Joint nociceptors are innervated by finely myelinated (group III) or unmyelinated (group IV) primary afferent fibers.

Arthritis is a common painful condition caused by inflammation of one or more joints. The nociceptors become sensitized by the release of a number of chemical substances from nerve endings, mast cells, and blood elements. These substances include neuropeptides (substance P, calcitonin gene–related peptide), histamine, bradykinin, serotonin, and prostaglandins. The sensitized nerve endings cause the joint to develop **hyperalgesia,** a condition in which the threshold for pain is lowered and the amount of pain produced by a given stimulus is increased. The joint also becomes swollen. This is caused by **neurogenic edema,** which is the collection of edema fluid that follows an increase in capillary permeability caused by the release of neuropeptides from joint nociceptors. These peptides also cause **vasodilation,** which increases the temperature of the joint. Arthritic pain is often treated successfully with substances that block the synthesis of prostaglandins, such as acetylsalicylic acid.

Viscera are also supplied with sensory receptors. Most of these are involved in reflexes and have little to do with sensory experience. However, some visceral mechanoreceptors are responsible for the sensation of distention, and visceral nociceptors produce visceral pain. Pacinian corpuscles are present in the mesentery and in the capsules of visceral organs, such as the pancreas; these presumably signal mechanical transients. Whether some forms of visceral pain result from overactivity of the mechanoreceptor afferents is still controversial. Some viscera, however, clearly have specific nociceptors.

Dermatomes, myotomes, and sclerotomes form embryonic segments of the body

Primary afferent fibers in the adult are distributed systematically, as determined during embryological development. The mammalian embryo becomes segmented, and each body segment is called a **somite.** A somite is innervated by an adjacent segment of the spinal cord or in the case of a somite of the head, by a cranial nerve. The portion of a somite destined to form skin is called a **dermatome.** Similarly, the part of a somite that forms muscle is a **myotome,** and the part that forms bone, a **sclerotome.** Viscera are also supplied by particular segments of the spinal cord or particular cranial nerves.

Many dermatomes become distorted during development, chiefly because of the way the upper and lower extremities are formed and because humans maintain an upright posture. However, the sequence of dermatomes can be understood if pictured on the body in a quadrupedal position (Figure 7-9).

Although a dermatome receives its densest innervation from the corresponding spinal cord segment, it is also innervated by several adjacent spinal segments. Thus transection of a dorsal root produces little sensory loss in the corresponding dermatome. Anesthesia of any given dermatome requires interruption of several successive dorsal roots.

Spinal roots and the spinal cord contribute to sensory pathways

Axons of the peripheral nervous system enter or leave the CNS through the spinal roots (or through cranial nerves). The dorsal root on one side of a given spinal segment is composed entirely of the central processes of **dorsal root**

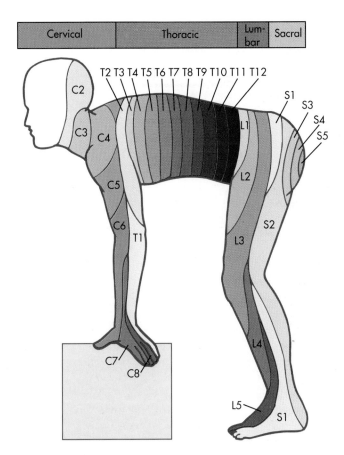

Figure 7-9 Dermatomes represented on a drawing of a person assuming a quadrupedal position.

ganglion cells. The **ventral root** consists chiefly of motor axons, including α-motor axons, γ-motor axons, and at certain segmental levels, autonomic preganglionic axons. Ventral roots also contain many primary afferent fibers, whose role is still unclear.

The spinal cord can be subdivided into gray matter and white matter (Figure 7-10). The gray matter includes the cell bodies and dendrites of the intrinsic neurons of the spinal cord. There, synaptic connections are made by primary afferent fibers and by pathways descending from the brain. The **gray matter** is subdivided into the **dorsal horn,** the **intermediate region,** and the **ventral horn.** The neurons of the gray matter form layers, or **laminae.**

The gray matter of the spinal cord is surrounded by **white matter** (Figure 7-10). The white matter between the dorsal midline of the spinal cord and the entry line of the dorsal roots is called the **dorsal funiculus.** The white matter between the dorsal root entry line and the ventral root is the **lateral funiculus.** The white matter found between the ventral root exit line and the ventral midline is the **ventral funiculus.** The **dorsolateral fasciculus** is a zone of fine nerve fibers that caps the dorsal horn. The white matter contains axons that belong to primary afferent fibers, spinal cord interneurons, and long ascending and descending pathways that connect the spinal cord and brain.

The trigeminal nerve transmits sensory information from the face and cranial cavities

The arrangement for primary afferent fibers that supply the face is comparable to that for fibers supplying the body. Peripheral processes of neurons in the **trigeminal ganglion** pass through the ophthalmic, maxillary, and mandibular divisions of the trigeminal nerve to innervate dermatome-like regions of the face (Figure 7-11, *A*). The trigeminal nerve also innervates the oral and nasal cavities and the dura mater.

The large myelinated fibers that supply the mechanoreceptors of the skin and structures of the oral and nasal cavities synapse in the **principal sensory nucleus** of the trigeminal nerve (Figure 7-11, *B*). Small myelinated and unmyelinated primary afferent fibers of the trigeminal nerve terminate in the nerve's **spinal nucleus** (Figure 7-11, *C*). Primary afferent fibers from stretch receptors have their cell bodies in the **mesencephalic nucleus** of the trigeminal nerve (Figure 7-11, *D*). This arrangement is exceptional because all other primary afferent cell bodies in the somatovisceral system are in peripheral ganglia. The central processes synapse in the **motor nucleus** of the trigeminal nerve.

The dorsal column–medial lemniscus pathway includes the fasciculus gracilis and fasciculus cuneatus

The ascending branches of many large myelinated nerve fibers travel rostrally in the dorsal column to the medulla (see a standard textbook of neuroanatomy). The dorsal column can be subdivided into two smaller components, the **fasciculus gracilis** and the **fasciculus cuneatus.** Axons that innervate sensory receptors of the lower extremity and the lower trunk (T7 segment and caudally) ascend in the gracile fasciculus, whereas fibers from receptors of the upper extremity and upper trunk ascend in the cuneate fasciculus (T6 segment and rostrally). These axons are the first-order neurons of the dorsal column–medial lemniscus pathway. The second-order neurons are in the nucleus gracilis and nucleus cuneatus, which are collections of neurons in the caudal medulla. These nuclei are often called collectively the **dorsal column nuclei.** Axons of the fasciculus gracilis synapse in the nucleus gracilis, and axons of the fasciculus cuneatus synapse in the nucleus cuneatus.

Many neurons in the dorsal column nuclei respond in much the same way as the primary afferent fibers that synapse on them. Some behave like rapidly adapting receptors, responding to hair movement or to mechanical transients applied to the glabrous skin. Others discharge at high frequencies when vibratory stimuli are applied to their receptive fields and thus resemble pacinian corpuscles. Still other neurons in the dorsal column nuclei have slowly adapting responses to cutaneous stimuli. In

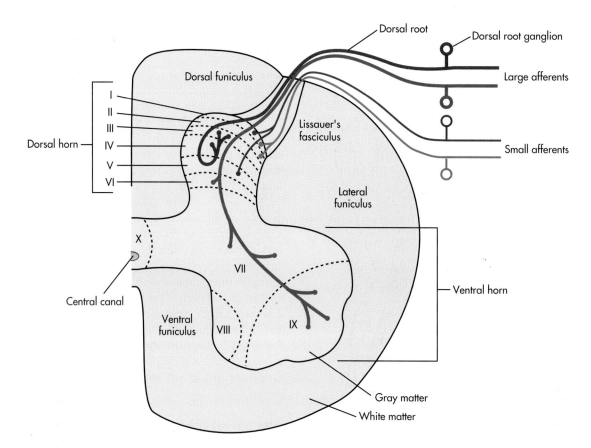

Figure 7-10 Distribution of large and small primary afferent fibers in the spinal cord. An outline of the gray matter on one side of the spinal cord and the boundaries between the laminae is shown. Laminae I to VI form the dorsal horn; parts of laminae VI and VII make up the intermediate region; and part of lamina VII, plus laminae VIII and IX, form the ventral horn; lamina X is the gray matter surrounding the central canal. Terminals of two large primary afferent fibers are shown. One, from a hair follicle receptor *(purple)*, synapses in laminae III to V. The other, from a muscle spindle *(blue)*, synapses in laminae VI, VII, and IX. Terminals from two fine afferent fibers are also shown. The small myelinated fiber (A-δ) from a cutaneous nociceptor *(red)* ends in laminae I and V, whereas the unmyelinated (C) afferent fiber *(green)* synapses in laminae I and II.

the cuneate nucleus, many neurons are activated by muscle stretch. The main differences between the responses of dorsal column neurons and those of the primary afferent fibers are that (1) dorsal column neurons have larger receptive fields because more than one primary afferent fiber synapses on a given dorsal column neuron, (2) they sometimes respond to more than one class of sensory receptors because of the convergence of several different types of primary afferent fibers on the second-order neurons, and (3) they often have inhibitory receptive fields mediated through interneuronal circuits in the dorsal column nuclei.

The dorsal column nuclei project to the contralateral thalamus by way of the **medial lemniscus.** The medial lemniscus terminates in the **ventral posterolateral (VPL) nucleus** of the thalamus. Neurons in the VPL nucleus in turn project to the **primary somatosensory (SI) cortex.**

Projections of trigeminal nuclei
As already mentioned, large myelinated primary afferent fibers that supply mechanoreceptors in the skin of the face synapse in the principal sensory nucleus of the trigeminal nerve. Second-order neurons in the principal

sensory nucleus project to the contralateral thalamus by way of the **trigeminothalamic tract** (Figure 7-11, *B*). Some neurons project ipsilaterally. The projections are to the **ventral posteromedial (VPM) thalamic nucleus.** Third-order neurons of the VPM nucleus project to the somatosensory cortex. This pathway of the trigeminal system is equivalent for the face to the dorsal column–medial lemniscus pathway for the body.

Other somatovisceral sensory pathways of the dorsal spinal cord
Three other pathways that carry somatovisceral sensory information ascend in the dorsal part of the spinal cord on the same side as the afferent input: the spinocervical tract, the postsynaptic dorsal column pathway, and the dorsal spinocerebellar tract.

The cells of origin of the **spinocervical tract** receive input largely from cutaneous mechanoreceptors, although some of these cells are also activated by cutaneous nociceptors. The cells of origin of the **postsynaptic dorsal column pathway** receive information similar to that reaching spinocervical tract neurons. In addition, some of these neurons are activated by nociceptors in

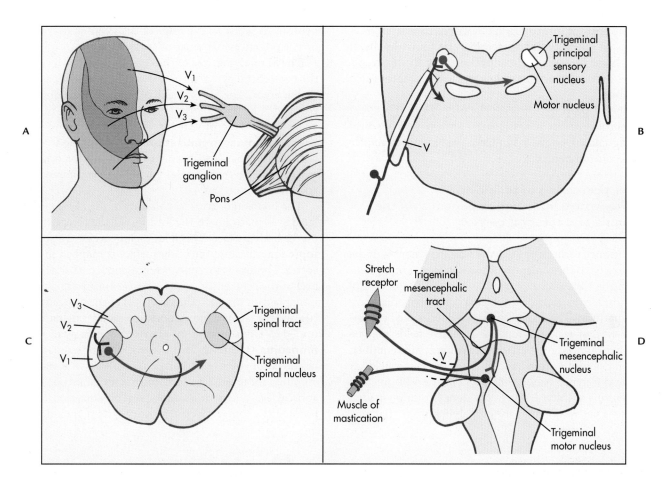

Figure 7-11 A, Dermatome-like areas of distribution of the ophthalmic *(V₁)*, maxillary *(V₂)*, and mandibular *(V₃)* divisions of the trigeminal nerve. **B,** Synaptic terminals of large myelinated primary afferent fibers of the trigeminal nerve in the main sensory nucleus and crossing of the trigeminothalamic tract. **C,** Descending branches of fine myelinated and unmyelinated primary afferent axons of the trigeminal nerve synapsing in the spinal nucleus and crossing in the trigeminothalamic tract. **D,** Location of cell bodies of primary afferent proprioceptive neurons of the trigeminal nerve in the mesencephalic nucleus. Synaptic connections of collaterals of these neurons are made with motor neurons in the trigeminal motor nucleus.

visceral organs. The information conveyed by these neurons is eventually conveyed to the VPL nucleus of the thalamus.

The **dorsal spinocerebellar tract** responds to input from muscle and joint receptors of the lower extremity. The main destination of the tract is the cerebellum, but it also provides proprioceptive information from the leg to the contralateral VPL nucleus of the thalamus after a relay in the medulla. Proprioceptive information from the arm is signaled by the dorsal column pathway.

Sensory functions of the dorsal spinal cord pathways

THE SENSORY QUALITIES MEDIATED BY THE ASCENDING PATHWAYS IN THE DORSAL PART OF THE SPINAL CORD INCLUDE FLUTTER-VIBRATION, TOUCH-PRESSURE, JOINT MOVEMENT, POSITION SENSE, AND VISCERAL DISTENTION. Each of these qualities of sensation depends on activity in a set of sensory neurons that collectively form a labeled-line sensory channel. A sensory channel may involve several parallel ascending pathways, and it includes particular afferent neurons and sensory-processing mechanisms at the levels of the spinal cord, brainstem, thalamus, and cerebrum.

Flutter-vibration is a complex sensation. **Flutter** refers to recognition of events that have low-frequency components. The sensory receptors that detect flutter include hair follicles and Meissner's corpuscles. Ascending sensory tracts that convey information needed for flutter sensation include the dorsal column–medial lemniscus pathway, the spinocervical tract, and the postsynaptic dorsal column pathway. High-frequency vibration is detected primarily by pacinian corpuscles. Branches of pacinian corpuscle afferents ascend in the dorsal column, and some postsynaptic dorsal column neurons respond to activation of pacinian corpuscles.

Touch-pressure sensation involves the recognition of skin indentation by Merkel cell endings and Ruffini's corpuscles. The ascending pathways that convey information from these receptors include the dorsal column–medial lemniscus and the postsynaptic dorsal column pathways.

Proprioception, the senses of joint movement and joint position, is complex and depends on sensory information that arises from muscle, joint, and cutaneous receptors. For some proximal joints, such as the knee, the most important information is derived from stretch receptors in the muscles that move the joint. In distal joints, however, such as those of the digits, Ruffini's corpuscles in the skin and nail beds and joint receptors also contribute.

Visceral pain depends on the activation of visceral nociceptors. It has recently been shown that visceral pain signals are conveyed in large part by postsynaptic dorsal column neurons.

Higher processing of tactile and proprioceptive information depends on the thalamus and cerebral cortex

As mentioned earlier, the medial lemniscus synapses in the VPL nucleus of the thalamus. The responses of many neurons in the VPL nucleus resemble those of the first- and second-order neurons of the dorsal column–medial lemniscus pathway. The responses may be dominated by a particular type of receptor, and the receptive fields may be small, although larger than that of a primary afferent fiber. Thalamic neurons often have inhibitory receptive fields. A notable difference between neurons in the VPL nucleus and neurons at lower levels of the dorsal column–medial lemniscus pathway is that the excitability of the thalamic

neurons depends on the stage of the sleep-wake cycle and on the presence or absence of anesthesia.

The SI receiving area of the cerebral cortex is located in the postcentral gyrus of the parietal lobe. Within any particular area of the SI cortex, all of the neurons along a line perpendicular to the cortical surface have similar response properties and receptive fields. The SI cortex is thus said to have a **columnar organization.** A comparable columnar organization has also been demonstrated for other primary sensory-receiving areas, including the primary visual and auditory cortices.

The location of cortical columns in the SI region is related systematically to the location of the receptive fields on the body surface. This relationship is called a **somatotopic map** because the body surface is mapped in the SI cortex. The lower extremity is represented in the medial aspect of the postcentral gyrus, whereas the upper extremity is mapped on the dorsolateral aspect of the postcentral gyrus, and the face is mapped dorsal to the lateral fissure (Figure 7-12). This somatotopic map for humans is called a **homunculus,** meaning "a little man." The somatotopic organization of the SI cortex is a means for encoding stimulus location. The somatotopic organization at the cortical level reflects the same type of organization at lower levels of the somatovisceral sensory system, including the

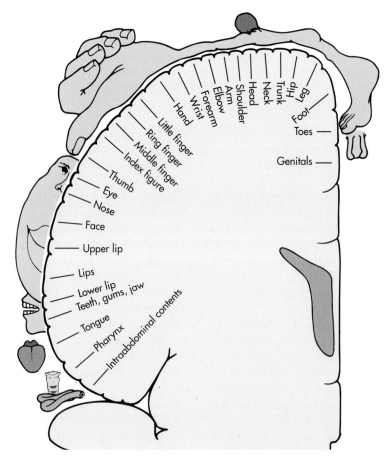

Figure 7-12 Sensory homunculus of the primary somatosensory cortex. One cerebral hemisphere is drawn as if it were sectioned in the coronal plane. The sizes of the different parts of the homunculus indicate the proportionate amounts of cortex dedicated to different parts of the body and head.

dorsal column nuclei and the VPL and VPM nuclei of the thalamus.

Besides being responsible for the initial processing of somatovisceral sensory information, the SI cortex also begins higher-order processing, such as **feature extraction,** the recognition of special features of a stimulus. For example, certain neurons in area 1 respond preferentially to a stimulus moving in one direction across the receptive field but not in the opposite direction (Figure 7-13). This response pattern is the result of the organization of inhibitory circuits in the cortex. Such neurons might contribute to the perceptual ability to recognize the direction of an applied stimulus.

The spinothalamic tract is responsible for somatic pain and temperature sensations

The **spinothalamic tract** originates from spinal cord neurons that project mainly to the contralateral thalamus. The place where the axon of a spinothalamic tract cell crosses is within the same segment as the cell body, and the axon ascends in the lateral or ventral funiculus. The spinothalamic tract terminates in several nuclei of the thalamus, including the VPL nucleus and several nuclei of the medial thalamus.

The cells of origin of the spinothalamic tract are found chiefly in spinal cord laminae I and V. Effective stimuli include noxious mechanical, thermal, and chemical stimuli. Some spinothalamic neurons are excited by activity in cold or warm thermoreceptors or sensitive mechanoreceptors.

Spinothalamic tract cells often receive a convergent excitatory input from several classes of sensory receptors. For example, a given spinothalamic tract neuron may be activated weakly by tactile stimuli but more powerfully by noxious stimuli (Figure 7-14). Such neurons are called **wide-dynamic-range** cells because they are activated by stimuli that have a wide range of intensities. Wide-dynamic-range neurons mainly signal noxious events, the weak response to tactile stimuli perhaps being ignored by higher centers. However, in pathological conditions, these neurons may be activated sufficiently by normally innocuous stimuli to evoke a sensation of pain. This would explain some pain states in which activation of mechanoreceptors causes pain. This condition is called **mechanical allodynia.** Other spinothalamic tract cells are activated only by noxious stimuli. Such neurons are often called **nociceptive-specific cells** or high-threshold cells (Figure 7-14).

> An example of a pathological state in which **allodynialy** is prominent is **central pain,** which can result from damage to the CNS. For example, a lesion involving the VPL nucleus may result in a central pain syndrome called **thalamic pain.** The quality of the pain is typically burning, although it can be sharp. Pain is often evoked by very weak stimulation, such as contact of the clothing with the skin. Patients with thalamic pain often prefer moistened clothing to dry clothing and sometimes wear a wet cotton glove on the affected side (the **Michael Jackson sign**).

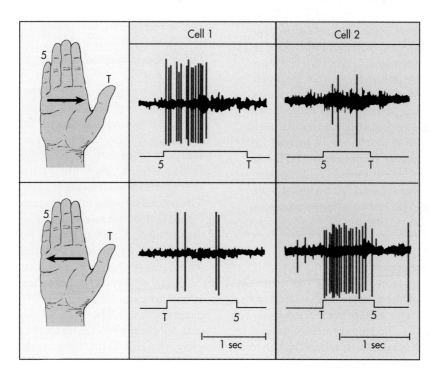

Figure 7-13 Feature extraction by cortical neurons. The responses of two cortical neurons to stimuli moved across the palm are shown. Cell 1 was excited strongly by movement of the stimulus toward the thumb *(T)* but only weakly by movements in the opposite direction. Cell 2 showed the converse behavior.

Spinothalamic tract cells often have inhibitory receptive fields. Inhibition may result from weak mechanical stimuli, but usually the most effective inhibitory stimuli are noxious ones. The nociceptive inhibitory receptive fields may be very large and include most of the body and face (Figure 7-14).

The **gate control theory of pain** explains how innocuous stimuli may inhibit the responses of dorsal horn neurons that transmit information about painful stimuli to the brain. In this theory, pain transmission is prevented by innocuous inputs mediated by large myelinated afferent fibers, whereas pain transmission is enhanced by inputs carried over fine afferent fibers. The inhibitory interneurons of lamina II serve as a gating mechanism. The circuit diagram originally proposed has been criticized, but the basic notion of a gating mechanism is still viable.

Many of the spinothalamic tract cells projecting to medial thalamic nuclei have very large receptive fields that often include much of the surface of the body and face. The large receptive fields of these spinothalamic neurons suggest that they trigger **motivational-affective responses** to painful stimuli rather than participate in **sensory discrimination.**

Various therapeutic techniques have been developed for the treatment of pain. Some of these involve the surgical interruption of nociceptive pathways, such as the spinothalamic tract. For example, an **anterolateral cordotomy** involves a surgical lesion in the ventrolateral white matter of the spinal cord at a level rostral to the spinal cord segments that receive the pain signals and in the white matter on the opposite side (because the spinothalamic tract crosses within the spinal cord). After such a lesion, pain and temperature sensations are lost on the opposite side of the body, below the level of the lesion. Cordotomies can be effective, at least for a few months. However, pain may recur, so cordotomies are of limited value when survival time is extended. In cases of chronic pain, other modalities of treatment, such as **transcutaneous electrical nerve stimulation (TENS)** or stimulation of the dorsal funiculus with an implanted electrode, are often tried. These approaches are based on the gate theory of pain and depend on inhibitory processing of nociceptive signals in the CNS.

Projection of trigeminal nuclei

Nociceptors and thermoreceptors of the face enter the brainstem with the trigeminal nerve and synapse in the spinal nucleus of the trigeminal nerve (Figure 7-11, C). Second-order neurons of the spinal nucleus project to the contralateral VPM thalamic nucleus and medial thalamus through the trigeminothalamic tract. Third-order thalamic neurons in turn project to the face area of the somatosensory cortex. This pathway for the face

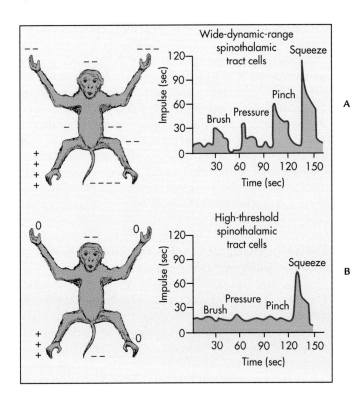

Figure 7-14   A, Responses of a wide-dynamic-range spinothalamic tract cell. **B,** Responses of a high-threshold spinothalamic tract cell. The figures at left indicate the excitatory *(plus signs)* and inhibitory *(minus signs)* receptive fields. The graphs at right show the responses to graded intensities of mechanical stimulation in the receptive field.

is equivalent to that involving the spinothalamic tract for the body. PAIN IN THE TRIGEMINAL DISTRIBUTION IS OF PARTICULAR IMPORTANCE BECAUSE IT INCLUDES BOTH TOOTH PAIN AND HEADACHES.

Other somatovisceral sensory pathways of the ventral spinal cord

Two other pathways, the spinoreticular tract and the spinomesencephalic tract, transmit somatovisceral sensory information and ascend in the ventral part of the spinal cord. The cells of origin of the **spinoreticular tract** are often difficult to activate, but when receptive fields are found, these are generally large, sometimes bilateral, and the effective stimuli include noxious ones. The reticular formation is located within the core of the brainstem, and it is involved in attentional mechanisms and arousal. Ascending fibers from the reticular formation extend to the medial thalamus and from there to wide areas of the cerebral cortex.

Many cells of the **spinomesencephalic tract** respond to noxious stimuli, and the receptive fields are generally small. The terminations of the tract are in several midbrain nuclei, including the **periaqueductal gray** (the area around the cerebral aqueduct), which is an important component of the endogenous analgesia system (see later discussion in this chapter). Information from the midbrain is also relayed to the **limbic sys-**

tem. This may provide one pathway by which noxious stimuli can trigger emotional responses. Motivation-affective responses may also result from activation of the periaqueductal gray and midbrain reticular formation. The latter is an important part of the arousal system, and stimulation in the periaqueductal gray causes vocalization and aversive behavior.

Sensory functions of the ventral spinal cord pathways

The most important sensory modalities mediated by ventral spinal cord pathways are pain and thermal sensations. Thermal sense depends on input from cold and warm receptors to spinothalamic tract neurons. Pain resulting from the stimulation of nociceptors is mediated partly by spinothalamic tract cells and partly by the spinoreticular and spinomesencephalic tracts.

THE MOTIVATIONAL-AFFECTIVE RESPONSES TO PAINFUL STIMULI INCLUDE ATTENTION AND AROUSAL, SOMATIC AND AUTONOMIC REFLEXES, ENDOCRINE RESPONSES, AND EMOTIONAL CHANGES. These collectively account for the unpleasant nature of painful stimuli. The motivational-affective responses depend on several ascending pathways, including the component of the spinothalamic tract that projects to the medial thalamus, the spinoreticular tract, and the spinomesencephalic tract. As indicated previously, these pathways have access to attentional, orientational, and arousal systems, as well as to the limbic system.

Pain that originates from the skin is generally well localized, presumably because spinothalamic tract cells have relatively discrete cutaneous receptive fields. Also, the ascending system through which they signal is somatotopically organized. However, pain that originates from deep structures, including muscle and viscera, is poorly localized and is often mistakenly attributed to superficial structures **(referred pain).**

Angina pectoris is a type of visceral pain that results from ischemia (inadequate blood flow) to the heart. The pain is often referred to the inner aspect of the left arm, although other regions of referral, such as the jaw, abdomen, or back, are not uncommon. The ischemia, generally caused by arteriosclerotic narrowing of one or more coronary arteries, releases algesic chemicals that sensitize visceral nociceptors supplying the heart. The nociceptors activate spinothalamic tract neurons in the left upper thoracic spinal cord. These neurons are also excited by sensory receptors supplying the left upper trunk and the T1 dermatome, which courses along the inner aspect of the arm (Figure 7-9). Presumably, activation of visceral nociceptors in the heart results in the excitation of spinothalamic neurons that also signal pain originating from the body wall. This in turn leads to a misinterpretation of the source of the pain. This concept is the basis of the **convergence-projection theory** of referred pain.

Centrifugal control of somatovisceral sensation allows the brain to control the sensory information that it receives

SENSORY EXPERIENCE IS NOT JUST THE PASSIVE DETECTION OF ENVIRONMENTAL EVENTS; INSTEAD, IT MORE OFTEN DEPENDS ON EXPLORATION OF THE ENVIRONMENT. Tactile cues are sought by moving the hand over a surface. Visual cues result from scanning visual targets with the eyes. Thus sensory information is often received as a result of activity in the motor system. Furthermore, sensory transmission in pathways to the sensory centers of the brain is regulated by descending control systems. This allows the brain to control its input by filtering the incoming sensory messages. Important information can be processed and unimportant information ignored.

The tactile and proprioceptive somatosensory pathways are regulated by descending pathways. However, of particular interest are the descending control systems that regulate the transmission of nociceptive information. These systems presumably reduce excessive pain under certain circumstances.

Soldiers on the battlefield, athletes in competition, accident victims, and others facing stressful circumstances often feel little or no pain at the time a wound occurs or a bone is broken. Later, however, pain may be severe. Although the descending regulatory pathways that control pain are part of the more general centrifugal system that modulates all forms of sensation, the pain-control system is so important that it is distinguished as a special **endogenous analgesia system.**

Several descending pathways contribute to the endogenous analgesia system. The activity of these descending pathways inhibits spinothalamic tract neurons. The **raphe nuclei,** which are located at the midline of the medulla, and the **periaqueductal gray,** which is located near the midline in the midbrain, give rise to direct and indirect projections to the medullary and spinal dorsal horns, and these pathways inhibit nociceptive neurons, including trigeminothalamic and spinothalamic tract cells (Figure 7-15, *A*).

The endogenous analgesia system can be subdivided into pathways that release one of the **endogenous opioids** and those that do not. The endogenous opioid substances are neuropeptides that activate one or more of the several forms of opiate receptors. Some of the endogenous opioids are **enkephalin, dynorphin,** and **β-endorphin.** Opioid analgesia can generally be antagonized with the narcotic antagonist **naloxone.** Therefore naloxone is used as a test of whether analgesia is mediated through an opioid mechanism.

Opiates typically inhibit neural activity in the nociceptive pathways. Two sites of action have been pro-

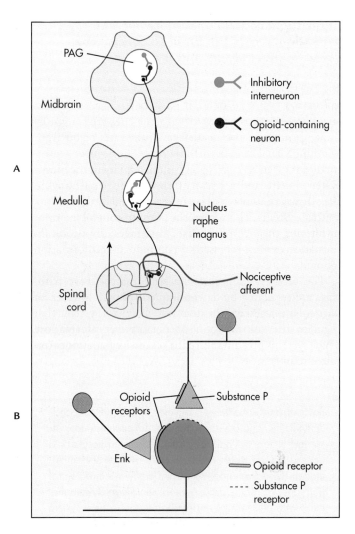

A

B

Figure 7-15 A, Neurons that play a role in the endogenous analgesia system. The periaqueductal gray *(PAG)* activates the raphe-spinal pathway, which in turn inhibits spinothalamic tract cells. Interneurons containing opioid neurotransmitters are at each level. **B,** Possible presynaptic and postsynaptic sites of action of enkephalin *(Enk)*. The presynaptic action prevents the release of substance P from nociceptors, and the postsynaptic action is inhibition of nociceptive neurons.

posed for opiate inhibition: presynaptic and postsynaptic (Figure 7-15, *B*). The presynaptic action of opiates on nociceptive afferent terminals is thought to prevent the release of excitatory transmitters, such as the neuropeptide **substance P.** The postsynaptic action produces an inhibitory postsynaptic potential. How can an inhibitory neurotransmitter activate descending pathways? One hypothesis is that the descending analgesia system is under tonic inhibitory control by inhibitory interneurons in both the midbrain and the medulla. The action of opiates would inhibit the inhibitory interneurons and thereby disinhibit the descending analgesia pathways. However, recent evidence indicates that another opioid action can be postsynaptic excitation.

Opiate receptors are found in the brain and spinal cord. At the spinal level, opiate receptors are located not only on the dorsal horn neurons but also on the terminals of nociceptors within the dorsal horn. Because of the presence of these opiate receptors, pain can sometimes be treated by the application of morphine to the spinal cord. This is done by the use of a **morphine pump** connected to a catheter introduced into the epidural space. The morphine can diffuse across the meninges and enter the spinal cord dorsal horn. The advantage of this route of delivery of morphine is that the morphine has a direct action on pain-processing circuits without seriously affecting thought processes, as may happen with systemically administered morphine. However, there is still a danger that morphine given by a morphine pump can depress respiration if the drug spreads rostrally in the cerebrospinal fluid.

The dose of morphine applied by the pump can be controlled by the patient **(patient-controlled analgesia).** The total dose of morphine that successfully minimizes pain is less when regulated by the patient than when regulated by the health care team.

Some endogenous analgesia pathways operate by neurotransmitters other than opioids and thus are unaffected by naloxone. One way of engaging a nonopioid analgesia pathway is through any of several types of stress. The analgesia so produced is called **stress-induced analgesia.**

Many neurons in the raphe nuclei release **serotonin** as a neurotransmitter. Serotonin is able to inhibit nociceptive neurons and presumably plays an important role in the endogenous analgesia system. Other brainstem neurons release catecholamines, such as **norepinephrine.** Catecholamines also inhibit nociceptive neurons, and therefore catecholaminergic neurons contribute to the endogenous analgesia system. Undoubtedly many other substances also participate in the analgesia system. Furthermore, there is evidence that endogenous opiate antagonists exist that can prevent opiate analgesia.

SUMMARY

- Sensory receptors respond to stimuli by various transduction mechanisms. The specific mechanism depends on the type of receptor.
- Transduction causes a receptor potential, which is usually a depolarization that may cause the sensory receptor's primary afferent fiber to discharge.
- In some sensory receptors, the primary afferent fiber develops a generator potential in response to the release of synaptic transmitter from a separate sensory receptor cell.

- The responses of sensory receptors can be rapidly or slowly adapting depending on the type of information to be signaled.
- A sensory receptor has a receptive field, which is the region that when stimulated, affects the discharge of the neuron. Central sensory neurons may have both excitatory and inhibitory receptive fields.
- Sensory information is encoded so that modality, spatial location, threshold, intensity, frequency, and duration are all recognized.
- Somatovisceral sensory receptors include mechanoreceptors, thermoreceptors, and nociceptors.
- Cutaneous sensory receptors include a number of types of mechanoreceptors, including hair follicle receptors, Meissner's corpuscles, pacinian corpuscles, Merkel cell endings, and Ruffini's corpuscles. The skin also contains cold and warm thermoreceptors and several kinds of nociceptors.
- Skeletal muscle contains stretch receptors as well as nociceptors. Joints and viscera are also supplied with mechanoreceptors and nociceptors.
- The dorsal column–medial lemniscus pathway mediates the sensations of flutter-vibration, touch-pressure, and proprioception. The path is somatotopically organized. The cortical representation of the body forms a sensory homunculus.
- The spinothalamic tract mediates pain and temperature sensations. The motivational-affective part of the pain response involves nonsomatotopic connections with the medial thalamus. Visceral pain is often referred to somatic structures.
- The somatovisceral sensory pathways, including the spinothalamic tract, are controlled by pathways that descend from the brain. The endogenous analgesia system regulates pain by releasing endogenous opioid substances and certain monoamines, such as serotonin and norepinephrine, as neurotransmitters in the spinal cord dorsal horn.

BIBLIOGRAPHY

Belmonte C, Cervero F: *Neurobiology of nociceptors,* Oxford, 1996, Oxford University Press.

Boivie J, Hansson P, Lindblom U, eds: *Touch, temperature, and pain in health and disease,* Seattle, 1994, IASP.

Fields HL, Besson JM, eds: *Pain modulation,* vol 77, *Progress in brain research,* Amsterdam, 1988, Elsevier.

Gebhart GF, ed: *Visceral pain,* Seattle, 1995, IASP.

Johnson KO, Hsiao SS: Neural mechanisms of tactual form and texture perception, *Annu Rev Neurosci* 15:227, 1992.

Mountcastle VB: Central nervous mechanisms in mechanoreceptive sensibility. In Brookhart JM, Mountcastle VB, section eds: *Handbook of physiology: the nervous system III,* Bethesda, Md, 1984, American Physiological Society.

Penfield W, Jasper H: *Epilepsy and the functional anatomy of the human brain,* Boston, 1954, Little, Brown.

Steriade M, Jones EG, McCormick DSA: *Thalamus,* vol 1, *Organization and function,* Amsterdam, 1997, Elsevier.

Steriade M, Jones EG, McCormick DSA: *Thalamus,* vol 2, *Experimental and clinical aspects,* Amsterdam, 1997, Elsevier.

Willis WD, Coggeshall RE: *Sensory mechanisms of the spinal cord,* New York, 1991, Plenum.

▷ CASE STUDIES

Case 7-1

A 74-year-old woman awakens with a feeling of numbness on the left side of her body. She also has difficulty moving her left arm and leg. Her physician finds that she cannot distinguish between a coin and a paper clip when these are placed in her left hand while her eyes are closed. Her ability to recognize that two separate points on the skin are stimulated simultaneously is much poorer on her left than on her right side. She fails to recognize the vibration of a tuning fork placed against her left wrist or ankle. Pin pricks feel duller on the left than on the right side. Several weeks after the initial incident, she begins to feel burning pain on the left side, and even gentle contact of objects with the skin of her left arm or leg causes additional pain.

1. **What is the most likely location of the lesion that produces her symptoms?**
    A. Central part of the right medulla
    B. Cerebral cortex around the right central sulcus
    C. Peripheral nerves of the left arm and leg
    D. Posterior thalamus and adjacent internal capsule on the right
    E. Right half of the spinal cord above C5

2. **The patient's ability to feel pin pricks is diminished, but she can perceive spontaneous pain and allodynia for what reason?**
    A. Her lesion has damaged the brainstem reticular formation pathways that project to the medial thalamus.
    B. The pain symptoms are imaginary and do not reflect changes in the nervous system.
    C. Spinothalamic input to the VPL nucleus is largely interrupted, but there are plastic changes in denervated cortical circuits.
    D. Nociceptive primary afferent fibers have been destroyed in peripheral nerves, but mechanoreceptive afferents become nociceptive.
    E. Spinal cord nociceptive neurons such as spinothalamic tract cells stop signaling pin-prick sensations but discharge spontaneously and in response to touch.

Case 7-2

A 46-year-old man develops cancer of the descending colon. As the disease progresses, he develops severe pelvic pain. Morphine is administered systemically to counteract the pain. However, unless the dose is so high that he becomes somnolent, he obtains insufficient pain relief. An alternative method for pain control in this patient is clearly desirable. The therapy chosen is a morphine pump to infuse morphine epidurally through a catheter placed over the lumbosacral spinal cord.

1. This approach is likely to be successful because of which reason?

    A. Morphine will reach the periaqueductal gray in the cerebrospinal fluid via the cerebral aqueduct.

    B. There are opiate receptors in the spinal cord dorsal horn, and activation of these will reduce nociceptive transmission.

    C. The morphine would act on the cancer cells in the pelvic region, preventing these cells from inducing pain.

    D. Nociceptors in the meninges are responsible for the pain, and morphine would block their activity.

    E. When morphine reaches the spinal cord, it will cause the release of substance P from the terminals of nociceptors in the dorsal horn.

2. Morphine is more likely than a local anesthetic to succeed in this case because of which reason?

    A. Morphine is unlikely to cause respiratory depression.

    B. Local anesthetic infusion may cause itching sensations.

    C. Tolerance will develop to the local anesthetic.

    D. Morphine will block all types of sensation.

    E. Morphine will block pain preferentially.

Special Senses

- Describe the visual system, including the eye and the central visual pathways.
- Describe the auditory system, including the cochlea and the central auditory pathways.
- Describe the vestibular system, including the labyrinth and the central vestibular pathways.
- Describe the chemical senses, including taste and smell.

In the evolution of the nervous system, an important trend has been **encephalization,** in which special sensory organs developed in the heads of animals and appropriate neural systems developed in the brains. These special sensory systems, which include the **visual, auditory, gustatory,** and **olfactory systems,** allowed the animal to detect and analyze light, sound, and chemical signals in the environment. In addition, the **vestibular system** evolved to signal the position of the head.

Visual System

The visual system detects and interprets photic stimuli. In vertebrates, effective photic stimuli are electromagnetic waves of lengths between 400 and 700 nm, which make up **visible light.** Light enters the eye and impinges on **photoreceptors** in a specialized sensory epithelium, the **retina.** The photoreceptors are the **rods** and **cones.** RODS HAVE LOW THRESHOLDS FOR DETECTING LIGHT, AND THEIR PHOTOPIGMENT BLEACHES IN STRONG LIGHT. THUS RODS OPERATE BEST UNDER CONDITIONS OF REDUCED LIGHTING (SCOTOPIC VISION). However, rods neither provide well-defined visual images nor contribute to color vision. CONES, IN CONTRAST, ARE NOT AS SENSITIVE TO LIGHT BUT OPERATE BEST UNDER DAYLIGHT CONDITIONS (PHOTOPIC VISION). CONES ARE RESPONSIBLE FOR HIGH VISUAL ACUITY AND COLOR VISION.

The structure of the eye is complex

The wall of the eye is formed of three concentric layers (Figure 8-1). The outer layer is the fibrous coat, which includes the transparent **cornea** with its epithelium, the **conjunctiva,** and the opaque **sclera.** The middle layer is the vascular coat, which includes the **iris** and **choroid.** The iris con-tains both radially and circularly oriented smooth muscle fibers, which constitute the **pupillary dilator** and **sphincter** muscles; the iris forms a diaphragm to control the size of the **pupil.** THE DILATOR IS ACTIVATED BY THE SYMPATHETIC NERVOUS SYSTEM AND THE SPHINCTER BY THE PARASYMPATHETIC NERVOUS SYSTEM (see Chapter 10). The choroid is rich in blood vessels that supply the outer layers of the retina. The inner retinal layers are nourished by tributaries of the central artery and veins of the retina; these vessels enter the eye through the optic nerve.

The inner layer of the eye is the neural coat, the **retina** (Figure 8-1). The functional part of the retina covers the entire posterior eye except for the **blind spot,** which is the optic nerve head. Visual acuity is highest in the central part of the retina, the **macula lutea.** The **fovea** is a pitlike depression in the middle of the macula where visual targets are focused; it is the **fixation point,** or point at which light rays are focused when the eyes are directed at a visual target of interest.

Besides the retina, the eye contains a **lens** to focus light on the retina, **pigment** to reduce light scatter, and fluids called **aqueous humor** and **vitreous humor** that help maintain the shape of the eye. Externally attached **extraocular muscles** aim the eye toward an appropriate visual target.

The lens is held in place behind the iris by the **suspensory ligaments** (or **zonule fibers**), which attach to the wall of the eye at the **ciliary body** (Figure 8-1). WHEN THE CILIARY MUSCLES ARE RELAXED, THE TENSION EXERTED BY THE SUSPENSORY LIGAMENTS TENDS TO FLATTEN THE LENS. WHEN THE CILIARY MUSCLES CONTRACT, TENSION ON THE SUSPENSORY MUSCLES IS REDUCED, ALLOWING THE LENS TO ASSUME A MORE SPHERICAL SHAPE BECAUSE OF ITS ELASTIC PROPERTIES. The ciliary muscles are activated by the parasympathetic nervous system via the oculomotor nerve.

Light scattering within the eye is minimized by pigment. The choroid contains an abundance of pigment. In addition, the outermost layer of the retina is a pigment-containing epithelium. Besides light absorption, the pigment cells of the **retinal pigment layer** are involved in the turnover of photoreceptor outer segments and the regeneration of **rhodopsin,** the photopigment found in the rods.

The space around the iris is filled with aqueous humor, which is a clear fluid resembling cerebrospinal fluid. The aqueous humor is actively secreted by the **ciliary pro-**

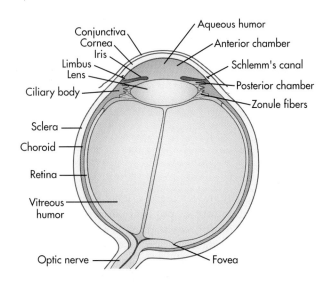

Figure 8-1 Right eye as viewed from above.

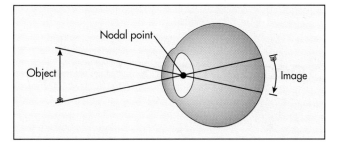

Figure 8-2 Image formation in the eye. The image is reversed as rays of light pass through the nodal point of the lens.

cesses, which form an epithelium that is posterior to the iris and that protrudes into a space called the **posterior chamber** (Figure 8-1). The aqueous humor circulates through the posterior chamber, out the pupil, and into the anterior chamber. It is then reabsorbed into the **Schlemm's canal** and returned to the venous circulation.

> Imbalance in the secretion and reabsorption of aqueous humor can increase the pressure in the eye, a condition that threatens the viability of the retina. This malady is known as **glaucoma.** Reabsorption can be increased surgically, and secretion can be reduced by medication therapy. Cholinergic medications, such as pilocarpine, which constrict the pupil, are helpful because they reduce the resistance to drainage of the aqueous humor.

The space behind the lens contains a gelatinous material, the **vitreous humor.** The vitreous humor turns over very slowly, so it does not contribute actively to glaucoma.

The extraocular muscles insert on the sclera from their origins on the bony orbit. Details concerning the organization and operation of the eye movement control system are described in Chapter 9.

Physical properties of the eye are termed physiological optics

The eye is often compared to a camera. Both devices capture images by using a lens system to focus light on a photosensitive surface. The quality of the image is enhanced by use of a diaphragm to reduce the effect of spherical aberrations of the lens and to increase depth of field. The diaphragm also controls the amount of entering light.

Like a camera, the eye produces an inverted image of an object (Figure 8-2). The inversion is caused by the fact that

light rays from the object cross at a nodal point within the lens. The image is inverted both from side to side and from above downward.

The ability of a lens to bend light is called its **refractive power.** The unit of refractive power is the **diopter.** For an image to be in focus on the retina, light coming from any point on the object and passing through the cornea and lens must be refracted just enough so that it falls on a corresponding point on the retina. THE CORNEA IS THE MAIN REFRACTIVE SURFACE OF THE EYE. It has a refractive power of 43 diopters. HOWEVER, THE LENS IS CRUCIAL FOR FOCUSING IMAGES ON THE RETINA because its refractive power can vary from 13 to 26 diopters. THE REFRACTIVE POWER OF THE LENS IS ALTERED BY CHANGES IN THE SHAPE OF THE LENS THROUGH RELAXATION OR CONTRACTION OF THE CILIARY MUSCLES. **Accommodation** is the process by which contraction of the ciliary muscle causes the lens to become more rounded. The result of accommodation is that images of nearby objects are brought into focus on the retina.

> During aging, the lens loses its elasticity. This loss reduces the ability of the eye to accommodate. This visual disturbance is called **presbyopia.** Other common defects in focusing ability are myopia, hypertropia, and astigmatism. In **myopia** (nearsightedness), images are focused in front of the retina because the eye is disproportionately long for the refractive system. In **hypermetropia** (farsightedness), images are focused behind the retina because the eye is short relative to the refractive system. **Astigmatism** is the result of asymmetrical focusing, usually because the cornea lacks radial symmetry.

Retina

The outermost of the 10 retinal layers is the **pigment epithelium.** The pigment cells capture stray light. They also phagocytize photoreceptor membrane shed from the outer segments of the rods and cones. Substances that move between the photoreceptors and the blood vessels within the choroid must pass through the pigment cell layer. Interactions between pigment cells and photoreceptor cells are very important in visual function.

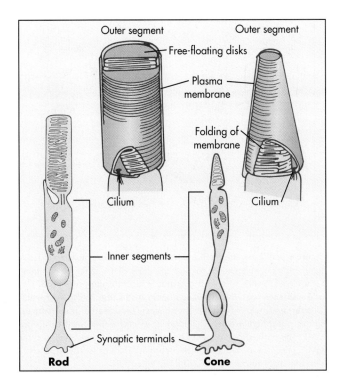

Figure 8-3 Structure of rods and cones. The inner and outer segments and the synaptic terminals are shown, as are details of the membranous discs in the outer segments.

Individual photoreceptor cells can be subdivided into three regions: the **outer segment,** the **inner segment,** and the **synaptic terminal** (Figure 8-3). The outer segment contains a stack of **membranous discs** that are rich in photopigment. The inner segment connects with the outer segment by way of a modified cilium. The inner segment of the photoreceptor cell contains the nucleus, mitochondria, and other organelles. The synaptic ending contacts one or more **bipolar cells.**

THE ROD IS SO SENSITIVE TO LIGHT THAT IT CAN RESPOND TO A SINGLE PHOTON. The greater sensitivity of rods than cones is partly caused by the long outer segments of rods. Consequently rods contain more photopigment, which is arranged in a monomolecular layer on each outer-segment disc. The pigment is **rhodopsin,** which is composed of a chromophore, retinal, and a protein, opsin. **Retinal** is the aldehyde form of **vitamin A.** In the dark, retinal is bound to opsin in the 11-*cis*-retinal form. Absorption of light causes a change to the all-*trans*-retinal form, which no longer binds to opsin. Before the photopigment can be regenerated, all-*trans* retinal must be transported to the pigment cell layer, reduced, isomerized, and esterified.

Cones also contain 11-*cis* retinal attached to an opsin. However, three different **cone opsins** are found in three different types of cones, each sensitive to a different part of the visible light spectrum. ONE CONE TYPE RESPONDS BEST TO BLUE LIGHT (420 NM), ANOTHER TO GREEN (531 NM), AND THE THIRD TO RED (558 NM). The presence of three types of cones gives the retina a mechanism for **trichromatic color vi-**

sion. Light causes a series of changes in the photopigment of cones; these changes resemble the sequence in rods, but the reactions and the recovery are quicker.

Color vision requires at least two photopigments. A single pigment absorbs light over much of the spectrum but absorbs best at a particular **wavelength.** The amount of light absorbed depends on its wavelength and **intensity.** The light of one wavelength and a given intensity could produce the same effect on a particular photoreceptor as another light of a different wavelength and intensity. Therefore the signal is ambiguous because intensity can substitute for wavelength. However, with at least two different photoreceptors that have different pigments, different wavelengths can be distinguished if the intensity of the light that falls on both photoreceptors is the same. Three different photoreceptor types reduce the ambiguity even more.

Color blindness is often based on a genetic defect that results in the loss of one or more of the cone mechanisms or in a change in the absorption spectra of one or more photopigments. People are normally **trichromats** because they have three cone mechanisms. **Dichromats** have two cone mechanisms and cannot distinguish between red and green. **Monochromats** generally lack all three cone mechanisms, but in rare instances, they lack two. **Protanopia** is the loss of the long-wavelength system; **deuteranopia,** the loss of the medium-wavelength system; and **tritanopia,** the loss of the short-wavelength system. Any of these causes a person to be a dichromat.

The most common type of color blindness is the red-green form. This occurs in 8% of the male population and is a sex-linked recessive trait because the genetic defect is on the X chromosome. The main difficulty experienced by people with red-green color blindness occurs when there is a serious need to distinguish these colors, such as at traffic lights.

THE CONES ARE MOST CONCENTRATED IN THE FOVEA, WHERE ALL OF THE PHOTORECEPTORS ARE CONES (Figure 8-4). This is the region of the retina that provides the greatest visual acuity. In the fovea the retina is thinned to just the four outer layers; thus the image there is of the highest quality. Rods are most concentrated in the parafoveal region.

NO PHOTORECEPTORS EXIST IN THE OPTIC DISC (Figure 8-4), which is where the ganglion cell axons collect to leave the eye as the **optic nerve.** The optic disc is therefore a **blind spot.** The optic disc is in the medial retina. Therefore the part of the visual field that would be imaged on the blind spot would be on the temporal side of the field of vision of that eye. The blind spot is not noticed in binocular vision because the region of the visual field that fails to be seen by the blind spot in one eye is seen by the opposite eye because the light falls on the temporal side of that retina.

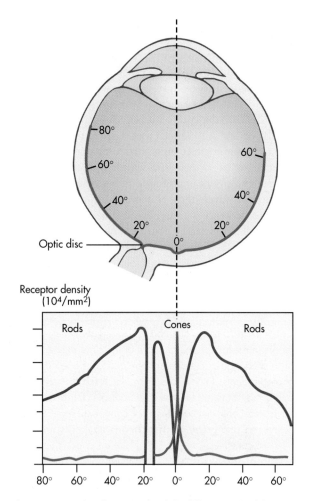

Figure 8-4 Density of cones and rods in different parts of the retina.

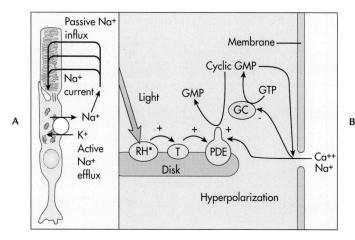

Figure 8-5 **A,** Dark current in a photoreceptor, which is caused by passive influx of Na$^+$, which is returned to the extracellular space by pumping. Light closes the Na$^+$ channels and thus reduces the dark current. **B,** Second messenger system underlying phototransduction. When light reacts with rhodopsin *(RH)*, G protein transducin *(T)* is activated. This in turn activates phosphodiesterase *(PDE)*, which breaks down cyclic GMP into GMP. The dark current depends on cyclic GMP, and thus a fall in cyclic GMP concentration reduces the dark current, which causes hyperpolarization of the photoreceptor. *GC,* Guanylyl cyclase.

Information processing in the retina

The most direct route for information flow through the retina is from **photoreceptors** to **bipolar cells** and then to **ganglion cells.** The ganglion cells provide the output of the retina to the **thalamus.**

The neural pathways in the retina can be subdivided into **rod pathways** and **cone pathways.** Convergence from photoreceptors onto bipolar cells is greater in the rod than in the cone pathways. This convergence enhances the sensitivity of the rod pathways. Cone pathways display much less convergence, in keeping with their role in visual acuity.

Because the photoreceptor cells and many of the retinal interneurons have short processes, action potentials are not required for transmitting information to the next cell in the circuit. Instead, local potentials alter neurotransmitter release, which in turn provides for information transfer. In darkness, photoreceptor cells have open Na$^+$ channels, which result in a **dark current** and consequently a tonic release of neurotransmitter onto bipolar cells and **horizontal cells** (Figure 8-5). When light is absorbed by photopigment in the outer segments of the photoreceptors, the Na$^+$ channels are closed, which leads to a hyperpolarization of the photo-

receptor cells and a decrease in the release of transmitter, probably glutamate.

This information processing involves an amplification mechanism that depends on a second messenger system. Cyclic GMP maintains the Na$^+$ channels in an open configuration (Figure 8-5). Light activates a G protein called **transducin** in the photoreceptor membrane. Transducin in turn activates a phosphodiesterase, which hydrolyzes cyclic GMP. This causes the sodium channels to close and the membrane to hyperpolarize.

The **receptive field** of a photoreceptor is generally a small circular area that is coextensive with the area of the retina occupied by the photoreceptor. Bipolar cells are of two types: **on-center** and **off-center** (Figure 8-6). An on-center bipolar cell is depolarized when light shines in the center of its receptive field and hyperpolarized when light shines in an annulus around the center of the receptive field. An off-center bipolar cell behaves in the converse manner. The different responses to stimulation of the center of the receptive field depend on differences in the receptors that respond to glutamate released from the synaptic endings of the photoreceptors on the bipolar cells. The responses to stimulation of the area surrounding the center of the receptive field are determined by interneuronal pathways involving horizontal cells.

Ganglion cells, like bipolar cells, may have center-surround antagonistic receptive fields (Figure 8-6), or like amacrine cells, they may have large receptive fields. The type of receptive field presumably reflects the dominant input. Ganglion cells can be classified as X-, Y-, and W-cells. Both X- and Y-cells have center-surround receptive fields. **X-cells** have smaller receptive fields than

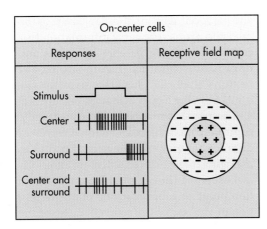
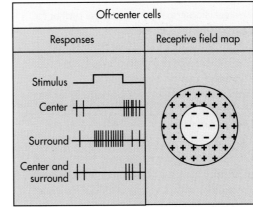

Figure 8-6 Center-surround receptive field organization of retinal ganglion cells. *Left,* Responses to light stimuli on the center or in a surrounding annulus for on- and off-center ganglion cells. The effect of stimulating the entire field is also shown. *Right,* Receptive fields. Plus signs indicate excitation, and minus signs, inhibition.

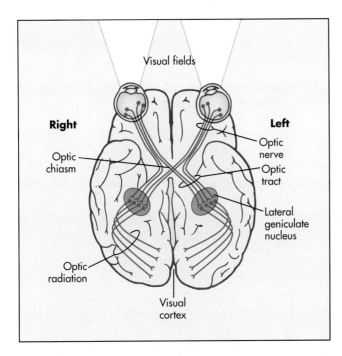

Figure 8-7 Main visual pathway as viewed from the base of the brain.

Y-cells, respond more tonically to stimuli, have slower axons, sum multiple responses in a linear fashion, and distinguish between colors. They are responsible for high visual acuity and color vision. **Y-cells** respond to complex stimuli in an unpredictable fashion. They are motion detectors. **W-cells** often have large, diffuse receptive fields. They signal the intensity of ambient light.

Central visual projections of the retina

The **optic nerves** from the two eyes converge at the optic chiasm (Figure 8-7). Some of the optic nerve fibers decussate in the chiasm and join the optic tract, and some continue posteriorly in the optic tract on the same side as the eye of origin. The fibers that cross orig-

inate from the **nasal hemiretinas** of the two eyes. The uncrossed fibers originate from the **temporal hemiretinas.** Because of this arrangement, each optic tract contains both uncrossed and crossed fibers. The optic tract fibers synapse in the lateral geniculate nucleus (Figure 8-7).

The lateral geniculate nucleus relays visual information to the cerebral cortex

Most neurons in the **lateral geniculate nucleus (LGN)** project to the visual cortex (Figure 8-7); however, some are interneurons. A given LGN neuron receives a dominant input from one or a few retinal ganglion cells, and the responses resemble those of the ganglion cells. Thus the LGN neurons can be classified as X- or Y-cells, and they have on- or off-center receptive fields. However, LGN neurons are subject to input from regions other than the retinas. These other regions include the visual cortex, several brainstem nuclei, and the reticular nucleus of the thalamus. Inhibitory actions that originate from the brainstem or thalamic reticular nucleus can prevent visual signals from reaching the cortex or can reduce these signals. In effect, the LGN serves as a filter for visual information before it accesses the visual cortex.

Visual field deficits result from interruption of the visual pathway

Because the central visual pathway extends from the base of the brain just above the pituitary gland through the temporal and parietal lobes to the occipital lobe, damage to a wide area of the brain can cause loss of vision. The visual loss can be in one eye if the retina or optic nerve on one side is involved, but the visual loss can be in both eyes if the optic chiasm, optic tract, LGN, optic radiation, or visual cortex is involved. The particular pattern of visual loss depends on the exact site and extent of damage.

A visual field defect is described in terms of the part of the visual world that a patient is unable to see. Each eye has a visual field that can be subdivided into a temporal and a nasal visual hemifield. The hemifield can be further subdivided into an upper and a lower quadrant.

Loss of vision in one eye is simply **blindness** in that eye or a **scotoma** (partial blindness in one visual field). A lesion affecting the optic chiasm causes loss of vision in the temporal fields of both eyes, a condition called **bitemporal hemianopsia.** This can happen, for example, because of a pituitary tumor. Destruction of an optic tract causes loss of vision in the contralateral half of the visual field of each eye, or **contralateral homonymous hemianopsia.** A similar visual field deficit results from destruction of an LGN, the entire optic radiation, or the primary visual cortex on one side. Macular vision may be spared in cortical lesions, perhaps because of the very large size of the macular representation or because of collateral circulation in the case of a vascular lesion.

The striate cortex is the primary visual receiving area

The optic radiation ends chiefly in layer IV of the **primary visual cortex.** The dense axon terminals form a white stripe (the **stripe of Gennari**) that can be seen grossly and that gives rise to the name **striate cortex** for this region of cortex. Projections from the magnocellular (large-celled)

and parvocellular (small-celled) layers of the LGN are separate, and axons that carry information from the two eyes end in alternating patches of cortex are called **ocular dominance columns** (Figure 8-8, *B*). Recordings from neurons in area 17 reveal that usually a given cell receives input from both eyes, although one eye is dominant.

The retina is mapped onto the striate cortex (**retinotopic map**). The macular region is represented at and for a distance anterior to the occipital pole. The remainder of the retina is represented still more anteriorly along the medial aspect of the occipital lobe. The macular representation occupies more cortical volume than the representation of the rest of the retina because of the requirements for visual acuity.

Most neurons in the striate cortex respond best to elongated stimuli. A rectangular visual target or an edge evokes a more vigorous response than a small spot. The orientation of the stimulus is an important factor. Neurons in a region of striate cortex perpendicular to the cortical surface all respond best to elongated stimuli having the same orientation (Figure 8-8, *B*). These neurons form **orientation columns.**

The higher processing of visual information depends on many cortical areas

The striate or primary visual cortex receives visual information from the LGN and begins analysis of that information. The striate cortex connects with many other cortical areas, known as the **extrastriate visual cortex,** which par-

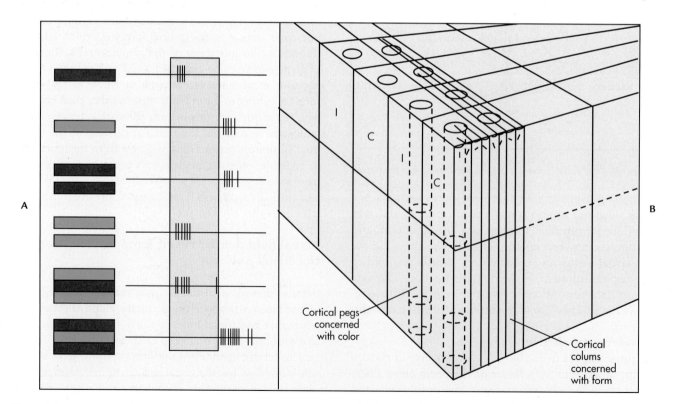

Figure 8-8 A, Responses of a simple cell in the striate cortex to various combinations of red and green bars. The cell responded best to a red bar flanked by two green bars. **B,** Diagram of the columns in the visual cortex. Ocular dominance columns are indicated by *I* (ipsilateral eye) and *C* (contralateral eye) and orientation columns by the short bars at various angles. The cortical pegs contain neurons that have double-opponent color fields.

ticipate in the further processing of visual information. These cortical areas are interconnected with other nuclei of the thalamus.

Stereopsis is binocular depth perception. It depends on slight differences in the images in the two eyes such that a given cortical neuron has its receptive field at points on the two retinas that are slightly out of correspondence. This provides the brain with a signal that can be used to judge differences in the distances of objects.

Color vision depends on the discrimination of wavelengths of light. Retinal ganglion cells and LGN neurons may respond selectively to one wavelength and be inhibited by another. These cells are called **spectral opponent neurons.** An example would be a neuron excited by a red light shone in the center of its receptive field and by a green light shone in the surrounding part of the field (Figure 8-8, *A*). Spectral opponent cells belong to the X-cell category. Neurons in the cortex discriminate wavelength and brightness; thus they permit the perception of true color. Such neurons are concentrated in **cortical pegs,** which are sets of neurons within the ocular dominance columns (Figure 8-8, *B*).

The superior colliculus mediates orienting reflexes

The **superior colliculus** is a layered midbrain structure that serves as a visual center and coordination center for orientation reflexes occurring in response to visual, auditory, and somatic stimuli. The dorsal three layers are involved in visual processing, whereas the deeper four layers also process other sensory input.

Retinal ganglion cells project to the upper layers of the superior colliculus. The ganglion cells include both Y- and W-cells. The superior colliculus also receives a projection from the cerebral cortex. The cortical neurons involved in this projection are activated by Y-cells. Thus the visual input to the superior colliculus is concerned with motion detection and light intensity. The output of the upper layers of the superior colliculus influences visual processing in the cortex. Experiments in animals suggest that the superior colliculus is important in determining the location of objects in visual space, whereas the cortex determines what the objects are. The deep layers of the superior colliculus are considered with the motor system (see Chapter 9).

Auditory System

The auditory system is designed to analyze sound. Audition is important not only for the recognition of environmental cues but also for communication, especially language in humans.

Sound is produced by pressure waves in the air

Sound is produced by alternating waves of pressure in the air. Sound waves are composed of the sum of a set of sinusoidal waves of the appropriate amplitudes, frequencies,

and phase. Thus sound can be regarded as a mixture of pure tones. THE HUMAN ACOUSTIC SYSTEM ACTS AS A FILTER THAT IS SENSITIVE TO PURE TONES WITHIN A RANGE OF FREQUENCIES FROM APPROXIMATELY 20 TO 15,000 HZ. Threshold varies with frequency. Sound intensity is measured in **decibels (dB),** which are expressed in terms of a reference level of sound pressure (P_r), often 0.0002 dyne/cm², which is the threshold for hearing. The formula for sound intensity follows:

$$\text{Sound pressure (decibels)} = 20 \log(P/P_r)$$

where *P* is pressure.

THE EAR IS MOST SENSITIVE TO TONES FROM **1000** TO **3000** HZ. At these frequencies, threshold is by definition zero. Threshold is higher at frequencies less than 1000 Hz and greater than 3000 Hz (Figure 8-9). For example, threshold at 100 Hz is approximately 40 dB. Speech has an intensity of about 65 dB. Damage to the acoustic apparatus can be produced by sounds that exceed 100 dB, and discomfort results from sound pressures that exceed 120 dB.

Structures of the external, middle, and inner ear all contribute to hearing

The ear can be subdivided into the **external ear, middle ear,** and **inner ear.** The external ear includes the **pinna** and the **external auditory meatus,** which leads by way of the **auditory canal** to the outer surface of the tympanic membrane (Figure 8-10, *A*). The auditory canal contains glands that secrete **cerumen,** a wax that guards the ear from invasion by insects.

The middle ear is a cavity that extends deep to the tympanic membrane. It contains a chain of ossicles, the **malleus, incus,** and **stapes** (Figure 8-10, *A*), which connect the tympanic membrane with another membrane that covers the **oval window,** an opening into the inner ear (Figure 8-10, *B*). A second opening between the middle and inner

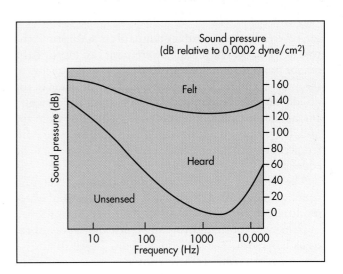

Figure 8-9 Sound levels for human hearing as a function of frequency. Below the range for hearing, sound is not sensed; above the hearing range, it is detected by both the auditory and the somatosensory systems.

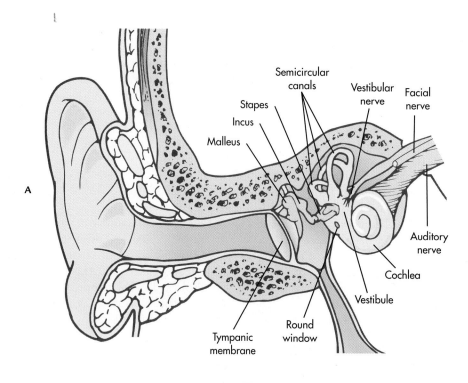

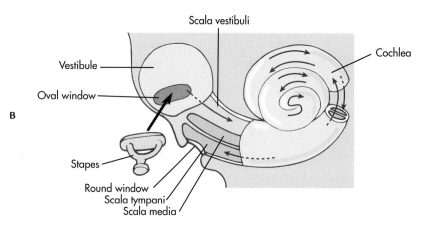

Figure 8-10 Structure of the cochlea. **A,** Components of the ear, including the membranous labyrinth. **B,** Cochlea in more detail. The arrows indicate the path of fluid movement that would result from movement of the stapes into the oval window.

ear, covered by the **secondary tympanic membrane,** is the **round window.** The middle ear contains two muscles, the **tensor tympani** and the **stapedius;** the former attaches to the malleus and the latter to the stapes. Contraction of the middle ear muscles dampens movements of the ossicular chain. The eustachian tube provides an opening from the middle ear to the nasopharynx. This permits pressure differences between the environment and the middle ear to be equalized.

The inner ear is a cavity within the temporal bone and contains the **cochlea** (Figure 8-10, *A*) and **vestibular apparatus.** The cochlea is the organ of hearing and is formed by elements of both the **bony labyrinth** and the **membranous labyrinth.** The space in the bony labyrinth just inside the oval window is the **vestibule.**

The cochlea is a coiled structure formed by the division of the bony labyrinth into two compartments. The partition between the compartments is formed by a component

of the membranous labyrinth; this component is called the **cochlear duct,** or **scala media.** The portion of the bony labyrinth in continuity with the vestibule is the **scala vestibuli.** This extends along the two and a half turns of the human cochlea to the end of the cochlear duct. At this point the scala vestibuli connects with the **scala tympani** by way of a space called the **helicotrema.** The scala tympani spirals back to the bony interface with the middle ear and ends at the **secondary tympanic membrane** that covers the **round window.** The base of the cochlea is near the oval and round windows (Figure 8-10, *B*), and the apex is at the helicotrema. The bony core of the cochlea is the **modiolus.**

The cochlear duct is a tube and is part of the membranous labyrinth (Figure 8-11, *A*). The **basilar membrane** forms the base of the cochlear duct and can be regarded as the main partition between the scala vestibuli and scala tympani. The basilar membrane is narrowest near the base

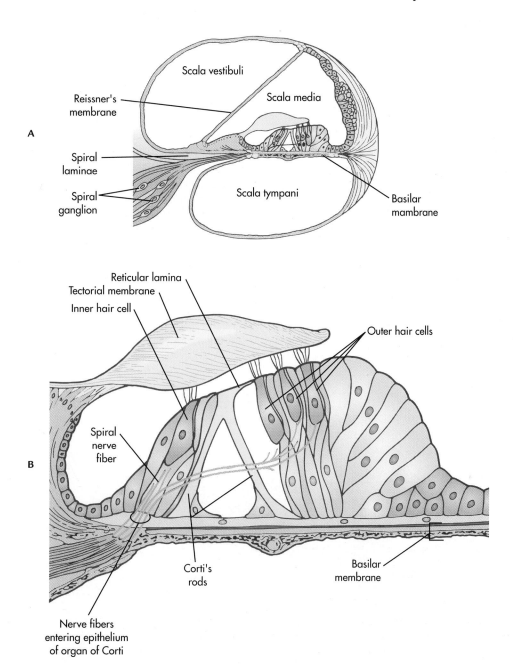

Figure 8-11 A, Organ of Corti within the cochlear duct (scala media). **B,** Enlargement of the organ of Corti.

of the cochlea and widest near the helicotrema. The basilar membrane is attached internally to a ledge, the **spiral lamina,** that arises from the modiolus. Externally the basilar membrane is anchored to the wall of the cochlea by the **spiral ligament.** Contained within the spiral ligament is a vascular structure, the **stria vascularis.** The roof over the cochlear duct is formed by **Reissner's membrane.** The cochlear duct contains **endolymph,** a fluid with a high concentration of K^+; the endolymph is secreted by the stria vascularis. The bony labyrinth contains **perilymph,** which resembles cerebrospinal fluid.

The **organ of Corti** is the sense organ for hearing (Figure 8-11, *B*). It lies within the cochlear duct along the basilar membrane. The organ of Corti consists of **hair cells,** the **tectorial membrane,** a stiff framework, and several types of supportive cells. The **stereocilia** of the hair cells

contact the tectorial membrane. The hair cells are innervated by primary afferent fibers and efferent fibers of the cochlear nerve. The cell bodies of the primary afferent fibers are in the **spiral ganglion,** which is contained in the modiolus. The spiral ganglion cells are bipolar neurons whose peripheral processes reach the hair cells through the spiral lamina. The central processes join the **cochlear nerve,** which projects into the brainstem.

Sound transduction depends on the organ of Corti

The external ear acts as a filter that is tuned to frequencies between 800 and 6000 Hz. The pinna serves little function in humans, although it is important in many animals. Pressure waves that reach the tympanic membrane cause it and the ossicular chain to vibrate at the frequency of sound. The ossicular chain in turn oscillates the oval window and the fluids within the cochlea. The round window completes the hydraulic pathway.

The middle ear mechanism serves as an **impedance matching device** to couple airborne sound waves with those conducted through the cochlear fluids (Figure 8-12, *A*). If sound waves were to be conducted directly from air to the oval window, most of the energy would be reflected and lost. With the mechanical advantage provided by the ratio of the area of the tympanic membrane to that of the oval window, plus that provided by the lever action of the ossicular chain, only 10 to 15 dB are lost in the impedance-matching process of the ear.

Within the cochlear duct, the maximal amplitude of the oscillations extends for various distances along the basilar membrane; the distance depends on the frequency of the sound (Figure 8-12, *B*). Although much of the basilar membrane oscillates in a **traveling wave** in response to a particular frequency of sound, high frequencies result in

movements that are largest in the basal part of the cochlea, whereas low frequencies induce movements that are largest near the apex of the cochlea.

As the basilar membrane oscillates, the stereocilia of the hair cells in the organ of Corti are subjected to shear forces at their junctions with the tectorial membrane (Figure 8-13). When the stereocilia are bent in a direction toward the longest cilia, a hair cell becomes depolarized because of an increased conductance of the apical membrane to cations. This depolarization is a **receptor potential,** and it causes the release of an excitatory transmitter that produces a **generator potential** in the primary afferent fibers synapsing on the hair cells. As the oscillations of the basilar membrane move in the opposite direction, the membrane of the hair cell is hyperpolarized, and less transmitter is released. The generator potential in the primary afferent terminals is thus an oscillatory one, and if its amplitude is sufficient during the depolarizing phases, it triggers action potentials in primary afferent nerve fibers.

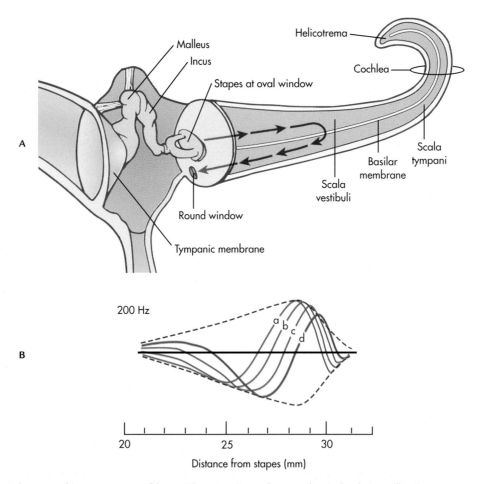

Figure 8-12 A, Impedance-matching arrangement of the ear. The tympanic membrane and ossicular chain oscillate in response to sound waves in the air. The movements of the stapes in the oval window produce comparable oscillations of the fluid columns within the cochlea. The distance along the basilar membrane at which the oscillation is maximal depends on the frequency of the sound. The largest displacements of the basilar membrane are near the base of the cochlea for high frequencies and near the apex for low frequencies. **B,** Traveling wave produced by a 200-Hz sound at four different times (*a* to *d*). The dashed line is the envelope of the peaks of the successive positions of the wave, showing a maximal deflection of the basilar membrane about 29 mm from the stapes.

The difference in potential between the endolymph and the intracellular fluid of the hair cells is unusually high. This potential difference is an important factor in the sensitivity of the auditory system. If the potential in the perilymph is considered the reference potential, the endolymph has a positive steady potential of about 85 mV. This is called the **endocochlear potential** and is the result of electrogenic pumping by the stria vascularis. The resting potential of the hair cells is approximately 85 mV with reference to the endolymph. Because of the positive potential in the endolymph, however, the transmembrane potential across the apical membrane of the hair cells can be as great as 170 mV. This increases the ionic driving forces across the transducer membrane.

An oscillatory potential called the **cochlear microphonic potential** can be recorded from the bony labyrinth of the cochlea. This potential results from the current flow associated with the activity of the hair cells in response to sound. The cochlear microphonic potential has the frequency of the sound stimulus, and its amplitude is graded with the sound intensity.

Cochlear nerve fibers that innervate hair cells at different points along the length of the organ of Corti are tuned to different frequencies of sound. The tuning properties of the primary afferent fibers can be demonstrated by constructing tuning curves that relate the threshold for activation of the fiber to the frequencies of sound stimuli (Figure 8-14). The frequency that activates the fiber at the lowest intensity is called the **characteristic frequency** of the fiber. Cochlear nerve fibers that innervate the organ of Corti near the base of the cochlea have high characteristic frequencies, whereas those innervating the apex have low characteristic frequencies. The organ of Corti is thus organized **tonotopically.**

For the lower part of the frequency range detected by the cochlea (<4000 Hz), the discharges of a given cochlear nerve fiber show **phase locking.** That is, they occur consistently at a particular phase of the sound oscillation. The discharges of a population of afferent nerve fibers could signal the stimulus frequency. This is **volley coding of acoustic signals.** However, cochlear afferent fibers with higher characteristic frequencies do not show phase locking. Coding in these depends on **place coding;** the afferent fibers that innervate regions near the base of the cochlea signal frequencies that depend on the site innervated. **Intensity coding** depends on the number of discharges evoked by sounds of different intensities and presumably also on the number of neurons that discharge.

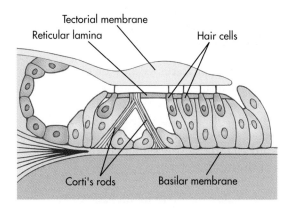

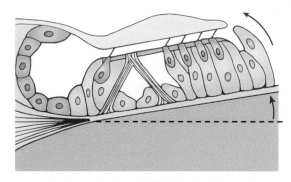

Figure 8-13 Transduction in the organ of Corti. An upward movement of the basilar membrane causes the development of shear forces between the stereocilia of the hair cells and the tectorial membrane, resulting in displacement of the cilia *(arrow).*

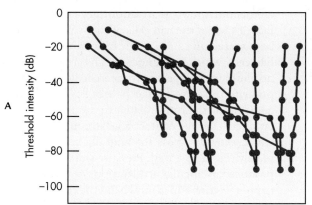

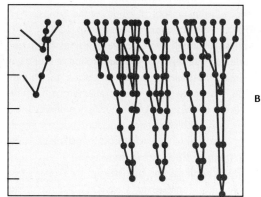

Figure 8-14 Tuning curves for neurons in the auditory pathway. **A,** Tuning curves for excitation of 7 neurons in the cochlear nerve. **B,** Tuning curves for 12 neurons in the inferior colliculus.

The central auditory pathway is responsible for sound localization and analysis of sound frequency

The **superior olivary complex** is concerned with **sound localization.** Neurons in the medial superior olivary nuclei compare the arrival times of sound in the two ears, whereas neurons in the lateral superior olivary nuclei compare differences in the intensity of sounds that reach the two ears. A sound originating from a source located to the left reaches the left ear first, and the head provides an acoustic shield that lowers the intensity of the sound reaching the right ear. By means of these **binaural cues,** signals from the superior olivary nuclei allow the central auditory pathways to judge the location of the sound source.

Binaural processing occurs also in the cerebral cortex, as shown by the presence of **summation** and **suppression columns** in the auditory cortex. The responses of the neurons in these columns depend on whether sounds are introduced into the left or right ear or both ears. In summation columns, neurons respond better when sounds reach both ears rather than only one. Neurons of suppression columns respond better to sound in one ear than to simultaneous sound in both.

Frequency analysis within the central auditory pathways is reflected in the **tonotopic maps** characteristic of many auditory structures. The tonotopic map of the cochlea is also reflected in tonotopic maps in the cochlear nuclei, inferior colliculus, medial geniculate nucleus, and several regions of the auditory cortex.

The degree of deafness and the frequencies affected can be determined by **audiometry.** The patient is tested in each ear with pure tones of different frequencies and intensities. When auditory thresholds for different sample frequencies are compared with those expected in normal subjects, hearing deficits can be described in terms of decibel losses for a certain range of frequencies or for the entire frequency spectrum.

The bilateral organization of the central auditory pathway is the reason that neurological lesions of the brainstem at levels rostral to the cochlear nuclei do not produce unilateral deafness (although large unilateral lesions of the auditory cortex do interfere with the localization of sounds in space). Unilateral deafness implies a defect in the sound-conduction system (e.g., tympanic membrane, ossicle chain) or in the initial stages of the auditory pathway (i.e., organ of Corti, cochlear nerve, cochlear nuclei). These conditions are called **conduction deafness** and **sensory-neural deafness,** respectively.

The type of deafness can be assessed by Weber's test and the Rinne test. For **Weber's test,** a vibrating tuning fork is placed on the forehead. Normally, the sound is not localized to either ear. In conduction deafness, the sound is localized to the deaf ear; in sensory-neural deafness, the sound is localized to the normal ear. For the **Rinne test,** the base of the tuning fork is placed against the mastoid process. In normal subjects, when the sound disappears, it can be heard again if the tuning fork is moved to a position in the air near the external auditory meatus (**air conduction** is better than **bone conduction**). In conduction deafness, bone conduction is better that air conduction, so sound is not restored when the tuning fork is moved.

Vestibular System

The vestibular apparatus is part of the membranous labyrinth of the inner ear. The sensory role of the vestibular system is a form of proprioception. THE VESTIBULAR APPARATUS DETECTS HEAD MOVEMENTS AND THE POSITION OF THE HEAD IN SPACE. To accomplish this, it uses two sets of sensory epithelia to transduce angular and linear accelerations of the head.

The vestibular apparatus includes the semicircular ducts and otolith organs

The **vestibular apparatus** is contained within the bony labyrinth, but unlike the cochlea, its function depends mainly on the membranous labyrinth. The vestibular apparatus is connected with the cochlear duct, contains endolymph, and is surrounded by perilymph. The vestibular apparatus includes three pairs of **semicircular canals** on each side: the **anterior, posterior,** and **horizontal canals** (Figure 8-15). The anterior and posterior canals are oriented in vertical planes perpendicular to each other as well as to the plane of the horizontal canals. Thus the canals are well positioned to sense events in the three dimensions of space. The superior canal on one side is parallel to the posterior canal on the other side; the horizontal canals are in the same plane.

Each of the semicircular canals has a dilation called an **ampulla** (Figure 8-15). Within the ampulla is a sensory epithelium known as an **ampullary crest.** The apical surface of each of the hair cells of the sensory epithelium has both **stereocilia** and a single **kinocilium** (unlike cochlear hair cells, which lack kinocilia). The arrangement of the kinocilium with respect to the stereocilia gives a **functional polarity** to the vestibular hair cells. The cilia are all oriented in the same way relative to the axis of the semicircular duct. The cilia contact a gelatinous mass, the **cupula,** which extends across the ampulla and occludes it completely (Figure 8-15, *A*). Pressure shifts in the endolymph produced by angular accelerations of the head distort the cupula (Figure 8-15, *B*) and bend the cilia of the ampullary crest.

The semicircular canals connect with the **utricle,** one of the otolith organs. The sensory epithelium of the utricle is

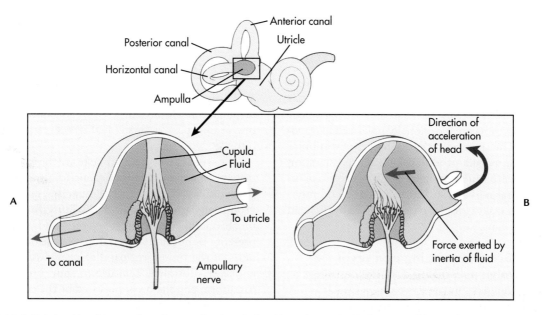

Figure 8-15 A, Relationship of the cupula to the ampulla when the head is stationary. **B,** Displacement of the cupula when the head is rotated.

the **utricular macula,** which is oriented horizontally along the floor of the utricle. The **otolithic membrane** is a gelatinous mass that contains numerous **otoliths** formed from crystals of calcium carbonate. The hair cells of the macula are oriented in relation to a groove called the **striola,** along the length of the macula. For example, the kinocilia in the utricle are on the striolar side of the hair cells. The **saccule** is a separate part of the membranous labyrinth, and the **saccular macula** is oriented vertically. Linear accelerations of the head shift the otolithic membranes with respect to the hair cells. This shift results in bending of the cilia and sensory transduction. Angular accelerations do not substantially affect the otolithic membranes because the otolithic membranes do not protrude into the endolymph.

Vestibular transduction depends on neuroepithelia containing hair cells

When the stereocilia on the vestibular hair cells are bent toward the kinocilium, the hair cell is depolarized because of an increased conductance of the hair cell membrane to cations (Figure 8-16). Bending of the cilia in the opposite direction leads to hyperpolarization. When vestibular hair cells are depolarized, they release more neurotransmitter (probably an excitatory amino acid such as glutamate), and when they are hyperpolarized, they release less. The neurotransmitter excites primary afferent fibers that end on the hair cells. In the absence of overt stimuli, vestibular primary afferent fibers are spontaneously active (Figure 8-16). The activity either increases or decreases depending on the direction in which the cilia are bent.

In the ampullary crest of the horizontal semicircular duct, the kinocilia are arranged so that they are on the

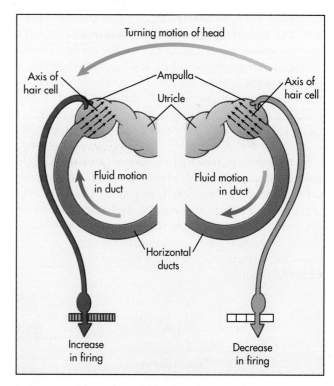

Figure 8-16 Effect of head movement on the hair cells in the ampullae of the horizontal semicircular ducts. The functional polarity of the hair cells is indicated by small arrows.

utricular side of the ampulla (Figures 8-16). If the head is rotated to the left, inertial forces shift the endolymph relatively to the right in both of the horizontal canals. In the left ear, this means that the stereocilia of the hair cells of the left horizontal canal bend toward the kinocilium (toward the utricle) and that the discharges of the primary afferent fibers supplying the left ampullary crest increase.

Conversely, the stereocilia in the crest of the right horizontal duct bend away from their kinocilia (away from the utricle), and thus the discharges of the primary afferent fibers of this crest are reduced.

The orientation of the kinocilia in the utricular macula is toward the striola. The orientation in the saccular macula is away from the striola. That is, hair cells on the two sides of the striola are functionally polarized in opposite directions. The changes in the discharges of vestibular afferents from a macula produced by linear acceleration of the head differ for different hair cells. The pattern of input to the central nervous system is analyzed and interpreted by the central vestibular pathways in terms of head position.

Central vestibular processing and vestibular sensation involve ascending and descending pathways

Primary afferent fibers from the vestibular apparatus reach the brainstem by way of the **vestibular nerve** (cranial nerve VIII). Most of the afferents terminate in the **vestibular nuclei.** The vestibular nuclei connect with the **cerebellum** and **reticular formation,** the **oculomotor nuclei,** and the **spinal cord.** These connections are very important for vestibular control of eye and head movements and posture. A pathway to the cerebral cortex by way of the thalamus is responsible for vestibular sensation.

Chemical Sensory System

The chemical senses include **taste (gustation)** and **smell (olfaction).** They permit the detection of chemical substances in food, water, and the atmosphere. Humans are less adept at chemical detection than many animals, but the chemical senses contribute substantially to the affective aspects of life, and their malfunction can be significant in disease.

Taste is mediated by taste buds

The human gustatory system recognizes many different taste stimuli. However, these can generally be classified as one of four primary taste qualities: sweet, salty, sour, and bitter.

The sensory receptors for taste are the **taste buds.** Most taste buds are on the tongue, but some are on the palate, pharynx, larynx, and upper esophagus. Taste buds occur in groups on papillae (Figure 8-17). **Fungiform papillae** are mushroomlike structures, several hundred of which are present on the anterior two thirds of the tongue. The taste buds of the fungiform papillae respond mainly to sweet and salty substances but also to sour. The taste buds on fungiform papillae are innervated by the **chorda tympani** branch of the **facial nerve. Foliate papillae** are folded structures on the posterior edge of the tongue, and their taste buds respond best to sour stimuli. **Circumvallate papillae** are large, round structures encircled by a depression; they are on the posterior tongue and respond to bitter substances. The foliate and circumvallate papillae are innervated by the **glossopharyngeal nerve.** Taste buds in the region of the epiglottis and upper esophagus are supplied by the **vagus nerve.**

A taste bud consists of a group of some 50 **gustatory receptor cells** in association with supporting cells and basal cells. The gustatory cells are continuously replaced by the differentiation of supporting cells from basal cells. The apical membranes of the gustatory cells have microvilli that protrude into a **taste pore,** where they come into contact with saliva.

Receptor molecules on the microvilli recognize chemical substances in the saliva. The gustatory cells are in syn-

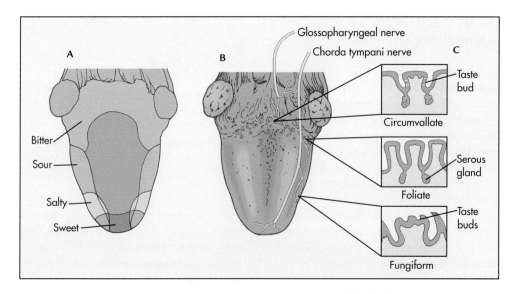

Figure 8-17 Peripheral sensory apparatus for gustation. **A,** Taste qualities associated with different regions of the tongue. **B,** Innervation of taste buds in the anterior two thirds and posterior one third of the tongue by the facial and glossopharyngeal nerves. **C,** Arrangement of the taste buds on the three types of papillae.

aptic contact with primary afferent nerve terminals. Gustatory signals apparently evoke a receptor potential in the gustatory cell, which leads to transmitter release, generator potential, and coded pattern of nerve impulses in the primary afferent fiber. Individual gustatory cells do not appear to be completely selective for a particular primary taste. Rather, they respond best to one type of taste stimulus and less well to others. The recognition of a particular taste quality depends on the activity of a population of gustatory cells. This is a modified labeled-line system.

The primary afferent fibers from the taste buds enter the brainstem and travel caudally in the **solitary tract,** ending in the **nucleus of the solitary tract.** Ascending gustatory fibers reach a special part of the **ventral posteromedial nucleus** of the thalamus. This nucleus projects to the **postcentral gyrus,** ending adjacent to the area representing the tongue. An unusual feature of the gustatory projection is that it is ipsilateral rather than crossed.

Smell depends on the olfactory mucosa and central olfactory pathways

The human olfactory system can recognize many odors. These are difficult to classify, but there are at least seven primary odors: camphoraceous, musk, floral, peppermint, ethereal, pungent, and putrid.

The sensory receptors for olfaction are located in the **olfactory mucosa,** a specialized area of about 2.5 cm^2 in each nasal mucosa. The **olfactory receptor cells** are themselves primary afferent neurons. They have an apical process with cilia that extend into a layer of mucus, in which are dissolved chemical substances that elicit olfactory responses. The base of the olfactory receptor cells gives rise to an axon that projects centrally to end in the **olfactory bulb.** Associated with the olfactory receptor cells are supporting and basal cells that replace olfactory receptor cells as they turn over.

Olfactory transduction depends on the binding of odorants (dissolved in the mucous layer) to receptor molecules on the cilia of olfactory receptor cells. The resulting receptor potential increases the firing rate of the primary afferent fiber. The firing rate is a function of the concentration of the odorant.

The coding mechanism for odors is a modified labelline system similar to that for taste. Olfactory receptors respond best to a particular type of odorant and less well to others. Olfactory receptors are grouped according to sensitivity to the class of odorant and are located in different regions of the olfactory mucosa. The central nervous system is presented with a spatially coded input that partly represents odor qualities.

The central olfactory pathway is complex. An unusual feature is that the primary afferent neurons synapse directly on neurons of the telencephalon, whereas in all other sensory systems, sensory processing occurs at several lower stages before information reaches the telencephalon. The primary afferent axons from olfactory receptors are unmyelinated axons that collect into filaments of the **olfactory nerve** (Figure 8-18). The olfactory nerve bundles pass through the base of the skull and synapse in the **olfactory bulb.** The main projections of the olfactory bulb form the **olfactory tract.** Terminations are made in a number of

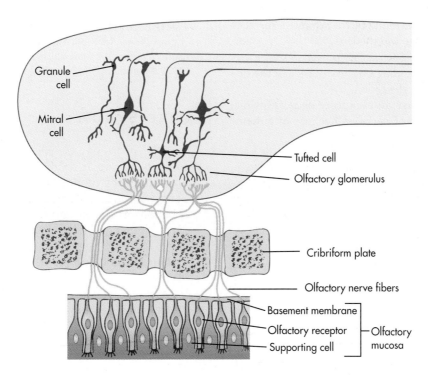

Figure 8-18 Initial part of the olfactory pathway, showing the olfactory receptor cells, their projection to the olfactory bulb, and their synapses in the glomeruli with projection cells known as *tufted* and *mitral cells.* Also shown are some of the granule cells, which serve as inhibitory interneurons.

structures at the base of the brain. The orbitofrontal region of the neocortex also receives olfactory information by way of the thalamus. Presumably, the limbic system projections of the olfactory system are involved in the affective responses to odors, whereas the neocortex is concerned with the discrimination of odors.

Important disturbances in olfaction include **anosmia,** the loss of olfaction, and **uncinate fits,** seizures originating in the temporal lobe that cause **olfactory hallucinations.** Head trauma can cause anosmia on one or both sides because olfactory nerve filaments can be torn as they enter the cranial cavity through the cribriform plate of the ethmoid bone or the cribriform plate may be fractured. Unilateral anosmia can be produced by compression of an olfactory bulb or tract by a tumor, such as an **olfactory groove meningioma.** Uncinate fits are epileptic seizures that originate in a region of the temporal lobe near the olfactory cortex. These seizures begin with a **sensory aura** in which the person undergoing the seizure has an olfactory hallucination of an unpleasant odor, such as burning rubber. After this there may be automatisms, such as movements of the lips and chewing.

SUMMARY

- Vision depends on the detection of visible light by photoreceptors in the eye. Rods are very sensitive but do not provide high-resolution images or information about color. Cones are less sensitive but have good resolving power and allow color vision.
- Light is focused on the retina by the refractive surfaces of the eye: the cornea and the lens.
- The lens has a variable refractory power so that focus can be changed depending on the distance of the object to be imaged on the retina.
- Photoreceptors release an excitatory neurotransmitter under conditions of darkness because of a membrane conductance for Na^+.
- Many photoreceptors and retinal ganglion cells have a center-surround receptive field organization. Some ganglion cells (X-cells) provide signals appropriate for high visual acuity and color; other cells (Y-cells) have nonlinear responses that are appropriate for motion detection. Still other cells (W-cells) may have diffuse receptive fields and signal brightness.
- The auditory system analyzes sound. Sound frequency determines pitch.
- Sound causes oscillatory movements of the tympanic membrane. These movements are transmitted to the oval window by a chain of ossicles.
- Oscillations of the oval window are transmitted to the fluids within the cochlea, resulting in oscillations of the basilar membrane.

- Transduction of sound occurs when movements of the basilar membrane cause the stereocilia on the hair cells of the organ of Corti to bend.
- Cochlear nerve fibers transit signals to the cochlear nuclei in the brainstem. Ascending connections are made bilaterally in the superior olivary complex, inferior colliculus, thalamus, and cortex.
- The semicircular ducts of the vestibular apparatus detect angular accelerations of the head because of an inertial shift in the endolymph, which causes the cilia of the hair cells to bend.
- The otolith organs (utricle and saccule) detect linear accelerations of the head because of shifts in the otolithic membrane in response to changes in gravitational forces.
- The vestibular apparatus sends signals to the brainstem that are used to control eye movements and posture and to evoke vestibular sensations.
- Taste receptors are most sensitive to one of the primary tastes: sweet, salty, sour, and bitter.
- Olfactory receptor cells in the nasal mucosa signal smell.

BIBLIOGRAPHY

Ehret G, Romand R: *The central auditory system,* New York, 1997, Oxford University Press.

Faurion A: Physiology of the sweet taste, *Progr Sensory Physiol* 8:130, 1987.

Merigan WH, Maunsell JHR: How parallel are the primate visual pathways? *Annu Rev Neurosci* 16:369, 1993.

Nicholls JG, Martin AR, Wallace BG: *From neuron to brain,* ed 3, Sunderland, Mass, 1992, Sinauer.

Shepherd GM: *The synaptic organization of the brain,* ed 3, New York, 1990, Oxford University Press.

Wässle H, Boycott BB: Functional architecture of the mammalian retina, *Physiol Rev* 71:447, 1991.

Wilson VJ, Jones GM: *Mammalian vestibular physiology,* New York, 1979, Plenum.

CASE STUDIES

Case 8-1

A 67-year-old woman awakens with impaired vision. On examination, she cannot see objects well in the right visual field of either eye. Some vision is retained in the central regions of the visual fields, but vision is absent in both the upper and lower quadrants.

1. **What is the name for this type of visual field defect?**
   - **A.** Bitemporal hemianopsia
   - **B.** Central scotoma
   - **C.** Homonymous hemianopsia with macular sparing
   - **D.** Inferior homonymous quadrantanopsia
   - **E.** Superior homonymous quadrantanopsia

2. Which artery is involved?
   A. Anterior cerebral
   B. Anterior choroidal
   C. Internal carotid
   D. Middle cerebral
   E. Posterior cerebral

3. Which part of the visual pathway has been damaged?
   A. LGN
   B. Occipital lobe
   C. Optic chiasm
   D. Optic tract
   E. Retina

Case 8-2
A 16-year-old boy notices that he has difficulty understanding what his English teacher is saying in class. He has been a good student, but his grades are falling. On interview by his physician, he admits an enthusiasm for loud rock music. Weber's test shows that sound does not localize to either ear. The Rinne test shows that air conduction is better than bone conduction bilaterally. Audiometry demonstrates a 40- to 60-dB loss of hearing at frequencies above 2500 Hz.

1. What is the boy's hearing deficit called?
   A. Bilateral conduction deafness
   B. Complete deafness
   C. Conduction deficit on the left
   D. Sensorineural deafness on both sides
   E. Sensorineural deficit on right

2. Which structure is most likely to be affected?
   A. Cerebral cortex of temporal lobe
   B. Cochlear nerve
   C. Hair cells of the cochlea
   D. Ossicular chain
   E. Tympanic membranes

Motor System

OBJECTIVES

■ Describe the properties of motor units and of motor neurons.

■ State the structure and function of the muscle stretch receptors (muscle spindles and Golgi tendon organs).

■ Indicate the role of motor neurons and interneurons in spinal cord reflexes.

■ Identify the changes in motor control that occur after transection of the spinal cord or upper brainstem.

■ Describe vestibular and other postural reflexes, locomotion, and the control of eye movements.

■ State the role of the cerebral cortex in motor control.

■ Describe the organization of the cerebellum and the motor consequences of cerebellar disease.

■ Identify disorders caused by damage to the basal ganglia and associated structures.

The term **motor system** refers to the neural pathways that control the sequence and pattern of contractions of skeletal muscles. Skeletal muscle contractions result in **posture, reflexes, rhythmic activity** (e.g., locomotion, respiration), and **voluntary movements.** A given motor act may involve several of these. Motor acts make up a substantial part of the readily observable behavior of an organism. Motor behaviors that are especially important in humans include speech and movements of the digits and eyes.

Motor control depends on sensory signals from muscle **stretch receptors** and the **reflex activity** of the spinal cord. The higher motor centers of the brain superimpose commands on spinal cord reflex activity. These centers include the **brainstem, motor cortex, cerebellum,** and **basal ganglia.** Voluntary movements are initiated by commands generated in the cerebral cortex in concert with activity in a number of cortical control systems. Motor programs are developed by these cortical areas so that muscles are contracted in a coordinated way. The cerebellum and basal ganglia help regulate activity in the motor regions of the cerebral cortex.

Spinal Cord Motor Organization

The motor unit is the basic element in motor control

The **motor unit** consists of an **α-motor neuron,** its **motor axon,** and all the skeletal muscle fibers that it innervates (see Chapter 13). A **muscle unit** is the set of skeletal muscle fibers in a motor unit. The discharge of an α-motor neuron normally results in the contraction of each of the muscle fibers that it supplies because the **endplate potential** in skeletal muscle fibers is normally suprathreshold (see Chapters 4 and 13). In mammals and other vertebrates, no inhibitory synapses exist on skeletal muscle fibers, although they do exist in many invertebrates. This means that all decisions about whether a skeletal muscle fiber will contract are normally made by the α-motor neuron. Furthermore, each time an α-motor neuron discharges, the entire muscle unit contracts. This means that the smallest gradation of force that can be generated by a muscle depends on the force of contraction of the weakest muscle units in that muscle.

A given skeletal muscle contains a number of motor units. The ratio of the total number of skeletal muscle fibers in a muscle to the number of α-motor neurons is the **innervation ratio.** This is the number of muscle fibers in the average motor unit. The innervation ratio is large for muscles that are used for coarse movements (e.g., 2000 fibers for the gastrocnemius muscle) and small for muscles that produce finely graded movements (e.g., 3 to 6 for the eye muscles). The muscle fibers in a motor unit are distributed widely in a muscle, and they are separated by fibers belonging to other motor units. All the skeletal muscle fibers in a motor unit are of the same histochemical type. That is, the muscle fibers are all of type I, type IIB, or type IIA. The contractile properties of these muscle fiber types are summarized in Table 9-1. The motor units that twitch slowly and resist fatigue are classified as **S (slow)** and have type I fibers. S motor units depend on oxidative metabolism for their energy supply and have weak contractions (Figure 9-1). The motor units with fast twitches are **FF (fast, fatigable)** and **FR (fast, fatigue resistant).** FF motor units have type IIB fibers, use glycolytic metabolism, and have strong contractions, but they fatigue easily. FR motor units have type IIA fibers and rely on oxidative metabolism; their contractions are of intermediate force, and these motor units resist fatigue (Figure 9-1).

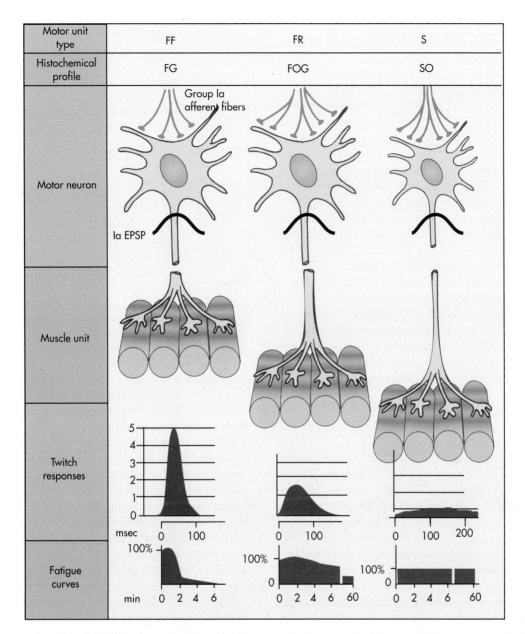

Motor unit type	FF	FR	S
Histochemical profile	FG	FOG	SO
Motor neuron			
Muscle unit			
Twitch responses			
Fatigue curves			

Figure 9-1 Summary of features of motor units in a mixed muscle (medial gastrocnemius muscle of a cat). Relative sizes are shown for motor neurons, muscle fibers, monosynaptic excitatory postsynaptic potentials *(EPSP)* evoked by volleys in group Ia afferent fibers, and twitch responses. *FF,* Fast, fatigable; *FG,* fast glycolytic; *FOG,* fast, oxidative-glycolytic; *FR,* fast, fatigue resistant; *S,* slow; *SO,* slow, oxidative.

α-Motor neurons form the final common pathway

The only way in which the central nervous system can cause skeletal muscle fibers to contract is by evoking discharges in α-motor neurons. Therefore all motor acts depend on neural circuits that eventually impinge on α-motor neurons. This is why these neurons are called the **final common pathway.**

The motor nucleus contains α-motor neurons

α-Motor neurons are large neurons found in lamina IX of the spinal cord ventral horn and in **cranial nerve motor**

Table 9-1	Muscle Fiber Contractile Properties			
Type	**Speed**	**Strength**	**Fatigability**	**Motor Unit**
I	Slow	Weak	Fatigue resistant	S
IIB	Fast	Strong	Fatigable	FF
IIA	Fast	Intermediate	Fatigue resistant	FR

nuclei that supply skeletal muscles. Each muscle or group of synergistic muscles (i.e., those having a similar action) has its own **motor nucleus.** α-Motor neurons that supply a given muscle are generally arranged as a longitudinal column of cells, often extending two or three segments in the spinal cord and several millimeters in the brainstem. The set of α-motor neurons that innervates a muscle is called the **motor neuron pool** of the muscle.

The motor nuclei of different muscles or muscle groups are located in different parts of the ventral horn. That is, motor nuclei have a **somatotopic organization.** Motor nuclei that supply the axial muscles of the body are in the medial part of the ventral horn in the cervical and lumbosacral enlargements and in the most ventral part of the ventral horn in the upper cervical, thoracic, and upper lumbar segments of the spinal cord. The innervation ratio for the motor units in these muscles is large because the role of the axial muscles includes gross activities such as maintenance of posture, support for limb movements, and respiration.

Motor nuclei that innervate the limb muscles are in the lateral part of the ventral horn in the cervical and lumbosacral enlargements. The most distal muscles are supplied by motor nuclei located in the dorsolateral part of the ventral horn, whereas more proximal muscles are innervated by motor nuclei in the ventrolateral ventral horn. The innervation ratios of these muscles are smaller for the distal muscles and larger for the proximal ones.

Motor neurons are large cells with several processes

The individual α-motor neuron (Figure 9-2) is a cell with a large soma (≤70 μm in diameter). Each of the 5 to 22 dendrites may be as long as 1 mm. The large myelinated axon has a diameter of 12 to 20 μm, and its conduction velocity is 72 to 120 m/sec. The axon of an α-motor neuron is often called an **α-motor axon.** It arises from an axon hillock on the soma or a proximal dendrite and has a short, unmyelinated **initial segment** before the myelin sheath begins. These axons collect in bundles that leave the ventral horn, pass through the ventral white matter of the spinal cord, and enter a filament of the ventral root. Just before leaving the ventral horn, some α-motor axons give off **recurrent collaterals.** Recurrent collaterals typically project dorsally and synapse on interneurons, called **Renshaw cells,** in the ventral part of lamina VII (see later section).

Synaptic integration depends on postsynaptic potentials

The dendrites and soma of the α-motor neuron are covered with synapses from primary afferent fibers, interneurons, and pathways that descend from the brain. Most of the synapses are from interneurons. Approximately half of the surface membrane lies beneath synaptic endings. Some of the synapses are excitatory, whereas others are inhibitory.

The part of the α-motor neuron membrane with the lowest threshold is thought to be the **initial segment,** which therefore serves as a **trigger zone** for the generation of action potentials. Excitatory synaptic currents depolar-

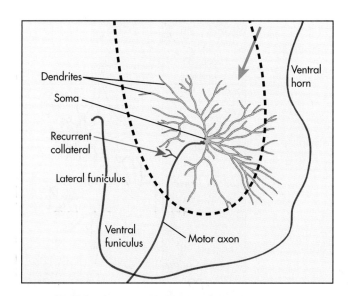

Figure 9-2 α-Motor neuron injected intracellularly with horseradish peroxidase. A small arrow indicates a recurrent collateral of the motor axon. The large arrow shows the direction followed by the microelectrode.

ize all parts of the membrane of the motor neuron, but in terms of the initiation of an action potential, the depolarization of the initial segment is crucial. The **excitatory postsynaptic potentials (EPSPs)** produced by activation of more than one excitatory pathway to a motor neuron may sum (Figure 9-3, *A*), and the summed EPSPs may exceed threshold for discharge **(spatial summation).** Alternatively, repetitive activation of an excitatory pathway can produce **temporal summation** (see Chapter 4). **Inhibitory postsynaptic potentials (IPSPs)** interfere with the excitatory ones and tend to prevent the discharge of an action potential (Figure 9-3, *B*). The interaction of excitatory and inhibitory synaptic currents in determining whether a neuron discharges is termed **synaptic integration.**

The location of a synapse on the membrane of a neuron such as an α-motor neuron may determine the effectiveness of that particular synapse in synaptic integration. Analysis of the **passive electrical properties** of α-motor neurons indicates that synaptic currents can reach the initial segment from even the most distant part of the dendritic tree. However, synaptic potentials produced by distal synapses are smaller and slower than those produced by proximal synapses. For example, if a synapse on a dendrite is one **length constant** (see Chapter 3) away from the initial segment, the size of the membrane potential change in the initial segment is only about one third (1/e) of that generated in the dendrite. Furthermore, synaptic potentials are considerably slowed.

In many neurons, inhibitory synapses, which prevent the generation of action potentials, tend to be located near the initial segment. Another arrangement is that excitatory and inhibitory synapses from neural pathways with antagonistic functions are located near each other on a given dendrite but away from the initial segment. This allows different pathways to influence the motor

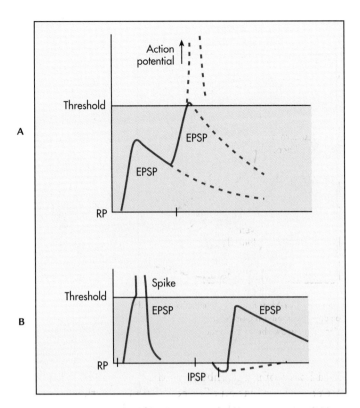

Figure 9-3 Synaptic integration. **A,** Summation of two EPSPs recorded from an α-motor neuron. The second EPSP exceeds threshold, so an action potential is triggered. The two EPSPs can result from the stimulation of separate pathways (spatial summation) or the repetitive activation of a single pathway (temporal summation). **B,** An EPSP and the action potential it triggers are shown at the left, and the interaction between the EPSP and an inhibitory postsynaptic potential *(IPSP)* at the right. Note that the IPSP prevents the EPSP from triggering the spike. *RP,* Resting potential.

neuron independently. In still another arrangement, excitatory synaptic endings of one pathway receive axoaxonal synapses from another. These axoaxonal synapses cause presynaptic inhibition, which can reduce the effectiveness of a pathway to the motor neuron without altering the excitability of the motor neuron, allowing it to participate in other pathways.

Action potentials generated by α-motor neurons have special features

When a motor neuron discharges in response to synaptic excitation, the potentials follow a characteristic sequence. A recording from the soma first reveals an EPSP (Figure 9-4, *A*). Arising from this is a spike potential with two phases: an initial small spike, on which is superimposed a slightly delayed but larger spike. The first small spike is believed to represent the action potential generated by the initial segment; it is small in a recording from the soma because of **electrotonic decrement.** The larger spike is thought to represent invasion of the soma by the action potential. The activation of a motor neuron in this fashion is called **orthodromic activation** because the sequence is in the normal, or orthograde, direction.

Under experimental conditions an action potential may be initiated in the motor axon and conducted retrogradely to the motor neuron. This is called **antidromic activation** (Figure 9-4, *B*). A recording from the soma of the motor neuron reveals that the antidromic action potential arises directly from the resting membrane potential and has the same series of small and larger spikes as the orthodromic action potential. The missing part of the potential sequence is the EPSP. After the spike, a long afterhyperpolarization occurs. This is also present in orthodromic action potentials, but it is often obscured by the EPSP.

The afterhyperpolarization is a very important feature of the motor neuronal action potential because it helps determine the characteristic firing rate of the neuron. Large α-motor neurons have shorter afterhyperpolarizations (≈50 msec long) than small α-motor neurons (≈100 msec long). Therefore large α-motor neurons tend to discharge at rates of up to about 20 Hz, whereas small ones discharge at approximately 10 Hz.

Muscle fibers contract with a twitch when a motor neuron discharges once. However, repetitive discharges result in a **tetanic contraction** of the muscle (see Chapter 13). The contractile force of a tetanic contraction increases with the rate of discharge of the motor neuron up to a limit imposed by the properties of the muscle. When the tetanic contraction is submaximal, muscle force increases with each motor neuronal discharge. This condition is called an **unfused** or **incomplete tetanus.** When the tetanic contraction is maximal, the contraction becomes a **fused** or **complete tetanus.** The motor neuronal firing rate that produces a fused tetanus in the motor unit causes the greatest contractile force possible for that motor unit.

The characteristic firing rates of α-motor neurons match the mechanical properties of the skeletal muscle fibers they innervate. For example, large motor neurons fire at fast rates and innervate fast-twitch muscle fibers; that is, the muscle units of large motor neurons are either the FF or the FR type (Table 9-1). Small motor neurons fire at low rates and innervate slow-twitch muscle fibers; the muscle units of small motor neurons are the S type.

The contraction of a muscle is regulated by the nervous system in two ways. The first is by altering the **firing rates** of α-motor neurons. As already indicated, the effects of changing the firing rate are limited by the firing rate at which a tetanus in a given motor unit becomes fused. The second means of regulating muscle tension is by changing the number of active α-motor neurons. This activation is called **recruitment.**

The recruitment of α-motor neurons is orderly. Small α-motor neurons are usually recruited more easily than large ones. This may be related to differences in the membrane properties of small and large α-motor neurons or may reflect the synaptic organization that controls their discharges. This difference is called the **size principle.** Not only are the small α-motor neurons recruited before the large ones during excitation, but the activity of the small α-motor neurons persists longer than that of the large

Orthodromic excitation

Antidromic activation and
recurrent inhibition

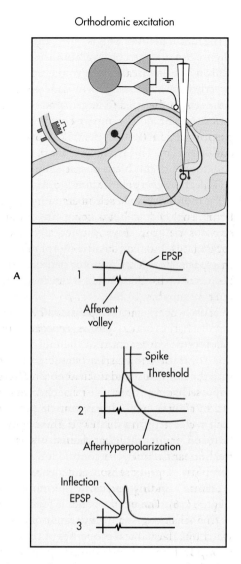

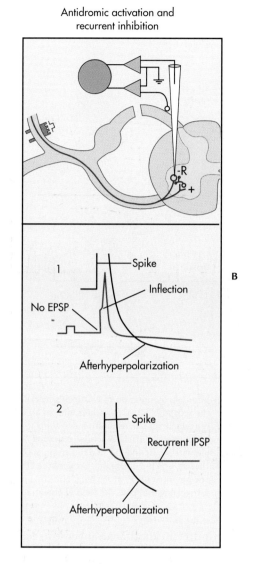

Figure 9-4 Orthodromic and antidromic action potentials recorded from motor neurons. **A,** Monosynaptic EPSP *(1),* a larger EPSP that reaches threshold on some trials *(2),* and a low-gain recording of an orthodromic action potential *(3).* In *3,* the arrows indicate the EPSP *(smaller crest)* and the inflection between the initial segment and the soma-dendritic spikes *(upper crest).* The drawing at the top shows the recording arrangement and the interruption of the ventral root to prevent antidromic activation. **B,** Recordings in *1* show an antidromic action potential in a motor neuron at high gain *(truncated spike)* and at low gain. Note the inflection on the rising phase of the spike. Also note that the spike is succeeded by a large afterhyperpolarization. This is best seen in the high-gain record. In *2,* most of the records are with the stimulus subthreshold for the motor axon, and thus the potentials recorded are IPSPs caused by the activity of Renshaw cells *(R)* excited by other motor axons. The drawing at the top shows the experimental arrangement. Note that the dorsal root is cut to prevent orthodromic excitation.

ones during inhibition. Because the diameters of the motor axons of large α-motor neurons are greater than the diameters of the axons of small α-motor neurons, the action potentials recorded extracellularly from the ventral root are greater for the large than for the small α-motor neurons (Figure 9-5). This allows evaluation of the recruiting sequence by recordings from the ventral root.

Because of the progressive and orderly recruitment of small and then large α-motor neurons, a weak activation of a motor neuronal pool discharges only the small α-motor neurons. This activity produces a weak, slow contraction of slow-twitch muscle fibers. This type of muscle activity is suited to the maintenance of posture and to slow movements, such as walking. The recruitment of large α-motor neurons activates powerful fast-twitch muscle fibers. The

contractions of these fibers add to the initial force evoked by the slow-twitch fibers, and the resulting movements are appropriate to vigorous activity, such as running and jumping.

Several diseases of the central nervous system cause weakness by destroying α-motor neurons. One of these is **poliomyelitis.** For unknown reasons, the poliovirus selectively kills α-motor neurons and thus paralyzes the muscles they supply. Usually, the α-motor neurons affected are concentrated in only a few motor nuclei of the spinal cord, but more widespread loss can occur, and sometimes cranial nerve motor nuclei are involved (bulbar polio). The

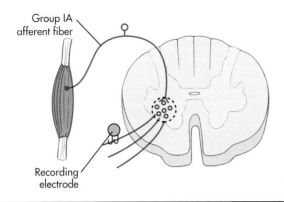

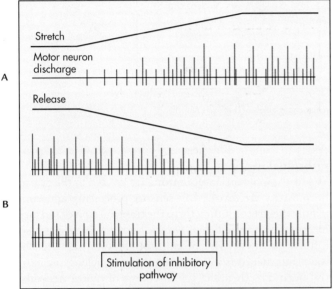

Figure 9-5 Size principle and motor neuron recruitment. *Top,* Arrangement of the electrode during the experiment. **A,** Stretching the muscle activates several motor neurons. The motor axon with the smallest action potential in the ventral root filament is activated first; then progressively larger units begin to discharge. The converse sequence is seen when the muscle is released from the stretch: the large units stop firing first. **B,** An inhibitory input causes cessation of discharge of the larger units but not of the small unit.

denervated muscle undergoes atrophy, although some muscle fibers may be reinnervated by collateral sprouts of the axons of α-motor neurons that did not die.

Another disease that affects α-motor neurons is **amyotrophic lateral sclerosis (ALS),** often called **Lou Gehrig's disease** after the baseball player of the New York Yankees who died of this disease. In ALS, α-motor neurons at all levels of the spinal cord and brainstem gradually die. As they die, they discharge erratically and cause **fasciculations** (visible contractions of motor units). After an α-motor neuron dies, the denervated muscle fibers of its motor unit **atrophy** and develop **fibrillations** (spontaneous contractions of individual muscle fibers that cannot be seen through the skin but that can be observed by **electromyography**). In ALS, cortical pyramidal cells that give rise to the corticospinal tract (see later section) also die, resulting in further weakness of voluntary movements and pathological reflexes.

Muscle stretch receptors are important sense organs

Skeletal muscles and their tendons contain specialized sensory receptors called **stretch receptors** that discharge when the muscles are stretched. These receptors include **muscle spindles** and **Golgi tendon organs.** These receptors are involved in sensory experience and contribute to proprioception (see Chapter 7). However, they are discussed here because of their importance in motor control.

The most complex muscle receptor is the muscle spindle. Muscle spindles are composed of elongated bundles of narrow muscle fibers called **intrafusal muscle fibers** enclosed within a connective tissue capsule. The spindles are richly innervated with both sensory and motor endings. Most of the muscle spindle lies freely within the spaces between the regular or **extrafusal muscle fibers,** but its distal ends merge with the connective tissue in the muscle. This parallel arrangement is important for the operation of the muscle spindle. When the whole muscle contracts, the muscle spindle is unloaded unless the intrafusal fibers also contract.

The intrafusal muscle fibers are of two main types: **nuclear bag fibers** and **nuclear chain fibers.** Their names are based on the arrangement of their nuclei (Figure 9-6). Nuclear bag fibers are larger than nuclear chain fibers and have a cluster of nuclei near the midpoint (resembling a "bag" of oranges). Nuclear chain fibers have a single row of nuclei near the midpoint.

The two types of sensory endings in a muscle spindle are a **primary ending** and one or more **secondary endings** (Figure 9-6). The primary ending has spiral terminals on both nuclear bag and nuclear chain fibers, and it is innervated by a large, myelinated afferent nerve fiber called a **group Ia fiber.** Secondary endings have spraylike terminals that are chiefly on nuclear chain fibers. The secondary endings are supplied by medium-sized **group II fibers.**

γ-Motor neurons provide the motor innervation of muscle spindles (Figure 9-6). The endings may be small endplates or elongated trail endings. There are two types of γ-motor neurons: **dynamic γ-motor neurons** innervate chiefly the nuclear bag intrafusal muscle fibers, and **static γ-motor neurons** supply nuclear chain fibers.

Primary endings respond to maintained muscle stretch with a slowly adapting discharge that has both a dynamic and a static component (Figure 9-7). The dynamic response signals the rate of stretch of muscle, and the static component signals muscle length. Secondary endings have only a static response; thus they signal muscle length. The dynamic response probably results from the property of nuclear bag fibers of elastic rebound after an initial rapid elongation during muscle stretch.

γ-Motor neurons regulate the sensitivity of muscle spindles to muscle stretch. They can also prevent the unloading effect of muscle shortening by contracting the intrafusal muscle fibers during or just before contracting the extrafusal muscle fibers (Figure 9-8). Dynamic γ-motor neurons enhance the dynamic responses of the primary

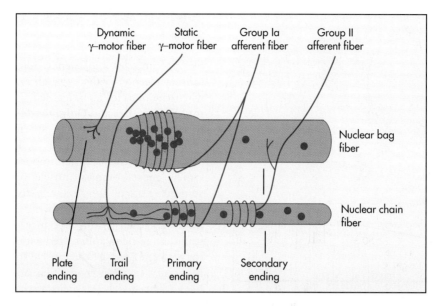

Figure 9-6 Innervation of nuclear bag and nuclear chain fibers of a muscle spindle.

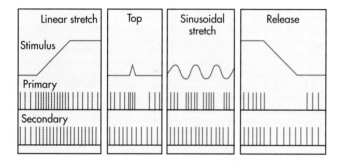

Figure 9-7 Responses of primary and secondary endings of a muscle spindle to linear stretch, tap, sinusoidal stretch, and release of the muscle.

endings, and static γ-motor neurons increase the static responses of both primary and secondary endings. THE CENTRAL NERVOUS SYSTEM CAN THUS INDEPENDENTLY REGULATE DYNAMIC AND STATIC RESPONSES OF MUSCLE SPINDLES.

Another type of muscle stretch receptor is the **Golgi tendon organ.** These receptors are found in tendons, in the connective tissue within skeletal muscles, and around joint capsules. Golgi tendon organs are supplied by large, myelinated primary afferent nerve fibers, called **group Ib fibers.** The terminals of group Ib fibers interdigitate with bundles of collagen fibers, an arrangement that allows the application of mechanical force to the terminals when the muscle is either contracted or stretched (Figure 9-9). Golgi tendon organs are therefore arranged in series with the muscle and its tendon.

Spinal cord interneurons form motor control circuits

As mentioned earlier, most of the synapses on α-motor neurons originate from spinal cord interneurons. **Interneurons** are neurons interposed between primary afferent neurons and motor neurons. Interneurons whose pro-

cesses are confined to the spinal cord are often called **propriospinal neurons.**

Most spinal cord interneurons are located in the dorsal horn. Many are involved in sensory processing and contribute directly or indirectly to the transmission of sensory information to the brain. Dorsal horn interneurons also influence reflex activity, often through polysynaptic pathways. Interneurons in the intermediate nucleus and ventral horn directly affect the discharge of motor neurons. Furthermore, axons in pathways that descend from the brain only rarely terminate directly on motor neurons. Instead they usually end on interneurons and alter motor output by changing the level of activity in spinal cord neural circuits.

Various types of interneurons involved in motor control have been well characterized. The Renshaw cell has already been mentioned. **Renshaw cells** are inhibitory interneurons located in the part of lamina VII that protrudes ventrally between the lateral part of lamina IX and lamina VIII. Recurrent collaterals from α-motor axons synapse on Renshaw cells. When the motor axons discharge, they release acetylcholine at the synapses on Renshaw cells and excite these cells. The Renshaw cells in turn synapse on and inhibit α-motor neurons; the discharge of α-motor neurons causes an inhibitory feedback via Renshaw cells. This is called **recurrent inhibition** (Figure 9-4, *B*).

Another well-studied interneuron is the **group Ia inhibitory interneuron.** These interneurons are located in the dorsal part of lamina VII. They are excited monosynaptically by group Ia primary afferent fibers from the primary endings of muscle spindles. The term **monosynaptic** implies a neural pathway in which there is only one synaptic interruption between one element of the pathway and the next. Group Ia inhibitory interneurons in turn synapse on the α-motor neurons that supply the muscle or muscle group that serves as the antagonist to the muscle that gives

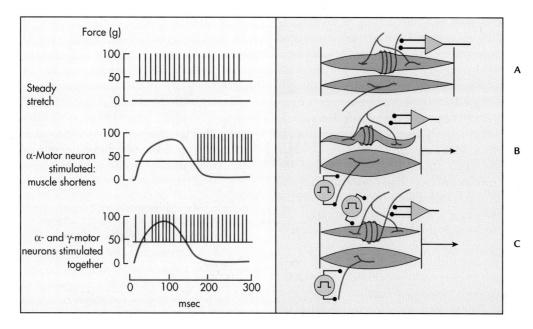

Figure 9-8 Effect of the activation of γ-motor neurons. **A,** Stretch of the muscle activates an afferent fiber supplying a muscle spindle. **B,** The discharge stops when a muscle contraction is produced by activity in α-motor neurons. **C,** The effect of unloading is avoided because α- and γ-motor neurons are coactivated.

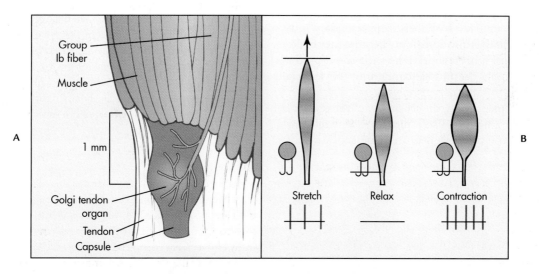

Figure 9-9 A, Structure of a Golgi tendon organ and its relationship to the tendon of a muscle. **B,** The recordings at the bottom show that a Golgi tendon organ can be activated by either muscle stretch or muscle contraction. The activity of Golgi tendon organs signals muscle tension.

rise to the group Ia afferent fibers. Thus a disynaptic pathway is formed that involves group Ia fibers from one muscle group, inhibitory interneurons, and α-motor neurons to the antagonist muscle group (Figure 9-10).

Spinal cord reflexes underlie motor responses

A **reflex** is a relatively simple, stereotyped motor response to a defined sensory input. Some of the reflexes mediated by spinal cord circuits are described here. However, many other reflexes are also organized at the level of either the spinal cord or the brain (see later section).

Stretch reflexes are responses to muscle spindle input

A particularly important spinal reflex is the **stretch reflex.** Stretching a muscle causes a reflex contraction of that muscle and a reflex relaxation of the antagonist muscles. The stretch reflex has the following components: phasic and tonic. The **phasic stretch reflex** is elicited by stretching the muscle quickly. This is often done clinically by tapping the tendon of the muscle with a reflex hammer. For example, when the patellar tendon is struck, a knee jerk reflex results. The **tonic stretch reflex** results from a slower stretch of a muscle, such as occurs during passive movement of a joint by an examining physician. THE TONIC STRETCH REFLEX IS IMPORTANT IN THE MAINTENANCE OF POSTURE.

Hinge joints, such as the knee and ankle, are extended or flexed by extensor and flexor muscles, which are antagonists because they produce opposite movements of the joint. A phasic stretch reflex produced by stretching an extensor muscle results in contraction of the extensor muscle and relaxation of the flexor muscle. Conversely, a phasic stretch reflex of the flexor muscle involves a concomitant relaxation of the extensor muscle. This organization of the stretch reflex pathways is called **reciprocal innervation.**

The neural basis of a spinal reflex is the reflex arc, a circuit that includes a set of primary afferent fibers, interneurons, and α-motor neurons. The reflex arc for the phasic stretch reflex of a particular muscle includes (1) group Ia afferent fibers from primary endings of muscle spindles located within that muscle, (2) monosynaptic excitatory connections of these afferents with α-motor neurons that innervate the muscle, and (3) a disynaptic inhibitory pathway involving group Ia inhibitory interneurons that synapse with α-motor neurons innervating the antagonistic muscles (Figure 9-10).

The reflex arc for the tonic stretch reflex involves the same connections just described for the phasic stretch reflex. However, group II afferent fibers from secondary endings of muscle spindles also contribute because they make monosynaptic excitatory connections with the α-motor neurons that supply the muscle containing the muscle spindles.

As previously mentioned, the sensitivity of the primary and secondary endings of muscle spindles is controlled by dynamic and static α-motor neurons. The activation of these neurons can result in a sufficiently strong excitatory input in group Ia afferent fibers to discharge the γ-motor neurons. However, the group Ia fibers in humans discharge after contractions of skeletal muscle. This pattern of discharge indicates that γ-motor neurons do activate muscle spindles during voluntary movements but at about the same time as the activation of α-motor neurons. Presumably the shortening of the muscle spindles prevents unloading. Thus voluntary and other movements depend on the coactivation of α- and γ-motor neurons.

In neurological examinations, a reflex hammer is commonly used to elicit **phasic stretch reflexes.** The limb to be examined is placed in a position that allows relaxation of the joint operated on by the muscle tested. The tendon of each muscle tested is struck briskly with the reflex hammer, and the subsequent contraction of the muscle is observed (or felt). Responses on the two sides are compared. The fact that tendons are struck gave rise to a misleading terminology for the stretch reflex *(deep tendon reflex);* this terminology should be avoided. The sensory receptors responsible for the phasic stretch reflex are muscle spindles located within the muscle and not receptors in the tendon. Muscles that are often tested include the biceps brachii, the quadriceps, and the triceps surae. When phasic stretch reflexes appear to be reduced, it is sometimes possible to enhance them by **Jendrassik's maneuver,** in which the subject interlocks the fingers of the two hands and pulls the hands apart against resistance. **Tonic stretch reflexes** are examined by flexing and extending joints.

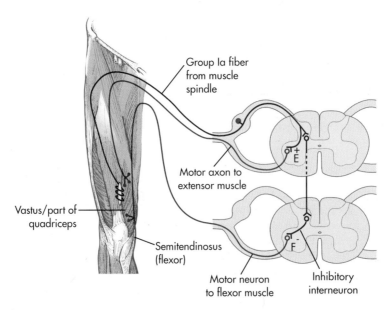

Figure 9-10 Reflex pathway for the stretch reflex. The illustration is for the quadriceps stretch reflex, but similar connections can be made for other muscles, including flexor muscles. A muscle spindle is shown to be supplied by a group Ia fiber that enters the spinal cord through a dorsal root and makes monosynaptic excitatory connections with an α-motor neuron to the quadriceps muscle in the same segment and a group Ia inhibitory interneuron in another segment. The inhibitory interneuron synapses with an α-motor neuron to the antagonistic flexor muscle, semitendinosus. *E,* Extensor motor neuron; *F,* flexor motor neuron.

In pathological conditions, the stretch reflexes may be either diminished or hyperactive. Causes of decreased stretch reflexes include the death of motor neurons as a result of motor neuron disease (e.g., poliomyelitis, ALS) and the interruption of peripheral nerves or spinal roots (such as occurs in peripheral neuropathy or after a herniated disk). Increased stretch reflexes are seen in diseases that affect the descending motor pathways, such as cerebrovascular accidents (strokes) that interrupt the internal capsule.

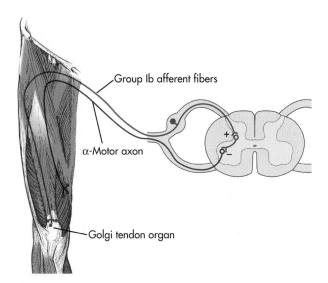

Figure 9-11 Pathway for the inverse myotatic reflex produced by Golgi tendon organs. A Golgi tendon organ is shown in the patellar tendon. Its group Ib afferent fiber enters the spinal cord through a dorsal root to terminate on an inhibitory interneuron that synapses on a motor neuron to the quadriceps muscle.

The inverse myotatic reflex depends on input from Golgi tendon organs

An important reflex whose afferent limb is group Ib afferent fibers from Golgi tendon organs is sometimes called the **inverse myotatic reflex.** Group Ib afferent fibers from extensor muscles synapse monosynaptically on inhibitory interneurons (Figure 9-11). The inhibitory interneurons in turn synapse on the α-motor neurons that supply the same and other extensor muscles in the limb. Flexor muscles are relatively unaffected by this pathway. This pathway is activated by increases in muscle force, which can be produced either by stretch or contraction of the muscle, rather than by stretch alone. Therefore the word *myotatic* (which refers to muscle stretch) is probably inappropriate.

Reflexes may form negative-feedback loops

The stretch and the group Ib (inverse myotatic) reflexes are examples of negative-feedback loops. In a **negative-feedback loop,** the output of the system is compared with the desired output (Figure 9-12). Any difference (error) is fed back to the input so that a corrective action can be made. The variable regulated by a negative-feedback system is the **controlled variable.** In the stretch reflex the controlled variable is the muscle length; in the group Ib pathway it is muscle force.

An example of how these negative-feedback loops might operate is the muscle behavior in a soldier at attention. The knees tend to flex because of gravitational forces. If slight flexion occurs, the knee extensor muscles are stretched, which activates the stretch reflex in these muscles. The result is restoration of knee extension. In terms of muscle length, gravitational forces tend to stretch

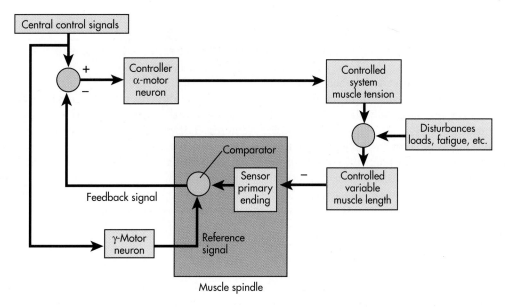

Figure 9-12 Operation of the stretch reflex as a negative-feedback system that regulates muscle length. Length is determined by the level of muscle tension, which depends on activity in α-motor neurons. Muscle length is detected by the muscle spindle, which has its sensitivity set by γ-motor neurons. If the muscle length is increased, such as by a changed load, feedback conveyed by the primary endings increases the discharges of α-motor neurons, which reduces muscle length through further contraction of the muscle.

the knee extensors; the stretch reflex acts as a negative-feedback mechanism to control muscle length, keeping it constant. On the other hand, if the knee extensor muscles begin to fatigue, the force that they exert on the patellar tendon decreases, causing the knee to flex. However, a reduction in the tension in the patellar tendon reduces the activity of Golgi tendon organs in the tendon. Decreased activity in group Ib afferent fibers reduces the inverse myotatic reflex (which inhibits α-motor neurons to the knee extensor muscles), which allows the knee extensor muscles to contract more vigorously. Thus a reduction in tension in the patellar tendon causes a negative feedback, which restores the tension toward its original level.

Reflexes control muscle stiffness

The concurrent regulation of muscle length and muscle force makes it possible to control muscle stiffness. Muscle has mechanical properties that resemble those of a spring. When a spring is slack, it exerts no force. When the spring is lengthened beyond a threshold point, known as the **set point** (or resting length), each increment of stretch is associated with the development of an increment of force. The relationship between length and force in an ideal spring is linear, and the slope of the length-force curve is the stiffness of the spring:

$$\text{Stiffness} = \text{Change in force} \div \text{Change in length}$$

The stiffness of different springs varies, being greater if more force is produced for a given increment of stretch.

Muscles also have characteristic **length-force relationships** (see Chapter 12). These are determined with the muscle relaxed or activated by nerve stimulation, and the curves that represent these relationships can be highly nonlinear. If a muscle is passively stretched, the muscle develops force as it is stretched beyond the set point (resting length). When the nerve to the muscle is stimulated, the length-force curve shifts, now having a lower set point and a greater slope. The increased slope indicates that contraction has increased the stiffness of the muscle. It is the interplay between length and force that regulates muscle stiffness and that sets joint position.

In a joint whose position is controlled by sets of agonist and antagonist muscles, a particular joint angle **(equilibrium point)** can actually be attained in several ways. Because the extensor and flexor muscles are reciprocally innervated, neural circuitry is available to cause one muscle to be activated and the antagonist to be relaxed. The combination of these two events determines the equilibrium point of the joint. Another possibility is **co-contraction** of the agonist and antagonist muscles. Although this mechanism requires more energy than the one using reciprocal innervation, co-contraction can provide stability in case of unanticipated changes in load because the stiffness of the joint is increased. One typically uses co-contraction to perform a new task un-

til the task is learned, when co-contraction is replaced by the strategy of relaxing the antagonist.

Flexion reflexes have several roles

Other important reflexes, such as the flexion reflex, also operate at the spinal cord level. In the flexion reflex the **physiological flexor muscles** of one or more joints in a limb contract and the **physiological extensor muscles** relax. THE PHYSIOLOGICAL FLEXOR MUSCLES ARE THOSE THAT TEND TO WITHDRAW THE LIMB FROM A NOXIOUS STIMULUS. The flexion reflex has several uses. The **flexor withdrawal reflex** consists of a defensive removal of a limb from a threatening or damaging stimulus. For example, if one steps on a nail, the foot is withdrawn reflexly by flexion of the ankle, knee, and hip. This reflex takes precedence over other reflexes. It may be accompanied by a **crossed extensor reflex,** which involves the contraction of the extensor muscles and the relaxation of the flexor muscles of the contralateral limb. The crossed extension serves as a postural adjustment to compensate for the loss of the antigravitational support by the limb that flexes. In quadrupeds the converse pattern can occur in the other pair of limbs. The flexion reflex is also involved in locomotion and in the scratch reflex.

The flexion reflex is initiated by the flexion reflex afferent fibers, which supply high-threshold muscle and joint receptors, many cutaneous receptors, and nociceptors. It seems likely that the lower-threshold receptors help modulate locomotion and that the nociceptors are crucial for evoking the flexor withdrawal reflex. The flexion reflex pathway from primary afferent fibers to the α-motor neurons is polysynaptic and involves both excitatory and inhibitory interneurons (Figure 9-13). There are both uncrossed and crossed components of the pathway. The α-motor neurons involved are those appropriate to the reflex movements already described.

Organization of Descending Motor Pathways

The descending motor pathways have traditionally been divided into pyramidal and extrapyramidal components. The **pyramidal system** includes the corticospinal and corticobulbar tracts. *Pyramidal* refers to the presence of at least part of these tracts in the medullary pyramid. THE PYRAMIDAL SYSTEM IS THE MAIN PATHWAY THAT MEDIATES VOLUNTARY MOVEMENTS OF THE DISTAL PARTS OF THE EXTREMITIES AS WELL AS MIMETIC MOVEMENTS OF THE FACE MUSCLES AND MOVEMENTS OF THE TONGUE. The **extrapyramidal system** originally referred to motor pathways other than the corticospinal and corticobulbar tracts. At present, however, *extrapyramidal* is most usefully applied to motor disorders associated with lesions involving the **basal ganglia,** without reference to the particular motor pathways affected.

A helpful classification of descending motor pathways is based on their site of termination in the spinal

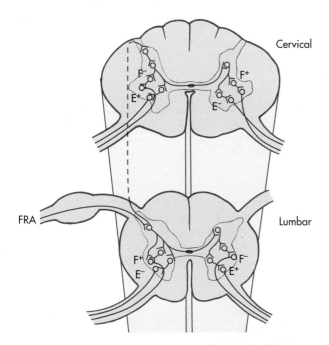

Figure 9-13 Flexion reflex pathway. The receptive field of flexion reflex afferents *(FRA)* on the lower extremity is not shown. The activation of these afferents leads to input over the dorsal roots of the lumbar enlargement. Via polysynaptic connections, flexor motor neurons *(F)* of the lower extremity on the side stimulated are activated and extensor motor neurons *(E)* inhibited, resulting in flexion of the lower extremity. Crossed connections activate extensor motor neurons and inhibit flexor motor neurons to the opposite lower extremity, the crossed extensor reflex. A reverse pattern of reflex activity may be produced in the upper extremities.

cord. One set of pathways ends on motor neurons in the lateral part of lamina IX or on the interneurons that project to them (Figure 9-14). THIS LATERAL SYSTEM OF DESCENDING PATHWAYS CONTROLS THE MUSCLES OF THE DISTAL PART OF THE LIMBS. THESE MUSCLES SUBSERVE FINE MOVEMENTS USED IN MANIPULATION AND OTHER PRECISE ACTIONS, ESPECIALLY OF THE DIGITS. A parallel control system ends in the brainstem and regulates the part of the facial motor nucleus that supplies the muscles of the lower part of the face as well as the hypoglossal nucleus, which innervates the tongue.

The other set of pathways ends on motor neurons in the medial part of lamina IX or on interneurons that project to them (Figure 9-14). THIS MEDIAL SYSTEM OF DESCENDING PATHWAYS CONTROLS AXIAL AND GIRDLE MUSCLES AS WELL AS MOST CRANIAL NERVE MOTOR NUCLEI. THE MUSCLES OF THE BODY THAT ARE REGULATED BY THE MEDIAL SYSTEM CONTRIBUTE TO POSTURE, BALANCE, AND LOCOMOTION. Muscles in the head are involved in activities such as closure of the eyelids, chewing, swallowing, and phonation.

The lateral system has a somatotopic organization

The lateral system includes two pathways from the brain to the spinal cord (Figure 9-14): the lateral corticospinal tract

and the rubrospinal tract. In addition, the part of the corticobulbar tract that controls the lower face and the tongue can be considered part of the lateral system.

The motor cortex has a somatotopic organization (Figure 9-15) resembling that of the somatosensory cortex (see Chapter 7). The cells of origin of the component of the **lateral corticospinal tract** controlling the upper extremity are in the dorsolateral precentral gyrus (arm representation), whereas neurons controlling the lower extremity are in the vertex and medial part of the precentral gyrus (leg area). **Corticobulbar tract** neurons that control the lower face and tongue are in the lateral precentral gyrus, just dorsal to the lateral fissure. These neurons project contralaterally to spinal cord motor nuclei or to the hypoglossal nucleus and part of the facial motor nucleus. Many of the terminations of the corticospinal tract are on interneurons, but some are directly on motor neurons, allowing a direct influence on the cerebral cortex on motor neurons that supply distal muscles, such as those controlling hand and digit movements.

The **rubrospinal tract** originates in the red nucleus. This tract appears to be much less significant in humans than in other animals.

The medial system can exert bilateral control

The **ventral corticospinal tract** projects bilaterally to influence motor neurons on both sides of the body. This is an important arrangement because the axial muscles on both sides often function together. Much of the **corticobulbar tract** belongs to the medial system and provides a bilateral innervation of many cranial nerve motor nuclei.

The **tectospinal tract** originates from the deep layers of the superior colliculus and helps control head movements. The **lateral** and **medial vestibulospinal tracts** originate from vestibular nuclei and help control posture and head movements. The **pontine** and **medullary reticulospinal tracts** arise from the reticular formation; they influence posture and control sensory transmission. The descending projections of monoaminergic nuclei in the brainstem form an additional modulatory system.

Brainstem Control of Posture and Movement

A hierarchic organization of the motor system can be demonstrated by the effects of lesions at different levels of the neuraxis. A lesion can result in a particular effect either (1) by abolishing functions subserved by a structure whose influence is removed by the lesion or (2) by allowing an action to appear through removal of an inhibitory influence. The latter responses are called **release phenomena.** Lesions that are particularly instructive include spinal cord transection and decerebration.

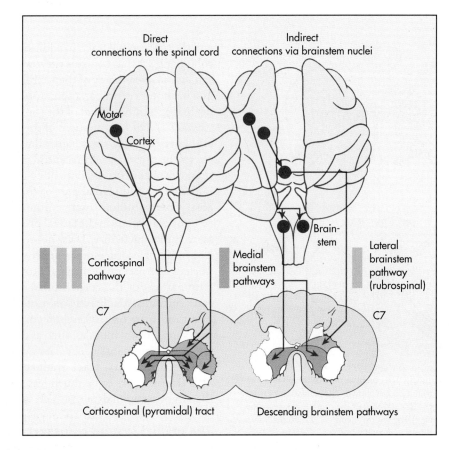

Figure 9-14 Lateral and medial motor control systems. Descending motor pathways in the lateral funiculus include the lateral corticospinal tract *(left)* and rubrospinal tract *(right)*. The lateral corticospinal tract projects directly to motor neurons innervating distal muscles, as well as to interneurons controlling these motor neurons. The rubrospinal tract projects onto lateral interneurons. Medial pathways include the ventral corticospinal tract *(left)* and several pathways from the medial brainstem *(right)*. These pathways end in the medial ventral horn and control motor neurons to axial and proximal muscles.

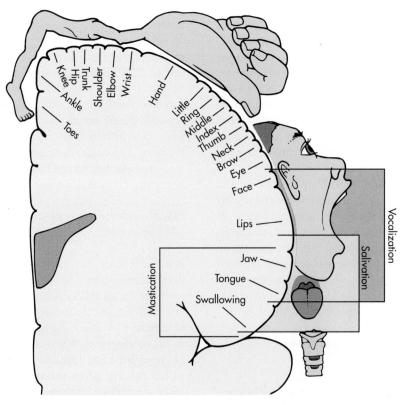

Figure 9-15 Somatotopic organization (homunculus) of the motor cortex.

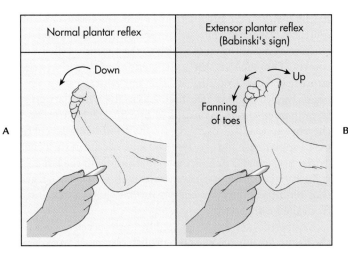

Normal plantar reflex	Extensor plantar reflex (Babinski's sign)
Down	Up / Fanning of toes

A **B**

Figure 9-16 Babinski's sign. **A,** The normal response to stroking the plantar surface of the foot. **B,** Babinski's sign (extensor plantar reflex) in a person with interruption of the corticospinal tract.

Spinal cord injury is unfortunately a relatively common occurrence and generally affects young adults. Frequent causes are automobile and motorcycle accidents and gunshot wounds. Although incomplete transections are more frequent than complete ones, incomplete lesions may nevertheless be disastrous. When spinal injuries affect the upper cervical spinal cord, they are often fatal because of the interruption of the respiratory control pathways that descend from the brainstem to the phrenic motor nucleus. A lesion below the phrenic nucleus may result in paralysis of all four extremities, **quadriplegia,** whereas a lesion of the thoracic spinal cord causes **paraplegia,** which is paralysis of the lower extremities.

Spinal cord transection produces characteristic deficits

Spinal cord transection at a cervical level caudal to the phrenic nucleus (thus sparing respiration) results in severe motor loss as well as in a complete loss of sensation from the body at dermatomal levels below that of the transection. The most important change is the loss of voluntary movements. IMMEDIATELY AFTER TRANSECTION, A PERIOD OF SPINAL SHOCK FOLLOWS IN WHICH REFLEXES ARE ABSENT. This presumably results from the loss of the excitatory actions of pathways descending from the brain. After a time, up to months, **hyperactive stretch** and **flexion reflexes** develop. Hyperactive stretch reflexes may result in **clonus,** alternating contractions of extensor and then flexor muscles. **Mass reflexes** are associated with hyperactive flexion reflexes and are characterized by flexion of one or both limbs and evacuation of the bladder and bowel. These changes may reflect the loss of descending inhibition and also rearrangements in spinal cord circuits, possibly because of the sprouting of primary afferent fibers and the formation of new synaptic connections within the spinal cord. Other release phenomena include the appearance of pathological reflexes, such as **Babinski's sign** (Figure 9-16), which follows interruption of the lateral corticospinal tract. Although locomotion is not regained in humans, a capability for locomotion reappears in experimental animals after spinal transection. This can be attributed to activation of a **locomotor pattern generator** within the neural circuitry of the spinal cord. A PATTERN GENERATOR IS A NEURAL CIRCUIT THAT CONTROLS A SPECIFIC TYPE OF MOTOR BEHAVIOR, OFTEN A RHYTHMIC BEHAVIOR SUCH AS LOCOMOTION OR RESPIRATION. In animals with chronic spinal transections, locomotion can be triggered by afferent signals rather than by pathways descending from the brain. It is hoped that a way will be found to activate the spinal cord locomotor pattern generator in humans with spinal cord injury.

Decerebrate rigidity results from transection of the brainstem

Transection of the brainstem at a midbrain level results in **decerebrate rigidity.** This condition develops immediately after the brainstem is transected. In experimental animals, the "rigidity" is expressed as an exaggerated extensor (antigravity) posture caused by hyperactive stretch reflexes. The term *decerebrate rigidity* is unfortunate because the condition more closely resembles spasticity than the rigidity that results from basal ganglion disease (see later discussion). Activation of γ-motor neurons is thought to be important in decerebrate rigidity because the hyperactive reflexes are lost after transection of the dorsal roots in experimental animals. Dorsal rhizotomies can interrupt input from muscle spindle afferents whose activity is increased in decerebrate rigidity because of an increased excitatory drive by pathways descending from the lower brainstem. The extensor posture can also be reduced or eliminated by lesions of the vestibular nuclei.

Postural reflexes include vestibular, tonic neck, and righting reflexes

Various reflexes assist in postural adjustments that occur as the head is moved or the neck is bent. The receptors that trigger these reflexes include the **vestibular apparatus** and **stretch receptors in the neck.** The visual system also contributes to postural adjustments, but the reflexes described here are elicited in the absence of visual cues.

Angular accelerations of the head activate the sensory receptors in the semicircular ducts and elicit reflexes that cause eye, neck, and limb movements that tend to oppose changes in position. For example, if the head is turned to the left (Figure 9-17), the eyes are reflexly rotated to the right through a similar angle. This action is called the **vestibuloocular reflex.** The two eyes move together in the same direction and through the same angle, so the eye movements are said to be **conjugate.** If head rotation exceeds the range of eye movement, the eyes are quickly deflected to the left and another visual target is found. If the

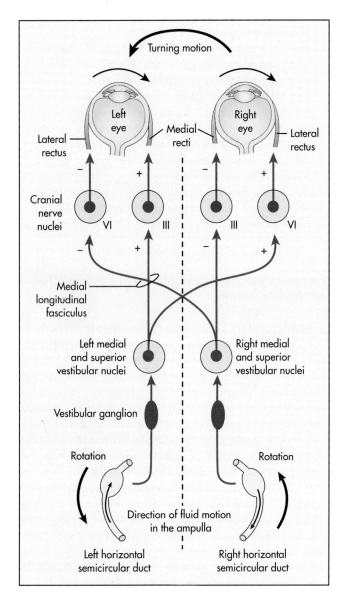

Figure 9-17 Neural circuit for the vestibuloocular reflex, a vestibular reflex that helps maintain a visual target despite head movement. The horizontal semicircular ducts, brainstem pathways, and eyes are viewed from above. Rotation of the head to the left is indicated by the thick black arrows. Fluid movement within the ducts is indicated by the thin black arrows. The neural activity produced by the vestibular system causes the eyes to move conjugately to the right. As the eyes reach the limit of their movement, they are quickly returned to the left.

head continues to rotate to the left, there is an alteration of slow eye movements to the right followed by rapid eye movements to the left. These alternating slow and fast eye movements are called **nystagmus.** A similar response pattern affects the neck muscles and is called the **vestibulo-collic reflex.** The same stimulus also tends to increase contractions of the extensor (antigravity) muscles on the left side of the body. This response opposes the tendency to fall to the left as the leftward head rotation continues.

The neural mechanism that underlies these reflexes depends on stimulation of sensory receptors in the semicircular ducts. In the case of rotation of the head in a plane parallel to the ground, the semicircular canals that are pri-

marily involved are the horizontal ones (Figure 9-17). The inertia of the endolymph within the horizontal semicircular canals causes the endolymph to lag behind as the head rotates. This relative shift of the endolymph deflects the cupulae of the ampullae of the horizontal canals and bends the stereocilia of the hair cells in the ampullary crest (see Chapter 7). The hair cells of one duct depolarize and thereby increase the discharges in the vestibular afferent fibers supplying that duct. The opposite occurs in the other horizontal canal. The mismatch in input from the left and right canals to the brainstem results in reflex discharges that tend to counteract the positional changes resulting from the head rotation.

Several reflexes can be elicited by linear accelerations of the head and activation of the otolith organs. If an experimental animal is dropped, the stimulation of the utricles leads to extension of the forelimbs, the **vestibular placing reaction.** The response is in preparation for landing. If the head is tilted, the otolith organs cause the eyes to rotate in the opposite direction, the ocular counter-rolling response. Ocular counter-rolling tends to keep the visual axes aligned with the horizon.

Other postural reflexes that depend on the vestibular apparatus tend to keep the body position normal despite tilting (without bending the neck). If the neck is bent, the **tonic neck reflexes** are triggered, resulting in postural adjustments that are opposite to those evoked by vestibular stimulation. **Righting reflexes** also tend to restore the position of the head and body in space to normal; these involve the vestibular apparatus, neck stretch receptors, and mechanoreceptors in the body wall.

Locomotion

As mentioned earlier, a pattern generator for locomotion is contained within the neural circuitry of the spinal cord. Actually, separate pattern generators exist for each limb. The activity of these is coupled so that the movements of the limbs are coordinated during locomotion.

The pattern generators for locomotion and for other rhythmic activities (e.g., respiration) are regarded as **biological oscillators.** Many biological oscillators operate on the basis of the reciprocal inhibition of circuits called **half-centers** that control antagonistic muscles. The details of how half-centers work and the factors that cause switching between the two half-centers vary with the particular oscillator being considered.

The locomotor pattern generator is normally activated by commands that descend from the brainstem. The midbrain locomotor center helps initiate locomotion by activating neurons in the pontomedullary reticular formation. These neurons transmit the descending commands. The locomotor pattern generator converts tonic activity in the descending pathways into rhythmic discharges of motor neurons to the muscles involved in locomotor activity. The midbrain locomotor center can be activated by voluntary commands from the motor cortex. It can also be engaged by afferent signals, as can the activity of the locomotor pattern

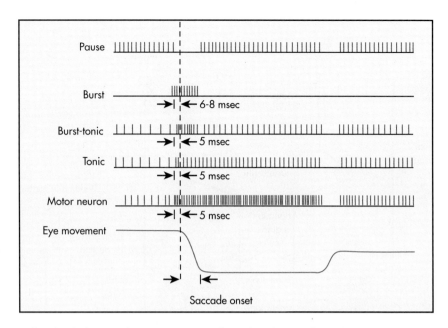

Figure 9-18 Types of neurons found in the horizontal gaze center. Pause cells are thought normally to inhibit burst cells. A saccade begins with a cessation of activity in pause cells and an explosion of activity in burst cells. Slightly later, burst-tonic and tonic cells discharge. Motor neurons to the muscles involved in the saccade are excited in the burst-tonic fashion, which causes the eye muscle to contract quickly and then to maintain its contraction. This results in the saccadic eye movement.

generator in the spinal cord. These afferent signals modify the ongoing motor program so that motor performance is altered in accord with environmental demands.

Control of eye position depends on brainstem circuits and the cerebral cortex

Movements of the eyes are generally **conjugate** (in the same direction), although sometimes they are **convergent** or **divergent** when they are targeted on nearby objects (as in reading) or on distant objects.

A rapid conjugate movement of the eyes is called a **saccade.** Usually a saccade causes a visual target to be imaged on the fovea. However, saccades can be made in the dark. Once the eyes have located a visual target, fixation is maintained by **smooth pursuit movements.** Smooth pursuit movements do not take place in the dark because they require a visual target. Actually, during fixation, the eyes drift somewhat and are returned to the target by microsaccades. Without these small movements, the retina would adapt and lose sight of the target.

> Misalignment of the two visual axes can cause double vision, or **diplopia.** Such misalignment, or **strabismus** (cross-eye), can result from weakness of the muscles of one eye, causing its visual axis to differ from that of the other eye. Over time the misaligned eye may lose visual acuity, a condition called **amblyopia.**

Horizontal eye movements are organized by the **horizontal gaze center,** which is located near the abducens nucleus in the pons. There is also a **vertical gaze center** in the midbrain pretectum. Neurons with response properties corresponding to different components of saccadic eye movements have been found in the horizontal gaze center (Figure 9-18). **Burst cells** discharge rapidly just before saccades occur, so they are thought to initiate these movements. **Tonic cells** discharge during slow pursuit movements and fixation. **Burst-tonic** cells show a burst discharge during saccades and tonic activity during fixation. **Pause cells** stop firing during saccades and seem to inhibit burst cells. Saccades occur when pause cells stop firing, resulting in a release of activity in burst cells and a discharge of eye muscle motor neurons. Feedback that occurs when the eye is on target inhibits the burst cells and reactivates the pause cells.

The vestibular nuclei and the gaze centers send direct projections to the motor nuclei that supply the eye muscle (Figure 9-17). The circuit is reciprocally organized so that a signal causing an eye movement excites a set of agonistic motor neurons and inhibits the antagonistic ones. For example, neurons in the horizontal gaze center send projections to abducens motor neurons of the ipsilateral eye as well as ascending projections through the medial longitudinal fasciculus to excite motor neurons to the contralateral medial rectus muscle (Figure 9-19). Appropriate connections are made to inhibit the motor neurons of the antagonistic muscles.

Neurons located in the deep layers of the superior colliculus and activated by visual, auditory, or somatosensory stimuli project to the horizontal gaze center (see Chapter 7). They produce saccadic eye movements that are part of an orientation response to a novel or threatening stimulus.

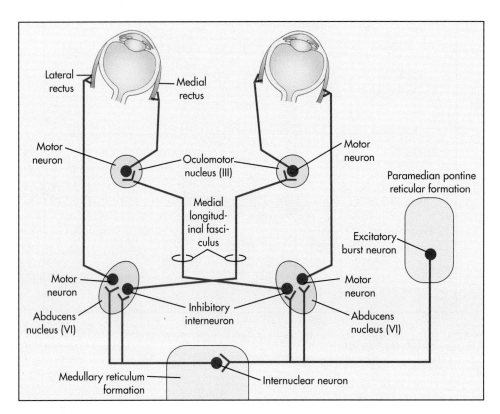

Figure 9-19 Organization of the horizontal gaze center. Activation of burst neurons in the right gaze center results in direct the excitation of abducens motor neurons on the right and oculomotor neurons to the medial rectus muscle on the left through an interneuronal pathway via the medial longitudinal fasciculus. Concurrently, the contralateral saccadic mechanism is inhibited by way of the reticular formation.

The **frontal eye fields** in the premotor region of the frontal lobe trigger voluntary saccadic eye movements via a projection to the contralateral horizontal gaze center. The **occipital eye fields** are involved in smooth pursuit movements, optokinetic nystagmus, and visual fixation. Adjustments for near vision include convergence, pupillary constriction, and accommodation of the lens. The occipital eye fields are connected with the superior colliculus and the pretectal region and influence the vertical and horizontal gaze centers.

Cortical Control of Voluntary Movement

The **corticospinal** and **corticobulbar tracts** are the most important pathways used in the initiation and execution of voluntary movements. THE LATERAL CORTICOSPINAL TRACT AND THE COMPARABLE PART OF THE CORTICOBULBAR TRACT CONTROL THE FINE MOVEMENTS PRODUCED BY THE MUSCLES OF THE CONTRALATERAL DISTAL EXTREMITIES, LOWER FACE, AND TONGUE. THE VENTRAL CORTICOSPINAL TRACT AND PART OF THE CORTICOBULBAR TRACT, AS WELL AS MORE INDIRECT PATHWAYS, PROVIDE FOR POSTURAL SUPPORT OF VOLUNTARY MOVEMENTS.

Corticospinal and corticobulbar neurons do not operate in isolation. Their discharges represent decisions based on input from many sources. The motor cortex receives projections from the **ventral lateral nucleus** of the thalamus, **postcentral gyrus, posterior parietal cortex, supplementary motor cortex,** and **premotor cortex.** The ventral lateral thalamic nucleus is part of the circuitry by which the cerebellum and basal ganglia regulate movements (see later discussion). The postcentral gyrus processes and then transmits somatosensory information to the motor cortex, which provides feedback about movements and contacts between the skin and objects being explored. The posterior parietal cortex, supplementary motor cortex, and premotor cortex help program movements.

Motor programs are developed in the sensorimotor cortex

Voluntary movements require contractions and relaxations in the proper sequence, not only of the muscles directly involved in the movements but also of the appropriate postural muscles. Therefore a mechanism is needed for programming these complex events. The cortical areas thought to be responsible for cortical motor programs include the **posterior parietal lobe, supplementary motor cortex,** and **premotor cortex** (Figure 9-20).

The posterior parietal lobe receives somatosensory information from the postcentral gyrus and visual information from the occipital cortex. The posterior parietal cortex connects with the supplementary motor cortex and premotor cortex (Figure 9-20) and is important for processing sensory information that leads to goal-directed movements.

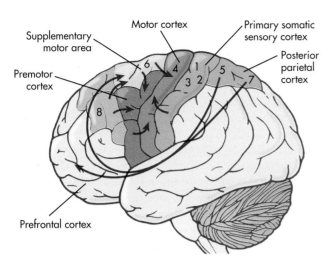

Figure 9-20 Cortical regions involved in the programming of movements. The arrows show some of the interconnections of these regions. The numbers refer to Brodmann's areas.

A lesion of the posterior parietal cortex causes deficits in visually guided movements. Humans may develop a **neglect syndrome** (especially if the lesion is in the nondominant hemisphere for language, generally the right hemisphere). In this syndrome, a patient is unable to recognize objects placed in the contralateral hand and unable to draw three-dimensional objects accurately. In fact, the patient may deny that the contralateral limbs even belong to him or her.

The supplementary motor cortex is concerned with complex, often bilateral, movements. A lesion in the supplementary motor cortex is likely to cause deficits in orientation during movements and impairment of bilateral coordination.

The premotor cortex is influenced by the cerebellum, posterior parietal lobe, and supplementary motor cortex, and it projects to the motor cortex. It is especially involved in the control of axial and proximal muscles. A lesion of the premotor cortex in humans or monkeys results in the appearance of the **grasp response,** in which touching the palm or extending the fingers elicits a grasping movement of the hand.

The motor cortex is the main motor output region

The motor cortex is recognizable microscopically by the presence of the **giant pyramidal,** or **Betz,** cells. However, many more projections of this area arise from small and medium-sized pyramidal cells than from Betz cells. The corticospinal and corticobulbar tracts originate from pyramidal cells in layer 5 of the motor cortex, as well as from other cortical regions, including the premotor cortex, supplementary motor cortex, and postcentral gyrus. The

somatotopic organization of the motor cortex has already been described (Figure 9-15).

The motor cortex controls both distal and proximal muscles. HOWEVER, THE CORTICOSPINAL AND CORTICOBULBAR PROJECTIONS OF THE LATERAL SYSTEM ARE ESPECIALLY IMPORTANT FOR CONTROL OF THE DISTAL MUSCLES OF THE CONTRALATERAL EXTREMITIES, LOWER FACE, AND TONGUE. A lesion that interrupts the corticospinal and corticobulbar tracts eliminates movements of distal muscles, but other pathways can still be used to activate proximal and axial muscles.

The lateral corticospinal tract makes monosynaptic excitatory connections with α-motor neurons, especially those that are located in the dorsolateral part of the ventral horn and that innervate distal muscles. The same pathway also excites γ-motor neurons. Thus when the lateral corticospinal tract commands a voluntary movement, it coactivates α- and γ-motor neurons. In addition, the corticospinal tract influences interneurons that regulate reflex transmission. During learned movements, some pyramidal tract neurons discharge just before a particular phase of the movement (e.g., flexion or extension of a joint). The activity encodes the force exerted by the muscles involved in the movement rather than the position of the joint. Some neurons encode the rate at which force is developed, whereas others encode the steady-state force.

When the corticospinal and corticobulbar tracts are completely interrupted, the distal muscles of the contralateral upper and lower extremities and muscles of the contralateral lower face and tongue are paralyzed **(hemiplegia).** Unless the lesion is restricted to these tracts, the deficit is a **spastic paralysis.** Spasticity usually accompanies hemiplegia produced by a lesion of the internal capsule or a lesion at other levels of the nervous system because the corticoreticulospinal pathway, along with the pyramidal tract, is interrupted. Spasticity is also present in spinal cord injuries when transection at an upper cervical level causes quadriplegia or transection below the cervical enlargement causes paraplegia. Spastic paralysis is associated with an increase in muscle tone and increased phasic stretch reflexes. The latter may lead to **clonus,** such as in the ankle, in response to a brisk passive movement. Interruption of the lateral corticospinal tract at any level causes an important release response, Babinski's sign (Figure 9-16).

Cerebellar Regulation of Posture and Movement

The cerebellum assists in the performance of coordinated movements by receiving sensory information about the status of movements and then adjusting the activity of the various descending motor pathways to optimize performance. These functions improve with practice; thus the cerebellum is involved in learning motor skills. Destruction of the cerebellum produces no sensory deficits; therefore it has no essential role in sensation.

The organization of the cerebellum is consistent throughout

Afferent fibers from other parts of the central nervous system approach the cerebellum through the cerebellar white matter. Two types of afferent fibers are found: **mossy fibers** and **climbing fibers** (Figure 9-21). Mossy fibers orig-

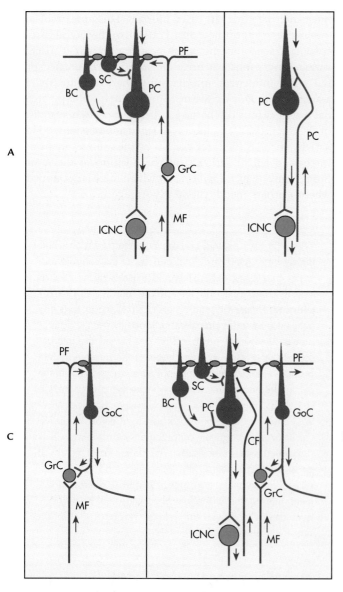

Figure 9-21 Excitatory and inhibitory circuits in the cerebellar cortex. Excitatory neurons are green; inhibitory neurons are blue. **A,** Connections made by mossy fibers *(MF)* through granule cells to Purkinje cells *(PC),* stellate cells *(SC),* and basket cells *(BC).* Purkinje cells inhibit neurons of the deep cerebellar nuclei. **B,** Climbing fiber *(CF)* input to a Purkinje cell. **C,** Excitation of a Golgi cell *(GoC)* by a mossy fiber through the granule cell *(GrC)* pathway, with inhibition of granule cells by the Golgi cell. **D,** Combination of these circuits. *ICNC,* Deep cerebellar nuclear cell; *PF,* parallel fiber.

inate from various sources, but all climbing fibers are derived from the contralateral **inferior olivary nucleus.** In the cerebellar cortex the mossy fibers synapse in the granular layer on the dendrites of **granule cells.** There is considerable divergence because a given mossy fiber branches repeatedly and synapses on many different granule cells. An individual climbing fiber synapses at many sites on the soma and dendritic tree of one or a few **Purkinje cells.** Thus the climbing fiber pathways show little divergence.

The granule cell axons form bundles of **parallel fibers** that synapse on the dendrites of Purkinje cells and of several classes of interneurons, including **Golgi cells, basket cells,** and **stellate cells.** Granule cells are the only excitatory interneurons in the cerebellar cortex; the other types are all inhibitory. The mossy fiber–granule cell pathway and the climbing fiber pathway are able to excite Purkinje cells; hence they may be regarded as the excitatory circuits of the cerebellar cortex. Mossy fiber–granule cell excitation typically elicits single action potentials in a set of Purkinje cells **(simple spike response),** whereas a climbing fiber evokes a high-frequency burst of action potentials in a Purkinje cell **(complex spike).** Other pathways in the cerebellar cortex feature inhibition: Golgi cells inhibit granule cells, basket cells inhibit Purkinje cell somas, and stellate cells inhibit Purkinje cell dendrites. All of these inhibitory interneurons are activated by the mossy fiber–granule cell pathway.

A surprising observation is that although Purkinje cells are the only output neurons of the cerebellar cortex, their synaptic actions are inhibitory. This inhibition modulates the discharges of the neurons of the deep cerebellar nuclei and lateral vestibular nucleus.

There are three functional systems of the cerebellum

The cerebellum can be considered on phylogenetic and functional grounds to be composed of the following major components: the archicerebellum, the paleocerebellum, and the neocerebellum. The **archicerebellum** is the earliest part of the cerebellum to evolve and is related in function primarily to the vestibular system. The archicerebellum is thus often referred to as the **vestibulocerebellum.** It corresponds in the human to the flocculonodular lobe and parts of the vermis in addition to the nodule. THE ARCHICEREBELLUM HELPS CONTROL AXIAL MUSCLES AND THUS BALANCE. IT ALSO COORDINATES HEAD AND EYE MOVEMENTS. A lesion of the archicerebellum can result in a "drunken" stagger called an **ataxic gait** and in **nystagmus.**

The **paleocerebellum** receives somatotopically organized information from the spinal cord; hence it is often called the **spinocerebellum.** The paleocerebellum regulates both movement and muscle tone. Lesions of the paleocerebellum produce deficits in coordination similar to those seen after damage to the neocerebellum.

The **neocerebellum** is the dominant component of the human cerebellum. It occupies the hemispheres of the cerebellum. The input is from wide areas of the cerebral cortex; hence this region is sometimes called the **cerebrocerebellum.** THE NEOCEREBELLUM MODULATES THE OUTPUT OF THE MOTOR CORTEX. Because the right side of the neocerebellum controls activity in the left cortex and because the left cortex influences movements of the right limbs, the neocerebellum regulates motor activity of the same side of the body. The neocerebellum probably interacts with neurons of the premotor cortex in programming movements.

Lesions of the neocerebellum affect chiefly the distal limbs. The neurological signs include delayed initiation of movements, **ataxia of the limbs** (incoordination), and reduced muscle tone. The limb ataxia results in **asynergy** (lack of synergy in movements), **dysmetria** (inaccurate movements), **intention tremor** (oscillations at the end of a movement), and **dysdiadochokinesia** (irregular performance of pronation and supination movements of the forearm). Reduced muscle tone leads to **pendular phasic stretch reflexes** in the lower extremity. Bilateral lesions of the neocerebellum may result in **dysarthria** (slow, slurred speech, synonymous with "scanning speech"). These classic neocerebellar signs are often seen in **multiple sclerosis.**

Regulation of Posture and Movement by the Basal Ganglia

As with the neocerebellum, THE BASAL GANGLIA HELP REGULATE THE ACTIVITY OF THE MOTOR CORTEX. Unlike the archicerebellum and paleocerebellum, the basal ganglia exert only a minor influence on descending motor pathways other than the corticospinal and corticobulbar tracts. Judging from the effects of lesions, the role of the basal ganglia is often opposed to that of the neocerebellum.

Organization of the basal ganglia

The basal ganglia are the deep nuclei of the telencephalon. They include the **caudate nucleus** and **putamen** (neostriatum) and the **globus pallidus** (paleostriatum). The caudate nucleus and putamen are often collectively called the **striatum** because of the "striations" formed by fibers that pass between these nuclei in the human. Brainstem nuclei that are closely associated with the basal ganglia are the **substantia nigra** and the **subthalamic nucleus.** The role of the basal ganglia in motor control has been inferred more on the basis of the effects of disorders of the basal ganglia than from experimental evidence.

Disturbances caused by basal ganglia diseases

Basal ganglia diseases can produce various motor disturbances. These can be categorized as disorders of movement and disorders of posture. Movement disturbances include

tremor (rhythmic, "pill-rolling" oscillations at rest), **chorea** (rapid flicking movements), **ballism** (violent, flailing movements), **athetosis** (slow, writhing movements of limbs), and **dystonia** (slow, twisting movements of the torso). Movements that are delayed in initiation and slow to reach completion are referred to as **bradykinesia.** The disorders of posture produced in basal ganglia disease are forms of rigidity. The rigidity may be the **cog-wheel** type. As the joint is moved, resistance occurs throughout the range of movement, although there may be repeated alterations in the amount of resistance. These alterations produce a ratchetlike effect as the joint is passively moved. Alternatively, **lead-pipe** rigidity may occur, in which resistance is constantly present through the range of motion of the joint. The rigidity of basal ganglia disease should be distinguished from "decerebrate rigidity," which is more similar to spasticity (see previous discussion).

Parkinson's disease is caused by a lesion of the substantia nigra and is characterized by tremor, rigidity, and bradykinesia. The loss of dopaminergic projections to the striatum is thought to be crucial. **Hemiparkinsonism** results when one substantia nigra is affected; the manifestations are then contralateral because they are caused by inappropriate regulation of the corticospinal tract. Destruction of part of the subthalamic nucleus on one side results in **hemiballism,** which is characterized by ballistic movements on the contralateral side. **Huntington's chorea** is a genetic disorder in which there is loss of striatopallidal and striatonigral neurons containing γ-aminobutyric acid; cholinergic striatal interneurons are also lost. Loss of inhibitory input to the globus pallidus is thought to underlie the choreiform movements characteristic of the disease. The cerebral cortex also degenerates, leading to severe mental retardation. In **cerebral palsy,** athetosis often occurs because of damage of the striatum and globus pallidus.

S UMMARY

- The basic element of motor control is the motor unit, which comprises an α-motor neuron and all of the muscle fibers that it innervates.
- Motor units have a variable number of muscle fibers depending on the coarseness or fineness of the movements made by the particular muscle.
- All of the muscle fibers of a motor unit are of the same histochemical type.
- α-Motor neurons form the final common pathway for movements.
- α-Motor neurons are found in motor nuclei of the spinal cord ventral horn and in cranial nerve motor nuclei. Spinal cord motor nuclei are arranged somatotopically.

- EPSPs can sum spatially or temporally, and the synaptic currents may reach threshold at the initial segment. IPSPs may prevent the threshold from being reached.
- The afterhyperpolarization in α-motor neurons is often quite large and helps regulate the discharge rate.
- Repetitive firing of α-motor neurons can produce an unfused or a fused tetanus of the muscle fibers that they innervate. Contractile force can therefore be increased by increasing the discharge rates of α-motor neurons up to the point that a fused tetanus is produced. Contractile force can also be increased by the recruitment of additional α-motor neurons.
- The recruitment of α-motor neurons is orderly. Small α-motor neurons are generally activated before large ones in most motor acts.
- Muscles and tendons contain stretch receptors; these include muscle spindles and Golgi tendon organs.
- The primary endings of muscle spindles signal the rate of change in muscle stretch as well as muscle length. The secondary endings signal muscle length.
- Golgi tendon organs are supplied by group Ib afferent fibers. They respond to both muscle stretch and muscle contraction and signal the tension in the tendon.
- Spinal cord reflexes are relatively simple, stereotyped responses to a defined sensory input.
- The stretch reflex involves a monosynaptic, excitatory connection between group Ia afferent fibers from muscle spindles in a muscle and the α-motor neurons that supply the muscle, as well as synergistic muscles; it also involves a disynaptic inhibitory connection to antagonist motor neurons.
- The inverse myotatic reflex involves a disynaptic pathway from Golgi tendon organs through inhibitory interneurons to α-motor neurons of the same muscle. This reflex controls muscle tension.
- Both the stretch reflex and the inverse myotatic reflex represent negative-feedback loops. The controlled variable of the stretch reflex is muscle length, and that of the inverse myotatic reflex is muscle tension.
- The flexion reflex involves afferent fibers that supply the skin, muscle, and joints. These excite α-motor neurons to flexor muscles and inhibit α-motor neurons to extensor muscles in the limb.
- The lateral corticospinal tract controls muscles of the distal extremities, lower face, and tongue.
- The ventral corticospinal tract controls the proximal limb and axial muscles and thus provides for postural support.
- Spinal cord transection causes sensory loss and paralysis below the level of the lesion. Stretch and flexion reflexes become hyperactive, and pathological reflexes, such as Babinski's sign, appear.
- Transection of the upper brainstem may lead to decerebrate rigidity, in which the stretch reflexes also become exaggerated.

- Locomotion is organized by a pattern generator in the spinal cord. Locomotion can be triggered by activity in the midbrain locomotor center, and it can be modified by segmental afferent input.
- Eye position is controlled by several motor systems.
- The motor cortex issues commands that are transmitted by the corticospinal and corticobulbar tracts and that evoke voluntary movements.
- The lateral corticospinal tract and the equivalent part of the corticobulbar tract control fine movements of distal muscles of the limbs and of the lower face and tongue.
- Interruption of the lateral corticospinal tract and the corticobulbar tract on one side in the brain results in a contralateral hemiplegia. If other descending pathways, such as the inhibitory corticoreticulospinal pathway, are also interrupted, the paralysis becomes spastic with hyperactive phasic stretch reflexes.
- The cerebellum helps coordinate movements and is involved in learning motor skills.
- The output of the cerebellum influences the activity of motor pathways descending from the brainstem and corticospinal and corticobulbar tracts.
- Damage to the vestibulocerebellum can produce an ataxic (staggering) gait and nystagmus.
- Damage to the neocerebellum causes tremor and incoordination of the limbs and reduced muscle tone, resulting in pendular stretch reflexes.
- Disturbances of the basal ganglia result in disorders of movement and posture, including resting tremor, chorea, ballism, athetosis, dystonia, bradykinesia, and rigidity.

BIBLIOGRAPHY

Binder MD, Mendell LM: *The segmental motor system,* New York, 1990, Oxford University Press.

Brooks VB: *The neural basis of motor control,* New York, 1986, Oxford University Press.

Donoghue JP, Sanes JN: Motor areas of the cerebral cortex, *J Clin Neurophysiol* 11:382, 1994.

Gilman S, Bloedel JR, Lechtenberg R: *Disorders of the cerebellum,* Philadelphia, 1981, FA Davis.

Hunt CC: Mammalian muscle spindle: peripheral mechanisms, *Physiol Rev* 70:643, 1990.

Jami L: Golgi tendon organs in mammalian skeletal muscle: functional properties and central actions, *Physiol Rev* 72:623, 1992.

Lüscher HR, Clamann HP: Relation between structure and function in information transfer in spinal monosynaptic reflex, *Physiol Rev* 72:71, 1992.

Moschovakis AK, Highstein SM: The anatomy and physiology of primate neurons that control rapid eye movements, *Annu Rev Neurosci* 17:465, 1994.

Thach WT, Goodkin HP, Keating JG: The cerebellum and the adaptive coordination of movement, *Annu Rev Neurosci* 15:403, 1992.

Wilson VJ, Jones GM: *Mammalian vestibular physiology,* New York, 1979, Plenum.

▷ **CASE STUDIES**

Case 9-1

A 74-year-old man suddenly found that he could not move his left arm and leg. Examination in the emergency department demonstrated weakness in the left arm and leg, especially in the distal parts of these extremities. The patient also had difficulty in using the muscles of his lower face, and the left side of his tongue was not as strong as the right side. Babinski's sign was present on the left side. In an examination 1 month later, the distribution of weakness had not changed, although the weakness was not quite as profound. The left biceps, triceps, patellar, and ankle jerk reflexes were markedly increased, and there was ankle clonus on the left. The ability of the patient to recognize tactile and vibratory stimuli was reduced on the left side of the face and body, and proprioception was impaired in the left arm and leg.

1. **Which part of the nervous system is most likely affected by the stroke?**
    - **A.** Basal ganglia on the right
    - **B.** Cerebellum on the left
    - **C.** Internal capsule on the right
    - **D.** Precentral and postcentral gyri on the right
    - **E.** Spinal cord on the left

2. **Which of the following provides evidence indicating that the paralysis is of the spastic type?**
    - **A.** Babinski's sign
    - **B.** Clonus and hyperactive phasic stretch reflexes
    - **C.** Deficits in somatic sensation
    - **D.** Paralysis of the tongue
    - **E.** Weakness of the arm and leg

Case 9-2

A 56-year-old woman noticed that her movements had slowed and that her hands shook when she was resting. These changes developed over several years. Her physician found that she had a pill-rolling tremor of her hands while the hands were at rest and that she initiated and executed movements slowly. Her face was not expressive. When her joints were passively bent, there was resistance to the movement, but the resistance gave way and then resumed repeatedly as the bending progressed. Phasic stretch reflexes were normal, as was muscle strength.

1. **Which structures of the central nervous system are most likely to be affected in this patient?**
    - **A.** Basal ganglia and substantia nigra
    - **B.** Brainstem reticular formation
    - **C.** Deep nuclei of the cerebellum
    - **D.** Primary motor cortex
    - **E.** Supplementary motor cortex

2. **Relief of some symptoms may be provided by replacement therapy for which of the following?**
    - **A.** Dopamine
    - **B.** Epinephrine
    - **C.** γ-Aminobutyric acid
    - **D.** Glutamate
    - **E.** Substance P

CHAPTER 10

Autonomic Nervous System and Its Control

OBJECTIVES

■ Describe and compare the organization of the sympathetic, parasympathetic, and enteric nervous systems.

■ Explain the operation and control of the autonomic nervous system and the neurotransmitters and receptors that are used.

■ Relate the activity of the hypothalamus and limbic system to autonomic and other functions.

The autonomic nervous system is a motor system concerned with the regulation of smooth muscle, cardiac muscle, and glands. It is not directly accessible to voluntary control. Instead, it operates in an automatic fashion on the basis of **autonomic reflexes** and central control. A MAJOR FUNCTION OF THE AUTONOMIC NERVOUS SYSTEM IS HOMEOSTASIS, WHICH IS THE MAINTENANCE OF THE INTERNAL ENVIRONMENT IN AN OPTIMAL STATE. For instance, the autonomic nervous system in cooperation with the somatic motor system helps keep the body temperature relatively constant. Another important role is making the appropriate adjustments in smooth muscle tone, cardiac muscle activity, and glandular secretion for different behaviors. For example, the autonomic activity that can be observed during digestion is very different from that seen during a sprint.

Organization of the Autonomic Nervous System

The sympathetic system innervates structures in the body wall and internal viscera

The **sympathetic nervous system** is a widely distributed motor system. It reaches not only the viscera contained in the body cavities but also the skin and muscles of the body wall. It does this through a sequential pathway consisting of two types of motor neurons called **preganglionic** and **postganglionic neurons.**

The cell bodies of the sympathetic preganglionic neurons are located in the thoracic and upper lumbar spinal cord (T1 to about L2) in the **intermediolateral** and **inter-mediomedial cell columns** (Figure 10-1). The motor axons of the sympathetic preganglionic neurons leave the spinal cord in the T1 to L2 ventral roots. The motor axons are small myelinated **B fibers** or in some cases unmyelinated **C fibers.** They pass from the spinal nerves into the **white communicating rami.**

When the sympathetic preganglionic axons in a given white ramus reach the **sympathetic paravertebral ganglion** of the same segment, they may (1) synapse in that ganglion, (2) turn rostrally or caudally to synapse in a paravertebral ganglion at another segmental level, or (3) continue through a splanchnic nerve to synapse in a **prevertebral ganglion** (Figure 10-1). In this way, preganglionic axons that originate from motor neurons limited to spinal cord segments T1 to L2 are able to synapse on postganglionic neurons located in the entire chain of paravertebral sympathetic ganglia (including the superior, middle, and inferior cervical sympathetic ganglia and the ganglia below L2 that do not receive white communicating rami) as well as in the prevertebral ganglia of the abdominal cavity (Figure 10-2). Preganglionic axons also directly innervate the chromaffin cells of the **adrenal medulla,** which are developmentally comparable to sympathetic ganglion cells.

Sympathetic postganglionic neurons are located in the paravertebral and prevertebral ganglia. The axons are unmyelinated **C fibers** that distribute either to the body wall or to the viscera in the body cavities (Figure 10-2). If they are destined for the body wall, they pass from a paravertebral ganglion into a spinal nerve via a **gray communicating ramus.** Gray rami are found in all ganglia of the sympathetic chain and connect with the appropriate spinal nerves. Sympathetic postganglionic axons destined for viscera in the body cavities enter **splanchnic nerves** and distribute to their targets. Postganglionic axons originating in prevertebral ganglia distribute to their targets through the sympathetic plexuses near the target organs.

The sympathetic preganglionic neurons that supply the head are in the upper thoracic segments. Their axons leave the spinal cord in the white communicating rami at T1 and T2, enter the **sympathetic chain,** and ascend to the superior cervical sympathetic ganglion, where they synapse on sympathetic postganglionic neurons. The postganglionic axons pass into the head through a plexus around the great

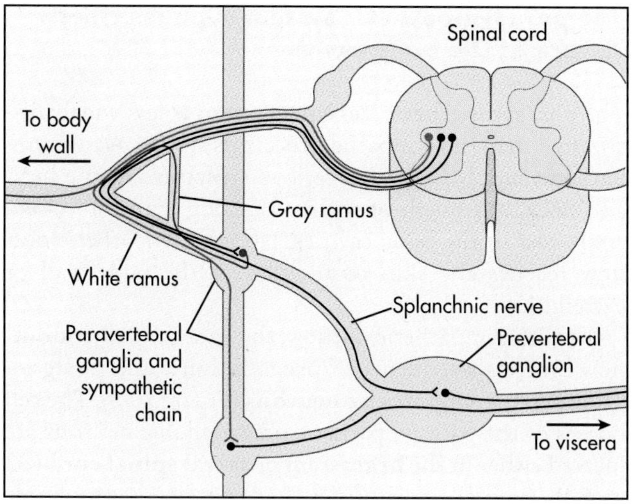

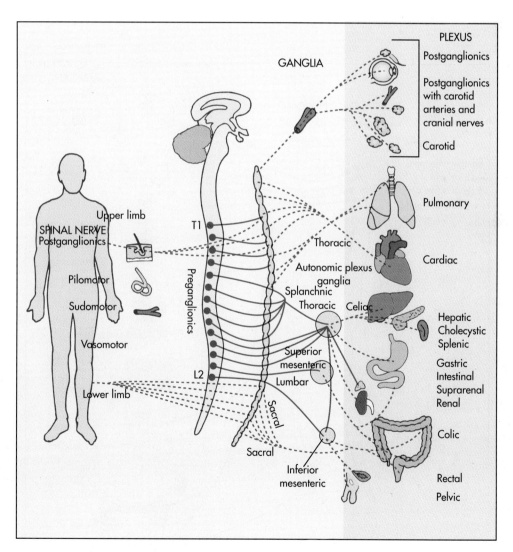

Figure 10-1 Distribution of sympathetic preganglionic projections to paravertebral and prevertebral ganglia.

Figure 10-2 Sympathetic nervous system.

vessels. They synapse on smooth muscle and glands of the face, eyes, and other structures of the head.

> Interruption of the sympathetic supply to the head (or of descending pathways from the hypothalamus that control sympathetic activity) results in **Horner's syndrome.** This syndrome consists of (1) a **partial ptosis** (drooping of the eyelid caused by paralysis of the superior tarsal muscle of the eyelid), (2) **pupillary constriction** (because the unopposed parasympathetic supply of the iris is intact), (3) **anhydrosis of the face** (caused by interruption of the innervation of the sweat glands of the face), and (4) **enophthalmos** (retraction of the globe of the eye because innervation of the smooth muscle of the orbit has been interrupted).

The parasympathetic system supplies chiefly viscera of the body cavities

The **parasympathetic nervous system** is less widely distributed than the sympathetic nervous system. A parasympathetic supply exists for various structures in the head and neck, but much of the distribution is to the viscera contained in the body cavities. No parasympathetic outflow reaches the skin or muscles of the body wall or extremities.

As with sympathetic outflow, the parasympathetic outflow involves a sequence of **preganglionic** and **postganglionic parasympathetic neurons** (Figure 10-3). The cell bodies of the parasympathetic preganglionic neurons are located either in the **brainstem** or **sacral spinal cord (S2 to S4).** Cranial nerve nuclei that contain preganglionic parasympathetic neurons include the **Edinger-Westphal**

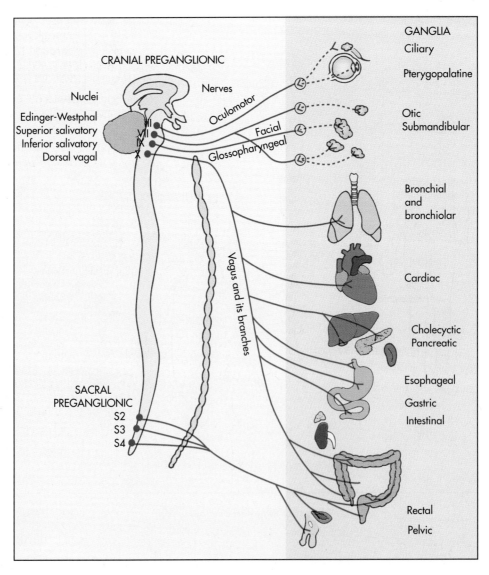

Figure 10-3 Parasympathetic nervous system.

nucleus (cranial nerve III), **superior salivatory nucleus** (cranial nerve VII), **inferior salivatory nucleus** (cranial nerve IX), and the **nucleus ambiguus** and **dorsal motor nucleus of the vagus** (cranial nerve X). Sacral parasympathetic neurons are located in the **sacral parasympathetic nucleus.** No lateral horn exists in the sacral spinal cord, but the parasympathetic nucleus is in a roughly similar position.

The cranial parasympathetic preganglionic axons leave the brainstem in the appropriate cranial nerves and synapse on ganglion cells in the appropriate **cranial parasympathetic ganglia** (Figure 10-3): the **ciliary ganglion** (cranial nerve III), **sphenopalatine** and **submaxillary ganglia** (cranial nerve VII), **otic ganglion** (cranial nerve IX), and **ganglia in or near the walls of target viscera** in the thoracic and abdominal cavities (cranial nerve X). For the gastrointestinal tract the vagal preganglionic axons synapse on neurons belonging to the **enteric nervous system** (see later discussion). The sacral parasympathetic preganglionic axons distribute to the abdominal and pelvic cavities and synapse on ganglion cells in these regions. The **splenic flexure** of the colon is the boundary between the gastrointestinal organs supplied by the vagus nerve and those supplied by the sacral parasympathetics. Parasympathetic postganglionic neurons directly innervate nearby target organs.

The parasympathetic preganglionic neurons that control pupil size are located in the **Edinger-Westphal nucleus,** which is near the midline just ventral to the cerebral aqueduct. The preganglionic axons leave the midbrain with the **oculomotor nerve** and synapse in the **ciliary ganglion,** which is in the orbit just behind the eye. Axons of the postganglionic neurons of the ciliary ganglion pass into the eye through short ciliary nerves, and some terminate on smooth muscle cells of the iris that form the **pupillary sphincter.**

> When there is a large **increase in intracranial pressure,** such as happens during a **cerebral hemorrhage** or because of a **brain tumor,** the brain may shift position, causing herniation of the uncus **(uncal herniation)** in the medial temporal lobe through the tentorial notch of the dura. This may compress the oculomotor nerve and cause a sudden unilateral dilation of the pupil. A **fixed, dilated pupil** is an indicator of impending death unless the high intracranial pressure is relieved by surgery.

The enteric nervous system controls functions of the gut wall

The **enteric nervous system** is a miniature nervous system within the wall of the gastrointestinal tract (see Chapter 32). Reflex networks in this system organize gut movements that can occur even when the gut is removed from the body. Afferent neurons, interneurons, and motor neurons are included in the system. Parasympathetic and sympathetic connections to the enteric nervous system permit autonomic control. The component of the enteric nervous system in **Auerbach's myenteric plexus** controls the activity of the muscular layers, and that in **Meissner's submucosal plexus** controls the muscularis mucosae and intestinal glands.

Autonomic Functions

The sympathetic nervous system actively regulates visceral function under normal circumstances. The parasympathetic nervous system often acts contrary to the sympathetic nervous system when a given organ is innervated by both systems. However, it is more appropriate to view concurrent control of organs by activity in the sympathetic and parasympathetic nervous systems as a means of coordinating visceral activity.

The preganglionic neurons of the autonomic nervous system, as with α-motor neurons of the somatic motor system, use **acetylcholine** as their neurotransmitter (Figure 10-4). Some of the **acetylcholine receptors** on postganglionic neurons, as with those of skeletal muscle, are of the nicotinic type. Nicotinic receptors are activated by low doses of nicotine and are blocked by curare. Other acetylcholine receptors on postganglionic neurons are of the muscarinic type. **Muscarinic receptors** are activated by **muscarine** and blocked by **atropine.**

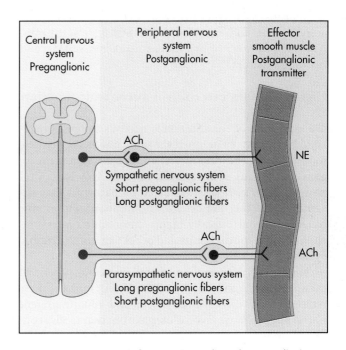

Figure 10-4 Transmitters of autonomic ganglia and postganglionic synapses. *Ach,* Acetylcholine; *NE,* norepinephrine.

Autonomic neurotransmission depends on cholinergic, adrenergic, and peptidergic receptors

Parasympathetic and some sympathetic postganglionic neurons also use acetylcholine as a neurotransmitter. The receptors on target organs are of the muscarinic type. The cholinergic sympathetic postganglionic axons include those that supply sweat glands, the **sudomotor fibers,** as well as **vasodilator fibers** in skin and skeletal muscle. Postganglionic parasympathetic neurons also release neuropeptides, such as **vasoactive intestinal polypeptide.**

Sympathetic postganglionic neurons generally use **norepinephrine** as their neurotransmitter (Figure 10-4), although as previously mentioned, some use acetylcholine. Receptors for norepinephrine include **α- and β-adrenergic receptors.** α-Receptors are more powerfully activated by norepinephrine than by isoproterenol; the converse is true of β-receptors. Phenoxybenzamine can be used to block α-adrenergic receptors, and propanolol can be used to block β-adrenergic receptors. However, selective antagonists are available for many of the subtypes of adrenergic receptors. Sympathetic postganglionic neurons also release neuropeptides, such as **neuropeptide Y,** and **ATP.**

The **adrenal medulla** is supplied by sympathetic preganglionic axons, which release acetylcholine as their neurotransmitter. The **chromaffin cells** of the adrenal medulla are developmentally similar to sympathetic postganglionic neurons, and they secrete **epinephrine** and **norepinephrine** into the circulation, where these agents act as hormones. In humans, the ratio of epinephrine to norepinephrine is 4:1.

Neurons of the enteric nervous system release not only acetylcholine and norepinephrine but also **serotonin,** ATP, and a variety of peptides as neurotransmitters and neuromodulators.

Higher centers can control autonomic function

The operation of the autonomic nervous system is regulated hierarchically in much the same way as the somatic motor system. The most direct neuron control of many organs is by means of **autonomic reflexes.** However, autonomic neurons are also regulated by pathways that descend from the brainstem. In addition, autonomic function is controlled by higher autonomic centers, including the **hypothalamus** and other parts of the **limbic system.**

Autonomic reflexes are mediated by neural circuits in the spinal cord and brainstem. The afferent limbs of these reflex pathways include both visceral and somatic afferent fibers. The pathways involve interneurons that receive convergent input from visceral and somatic sensory receptors. The efferent limbs are formed by sympathetic and parasympathetic preganglionic and postganglionic neurons.

The actions of the two autonomic systems are generally reciprocal.

Brainstem pathways that regulate the activity of autonomic preganglionic neurons originate from several sites, including the **reticular formation, raphe nuclei,** and **locus ceruleus complex.** These brainstem structures receive information about the visceral activities that they regulate via ascending tracts. Some autonomic functions depend strongly on these brainstem pathways. For example, **micturition** and **defecation** depend on the integrity of pathways that interconnect the sacral spinal cord and the pons.

The urinary bladder is emptied by means of the **micturition reflex,** which involves both the sympathetic and parasympathetic nervous systems and a descending control system (see also Chapter 32). As the bladder fills to near its capacity, receptors in the bladder wall are activated. Signals ascend to the **micturition center** in the pons, activating descending pathways that cause a parasympathetic contraction of the **detrusor muscle** of the bladder and relaxation of the **internal** and **external sphincters.** Simultaneously, the sympathetic system relaxes the neck of the bladder and no longer causes constriction of the internal sphincter. The bladder can thus begin to empty. The receptors in the bladder wall also respond to contraction of the bladder wall musculature and ensure complete emptying.

> After spinal cord injury, the micturition reflex is disturbed by disruption of the long pathways connecting the sacral spinal cord and the micturition center in the pons. The bladder now fills excessively **(atonic neurogenic bladder)** and must be drained by catheterization. Later, a spinal reflex pathway becomes operative, but it is overactive **(spastic bladder).** However, the bladder does not empty completely, so it is predisposed to **infection,** and there is frequent **incontinence.**

Higher centers that regulate autonomic function include the hypothalamus and other components of the limbic system. Limbic structures are interconnected with nonlimbic parts of the nervous system, including the neocortex, cerebellum, and basal ganglia. The hypothalamus projects to the brainstem (e.g., to the reticular formation) and to the spinal cord. The limbic system controls motivation directly through neural pathways and indirectly through the endocrine system.

Functions of the Hypothalamus

The hypothalamus (see Chapter 44) has several broadly defined functions, which include the regulation of homeostasis, motivation, and emotional behavior. These functions are mediated through hypothalamic control of autonomic and endocrine activity as well as by interactions between the hypothalamus and other parts of the limbic system.

If the hypothalamus is stimulated electrically, particular regions can be shown to relate to particular autonomic responses. For example, stimulation in the lateral and posterior hypothalamus produces responses mediated by the sympathetic nervous system. Stimulation in the anterior hypothalamus activates parasympathetic output. The responses include changes in heart rate and blood pressure. Other global functions controlled by the hypothalamus include food and water intake, emotional behavior, and regulation of the immune system.

Neuroendocrine cells of the hypothalamus regulate neuronal circuits and endocrine functions

The neurons in some hypothalamic nuclei release peptides, either as hormones or as neuromodulator substances. Such neurons are classified as **neuroendocrine cells.** Neuroendocrine structures include the **paraventricular** and **supraoptic nuclei,** which give rise to the **hypothalamohypophysial tract** from the hypothalamus to the **posterior pituitary gland.** This tract releases the peptide hormones **oxytocin** and **vasopressin** into the circulation (see Chapter 44). The paraventricular nucleus also sends peptide-containing axons to various sites within the central nervous system, including the solitary nucleus, the dorsal motor nucleus of the vagus, and the intermediolateral cell column of the spinal cord. Oxytocin and vasopressin apparently are used both as hormones and as neuromodulators in autonomic neural circuits.

Neuroendocrine cells in a number of hypothalamic nuclei secrete hormones into the **portal system** that supplies the **anterior pituitary gland** (see Chapter 44). These hormones trigger or inhibit the release of pituitary hormones into the circulation, and they are very important in endocrine regulation. As in the case of oxytocin and vasopressin, the same hypothalamic substances can be used as neuromodulatory substances at synaptic terminals within the central nervous system.

An important hypothalamic function is temperature regulation

Homeothermic animals regulate their body temperature. WHEN THE ENVIRONMENTAL TEMPERATURE DECREASES, THE BODY ADJUSTS BY REDUCING HEAT LOSS AND INCREASING HEAT PRODUCTION. CONVERSELY, WHEN THE TEMPERATURE INCREASES, THE BODY INCREASES ITS HEAT LOSS AND REDUCES HEAT PRODUCTION.

Information about the external temperature is provided by **thermoreceptors** in the skin (and probably other organs such as muscle). Internal temperature is monitored by **central thermoreceptive neurons** in the anterior hypothalamus. The central thermoreceptors monitor the temperature of the blood. The system acts as a servomechanism with a set point at the normal body temperature. Error signals, representing deviations from the set point, lead to responses that tend to restore body temperature toward the set point. These responses are mediated by the autonomic nervous system, somatic nervous system, and endocrine system.

Cooling causes **shivering,** which consists of asynchronous muscle contractions that lead to increased heat production. There is also an increase in the activity of the thyroid gland and sympathetic nervous system, both of which tend to raise heat production metabolically. Heat loss is reduced by **cutaneous vasoconstriction** and by **piloerection.** (Piloerection is effective in animals with fur, although not in humans; in the latter, the result is goose bumps.)

Warming the body has the opposite effects. The activity of the thyroid gland decreases, which leads to reduced metabolic activity and less heat production. Heat loss is increased by **sweating** and **cutaneous vasodilation.**

The hypothalamus serves as the temperature servomechanism. The heat loss responses are organized by the **heat loss center,** which is thought to be composed of neurons in the preoptic region and anterior hypothalamus. Lesions here prevent sweating and cutaneous vasodilation; this results in **hyperthermia** when the individual is placed in a warm environment. Conversely, electrical stimulation here causes cutaneous vasodilation and sweating. Neurons in the posterior hypothalamus form a **heat-production and heat-conservation center.** Lesions in the area dorsolateral to the mammillary bodies eliminate heat production and conservation, leading to **hypothermia** in a cold environment. Electrical stimulation in this region evokes shivering.

> In **fever,** the set point for body temperature is elevated. An example mechanism is the release of a **pyrogen** by certain bacteria. The pyrogen changes the set point, which leads to increased heat production by shivering and to heat conservation by cutaneous vasoconstriction.

Limbic System

The limbic system includes the **limbic lobe** of the telencephalon as well as the **hypothalamus** and several **thalamic** and **midbrain nuclei.** The limbic components of the telencephalon include the **cingulate, parahippocampal,** and **subcallosal gyri** as well as the **hippocampal formation** (hippocampus, dentate gyrus, and subiculum).

The functions of the limbic system include the regulation of aggressive behavior and sexuality. More generally, the limbic system appears to be concerned with motivational states, which in turn are vital for the survival of both the individual and the species.

> Bilateral removal of temporal lobe structures, including the amygdaloid nuclei, results in a complex set of changes in behavior called the **Klüver-Bucy syndrome.** Animals previously wild become tame, they develop a pronounced tendency to put objects into their mouths, and they become sexually hyperactive. These changes result chiefly from damage to the amygdaloid nuclei.

The **hippocampus** appears to be important for the storage of recent memory (see also Chapter 11). MEMORIES ARE STORED IN THE FOLLOWING SEQUENCE: SHORT-TERM MEMORY, RECENT MEMORY, AND LONG-TERM MEMORY. Short-term memory is easily disrupted and is presumed to depend on ongoing neural events. Long-term memory seems to result from a permanent functional or structural change in the nervous system. Bilateral lesions of the hippocampus may not interfere with either short- or long-term memory but may prevent the process by which short-term memories are permanently stored. The process of recollection of memories may also be disrupted, resulting in **amnesia.**

> Bilateral lesions of the temporal lobes that damage the hippocampus, and degenerative diseases that destroy hippocampal circuits, notably **Alzheimer's disease,** can lead to deficits in the consolidation of recent memory. A patient with such disturbances may be able to remember a conversation for a short time, but minutes later may repeat the same conversation as if it had never happened. However, memories of childhood events may still be relatively clear.

SUMMARY

- Sympathetic preganglionic neurons are located in the intermediolateral (and intermediomedial) cell columns of the T1 to L2 segments of the spinal cord. Their axons leave the spinal cord through ventral roots and enter the sympathetic chain through white communicating rami.
- Sympathetic preganglionic neurons synapse on postganglionic neurons in the paravertebral or prevertebral ganglia. Postganglionic axons synapse in target organs.
- Parasympathetic preganglionic neurons are located in cranial nerve nuclei and the sacral preganglionic nucleus. Postganglionic axons synapse in target organs.
- The enteric nervous system is in the wall of the gastrointestinal tract in the myenteric and submucosal plex-

uses. It coordinates the movements and glandular secretions of the gut.
- The sympathetic and parasympathetic nervous systems regulate the activity of smooth muscle, cardiac muscle, and glands. Often, these components of the autonomic nervous system act in a reciprocal fashion.
- Preganglionic sympathetic and parasympathetic neurons release acetylcholine as their neurotransmitter. This neurotransmitter acts on nicotinic cholinergic receptors (and also on muscarinic receptors) on postganglionic neurons. These receptors are blocked by curare.
- Parasympathetic and some sympathetic postganglionic neurons (sudomotor and vasodilator neurons) also release acetylcholine. The postsynaptic receptors on target cells in this case are muscarinic and can be blocked by atropine.
- Most sympathetic postganglionic neurons release norepinephrine, which acts on α- and β-adrenergic receptors.
- The adrenal medulla receives sympathetic preganglionic input and releases epinephrine and norepinephrine into the general circulation.
- The autonomic nervous system operates reflexly and in response to descending control systems, especially the hypothalamus and other parts of the limbic system.
- The hypothalamus regulates homeostasis, motivation, and emotional behavior through control of the autonomic nervous system, endocrine system, and somatic nervous system. Some of the functions regulated include body temperature, cardiovascular activity, appetite, water intake, and immune responses.
- The hypothalamus controls endocrine function both by the direct release of hormones in the posterior pituitary gland and by the release of peptides into the portal circulation of the anterior pituitary gland.
- The limbic system includes not only the hypothalamus but also a number of forebrain structures, including the hippocampus and several nuclei in the midbrain. Functions of the limbic system include the regulation of aggressive behavior and sexuality. The hippocampus is involved in the storage of recently acquired memories and in memory consolidation.

BIBLIOGRAPHY

Bannister R: *Autonomic failure: a textbook of clinical disorders of the autonomic nervous system,* New York, 1983, Oxford University Press.

Blessing WW: *The lower brainstem and bodily homeostasis,* New York, 1997, Oxford University Press.

Dampney RAL: Functional organization of central pathways regulating the cardiovascular system, *Physiol Rev* 74:323, 1994.

Davis M: The role of the amygdala in fear and anxiety, *Annu Rev Neurosci* 15:353, 1992.

Elfin LG, Lindh B, Hökfelt T: The chemical neuroanatomy of sympathetic ganglia, *Annu Rev Neurosci* 16:471, 1993.

Loewy AD, Spyer KM: *Central regulation of autonomic functions,* New York, 1990, Oxford University Press.

Lopes da Silva FH et al: Anatomic organization and physiology of the limbic cortex, *Physiol Rev* 66:235, 1990.

▷ CASE STUDY

Case 10-1

A 24-year-old man was rescued from a car wreck. After his neck was stabilized by paramedics, he was taken to the emergency department. Imaging studies showed that he had a fracture of the C5 vertebra with likely damage to the spinal cord. Although he could breathe adequately, he could not move his arms or legs. Phasic stretch reflexes were absent in all extremities, and he could feel no form of stimulus to the skin below his shoulders. Babinski's sign was observed bilaterally. The systemic arterial blood pressure was 116/76 mm Hg. The urinary bladder was full, so the patient's bladder was catheterized. On follow-up examination several weeks later, the phasic stretch reflexes were hyperactive in all four extremities, and there was ankle clonus bilaterally. The basal blood pressure remained lower than normal, and plasma norepinephrine and epinephrine levels were also below normal. However, the blood pressure periodically became elevated until the bladder was emptied after stimulation of the lower abdominal wall.

1. **The blood pressure increased in this patient when the bladder became distended for which of the following reasons?**

   A. Activity in the hypothalamospinal tract was increased by the visceral afferent input from the bladder.

   B. Bladder distention was excessive because of hypotonus of the bladder wall and thus became painful.

   C. Infection of the bladder resulted in a buildup of bacterial products that caused vasoconstriction.

   D. Responses to plasma catecholamines were increased because of α-adrenoreceptor upregulation after denervation.

   E. Spinal autonomic reflexes were enhanced after recovery from spinal shock.

2. **If this patient were placed in a cold or hot environment, which of the following would occur?**

   A. His body could not thermoregulate, he so would tend to become hypothermic or hyperthermic.

   B. Excessive vasodilation in a hot environment would cause him to become hypothermic.

   C. Exaggerated shivering in a cold environment would result in hyperthermia.

   D. Peripheral and central thermoreceptors would become hyperactive, which would enhance thermoregulation.

   E. Lack of hypothalamic control of sweating and shivering would balance out, so he would have no problem with thermoregulation.

Higher Functions of the Nervous System

- Describe the electroencephalogram and evoked potentials and their relationship to states of consciousness and epilepsy.
- Explain learning and memory.
- Relate cerebral dominance to language function.

The central nervous system is responsible for the higher functions that characterize humans. These functions include consciousness, thought, perception, learning, memory, and language. States of consciousness, including the sleep-wake cycle, are generally studied with the help of neurophysiological techniques such as the electroencephalogram and evoked potentials.

Learning and memory depend on alterations in neural functions and even in structure. The human brain is actually two brains. The left hemisphere is dominant for certain functions, including handedness and language, and the opposite hemisphere is dominant for other functions, such as spatial relations and music.

Electroencephalogram

The higher functions of the human brain are expressed on the background of continuous thalamocortical interactions. Neurons of nearly all the nuclei of the thalamus project to the cerebral cortex, and the cerebral cortex projects back to the thalamus.

Recordings from the surface of the cerebral cortex (**electrocorticogram**) or from the scalp (**electroencephalogram [EEG]**) reveal the incessant oscillations of extracellular potentials caused by membrane potential oscillations in large numbers of cortical neurons. The oscillations are produced in response to the rhythmical alterations of activity in thalamocortical circuits. On a single-neuron level, activity corresponding to the EEG consists of alternating **excitatory** and **inhibitory postsynaptic potentials.** The excitatory potentials often result in discharges of cortical neurons.

The normal EEG can be described in terms of its frequency composition. Several characteristic frequency ranges can be recognized (Figure 11-1). These are called **alpha waves** (8 to 13 Hz), **beta waves** (>13 Hz), **theta waves** (4 to 7 Hz), and **delta waves** (<4 Hz). Other transient waves are also seen. The dominant frequency depends on several factors, including age, state of consciousness, recording site, action of drugs, and presence of disease. During the early years of life, the EEG is dominated by low frequencies. In mature individuals at rest with the eyes closed, the EEG recorded from the posterior region of the brain shows an alpha rhythm, whereas that recorded from the anterior part of the brain has a beta rhythm. If the individual is aroused, lower-voltage, higher-frequency beta rhythms take the place of the lower-frequency alpha waves (Figure 11-1). Slower waves of theta and delta frequencies are associated with deeper levels of sleep. BRAIN DEATH IS A PERSISTENT ISOELECTRIC EEG IN THE ABSENCE OF DEPRESSANT DRUGS.

Evoked Potentials

The EEG represents spontaneous activity that is not linked to a particular event. Similar activity can be evoked in response to a stimulus that activates a neural pathway to the thalamus and circuits within the cerebral cortex. Such stimulus-linked activity is called a **cortical evoked potential.** Evoked potentials can easily be produced in humans by stimulating a peripheral nerve with electric shocks, the retina with flashes of light, or the ear with an acoustic stimulus such as a click. The recorded waveform is largest over the appropriate region of the brain.

States of Consciousness

Mental processes occur in the brains of conscious subjects. Consciousness is not understood, but it is required for perception, thought, and use of language. The conscious state appears to depend on an interaction between the **brainstem reticular formation** and **thalamocortical circuits.** When consciousness is depressed, the EEG becomes more synchronous and slowed in frequency. During behavioral arousal, as in response to a painful stimulus, the EEG changes to a low-voltage, high-frequency pattern (EEG arousal).

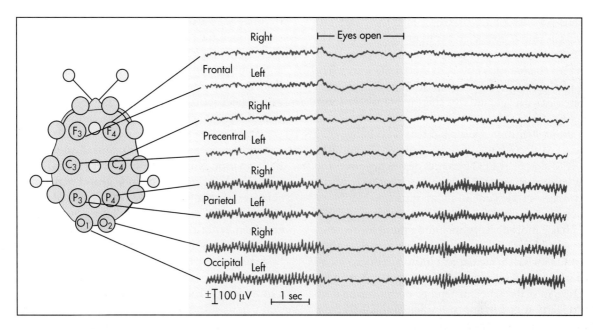

Figure 11-1 EEG recorded from a normal human. Recordings are from eight sites on the scalp. In the resting condition an alpha rhythm is prominent over the parietal and occipital lobes. When the eyes are opened, the alpha rhythm is blocked and replaced by a beta rhythm.

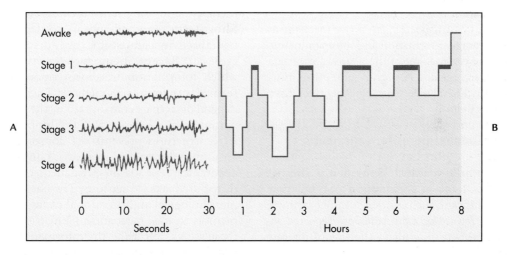

Figure 11-2 Stages of sleep and changes during the night. **A,** EEG recordings during the waking state and progressively deeper levels of non-REM sleep. The EEG in REM sleep would resemble that shown for the awake individual. **B,** Different sleep stages experienced during a typical night for a young adult. The bars represent periods of REM sleep.

Sleep is active, not the absence of brain activity

Sleep is an alteration rather than a loss of consciousness. This is shown by the ease with which sleep is interrupted by significant environmental events such as a baby's cry. Sleep has a circadian rhythm as well as a more rapid oscillation. **Circadian rhythms** repeat at approximately daily intervals. The sleep rhythm, along with many other biological rhythms, is normally entrained by the **light-dark cycle.** When a person rapidly changes location to a different time zone, it takes days for the circadian rhythms to be reentrained. The sleep disturbance and other disorders that result are collectively known as **jet lag.**

The various stages of sleep are characterized by different types of motor, autonomic, EEG, and psychological activity. The major distinction is between **rapid-eye-movement (REM) sleep** and **non-REM sleep.** When an individual falls asleep, the initial type is non-REM sleep. The EEG becomes more synchronized and slows (Figure 11-2, *A*). There are four levels of non-REM sleep. In the first level **(stage 1),** the person is drowsy, and the EEG shows 7- to 10-Hz rhythms. Over time the depth of non-REM sleep increases; that is, the EEG becomes progressively slower, and the person becomes difficult to arouse. In **stage 2,** or light sleep, a person is easily aroused; the dominant EEG frequencies are 3 to 7 Hz, with bursts of 12- to 14-Hz sleep spindles. During **stage 3** sleep, muscle tone and reflex activity are depressed, blood pressure falls, the heart rate slows, and the pupils constrict; the EEG shows 1- to 2-Hz, high-voltage waves. **Stage 4** is the deepest level of sleep, and it is also characterized by 1- to 2-Hz EEG waves. The amount of time spent in the deepest stage of non-REM sleep decreases with age, and this stage may entirely disappear after age 60.

After about 90 minutes, sleep lightens and changes to a period of REM sleep that lasts approximately 20 minutes. During REM sleep, the EEG becomes desynchronized and has a low voltage; the pattern is similar to that seen during arousal (Figure 11-2). Tone in many muscles disappears, and reflexes are inhibited. Interrupting this tonic inhibition are phasic motor events, including rapid movements of the eyes and brief contractions of other muscles. Autonomic events include irregular respiration, reduced blood pressure interrupted by episodes of hypertension, and penile erection in males. Dreams tend to occur during deep non-REM sleep. It is difficult to awaken individuals from REM sleep, but spontaneous awakening often occurs. REM sleep recurs about six times in a night. The proportion of time spent in REM sleep is greatest in the fetus and newborn, but it declines sharply during early infancy and then further with aging.

Sleep appears to be triggered by an active mechanism that involves the reticular formation and monoaminergic neurons in the brainstem. Some of the neurotransmitters associated with sleep include serotonin, norepinephrine, and acetylcholine. Several sleep-inducing peptides have been discovered as well.

Attention depends on neural mechanisms

Attention is the process by which perception is directed at particular events. It involves orientation to stimuli that are potentially significant, such as novel stimuli or stimuli likely to lead to a reward or a punishment. Repeated attention to a stimulus may result in the loss of interest in or **habituation** to the stimulus. Application of a threatening stimulus enhances attention; this process is termed **sensitization.**

There are several forms of epilepsy

Epilepsy refers to disease states characterized by behavioral and EEG seizures. The seizures may be partial or generalized. In **partial seizures,** only part of the brain shows abnormal activity. Consciousness is retained in partial simple seizures but lost in partial complex seizures. In **generalized seizures,** large regions of the brain are involved, and consciousness is lost.

Partial seizures may originate in a damaged area of the motor cortex. Such seizures are characterized by contractions of muscles in the somatotopically appropriate region on the contralateral side and a focal EEG spike train. (An EEG spike is a synchronous wave that results from simultaneous activity in many neurons.) The seizures often spread to adjacent areas in a **march** of convulsive activity to other contralateral parts of the body. For example, the seizure may start with contractions of the fingers, but the movements may then spread to the arm, shoulder, face, and lower extremities. Partial seizures may also originate from the somatosensory cortex and produce focal sensory experiences contralaterally. Psychomotor seizures are partial seizures that originate in the limbic lobe. These are characterized by semipurposeful movements, changes in consciousness, hallucinations, and illusions. A common hallucination is an unpleasant odor **(uncinate fit).**

Generalized seizures include **grand mal** and **petit mal seizures.** Grand mal attacks may be preceded by an **aura.** Consciousness is soon lost, followed by tonic and clonic contractions of muscles on both sides of the body. Petit mal attacks are brief losses of consciousness, accompanied by a characteristic EEG pattern.

Learning and Memory

Learning is a process by which behavior is modified on the basis of experience. **Memory** is the storage of information that has been learned. There are several stages of memory, including short-term memory, recent memory, and long-term memory (see Chapter 10). **Short-term memory** appears to depend on ongoing neural activity because it is easily disrupted (e.g., by anesthesia). **Recent memory** refers to the process by which information in short-term memory is transformed into long-term memory. This process seems to depend on activity transmitted by the hippocampal formation because damage to the hippocampus and related structures prevents the consolidation of short-term into long-term memory. **Long-term memory** apparently depends on permanent changes in widely distributed sets of neurons. The changes may include morphological and functional changes. In addition to memory stores, mechanisms must exist for accessing these stores, retrieving the information, recalling it to consciousness, comparing it to other information, and using the information for decisions.

Experiments are being performed to elucidate the mechanisms of learning and memory. Simple forms of learning have been studied in the simple nervous systems of invertebrates. Habituation and sensitization are examples of **nonassociative learning** because they do not require learning an association between two events. In habituation a response to a particular stimulus diminishes with repetition of the stimulus. Habituation is thus the process of learning that a stimulus is unimportant. Conversely, sensitization is the process by which a person learns that a stimulus is important. For example, with repetition of a painful stimulus, an individual quickly learns to respond.

In **associative learning** the relationship between two different stimuli is learned. In **classic conditioning** a conditioned stimulus is paired with an unconditioned stimulus. The latter initially produces an unconditioned response; for example, food produces salivation in a hungry dog. After conditioning, the conditioned stimulus may produce the same response; for example, ringing a bell at the time food is presented ultimately causes salivation even if the food is omitted. In **operant conditioning,** reinforcement of a response changes the probability of the response. Operant behaviors are not reflexes but rather spontaneous actions. An example of operant conditioning would be an animal's avoidance of a wire grid that induces an electric shock when the animal happens to step on the grid. In this case the conditioning stimulus provides **negative reinforcement.**

Habituation, sensitization, and classic conditioning have all been demonstrated in invertebrate models, and the neural mechanisms that underlie both nonassociative and associative learning are being investigated. A major theme of such work is that synaptic efficacy changes during these simple forms of learning. These changes depend on the activation of second messenger systems. Long-term changes are accompanied by structural as well as functional changes. A parallel experimental approach in mammals involves the enhancement or depression of synaptic transmission for hours to days or even longer after the activation of particular pathways in the hippocampus and cerebellum. The mechanisms that underlie **long-term potentiation** and **long-term depression** are under active study.

Cerebral Dominance

The two halves of the human brain are not equivalent. IN A REAL SENSE, THE HUMAN HAS TWO BRAINS THAT COMMUNICATE WITH EACH OTHER VIA THE CEREBRAL COMMISSURES. The left hemisphere is dominant in most individuals with respect to control of the preferred hand (right in most people) and to language. However, the right hemisphere can be considered dominant for other functions (e.g., music, spatial relationships).

Cerebral dominance has been studied best in patients whose left and right hemispheres have been disconnected by surgical division of the corpus callosum. Visual images can be shown separately to the left and right visual fields of such individuals, and they can be asked to identify objects placed in the right or left hand (Figure 11-3). If a picture of an object, such as a ring, is presented to the left hemisphere, the subject can identify the object verbally as a ring. If a picture of a key is presented to the right hemisphere, the subject cannot identify it verbally. This is because information about the key that reaches the right hemisphere does not gain access to the language centers of the left hemisphere. However, the subject can identify the picture in another way, by picking up a key with the left hand after feeling a group of objects.

Language is processing by certain cortical areas

Language depends on activity in the left hemisphere in most people. This can be demonstrated by injecting local

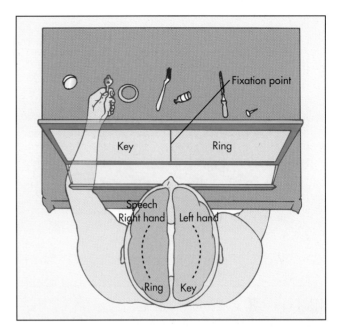

Figure 11-3 Technique for investigating a patient with a disconnection syndrome caused by transection of the corpus callosum. The subject is asked to look at a fixation point at the center of the screen. Pictures are projected on the screen. If the picture is in the left visual field, the image is processed in the right hemisphere (key in this instance). The subject can also reach under the screen to find objects that can be identified by tactile cues. (See also text.)

anesthetic into the carotid circulation on the left while an individual is speaking. The anesthetic stops speech (causes **aphasia**).

Analysis of aphasia that occurs after damage to the left hemisphere of adults has revealed that several major zones are important for language. One of these is called **Broca's area,** which is located in the inferior frontal gyrus just anterior to the face representation in the motor cortex (Figure 11-4). The other important region for the control of language is **Wernicke's area,** which is in the supramarginal and angular gyri of the temporal lobe and the posterior part of the superior temporal gyrus. A structural correlate of cerebral dominance for language is the greater size of the left than of the right **planum temporale** (temporal plane, the superior surface of the temporal lobe [Figure 11-4]).

Damage to Broca's area diminishes the ability of the individual to speak and write. The person understands spoken or written words, and there is nonfluent speech. Although the lesion may also result in hemiplegia, there is not necessarily an impediment to sound production. Vocabulary is often reduced to expletives. This type of aphasia is called **expressive** or **Broca's aphasia.** Damage to Wernicke's area diminishes the comprehension of spoken or written language. However, the person has fluent speech, much of which is meaningless, with frequent **paraphasias** and **neologisms.** This type of aphasia is called **receptive** or **Wernicke's aphasia.**

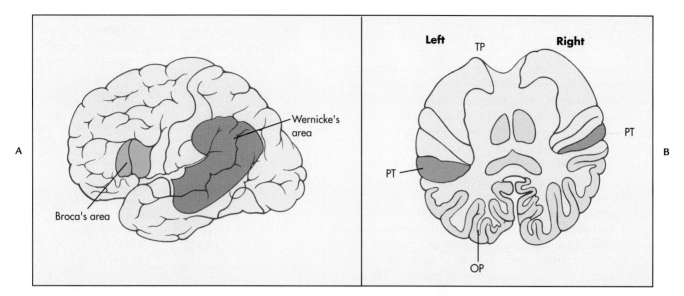

Figure 11-4 Areas of the cerebral cortex important for language. **A,** Broca's and Wernicke's areas. **B,** The relative size of the planum temporale *(PT)* on the two sides of the brain. *OP,* Occipital pole; *TP,* temporal pole.

SUMMARY

- The EEG can be recorded from scalp electrodes, and it is produced by ongoing activity in thalamocortical neural circuits. It represents the summed synaptic potentials of numerous cerebral cortical neurons.
- The EEG has waves of different characteristic frequencies, which range from more than 13 Hz (beta waves) to 8 to 13 Hz (alpha waves), 4 to 7 Hz (theta waves), and less than 4 Hz (delta waves). Beta waves are observed in the aroused state and in REM sleep, alpha waves in quiet wakefulness, and delta waves in non-REM sleep.
- Events in cortical neurons can be triggered by the stimulation of sensory pathways. When recorded in a way similar to that used for the EEG, these events are called evoked potentials.
- Consciousness is a state resulting from activity of the brain. It may be impaired or lost in disease states.
- Sleep is an alteration of consciousness and occurs with a circadian rhythm. Sleep is subdivided into REM and non-REM forms.
- Learning and memory allow the modification of behavior based on experience. Memory includes short-term, recent, and long-term stages. Learning can be nonassociative or associative depending on whether conditioned and unconditioned stimuli are paired.
- The two cerebral hemispheres differ in that one is dominant for some functions and the second is dominant for other functions.
- Damage to Broca's or Wernicke's area results in the loss of the ability to use language.

BIBLIOGRAPHY

Baudry M, Davis JL, eds: *Long-term potentiation,* Cambridge, Mass, 1991, MIT Press.

Thompson RF, Krupa DJ: Organization of memory traces in the mammalian brain, *Annu Rev Neurosci* 17:519, 1994.

Werker JF, Tees RC: The organization and reorganization of human speech, *Annu Rev Neurosci* 15:547, 1993.

Zola-Morgan S, Squire LR: Neuroanatomy of memory, *Annu Rev Neurosci* 16:547, 1993.

CASE STUDY

Case 11-1

A 78-year-old man suddenly developed a right-sided hemiplegia. He was unable to give a satisfactory history because the only words that he could speak were curse words. However, he did nod his head appropriately in response to questions.

1. **Which part of the brain produced the speech disorder in this patient?**
   A. Corpus callosum
   B. Inferior frontal gyrus on the left
   C. Inferior frontal gyrus on the right
   D. Posterior part of the superior temporal gyrus on the left
   E. Posterior part of the superior temporal gyrus on the right

2. **What other neurological deficit is this patient likely to have?**
   A. Difficulty writing
   B. Intention tremor on the right
   C. Left homonymous hemianopsia
   D. Loss of hearing in the left ear
   E. Babinski's sign on the left

MUSCLE

III

Richard A. Murphy

CHAPTER 12

Molecular Basis of Contraction

OBJECTIVES

- Describe the molecules and their interactions that generate force and movement in muscle.
- Describe how conformational changes in molecules are linked to generate large forces and movements.
- Describe contraction in terms of forces generated and rates of movement.
- Indicate how the combination of structural and mechanical data can explain contraction in terms of the sliding filament–cross-bridge mechanism.

Movement is perhaps the most striking difference between plants and animals and is made possible by muscle. Muscle allows humans to walk and talk and is required for the function of most organs. This section introduces the basic concepts of muscle, the largest tissue mass of the human body. Chapter 12 focuses on the biological energy transformation termed **chemomechanical transduction;** the molecular basis of energy transformation is identical in all muscles. Chapter 13 focuses on muscles under voluntary control, and Chapter 14 discusses involuntary muscles that are involved in organ function.

Contractile Unit

The basic structure involved in contraction consists of organized arrays of insoluble proteins. One set of proteins forms a **cytoskeleton** that serves as an anchor and as a force-transmitting structure for the contractile proteins, which are organized in the **myofilaments.** The contractile unit in **striated muscle** cells is called a **sarcomere** (see Figures 12-1 and Figure 13-2). Enormous numbers of sarcomeres are linked by the cytoskeleton. **Z disks** mechanically link sarcomeres end to end. **Intermediate filaments** connect the Z disks of adjacent **myofibrils** (see Figure 13-2) within a striated muscle cell. The transverse alignment of sarcomeres and their constituent myofilaments gives these cells their striated appearance.

Thin filaments are connected to the cell cytoskeleton that transmits force

Thin filaments are ubiquitous cell structures that always contain **actin** and **tropomyosin** (Figure 12-2). The thin filaments in vertebrate striated muscle are anchored in the Z disks, and a molecule of **troponin** is bound to each tropomyosin molecule. Troponin, a regulatory protein, contains Ca^{++} binding sites that are involved in the control of contraction and relaxation in vertebrate striated muscle (see Chapter 13).

Thick filaments are aggregates of the molecules that generate force

Myosin is a large, complex molecule consisting of tail and head regions (Figure 12-2). The tails aggregate to form thick filaments, with the heads projecting out toward the thin filaments. Each head, termed a **cross-bridge,** contains two actin binding sites and two enzymatic sites that can hydrolyze ATP to ADP and inorganic phosphate (P_i). These sites are involved in chemomechanical transduction. The interactions between the cross-bridges and the thin filaments draw the thin filaments toward the sarcomere's center and thereby shorten the sarcomere as the Z disks come closer together in the **sliding filament–cross-bridge mechanism** (Figure 12-1).

Cross-Bridge Cycling Produces Muscle Contraction

The hydrolysis of ATP occurs when purified myosin and thin filaments are mixed in a solution that approximates the ionic content of the cytoplasm, which is often called the **myoplasm** in muscle cells (Figure 12-3, *A*). This cycle can be represented by the following steps.

1. ATP binds to myosin and is hydrolyzed to form the myosin-ADP-P_i complex. This complex, characterized by a high level of free energy, has a great affinity for actin and rapidly binds to the thin filament.
2. P_i and ADP are released after myosin attaches to the thin filament, and the myosin head undergoes

a conformational change. The resulting actin-myosin complex has a low level of free energy.

3. The actin-myosin complex then binds ATP. The resulting actin-myosin-ATP complex has a low actin binding affinity, so the cross-bridge dissociates from the thin filament.

4. Internal hydrolysis of the bound ATP regenerates the high-energy myosin-ADP- P_i complex to complete the cycle.

In this biochemical cycle the release of free energy occurring in the overall reaction, ATP to ADP plus P_i, is lost as heat. The conversion of part of this energy into mechanical work depends on the filament organization of the muscle cells. The orientation of the myosin heads incorporated into a thick filament is constrained. The preferred orientation of the high-energy complexes (myosin-ADP- P_i and actin-myosin-ADP- P_i) is perpendicular (90 degrees) to the thick filament (Figure 12-3, B). However, the preferred (i.e., lowest level of free energy) conformation of the actin-myosin complex after the release of ADP and P_i occurs when the cross-bridge is oriented 45 degrees to the filaments. Thus part of the energy from ATP is translated into conformation changes in the cross-bridges. This "bending" of the cross-bridges generates forces that draw the thin filaments past the thick filaments and toward the center of the sarcomere. The force is transmitted by the cytoskeleton to the ends of the cell and thereby exerts a force on the skeleton. A single cross-bridge cycle moves a thin filament only 10 nm (10^{-8} m) and develops a minute force estimated to be around 5×10^{-12} N. Nevertheless, MILLIONS OF CROSS-BRIDGES CYCLING ASYNCHRONOUSLY CAN GENERATE GREAT FORCES AND CAN CONSIDERABLY SHORTEN MUSCLE CELLS.

Several factors determine cross-bridge cycling

The cross-bridge cycle illustrated in Figure 12-3 continues until all the ATP is consumed and the cycle is arrested (after step 2). This occurs after death, when the ATP supplies are not replenished, and is characterized by **rigor mortis,** or muscular rigidity, because the cross-bridges are permanently attached.

Resting or relaxed muscle contains detached cross-bridges in the myosin-ADP- P_i state, and the muscle is freely extensible. These cross-bridges are prevented from attaching to the thin filaments by Ca^{++}-dependent regulatory systems, which differ among muscle types (see Chapters 13 and 14).

Cross-bridge cycling rates determine how fast a muscle shortens. The maximum shortening velocities occur when

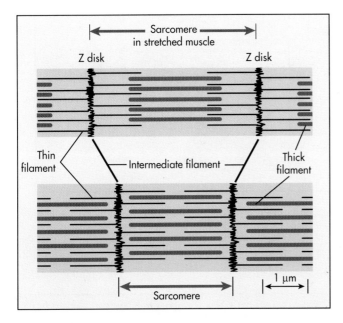

Figure 12-1 Sarcomere. The contractile proteins are found in interdigitating arrays of thick and thin filaments that slide past one another during contraction and relaxation. Thin filaments are attached to the Z disks. Other cytoskeletal proteins stabilize the filaments.

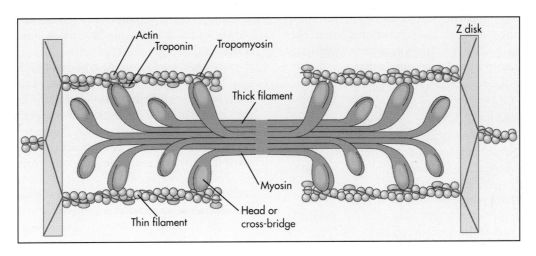

Figure 12-2 The core of the thin filament is a twisted, two-stranded chain of polymerized actin molecules. Each molecule of the long, rigid tropomyosin binds with six or seven actin monomers plus one troponin in striated muscle. Thick filaments are composed of 300 to 400 myosin molecules. Note the central zone lacking cross-bridges that divides the thick filament into two halves, where the cross-bridges have opposite orientations.

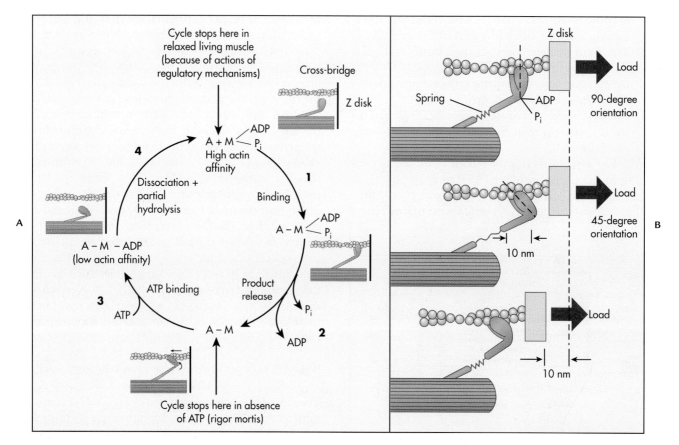

Figure 12-3 Steps in the cross-bridge cycle. **A,** Relationship among the steps (*1* to *4*) of the hydrolysis of ATP and cross-bridge conformations. **B,** Preferred or minimal free energy conformations of attached cross-bridges. The transition from the 90- to the 45-degree conformation that occurs on the release of P_i and ADP generates a force in the cross-bridge represented by the stretched spring. This force can be translated into shortening by the movement of the thin filament past the thick filament if the load is not too great. *A,* Actin; *M,* myosin.

no load opposes filament sliding. A load on a muscle cell is transmitted by the cytoskeleton to the sarcomere and opposes bending of the cross-bridges (Figure 12-3, *B*). Increasing the load slows cross-bridge cycling. The velocity of muscle contraction falls to zero when the load prevents the transition from the 90- to the 45-degree conformation. Different types of unloaded muscle cells vary in their maximum shortening velocities. Such functional differences are determined by the specific isoenzymatic variant of myosin expressed in a particular muscle cell.

> Contractile protein isoform expression changes during development. Fetal, neonatal, and adult myosin isoforms constitute a normal progression. Pathological conditions can lead to changes in the expression of myosin genes and thereby can alter muscle performance. Injuries or diseases such as **amyotrophic lateral sclerosis** or **poliomyelitis** can destroy the innervation of skeletal muscle cells and produce muscle paralysis. The denervated muscle cells subsequently express neonatal and fetal myosin isoforms and eventually **atrophy.**

Contraction Can Produce Several Actions

Contracting muscle cells may develop a force without shortening, may shorten at various velocities, or may lengthen while opposing a force larger than the muscle can generate. The response depends on the loading. A simple mechanical analysis of contraction describes the output of the muscle cells and helps show how muscle functions.

ONLY THREE VARIABLES ARE NEEDED TO DESCRIBE THE OUTPUT OF A MUSCLE: FORCE, LENGTH, AND TIME (Table 12-1). The analysis is simplified by experimentally holding one of the three variables constant and determining the relationship between the other two. This experimental constraint yields two types of contractions: **isometric** (constant length) and **isotonic** (constant force or load).

In isometric contractions, force generation depends on sarcomere length

A muscle cell develops a characteristic force when it is maximally stimulated at a fixed length. The force-length relationship depicts this steady-state behavior (Figure

Table 12-1	Basic Mechanical Variables in Muscle Contraction	
Parameter	**Units**	**Definition**
Force (F)	Newton (N)	
Length (L)	Meter (m)	
Time (T)	Second (sec)	
Derived Variables		
Velocity (V)	m/sec	Change in length ÷ change in time
Work (W)	N × m	Force × distance

12-4). Stimulated skeletal muscle cells develop no force if they are first stretched to sarcomere lengths greater than 3.7 μm. At shorter lengths, FORCE IS PROPORTIONAL TO THE NUMBER OF CROSS-BRIDGES THAT INTERACT WITH THE THIN FILAMENT IN EACH HALF-SARCOMERE. Force generation is also lower when the muscle lengths are less than the optimum length (L_o). Disturbances of the sarcomeric structure and failure of the activation processes are responsible.

The forces generated depend on the size of the muscle cell and the number of filaments. When force is normalized for size by expressing it as force per cell cross-sectional area, vertebrate muscle cells generate about 3×10^5 N/m² when the cells are at their L_o. These remarkable forces are attributed to high concentrations of cross-bridges that individually generate very small forces. INCREASES IN STRENGTH ASSOCIATED WITH GROWTH OR EXERCISE RESULT FROM THE SYNTHESIS OF MORE THICK AND THIN FILAMENTS AND AN INCREASE IN THE CROSS-SECTIONAL AREA OF MUSCLE CELLS.

In isotonic contractions, velocities depend on the load

A lever simplifies the measurement of shortening of a muscle at a constant load (Figure 12-5, A). The relaxed muscle is adjusted to the L_o for force development (Figure 12-4), and different loads are attached to the lever before the muscle is stimulated. If the load is greater than the muscle can lift, the force developed is maximum (F_o), and the contraction is isometric, as just discussed. If the load is somewhat smaller, force develops without shortening until the force developed by the muscle is equal to the load. The muscle then begins to shorten isotonically (Figure 12-5, B). The slope of the length-versus-time record equals the shortening velocity. A third contraction with an even lighter load has a higher shortening velocity. The complete dependence of velocity on load obtained from many contractions is shown in Figure 12-5, C.

THE VELOCITY-FORCE RELATIONSHIP IS THE MECHANICAL MANIFESTATION OF THE SUM OF ALL THE CROSS-BRIDGE INTERACTIONS IN THE CELL. SHORTENING VELOCITY IS PROPORTIONAL TO THE AVERAGE CROSS-BRIDGE CYCLING RATE. A maximum velocity (V_o)

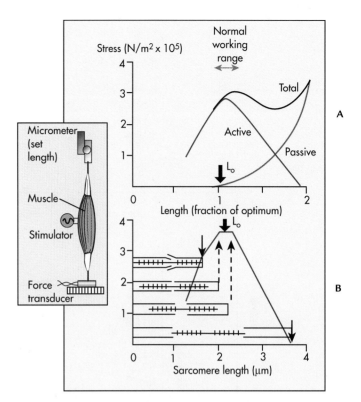

Figure 12-4 A, Relaxed muscles behave like a rubber band as the cell is lengthened (passive curve). This elasticity is due to connective tissue fibrils of collagen and elastin surrounding the muscle and individual muscle cells, although intracellular cytoskeletal elements contribute. Contracting muscles develop greater forces; this curve is known as the *total force–length relationship*. The difference between the total force and the passive force curves is the active force–length relationship and represents the force-generating properties of the cross-bridges. The inset shows an experimental setup. **B,** A sophisticated analysis of single cells or sarcomeres reveals that the generated force depends on the overlap of thick and thin filaments. At L_o the cell can develop the most force because all the cross-bridges can interact with the thin filaments in each half of a sarcomere.

occurs with zero load. A load slows the average cycling rate as it opposes the cross-bridge transition from the 90- to the 45-degree conformation, thereby slowing step 2 in Figure 12-3, A, in the cross-bridge cycle.

Contracting muscles may lengthen while resisting imposed loads

Cross-bridge cycling produces force development and shortening. Nevertheless, the force of gravity, the contraction of opposing muscles, or other external forces can impose large loads that may lengthen contracting muscle cells. A contracting muscle cell can briefly resist imposed loads that are 60% greater than the force the cell can develop (Figure 12-5, B). High forces are required to break the cross-bridge attachments to the thin filaments. Heavily loaded cross-bridges cannot undergo a conformational change to 45 degrees. After the link is broken, the cross-bridges reattach and thereby resist further lengthening. The cross-bridge cycle, with release of P_i and ADP and

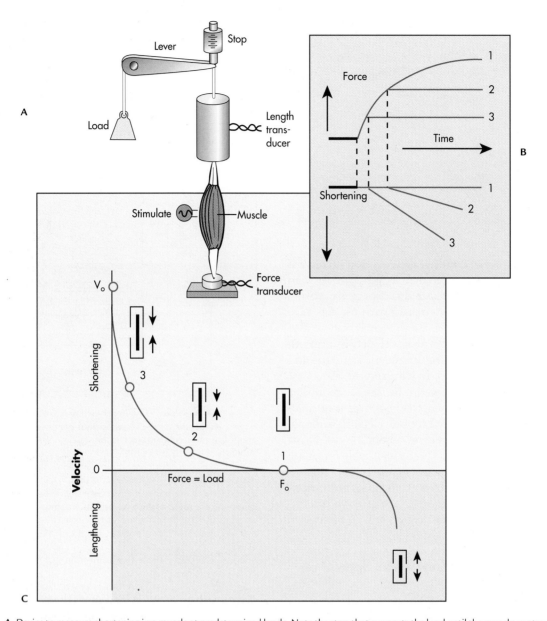

Figure 12-5 A, Device to measure shortening in a muscle at predetermined loads. Note the stop that supports the load until the muscle contracts. **B,** Transducers in the apparatus detecting force and length show the response to stimulation at very high *(1)*, moderate *(2)*, and low *(3)* loads. **C,** The velocity-force relationship for a shortening muscle is hyperbolic. The cell can either shorten rapidly or develop high forces. Contracting muscles can withstand higher forces than they develop (loads > maximum force [F_o]). High imposed loads are associated with a slow lengthening. At a load of approximately 1.6 F_o, the contractile system yields, and rapid lengthening occurs. The relative rates of movement at various loads are indicated by the lengths of the arrows beside the four sarcomere diagrams. V_o, Maximum shortening velocity at zero load.

binding of ATP, is never completed when the muscle is stretched (Figure 12-3). The work is done on the muscle cells rather than by the muscle cells, and no ATP cost is incurred.

Large external forces on the musculoskeletal system can cause bones to break, tendons to rupture, and muscles to tear. Such injuries may occur when the muscles are relaxed if the musculoskeletal system is forced beyond its

normal range of movements. However, most injuries happen when muscles are maximally contracted, as may occur when the weight of the body is concentrated on one extended arm in a fall. The highest forces that occur in a muscle are the result of imposed external loads (Figure 12-5) that stretch contracting muscle cells and are transmitted by the tendons to joints and bones. Stretching contracting muscle cells is a normal occurrence and does not usually result in injury. Nevertheless, such situations occasionally push the musculoskeletal system beyond its limits.

Vertebrate muscle can be divided into two broad classes. One consists of rapidly contracting muscle cells characterized by high rates of work, high ATP consumption, and high efficiencies in converting the energy of ATP into mechanical work (see Chapter 13). These cells are typically attached to the skeleton and are striated. The other class of muscle contains slowly contracting muscle cells, which are specialized to contract more or less continuously and which use little ATP (see Chapter 14). These smooth muscle cells are typically part of the walls of hollow organs.

SUMMARY

- The elementary contractile unit has an array of thick filaments containing myosin. The thick filaments interdigitate with thin filaments that consist of actin, tropomyosin, and other proteins attached to cytoskeletal elements.
- Contraction is produced by cross-bridges that consist of the heads of myosin molecules projecting from thick filaments. The cross-bridges cyclically interact with the thin filaments.
- Each cross-bridge cycle converts part of the free energy associated with the hydrolysis of an ATP molecule into a conformational change in the cross-bridge.
- Muscles are organized to link enormous numbers of contractile units such that the summed contributions of individual cross-bridges generate very high forces or large movements.
- Shortening velocities are determined by cross-bridge cycling rates. These rates vary with the isoform of myosin expressed in a cell and with the load.
- Contracting muscles sometimes lengthen while decelerating the body or stabilizing complex motions.

BIBLIOGRAPHY

Cooke R: Actomyosin interaction in striated muscle, *Physiol Rev* 77:671, 1997.

Eisenberg E, Hill TL: Muscle contraction and free energy transduction in biological systems, *Science* 227:999, 1985.

Gordon AM, Huxley AF, Julian FJ: The variation in isometric tension with sarcomere length in vertebrate muscle fibres, *J Physiol* 184:170, 1966.

Hochachka PW: *Muscles as molecular and metabolic machines,* Boca Raton, Fla, 1994, CRC.

Ishijima A et al: Simultaneous observation of individual ATPase and mechanical events by a single myosin molecule during interaction with actin, *Cell* 92:161, 1998.

Josephson RK: Contraction dynamics and power output of skeletal muscle, *Annu Rev Physiol* 55:527, 1993.

Millman BM: The filament lattice of striated muscle, *Physiol Rev* 78:359, 1998.

Obinata T: Contractile proteins and myofibrillogenesis, *Int Rev Cytol* 143:153, 1993.

Peachey LD, Adrian RH, eds: *Handbook of physiology,* section 10, *Skeletal muscle,* Bethesda, Md, 1983, American Physiological Society.

Rayment I, Smith C, Yount RG: The active site of myosin, *Ann Rev Physiol* 58:671, 1996.

Ruppel KM, Spudich JA: Structure-function analysis of the motor domain of myosin, *Ann Rev Cell Dev Biol* 12:543, 1996.

Trinick J: Titin and nebulin: protein rulers in muscle, *Trends Biochem Sci* 19:405, 1994.

CASE STUDY

Case 12-1

In a fitness test a subject repeatedly stepped up using the right leg while the left leg was used to oppose the effect of gravity in the step down. Muscle pain was experienced several hours after the test. The soreness reached a peak in 1 to 2 days and persisted for about a week. The presence of proteins specific for muscle in the subject's serum provided evidence for muscle cell injury. Structural damage was apparent in biopsy samples from the affected muscles.

1. **Which circumstances are most likely to impose excessively high forces and might injure muscle cells?**
   - **A.** Isometric contraction when no shortening occurs
   - **B.** Overstretching of inactive muscle cells
   - **C.** Excessive shortening of contracting muscle cells
   - **D.** Stretching of contracting muscle cells by gravitational or other loads imposed during exercise
   - **E.** Rapid shortening at low loads

2. **Why are metabolic limitations that lead to ATP depletion not responsible for delayed-onset muscle soreness?**
   - **A.** ATP depletion would lead to rigor (attached, noncycling cross-bridges).
   - **B.** Any metabolic effect should have a rapid onset.
   - **C.** ATP consumption is highest in rapidly shortening muscles, where forces are modest.
   - **D.** ATP production was not impaired in the test in which brief contractions did not limit blood flow.
   - **E.** All of the above.

3. **If injury was responsible for the development of soreness, which muscles would be most affected?**
   - **A.** All the muscles in both legs
   - **B.** All the muscles that contracted during the fitness test
   - **C.** The muscles that contracted in the left leg
   - **D.** Primarily the muscles in the right leg that were actively shortening
   - **E.** The relaxed muscles that were passively stretched

Muscles Acting on the Skeleton

- Quantify the output of muscle cells acting via skeletal connections.
- Describe the distinctive structure-function relationship of skeletal muscle cells.
- Describe how motor nerves recruit and control skeletal muscle cells.
- Characterize the steps linking action potentials to cross-bridge cycling.
- Explain how the specialization of muscle cells allows varied types of contractile function.
- Describe developmental changes and adaptive responses to exercise and disease.

Humans make a voluntary decision to talk, walk, stand up, or sit down. The muscles that make these actions possible are skeletal muscles. A muscle cell acting on a skeleton to produce movement has a specific role that dictates many of its properties. These properties are examined in this chapter beginning with the structure of skeletal muscle.

Skeletal Muscle Usually Acts on the Skeleton

The skeleton serves as a supporting lever system on which most skeletal muscle cells act (Figure 13-1). Exceptions include striated muscle in the lips and esophagus, where the muscles participate in the voluntary acts of speaking and swallowing. Characteristically, striated muscle cells in the limbs bridge two joints before they attach to the skeleton via tendons or other mechanical connections that contain inextensible collagen fibrils.

The relationship between the muscle cells and the skeleton dictates the following important characteristics of skeletal muscle:

1. Individual skeletal muscle cells connect two tendons and contract independently in response to a nerve impulse.
2. The force of contraction can be increased by recruiting more cells.

3. Skeletal muscle cells are usually relaxed, and the skeleton bears most gravitational loads.
4. Skeletal muscle cells typically act on the short end of the skeletal lever system (Figure 13-1). Thus they must develop forces that are much greater than the load moved. However, large movements can result from limited cell shortening.
5. Most contractions produce movement and do mechanical **work** (work = force × distance). The rate of doing work, **power** (power = work ÷ time), can be great.
6. Skeletal muscles are characterized by a high **efficiency** (efficiency = work done ÷ ATP consumed).

Skeletal muscle cells are multinuclear giants formed by the fusion of embryonic precursors

Muscles such as the biceps consist of bundles of muscle cells that are separated from other muscles by connective tissues. The contraction of some or all of the cells in a muscle yields complex movements. Mammals typically have more than 400 muscles, with several attached to one bone. (An elephant's trunk is a notable exception, with thousands of muscles and no bones.) Discrete movements are the result of coordinated contractions involving many muscles. Muscles may act together as **synergists** to produce the same movement, or they may function as **antagonists** to other muscles to decelerate a motion. The summed actions of several muscles stabilize joints and produce precisely controlled movements. Both **flexors** and **extensors** (antagonist muscles that act on the limb joints) are normally involved in a movement. Individuals vary in the muscles they use to accomplish a specific motion. These patterns reflect differences in neuromuscular learning or training and are a factor in coordination and athletic performance.

Embryonic myoblasts fuse to form the enormous multinucleated, differentiated skeletal muscle cells. Although their diameter is that of a fine thread (50 to 100 μm), these multinucleated cells may be many centimeters long. The contractile units, or sarcomeres (see Chapter 12), of skeletal muscle are linked in series along a **myofibril** (Figure 13-2). The cytoskeleton links the Z disks of the

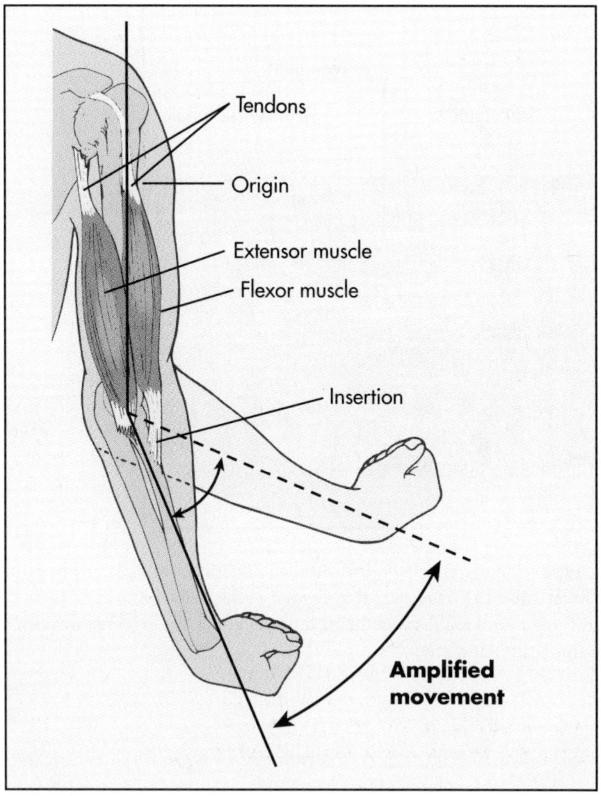

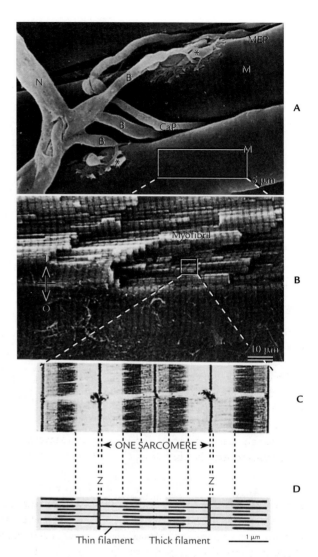

Figure 13-1 Groups of skeletal muscle cells form discrete muscles. The cells span anchor sites on the skeletal lever system.

Figure 13-2 A, Scanning electron micrograph of segments of three mammalian skeletal muscle cells *(M)* showing striations. Each cell receives a branch *(B)* of a motor nerve *(N)* in a complex structure termed the *motor endplate (MEP)* or neuromuscular junction *(asterisks).* Note the close association of the giant cells with the capillaries *(cap).* **B,** Scanning electron micrograph of skeletal muscle cell that was broken open to show the interior packed with large numbers of striated myofibrils. *I,* Interior; *O,* extracellular space. **C,** Higher-magnification transmission electron micrograph of a thin section through two myofibrils. Individual filaments are difficult to discern at this magnification. **D,** Structure of the sarcomere arising from thin filaments attached to Z disks *(Z)* interdigitating with a central lattice of thick filaments. *(A from Desaki J, Uehara Y: J Neurocytol 10:107, 1981. **B** from Swada H, Ishikawa H, Yamada E: Tissue Cell 10:183, 1978. **C** from Huxley HE: Sci Am 213:18, 1965.)*

myofibrils so that the sarcomeres are aligned. The resulting alternating dark and light stripes correspond to regions that contain thick filaments separated by regions containing only thin filaments. These stripes are clearly visible when viewed through the light microscope. Enormous numbers of sarcomeres may be present. For example, a 10-cm-long cell would have more than 45,000 sarcomeres.

Four structurally and functionally distinct membranes in the cell are involved in activating skeletal muscle cells

The **neuromuscular junction,** or **motor endplate,** is a specialized region of the plasma membrane (Figures 13-2 and 13-3). The plasma membrane, or **sarcolemma,** along which action potentials are propagated, is the second membrane (see Chapter 3). Tiny openings in the sarcolemma lead into the **transverse-tubular (T-tubular) network** located near the Z disks in mammals. This network defines an extracellular space within the cell (Figure 13-3). The extensive T-tubular network virtually encircles each myofibril. DEPOLARIZATION SPREADS INTO THE CELL VIA THIS SYSTEM WHEN THE ACTION POTENTIAL TRAVELS DOWN THE SARCOLEMMA. BY THIS MEANS, EXCITATION SPREADS TO THE LEVEL OF THE MYOFIBRILS. The **sarcoplasmic reticulum,** a distinct membrane system, is closely apposed to the T tubules (Figure 13-3). The sarcoplasmic reticulum surrounds an intracellular compartment that forms a sleeve around each myofibril.

Each motor neuron controls many muscle cells

The basic neuromuscular relationships are described in Chapter 9. Each skeletal muscle cell has one **neuromuscular junction** with a branch of one motor neuron. The resulting functional grouping of a nerve and its associated muscle cells is called a **motor unit.** Motor units may contain from a few muscle cells to many thousands of cells.

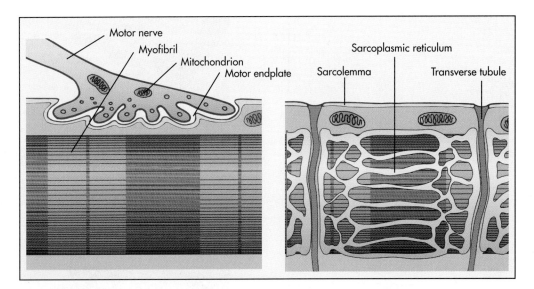

Figure 13-3 Membranes of skeletal muscle. The plasma membrane separating the extracellular space from the intracellular space (myoplasm) has three specialized portions. These are the motor endplate, the sarcolemma, and the transverse tubules (T tubules) that form a network at the ends of each sarcomere in mammals and are contiguous with the extracellular space. The sarcoplasmic reticulum is a distinct membrane system enclosing a separate intracellular compartment surrounding each myofibril and is intimately associated with the T-tubular system.

Muscle weakness or hyperactivity **(spasms)** is usually symptomatic of problems in the central or peripheral neural motor systems. The effect is to block or enhance excitatory or inhibitory neurotransmitter release at synapses and ultimately to determine acetylcholine release at the neuromuscular junction. For example, food poisoning resulting from the toxin produced by *Clostridium botulinum* leads to weakness and paralysis, which are mediated in part by a reduced acetylcholine release. Another bacterium, *Clostridium tetani*, causes **tetanus,** an infectious disease characterized by muscular spasms. Although the tetanus toxin can experimentally block neuromuscular transmission, its main effect is to block transmitter release at inhibitory synapses in the central motor pathways. This blockade evokes repeated action potentials in the motor axons that cause the spasms.

An action potential is elicited in a motor nerve when the sum of the excitatory and inhibitory synaptic inputs to the cell body produces a critical depolarization (see Chapters 3 and 9). That action potential releases sufficient acetylcholine at the neuromuscular junction to produce an endplate potential and generate an action potential in all the muscle cells in the motor unit, and synchronous contractions result. MOTOR UNITS RATHER THAN CELLS ARE THE BASIC FUNCTIONAL CONTRACTILE ELEMENTS THAT CAN BE RECRUITED INDIVIDUALLY.

Myasthenia gravis is a serious, progressive disease characterized by extreme muscle weakness. An autoimmune mechanism is typically involved. Circulating antibodies to the acetylcholine receptors in the endplate mem-

brane markedly reduce the number of receptors, and neuromuscular transmission fails. The symptoms of weakness can be alleviated by anticholinesterase medications, such as **neostigmine.** Acetylcholine released at the endplate persists after treatment, and its concentration rises to a level that restores neuromuscular transmission.

Ca^{++} Mobilization Regulates Skeletal Muscle Contraction

The process that links the action potential to cross-bridge cycling and contraction is called **excitation-contraction coupling** (Figure 13-4). The events involved are (1) neuromuscular transmission and depolarization of the endplate membrane, sarcolemma, and T tubules; (2) the mobilization of Ca^{++}; and (3) the action of Ca^{++} on myofibrillar regulatory mechanisms that control cross-bridge cycling. Excitation-contraction coupling in skeletal muscle is comparatively simple in the sense that only one event is critical in each of the three steps.

Ca^{++} is the messenger that couples signals at the cell membrane to cycling of the cross-bridges

Skeletal muscle cells are too large and contract too rapidly for Ca^{++} to diffuse through channels in the sarcolemma from the extracellular space to the myofibrils. The cellular compartment enclosed by the sarcoplasmic reticulum (Figure 13-3) contains the Ca^{++} pool involved in activation. Signal transduction in skeletal muscle cells is the process by which an action potential triggers Ca^{++} release from the sarcoplasmic reticulum. Depolarization of T tu-

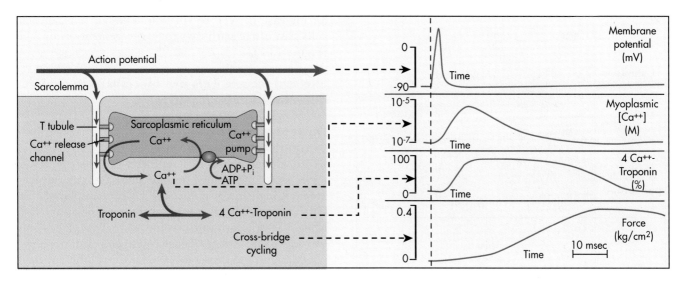

Figure 13-4 Excitation-contraction coupling in skeletal muscle.

bules opens anatomically coupled channels in the sarcoplasmic reticulum. Channel opening allows Ca^{++} ions to diffuse down their electrochemical gradient into the myoplasm (Figure 13-4). This process requires only a few milliseconds because the Ca^{++} concentration gradient is huge ($\approx 10^5$) and the distances are short (<1 μm).

In addition to the voltage-sensitive Ca^{++} channels, the sarcoplasmic reticular membrane contains large amounts of a protein complex that pumps Ca^{++} from the myoplasm back into the sarcoplasmic reticulum. This active transport depends on the hydrolysis of ATP (Figure 13-4).

Ca^{++} pumping and cross-bridge cycling account for the hydrolysis of a large fraction of an estimated 40 kg of ATP that is hydrolyzed by a 68-kg man during a restful day. (In vivo, a small pool of ATP is continuously resynthesized from ADP.) This generates considerable heat that normally must be dissipated by sweating and other mechanisms. However, muscle plays a key role in thermoregulation. Exposure to cold causes shivering, which produces heat but no useful work.

Cross-bridge attachment to actin requires Ca^{++}

A Ca^{++} switch effectively allows the transition from an **off state,** in which cross-bridges cannot attach in a relaxed muscle, to an **on state,** in which attachment and cycling are possible (Figure 13-5). **Troponin,** a regulatory protein bound to tropomyosin in the thin filament, has four high-affinity Ca^{++} binding sites. These sites are filled very rapidly when Ca^{++} is released from the sarcoplasmic reticulum (Figure 13-4). The result is that all the thin filaments are quickly turned on (Figure 13-5). The cross-bridges can then cycle until the transport pump lowers the Ca^{++} concentration so that Ca^{++} dissociates from troponin (Figure 13-4). The thin filaments return to the off state, and the cell relaxes. ACTIVATION IN SKELETAL MUSCLE IS AN ALL-OR-NONE PROCESS. Action potentials give uniform Ca^{++} transients.

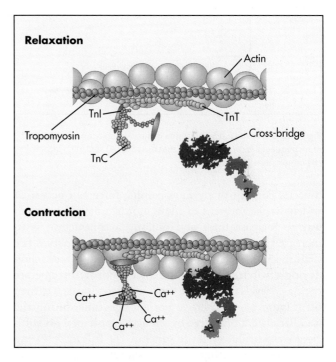

Figure 13-5 Ca^{++} enables cross-bridge cycling by reversible binding to the regulatory protein troponin. Troponin has three subunits (TnI, TnT, and TnC). The binding of four Ca^{++} ions to TnC induces a conformational change in a segment of a thin filament enabling cross-bridge attachment. Only the myosin head that normally projects from a thick filament is illustrated. *(Courtesy R.J. Solaro.)*

This switches all of the thin filaments to the on state for a brief period and leads to a consistent mechanical response called a **twitch** (Figure 13-6).

The motor system grades contractile force

Skeletal muscles must generate different forces, sometimes for considerable periods. Two mechanisms control the amount of force generated by a muscle. First, because

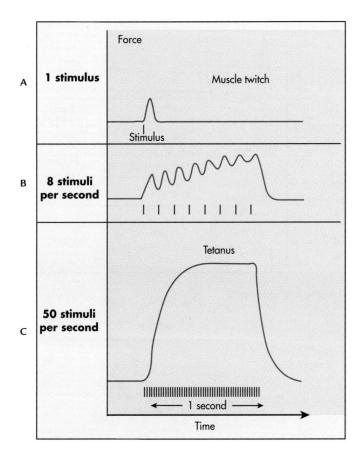

Figure 13-6 The force of contraction of a motor unit can be increased by more frequent action potentials so that twitches **(A)** sum in an incomplete **(B)** or complete **(C)** tetanus.

muscles contain many motor units, force can be varied widely by recruitment of more motor units. The second way to increase force and prolong a contraction is to increase the frequency with which the motor nerves fire (Figure 13-6). Even though all the cross-bridges are cycling during a twitch, the maximum force is not attained before the Ca^{++} levels fall and the contractile apparatus is turned off (Figure 13-4). There is not enough time during the Ca^{++} transient produced by one action potential for sufficient cross-bridge cycles to generate the full force. Firing the motor nerves at higher frequencies elicits further Ca^{++} transients. This allows the mechanical responses to summate and produce a greater, prolonged contraction termed a **tetanus.** (Note that this is not the same as the disease termed *tetanus.*) The maximum tetanic force may be up to eightfold greater than the twitch force.

Several factors contribute to finely graded contractions. The motor units recruited for weak contractions yield only small increments in force. THE PRESENCE OF LARGE NUMBERS OF MOTOR UNITS AND OF TETANIZATION IN A MUSCLE ALLOW CONTINUOUS GRADATIONS IN FORCE GENERATION OVER A WIDE RANGE.

Skeletal Muscle Is Functionally Diverse

The transition from rest to contraction in skeletal muscle triggers an extraordinary jump in ATP consumption. This must be matched instantaneously by an increase in ATP resynthesis. Like all cells, muscle cells have three pathways for the regeneration of ATP (Figure 13-7).

Skeletal muscle cells are specialized to exploit different metabolic pathways

Direct phosphorylation of ADP from creatine phosphate by creatine phosphotransferase constitutes a transfer of phosphate and not net ATP synthesis. Creatine phosphate serves as a large storage pool of almost instantaneously available high-energy phosphate. Direct phosphorylation buffers the cellular ATP levels at the onset of contraction while synthetic pathways become active. The cell has only two ways to synthesize ATP (glycolysis and oxidative phosphorylation), and these processes have very different characteristics (Figure 13-7).

Glycolysis can supply ATP at very high rates, even though the yield per mole of glucose is low. However, this pathway fails when the cellular glycogen stores are depleted (seconds to minutes in muscles). **Oxidative phosphorylation** in the mitochondria uses O_2 and substrates that diffuse into the cell from the capillaries to generate ATP continuously and very efficiently. The disadvantage is that this pathway is much slower than glycolysis. Oxidative phosphorylation cannot meet the demands of very rapid cross-bridge cycling rates.

Fiber types match ATP production and consumption rates

Two main types of skeletal muscle cells occur in humans and other primates. This specialization allows either high-power output or long contractions. The two cell classes are differentiated on the basis of whether the gene for a slow or a fast myosin is expressed (Table 13-1). The isoenzymes differ in having moderate or high ATPase activity or cycling rate. **Slow fibers** are characterized by moderate shortening velocities and power outputs, and they consume ATP at moderate rates. Slow fibers have a large blood supply (high capillary density), many mitochondria, and a moderate diameter. These characteristics minimize diffusion distances for O_2 and substrates. Slow fibers are sometimes called **red fibers** because of the distinct coloration provided by the iron-containing hemoglobin in the blood vessels, myoglobin in the myoplasm, and cytochromes in the mitochondria. If the blood supply is adequate, slow fibers provide great endurance.

The maximum ATP consumption rate of **fast fibers** can be met only by glycolysis. These large, pale **(white)** cells have a more extensive sarcoplasmic reticulum, and therefore rapid contraction is matched by rapid relaxation. These cells are pale because they contain few O_2-binding proteins. Fast fibers fatigue rapidly as glycogen is depleted.

The motor unit rather than the cell is the functional group. Fast and slow motor units differ by more than their exclusive composition of either slow or fast fibers (Figure 13-8). Slow motor units usually generate low forces be-

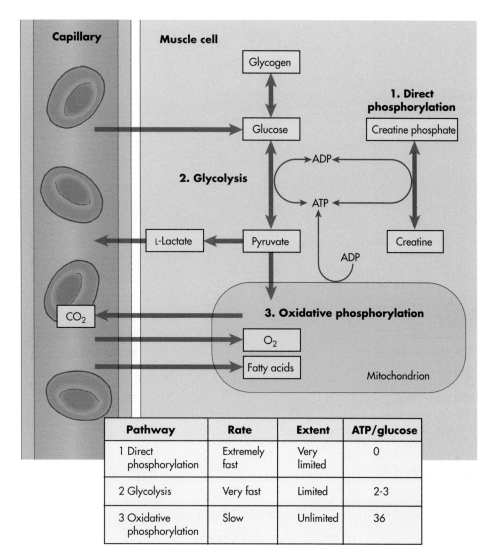

Figure 13-7 Comparison of the three pathways for ATP production.

Pathway	Rate	Extent	ATP/glucose
1 Direct phosphorylation	Extremely fast	Very limited	0
2 Glycolysis	Very fast	Limited	2-3
3 Oxidative phosphorylation	Slow	Unlimited	36

Table 13-1 Fiber Types in Primate Skeletal Muscle		
	Slow, Oxidative (Red)	**Fast, Glycolytic (White)**
Myosin isoenzyme (ATPase rate)	Moderate	Fast
Sarcoplasmic reticular Ca^{++} pumping rate	Moderate	Fast
ATP consumption rate	Moderate	Extremely high
Diameter (diffusion distance)	Moderate	Large
Oxidative capacity: mitochondrial content, capillary density	High	Low
Glycolytic capacity	Moderate	High

cause of the smaller average fiber diameter and the comparatively few cells. The motor nerve determines the physiological characteristics of a motor unit (see Chapter 9). Nerves with small cell bodies and narrow axons can synthesize limited amounts of acetylcholine, and they form small motor units. Small motor axons are readily excitable; relatively few excitatory postsynaptic potentials at the small cell body are needed to depolarize the cell to the critical potential required to fire an action potential. The large axons of fast motor units are less excitable. The largest motor units may contain more than a thousand cells, and they develop hundreds of grams of force in humans.

Fatigue is a state of disturbed homeostasis

Most muscles can carry out various types of activities. For instance, moderate workloads can be sustained with little fatigue. THE INITIAL MOTOR UNITS RECRUITED ARE THE MORE EXCITABLE SLOW UNITS, WHICH ARE FATIGUE RESISTANT. THE FAST MOTOR UNITS ARE ALSO RECRUITED FOR RAPID, FORCEFUL CON-

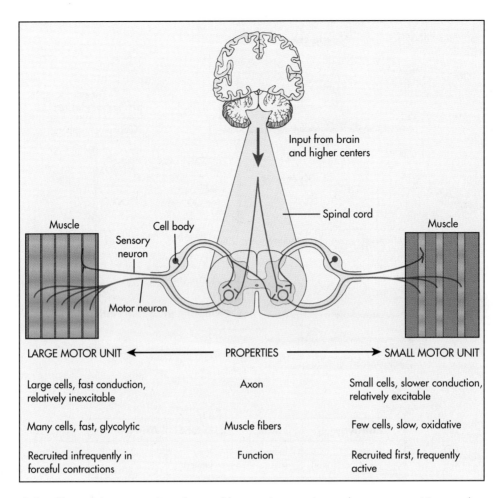

Input from brain and higher centers

Spinal cord

Muscle

Cell body

Sensory neuron

Motor neuron

Muscle

LARGE MOTOR UNIT ←	PROPERTIES	→ SMALL MOTOR UNIT
Large cells, fast conduction, relatively inexcitable	Axon	Small cells, slower conduction, relatively excitable
Many cells, fast, glycolytic	Muscle fibers	Few cells, slow, oxidative
Recruited infrequently in forceful contractions	Function	Recruited first, frequently active

Figure 13-8 Characteristics of fast and slow motor units and some of the synaptic connections to the motor axons. Most muscles contain a mix of many slow (red) motor units with smaller numbers of fast (white) motor units. The cells of a motor unit are not anatomically discrete groups but are dispersed among the cells of other motor units.

TRACTIONS WITH A HIGH POWER OUTPUT. THESE MAXIMAL EFFORTS CANNOT BE SUSTAINED, AND THE FAST UNITS FATIGUE RAPIDLY.

Surprisingly, little is known about the causes of the **general physical fatigue** one experiences after vigorous exercise. Fatigue occurs before cells fail to contract. Cellular creatine phosphate and glycogen contents decrease during activity, even in slow motor units. However, individuals stop using their motor units before the cellular ATP concentration falls. Metabolic changes, such as an increased blood lactate concentration and a fall in pH, may contribute to the perception of fatigue, but they do not fully explain the phenomenon. An elevated oxidative metabolism resynthesizes the metabolic stores within a brief period after the cessation of exercise even though fatigue persists.

Muscle Fibers Grow and Adapt with Exercise

The growth of muscle involves the addition of new sarcomeres at the ends of myofibrils and the formation of additional myofibrils within the cells. The differentiation of skeletal muscle cells depends on their pattern of contractile activity. Motor units that are frequently active express the slow myosin isoenzyme and develop a high oxidative capacity. Motor units that contract infrequently differentiate into the fast fiber phenotype. Thus differentiation depends on innervation.

Skeletal muscle atrophies if not used. Cell diameter and the number of myofibrils decrease. Such changes can be initiated after only 2 days of bed rest. If the motor nerve is destroyed by injury or disease, the denervated muscle cells first atrophy, and most degenerate within a few months. This occurs in severe cases of **poliomyelitis** in which the viral infection in the central nervous system damages the motor neurons. These processes are reversible if reinnervation occurs. The fiber type changes if a cell in a formerly fast motor unit is reinnervated by a small motor nerve, and vice versa.

Activity has large and diverse effects on muscle. These changes depend on the type of activity (Table 13-2). The responses are adaptive and include neuro-

Table 13-2	Effects of Exercise	
Type of Training	**Example**	**Major Adaptive Response**
Learning and coordination	Typing	Increased rate and accuracy of motor skills (central nervous system)
Endurance (submaximal, sustained efforts)	Marathon running	Increased oxidative capacity in all involved motor units, with limited cellular hypertrophy
Strength (brief, maximal efforts)	Weight lifting	Hypertrophy and enhanced glycolytic capacity of motor units used

muscular learning, increased endurance, and increased strength. The learned ability to carry out complex movements, such as riding a bicycle, persists for years even without practice. However, regular exercise is required to maintain changes in the muscle cells. The increased physical well-being that results from moderate endurance exercise is mainly caused by the enhanced capacity of the respiratory and cardiovascular systems rather than by the effects on the skeletal muscle fibers (see Chapter 26). Strength training also has broader effects, including growth in bones and tendons to bear the greater forces.

Although exercise can have profound effects on the involved motor units, weight lifting does not convert slow units into fast units or induce the formation of new muscle cells. The transformation of slow fibers to fast fibers and the reverse can occur, as shown by cross-innervation experiments or reinnervation after injury. However, no exercise regimen changes activity patterns sufficiently to alter the expression of the myosin isoenzymes.

Testosterone promotes the hypertrophy of skeletal muscle cells by inducing the formation of more myofibrils. This hormone contributes to the greater muscularity and strength of men than women. **Anabolic steroids,** compounds that are structurally similar to testosterone, are taken by many athletes to increase muscle bulk and to improve performance in sports that require strength. However, these hormones have diverse actions (see Chapter 49) and cause many deleterious side effects at the doses required to amplify the effects of strength training alone. The risks are increased by the variety and impurity of illicit drugs.

Summary

- Skeletal (voluntary) muscle cells are controlled by the motor system, and most act on the skeleton to generate force and movement.
- The following specialized membranes help regulate contraction: (1) the motor endplate, where action potentials are generated; (2) the sarcolemma, which propagates action potentials; (3) the T tubules, which transmit depolarization from the sarcolemma to the sarcoplasmic reticulum; and (4) the sarcoplasmic reticulum, which is an intracellular Ca^{++}-storage compartment.
- Excitation-contraction coupling includes (1) the acetylcholine-induced action potential, (2) the voltage-dependent opening of Ca^{++} channels in the sarcoplasmic reticulum, (3) Ca^{++} diffusion and binding to troponin, and (4) a conformational change of the thin filament to allow cross-bridge attachment and cycling.
- In a motor unit, one nerve action potential induces a twitch in all the muscle fibers that receive branches from the nerve. Contractile force is graded by the recruitment of more motor units and by tetanization with trains of nerve impulses.
- Slow, oxidative, fatigue-resistant motor units are involved in all muscular activity. Fast, glycolytic motor units are also recruited to increase force and power output for brief periods before fatigue induces systemic changes that lead to the cessation of muscular activity.
- The phenotype of a muscle cell depends on its activity patterns. Strength-promoting exercise can induce cell hypertrophy with the synthesis of additional myofibrils. Cells atrophy if they are not recruited, and they degenerate after denervation.

BIBLIOGRAPHY

Block BA: Thermogenesis in muscle, *Annu Rev Physiol* 56:535, 1994.

Buckingham M: Skeletal muscle development and the role of the myogenic regulatory factors, *Biochem Soc Trans* 24:506, 1996.

Cope TC, Pinter MJ: The size principle: still working after all these years, *News Physiol Sci* 10:280, 1995.

Fitts RH: Cellular mechanisms of muscle fatigue, *Physiol Rev* 74:49, 1994.

Franzini-Armstrong C, Protasi F: Ryanodine receptors of striated muscles: a complex channel capable of multiple interactions, *Physiol Rev* 77:699, 1997.

Hochachka PW: *Muscles as molecular and metabolic machines,* Boca Raton, Fla, 1994, CRC.

Holmes KC: The actomyosin interaction and its control by tropomyosin, *Biophys J* 68:2S, 1995.

Josephson RK: Contraction dynamics and power output of skel-etal muscle, *Annu Rev Physiol* 55:527, 1993.

Lieber RL: *Skeletal muscle structure and function: implications for reha-bilitation and sports medicine,* Baltimore, 1992, Williams & Wilkins.

Mintz E, Guillain F: Ca^{2+} transport by the sarcoplasmic reticu-lum ATPase, *Biochim Biophys Acta* 1318:52, 1997.

Netter FH: Musculoskeletal system. In Dingle RV, ed: *The CIBA collection of medical illustrations,* vol 8, Summit, NJ, 1987, Ciba-Geigy.

Rome LC, Lindstedt SL: Mechanical and metabolic design of the muscular system in vertebrates. In Dantzler WH, ed: *Handbook of physiology,* Section 13, New York, 1997, Oxford University Press.

Rüegg JC: *Calcium in muscle contraction,* ed 2, Berlin, 1992, Springer-Verlag.

Schiaffino S, Reggiani C: Molecular diversity of myofibrillar pro-teins: gene regulation and functional significance, *Physiol Rev* 76:371, 1996.

▷ CASE STUDIES

Case 13-1

A pediatrician noted slow muscular development in a young boy. By the time the boy was age 5 a pattern of progressive muscular weakness was evident. Laboratory tests showed high concentrations of soluble proteins characteristic of skeletal muscle cells in the serum. A muscle biopsy revealed a pattern of necrosis and phago-cytosis of both fast and slow muscle fibers. DNA analysis revealed the absence of a gene for a cytoskeletal protein, called **dystrophin.** This finding led to a diagnosis of **Duchenne's muscular dystrophy.**

1. What is the significance of myoplasmic proteins in the serum?

    A. Their presence is diagnostic of muscular dystro-phy.

    B. The results imply that there is either injury or ne-crosis of skeletal muscle cells.

    C. Their presence demonstrates that these proteins are being inappropriately synthesized and secreted into the vascular system along with the normal serum proteins.

    D. This is a normal occurrence after exercise.

    E. The condition results from muscle cell atrophy.

2. Why do girls not develop Duchenne's muscular dystrophy?

    A. The defective gene is recessive, sex linked, and nor-mally lethal by adolescence.

    B. Testosterone is required for the expression of dys-trophin.

    C. The cytoskeletal role of dystrophin is filled by a dif-ferent protein in girls.

    D. The defective gene is lethal during early fetal devel-opment in girls.

    E. Girls are always heterozygous for the dystrophin gene.

3. What is the best therapy for this patient?

    A. Dietary supplements of dystrophin

    B. Introduction of a functional allele of the dystro-phin gene into the skeletal muscle

    C. Chemotherapy to prevent the replication of af-fected skeletal muscle cells

    D. Exercise and physical therapy

    E. Intravenous injection of dystrophin

Case 13-2

Before surgery, a patient received a muscle relaxant (which blocks acetylcholine receptors in the motor end-plate) and a general anesthetic (which acts by affecting cell membrane properties). Unexpectedly massive spon-taneous muscular contractions were followed by pro-longed contractures causing muscular and joint rigidity. The heartbeat and respiratory rates accelerated, and the blood pressure was elevated. Body temperature rose to 44° C. Malignant hyperthermia was diagnosed. The cri-sis subsided after treatment with **dantrolene,** a medica-tion that blocked Ca^{++} release from the sarcoplasmic reticulum. Subsequent investigation revealed a familial history of similar episodes, a condition associated with mutation in the gene for the Ca^{++}-release channel.

1. What might be the cause of such massive contrac-tions?

    A. Hyperexcitability in the motor systems leading to sustained trains of action potentials to all muscles

    B. Inhibition of acetylcholine esterase

    C. Pathological elevations in muscle myoplasmic Ca^{++} concentrations caused by a leaky sarcolemma

    D. A sustained increase in myoplasmic Ca^{++} levels caused by increased conductance of the sarcoplas-mic reticulum Ca^{++} channels

    E. A blockade of inhibitory synaptic input to the mo-tor neurons

2. What is the major cause of the rise in body tem-perature?

    A. Heat produced as a result of cross-bridge cycling and ATP hydrolysis

    B. Heat produced as a result of ATP hydrolysis by Ca^{++} pumps in the sarcoplasmic reticulum

    C. Reduced heat dissipation from the body

    D. Rapid metabolic rates

    E. The presence of a mutant gene for the sarcoplas-mic reticulum Ca^{++} pump

Case 13-3

Space flight imposes a microgravity environment and a lack of normal loading of muscles, tendons, and bones in astronauts. A knowledge of the effects of microgravity becomes essential as manned space flights grow longer.

The available information documents a loss of muscle mass, strength, and endurance. Tendon strength is diminished, and bone resorption occurs as reflected in a negative calcium balance and decreased bone mineral density. An underlying cellular cause is atrophy of the muscle fibers, particularly the slow, oxidative motor units that are most frequently recruited. There is also a phenotypic conversion of slow, oxidative motor units into fast, glycolytic motor units.

1. **What problem do astronauts *not* face in prolonged space flight?**
   A. An impaired ability to carry out the mission in space
   B. An enhanced susceptibility to injury during reentry into the earth's gravitational field
   C. A compromised ability to land the space shuttle
   D. An extended postflight weakness
   E. A susceptibility to postflight musculoskeletal injury

2. **The changes produced by microgravity do *not* result from some of the same causes as which of the following?**
   A. Disuse atrophy when an individual is paralyzed
   B. Weakness associated with bed rest, particularly in elderly individuals

   C. Reinnervation of a formerly slow, oxidative fiber by a large, inexcitable motor neuron after nerve injury
   D. Stopping of an intense weight-lifting program
   E. Weakness in an individual with Duchenne's muscular dystrophy

3. **What is an ineffective strategy for protecting crews and enabling prolonged space flight?**
   A. Developing exercise regimens to increase the work output of muscles most subject to disuse atrophy in microgravity
   B. Undertaking research on changes in the musculoskeletal system of laboratory rodents in space
   C. Developing automatic landing systems for space vehicles
   D. Developing devices to recruit motor units by stimulating the motor nerves
   E. Replacing manned missions with unmanned missions

CHAPTER 14

Muscle in the Walls of Hollow Organs

OBJECTIVES

■ Describe the structure and function of muscle in hollow organs.

■ Explain the control systems that act on smooth muscle cells.

■ Describe the regulatory systems that determine cross-bridge attachment and the kinetics of cross-bridge cycling.

A distinct type of muscle plays important roles in the vascular, airway, gastrointestinal, urogenital, and other organ systems. This type of muscle lacks striations and is termed **smooth muscle.** Smooth muscles have great medical significance because of their involvement in many diseases, including asthma, hypertension, and atherosclerosis. Smooth muscle contraction is involuntary, and its function is regulated by autonomic nerves and various types of hormonal signals that integrate organ function.

Muscle Regulates the Volume of Hollow Organs

The load on the cells in hollow organs is imposed by pressure in the organ. If the muscle cells are relaxed, the volume of the organ increases with the volume of its contents until the connective tissue matrix within the organ wall limits further expansion. The muscle may shorten in what is termed a **phasic contraction** to empty the hollow organ by briefly increasing the pressure. However, the muscle may contract isometrically for long periods to maintain the dimensions of the organ: this sustained force is called a **tonic contraction.** In such cases the muscle serves as an "adjustable skeleton." The economy of force maintenance (force × time/ATP consumption) is critical in muscles that are always contracting. In fact, THE ECONOMY OF SOME SMOOTH MUSCLES IS MORE THAN 300 TIMES THAT OF STRIATED MUSCLE.

The cells in hollow organs do not individually link two bones but are connected to one another and to extracellular connective tissue. Thus they cannot be recruited individually to increase force. Each cellular link in the chain must be equally activated and develop the same force. Contraction in one part of an organ changes the pressure throughout, so muscle cell function must be coordinated.

No scheme to classify the types of smooth muscle has been satisfactory, although the functional distinction between phasic and tonic muscles is useful. Most of the smooth muscles in the gastrointestinal tract and urogenital organs are phasic: such muscles are either normally relaxed or rhythmically active. The smooth muscles in the walls of blood vessels, airways, and sphincters, in contrast, are typically tonic: they are always contracted to some degree. Such sustained active force is called **tone.** This chapter emphasizes the basic mechanisms that underlie such behavior. Other chapters describe smooth muscle function in specific organ systems.

The structure of smooth muscle in organs is complex

The simplest hollow organ may be an **arteriole** (Figure 14-1), which consists of the following main elements: an endothelial cell lining, a single smooth muscle cell layer encircling the endothelial cells, and connective tissue (see Chapters 22 and 23). In the intestinal tract the mucosal lining of the tube participates in the digestion and absorption of nutrients. The muscle in the walls mixes and propels the contents (see Chapter 32). The following muscle layers exist: an inner circular layer to determine circumference and an outer longitudinal layer to control length. Mixing and propelling of the contents are coordinated by an elaborate neural network that originates from plexuses between the two muscle layers (see Chapter 32).

In some organs the smooth muscle is in the form of a sack. Normally the sack is relaxed, and its volume increases with its content. Contraction of the muscle empties the sack in coordination with the relaxation of a smooth muscle valve, or **sphincter,** at its orifice. Examples are the urinary bladder, the uterus, and the gallbladder. Contraction of the anatomically complex layers of smooth muscle enable the organ to empty its content.

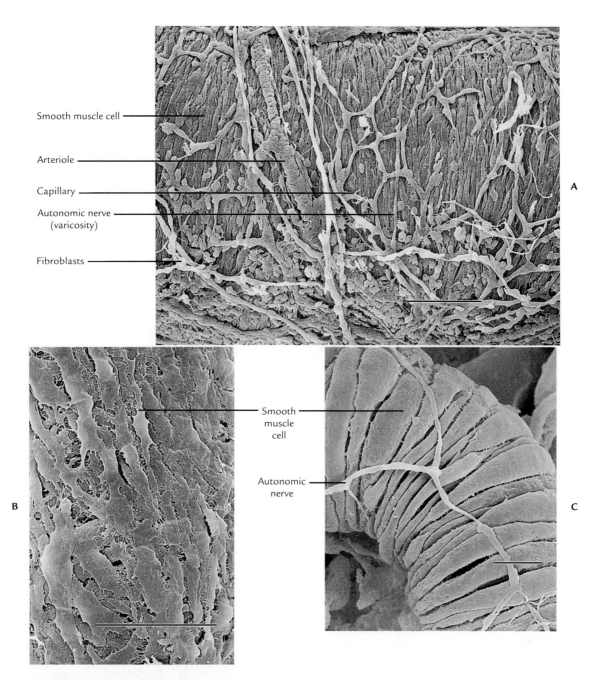

Figure 14-1 Scanning electron micrographs of smooth muscle in the oviduct **(A)**, the outer layer of the epididymis **(B)**, and a small arteriole **(C).** Note the irregular and varied shape of the smooth muscle cells, their link into muscular sheets, and an extracellular matrix that is typically the product of smooth muscle cells. (Bar = 5 μm.) *(From Uehara Y et al. In Motta PM, ed: Ultrastructure of smooth muscle, Norwell, Mass, 1990, Kluwer Academic.)*

CONTROL AND COORDINATION OF THE MUSCLE DEPEND ON (1) INTRINSIC AND EXTRINSIC INNERVATION, (2) THE BLOOD SUPPLY THAT PROVIDES NUTRIENTS AND HORMONES, AND (3) CELL JUNCTIONS THAT ALLOW ELECTRICAL, CHEMICAL, AND MECHANICAL INTERACTIONS. The nature and relative importance of these elements are highly variable. In brief, the functional requirements for muscles in the walls of hollow organs are very different from those of muscles attached to the skeleton. These differences in function are responsible for the differences in the properties of the smooth muscle (Table 14-1).

Cellular Structure Is Linked to Function

Most smooth muscle cells are 2 to 5 μm in diameter and up to 400 μm long at the optimum length (L_o) for force generation, although cells may have very irregular shapes (Figure 14-1). All cells have a single central nucleus, and most cells taper toward the ends. The cells are comparatively featureless when viewed with a light microscope, and the general characteristics of the membranes, contractile apparatus, and cytoskeleton differ from the respective characteristics in skeletal muscle.

Table 14-1 Functional Comparison of Skeletal and Smooth Muscle

Property	Skeletal Muscle	Smooth Muscle
Usual role	Movement (work)	Movement and dimensional control
Structure and function	Quite uniform	Highly diverse
Power output and ATP consumption	Very high	Low
Activity pattern	Normally relaxed	Normally contracting
Cell recruitment	Individually (as motor units)	Uniformly (cells coupled)
Cross-bridge recruitment	Thin filament regulated, all-or-none	Myosin regulated, variable cross-bridge attachment rates
Cross-bridge kinetics	Fixed by myosin isoform and load	Regulated cycling rates

Three membranes (sarcolemma, caveola, and sarcoplasmic reticulum) are involved in coupling extracellular signals to the contractile apparatus and in defining the Ca^{++} compartments (Figure 14-2, A). The *caveolae* are tiny saclike invaginations of the sarcolemma, and they are arranged in rows along the cell. In smooth muscle the sarcoplasmic reticulum is a continuous, irregular tubular network that branches throughout the cell. The sarcoplasmic reticulum is closely associated with the sarcolemma and the caveola, but it lacks the specialized junctions that couple the T tubules to the sarcoplasmic reticulum of skeletal muscle. There are no anatomically defined motor endplates. Neurotransmitters released from the enlarged **varicosities** spaced along the autonomic nerves (Figure 14-1) diffuse to receptors distributed in the sarcolemma.

The contractile apparatus lacks a myofibrillar structure

Contractile units consist of thin filaments attached to a cytoskeleton; they overlap with a much smaller number of myosin-containing thick filaments (Figure 14-3). The filaments are approximately aligned in the cell's long axis, along which force is generated. However, shortening of the cells can lead to angular displacements of the myofilaments. Nevertheless, the three-dimensional organization of the thick and thin filaments and the cytoskeleton is uncertain.

The forces produced by cross-bridges bound to the thin filaments are transmitted by the cytoskeleton. Thin filament attachment sites are **dense bodies** scattered throughout the myoplasm and **membrane dense areas** located at intervals along the sarcolemma (Figure 14-3). These structures are analogous to Z disks of skeletal muscle. Dense bodies and membrane dense areas are linked by cytoskeletal **intermediate filaments.**

The cells must be coupled to one another to generate force. A variety of junctions (Figure 14-2, B) provide for electrical and chemical communication and mechanical links between smooth muscle cells. Junctions essential to organ function are also formed with other cells, such as the vascular endothelium or airway epithelial cells. The type and density of junctions vary with the tissue. **Gap junctions** are most prominent in phasic smooth muscles, in which contraction is initiated by trains of action potentials propagated from cell to cell. IN SMOOTH MUSCLE THE FUNCTIONAL UNITS, WHICH ARE EQUIVALENT TO SKELETAL MUSCLE MOTOR UNITS, ARE BUNDLES OR LAYERS OF CELLS. THE CONTRACTILE SYSTEM IS ANATOMICALLY COUPLED ACROSS THE PLASMA MEMBRANES OF SMOOTH MUSCLE CELLS (Figure 14-3).

Smooth muscle cells synthesize and secrete elastin and collagen fibrils. The highly extensible elastin and inextensible collagen in the extracellular matrix oppose increases in the volume of hollow organs. The organization of the contractile system and force-transmitting structures probably facilitates the considerable shortening capacity of smooth muscles.

When a blood vessel wall is weakened, the internal pressure causes the wall to bulge; the enlarged region is called an **aneurysm.** Aneurysms may be congenital, or they may result from vascular disease, such as **atherosclerosis** or **syphilis.** Sudden death is likely when an aneurysm ruptures in a large artery. Rupture is likely because the internal pressure puts a greater distending force on the enlarged segment of a vessel than it does on adjacent normal-sized regions (see Chapter 22).

Chemomechanical transduction is the same in smooth and striated muscle

Although the organization of the contractile proteins into filaments and the organization of filaments in the contractile apparatus are poorly understood in smooth muscle, the mechanical output is very similar to that in striated muscle. Maximum forces are comparable, and force exhibits a similar dependence on length (see Figure 12-4). Although maximal shortening velocities in smooth muscle cells are much slower than in skeletal muscles, shortening or lengthening velocities exhibit the same dependence on load (see Figure 12-5).

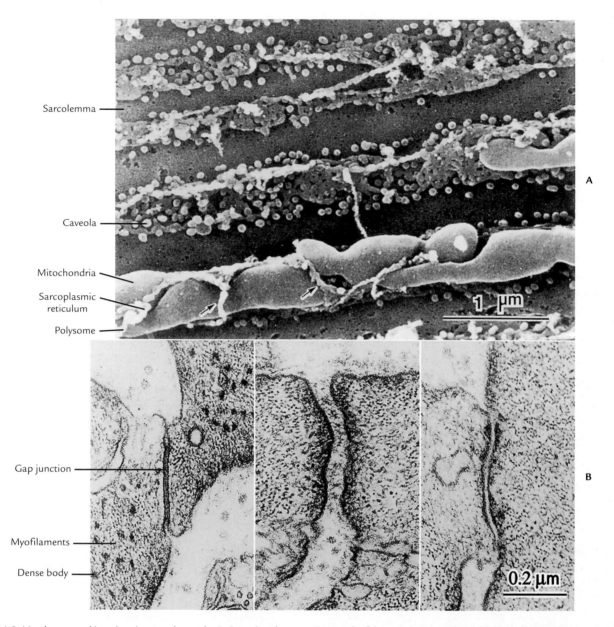

Figure 14-2 Membranes and junctions in smooth muscle. **A,** Scanning electron micrograph of the cytoplasmic surface of the sarcolemma of an intestinal smooth muscle cell. Rows of caveolae project into the cytoplasm but are open to the extracellular space. The intervening space is normally where junctions with other cells are formed on the outside surface and where dense areas of the cytoskeletal membrane anchor thin filaments on the inner surface. Elements of the sarcoplasmic reticulum *(arrows)* snake around the caveola and mitochondria. Polysomes consisting of clusters of ribosomes, sites of protein synthesis, are associated with the sarcoplasmic reticulum. **B,** Transmission electron micrographs of various types of junctions between intestinal smooth muscle cells. Left panel shows a gap junction where ions and small molecules can diffuse between cells (see also Figure 4-1). Other junctions that mainly provide mechanical links have wider separation of the cells with darkly staining extracellular proteins in the cleft. *(A from Inoué T. In Motta PM, ed:* Ultrastructure of smooth muscle, *Norwell, Mass, 1990, Kluwer Academic.* **B** *from Gabella G. In Motta PM, ed:* Ultrastructure of smooth muscle, *Norwell, Mass, 1990, Kluwer Academic.)*

The contractile proteins of smooth muscle are also similar to the proteins in skeletal muscle except that the myosin isoforms have lower inherent detachment rates. This feature contributes to the slow cycling and ATPase activities. THESE PROPERTIES SHOW THAT THE MYOSIN CROSS-BRIDGES IN BOTH TYPES OF MUSCLE CONVERT THE ENERGY DERIVED FROM ATP INTO FORCE OR MOVEMENT IN THE SAME WAY AND THAT A SLIDING-FILAMENT MECHANISM IS RESPONSIBLE FOR CONTRACTION. THE SPECIAL PROPERTIES OF SMOOTH MUSCLE (TABLE 14-1) ARE MAINLY THE RESULT OF COMPLEX MECHANISMS THAT CONTROL THE CELLULAR Ca^{++} CONCENTRATION AND THAT REGULATE THE RATES OF CROSS-BRIDGE ATTACHMENT AND CYCLING.

Extracellular Signals Influence Ca^{++} Mobilization

The Ca^{++} concentration ($[Ca^{++}]$) is the primary determinant of cross-bridge cycling in smooth muscle. However, the force of contraction is increased by recruiting more cross-bridges in the cells rather than by recruiting

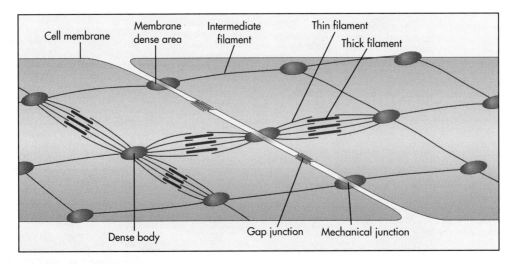

Figure 14-3 Possible organization of the cytoskeleton and myofilaments in smooth muscle. Three-dimensional imaging techniques are needed to reconstruct the structure of cells where the filaments are not organized into parallel arrays. Smooth muscle has many thin filaments and few thick filaments compared with striated muscle.

more cells, as in skeletal muscle. This type of regulation requires precise control of the myoplasmic [Ca^{++}]. A diverse array of excitatory and inhibitory signals to the sarcolemma and various Ca^{++}-mobilization mechanisms regulate the activation of the smooth muscle tissues. These signals are transmitted by nerves, circulating hormones or drugs, local hormones, ions, and metabolites. Signals are also received from other cell types, such as endothelial cells and coupled smooth muscle cells. Specific details on the key mechanisms are described in the chapters devoted to individual organ systems.

Nerves provide the most important control of smooth muscle

Several factors influence neural control. Most smooth muscle tissues have more than one type of innervation, typically parasympathetic and sympathetic. Many new neurotransmitters, including a variety of peptides and the gas nitric oxide, have been discovered.

The neurotransmitter-releasing sites (varicosities) of the nerves make intimate contacts with each smooth muscle cell in some tissues. However, in other tissues, neural contact may involve long diffusion paths for the transmitters. The action of a particular class of nerve and its neurotransmitter on a specific smooth muscle cell depends on the receptors expressed for that neurotransmitter. Some smooth muscle cells respond to norepinephrine by contracting, whereas others relax. These different responses allow coordinated adjustments within the body. Under conditions of stress, for example, epinephrine is released from the adrenal gland. The vascular smooth muscle of the gut constricts and shunts blood to the cardiac and skeletal muscle, where the vascular beds dilate.

Despite the importance of the innervation, the smooth muscle in virtually all organs continues to function more or less appropriately after the central autonomic connections (**extrinsic innervation**) are severed. Some smooth muscles receive no innervation. The ability of denervated smooth and cardiac muscle to maintain organ function without atrophy is a major distinction from skeletal muscle. Contributing factors include the maintenance of contractile activity in response to intrinsic neural activity, local or circulating hormones, and signals propagated among smooth muscle cells.

> The potential independence of smooth and cardiac muscle from the central nervous system is essential for successful organ transplantation. A good example is the transplanted heart with its endogenous coronary vasculature that functions successfully without innervation (see Chapter 19).

Both the sarcoplasmic reticulum and the sarcolemma regulate the intracellular Ca^{++} concentration

Ca^{++} mobilization is illustrated for phasic and tonic contractions in Figure 14-4. Phasic contractions last a few seconds or minutes and are elicited by brief periods of activation, which can be mediated by a burst of action potentials or by a short period of receptor occupancy by an activating neurotransmitter or hormone. The result is either a transient increase in the intracellular [Ca^{++}] with a small contraction or a series of transient increases in [Ca^{++}] with a larger contraction, analogous to a tetanus in skeletal muscle (Figure 14-4, *A*). Ca^{++} release from the sarcoplasmic reticulum and Ca^{++} influx through the sarcolemma from the extracellular fluid may both contribute to the transient increase in [Ca^{++}]. When stimulation ends, the myoplasmic Ca^{++} is pumped out of the cell or is sequestered in the sarcoplasmic reticulum (Figure 14-5).

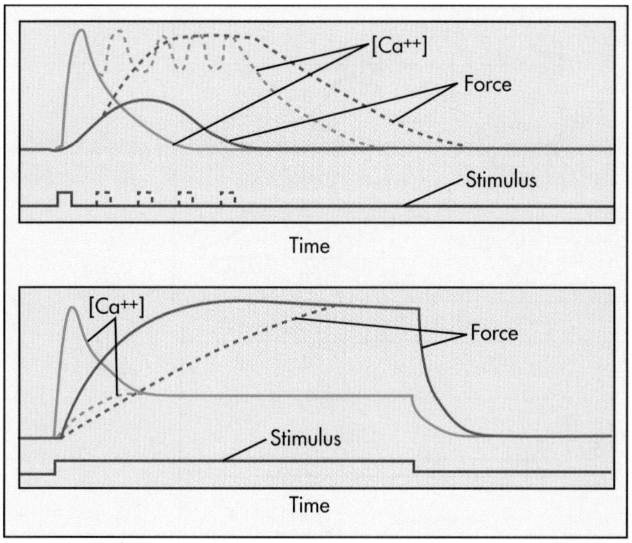

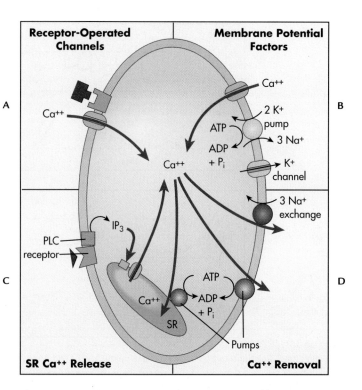

Figure 14-4 Patterns of Ca^{++} mobilization in phasic and tonic contractions of smooth muscle. **A,** Phasic contractions result from brief stimuli that elicit only a transient increase in Ca^{++} and a small contraction (solid lines). Repeated brief stimuli can lead to the summation of individual contractions and greater force (dashed lines). **B,** In tonic contractions, activation is maintained with continued receptor occupancy by neurotransmitters or other agents. An initial Ca^{++} release from the sarcoplasmic reticulum induces rapid force development (solid lines). However, the peak $[Ca^{++}]$ is not maintained. During the sustained tonic contraction, the force depends on Ca^{++} diffusing into the cells from the extracellular space, where the $[Ca^{++}]$ is about 1.6 mM. If the initial high Ca^{++} peak is blocked, the same force is developed, although the rates of the contraction are much slower (dashed lines). Thus $[Ca^{++}]$ can affect the rate as well as the force of a contraction.

Figure 14-5 Mechanisms regulating myoplasmic $[Ca^{++}]$ in smooth muscle. **A,** Receptor-operated Ca^{++} channels. **B,** Membrane K^+ channels and electrogenic Na^+-K^+ pumps modulate membrane potential and regulate Ca^{++} influx through voltage-dependent channels. **C,** Ca^{++} is released from the sarcoplasmic reticulum (SR) in response to the second messenger, inositol 1,4,5-trisphosphate (IP$_3$) generated by the receptor-coupled membrane enzyme phospholipase C (PLC). **D,** Ca^{++} pumps and passive Na^+-Ca^{++} exchange lower myoplasmic $[Ca^{++}]$. P$_i$, Inorganic phosphate.

If the stimulus is prolonged, the conductance of Ca^{++} channels in the sarcolemma remains elevated, and the myoplasmic $[Ca^{++}]$ remains above threshold values after an initial transient increase (Figure 14-4, B). The muscle contracts rapidly, and the contraction may be sustained at or near peak levels despite the falling $[Ca^{++}]$. The initial transient increase in the Ca^{++} level occurs in the absence of extracellular Ca^{++}. This finding indicates that the transient increase in $[Ca^{++}]$ is induced by the release of Ca^{++} from the sarcoplasmic reticulum. On the other hand, the sustained modest elevation in $[Ca^{++}]$ totally depends on the extracellular Ca^{++}, and the $[Ca^{++}]$ is regulated by the sarcolemma (dashed line in Figure 14-4, B). The contraction is much slower in the absence of an initial Ca^{++} transient from the sarcoplasmic reticulum. The slower rate of force development is due to reduced cross-bridge cycling rates and results in a lower ATP consumption rate.

Signals acting on the sarcolemma regulate the myoplasmic Ca^{++} concentrations

The following mechanisms regulate $[Ca^{++}]$: (1) membrane potential–dependent Ca^{++} influx through Ca^{++} channels from the extracellular space, (2) receptor-activated Ca^{++} channels in the sarcolemma, (3) control of Ca^{++} release from the sarcoplasmic reticulum, (4) sequestration and extrusion of Ca^{++} by pumps in both membranes, and (5) Na^+-Ca^{++} exchange across the sarcolemma, where the concentration gradients usually lead to the removal of Ca^{++} and an associated Na^+ movement into the cell (Figure 14-5) (see Chapter 18).

The membrane potential in smooth muscle is caused by the same mechanisms described for skeletal muscle and nerves in Chapter 2. However, the contribution of the electrogenic Na^+-K^+ pump to the membrane potential is much greater. The activity of this pump is regulated and can contribute approximately −20 mV to the total membrane potential of approximately −60 mV in unstimulated smooth muscle cells. The conductance of a variety of K^+ channels is also regulated in smooth muscle. Stimuli that lead to increased g_K hyperpolarize the cells (Figure 14-5).

Changes in the activity of the Na^+-K^+ pump and in K^+ channel conductance are responsible for slow oscillations in the membrane potential (Figure 14-6). The ion channels in the sarcolemma that open in response to depolarization in smooth muscle are mainly permeable to Ca^{++}; that is, they are **potential-dependent Ca^{++} channels.** Increases in the Na^+-K^+ pump activity also lower myoplasmic $[Ca^{++}]$. Because the Na^+ concentration gradient across the sarcolemma is increased, more Na^+ enters in exchange for Ca^{++}.

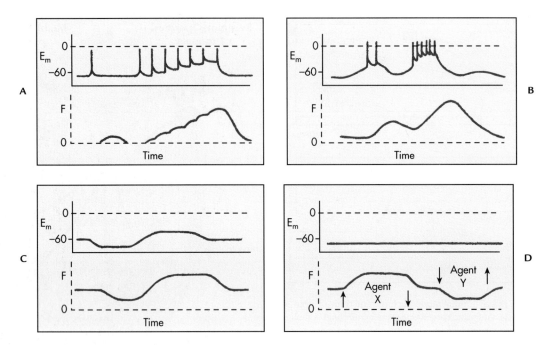

Figure 14-6 Relationship between membrane potential (E_m) and force (F) in various types of smooth muscle. **A,** Action potentials may be generated by pacemaker cells and propagated through the tissue. **B,** Slow waves can trigger bursts of action potentials and rhythmic contractile activity. **C,** Tone varies with membrane potential in tonic tissues that do not normally generate action potentials. **D,** Neurotransmitters and hormones acting through receptor-mediated mechanisms *(arrows)* can alter cell $[Ca^{++}]$ without detectable changes in the membrane potential.

Certain smooth muscles (mainly phasic) generate action potentials at some critical level of depolarization (Figure 14-6, *A* and *B*). Ca^{++} is the current-carrying ion in these action potentials. Other smooth muscles (functionally tonic) do not generate action potentials. Nevertheless, these cells have potential-dependent Ca^{++} channels. Graded depolarization caused by reduced electrogenic Na^+-K^+ pumping or by decreased K^+ channel conductance increases Ca^{++} influx (Figure 14-6, *C*).

Receptors mediate two paths for Ca^{++} mobilization (Figure 14-5). The binding of an agonist to a receptor can increase the Ca^{++} permeability of the sarcolemma by opening **receptor-activated channels.** This allows the influx of Ca^{++} from the extracellular pool. Receptor occupancy can also release Ca^{++} from the sarcoplasmic reticulum. Such receptor-mediated mechanisms can increase or decrease myoplasmic $[Ca^{++}]$ and thereby alter tone without changing the membrane potential (Figure 14-6, *D*). **Pharmacomechanical coupling** refers to activation mechanisms that do not change the membrane potential, in contrast to the alterations in membrane potential in **excitation-contraction coupling.**

A chemical messenger is implicated in Ca^{++} release from the sarcoplasmic reticulum in smooth muscle. Phospholipase C is activated by the occupancy of specific receptors. Phospholipase C hydrolyzes membrane phosphatidylinositol to yield **inositol 1,4,5-trisphosphate (IP$_3$)** and **diacylglycerol.** IP$_3$ diffuses to receptors in the sarcoplasmic reticulum to release Ca^{++}.

The mechanisms that reduce myoplasmic $[Ca^{++}]$ are the membrane pumps that actively transport Ca^{++} back into the sarcoplasmic reticulum or that extrude it into the extracellular space and the Na^+-Ca^{++} exchangers in the sarcolemma (Figure 14-5). Drugs, neurotransmitters, or hormones that inhibit contraction and induce relaxation in smooth muscle act by various mechanisms, including the reduction of extracellular Ca^{++} influx, the reduction of Ca^{++} release from the sarcoplasmic reticulum, or the enhancement of Ca^{++} pump activity.

Pathological excitatory signals that increase cell $[Ca^{++}]$ cause various life-threatening conditions. In **asthma,** for example, airborne irritants or antigens can act on the airway epithelial cells to activate mechanisms that increase $[Ca^{++}]$ in airway smooth muscle cells, constrict the airways, and make breathing difficult. Some cases of **myocardial infarction** (death of cardiac muscle cells because of impaired blood flow) and **strokes** result from arterial vasospasm.

Ca^{++} Regulates Cross-Bridge Cycling in Smooth Muscle

The force generated by a muscle is proportional to the number of cross-bridges acting on the thin filaments, and the rates of force development or shortening velocities depend on cross-bridge cycling rates (see Chapter 12). IN SMOOTH MUSCLE, BOTH FORCE AND CYCLING RATES ARE PHYSIOLOGICALLY REGULATED BY CHANGES IN CELL Ca^{++} (Figure 14-4). Contraction rates in smooth muscle are slower

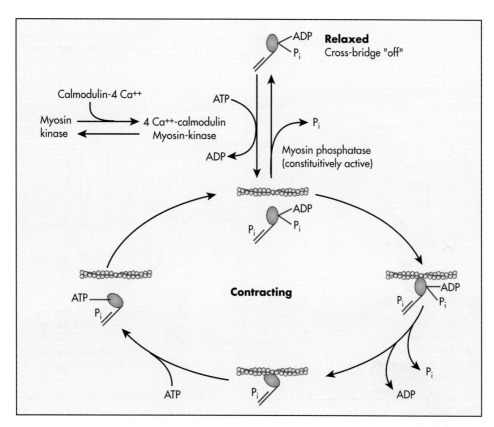

Figure 14-7 Ca^{++}-dependent phosphorylation of the cross-bridges by myosin kinase regulates the attachment to actin and the ATPase activity of smooth muscle myosin. Phosphorylated cross-bridges undergo the same cyclic interaction with actin as skeletal muscle myosin (see Figure 12-3). If the myoplasmic $[Ca^{++}]$ is lowered, Ca^{++} and calmodulin dissociate from myosin kinase, and the cross-bridges are dephosphorylated by myosin phosphatase. Note that the inorganic phosphate group attached to the cross-bridge by myosin kinase is at a different site from the inorganic phosphate group released during the cross-bridge cycle.

than in skeletal muscle, but phasic contractions require moderate cycling rates. However, the capacity to slow cross-bridge cycling by lowering cross-bridge detachment rates from the thin filament minimizes ATP consumption in a tonic contraction. In this situation the muscle is resisting imposed loads without shortening. Long cross-bridge interactions with the thin filaments are advantageous. The mechanisms by which the cross-bridge attachment rates are regulated to vary force and by which the cross-bridge detachment rates are regulated to determine cycling rates are the subject of current research.

Although Ca^{++} is a crucial link between the signals to the sarcolemma and cross-bridge cycling, the role of Ca^{++} is indirect in smooth muscle, which lacks the thin filament regulatory protein troponin. The available evidence suggests that regulation occurs at the cross-bridge itself. The mechanism is not allosteric (i.e., reversible binding of Ca^{++} to a regulatory site to induce conformational changes), but it involves phosphorylation of the cross-bridge at a specific serine residue (Figure 14-7). This **covalent regulatory mechanism** (the cross-bridge is chemically altered) uses ATP as the phosphate donor.

Myosin isolated from smooth muscle cannot bind to actin in the thin filament unless it is phosphorylated by a specific enzyme, **myosin kinase.** The active form of myosin kinase is a complex of the kinase with Ca^{++} and calmodulin (Figure 14-7). **Calmodulin** is a cytoplasmic protein that has four high-affinity Ca^{++} binding sites, and it participates in the activation of several Ca^{++}-dependent enzymes. The phosphorylated cross-bridge can cycle with no further need for Ca^{++} until it is dephosphorylated by **myosin phosphatase.** The regulatory scheme depicted in Figure 14-7 explains the biochemical evidence that cross-bridge attachment and cycling depend on phosphorylation of the cross-bridge. However, this scheme cannot account for variations in the rates of contraction associated with differences in the myoplasmic $[Ca^{++}]$ (Figure 14-4). IN SMOOTH MUSCLE, THE CROSS-BRIDGE CYCLING RATES DETERMINE THE RATES OF FORCE DEVELOPMENT OR SHORTENING VELOCITIES. THESE RATES DEPEND DIRECTLY ON THE CROSS-BRIDGE PHOSPHORYLATION LEVELS, WHICH DEPEND ON $[Ca^{++}]$.

The dual elements of variable cell force generation (which depends on control of cross-bridge attachment) and variable cell shortening velocities (which depend on control of cross-bridge detachment and thus of cycling rates) are unique to smooth muscle. They appear to be conferred by covalent cross-bridge regulation in which

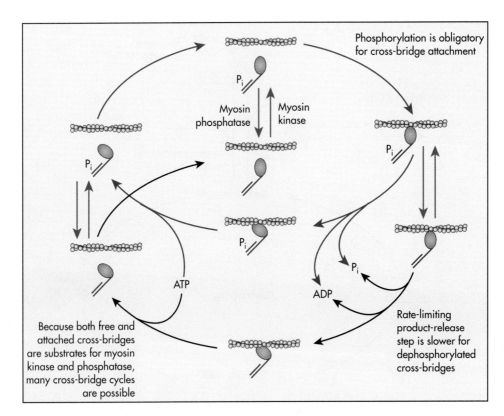

Figure 14-8 The behavior illustrated in Figure 14-4 can be explained if both free and attached cross-bridges are substrates for myosin kinase and myosin phosphatase. This allows a variety of cross-bridge cycles with the regulation of both force and velocity. When [Ca^{++}] is high, the myosin kinase activity is high relative to the phosphatase activity, and most cross-bridges traverse the rapid cycle (*red arrows*). If Ca^{++} levels fall, as in prolonged tonic contractions, force can be maintained with reduced cycling rates as more cross-bridges are dephosphorylated (cycles involving black cross-bridge states). ATP used for cross-bridge phosphorylation and dephosphorylation (*blue arrows* in Figure 14-7) is not illustrated in this figure.

the rates of cross-bridge phosphorylation and dephosphorylation rival those of ATP hydrolysis by the cross-bridge cycle in chemomechanical transduction. Figure 14-8 shows how myosin kinase and myosin phosphatase, acting on both free and attached cross-bridges, can account for the complex mechanical and energetic properties of smooth muscle. The Ca^{++}-dependent activation of myosin kinase and cross-bridge phosphorylation is obligatory to initiate cross-bridge attachment and cycling. However, myosin phosphatase can subsequently dephosphorylate a cross-bridge at other stages in the cycle, slowing detachment. Any cross-bridge may undergo many different cycles. If the cross-bridge remains phosphorylated, it undergoes a rapid cycle, as depicted in Figure 14-8. However, a cross-bridge can be dephosphorylated by myosin phosphatase after attachment. Dephosphorylation results in a slower detachment rate and a slower average cycle.

The [Ca^{++}] determines the typical cross-bridge cycle. If the [Ca^{++}] is high, the myosin kinase–myosin phosphatase activity ratio is high, and most cross-bridges are phosphorylated and cycle rapidly. Thus a high [Ca^{++}] is associated with rapid contractions (Figure 14-4). If the cell [Ca^{++}] levels rise only modestly or fall from high levels, the myosin kinase–myosin phosphatase activity ratio is reduced, and the probability increases that a

cross-bridge is dephosphorylated and that cycling is slowed.

The physiological advantages of this covalent regulatory mechanism are that it enables smooth muscle to develop force or to shorten rapidly in phasic contractions and to sustain forces and organ dimensions against imposed loads with diminished ATP consumption. ATP use is associated with cross-bridge phosphorylation and dephosphorylation, but the overall ATP savings in a muscle type where rapid contractions are unnecessary is very high.

> When organs becomes overstretched, the smooth muscle is rendered less able to contract fully. This can occur in the urinary bladder in men when the urethra is obstructed by an enlarged prostate, as in **benign prostatic hypertrophy.** Such patients cannot empty their urinary bladders.

Cardiac Muscle Has Unique Characteristics

Cardiac muscle cells are striated, and their thin filaments possess a troponin-based regulatory system (see

Table 14-2   Mechanisms for Grading Contractile Force

General Mechanism	Skeletal	Cardiac	Smooth*
Recruitment of more cells (motor units)	+	−	(+)
Summation of twitches by increasing stimulation frequency (tetanus)	+	−	+
Alteration of filament overlap by stretch	(+)	+	+
Variation of twitch by changing Ca^{++} transient	−	+	+
Alteration of Ca^{++} sensitivity of regulatory systems	−	+	+
Tonic depolarization and activation of potential-dependent Ca^{++} channels without action potentials	−	−	+
Receptor-activated channels (pharmacomechanical coupling)	−	−	+

*The relative importance of these mechanisms varies greatly with the type of smooth muscle. Parentheses indicate the possibility of little physiological importance.

Chapter 18). The myosin isoenzymes differ from striated muscle. However, the metabolic and contractile properties of the myocytes are comparable to those of slow skeletal muscle, and ATP consumption is met by oxidative phosphorylation. Like smooth muscle cells, cardiac muscle cells are small and have one central nucleus. They are connected to one another by specialized junctions that provide both electrical and mechanical coupling. Action potentials are propagated from cell to cell, and their contractions are thereby synchronized (see Chapter 18).

Cardiac muscle is well suited for the special function of the heart. This organ is a pump that must contract and relax rapidly. Each heartbeat is a response to a single action potential, and it is analogous to a twitch in skeletal muscle. The heart must generate substantial power during shortening to eject blood, and the efficiency of chemomechanical transduction is important.

Table 14-2 compares the mechanisms for grading the force of contraction in skeletal, cardiac, and smooth muscle.

Summary

- Smooth (involuntary) muscle is mainly a component of the walls of hollow organs, and it serves to stabilize organ dimensions by tonic contractions or to mix, propel, or expel organ contents by phasic contractions.
- Smooth muscle cells are anatomically discrete. A variety of junctions between cells coordinate communication, synchronous contraction, and force transmission.
- The contraction of smooth muscle is based on a sliding filament–cross-bridge mechanism, as is skeletal muscle, although the thick (myosin) and thin (actin) filaments of smooth muscle are not organized into sarcomeres and myofibrils.
- Smooth muscle is controlled by autonomic nerves (both excitatory and inhibitory), circulating hormones, locally generated hormones or metabolites from associated cell types, and electrical or chemical signals that couple cells via gap junctions.
- The sarcolemma in smooth muscle regulates cell $[Ca^{++}]$ in response to extracellular signals. The summed actions of the signals determine Ca^{++} influx via receptor-operated or voltage-gated channels and Ca^{++} efflux via Ca^{++} pumps and Na^{+}-Ca^{++} exchanges.
- The sarcoplasmic reticulum is an intracellular Ca^{++} compartment that generates Ca^{++} transients.
- Ca^{++} regulates contraction in smooth muscle by the formation of an active myosin kinase–calmodulin–Ca^{++} complex.
- Activated myosin kinase uses ATP to phosphorylate cross-bridges. This process enables the cross-bridges to attach to the thin filament and cycle.
- Dephosphorylation of attached cross-bridges by myosin phosphatase slows their detachment rate and thereby slows cross-bridge cycling rates and ATP consumption during sustained contractions.

BIBLIOGRAPHY

Arner A, Pfitzer G: Regulation of cross-bridge cycling by Ca^{2+} in smooth muscle, *Rev Physiol Biochem Pharmacol* 134:63, 1998.

Bárány M, ed: *Biochemistry of smooth muscle contraction,* San Diego, 1996, Academic.

Frank GB, Bianchi CP, ter Keurs HEDJ, eds: *Excitation-contraction coupling in skeletal, cardiac and smooth muscle,* New York, 1992, Plenum.

Horowitz A et al: Mechanisms of smooth muscle contraction, *Physiol Rev* 76:967, 1996.

Kao CY, Carsten ME, eds: *Cellular aspects of smooth muscle function,* Cambridge, 1997, Cambridge University Press.

Karaki H et al: Calcium movements, distribution, and functions in smooth muscle, *Pharmacol Rev* 49:157, 1997.

Kotlikoff MI et al: Calcium permeant ion channels in smooth muscle, *Rev Physiol Biochem Pharmacol* 134:147, 1998.

Kuriyama H et al: Physiological features of visceral smooth muscle cells, with special reference to receptors and ion channels, *Physiol Rev* 78:811, 1998.

McDonald TF et al: Regulation and modulation of calcium channels in cardiac, skeletal, and smooth muscle cells, *Physiol Rev* 74:365, 1994.

Motta PM, ed: *Ultrastructure of smooth muscle,* Norwell, Mass, 1990, Kluwer Academic.

Murphy RA: What is special about smooth muscle? The significance of covalent cross-bridge regulation, *FASEB J* 8:311, 1994.

Owens GK: Regulation of differentiation of vascular smooth muscle cells, *Physiol Rev* 75:487, 1995.

Quayle JM, Nelson MT, Standen NB: ATP-sensitive and inwardly rectifying potassium channels in smooth muscle, *Physiol Rev* 77:1165, 1997.

Szurszewski JH: A 100-year perspective on gastrointestinal motility, *Am J Physiol* 274:G447, 1998.

▷ CASE STUDIES

Case 14-1

A 19-year-old woman had severe respiratory distress and exhibited intense anxiety, cyanosis, sweating, and wheezing and had a heart rate of 120 beats/min. The emergency department physician administered O_2 and epinephrine. The patient's symptoms subsided, although wheezing and crackling sounds were audible by auscultation. The patient complained of severe fatigue.

1. **What was the physical cause for the difficulty in breathing?**

    A. Fatigue of the voluntary skeletal muscles involved in respiration

    B. Narrowing of the airways caused by edema

    C. Narrowing of the airways caused by smooth muscle contraction (hypersensitivity)

    D. Impaired airway smooth muscle metabolism

    E. Aspirated food in the trachea

2. **Which kind or kinds of muscle are involved in an asthmatic attack?**

    A. Cardiac, skeletal, and smooth

    B. Cardiac and skeletal

    C. Cardiac and smooth

    D. Voluntary

    E. Involuntary

3. **Which of the following does the physiological role of airway smooth muscle *not* involve?**

    A. Relaxation to reduce airway resistance

    B. Phasic contraction to increase airway resistance

    C. Tonic contraction to maintain airway dimensions

    D. Rhythmical contractions to enhance airflow

    E. Contraction and relaxation in different airways to shift airflow to different parts of the lungs

Case 14-2

A 38-year-old woman told her physician of recurring episodes of cold-induced paleness in her hands, followed by cyanosis and redness, with throbbing pain that gradually disappeared. The diagnosis was primary Raynaud's disease which occurs in about one of every six women.

1. **The symptoms were caused by which of the following?**

    A. Reduced O_2 content in the blood supply

    B. ATP consumption by the skeletal muscles in the hands that exceeded the oxidative capacity

    C. Transient localized arterial smooth muscle contraction with inadequate blood flow

    D. Thrombosis with blockage of blood flow to the hands

    E. Low temperature, reducing the O_2 binding capacity of hemoglobin

2. **The redness of the hands was caused by which of the following?**

    A. Restoration of normal blood flow after vasoconstriction

    B. Accumulation of vasodilators during hypoxia

    C. Hemoglobin, cytochromes, and myoglobin turning red in the absence of O_2

    D. Increased vascular sympathetic nerve activity

    E. Increased venous return

3. **Precipitation of an attack when the patient's hands are immersed in cold water is diagnostic of Raynaud's disease. What does it suggest?**

    A. The pain was the direct result of low temperature.

    B. The cooling is a trigger for peripheral vasospasm but is not necessarily a direct effect on arterial smooth muscle.

    C. A drop in the body's core temperature triggers the shunting of blood flow from the extremities.

    D. Reduced metabolism associated with cooling induces vasoconstriction.

    E. Raynaud's disease is due to the accumulation of metabolites.

IV

CARDIOVASCULAR SYSTEM

Robert M. Berne and Matthew N. Levy

CHAPTER 15

Overview of Circulation

- Describe the compositions and functions of the blood vessels.
- Define the relationship of the vascular cross-sectional area to the velocity of blood flow in the various vascular segments.
- Explain the pressure changes and pathways of blood flow throughout the vasculature.

The circulatory, endocrine, and nervous systems constitute the principal coordinating and integrating systems of the body. Whereas the nervous system is concerned primarily with communication and the endocrine system with the regulation of specific body functions, the circulatory system transports and distributes essential substances to the tissues and removes the by-products of metabolism. The circulatory system also participates in homeostatic mechanisms such as the regulation of body temperature, humoral communication throughout the body, and adjustments of O_2 and nutrient supply in different physiological states.

The cardiovascular system is made up of a pump, a series of distributing and collecting tubes, and an extensive system of thin-walled vessels

The heart consists of two pumps in series: (1) the right ventricle, which propels blood through the lungs for the exchange of O_2 and CO_2, and (2) the left ventricle, which propels blood to all other tissues of the body. Unidirectional flow through the heart is achieved by the appropriate arrangement of effective flap valves.

Although cardiac output is intermittent, continuous flow to the periphery is accomplished by distention of the aorta and its branches during ventricular contraction (**systole**) and the elastic recoil of the walls of the large arteries with forward propulsion of the blood during ventricular relaxation (**diastole**). Blood moves rapidly through the aorta and its arterial branches. The branches become narrower, and their walls become thinner and change histologically toward the periphery. The aorta is predominantly an elastic structure. However, the peripheral arteries are more muscular, and in the arterioles the muscular layer predominates (Figure 15-1).

In the aorta and the large arteries, frictional (viscous) resistance to blood flow is relatively small, and the pressure drop from the root of the aorta to the small arteries is also relatively small (Figure 15-2). However, IN THE SMALL ARTERIES AND ARTERIOLES, RESISTANCE TO BLOOD FLOW IS LARGE, AND THE PRESSURE DROP ACROSS THESE VESSELS IS ALSO LARGE. The greatest resistance is in the arterioles, which are sometimes referred to as the *stopcocks* of the circulatory system. The degree of contraction in the circular muscle of these small vessels regulates tissue blood flow and aids in controlling the arterial blood pressure.

In addition to a sharp reduction in pressure across the arterioles, flow changes from pulsatile to steady. THE PULSATILE ARTERIAL BLOOD FLOW, WHICH IS CAUSED BY INTERMITTENT CARDIAC EJECTION, IS DAMPED AT THE CAPILLARY LEVEL BY THE COMBINATION OF THE DISTENSIBILITY OF THE LARGE ARTERIES AND THE FRICTIONAL RESISTANCE IN THE SMALL ARTERIES AND ARTERIOLES. Many capillaries arise from each arteriole. Hence the total cross-sectional area of the capillary bed is very large despite the fact that the cross-sectional area of each capillary is less than that of each arteriole. As a result of the large total cross-sectional area, blood flow velocity slows considerably in the capillaries, just as the flow velocity decreases at the wide regions of a river. Note that the velocity of blood flow and the cross-sectional area at each level of the vasculature are essentially mirror images of each other (Figure 15-3). Because the capillaries consist of short tubes with walls only one cell thick and because flow velocity is slow, conditions in the capillaries are ideal for the exchange of diffusible substances between blood and tissue.

On its return to the heart from the capillaries, blood passes through venules and then through veins of increasing caliber and decreasing number. The thickness and composition of the vein walls change (Figure 15-1), the total cross-sectional area of the veins diminishes, and the velocity of blood flow in the veins increases (Figure 15-3). Also, most of the blood in the systemic circulation is located in the venous vessels. Conversely, the blood in the pulmonary vascular bed is about equally divided among the arterial, capillary, and venous vessels.

Blood entering the right ventricle from the right atrium is pumped through the pulmonary arterial system at a mean pressure about one seventh that in the systemic arteries. The blood then passes through the

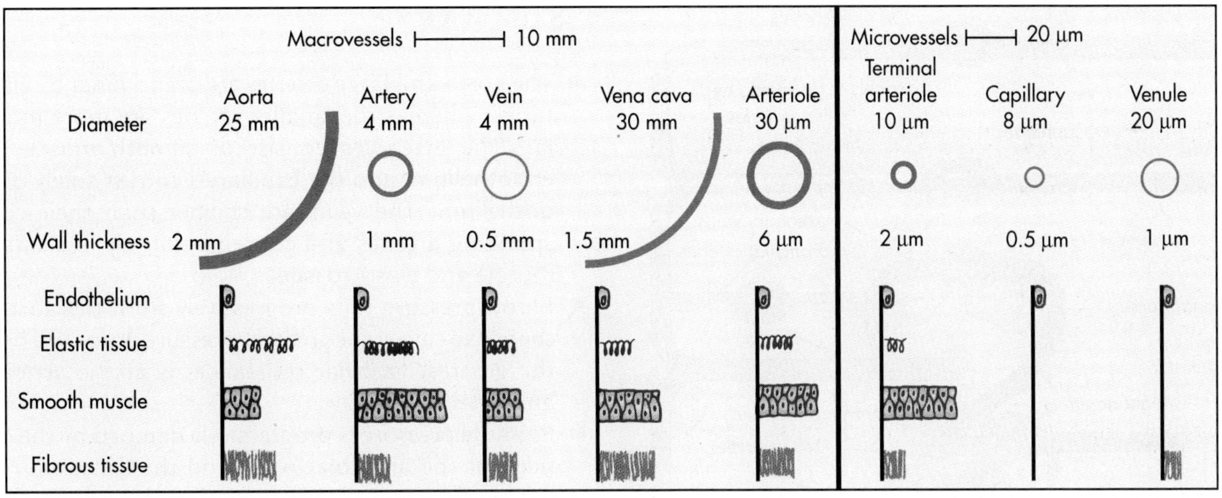

Figure 15-1 Internal diameter, wall thickness, and relative amounts of the principal components of the vessel walls of the various blood vessels that make up the circulatory system. Cross sections of the vessels are not drawn to scale because of the huge range from the aorta and venae cavae to the capillaries. *(Redrawn from Burton AC:* Physiol Rev *34:619, 1954.)*

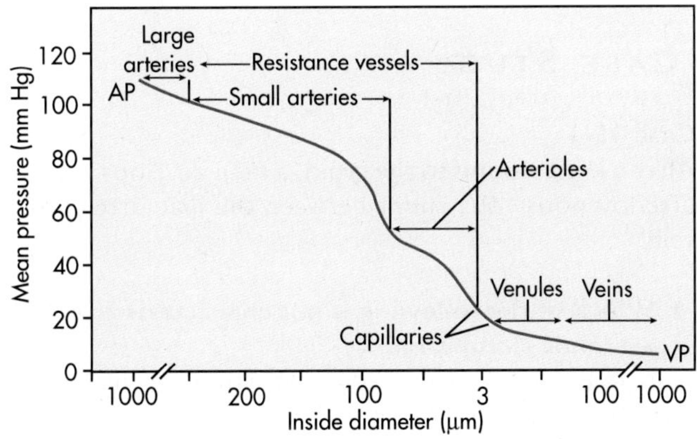

Figure 15-2 Pressure drop across the vascular system in the hamster cheek pouch. *AP,* Mean arterial pressure; *VP,* venous pressure. *(Redrawn from Davis MJ et al:* Am J Physiol *250:H291, 1986.)*

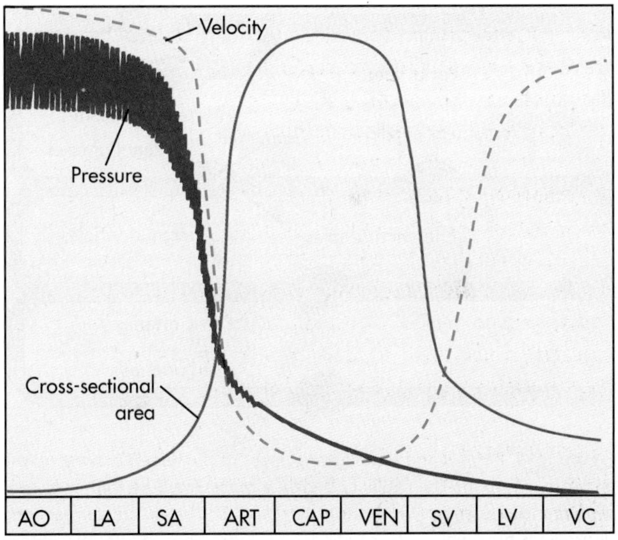

Figure 15-3 Phasic pressure, velocity of flow, and cross-sectional area of the systemic circulation. THE IMPORTANT FEATURES ARE THE INVERSE RELATIONSHIP AMONG VELOCITY AND THE CROSS-SECTIONAL AREA, THE MAJOR PRESSURE DROP ACROSS THE SMALL ARTERIES AND ARTERIOLES, AND THE MAXIMAL CROSS-SECTIONAL AREA AND MINIMAL FLOW RATE IN THE CAPILLARIES. *AO,* Aorta; *ART,* arterioles; *CAP,* capillaries; *LA,* large arteries; *LV,* large veins; *SA,* small arteries; *SV,* small veins; *VC,* venae cavae; *VEN,* venules.

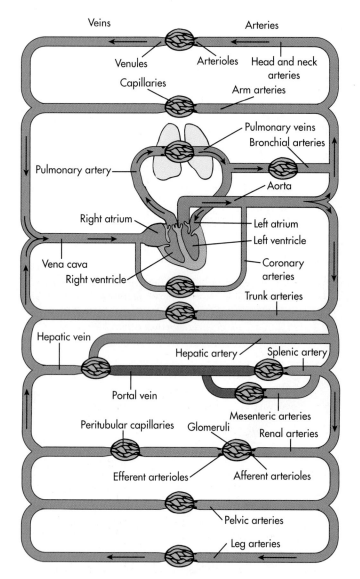

Figure 15-4 Parallel and series arrangement of the vessels making up the circulatory system. The capillary beds are represented by thin lines connecting the arteries *(red)* with the veins *(blue)*. The black, crescent-shaped thickenings proximal to the capillary beds represent the arterioles (resistance vessels). *(Redrawn from Green HD. In Glasser O, ed: Medical physics, vol 1, Chicago, 1944, Mosby.)*

lung capillaries, where CO_2 is released and O_2 is taken up. The O_2-rich blood returns via the pulmonary veins to the left atrium and ventricle to complete the cycle. The systemic and pulmonary circulation systems are diagrammed in Figure 15-4.

SUMMARY

- The aorta and large arteries are predominantly elastic tubes, whereas the smaller arteries are more muscular. The arterioles consist of smooth muscle and endothelium, and the capillaries consist solely of endothelium. The veins are thinner than their corresponding arteries and contain relatively less smooth muscle and elastic tissue.
- Blood pressure falls progressively from the aorta to the venae cavae; the greatest pressure drop, and hence the greatest vascular resistance, is at the arterioles and small arteries.
- Pulsatile pressure is progressively damped by the elasticity of the arteriolar walls and the frictional resistance of the arterioles, so capillary blood flow is essentially nonpulsatile.
- Blood velocity decreases from the aorta to the capillaries and then increases from the capillaries to the venae cavae. The velocity of blood flow in each segment of the circulatory system is inversely related to the total vascular cross-sectional area of that segment.
- Most of the blood in the vasculature is in the veins.
- The circulatory system consists of conduits arranged in series and in parallel.

CASE STUDY

Case 15-1
After a knife wound to the groin, a man develops a large arteriovenous (AV) shunt between the iliac artery and vein.

1. **Which of the following is *not* characteristic of his systemic circulation?**
    A. Blood flow in the capillaries of the finger nail bed is pulsatile.
    B. The circulation time (antecubital vein to tongue) is increased.
    C. The arterial pulse pressure (systolic pressure minus diastolic pressure) is increased.
    D. The greatest velocity of blood flow prevails in the aorta.
    E. Pressure in the right atrium is less than in the inferior vena cava.

CHAPTER 16

Blood and Hemostasis

- Describe the constituents of blood.
- Explain the functions of the cellular elements of blood.
- Describe the importance of blood group matching before blood transfusions.
- Explain the factors involved in hemostasis, blood coagulation, and clot lysis.

The main function of the circulating blood is to carry O_2 and nutrients to the tissues and remove CO_2 and waste products. However, blood also transports other substances (e.g., hormones) from their sites of formation to their sites of action and white blood cells and platelets to where they are needed. In addition, blood aids in the distribution of water, solutes, and heat and thus contributes to **homeostasis,** a constancy of the body's internal environment. Hence blood helps coordinate many of the body's functions.

Blood Is a Suspension of Red Cells, White Cells, and Platelets in a Complex Solution (Plasma) of Gases, Salts, Proteins, and Lipids

The circulating blood volume is about 7% of body weight. Approximately 55% of the blood is plasma, whose protein content is 7 g/dl ($\approx$4 g/dl of albumin and 3 g/dl of immunoglobulins).

Erythrocytes

Erythrocytes (red blood cells) are anuclear, flexible, biconcave disks that transport O_2 to body tissues. They average 7 μm in diameter, and there are 5 million per microliter in the blood. They arise from stem cells in the bone marrow, and during maturation, they lose their nuclei before entering the circulation, where their average life span is 120 days.

The main protein in erythrocytes is hemoglobin ($\approx$15 g/dl of blood) which consists of **heme,** an iron-containing tetrapyrrole, linked to **globin,** a protein composed of four polypeptide chains (two α and two β in the normal adult). The iron moiety of hemoglobin binds loosely and reversibly to O_2 to form **oxyhemoglobin.** The affinity of hemo-

globin for O_2 is affected by pH, temperature, and the concentration of 2,3-diphosphoglycerate. These factors facilitate O_2 uptake in the lungs and its release in the tissues (see Chapter 30).

Changes in the polypeptide subunits of globin can also affect the affinity of hemoglobin for O_2; for example, fetal hemoglobin has two γ chains instead of two β chains and has greater affinity for O_2. Changes can also result in disease states such as **sickle cell anemia** or **thalassemia.**

The number of circulating red blood cells is fairly constant under normal conditions. The production of erythrocytes **(erythropoiesis)** is regulated by the glycoprotein **erythropoietin,** which is secreted mainly by the kidneys. Erythropoietin accelerates the differentiation of stem cells in the bone marrow.

Anemia and chronic hypoxia (e.g., that resulting from living at high altitudes) stimulate erythrocyte production and can produce **polycythemia** (an increased number of red blood cells). When the hypoxic stimulus is removed in subjects with altitude polycythemia, the high red cell concentration in the blood inhibits erythropoiesis. The red cell count is also greatly increased in **polycythemia vera,** a disease of unknown cause. The elevated erythrocyte concentration increases blood viscosity, often to a degree that blood flow to vital tissues becomes impaired.

Leukocytes

There are normally 4000 to 10,000 leukocytes (white blood cells) per microliter of blood. Leukocytes include granulocytes (65%), lymphocytes (30%), and monocytes (5%). Of the granulocytes, about 95% are neutrophils, 4% are eosinophils, and 1% are basophils. White blood cells originate from the primitive stem cells in the bone marrow. After birth, granulocytes and monocytes in humans continue to originate in the bone marrow, whereas lymphocytes originate in the lymph nodes, spleen, and thymus.

Granulocytes and monocytes are motile, nucleated cells that contain **lysosomes,** which in turn contain enzymes capable of digesting foreign material such as microorganisms, damaged cells, and cellular debris. Thus leukocytes constitute a major defense mechanism against infections. Microorganisms or the products of cell destruction release

chemotactic substances that attract granulocytes and monocytes. When migrating leukocytes reach the foreign agents, they engulf them **(phagocytosis)** and then destroy them by the action of enzymes that form O_2-**derived free radicals** and **hydrogen peroxide.**

Lymphocytes

Lymphocytes vary in size. They have large nuclei, and most lack cytoplasmic granules. The two main types are **B cells,** which confer humoral immunity, and **T cells,** which confer cell-mediated immunity. When stimulated by an **antigen,** B cells are transformed into **plasma cells,** which synthesize and secrete antibodies (γ-globulin), which are carried by the bloodstream to their site of action.

> The main T cells are cytotoxic and are responsible for long-term protection against some viruses, bacteria, and cancer cells. They are also responsible for the rejection of transplanted organs.

Other T cells are **helper T cells,** which activate B cells, and **suppressor T cells,** which inhibit B cell activity. Special B and T cells, called **memory cells,** "remember" specific antigens. These cells can quickly generate an immune response when exposed to the same antigen after the first time.

> Protection against several infectious diseases has been achieved by injecting the appropriate antigen. Also, **vaccines** have been developed for certain diseases by injecting killed or attenuated organisms (antigens) into suitable hosts (e.g., horses, sheep).

Platelets

Platelets are small (3 mm), anuclear cell fragments of **megakaryocytes.** The megakaryocytes reside in the bone marrow and when mature, break up into platelets, which enter the circulation. Platelets are important in hemostasis, as discussed later.

Blood Groups Are Important in Matching Blood for Transfusions

In humans, there are four principal blood groups, designated O, A, B, and AB. The plasma of group O blood contains antibodies to red cells of groups A, B, and AB. Group A plasma contains antibodies to red cells of group B, and group B plasma contains antibodies to red cells of group A. Group AB plasma has no antibodies to red cells of group O, A, or B. In blood transfusions, cross-matching is necessary to prevent the agglutina-

tion of donor red cells by antibodies in the plasma of the recipient. Because the plasma of groups A, B, and AB has no antibodies to group O red cells, people with group O blood are called **universal donors.** Conversely, people with AB blood are called **universal recipients** because their plasma has no antibodies to red cells of the other three groups.

In addition to the ABO blood grouping, there are **rhesus factor–positive (Rh-positive)** and **Rh-negative groups.**

> An Rh-negative person can develop antibodies to Rh-positive red cells if exposed to Rh-positive blood. This can occur during pregnancy if the mother is Rh negative and the fetus is Rh positive (inherited from the father). In this case, Rh-positive red cells from the fetus enter the maternal bloodstream at the time of placental separation and induce Rh-positive antibodies in the mother's plasma. The Rh-positive antibodies from the mother can also reach the fetus via the placenta and agglutinate and hemolyze fetal red cells (**erythroblastosis fetalis,** a hemolytic disease of the newborn). Red cell destruction can also occur in Rh-negative individuals who have previously had transfusions of Rh-positive blood and have developed Rh antibodies. If these individuals are given a subsequent transfusion of Rh-positive blood, the transfused red cells will be destroyed by the Rh antibodies in their plasma.

Hemostasis Is Accomplished by Vasoconstriction, Platelet Aggregation, and Blood Coagulation

Vasoconstriction

Physical injury to a blood vessel elicits a contractile response of the vascular smooth muscle and thus a narrowing of the vessel. Vasoconstriction in severed arterioles or small arteries can completely obliterate the lumen of the vessel and stop the flow of blood. The contraction of the vascular smooth muscle is probably caused by direct mechanical stimulation by the penetrating object as well as by mechanical stimulation of the perivascular nerves.

Platelet aggregation

Damage to the endothelium of a blood vessel engenders platelet adherence at the site of injury. The adherent platelets release **ADP** and **thromboxane A_2,** which cause the adherence of additional platelets. The aggregation of platelets may continue in this manner until some of the small blood vessels become blocked by the mass of aggregated platelets. Extension of the platelet aggregate along the vessel is prevented by the antiaggregation action of **prostacyclin.** This substance is released from the normal endothelial cells in

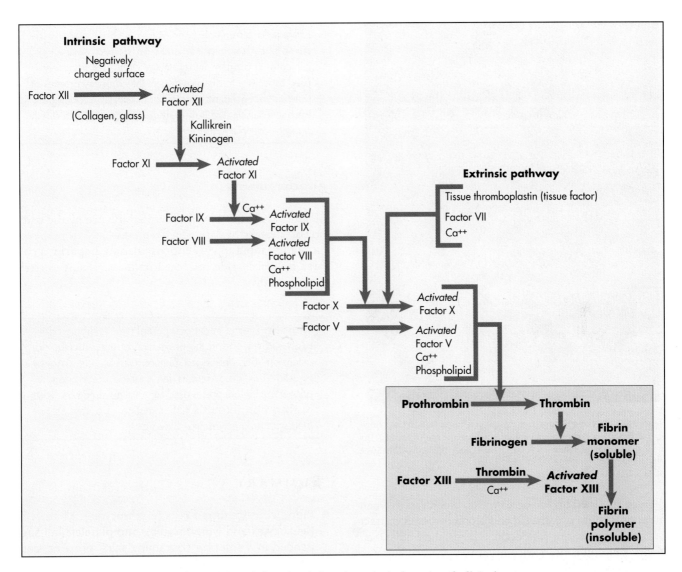

Figure 16-1 Intrinsic and extrinsic pathways in the formation of a fibrin clot.

the adjacent, uninjured part of the vessel. Platelets also release **serotonin (5-hydroxytryptamine),** which enhances vasoconstriction, and **thromboplastin,** which hastens blood coagulation.

Bleeding of one form or another is an important clinical problem. Trauma is the most common cause of bleeding. Gastrointestinal bleeding can cause severe anemia or even cardiovascular shock, and occult blood in the stool can be the first clue of cancer of the bowel or peptic ulcer.

When the platelet count is low, as in **thrombocytopenic purpura,** tiny hemorrhages **(petechiae)** or larger hemorrhages **(ecchymoses)** may appear in the skin and mucous membranes. Bleeding occurs into the tissues (especially joints) in **hemophilia,** a hereditary disease that afflicts humans. This disease occurs only in male patients, but the genetic abnormality is carried by females.

Blood coagulation

Clotting of blood is a complex process consisting of the sequential activation of various factors in the blood. The cascade of reactions in which one activated factor activates another, and so on, is depicted in Figure 16-1. Several of the factors are synthesized in the liver, as is vitamin K, which is essential for the synthesis of these liver-derived clotting factors.

THE KEY STEP IN BLOOD CLOTTING IS THE CONVERSION OF FIBRINOGEN TO FIBRIN BY THROMBIN. The clot formed by this reaction consists of a dense network of fibrin strands in which blood cells and plasma are trapped (Figure 16-2). The two blood coagulation pathways, the **extrinsic pathway** and the **intrinsic pathway,** converge on the activation of factor X, which catalyzes the cleavage of prothrombin to thrombin (Figure 16-1). Blood clotting via the extrinsic pathway is initiated by tissue damage and the release of tissue thromboplastin. Blood clotting via the intrinsic pathway is initiated by exposure of the blood to a negatively

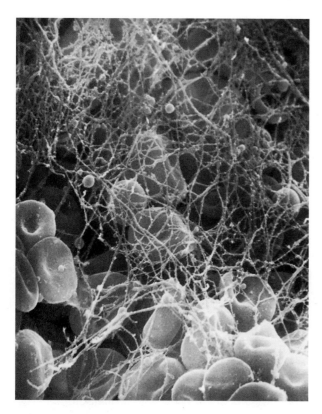

Figure 16-2 Scanning electron micrograph of a human blood clot, showing red blood cells immobilized within a network of fibrin threads. The small spheres are platelets. (×9000.) *(From Shelly WB: JAMA 249:3089, 1983.)*

charged surface. This can occur within blood vessels when the endothelium is damaged and blood comes in contact with collagen. It can also occur outside the body when blood comes in contact with negatively charged surfaces such as glass. If blood is carefully drawn into a syringe coated with silicone, clotting is greatly delayed.

After a clot is formed, the actin and myosin of the platelets trapped in the fibrin mesh interact in a manner similar to that in muscle. The resultant contraction pulls the fibrin strands toward the platelets and thereby extrudes the **serum** (plasma without fibrinogen) and shrinks the clot. The process is called **clot retraction.** The function of clot retraction is not clear, but it may serve to approximate the edges of severed blood vessels.

Several cofactors are required for blood coagulation (Figure 16-1); the most important is Ca^{++}. If Ca^{++} in the blood is removed or bound, coagulation does not occur.

Blood Clots Can Be Lysed, and Blood Coagulation Can Be Prevented

Clot lysis

Normal blood contains **plasminogen,** an inactive precursor of the proteolytic enzyme **plasmin.** Activators of the conversion of plasminogen to plasmin are found in tissues, plasma, and urine **(urokinase).**

Exogenous plasminogen activators such as **streptokinase** and **tissue plasminogen activator** are used clinically to dissolve intravascular clots. This treatment is used especially to dissolve clots in the coronary arteries of patients with acute **myocardial infarction** (damage to the heart muscle that is most frequently caused by a clot in a major coronary artery).

Anticoagulants

Blood coagulation can be prevented in vitro by the addition of citrate or oxalate, which removes Ca^{++} from the solution. For rapid in vivo anticoagulation, **heparin,** a sulfated polysaccharide produced by mast cells, is injected intravenously.

Heparin is used in extracorporeal circuits during open-heart surgery and in the prevention of intravascular clot extension. For prolonged anticoagulation, **dicumarol** is used. This drug inhibits the synthesis of vitamin K–dependent factors and is used for treating conditions such as **thrombophlebitis** (inflammation of a vein associated with an intravascular blood clot).

SUMMARY

- Blood consists of red cells (erythrocytes), white cells (leukocytes and lymphocytes), and platelets, all suspended in a solution containing salts, proteins, carbohydrates, and lipids.
- There are four major blood groups: O, A, B, and AB. Type O blood can be given to people with any of the blood groups because the plasma of all of the blood groups lacks antibodies to type O red cells. Hence people with type O blood are referred to as *universal donors.* By the same token, people with AB blood are referred to as *universal recipients* because their plasma lacks antibodies to red cells of all of the blood groups. In addition to O, A, B, and AB blood groups, there are Rh-positive and Rh-negative blood groups.
- A cascade of reactions that constitute an intrinsic pathway and an extrinsic pathway is involved in blood coagulation. The final steps in which the two pathways join are the conversion of prothrombin to thrombin and the conversion of fibrinogen to fibrin, a reaction catalyzed by thrombin.
- Blood clots may be liquefied by plasmin, a proteolytic enzyme whose formation from plasminogen is catalyzed by tissue activators (e.g., urokinase) or exogenous activators (e.g., streptokinase, tissue plasminogen activator).

BIBLIOGRAPHY

Jackson CM, Nemerson Y: Blood coagulation, *Annu Rev Biochem* 49:765, 1980.

Le DT et al: Hemostatic factors in rabbit limb lymph: relationship to mechanisms regulating extravascular coagulation, *Am J Physiol* 274:H769, 1998.

Ogston D: *The physiology of hemostasis,* Cambridge, Mass, 1983, Harvard University Press.

Ratnoff OD, Forbes CE, eds: *Disorders of hemostasis,* Orlando, Fla, 1984, Grune & Stratton.

Shattil SJ, Bennett JS: Platelets and their membranes in hemostasis: physiology and pathophysiology, *Ann Intern Med* 94:108, 1981.

▷ CASE STUDIES

Case 16-1

A 30-year-old man has a long history of epigastric pain that is relieved by eating food, drinking milk, or taking antacid tablets. He went to see his physician because of 3 weeks of progressive fatigue and shortness of breath on exertion. Physical examination revealed only severe pallor and a rapid heart rate. A stool sample was black and guaiac positive (indicative of blood in stool).

1. A peripheral blood examination showed which of the following?
   A. Red cells of uniform size
   B. A hematocrit of 45%
   C. A red cell count of 5 million cells/mm^3
   D. Blood hemoglobin of 6 g/dl
   E. A normal hemoglobin/red cell ratio

Case 16-2

A married woman was shot in the thigh during a domestic quarrel, and the bullet pierced the femoral artery. She lost a lot of blood before her spouse applied a tourniquet and rushed her to the hospital, where she received several units of blood. The patient's blood type is O, and she is Rh positive.

1. Which of the following blood types can she receive with safety?
   A. Group A and Rh positive
   B. Group AB and Rh positive
   C. Group AB and Rh negative
   D. Group O and Rh negative
   E. Group B and Rh negative

Electrical Activity of the Heart

OBJECTIVES

- Explain the types of cardiac action potentials.
- Define the ionic basis of cardiac action potentials.
- Explain the temporal changes in cardiac excitability.
- Explain the basis of automaticity.
- Describe the spread of excitation of the heart.
- Explain the basis of reentry.
- Describe the components of the electrocardiogram.

Action Potentials in the Heart Are Prolonged

The electrical behavior of cardiac cells differs considerably from that of nerve cells or of smooth or skeletal muscle cells (see Chapters 3, 13, and 14). In general, the durations of action potentials are much longer in cardiac cells than in nerve cells or in smooth or skeletal muscle cells. Furthermore, the action potentials differ substantially among various types of cardiac cells depending on the function and location of those cells.

Figure 17-1, *A*, shows the potential changes recorded from a ventricular muscle cell immersed in an electrolyte solution. When a microelectrode and a reference electrode are placed in the solution near the quiescent cell, no measurable potential difference (point a in Figure 17-1, *A*) exists between the two electrodes. At point b in Figure 17-1, *A*, the microelectrode is inserted into the interior of the cell. Immediately a potential difference is recorded across the cell membrane; the potential of the cell interior is about 90 mV lower than that of the surrounding medium. Such electronegativity of the cell interior is also characteristic of skeletal and smooth muscle cells, nerve cells, and indeed, most cells within the body (see Chapter 2).

At point c in Figure 17-1, *A*, the cell is stimulated artificially, usually by an electrical current. The cell membrane rapidly **depolarizes;** that is, the potential difference across the cell membrane tends to disappear. In most cardiac cells, the potential difference across the cell membrane reverses slightly, such that the potential of the interior of the cell exceeds the outside potential by about 20 mV. The rapid upstroke of the **action potential** is designated **phase 0.** A brief period of partial repolarization **(phase 1)** occurs immediately after the upstroke, and it is followed by a plateau **(phase 2)** that persists for about 0.2 second. The internal potential then becomes progressively more negative **(phase 3)** until the resting potential (V_m) is again attained (at point e in Figure 17-1, *A*). This **repolarization** (phase 3) proceeds more slowly than the **depolarization** (phase 0). The interval from the completion of repolarization until the beginning of the next action potential is designated **phase 4;** the potential that prevails during this period is called the **resting membrane potential.**

The cardiac action potential types are either fast or slow response

Two main types of action potentials may be recorded in the heart. **Fast-response action potentials** (Figure 17-1, *A*) occur in atrial and ventricular myocardial fibers and specialized conducting fibers **(Purkinje fibers)** that exist mainly in the endocardial surfaces of the ventricles. **Slow-response action potentials** (Figure 17-1, *B*) occur in the **sinoatrial (SA) node,** which is the natural pacemaker region of the heart, and the **atrioventricular (AV) node,** which is the specialized tissue that conducts the cardiac impulse from the atria to the ventricles.

Figure 17-1 shows that the resting membrane potential of the slow response is considerably less negative than that of the fast response. Also, the slope of the upstroke (phase 0) and the amplitude and overshoot of the slow-response action potentials are less than the corresponding values for the fast-response action potentials. The amplitude of the action potential and the rate of rise of the upstroke are important determinants of the conduction velocity, as described later.

Fast responses may change to slow responses under certain pathological conditions. For example, when the blood supply to a region of cardiac muscle is deficient in a patient with coronary artery disease, the K^+ concentration in the interstitial fluid bathing the affected muscle cells rises because K^+ is lost from the inadequately perfused **(ischemic)** cells. The action potentials in some of these cells

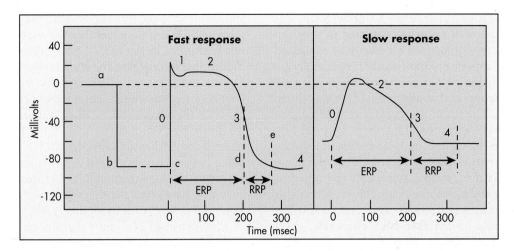

Figure 17-1 Changes in transmembrane potential recorded from a fast-response *(left)* and a slow-response *(right)* cardiac fiber in isolated cardiac tissue immersed in an electrolyte solution. The numbers refer to the various phases of the action potentials. *ERP,* Effective refractory period; *RRP,* relative refractory period.

may then be converted from fast to slow responses. In cardiac tissues composed of slow-response fibers, ischemia is more likely to retard or halt conduction than in tissues composed of fast-response fibers.

The Cardiac Transmembrane Potential Depends Mainly on K^+, Na^+, and Ca^{++}

The various phases of the cardiac action potential are associated with changes in the conductance of the cell membrane, mainly to Na^+ (g_{Na}), K^+ (g_K), and Ca^{++} (g_{Ca}). The conductance to an ion is an index of the permeability of the membrane to that ion, as explained in Chapter 2. Each phase of the action potential is associated with a change in conductance to one or more ions.

Resting potential

The V_m during phase 4 depends mainly on g_K. Just as with all other cells in the body, the concentration of K^+ inside a cardiac muscle cell, $[K^+]_i$, greatly exceeds the concentration outside the cell, $[K^+]_o$ (Figure 17-2). The direction of the concentration gradients for Na^+ and Ca^{++} in the cardiac cell is opposite to that for K^+. Estimates of the extracellular and intracellular concentrations of Na^+, K^+, and Ca^{++} and of the **Nernst equilibrium potentials** (see Chapter 2) for these ions are shown in Table 17-1. The ability of the resting cell membrane to conduct K^+ greatly exceeds its ability to conduct Na^+ or Ca^{++}. Thus THE RESTING MEMBRANE POTENTIAL IS DETERMINED MAINLY BY THE RATIO OF INTRACELLULAR TO EXTRACELLULAR CONCENTRATION OF K^+: $[K^+]_i/[K^+]_o$. Two specific types of K^+ channels account for the g_K of the resting myocardial cell; these channels conduct the so-called **delayed rectifier K^+ current** (i_K) and the **inwardly rectified K^+ current** (i_{K1}).

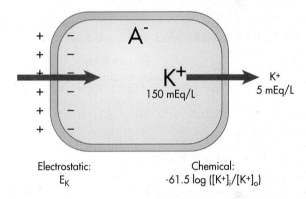

Figure 17-2 Balance of chemical and electrostatic forces that act across a resting cardiac cell membrane. The balance is based on a 30:1 ratio of $[K^+]_i$ to $[K^+]_o$ and the presence of a nondiffusible anion (A^-) inside, but not outside, the cell.

This assertion has been verified experimentally. Changes in the extracellular concentrations of Na^+ ($[Na^+]_o$) or Ca^{++} ($[Ca^{++}]_o$) scarcely affect V_m. However, when $[K^+]_i/[K^+]_o$ is decreased experimentally by raising $[K^+]_o$, the measured value of V_m approximates that predicted by the Nernst equation for K^+ (equilibrium potential for K^+ [E_K]) (Figure 17-3). For $[K^+]_o$ above 5 mM, the measured values of V_m correspond closely with the predicted values. The measured values are slightly less negative than those predicted by the Nernst equation because of the small but finite g_{Na}.

Fast-response action potentials occur in myocardial and Purkinje fibers

The upstroke depends on Na^+ flux
Fast-response cardiac fibers, notably myocardial fibers, do not ordinarily initiate cardiac impulses. The impulses that initiate each cardiac contraction usually

originate in specialized cells in the SA node. Such cells possess the property of **automaticity;** that is, they can generate action potentials spontaneously, as explained later. Therefore a given myocardial fiber is generally excited when an action potential originating in a distant automatic cell arrives at that myocardial fiber via cell-to-cell conduction. The traveling action potential (i.e., the **cardiac impulse**) is a wave of relative negativity (see Figure 3-11). When the cardiac impulse arrives at myocardial fibers adjacent to the given resting fiber, the negative potential at the external surface of the adjacent fibers decreases the V_m in the resting fiber. When this change in V_m attains a threshold value, certain voltage-sensitive channels, called **fast Na^+ channels,** open quickly; they are said to be **activated.** Na^+ then quickly enters the myocardial cell. The process is very rapid because (1) the g_{Na} of the abundant fast Na^+ channels in the cell membrane increases substantially, (2) the interior of the cell is negatively charged and therefore Na^+ is

pulled into the cell by the powerful electrostatic attraction, and (3) the transmembrane concentration gradient for Na^+ is large (Table 17-1) and therefore the net diffusional forces favor the inward movement of Na^+.

THE CHARACTERISTICS OF THE UPSTROKE OF THE ACTION POTENTIAL IN FAST-RESPONSE CARDIAC FIBERS DEPEND ALMOST ENTIRELY ON THE INFLUX OF Na^+. Other ions are unimportant. As shown by the upper curve in Figure 17-4, the amplitude of the cardiac action potential (i.e., the maximum value of the action potential during phase 0) varies linearly with the logarithm of $[Na^+]_o$. Conversely, changes in $[Na^+]_o$ have very little effect on the resting membrane potential (lower curve in Figure 17-4).

The inrush of Na^+ into the myocardial cell ceases within 1 or 2 msec after the excitation of the cell for two reasons. First, as the V_m becomes less negative and approaches the Nernst equilibrium potential for Na^+ (E_{Na}) (Table 17-1), the electrostatic force that tends to pull Na^+ into the cell progressively diminishes and then

Table 17-1	Ion Concentrations and Equilibrium Potentials in Cardiac Muscle Cells		
Ion	Extracellular Concentration (mM)	Intracellular Concentration (mM)	Equilibrium Potential (mV)
Na^+	145	10	70
K^+	4	135	−94
Ca^{++}	2	10^{-4}	132

Modified from ten Eick RE et al: *Prog Cardiovasc Dis* 24:157, 1981.

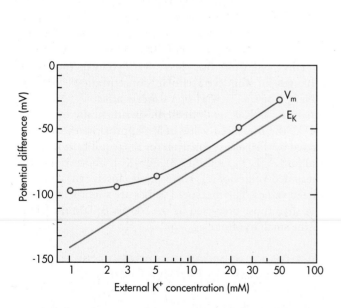

Figure 17-3 The V_m of a cardiac muscle fiber varies inversely with the K^+ concentration of the external medium. The oblique blue line represents the E_K predicted by the Nernst equation.

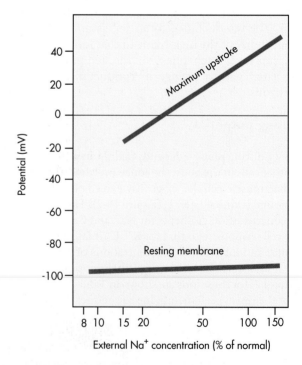

Figure 17-4 The concentration of Na^+ in the external medium is the main determinant of the peak value of the upstroke of the action potential (*upper curve*) in cardiac muscle, but it has little influence on the resting membrane potential (*lower curve*).

tends to repel the influx of Na^+ as the V_m becomes positive. Second, and even more important, the fast Na^+ channels close (i.e., they are **inactivated**) very soon after they open (see Chapter 3). Hence g_{Na} quickly returns to its low preactivation value (Figure 17-5). The Na^+ channels do not recover quickly from inactivation, and hence the cardiac cell remains inexcitable until the cell membrane has almost fully repolarized, as explained later.

The notch depends on K^+

In fast-response cardiac cells, phase 1 is a brief period of limited repolarization that occurs immediately after the action potential upstroke; this limited repolarization may be accompanied by a notch between the action potential upstroke and the plateau. For example, action potentials recorded from myocardial cells in the endocardial regions of the ventricles do not display a notch, whereas those recorded from the epicardial regions display a prominent notch (Figure 17-6). Two mechanisms are responsible for phase 1. When a distinct notch is not evident, phase 1 mainly reflects the initial inactivation of the fast Na^+ channels (Figure 17-5). In cells characterized by a prominent notch, phase 1 reflects not only the inactivation of fast Na^+ channels but also the activation of a specific K^+ current (the so-called **transient outward current [i_{to}]**). These K^+ channels open briefly, and the transient efflux of K^+ produces the notch at the very beginning of the plateau.

The plateau depends on Ca^{++} and K^+

During the plateau (phase 2) of the action potential, V_m is slightly positive, and it remains fairly constant for about 100 to 300 msec, depending on the type of fiber (Figure 17-1, A). The relative constancy of the membrane potential plateau indicates that any efflux of certain cations has been balanced electrically by an influx of other cations. THE PRINCIPAL MOVEMENTS OF CATIONS ACROSS THE CELL MEMBRANE DURING PHASE 2 ARE A NET EFFLUX OF K^+ AND A NET INFLUX OF CA^{++}.

In the resting cell (phase 4), relatively little K^+ leaves the cell because the electrical and chemical forces across the cell membrane are almost balanced (Figure 17-2). During the plateau, however, V_m is positive; therefore both chemical and electrical forces act to expel K^+ from the cell. The efflux of K^+ is minimized, however, because the conductance of the relevant K^+ channels (those that conduct the i_K and i_{K1} currents) is much less when V_m is positive than negative. This dependence of the conductance on the polarity of the cell membrane is referred to as **rectification;** of course, this property accounts for the names of the channels that conduct the relevant K^+ currents. Such a reduction in g_K during the action potential plateau (Figure 17-5) protects the cell from an excessive loss of K^+ during this long phase of the cardiac action potential.

During the plateau, the efflux of K^+ from the cell is balanced electrically by the influx of Ca^{++}, which enters the cell through specific Ca^{++} channels; these are called **L-type Ca^{++} channels** because their activation is long-lasting. These Ca^{++} channels are activated during the upstroke of the action potential when V_m reaches a voltage of about -35 mV. The opening of these channels is reflected by an increased g_{Ca}, which begins shortly after the upstroke of the action potential (Figure 17-5). A substantial amount of Ca^{++} enters the cardiac cell throughout the plateau because (1) g_{Ca} is increased, (2) the Ca^{++} concentration is much less inside than outside the cardiac cell (Table 17-1), and (3) the positive potential (≈ 20 mV) inside the cell during the plateau is much less than the equilibrium potential for Ca^{++} (Table 17-1). THIS INFLUX OF CA^{++} DURING THE PLATEAU IS A CRUCIAL FACTOR IN **EXCITATION-CONTRACTION COUPLING,** as described in Chapters 12 and 18.

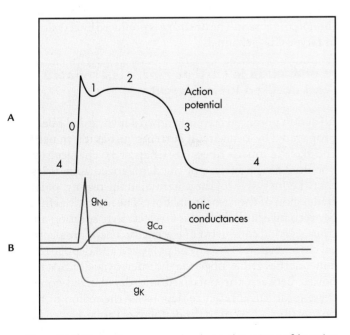

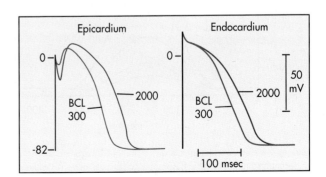

Figure 17-5 Changes in g_{Na}, g_{Ca}, and g_K during phases 0 to 4 of the action potential **(A)** of a fast-response cardiac cell. The conductance diagrams **(B)** are qualitative, not quantitative.

Figure 17-6 Action potentials recorded from myocardial cells in the epicardial and endocardial regions of the left ventricles. The preparations were driven at basic cycle lengths (*BCL*) of 300 and 2000 msec. (*Redrawn from Litovsky SH, Antzelevitch C: J Am Coll Cardiol 14:1053, 1989.*)

Various medications and neurotransmitters may influence the Ca^{++} current in cardiac cells. Increased Ca^{++} influx during the action potential plateau is a crucial step in the mechanism by which circulating or neurally released **catecholamines** (principally **epinephrine** and **norepinephrine**) strengthen myocardial contraction. Conversely, **Ca^{++} channel antagonists,** such as **verapamil, nifedipine,** and **diltiazem,** impede the Ca^{++} current. By reducing the amount of Ca^{++} that enters the myocardial cells, these antagonists weaken the cardiac contraction (Figure 17-7), diminish the firing frequency of SA node cells, and retard conduction in AV nodal fibers. Also, by altering the balance between Ca^{++} influx and K$^+$ efflux, the Ca^{++} channel antagonists diminish the level of V$_m$ during the plateau and abridge the duration of the plateau (Figure 17-7). The Ca^{++} channel antagonists are in wide use clinically in the treatment of **cardiac rhythm disturbances** and **hypertension.**

Repolarization depends on K$^+$

Final repolarization (phase 3) is achieved by a greater efflux than influx of relevant cations across the cardiac cell membrane. This imbalance is achieved by a decrease

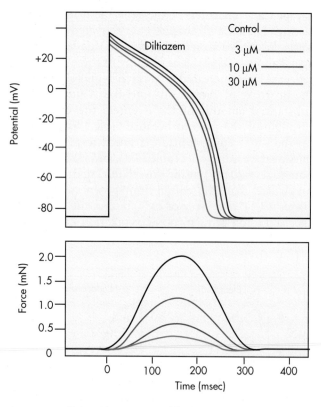

Figure 17-7 Effects of diltiazem, a Ca^{++} channel antagonist, on the action potentials (in millivolts) and isometric contractile forces (in millinewtons) recorded from an isolated papillary muscle of a guinea pig. The tracings were recorded under control conditions *(black line)* and in the presence of diltiazem in concentrations of 3 (M/L *(blue line)*, 10 (M/L *(red line)*, and 30 (M/L *(green line)*. *(Redrawn from Hirth C, Borchard U, Hafner D: J Mol Cell Cardiol 15:799, 1983.)*

in Ca^{++} influx by virtue of a reduction in g$_{Ca}$ and an increase in K$^+$ efflux by virtue of the return of g$_K$ back toward the level that prevails in the resting cell membrane (Figure 17-5). The reduction in g$_{Ca}$ principally reflects the inactivation of the L-type Ca^{++} channels. The increase in g$_K$ is mediated by changes in at least three types of specific K$^+$ channels. An important component of the change in g$_K$ is the K$^+$ channel rectification previously described. As repolarization proceeds and V$_m$ changes progressively from positive to negative, the conductances of the i$_K$ and i$_{K1}$ channels increase substantially because of the rectification. The efflux of K$^+$ during phase 3 rapidly restores the resting level (phase 4) of the membrane potential.

Any alterations in [Na$^+$]$_i$ and [K$^+$]$_o$ produced by the ionic fluxes occurring during the various phases of the action potential are corrected principally by the activity of Na$^+$-K$^+$-ATPase as described in Chapter 2. Similarly, alterations in [Ca^{++}]$_i$ are corrected mainly by the Na$^+$-Ca^{++} exchanger (see also Chapters 2 and 18).

Slow-response action potentials occur in sinoatrial and atrioventricular nodal fibers

Fast-response action potentials (Figure 17-1, *A*) consist of the following components: a spike (a very steep upstroke often accompanied by a notch), a plateau (phase 2), and a repolarization (phase 3). The upstroke is produced by the activation of fast Na$^+$ channels. In contrast, in slow-response fibers (Figure 17-1, *B*), such as those in the SA and AV nodes, the resting membrane potential is much less negative than in fast-response fibers, the upstroke rises much more gradually to the plateau, the plateau is not as prolonged, the action potential amplitude is smaller, and the notch is absent. The upstroke is produced by activation of L-type Ca^{++} channels.

Conduction in Cardiac Fibers Is Mediated by Localized Ionic Currents

An action potential traveling down a myocardial fiber is propagated by local circuit currents, just as it is in nerve and skeletal muscle fibers (see Chapter 3). The electrical potential at the surface of the depolarized zone is less than (i.e., negative to) the potential in the resting, polarized region of the myocardial fiber. The interstitial fluid between myocardial fibers is an electrolyte solution and thus is a good conductor of electricity. Therefore electrical currents flow between the polarized and depolarized zones of the cardiac fibers via the interstitial fluid. At the border between the polarized and depolarized zones, these local currents act to depolarize the region of the resting fiber adjacent to the depolarized zone. Hence THE MARGIN BETWEEN THE DEPOLARIZED AND POLARIZED ZONES MOVES IN THE DIRECTION FROM THE DEPOLARIZED TO THE POLARIZED ZONE. THIS MOVEMENT CONSTITUTES THE PROPAGATION OF THE ACTION POTENTIAL.

In fast-response fibers, the fast Na^+ channels are activated when the transmembrane potential is suddenly brought to the threshold value of about -70 mV. The inward Na^+ current then depolarizes the marginal cells very rapidly, and this repetitive process moves rapidly down the fiber as a wave of depolarization (see Chapter 3). The fast-response conduction velocities are about 0.3 to 1 m/sec for myocardial cells and about 1 to 4 m/sec for the specialized conducting (Purkinje) fibers in the ventricles.

Local circuits also propagate the cardiac impulse in slow-response fibers. However, the characteristics of the conduction process differ from those of the fast response. The threshold potential is about -40 mV for activating the Ca^{++} channels in the resting slow-response fiber. The consequent influx of Ca^{++} depolarizes the stimulated region of the fiber, and the consequent potential difference between the stimulated and resting regions of the fiber excites the adjacent polarized region. This process continues in that the moving depolarized region continuously excites the adjacent resting region of the fiber. However, the conduction is much slower because the kinetics of Ca^{++} influx in slow-response fibers are much slower than the kinetics of Na^+ influx in fast-response fibers. The conduction velocities of the slow responses in the SA and AV nodes are only about 0.02 to 0.1 m/sec.

> Slow-response fibers are more likely to be blocked by certain medications (such as digitalis and Ca^{++} channel antagonists) and by certain pathological processes (such as those induced by an inadequate blood supply) than fast-response fibers. Also, slow-response fibers cannot conduct as many impulses per second as fast-response fibers.
>
> The fast and slow fiber types are affected differentially by certain types of medications. For example, conduction in fast-response fibers is inhibited by Na^+ channel antagonists such as **quinidine, lidocaine,** and **procainamide,** whereas conduction in slow-response fibers is inhibited by Ca^{++} channel antagonists such as **verapamil** and **nifedipine.** Many of the medications used clinically to treat cardiac rhythm disturbances are Na^+ or Ca^{++} channel antagonists.

Cardiac Excitability Varies Throughout the Action Potential

The excitability of a cardiac cell is the ease with which it can be activated. One way to measure the excitability of a cardiac cell is to measure how much electrical current is necessary to induce an action potential. CHANGES IN CARDIAC EXCITABILITY ARE IMPORTANT BECAUSE THEY MAY GENERATE CERTAIN CARDIAC RHYTHM DISTURBANCES AND BECAUSE SUCH CHANGES MUST BE CONSIDERED IN THE DESIGN OF ARTIFICIAL PACEMAKERS AND OTHER ELECTRICAL DEVICES FOR CORRECTING LIFE-THREATENING RHYTHM ABNORMALITIES. The excitability of fast- and slow-response fibers differ substantially.

Fast-response fibers regain their excitability when they repolarize fully

Once a fast-response action potential has been initiated, the depolarized cell will no longer be excitable until the middle of phase 3, the period of final repolarization (Figure 17-1, *A*). The interval from the beginning of the action potential until the time the fiber can conduct another action potential is called the **effective refractory period.** In the fast response, this period extends from the beginning of phase 0 to the time in phase 3 at which V_m has reached about -50 mV (c to d in Figure 17-1, *A*). At this value of V_m, some of the fast Na^+ channels have begun to recover from inactivation.

Full excitability is not regained until the cardiac fiber has been fully repolarized (point e in Figure 17-1, *A*). During period d to e, an action potential may be evoked but only when the stimulus is stronger than that which elicits a response during phase 4. This period is called the **relative refractory period.**

> One of the most common disturbances of cardiac rhythm is an atrial or ventricular depolarization that occurs earlier than expected in the cardiac cycle. Such premature depolarizations happen occasionally in healthy individuals, but they appear more frequently in patients with certain cardiac diseases. When a premature depolarization arises during the relative refractory period of an antecedent excitation, its characteristics vary with the membrane potential that exists at that time, as explained later (Figure 17-8). Depolarizations that appear early in the relative refractory period may lead to more serious disturbances of rhythm, whereas those that appear very late in the relative refractory period or during the resting phase (phase 4) of the cardiac cycle are usually benign.

The dependency of premature depolarization on the prevailing transmembrane potential is illustrated in Figure 17-8. As a myocardial fiber is stimulated later and later in its relative refractory period, the amplitude and rate of rise of the upstroke of the premature action potential progressively increase. These changes develop because the number of fast Na^+ channels that have recovered from inactivation increases as repolarization proceeds during phase 3. Therefore the later in the relative refractory period the premature cardiac impulse appears, the greater its propagation velocity. Once the fiber is fully repolarized, its excitability has been fully restored, and an evoked response is not affected by the time in phase 4 at which the premature depolarization arises.

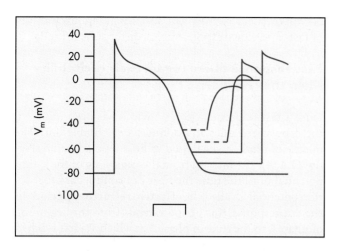

Figure 17-8 Changes in action potential amplitude and slope of the upstroke as premature action potentials are initiated at different stages of the relative refractory period of the preceding excitation in a fast-response fiber. *(Redrawn from Rosen MR, Wit AL, Hoffman BF:* Am Heart J *88:380, 1974.)*

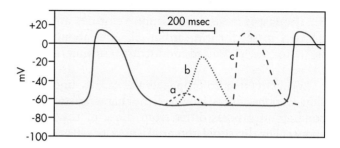

Figure 17-9 Effects of excitation at various times after the initiation of an action potential in a slow-response cardiac fiber. *(Modified from Singer DH et al:* Progr Cardiovasc Dis *24:97, 1981.)*

Slow-response fibers are not fully excitable at the time they achieve full repolarization

THE RELATIVE REFRACTORY PERIOD IN SLOW-RESPONSE FIBERS FREQUENTLY EXTENDS WELL BEYOND THE TIME THAT FULL REPOLARIZATION HAS BEEN RESTORED (Figure 17-1, *B*). This prolonged refractoriness has been termed **postrepolarization refractoriness.** Even after the cell has repolarized completely (phase 4), a relatively strong stimulus may be required to evoke a propagated response. Hence full excitability is achieved much more gradually in a slow- than in a fast-response fiber.

Until excitability is fully restored, the characteristics of the evoked action potentials and the velocity of the propagated impulses vary with the excitability (Figure 17-9). Action potentials that are induced in a slow-response fiber early in the phase of postrepolarization refractoriness (e.g., point a in Figure 17-9) are small and may not be propagated even though the fiber might be fully repolarized. An action potential induced later in this period (e.g., point b in Figure 17-9) would have a greater but still subnormal amplitude and upstroke, it would be propagated very slowly, and perhaps conduction would subsequently fail. Finally, at some time later in the postrepolarization period (e.g., point c in Figure 17-9), the amplitude and upstroke would be normal, and the induced action potential would be conducted at the normal velocity for that slow-response fiber.

Changes in cycle length alter the duration of the action potential

Changes in cycle length alter cardiac cells' duration of action potential and thus their refractory periods. Consequently, THE TIME BETWEEN CONSECUTIVE DEPOLARIZATIONS IS OFTEN AN IMPORTANT FACTOR IN INITIATING OR TERMINATING CERTAIN ARRHYTHMIAS. The magnitude of the change in ac-

tion potential duration evoked by a given change in cycle length varies substantially in different types of cardiac cells. For example, a change in the cycle length from 300 to 2000 msec prolongs the action potential more in a ventricular epicardial cell than in a ventricular endocardial cell (Figure 17-6).

The mechanism responsible for the correlation between action potential duration and cycle length is not fully understood. Changes in g_K that involve two specific types of K^+ channels, namely those that **conduct** i_K and i_{to}, appear to be involved. i_K activates and inactivates very slowly. Thus the shorter the time between consecutive depolarizations, the earlier a given depolarization falls within the inactivation period of the i_K from the preceding depolarization. Hence the persistence of an increased g_K from one depolarization to the next tends to hasten the repolarization of the next depolarization and thereby diminish the duration of its action potential.

The second K^+ current that contributes to the relationship between cycle length and action potential duration is i_{to}. This is the same current that produces the notch in the action potentials of certain types of cardiac cells, notably Purkinje fibers and ventricular epicardial cells (Figure 17-6). A strong correlation exists between the magnitude of i_{to} and the rate dependency of action potential duration in cardiac cells. The greater the efflux of K^+ during the action potential plateau, the shorter the action potential duration.

Natural Excitation of the Heart

The properties of **automaticity** (the ability to initiate a heartbeat) and of **rhythmicity** (the frequency and regularity of such pacemaking activity) are intrinsic to cardiac tissue. THE HEART CONTINUES TO BEAT FOR SOME TIME EVEN WHEN IT IS COMPLETELY REMOVED FROM THE BODY; THEREFORE THE AUTOMATIC BEHAVIOR CAN OCCUR EVEN WHEN THE HEART IS DEVOID OF ANY NEURAL OR HUMORAL REGULATION. If the coronary vessels of a recently excised heart are perfused with an appropriate solution, the heart contracts rhythmically for many hours. At least some cells in each cardiac chamber can initiate beats; such automatic cells reside mainly in the nodal and specialized conducting tissues. The nervous system affects the frequency at which the heart beats and influences other important cardiac functions. A large number of patients who have had cardiac transplants lead relatively normal lives despite the prolonged absence of normal innervation. This finding has irrefutably established that intact nervous pathways are not essential for effective cardiac function.

In the mammalian heart the automatic cells that ordinarily fire at the highest frequency are located in the **SA node;** this structure is the natural pacemaker of the heart. Other regions of the heart that can initiate beats under special circumstances are called **ectopic pacemakers.** Ectopic pacemakers may become dominant when (1) their own rhythmicity is enhanced, (2) the more rhythmic pacemakers are depressed, or (3) all conduction pathways between the ectopic focus and the more rhythmic foci are blocked.

When the SA node is destroyed, automatic cells in the **AV node** usually have the next highest level of rhythmicity, and they become the pacemakers for the entire heart. After some time, which may vary from minutes to days, automatic cells in the atria usually then become dominant. **Purkinje fibers** in the specialized conduction system of the ventricles are also automatic. Characteristically, these **idioventricular pacemakers** fire at a very slow rate ($\approx$35 beats/min). Ordinarily, they do not fire at all because impulses that originate in the SA node depolarize the Purkinje fibers at a frequency that is much greater than their intrinsic frequency. Thus the automaticity of the Purkinje fibers is inhibited by the process of **overdrive suppression,** which is explained later.

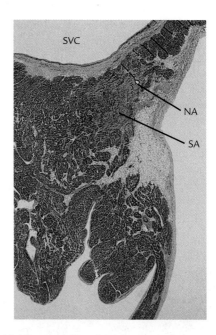

Figure 17-10 Micrograph from the right atrium of a human. *NA,* Nodal artery; *SA,* sinoatrial node; *SVC,* superior vena cava. *(From Stevens A, Lowe J: Human histology, St Louis, 1997, Mosby.)*

The sinoatrial node is the natural pacemaker of the heart

The SA node is the phylogenic remnant of the sinus venosus of lower vertebrate hearts. In humans it is about 15 mm long, 5 mm wide, and 2 mm thick. It lies in the terminal sulcus on the posterior aspect of the heart, at the junction of the superior vena cava and the right atrium (Figures 17-10 and 17-11).

Typical transmembrane action potentials recorded from an SA node cell are depicted in Figure 17-12. In general, the action potentials are characteristic of the slow response, as shown in Figure 17-1, *B*. The principal distinguishing feature of an automatic fiber in the SA node (as in all automatic fibers) resides in phase 4. Whereas the transmembrane potential remains constant during phase 4 in nonautomatic cells, AN AUTOMATIC FIBER IN THE HEART DISPLAYS A GRADUAL **DIASTOLIC DEPOLARIZATION** (ALSO CALLED THE PACEMAKER POTENTIAL) DURING PHASE 4 (Figure 17-12). Diastolic depolarization (phase 4) proceeds at a steady rate until the threshold for firing is attained, and then an action potential is triggered (phase 0).

The firing frequency of an automatic cell is varied by changing the slope of the slow diastolic depolarization (Figure 17-12, *A*), the maximum negativity during phase 4 (Figure 17-12, *B*), or the value of the triggering threshold (Figure 17-12, *C*). When the slope of the diastolic depolarization is decreased, more time is required for the transmembrane potential to reach threshold (Figure 17-12, *A*), so the firing frequency diminishes. Similarly, if a more negative transmembrane potential is achieved at the beginning of phase 4 (i.e., if the membrane becomes **hyperpolarized**), more time is required for the slow dia-

Various processes may interfere temporarily or permanently with the conduction of the cardiac impulse from atria to ventricles. Such processes include intense neural activity in the vagus nerves, the action of certain medications (such as **digitalis, adenosine,** and **Ca^{++} channel antagonists**), and certain pathological processes (such as **coronary artery occlusion** and **degeneration of the cardiac conducting fibers**). When the AV junction fails to conduct the cardiac impulse from the atria to the ventricles, the Purkinje fibers in the ventricles serve as idioventricular pacemakers that initiate ventricular contractions. However, they ordinarily generate impulses at such a low frequency that the heart cannot pump enough blood to support normal body function. Implantation of an artificial pacemaker may then be required to correct this deficiency.

stolic depolarization to reach threshold (Figure 17-12, *B*), so the firing frequency diminishes. Finally, if the firing threshold is increased, more time is required to attain the threshold value (Figure 17-12, *C*), so firing frequency diminishes. Of course, any combination of these three mechanisms can determine the firing frequency.

Automaticity depends on the flux of K⁺, Na⁺, and Ca⁺⁺

Several ionic currents contribute to the slow diastolic depolarization that characterizes automatic cardiac cells. In the SA node, diastolic depolarization is implemented by changes in at least three ionic currents: an inward "funny" current (i_f), an inward Ca^{++} cur-

rent (i_{Ca}), and an outward K^+ current (i_K) (Figure 17-13).

i_f is carried mainly by Na^+. This *funny current* was so named because its presence was contrary to the hypothesis of the investigators who named it. It is activated as the membrane potential becomes more negative than about -50 mV during repolarization (phase 3). The more negative the membrane potential at the end of repolarization, the greater the magnitude of i_f.

i_{Ca} is activated toward the end of phase 4, as the transmembrane potential becomes about -55 mV (Figure 17-13, *B*). The influx of Ca^{++} accelerates depolarization, which quickly leads to the upstroke of the action potential. A decrease in $[K^+]_o$ or the addition of a Ca^{++} channel antagonist (e.g., nifedipine) diminishes the amplitude of the action potential and the slope of the slow diastolic depolarization in the cells of the SA node.

Slow diastolic depolarization is mediated by the two inward currents i_f and i_{Ca} through well-characterized ion channels (Figure 17-13, *B*) and by a continuous inward "leak" of Na^+ through nonselective channels (not shown in Figure 17-13, *B*). The slow diastolic depolarization is opposed by a third, outward current, i_K. This current is activated during the action potential plateau, and it slowly inactivates during repolarization and throughout phase 4 (Figure 17-13, *B*). The efflux of K^+ tends to oppose the depolarizing effects of i_f and i_{Ca} and the inward leak of Na^+. However, the outward current i_K decays steadily throughout phase 4 (Figure 17-13, *B*) because of its gradual inactivation. Hence its opposition to the depolarizing effects of the inward currents of the other cations gradually diminishes. The diminishing opposition of the outward i_K to the depolarizing effects of the various inward currents thus contributes to the slow diastolic depolarization.

The ionic basis for automaticity in the AV node pacemaker cells is identical to that in the SA node cells. Similar ionic fluxes probably also account for automaticity in Purkinje fibers, except that the Ca^{++} current does not contribute appreciably to the slow diastolic depolarization or the action potential upstroke. Hence the slow diastolic depolarization in Purkinje fi-

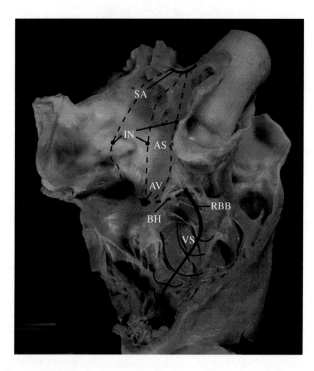

Figure 17-11 Conducting system of the human heart, trimmed to expose the right sides of the atrial septum *(AS)* and ventricular septum *(VS)*. *AV,* Atrioventricular bundle; *BH,* bundle of His; *IN,* internodal atrial muscle; *RBB,* right bundle branch; *SA,* sinoatrial node. *(From Stevens A, Lowe J: Human histology, St Louis, 1997, Mosby.)*

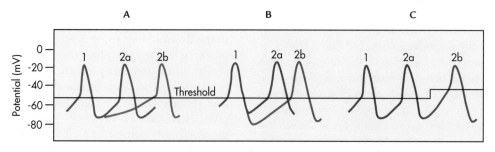

Figure 17-12 Effects of changes in the slope of the pacemaker potential **(A),** in the maximal diastolic potential **(B),** and in the firing threshold **(C)** on the cardiac cycle length of an SA nodal cell. In each panel the basic cycle length is equal to the times between action potentials 1 and 2a. The effects (a) of a reduction in the slope of slow diastolic depolarization are denoted by the time between action potentials 1 and 2b in **A;** (b) of hyperpolarization at the beginning of slow diastolic depolarization are denoted by the time between action potentials 1 and 2b in **B;** and (c) of an increase in the threshold for depolarization are denoted by the time between action potentials 2a and 2b in **C.**

bers is mediated principally by the balance among the hyperpolarization-induced inward current i_f, the inward leak of Na^+, and the gradually diminishing i_K.

The autonomic nerves regulate the heart rate

Neurotransmitters released by the autonomic nerves affect automaticity by altering the ionic currents across the pacemaker cell membranes. Through the release of **norepinephrine,** increased sympathetic nervous activity raises the heart rate by increasing the slope of slow diastolic depolarization. This increase is achieved mainly by augmenting i_f and i_{Ca} (Figure 17-13, B) in the membranes of the SA node cells.

Through the release of **acetylcholine,** increased parasympathetic activity diminishes the heart rate by reducing the slope (Figure 17-12, A) and by increasing the maximum negativity (Figure 17-12, B) of slow diastolic depolarization. The increase in maximum negativity is accomplished by the interaction of acetylcholine with **cholinergic receptors (muscarinic type)** that activate specific **acetylcholine-regulated K^+ channels** in the membranes of the automatic cells. The diminution in the slope of slow diastolic depolarization is achieved by a reduction in the ionic currents through the i_f and i_{Ca} channels. Changes in the firing threshold

(Figure 17-12, C) occur in response to certain medications and to changes in the ionic composition of the myocardial interstitial fluid.

Overdrive suppresses pacemaker cell automaticity

The automaticity of pacemaker cells is suppressed temporarily after they have been driven at a critically high frequency. This phenomenon is known as **overdrive suppression.** Because the SA node cells usually fire at a greater frequency than the automatic cells in the other latent pacemaking sites in the heart, the firing of the SA node cells at their greater frequency tends to suppress the automaticity in the other **(ectopic)** sites.

In certain disturbances, such as the **sick sinus syndrome,** the SA node cells periodically cease firing for many seconds. Although automatic cells are abundant in various ectopic sites in the heart, such cells often do not immediately become functional pacemakers. These ectopic pacemakers are temporarily suppressed because the cells in the normal pacemaking site, the SA node, normally fire at a much greater rate than the ectopic pacemaker cells. Such rapid firing delays the firing of the ectopic pacemaker cells by the phenomenon of overdrive suppression. Hence if the pacemaker activity of the ectopic cells is delayed for more than a few seconds, the subject might lose consciousness because of the virtual cessation of cerebral blood flow.

The mechanism responsible for overdrive suppression involves the membrane pump (Na^+-K^+-ATPase) that actively extrudes Na^+ from the cell in partial exchange for K^+; the ratio is $3\,Na^+$ to $2\,K^+$ (see Chapter 1). During each depolarization of an automatic Purkinje fiber, for example, a certain amount of Na^+ enters the cell during phase 0 of the action potential. Therefore the more frequently the cell is depolarized, the greater the amount of Na^+ that enters the cell per minute. During the overdrive, Na^+-K^+-ATPase expends more energy to extrude this larger quantity of Na^+ from the cell interior. The quantity of Na^+ extruded by Na^+-K^+-ATPase exceeds the quantity of K^+ that enters the cell. This enhanced activity of the pump hyperpolarizes the cell membrane because there is a net loss of cations from the cell interior. Hence the pump is said to be **electrogenic.** As a result of hyperpolarization, the transmembrane potential during phase 4 requires more time to reach threshold (Figure 17-12, B). Furthermore, when the overdrive suddenly ceases, the activity of Na^+-K^+-ATPase usually does not diminish instantaneously but remains overactive for some time. The consequent excessive extrusion of Na^+ retards the gradual depolarization of the pacemaker cell during phase 4 and thereby temporarily suppresses its automaticity.

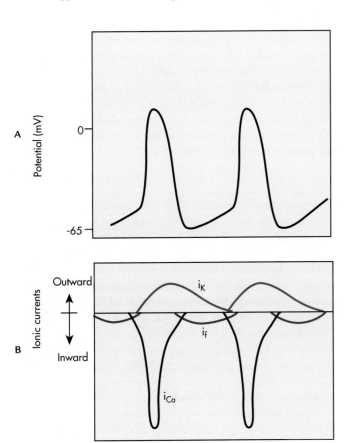

Figure 17-13 The transmembrane potential changes **(A)** that occur in SA node cells are produced by the following currents **(B):** i_{Ca} *(black),* i_f *(red),* and i_K *(blue). (Redrawn from Brown HF: Physiol Rev 61:644, 1981.)*

Atrial myocytes conduct the cardiac impulse from the sinoatrial to the atrioventricular node

From the SA node, the cardiac impulse spreads radially throughout the right atrium (Figure 17-11) along ordinary atrial myocardial fibers at a conduction velocity of approximately 1 m/sec. A special pathway, the **anterior interatrial band** (or **Bachmann's bundle**), conducts the impulse most directly from the SA node to the left atrium. However, even if this direct pathway is destroyed experimentally, conduction proceeds expeditiously from the right to the left atrium along ordinary myocardial fibers. Some of the action potentials that proceed inferiorly through the right atrium ultimately reach the AV node (Figures 17-11 and 17-14), which is normally the sole source of entry of the cardiac impulse from the atria to the ventricles.

Atrioventricular conduction

The AV node in adult humans is approximately 22 mm long, 10 mm wide, and 3 mm thick. It is situated posteriorly, on the right side of the interatrial septum near the ostium of the coronary sinus (Figure 17-11). The AV node is divided into the following functional regions: (1) the **A-N region,** which is the transitional zone between the atrium and the remainder of the node; (2) the **N region,** which is the midportion of the AV node; and (3) the **N-H region,** in which the nodal fibers gradually merge with the **bundle of His,** which is the beginning of the **specialized conducting system** for the ventricles.

Several features of AV conduction are physiologically and clinically significant. The principal delay in the passage of impulses from the atrial to the ventricular myocardial cells occurs in the A-N region of the node. The conduction velocity is actually less in the N region than in the A-N region, but the path length is substantially greater in the A-N than in the N region.

Conduction times through the A-N and N zones account for a considerable fraction of the **PR interval,** which signifies the delay between atrial and ventricular excitation in the electrocardiogram (see Figure 17-17). Functionally, this delay permits atrial contraction to contribute optimally to ventricular filling.

CELLS IN THE N REGION ARE CHARACTERIZED BY SLOW-RESPONSE ACTION POTENTIALS. The V_m is about -60 mV, the upstroke is not very steep, and the conduction velocity is about 0.05 m/sec. Tetrodotoxin, which blocks the fast Na^+ channels, has almost no effect on the action potentials in this region. Conversely, diltiazem, a Ca^{++} channel antagonist, decreases the amplitude and duration of action potentials and retards AV conduction. The action potentials of cells in the A-N region are intermediate in shape between those of cells in the N region and the atria. Similarly, the action potentials of cells in the N-H region are transitional between those of cells in the N region and those in the bundle of His. The entire conduction system between atria and ventricles, including the various transitional zones, is often referred to as the **AV junction.**

Cells in the N region display postrepolarization refractoriness (Figure 17-9). As the time between successive atrial depolarizations is decreased, the conduction time through the AV junction becomes prolonged. For example, when the atria are paced electrically in a group of humans, the conduction time (AH interval) from the atria to the bundle of His increases progressively as the interval between pacing stimuli decreases (Figure 17-15).

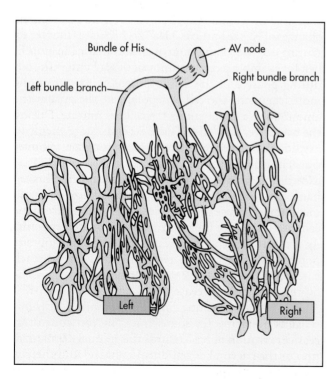

Figure 17-14 AV and ventricular conduction system of the calf heart.

Impulses tend to be blocked in the AV junction at cardiac cycle lengths that are easily accommodated in other regions of the heart. This often has a beneficial effect in certain clinical rhythm disturbances. For example, in **atrial tachycardia** (an abnormally fast heart rate that originates in the atria), the atria might be depolarized at a frequency of about 200 times per minute. Under such circumstances, some of the atrial impulses are usually blocked in the AV node. For example, if only alternate atrial impulses were conducted through the AV node, the ventricles would be depolarized only 100 times per minute. This AV nodal conduction pattern, which is referred to as **2:1 AV block,** tends to protect the ventricles from excessively high contraction frequencies. At frequencies as high as 200 times per minute, the time available for ventricular filling between contractions would be inadequate; therefore the heart would be unable to pump a sufficient volume of blood per minute (see Chapter 24). Thus when the atria contract at an abnormally rapid rate, the ventricles can pump more blood per minute when some of the atrial depolarizations are blocked in the AV junction than when all the atrial impulses can excite the ventricles. When the ventricles respond at too high a frequency, the physician usually attempts to reduce the number of atrial impulses conducted to the ventricles. The physician may attempt to block AV conduction partially by increasing vagal activity reflexly or by administering certain inhibitory medications (e.g., **adenosine, digitalis**).

The autonomic nerves regulate atrioventricular conduction

The vagus nerves release acetylcholine, which prolongs AV conduction. Moderate vagal activity may simply prolong AV conduction time. In a study on how the length of atrial pacing cycle affects AV conduction time (Figure 17-15), vagal activity to the heart was increased reflexly in human subjects by infusing **phenylephrine** (an adrenergic vasoconstrictor medication) to raise arterial blood pressure. For any given length of pacing cycle, the atrial to bundle of His (AH) conduction time was greater when vagal activity was increased than under control conditions. More intense vagal activity (not shown in Figure 17-15) could prevent the conduction of some of the atrial impulses through the AV node to the ventricles. The delayed conduction or conduction failure occurs largely in the N region.

The cardiac sympathetic nerves, on the other hand, facilitate AV conduction. They decrease the AV conduction time and enhance the rhythmicity of the latent pacemakers in the AV junction. The norepinephrine released at the sympathetic nerve terminals increases the amplitude and slope of the upstroke of the AV nodal action potentials, principally in the N region.

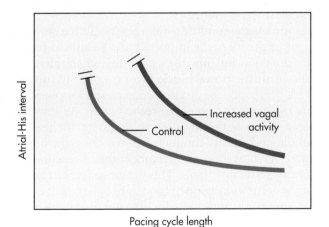

Figure 17-15 Changes in atrial-His intervals induced by pacing the atria at various cycle lengths in a group of eight humans under control conditions *(blue)* and during increased vagal activity *(red)* produced by intravenous infusions of phenylephrine. *(Redrawn from Page RL et al:* Circ Res *68:1614, 1991.)*

Conduction is rapid in ventricular tissue

The bundle of His is the beginning of the **specialized conduction system** for the ventricles (Figures 17-11 and 17-14). It passes subendocardially down the right side of the interventricular septum for approximately 12 mm and then divides into the right and left **bundle branches.** The right bundle branch, a direct continuation of the bundle of His, proceeds down the right side of the interventricular septum. The left bundle branch is considerably thicker than the right. It arises almost perpendicularly from the bundle of His and perforates the interventricular septum.

The bundle branches ultimately subdivide into a complex network of conducting fibers, called **Purkinje fibers,** which ramify over the subendocardial surfaces of both ventricles (Figure 17-14). Purkinje fibers are the broadest cells in the heart, 70 to 80 μm in diameter, compared with 10 to 15 μm for ventricular myocardial cells. The larger diameter of the Purkinje fibers accounts in part for their greater conduction velocity than that of myocardial fibers. The conduction velocity of the cardiac impulse over the Purkinje fiber system is the fastest of any tissue within the heart; estimates vary from 1 to 4 m/sec. This permits rapid activation of the entire endocardial surface of the ventricles. The wave of excitation spreads from the endocardium to the epicardium more slowly, about 0.3 to 0.4 m/sec.

The action potentials recorded from Purkinje fibers differ slightly from those obtained from ordinary ventricular myocardial fibers. In general, Purkinje fiber action potentials have a prominent notch (phase 1), and the duration of the plateau (phase 2) is substantially longer in Purkinje fibers. The prolonged plateau in the Purkinje fibers confers a long refractory period in these cells. Hence many premature atrial depolarizations may be conducted through the AV junction only to be blocked by the Purkinje fibers. This function of protecting the ventricles against the effects of premature atrial depolarizations is especially pronounced when the cardiac cycle length is prolonged because the duration of the action potential and hence the effective refractory period of the Purkinje fibers vary directly with the cycle length, just as they do in ventricular myocytes (Figure 17-6). However, in the AV node, the effective refractory period does not change appreciably over the normal range of heart rates, but it actually increases when the heart beats at very short cycle lengths. Therefore when the cycle lengths are very short, it is the AV node, rather than the Purkinje fibers, that protects the ventricles from excitation at excessive contraction frequencies.

Reentry Is the Basis of Many Rhythm Disturbances

Under appropriate conditions, a cardiac impulse may reexcite some region through which the impulse had previously passed. This reexcitation phenomenon, known as **reentry,** is responsible for many clinical disturbances of cardiac rhythm. When a reentrant circuit is fixed anatomically, the repetitive circling of the reentrant loop can lead to sudden, sustained tachycardias (such as **paroxysmal supraventricular** or **ventricular tachycardias**). However, if the reentry consists of multiple, highly irregular, continuously moving reentrant circuits, the consequent rhythm disturbances are **atrial** or **ventricular fibrillation.** Although patients can survive with atrial fibrillation for many years, proper treatment is important because the cardiac rhythm is highly irregular, patients are susceptible to the formation of blood clots in the atria, and the condition may lead to cerebral strokes and other serious consequences. Ventricular fibrillation is a rapidly lethal phenomenon because the ventricles immediately cease pumping blood. Immediate **defibrillation** by electrical countershock is essential to prevent death.

Figure 17-16 depicts a potential reentry loop that consists of a single bundle of cardiac fibers that splits into left and right branches. A connecting bundle runs between these branches. When all components of this reentry loop conduct normally (Figure 17-16, *A*), the descending impulse in the single bundle is conducted down the left and right branches. As the impulse reaches the connecting branch, it enters the branch from both sides and becomes extinguished at the point of collision. The impulse from the left branch cannot proceed beyond the point of collision in the connecting branch because the tissue distal to this point is refractory; it had just been depolarized from the other direction. Similarly, the impulse from the right branch cannot pass leftward through the point of collision in the connecting branch because the tissue to the left of the point of collision had just been depolarized. It is obvious from Figure 17-12, *B*, that the impulse cannot make a complete circuit if an antegrade block exists in the two branches of the fiber bundle.

If **bidirectional block,** the inability of a bundle of myocardium to conduct an impulse that arrives from either direction, exists at any point in the loop (e.g., in the right branch), reentry does not occur (Figure 17-16, *C*). To illustrate, the impulse originating in the single bundle can enter the left and right branches, as previously described. The impulse that enters the right branch from above is stopped in that branch as soon as it reaches the block. The impulse that travels down the left branch continues down that branch, but it also travels rightward in the connecting branch, When this impulse reaches the right branch, it travels upward and downward in this branch. The upwardly directed impulse soon arrives at the region of bidirectional block, where conduction is terminated. Therefore the impulse that originates in the single branch is unable to travel around a complete loop and thereby reenter the single branch regardless of the path that the impulse follows. Such a bidirectional block might be the consequence of severe ischemia (inadequate

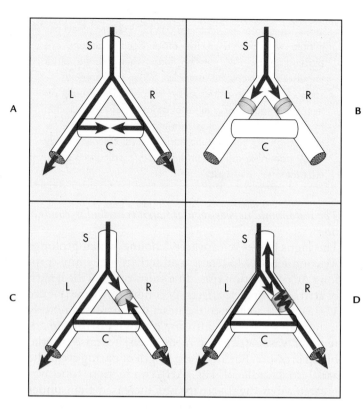

Figure 17-16 Role of unidirectional block in reentry. **A,** An excitation wave travels down a single bundle *(S)* of fibers and continues down the left *(L)* and right *(R)* branches. The depolarization wave enters the connecting branch *(C)* from both ends and is extinguished at the zone of collision. **B,** The wave is blocked in the *L* and *R* branches. **C,** The antegrade and retrograde impulses in branch *R* are both blocked. **D,** Unidirectional block exists in branch *R*. The antegrade impulse that travels downward from *S* to *R* cannot be conducted antegrade because the region of unidirectional block has not regained its excitability. The retrograde impulse in *R* arrives at this region later, after excitability has been regained.

blood circulation) to some region of tissue within the potential reentry loop.

A necessary condition for reentry is that at some point in the loop, the impulse must be able to pass in one direction but not the other; this phenomenon is called **unidirectional block.** Most commonly, this type of block is produced by a prolonged refractory period in one region of the potential reentry loop. As shown in Figure 17-16, *D*, the impulse that originates in the single bundle and that is conducted down the right branch travels a relatively short distance before it reaches temporarily refractory tissue. This prolonged refractoriness might occur in a region of moderate ischemia. It causes the antegrade impulse, which passes from the single bundle directly to the right segment, to be stopped in the region of unidirectional block.

In contrast, the impulse that had originated in the single bundle is also conducted down the left branch, through the connecting branch, and finally up and down the right branch (Figure 17-16, *D*). The impulse that travels upward in this branch may be able to be conducted retrogradely through the previously depressed region. The conduction path from the single bundle to the left branch to the connecting branch and then upward in the right branch to the region of potential block is much longer than the conduction path directly from the single bundle to the right branch. This longer conduction path might allow the previously refractory tissue to recover its excitability and might thereby permit retrograde conduction through the upper region of the right branch and thereby reenter and reexcite the single bundle.

Therefore in this example, unidirectional block is a temporal phenomenon. The antegrade impulse in the right branch travels only a short distance and arrives at the partially depressed region while it is still refractory; therefore the impulse is blocked. The same impulse that originated in the single bundle but that traveled the much longer path through the left and connecting branches and the lower region of the right branch is more likely to be conducted through the region of potential block than the impulse that traveled the shorter, more direct path. The longer conduction path allows more time for the partially depressed region to recover its excitability.

UNIDIRECTIONAL BLOCK IS A NECESSARY, BUT NOT A SUFFICIENT, CONDITION FOR REENTRY. THE EFFECTIVE REFRACTORY PERIOD OF THE REENTERED REGION MUST ALSO BE LESS THAN THE PROPAGATION TIME AROUND THE LOOP. In Figure 17-16, *D,* the retrograde impulse is conducted through the depressed zone in the right branch and if the tissue just beyond is still refractory from the initial antegrade depolarization, the single bundle is not reexcited. Therefore THE CONDITIONS THAT PROMOTE REENTRY ARE THOSE THAT PROLONG THE CONDUCTION TIME OR SHORTEN THE EFFECTIVE REFRACTORY PERIOD SUFFICIENTLY.

The **Wolff-Parkinson-White** syndrome is a common cause of reentrant rhythm disturbances in humans. In patients with this syndrome, an extraneous **bypass tract** parallels the normal AV junction structures (AV node and bundle of His), and it thereby constitutes a secondary conduction pathway between the atria and ventricles. The cardiac fibers that constitute the bypass tract are ordinary myocardial fast-response fibers, whereas the critical conduction fibers in the AV node are slow-response fibers. Usually, a patient with this syndrome is unaware of any functional problems because the natural atrial impulses traverse the normal and bypass pathways to the ventricles concomitantly (although conduction is faster in the bypass than in the nodal pathway). At times, however, the atrial impulse may travel to the ventricles exclusively via one of the parallel pathways (usually the normal AV junction route), and the impulse may then travel retrogradely via the secondary pathway (usually the bypass tract) to reex-

cite the atria. The impulse may then continue to travel around this reentry loop for minutes or hours; one conduction pathway mediates antegrade conduction, and the other mediates the retrograde conduction. Conduction time around the reentry loop is usually much less than the duration of a normal cardiac cycle. Hence the heart beats at an excessively fast rate. Such a rapid rate diminishes the ability of the heart to propel a normal cardiac output. Interruption of the reentry loop may be achieved by giving medication (e.g., adenosine, Ca^{++} channel blocker) that suppresses conduction through the normal AV node pathway (which mainly includes slow-response fibers) but does not impair conduction through the bypass tract (which comprises only fast-response fibers). If the presence of a bypass tract is very troublesome to the patient, the cardiologist can destroy the tract by applying a high-intensity electrical current directly to it via an electrode catheter.

Electrocardiography Is an Important Clinical Tool

The **electrocardiograph** is a valuable instrument because it enables the physician to record the variations in electrical potential at various loci on the body surface and thereby to derive vital information about the propagation of the cardiac impulse. By analyzing the details of these fluctuations, the physician gains valuable insight concerning (1) the anatomical orientation of the heart; (2) the relative sizes of its chambers; (3) various disturbances of rhythm and conduction; (4) the extent, location, and progress of ischemic injury to the myocardium; (5) the effects of altered electrolyte concentrations; and (6) the influence of certain medications on the heart. The science of electrocardiography is extensive and complex, but only the elementary features of the electrocardiogram are presented here.

The electrocardiogram reflects the temporal changes in the electrical potential between pairs of points on the skin surface. The cardiac impulse progresses through the heart in a complex three-dimensional pattern. Hence the precise configuration of the electrocardiogram varies from person to person, and in any given individual the pattern varies with the anatomical location of the recording electrodes.

In general, the pattern consists of **P, QRS,** and **T** waves (Figure 17-17). The **PR interval** is the time from the beginning of atrial activation to the beginning of ventricular activation; it normally ranges from 0.12 to 0.20 second. Most of this conduction time involves the passage of the impulse through the AV conduction system. PATHOLOGICAL PROLONGATIONS OF THE PR INTERVAL ARE ASSOCIATED WITH AV CONDUCTION DISTURBANCES PRODUCED BY INFLAMMATORY, CIRCULATORY, PHARMACOLOGICAL, OR NERVOUS MECHANISMS.

The configuration and amplitude of the **QRS com-**

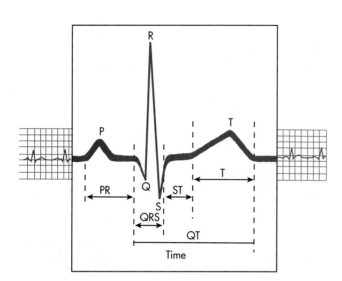

Figure 17-17 Important deflections and intervals of a typical electrocardiogram.

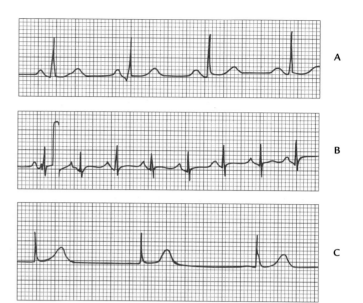

Figure 17-18 Electrocardiograms recorded from humans with various SA rhythms. **A,** Normal sinus rhythm. **B,** Sinus tachycardia. **C,** Sinus bradycardia.

plex vary considerably among individuals. The duration is usually between 0.06 and 0.10 second. ABNORMAL PROLONGATION OF THE QRS COMPLEX MAY INDICATE A BLOCK IN THE NORMAL CONDUCTION PATHWAYS THROUGH THE VENTRICLES (SUCH AS A BLOCK OF THE LEFT OR RIGHT BUNDLE BRANCH).

The **QT interval** is sometimes referred to as the period of **electrical systole** of the ventricles; it reflects the action potential duration of the ventricular myocardial cells. The duration of the QT interval is about 0.4 second, but it varies inversely with the heart rate, mainly because the action potential duration varies inversely with the heart rate (Figure 17-6).

During the **ST interval,** the entire ventricular myocardium is depolarized. Because all of the myocardial cells are at about the same electrical potential, the ST segment lies on the **isoelectric line** (which is the line that reflects that virtually all regions of the cardiac surface are at the same electrical potential).

The **T wave** reflects the repolarization of the ventricular myocardial cells. The T wave is usually deflected in the same direction from the isoelectric line as is the major component of the QRS complex. Deviation of the T wave and QRS complex in the same direction from the isoelectric line indicates that the propagation of repolarization does not follow the same route as the propagation of depolarization. Normally, depolarization proceeds from the endocardium to the epicardium, whereas repolarization proceeds in the opposite direction. The reason for this difference in the direction of propagation is related to disparities in the duration of the action potentials generated in the endocardial and epicardial regions of the ventricles. Endocardial cells are depolarized earlier than epicardial cells because the specialized conduction fibers lie in the ventricular endocar-

dium. However, epicardial cells usually begin to repolarize earlier than endocardial cells because the duration of the epicardial action potentials is shorter than that of the endocardial cells, especially when the heart beats at normal or short cardiac cycle lengths (Figure 17-6).

Electrocardiographic tracings of a normal sinus rhythm, sinus tachycardia, and sinus bradycardia are shown in Figure 17-18. These tracings show the sequence of P, QRS, and T waves that were recorded in normal individuals with different heart rates. A longer tracing of a vagally induced bradycardia in a paraplegic patient is shown in Figure 19-9.

SUMMARY

- The transmembrane action potentials recorded from cardiac myocytes consist of the following phases:

Phase 0 (upstroke)	Activation of fast Na^+ channels
Phase 1 (early partial repolarization)	Efflux of K^+ through i_{to} channels
Phase 2 (plateau)	Balance between influx of Ca^{++} through L-type Ca^{++} channels and efflux of K^+ through several types of K^+ channels
Phase 3 (final repolarization)	Inactivation of the Ca^{++} channels and increased conductance of several types of K^+ channels
Phase 4 (V_m)	Determination made mainly by the membrane g_K

- Fast-response action potentials are recorded from atrial and ventricular myocardial fibers and from specialized conducting (Purkinje) fibers. These action potentials have a steep upstroke and large amplitude. The upstroke is achieved by the activation of fast Na^+ channels. The effective refractory period extends from upstroke to midway through phase 3, and the relatively refractory extends to the end of the phase.

- Slow-response action potentials are recorded from SA and AV nodal cells. The V_m is less negative, the amplitude is smaller, and the upstroke is less steep than in a fast-response action potential. The upstroke is produced by the activation of Ca^{++} channels. The effective refractory period extends from the beginning of the upstroke until near the end of and sometimes beyond the end of phase 3. Full excitability is not regained until after the fiber is fully repolarized.

- Automaticity is characteristic of certain cells in the SA and AV nodes and in the specialized conducting system, and it is achieved by a slow depolarization of the membrane during phase 4.

- Normally, the SA node initiates the impulse that induces cardiac contraction. This impulse is propagated from the SA node to the atria, and the wave of excitation ultimately reaches the AV node.

- The cardiac impulse travels very slowly through the slow-response fibers in the AV node. The consequent delay between atrial and ventricular depolarization provides adequate time for atrial contraction to help fill the ventricles.

- Ectopic automatic cells in the atrium, AV node, or His-Purkinje system may initiate propagated cardiac impulses either because the normal pacemaker cells in the SA node are suppressed or the firing rate of the ectopic focus is abnormally enhanced.

- Propagation of a cardiac impulse may fail as the result of certain disease processes (e.g., ischemia, inflammation) or medications (e.g., Na^+ or Ca^{++} channel antagonists).

- A cardiac impulse may traverse a loop of cardiac fibers and reenter previously excited tissue when the impulse is conducted slowly enough around the loop and the impulse is blocked unidirectionally in some section of the loop.

- The electrocardiogram is recorded from the surface of the body, and it traces the conduction of the cardiac impulse through the heart.

- The component waves of the electrocardiogram are as follows:

P wave	Spread of excitation over the atria
QRS interval	Spread of excitation over the ventricles
T wave	Spread of repolarization over the ventricles

BIBLIOGRAPHY

Armour JA, Ardell JL: *Neurocardiology,* New York, 1994, Oxford University Press.

Armstrong CM: Voltage-dependent ion channels and their gating, *Physiol Rev* 72:S5, 1992.

Delmar M: Role of potassium currents on cell excitability in cardiac ventricular myocytes, *J Cardiovasc Electrophys* 3:474, 1992.

DiFrancesco D, Zaza A: The cardiac pacemaker current i_f, *J Cardiovasc Electrophys* 3:334, 1992.

Irisawa H, Brown HF, Giles W: Cardiac pacemaking in the sino-atrial node, *Physiol Rev* 73:197, 1993.

Levy MN, Schwartz PJ: *Vagal control of the heart: experimental basis and clinical implications,* Mt Kisco, NY, 1994, Futura.

Levy MN, Yang T, Wallick DW: Assessment of beat-by-beat control of heart rate by the autonomic nervous system: molecular biology techniques are necessary, but not sufficient, *J Cardiovasc Electrophysiol* 4:183, 1993.

Liu D-W, Gintant GA, Antzelevitch C: Ionic bases for electrophysiological distinctions among epicardial, midmyocardial, and endocardial myocytes from the free wall of the canine left ventricle, *Circ Res* 72:671, 1993.

Mazgalev T, Dreifus LS, Michelson EL: *Electrophysiology of the sino-atrial and atrioventricular nodes,* New York, 1988, Alan R Liss.

Pallotta BS, Wagoner PK: Voltage-dependent potassium channels since Hodgkin and Huxley, *Physiol Rev* 72:S49, 1992.

Rosen MR, Janse MJ, Wit AL: *Cardiac electrophysiology: a textbook,* Mt Kisco, NY, 1990, Futura.

Sicoura S, Antzelevitch C: Electrophysiological characteristics of M cells in the canine left ventricular free wall, *J Cardiovasc Electrophysiol* 6:591, 1995.

Spach MS, Josephson ME: Initiating reentry: role of nonuniform anisotropy in small circuits, *J Cardiovasc Electrophysiol* 5:182, 1994.

Sperelakis N: *Physiology and pathophysiology of the heart,* ed 3, Boston, 1995, Kluwer Academic.

Zipes DP, Jalife J: *Cardiac electrophysiology: from cell to bedside,* ed 2, Philadelphia, 1995, WB Saunders.

CASE STUDY

Case 17-1

A 63-year-old man suddenly felt a crushing pain beneath his sternum. He became weak, began to sweat profusely, and noticed that his heart was beating rapidly. He called his physician, who made the diagnosis of myocardial infarction. The tests made at the hospital confirmed his physician's suspicion that the patient had suffered a "heart attack"; that is, a major coronary artery to the left ventricle had suddenly become occluded. An electrocardiogram indicated that the SA node was the source of the rapid heart rate. Two hours after admission to the hospital, the patient suddenly became much weaker. His arterial pulse rate was only about 40 beats/min. An electrocardiogram at this time revealed that the atrial rate was about 90 beats/min and that conduction through the AV junction was completely blocked, undoubtedly because the infarct affected the AV conduction system. Electrodes of an artificial pacemaker were inserted into the patient's right ventricle, and the ventricular contractions were paced at a frequency of 75 beats/min. The patient felt stronger and more comfortable almost immediately.

1. **Soon after coronary artery occlusion, the interstitial fluid K^+ concentration rose substantially in the flow-deprived region. What does the high $[K^+]_o$ in this region mean?**

    A. It increases the propagation velocity of the myocardial action potentials.

    B. It decreases the postrepolarization refractoriness of the myocardial cells.

    C. It increases the resting (phase 4) transmembrane potential to a less negative value.

    D. It diminishes the automaticity of the myocardial cells.

    E. It decreases the likelihood of reentry arrhythmias.

2. **The mechanism by which the SA node generated impulses at a rapid rate during the early stages of the coronary artery occlusion involves which of the following?**

    A. An increased slope of the action potential upstroke (phase 0) of the automatic cells

    B. An increased slope of the slow diastolic depolarization of the automatic cells

    C. An increased firing threshold of the automatic cells

    D. An increased negativity (hyperpolarization) of the initial portion of the slow diastolic depolarization

    E. An increased action potential amplitude of the automatic cells

3. **What is the mechanism most likely responsible for the patient's arterial pulse rate of about 40 beats/min after impulse conduction through the AV junction was blocked?**

    A. Excitation of the ventricles via an AV bypass tract

    B. Conversion of ventricular myocardial fibers to automatic cells

    C. Firing of ventricular ectopic cells that have the same electrophysiological characteristics as SA node cells

    D. Firing of automatic cells (Purkinje fibers) in the specialized conduction system of the ventricles

    E. Excitation of ventricular cells by the rhythmic activity in the autonomic neurons that innervate the heart

4. **When the heart was being paced, the cardiologist discontinued ventricular pacing periodically to test the patient's cardiac status. The cardiologist found that the ventricles did not begin beating spontaneously until about 5 to 10 seconds after cessation of pacing because the preceding period of pacing led to which of the following?**

    A. Overdrive suppression of the automatic cells in the ventricles

    B. The release of norepinephrine from the cardiac sympathetic nerves

    C. The release of neuropeptide Y from the cardiac sympathetic nerves

    D. Fatigue of the ventricular myocytes

    E. The release of acetylcholine from the cardiac parasympathetic nerves

CHAPTER 18

Cardiac Pump

OBJECTIVES

- Describe how the microscopic and gross anatomy of the heart enable it to pump blood through the systemic and pulmonary circulations.
- Explain how electrical excitation of the heart is coupled to its contractions.
- List the factors that determine cardiac contractile force.
- Describe and explain the pressure changes in the heart chambers and great vessels during a complete cardiac cycle.

The heart exhibits a wide range of activity and functional capacity and performs a staggering amount of work over the lifetime of an individual. The heart can function independently of extracardiac stimuli, but its performance is influenced by humoral and neural factors. This chapter considers some of the basic intrinsic mechanisms that affect cardiac activity, and the effects of extracardiac factors are discussed in subsequent chapters.

The Gross and Microscopic Structures of the Heart Are Uniquely Designed for Optimal Function

Several important morphological and functional differences exist between myocardial and skeletal muscle cells (see Chapters 13 and 14). However, the contractile elements within the two types of cells are quite similar; each skeletal or cardiac muscle cell is made up of sarcomeres that contain thick filaments composed of myosin and thin filaments composed of actin. As in skeletal muscle, shortening of the cardiac sarcomere occurs via the sliding-filament mechanism. Actin filaments slide along adjacent myosin filaments via cycling of the intervening cross-bridges, and thereby the Z lines are brought closer together.

A striking difference in the appearance of cardiac and skeletal muscle is that cardiac muscle appears to be a syncytium (a single multinucleated cell formed from many fused cells) with branching and interconnecting fibers, whereas skeletal muscle cells do not interconnect. However, the myocardium is not a true anatomical syncytium because the myocardial fibers are separated laterally from adjacent fibers by their respective **sarcolemmas,** and the end of each fiber is separated from its neighbor by dense structures, **intercalated disks,** that are continuous with the sarcolemma (Figure 18-1). Nevertheless, cardiac muscle functions as a syncytium because a wave of depolarization, followed by contractions of the atria and ventricles **(an all-or-none response),** occurs when a suprathreshold stimulus is applied (see also Chapter 17).

As the wave of excitation approaches the end of a cardiac cell, the spread of excitation to the next cell depends on the electrical conductance of the boundary between the two cells. **Gap junctions (nexuses)** with high conductances are present in the intercalated disks between adjacent cells (Figure 18-1). These gap junctions, which facilitate the conduction of the cardiac impulse from one cell to the next, are made up of **connexons,** which are hexagonal structures that connect the cytosol of adjacent cells. Each connexon consists of six polypeptides surrounding a core channel that serves as a low-resistance pathway for cell-to-cell conductance. Impulse conduction in cardiac tissue progresses more rapidly in a direction parallel to, rather than perpendicular to, the long axes of the constituent fibers.

Another difference between cardiac and fast skeletal muscle fibers is in the number of mitochondria **(sarcosomes)** in the two tissues. Fast skeletal muscle has relatively few mitochondria, is called on for relatively short periods of repetitive or sustained contraction, and can metabolize anaerobically and build up a substantial O_2 debt. In contrast, cardiac muscle is richly endowed with mitochondria (Figure 18-1), must contract repetitively for a lifetime, and is incapable of developing a significant O_2 debt. Rapid oxidation of substrates with the synthesis of ATP can keep pace with the myocardial energy requirements because of the large number of mitochondria, which contain the respiratory enzymes necessary for oxidative phosphorylation (see also Chapter 14).

To provide adequate O_2 and substrate for its metabolic machinery, the myocardium is also endowed with a rich capillary supply, about one capillary per fiber. Thus diffusion distances are short, and O_2, CO_2, substrates, and waste material can move rapidly between myocardial cell and capillary. With respect to such exchanges, electron micrographs of the myocardium show deep invaginations of the sarcolemma into the fi-

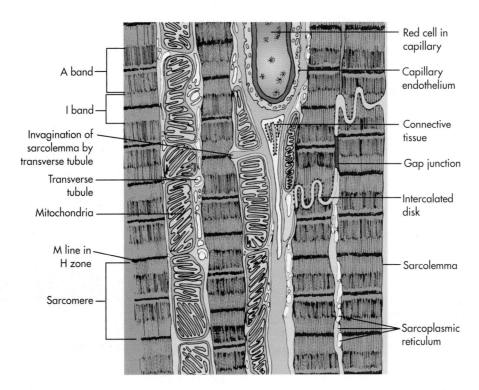

Figure 18-1 Diagram of an electron micrograph of cardiac muscle. Note the large number of mitochondria and the intercalated disks with nexuses (gap junctions), transverse tubules, and longitudinal tubules.

ber at the Z lines (Figure 18-1). These sarcolemmal invaginations constitute the **transverse-tubular (T-tubular) system.** The lumina of these T tubules are continuous with the bulk of interstitial fluid, and they play a key role in excitation-contraction coupling.

A network of sarcoplasmic reticulum consists of small-diameter sarcotubules that surround the myofibrils. The sarcoplasmic reticulum releases and takes up Ca^{++} and hence is important in myocardial contraction and relaxation.

The force of cardiac contraction is largely determined by the resting length of the myocardial fibers

Skeletal muscle and cardiac muscle show similar length-force relationships. The developed force is maximal when cardiac muscle begins contracting at resting sarcomere lengths of 2.0 to 2.4 μ. At such lengths, overlap of the thick and thin filaments is optimal, and the number of cross-bridge attachments is maximal. The developed force of cardiac muscle is less than maximal when the sarcomeres are stretched beyond the optimum length because the overlap of the filaments is less, and thus the cycling of the cross-bridges is less. At resting sarcomere lengths shorter than optimal, the thin filaments that extend from adjacent Z lines overlap one another in the central region of the sarcomere. This arrangement of the thin filaments diminishes contractile force.

The length-force relationship for the intact heart may be expressed graphically, as in the upper curve in Figure 18-2. Developed force (the force attained during contrac-

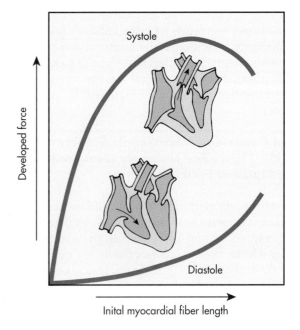

Figure 18-2 Relationship of the myocardial resting fiber length (sarcomere length), or end-diastolic volume, to the developed force, or peak systolic ventricular pressure, during ventricular contraction in the intact dog heart. *(Redrawn from Patterson SW et al: J Physiol 48:465, 1914.)*

tion) may be expressed as ventricular systolic pressure, and myocardial resting fiber length may be expressed as end-diastolic ventricular volume. The lower curve in Figure 18-2 depicts the ventricular pressure produced by increments in ventricular volume during diastole (at rest). The upper curve represents the peak pressure developed by the ventricle during systole at each filling volume. THE

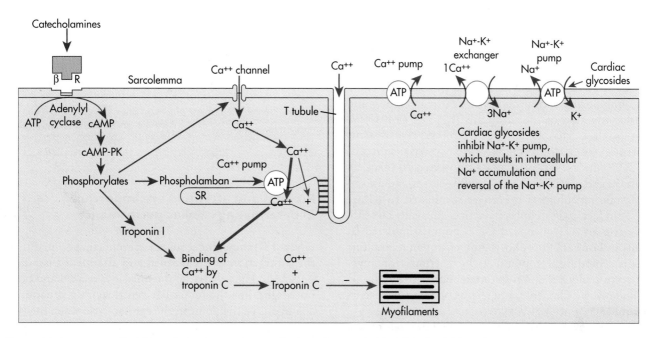

Figure 18-3 Movements of Ca^{++} in excitation-contraction coupling in cardiac muscle. The influx of Ca^{++} from the interstitial fluid during excitation triggers the release of Ca^{++} from the sarcoplasmic reticulum *(SR)*. The free cytosolic Ca^{++} activates contraction of the myofilaments (systole). Relaxation (diastole) occurs as a result of the uptake of Ca^{++} by the sarcoplasmic reticulum and the extrusion of intracellular Ca^{++} by an Na$^+$-Ca^{++} exchange and to a limited degree by the Ca^{++} pump. Negative signs indicate inhibition; positive signs indicate activation. β*R*, β-Adrenergic receptor; *cAMP*, cyclic adenosine monophosphate; *cAMP-PK*, cyclic AMP–dependent protein kinase.

GRAPH ILLUSTRATES THE RELATIONSHIP OF FORCE (OR PRESSURE) DEVELOPMENT BY THE VENTRICLE AS A FUNCTION OF INITIAL FIBER LENGTH (OR INITIAL VOLUME). This is known as the **Frank-Starling relationship,** named after the scientists who first described it.

Stretch of the myocardium by greater ventricular filling increases the level of cyclic AMP and Ca^{++} in the cardiomyocytes and enhances the affinity of troponin C for Ca^{++} (Figure 18-3). These two effects increase developed force and thereby contribute to the increase in force when the cardiac muscle fiber length increases.

The pressure-volume curve in diastole is quite flat at low volumes. Thus large increases in volume can be accommodated with only small increases in pressure; that is, the ventricle is very compliant. Nevertheless, the systolic pressure is considerable at the lower filling pressures. The ventricle becomes much less compliant with greater filling, however, as evidenced by the sharp rise of the diastolic curve at large intraventricular volumes. The normal heart operates only on the ascending portion of the Frank-Starling curve depicted in Figure 18-2 *(upper curve)*.

Excitation-contraction coupling is mediated principally by Ca^{++}

The heart requires optimum concentrations of Na$^+$, K$^+$, and Ca^{++} to function normally. In the absence of Na$^+$ the heart is not excitable and does not beat because the action potential of myocardial fibers depends on extracellular Na$^+$. In contrast, the resting membrane potential is independent of the Na$^+$ gradient across the membrane (see

Figure 17-4). Under normal conditions the extracellular K$^+$ concentration is about 4 mM. An increase in extracellular K$^+$, if great enough, produces depolarization, loss of excitability of the myocardial cells, and cardiac arrest in diastole. Ca^{++} is also essential for cardiac contraction. Removal of Ca^{++} from the extracellular fluid decreases contractile force and eventually causes arrest in diastole. Conversely, an increase in the extracellular Ca^{++} concentration enhances contractile force, but very high Ca^{++} concentrations induce cardiac arrest in systole (rigor). THE LEVEL OF THE FREE INTRACELLULAR CA^{++} CONCENTRATION IS MAINLY RESPONSIBLE FOR THE CONTRACTILE STATE OF THE MYOCARDIUM.

Initially a wave of excitation spreads rapidly along the myocardial sarcolemma from cell to cell via the gap junctions, and graded depolarization spreads into the interior of the cells via the T tubules. During the plateau (phase 2) of the action potential, the Ca^{++} permeability of the sarcolemma increases (see Chapter 17). Ca^{++} flows down its electrochemical gradient and enters the cell through Ca^{++} channels in the sarcolemma and in the invaginations of the sarcolemma, the T tubules (Figure 18-3). Channel opening is attributed to phosphorylation of the channel proteins by a cyclic AMP–dependent protein kinase. The primary source of extracellular Ca^{++} is the interstitial fluid (2 mM Ca^{++}).

The amount of Ca^{++} that enters the cell from the extracellular space is not sufficient to induce contraction of the myofibrils, but it serves as a trigger (**trigger Ca^{++}**) to release Ca^{++} from the intracellular Ca^{++} stores in the sarcoplasmic reticulum. The cytosolic free Ca^{++} concentration increases from a resting level of less than 0.1 μM to levels of 1.0 to 10 μM during excitation, and the Ca^{++} binds to the protein **troponin C** (see Chapter 12). The Ca^{++}-troponin complex interacts with tropomyosin to unblock active sites between the actin and myosin filaments (Figure 18-3). This unblocking action allows cross-bridge cycling and thus contraction of the myofibrils (systole). MECHANISMS THAT RAISE THE CYTOSOLIC CA^{++} CONCENTRATION INCREASE THE DEVELOPED FORCE, AND MECHANISMS THAT LOWER THE CYTOSOLIC CA^{++} CONCENTRATION DECREASE THE DEVELOPED FORCE.

At the end of systole the Ca^{++} influx ceases, and the sarcoplasmic reticulum is no longer stimulated to release Ca^{++}. In fact, the sarcoplasmic reticulum avidly takes up Ca^{++} via an ATP-energized Ca^{++} pump stimulated by **phospholamban.** Phosphorylation of troponin I inhibits the Ca^{++} binding of troponin C, which permits tropomyosin to again block the sites for interaction between the actin and myosin filaments, and relaxation (diastole) occurs (Figure 18-3).

The release of norepinephrine at the terminals of cardiac sympathetic nerves (as may occur during emotional stress) accelerates the rate of contraction and relaxation of the heart as well as the force of cardiac contraction. The norepinephrine activates adenylyl cyclase, and the resulting increase in cyclic AMP in turn activates cyclic AMP–dependent protein kinase. The kinase phosphorylates the Ca^{++} channels to enhance the rate and magnitude of Ca^{++} uptake. It also phosphorylates phospholamban, which enhances Ca^{++} uptake by the sarcoplasmic reticulum. Thus the phosphorylations by the cyclic AMP–dependent kinase increase both the speed of contraction and the speed of relaxation.

The Ca^{++} that enters the cell to initiate contraction must be removed during diastole. The removal is accomplished primarily by an electroneutral exchange of 3 Na^+ for 1 Ca^{++} (Figure 18-3). Ca^{++} is also removed from the cell by an electrogenic pump that uses energy to transport Ca^{++} across the sarcolemma (Figure 18-3).

Digitalis, a medication used in the treatment of heart failure, also increases contractile force by elevating the level of intracellular Ca^{++}. Digitalis inhibits Na^+-K^+-ATPase; hence less Na^+ is pumped out of the myocytes. This results in a decreased Na^+ gradient across the cell membrane, so that less Na^+ can enter the cell, and therefore less Ca^{++} can leave the cell by Na^+-Ca^{++} exchange (Figure 18-3).

Preload and afterload are important in determining cardiac performance

Figure 18-4 shows the sequence of events that occur during the contraction of a preloaded and afterloaded papillary muscle. In Figure 18-4, *A*, the muscle is relaxed and bears no weight. For the intact left ventricle, this situation is analogous to the point in the cardiac cycle when the ventricle has relaxed after ejection has terminated, the aortic valve is closed, and the mitral valve is about to open (the end of isovolumic relaxation in Figure 18-8). In Figure 18-4, *B*, the resting muscle is stretched by a preload, which in the intact heart represents the end of filling of the left ventricle during ventricular diastole; in other words, it represents the **end-diastolic volume.** In Figure 18-4, *C*, the resting muscle is still stretched by the preload, but a supported afterload has been added without allowing the muscle to be stretched further. In the intact heart, this situation is analogous to the point in the cardiac cycle at which ventricular contraction has started and the mitral valve has closed. The aortic valve has not yet opened because the ventricle has not developed enough intraventricular pressure to force it open (isovolumic contraction phase [see later section and Figure 18-8]). In Figure 18-4, *D*, the muscle has contracted and lifted the afterload. In the intact heart, this situation represents left ventricular ejection into the aorta. During ejection, the afterload is represented by aortic and

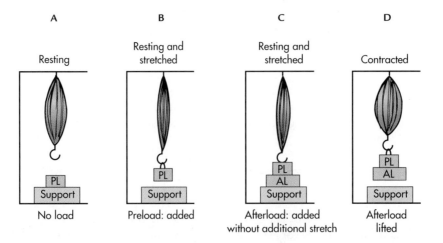

A	B	C	D
Resting	Resting and stretched	Resting and stretched	Contracted
No load	Preload: added	Afterload: added without additional stretch	Afterload lifted

Figure 18-4 Preload and afterload in a papillary muscle. **A,** Resting stage in the intact heart just before opening of the AV valves. **B,** Preload in the intact heart at the end of ventricular filling. **C,** Supported preload plus afterload in the intact heart just before opening of the aortic valve. **D,** Lifting preload plus afterload in the intact heart: ventricular ejection with decreased ventricular volume. *AL,* Afterload; *PL,* preload; *PL and AL,* total load.

intraventricular pressures, which are virtually equal to each other (see Figure 18-8).

The preload can be increased by greater filling of the left ventricle during diastole (Figure 18-2). At lower end-diastolic volumes, increments in filling pressure during diastole elicit a greater systolic pressure during the subsequent contraction. Systolic pressure increases until a maximum systolic pressure is reached at the optimum preload (Figure 18-1). If diastolic filling continues beyond this point, no further increase in developed pressure occurs. At very high filling pressures, peak pressure development in systole is reduced.

At a constant preload, a higher systolic pressure can be reached during ventricular contractions by raising the afterload (e.g., increasing aortic pressure by restricting the runoff of blood to the peripheral vessels). Increments in afterload produce progressively higher peak systolic pressures (Figure 18-5). If the afterload continues to increase, it becomes so great that the ventricle can no longer generate enough force to open the aortic valve (Figure 18-5). At this point, ventricular systole is totally isometric; there is no ejection of blood and thus no change in the volume of the ventricle during systole. The maximum pressure developed by the left ventricle under these conditions is the maximum isometric force the ventricle is capable of generating at a given preload.

Force and velocity are functions of the intracellular concentration of free Ca^{++}. When velocity is constant, force equals the afterload during contraction of the muscle. FORCE AND VELOCITY ARE INVERSELY RELATED. WITH NO LOAD, THE VELOCITY OF THE MUSCLE CONTRACTION IS MAXIMUM, WHEREAS WITH A MAXIMUM LOAD (WHEN CONTRACTION CAN NO LONGER SHORTEN THE MUSCLE), VELOCITY IS ZERO (Figure 18-6).

Preloads and afterloads depend on certain characteristics of the vascular system and the behavior of the heart. With respect to the vasculature, the degree of venomotor tone and peripheral resistance influence pre-

load and afterload. With respect to the heart, a change in the rate or stroke volume can also alter preload and afterload. Hence cardiac and vascular factors interact to produce effects on preload and afterload (see Chapter 24 for a full explanation).

> In **heart failure** the preload can be substantially increased because of the poor ventricular ejection and increased blood volume caused by fluid retention. In **essential hypertension** the high peripheral resistance augments the afterload by decreasing the peripheral runoff of the blood from the arterial system.

Contractility represents the performance of the heart at a given preload and afterload. CONTRACTILITY MAY BE DETERMINED EXPERIMENTALLY AS THE CHANGE IN PEAK ISOMETRIC FORCE (ISOVOLUMIC PRESSURE) AT A GIVEN INITIAL FIBER LENGTH (END-DIASTOLIC VOLUME). Contractility can be augmented by certain medications, such as norepinephrine or digitalis, and by an increase in contraction frequency **(tachycardia).** The increase in contractility **(positive inotropic effect)** produced by any of these interventions is reflected by increments in developed force and velocity of contraction.

> In rare instances, patients with asthma have accidentally received excessive doses of epinephrine subcutaneously. The patients develop marked tachycardia and increases in myocardial contractility, cardiac output, and total peripheral resistance. The result is dangerously high blood pressure. Treatment consists of a tourniquet on the injected limb with intermittent brief releases of the tourniquet and the use of adrenergic-blocking medications.

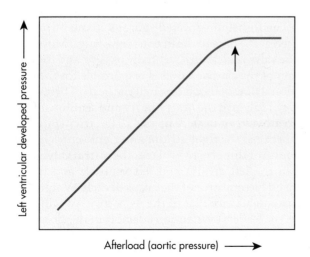

Figure 18-5 Effect of increasing afterload on developed pressure at constant preload. At the arrow, the maximum developed pressure is reached. Further increments in afterload prevent opening of the aortic valve.

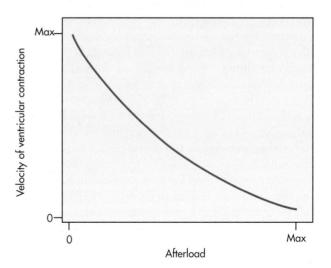

Figure 18-6 Effect of increasing afterload on the velocity of contraction at constant preload. *Max,* Maximum.

A reasonable index of myocardial contractility can be obtained from the contour of ventricular pressure curves (Figure 18-7). A hypodynamic heart is characterized by an elevated end-diastolic pressure, a slowly rising ventricular pressure, and a somewhat reduced ejection phase (curve C in Figure 18-7). A hyperdynamic heart (such as a heart stimulated by norepinephrine) shows a reduced end-diastolic pressure, a fast-rising ventricular pressure, and a brief ejection phase (curve B in Figure 18-7). The slope of the ascending limb of the ventricular pressure curve indicates the maximum rate of force development by the ventricle (maximum rate of change in pressure with time, **maximum dP/dt,** as illustrated by the tangents to the steepest portion of the ascending limbs of the ventricular pressure curves in Figure 18-7). The slope is maximal during the isovolumic phase of systole (Figure 18-8). At any given degree of ventricular filling, the slope provides an index of the initial contraction velocity and hence contractility.

A similar indication of the contractile state of the myocardium can be obtained from the maximum velocity of blood flow in the ascending aorta during the cardiac cycle (i.e., the initial slope of the aortic flow curve [Figure 18-8]). Also, the **ejection fraction,** which is the ratio of the volume of blood ejected from the left ventricle per beat **(stroke volume)** to the volume of blood in the left ventricle at the end of diastole (end-diastolic volume), is widely used clinically as an index of contractility. Other measurements (or combinations of measurements) that reflect the magnitude or velocity of the ventricular contraction have been used to assess the contractile state of the cardiac muscle. No index is entirely satisfactory, which undoubtedly accounts for the several indices in use.

The cardiac chambers consist of two atria, two ventricles, and four valves

The atria are thin-walled, low-pressure chambers that function more as large reservoirs and conduits of blood for their respective ventricles than as important pumps for ventricular filling. The ventricles are formed by a continuum of muscle fibers that originate from the fibrous skeleton at the base of the heart, primarily around the aortic orifice. These fibers sweep toward the apex at the epicardial surface. They also pass toward the endocardium as they gradually undergo a 180-degree change in direction to lie parallel to the epicardial fibers and form the endocardium and papillary muscles. At the apex of the heart the fibers twist and turn inward to form papillary muscles. At the base of the heart and around the valve orifices, the myocardial fibers form a thick, powerful muscle that decreases the ventricular circumference to aid in the ejection of blood, and narrow the atrioventricular (AV) valve orifices as an aid to valve closure. Ventricular ejection is implemented not only by a reduction in circumference but also by a decrease in the longitudinal axis; the decrease is

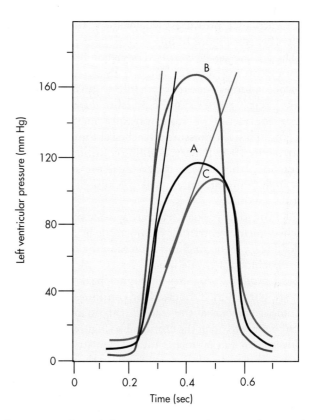

Figure 18-7 Left ventricular pressure curves with tangents drawn to the steepest portions of the ascending limbs to indicate the maximum dP/dt value. *A,* Control. *B,* Hyperdynamic heart, such as that which occurs after the administration of norepinephrine. *C,* Hypodynamic heart, such as that which occurs during cardiac failure. (See text for details.)

accomplished by a descent of the base of the heart. The early contraction of the ventricular apex, coupled with approximation of the ventricular walls, propels the blood toward the outflow tracts.

Cardiac valves

The cardiac valves consist of thin flaps of tough, flexible, endothelium-covered fibrous tissue firmly attached at the base to the fibrous valve rings. Movements of the valve leaflets are essentially passive, and the orientation of the cardiac valves is responsible for the unidirectional flow of blood through the heart. There are two types of valves in the heart: the AV and semilunar valves.

ATRIOVENTRICULAR VALVES.   The **tricuspid valve** lies between the right atrium and right ventricle and is made up of three cusps, whereas the **mitral valve** lies between the left atrium and left ventricle and has two cusps. The total area of the cusps of each AV valve is approximately twice that of the respective AV orifice, and thus the leaflets overlap considerably in the closed position. Attached to the free edges of these valves are fine, strong filaments **(chordae tendineae),** which arise from the powerful papillary muscles of the respective ventricles and prevent eversion of the valves during ventricular systole.

In the normal heart the valve leaflets are relatively close to one another during ventricular filling and provide a funnel for the transfer of blood from atrium to ventricle. This partial approximation of the valve surfaces during diastole is caused primarily by eddy currents behind the leaflets. Also, the chordae tendineae and papillary muscles are stretched by the filling ventricle and exert tension on the free edges of the valve leaflets.

Movements of the mitral valve leaflets throughout the cardiac cycle are shown in Figure 18-9. In **echocardiography,** short pulses of high-frequency sound waves (ultrasound) are sent through the chest tissues and heart, and the echoes reflected from the various cardiac structures are recorded. The timing and the pattern of the reflected waves provide important clinical information, such as the diameter of the heart, ventricular wall thickness, and magnitude and direction of the movements of various components of the heart, including the valves.

In Figure 18-9 the echocardiographic transducer is positioned to depict movement of the anterior leaflet of the mitral valve. The posterior leaflet moves in a pattern that is a mirror image of the anterior leaflet, except that in the projection shown in Figure 18-9 the excursions of the leaflet appear to be much smaller. At point D in Figure 18-9 the mitral valve opens, and during rapid filling (points D to E) the anterior leaflet moves toward the ventricular septum. During the reduced filling phase (points E to F), the valve leaflets float toward each other, but the valve does not close. The ventricular filling contributed by atrial contraction (points F to A) forces the leaflets apart, and a second approximation of the leaflets follows (points A to C). At point C the valve is closed by ventricular contraction. The valve leaflets, which bulge toward the atrium, stay pressed together during ventricular systole (points C to D).

SEMILUNAR VALVES. The valves between the right ventricle and pulmonary artery and between the left ventricle and aorta consist of three cuplike cusps attached to the valve rings. At the end of the reduced ejection phase of ventricular systole, blood flow reverses briefly toward the ventricles (shown as a negative flow in the phasic aortic flow curve in Figure 18-8). This flow reversal snaps the cusps together and prevents regurgitation of blood into the ventricles. During ventricular systole, the cusps do not lie back against the walls of the pulmonary artery and aorta; rather, they float in the bloodstream approximately midway between the vessel walls and their closed position. Behind the semilunar valves are small outpocketings **(sinuses of Valsalva)** of the pulmonary artery and aorta. Eddy currents develop in these sinuses and keep the valve cusps away from the vessel walls. The orifices of the right and left coronary arteries are located behind the right and left cusps, respectively, of the aortic valve. Were it not for the presence of the sinuses of Valsalva and the eddy currents de-

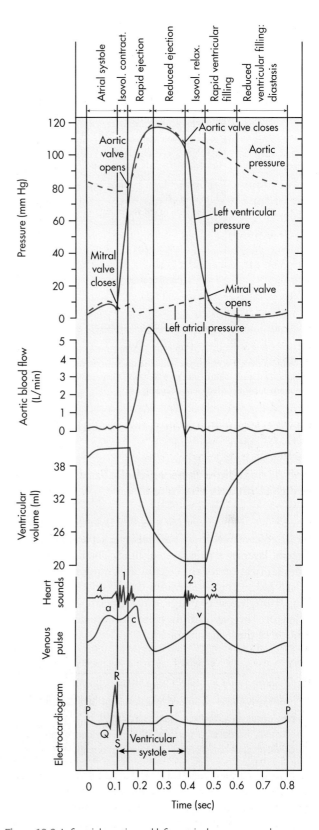

Figure 18-8 Left atrial, aortic, and left ventricular pressure pulses correlated in time with aortic flow, ventricular volume, heart sounds, venous pulse, and the electrocardiogram for a complete cardiac cycle in the dog (see text for details).

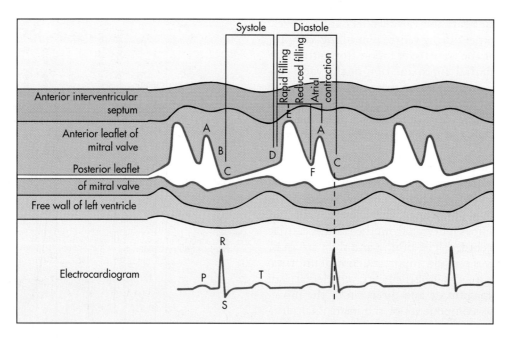

Figure 18-9 *Top,* Drawing made from an echocardiogram showing movements of the mitral valve leaflets (particularly the anterior leaflet), changes in the diameter of the left ventricular cavity, and thickness of the left ventricular walls during the cardiac cycles in a healthy person. The mitral valve closes at *C* and opens at *D. C* to *D,* Ventricular systole; *D* to *C,* ventricular diastole; *D* to *E,* rapid filling; *E* to *F,* reduced filling (diastasis); *F* to *A,* atrial contraction. *Bottom,* Simultaneously recorded electrocardiogram.

veloped therein, the coronary ostia could be blocked by the valve cusps.

The pericardium is an epithelialized fibrous sac that invests the heart

The pericardium consists of a visceral layer that is adherent to the epicardium and a parietal layer separated from the visceral layer by a thin layer of fluid. The fluid layer provides lubrication for the continuous movement of the enclosed heart. The pericardium is not very distensible and thus strongly resists a large, rapid increase in cardiac size. Therefore the pericardium helps prevent sudden overdistention of the heart chambers.

> In contrast to an acute change in intracardiac pressure, progressive and sustained enlargement of the heart (as can occur in **cardiac hypertrophy**) or a slow progressive increase in pericardial fluid (as can occur with **pericardial effusion**) gradually stretches the intact pericardium.

The two major heart sounds are produced mainly by closure of the cardiac valves

Four sounds are usually produced by the heart, but only two are ordinarily audible through a stethoscope. With electronic amplification the heart sounds, even the less intense sounds, can be detected and recorded graphically as a **phonocardiogram.**

The first heart sound is initiated at the onset of ventricular systole (Figure 18-8) and consists of a series of vibrations of mixed, unrelated low frequencies (a noise). It is the loudest and longest of the heart sounds and has a crescendo-decrescendo quality. The first heart sound is caused primarily by the oscillation of blood in the ventricular chambers and vibration of the chamber walls. The vibrations are engendered in part by the abrupt rise in ventricular pressure with acceleration of blood back toward the atria. However, the sound is produced mainly by sudden tension and recoil of the AV valves and adjacent structures when the blood is decelerated by closure of the AV valves.

The second heart sound, which occurs with closure of the semilunar valves (Figure 18-8), is composed of higher-frequency vibrations (higher pitch), is of shorter duration and lower intensity, and has a more snapping quality than the first heart sound. This sound is caused by abrupt closure of the semilunar valves, which initiates oscillations of the columns of blood and the tensed vessel walls by the stretch and recoil of the closed valves.

The third heart sound is usually not audible, but it is sometimes heard in children with thin chest walls or in patients with left ventricular failure. This sound consists of a few low-intensity, low-frequency vibrations heard best in the region of the apex. It occurs in early diastole and is believed to be the result of vibrations of the ventricular walls caused by the abrupt cessation of ventricular distention and deceleration of blood entering the ventricles.

A fourth, or atrial, sound, consisting of a few low-frequency oscillations, is occasionally heard in healthy individuals. It is caused by the oscillation of blood and cardiac chambers resulting from atrial contraction (Figure 18-8).

Asynchronous valve closures can produce **split sounds** over the apex of the heart for the AV valves and over the base for the semilunar valves. Deformities of the valves can produce cardiac **murmurs.** Valve lesions (stenosis or incompetence) may be congenital or produced by disease (e.g., **rheumatic fever**), and the timing (systolic or diastolic) and the character of the murmur provide clues regarding the type of valve damage.

The Sequential Relaxation and Contraction of the Atria and Ventricles Constitute the Cardiac Cycle

Ventricular systole

Isovolumic contraction
The onset of ventricular contraction coincides with the peak of the R wave of the electrocardiogram and the initial vibration of the first heart sound. It is indicated on the ventricular pressure curve as the earliest rise in ventricular pressure after atrial contraction (Figure 18-8). The interval between the start of ventricular systole and the opening of the semilunar valves (when ventricular pressure rises abruptly) is called **isovolumic contraction** because ventricular volume is constant during this brief period (Figure 18-8).

Ejection
Opening of the semilunar valves marks the onset of the **ejection phase,** which may be subdivided into an earlier, slightly shorter phase **(rapid ejection)** and a later, longer phase **(reduced ejection).** The rapid-ejection phase is characterized by the sharp rise in ventricular and aortic pressures that terminates at the peak ventricular and aortic pressures, an abrupt decrease in ventricular volume, and a large aortic blood flow (Figure 18-8). During the reduced ejection period, runoff of blood from the aorta to the periphery exceeds ventricular output, so aortic and ventricular pressures decline. Throughout ventricular systole the blood returning to the atria progressively increases atrial pressure.

During rapid ventricular ejection, left ventricular pressure slightly exceeds aortic pressure, and flow accelerates (continues to increase), whereas during reduced ventricular ejection, the reverse holds true. This reversal of the ventricular/aortic pressure gradient in the presence of the continued flow of blood from the left ventricle to the aorta (caused by the momentum of the forward blood flow) results from the storage of potential energy in the stretched arterial walls, which decelerates the flow of blood into the aorta.

The effect of ventricular systole on left ventricular di-ameter is shown in Figure 18-9. During ventricular systole (Figure 18-9, points C to D), the interventricular septum and the free wall of the left ventricle become thicker and move closer to each other.

At the end of ejection a volume of blood approximately equal to that ejected during systole remains in the ventricular cavities. This **residual volume** is fairly constant in normal hearts. However, it is smaller when heart rate increases or when outflow resistance is reduced, and it is larger when the opposite conditions prevail.

An increase in myocardial contractility may decrease residual volume, especially in the depressed heart. In severely hypodynamic and dilated hearts, as in **heart failure,** the residual volume can become much greater than the stroke volume.

Ventricular diastole

Isovolumic relaxation
Closure of the aortic valve produces the **incisura** (a notch) on the descending limb of the aortic pressure curve; it marks the end of ventricular systole. The period between closure of the semilunar valves and opening of the AV valves is called **isovolumic relaxation.** It is characterized by a precipitous fall in ventricular pressure without a change in ventricular volume (Figure 18-8).

Rapid filling phase
Most ventricular filling occurs immediately after the AV valves open. The blood that had returned to the atria during the previous ventricular systole is abruptly released into the relaxing ventricles. This period of ventricular filling is called the **rapid filling phase** (Figure 18-8). The atrial and ventricular pressures decrease despite the increase in ventricular volume because the relaxing ventricles are exerting less and less force on the blood in their cavities.

Diastasis
The rapid filling phase is followed by a phase of slow filling called **diastasis.** During diastasis, blood returning from the periphery flows into the right ventricle, and blood from the pulmonary circulation flows into the left ventricle. This small, slow addition to ventricular filling is indicated by gradual increases in atrial, ventricular, and venous pressures and in ventricular volume (Figure 18-8).

Atrial systole
The onset of atrial systole occurs soon after the beginning of the P wave of the electrocardiogram (curve of atrial depolarization). The transfer of blood from atrium to ventricle, accomplished by the peristalsis-like

wave of atrial contraction, completes the period of ventricular filling (Figure 18-8). Throughout ventricular diastole, atrial pressure barely exceeds ventricular pressure. This small pressure gradient indicates that the resistance of the pathway through the open AV valves during ventricular filling is normally very low.

Because there are no valves at the junctions of the venae cavae and right atrium or junctions of the pulmonary veins and left atrium, atrial contraction can force blood in both directions. Little blood is pumped back into the venous tributaries during the brief atrial contraction, mainly because of the inertia of the inflowing blood.

> Atrial contraction is not essential for ventricular filling. Adequate filling is often observed in patients with **atrial fibrillation** or **complete heart block** despite the absence of atrial contraction.

The contribution of atrial contraction is governed to a great extent by the heart rate and the structure of the AV valves. At slow heart rates, filling practically ceases toward the end of diastasis, and atrial contraction contributes little additional filling. When the heart rate is rapid, diastasis is abbreviated, and the atrial contribution can become substantial, especially if the atrium

contracts immediately after the rapid filling phase, when the AV pressure gradient is maximal.

> When the heart rate becomes so rapid that the period of ventricular relaxation becomes markedly abbreviated, ventricular filling is seriously impaired despite the contribution of atrial contraction. In certain diseases (e.g., **mitral stenosis**), the AV valves may be severely narrowed, and atrial contraction can become more important to ventricular filling than it is in the normal heart.

A graph of the pressure-volume relationship illustrates the sequential dynamic changes in a single cardiac cycle

The changes in left ventricular pressure and volume throughout the cardiac cycle are summarized in Figure 18-10. The element of time is not considered in this pressure-volume loop. Diastolic filling starts at point A in Figure 18-10 and terminates at point C, when the mitral valve closes. The initial decrease in left ventricular pressure (points A to B) despite the rapid inflow of blood from the atrium results from progressive ventricular relaxation and increased distensibility. During the remainder of diastole (points B to C) the increase in ventricular pressure reflects ventricular filling and the passive elastic characteristics of

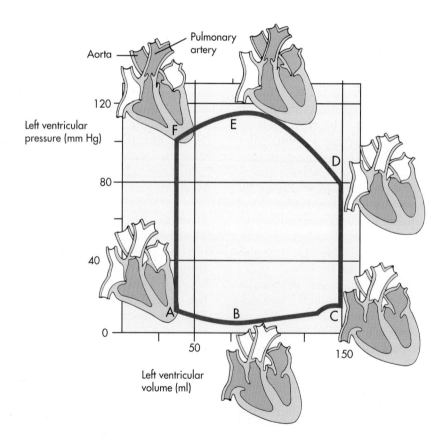

Figure 18-10 Pressure-volume loop of the left ventricle for a single cardiac cycle (*A* to *F*) (see text for details).

the ventricle. After the initial phase of ventricular diastole, only a small increase in pressure occurs with the increase in ventricular volume (points B to C), and atrial systole (the small upward deflection just to the left of point C) contributes to ventricular volume and pressure. With isovolumic contraction (points C to D), pressure rises steeply and ventricular volume remains constant. At point D the aortic valve opens. During the first phase of ejection (rapid ejection [points D to E]), the large reduction in volume is associated with a progressive increase in ventricular pressure that is less than the increase occurring during isovolumic contraction. This phase is followed by reduced ejection (points E to F) and a small decrease in ventricular pressure. The aortic valve closes at point F; this is followed by isovolumic relaxation (points F to A), which is characterized by a sharp drop in pressure and no change in volume. The mitral valve opens at point A to complete one cardiac cycle.

The Fick principle is used to determine cardiac output

Adolph Fick contrived the first method for measuring cardiac output in intact animals and humans. The basis for this method, called the **Fick principle,** is simply an application of the law of conservation of mass. It is derived from the fact that the quantity of O_2 delivered to the pulmonary capillaries via the pulmonary artery plus the quantity of O_2 that enters the pulmonary capillaries from the alveoli must equal the quantity of O_2 carried away by the pulmonary veins.

The rate, q_1, of O_2 delivery to the lungs equals the O_2 concentration in the pulmonary arterial blood, $[O_2]_{pa}$, multiplied by the pulmonary arterial blood flow, Q, which equals the cardiac output, as follows:

$$q_1 = Q[O_2]_{pa} \qquad \textbf{18-1}$$

At equilibrium, q_2, the net rate of O_2 uptake by the pulmonary capillaries from the alveoli equals the O_2 consumption of the body. The rate at which O_2 is carried away by the pulmonary veins, q_3, equals the O_2 concentration in pulmonary venous blood, $[O_2]_{pv}$, multiplied by the total pulmonary venous flow, which is virtually equal to the pulmonary arterial blood flow, Q, as follows:

$$q_3 = Q[O_2]_{pv} \qquad \textbf{18-2}$$

From the conservation of mass, the following occurs:

$$q_1 + q_2 = q_3 \qquad \textbf{18-3}$$

Therefore from Equations 18-1 to 18-3, the following occurs:

$$Q[O_2]_{pa} + q_2 = Q[O_2]_{pv} \qquad \textbf{18-4}$$

Solving for cardiac output, one finds the following:

$$Q = q_2/([O_2]_{pv} - [O_2]_{pa}) \qquad \textbf{18-5}$$

Equation 18-5 is the statement of the Fick principle.

In the clinical determination of cardiac output, O_2 consumption is computed from measurements of the volume and O_2 content of expired air over a given interval. Because the O_2 concentration of peripheral arterial blood is essentially identical to that in the pulmonary veins, $[O_2]_{pv}$, it is determined on a sample of peripheral arterial blood withdrawn by needle puncture. Pulmonary arterial blood represents mixed systemic venous blood. Samples for O_2 analysis are obtained from the pulmonary artery or right ventricle through a cardiac catheter.

An example of the calculation of cardiac output in a normal, resting adult is illustrated in Figure 18-11. With an O_2 consumption of 250 ml/min, an arterial (pulmonary venous) O_2 content of 0.20 ml of O_2 per milliliter of blood, and a mixed venous (pulmonary arterial) O_2 content of 0.15 ml of O_2 per milliliter of blood, the cardiac output would be $250/(0.20 - 0.15) = 5000$ ml/min.

The Fick principle is also used for estimating the O_2 consumption of organs in situ, when blood flow and the O_2 contents of the arterial and venous blood can be determined. Algebraic rearrangement of Equation 18-5 reveals that O_2 consumption equals the blood flow multiplied by the arteriovenous O_2 concentration difference. For example, if the blood flow through one kidney is 700 ml/min, arterial O_2 content

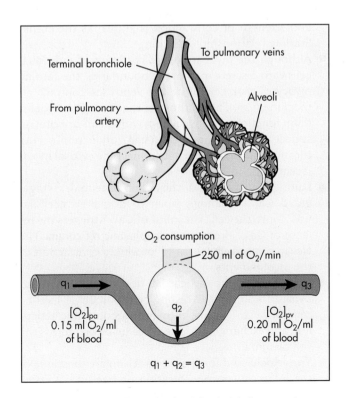

Figure 18-11 Diagram illustrating the Fick principle for measuring cardiac output. The change in color from pulmonary artery to pulmonary vein represents the change in color of the blood as venous blood becomes fully oxygenated.

is 0.20 ml of O_2 per milliliter of blood, and renal venous O_2 content is 0.18 ml of O_2 per milliliter of blood, then the rate of O_2 consumption by that kidney must be $700(0.20 - 0.18) = 14$ ml/min.

The indicator dilution technique is a relatively simple method for measuring cardiac output

The **indicator dilution technique** has been widely used to estimate cardiac output in humans. A measured quantity of some indicator (a dye or isotope that remains within the circulation) is injected rapidly into a large central vein or into the right side of the heart through a catheter. Arterial blood is continuously drawn through a detector (densitometer or isotope rate counter), and a curve of indicator concentration is recorded as a function of time. The greater the blood flow (cardiac output), the greater the dilution of the injected dye. The most common indicator is a bolus of cold saline injected into the pulmonary artery via a cardiac catheter. The cardiac output can be calculated from the change in the temperature of the blood flowing past the temperature detector at the tip of the catheter.

SUMMARY

- An increase in myocardial fiber length, such as that occurring with an augmented ventricular filling during diastole (preload), produces a more forceful ventricular contraction. This relationship between fiber length and strength of contraction is known as the Frank-Starling relationship or Starling's law.
- Although the myocardium is made up of individual cells with discrete membrane boundaries, the cardiac myocytes that constitute the ventricles contract almost in unison, as do those of the atria. The myocardium functions as a syncytium with an all-or-none response to excitation. Cell-to-cell conduction occurs through gap junctions that connect the cytosol of adjacent cells.
- During the upstroke of the action potential, voltage-gated Ca^{++} channels open to admit extracellular Ca^{++} into the cell. The influx of Ca^{++} triggers the release of Ca^{++} from the sarcoplasmic reticulum. The elevated intracellular Ca^{++} produces contraction of the myofilaments.
- Relaxation of the myocardial fibers is accomplished by restoration of the resting cytosolic Ca^{++} level by pumping Ca^{++} back into the sarcoplasmic reticulum and exchanging it for extracellular Na^+ across the sarcolemma.
- The velocity and force of contraction are functions of the intracellular concentration of free Ca^{++}. Force and velocity are inversely related, so with no load, force is negligible, and velocity is maximal. In an isometric contraction, in which no external shortening occurs, force is maximal, and velocity is zero.

- In the ventricles the preload is the stretch of the fibers caused by blood during ventricular filling, and the afterload is the aortic pressure against which the left ventricle ejects blood.
- Contractility is an expression of cardiac performance at a given preload and afterload. Contractility is increased mainly by interventions that increase intracellular Ca^{++} levels and decreased by interventions that decrease intracellular Ca^{++} levels.
- Simultaneous recording of the left atrial, left ventricular, and aortic pressures; ventricular volume; heart sounds; and electrocardiogram graphically portray the sequential and related electrical and cardiodynamic events throughout a cardiac cycle.
- Cardiac output can be determined, according to the Fick principle, by dividing the O_2 consumption of the body by the difference between the O_2 content of arterial and mixed venous blood. It can also be measured by dye dilution or thermodilution techniques.

BIBLIOGRAPHY

Bers DM, Lederer WJ, Berlin JR: Intracellular Ca transients in rat cardiac myocytes: role of Na-Ca exchange in excitation-contraction coupling, *Am J Physiol* 258:C944, 1990.

Brady AJ: Mechanical properties of isolated cardiac myocytes, *Physiol Rev* 71:413, 1991.

Carafoli E: Calcium pump of the plasma membrane, *Physiol Rev* 71:129, 1991.

Elzinga G, Westerhof N: Matching between ventricle and arterial load, *Circ Res* 68:1495, 1991.

Gibbons WR, Zygmunt AC: Excitation-contraction coupling in the heart. In Fozzard HA et al, eds: *The heart and cardiovascular system,* ed 2, New York, 1991, Raven.

Katz AM: Interplay between inotropic and lusitropic effects of cyclic adenosine monophosphate on the myocardial cell, *Circulation* 82:I-7, 1990.

Lakatta EG: Length modulation of muscle performance: Frank-Starling law of the heart. In Fozzard HA et al, eds: *The heart and cardiovascular system,* ed 2, New York, 1991, Raven.

Lorenz JN, Kranias EG: Regulatory effects of phospholamban on cardiac function in intact mice, *Am J Physiol* 273:H2826, 1997.

Luo W et al: Targeted ablation of the phospholamban gene is associated with markedly enhanced myocardial contractility and loss of β-agonist stimulation, *Circ Res* 75:401, 1994.

Lytton J, MacLennan DH: Sarcoplasmic reticulum. In Fozzard HA et al, eds: *The heart and cardiovascular system,* ed 2, New York, 1991, Raven.

Sheu SS, Blaustein MP: Sodium/calcium exchange and control of cell calcium and contractility in cardiac muscle and vascular smooth muscle. In Fozzard HA et al, eds: *The heart and cardiovascular system,* New York, 1991, Raven.

Smith JS, Rousseau E, Meissner G: Single sarcoplasmic reticulum Ca^{2+}-release channels from calmodulin modulation of cardiac and skeletal muscle, *Circ Res* 64:352, 1989.

Todaka K et al: Effect of ventricular stretch on contractile strength, calcium transient, and cAMP in intact canine hearts, *Am J Physiol* 274:H990, 1998.

CASE STUDY

Case 18-1

A 60-year-old woman entered the hospital complaining of shortness of breath, fatigue, and swelling of her ankles and lower legs. She had these symptoms for about 3 years but refused medical treatment until they became severe. As a child she had rheumatic fever and developed a murmur, which was diagnosed as mitral stenosis. Physical examination revealed a dyspneic, slightly cyanotic women with ankle and pretibial edema, distended neck veins, an enlarged tender liver, ascites, and rales at the lung bases. The electrocardiogram showed atrial fibrillation and right axis deviation. A chest x-ray film showed an enlarged heart and shadows at the lung bases that were compatible with pulmonary edema. A cardiac workup revealed a low cardiac output. After a week of treatment for congestive heart failure, her symptoms abated, and she was sent home with a prescription for medication.

1. **What did auscultation of the heart reveal?**
   A. Harsh systolic murmur heard best at the cardiac apex
   B. Harsh systolic murmur heard best in the second interspace to the left of the sternum
   C. Soft, high-pitched diastolic murmur heard best in the second interspace to the left of the sternum
   D. Rumbling, low-pitched diastolic murmur heard best at the cardiac apex
   E. High-pitched systolic murmur heard best in the second interspace to the right of the sternum

2. **Which of the following is *not* observed in atrial fibrillation?**
   A. An irregular heartbeat
   B. A heart rate measured by auscultation over the precordium greater than that measured by palpation of the radial artery
   C. A very rapid regular pulse
   D. A variation in the strength of the heartbeats as palpated at the wrist
   E. A lack of P waves in the electrocardiogram

3. **Which of the following therapeutic measures would help this patient?**
   A. Insertion of a pacemaker to correct the arrhythmia
   B. Phlebotomy (blood removal via a peripheral vein)
   C. Saline infusion to increase preload and hence cardiac output
   D. Intravenous administration of adenosine to restore normal cardiac rhythm
   E. Administration of a Ca^{++}-uptake blocker such as diltiazem

4. **Which of the following findings would be true for this patient?**
   A. Increased serum albumin level
   B. Increased pulmonary wedge pressure (obtained by threading a catheter via a peripheral vein as far as it will go into a branch of the pulmonary artery)
   C. Increased Na^+ excretion
   D. Reduced peripheral resistance
   E. Increased pulse pressure

5. **Which of the following medications would *not* be prescribed for this patient?**
   A. Dicumarol
   B. Digoxin
   C. Procainamide
   D. Hydrochlorothiazide
   E. Nitroglycerin

6. **The patient's whole-body O_2 consumption was 300 ml/min, and the pulmonary artery and the brachial artery blood O_2 content were, respectively, 8 ml/dl and 18 ml/dl. What was the patient's cardiac output?**
   A. 2.0 L/min
   B. 4.8 L/min
   C. 3.0 L/min
   D. 1.3 L/min
   E. 1.2 L/min

Regulation of the Heartbeat

- Describe the neural control of heart rate.
- Explain the role of preload in the regulation of myocardial contraction.
- Describe the neural regulation of myocardial contraction.
- Explain the effects of hormones on myocardial contraction.
- Explain the effects of blood gases on myocardial contraction.

The preceding chapters in this section dealt with the important constituents of blood, the electrical activity of the heart and the fluxes of critical ions across cardiac cell membranes, and the mechanical and chemical aspects of cardiac contraction. This chapter deals with the factors that regulate contraction of the heart and the heart's ability to pump blood around the body. The quantity of blood pumped by the heart each minute **(cardiac output)** equals the volume of blood pumped each beat **(stroke volume)** multiplied by the number of heartbeats per minute **(heart rate).** Thus the cardiac output may be varied by changing the heart rate or stroke volume. A discussion of the control of cardiac activity may therefore be subdivided into regulation of pacemaker activity and regulation of contractile strength. The control of pacemaker activity is mediated mainly by the autonomic nervous system. The cardiac nerves also regulate contractile strength, but a number of mechanical and humoral factors are also important.

The Heart Rate Is Under Nervous Control

In normal adults the average heart rate at rest is about 70 beats/min, but the rate is significantly greater in children. During sleep, the heart rate diminishes by 10 to 20 beats/min, but during exercise or emotional excitement, it may rise to well above 100 beats/min. In various types of heart failure and febrile diseases, the heart rate may also be high. In well-trained athletes at rest, it is often very slow: about 45 or 50 beats/min.

The sinoatrial (SA) node is usually under the tonic influence of both divisions of the autonomic nervous system. STIMULATION OF THE SYMPATHETIC SYSTEM INCREASES HEART RATE, WHEREAS STIMULATION OF THE PARASYMPATHETIC SYSTEM DECREASES IT. Changes in heart rate usually involve a reciprocal action of the two divisions of the autonomic nervous system. Thus an increased heart rate is usually achieved by a waning of parasympathetic activity and a concomitant increase in sympathetic activity; deceleration is usually accomplished by the opposite changes in neural activity.

Ordinarily, in healthy, resting individuals, parasympathetic activity predominates. Abolition of the parasympathetic regulation by the medication **atropine** (a **muscarinic receptor antagonist**) usually increases the heart rate substantially (Figure 19-1). Conversely, abolition of sympathetic regulation by the medication **propranolol** (a **β-adrenergic receptor antagonist**) usually slows the heart rate only slightly (Figure 19-1). Thus IN HEALTHY, RESTING PEOPLE THE INHIBITORY PARASYMPATHETIC EFFECTS ON HEART RATE USUALLY PREDOMINATE OVER THE FACILITATORY SYMPATHETIC EFFECTS. When the effects of both divisions of the autonomic nervous system are blocked by the combination of these two medications, the heart rate of adults averages about 100 beats/min. The rate that prevails after complete autonomic blockade is called the **intrinsic heart rate.**

Nervous control

Sympathetic effects are facilitatory

Cardiac sympathetic fibers originate in the upper five or six thoracic and lower one or two cervical segments of the spinal cord (see also Chapter 10). These preganglionic fibers emerge from the spinal column through the white communicating branches and enter the paravertebral chains of ganglia. Most of the preganglionic fibers ascend the paravertebral chains and synapse with postganglionic neurons, mainly in the stellate and middle cervical ganglia. Postganglionic sympathetic fibers then join with parasympathetic fibers to form the **cardiac plexus,** which is a complex network of nerve trunks that contain sympathetic and parasympathetic efferent nerves to the heart and afferent nerves from sensory receptors in the heart and great vessels.

Sympathetic fibers from the right and left sides of the body are distributed asymmetrically to the various structures in the heart. In the dog, for example, stimulation of the right cardiac sympathetic nerve increases the

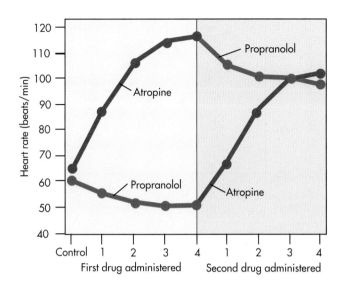

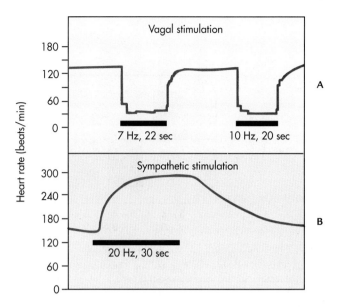

Figure 19-1 Mean effects of four equal doses of atropine *(red)* and propranolol *(blue)*, given sequentially, on the heart rates of 10 healthy young men. In half the trials, atropine was given first *(top curve)*; in the other half, propranolol was given first *(bottom curve).* *(Redrawn from Katona PG et al:* J Appl Physiol *52:1652, 1982.)*

Figure 19-2 Changes in heart rate evoked by stimulation *(horizontal bars)* of the vagus **(A)** and sympathetic **(B)** nerves in an anesthetized dog. *(Redrawn from Warner HR, Cox A:* J Appl Physiol *17:349, 1962.)*

heart rate more than equivalent stimulation of sympathetic fibers on the left side; the asymmetry is reversed for control of ventricular contractile force.

The facilitatory effects of sympathetic stimulation on heart rate develop much more slowly than the inhibitory effects of vagal stimulation (Figure 19-2). The onset of the cardiac response to sympathetic stimulation is gradual for two reasons. First, the sympathetic neurotransmitter norepinephrine is released relatively slowly from the cardiac sympathetic nerve terminals. Second, norepinephrine achieves its cardiac effects via a slow second messenger system, principally the adenylyl cyclase system (see Chapter 5). Furthermore, the sympathetic effects decay very gradually after the cessation of stimulation, in contrast to the abrupt termination of the response after the cessation of vagal activity (Figure 19-2). Most of the norepinephrine released during sympathetic stimulation is taken back up by the nerve terminals, and much of the remaining neurotransmitter is carried away by the bloodstream; these processes are slow. Hence sympathetic activity alters heart rate much more gradually than vagal activity.

The adrenergic receptors in the cardiac tissues are predominantly of the β-adrenergic receptor type; that is, they are responsive to specific **β-adrenergic receptor agonists** such as **isoproterenol** and are inhibited by specific **β-adrenergic receptor antagonists** such as **propranolol.**

Parasympathetic effects are inhibitory

The preganglionic parasympathetic fibers to the heart originate in the medulla oblongata in cells that lie in the **dorsal motor nucleus of the vagus** or the **nucleus am-**

biguus (see also Chapter 10). The precise location varies from species to species. Centrifugal fibers from these nuclei pass inferiorly through the neck via the vagus nerves (the tenth cranial nerves), which lie close to the common carotid arteries. The nerve fibers then travel through the mediastinum to synapse with postganglionic cells located on the epicardial surface of the heart or within the walls of the heart itself. Many of the cardiac ganglion cells are located in epicardial fat pads near the SA and atrioventricular (AV) nodes.

The right and left vagi are usually distributed differentially to the various cardiac structures. The right vagus nerve affects the SA node predominantly; stimulation decreases the firing rate. The left vagus nerve mainly retards AV conduction and may interrupt impulse conduction from the atria to the ventricles. However, the bilateral innervation overlaps considerably; left vagal stimulation inhibits the SA node, and right vagal stimulation impedes AV conduction.

The effects of vagal activity are mediated mainly by the neurotransmitter **acetylcholine,** which is released from the postganglionic vagus nerve endings in the cardiac tissues. Acetylcholine interacts with specific **cholinergic receptors (muscarinic type)** in the cardiac cell membranes. The action of the released acetylcholine can be blocked by the muscarinic receptor antagonist **atropine.** The cardiac tissues are rich in the enzyme **acetylcholinesterase,** which rapidly hydrolyzes the neurally released acetylcholine. Hence after vagal activity ceases, the effects decay quickly (Figure 19-2, *A*). Furthermore, the effects of vagal activity on heart rate have a very short latency (<100 msec) and attain their steady-state effects very quickly because the released acetylcho-

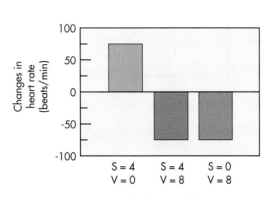

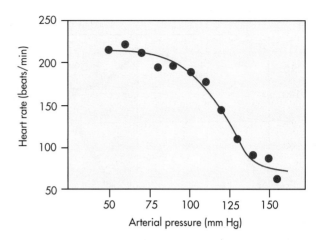

Figure 19-3 Changes in heart rate evoked by cardiac sympathetic *(S)* and vagal *(V)* stimulation in an anesthetized dog. The numerical values of *S* and *V* represent the stimulation frequencies in hertz.

Figure 19-4 Heart rate as a function of mean arterial pressure in a group of five conscious, chronically instrumented monkeys. Arterial pressure was increased by phenylephrine infusions and decreased by nitroprusside infusions. *(Redrawn from Cornish KG et al: Am J Physiol 257:R595, 1989.)*

line activates special **acetylcholine-regulated K⁺ channels** in the cardiac cells. Opening of these channels is so prompt because this action does not require an intermediate second messenger system such as the adenylyl cyclase system. THE COMBINATION OF THE BRIEF LATENCY AND RAPID DECAY OF THE RESPONSE PROVIDES THE POTENTIAL FOR THE VAGUS NERVES TO EXERT A BEAT-BY-BEAT CONTROL OF HEART RATE AND AV CONDUCTION.

The parasympathetic effects preponderate over sympathetic effects at the SA node. In an experiment in an anesthetized dog (Figure 19-3), the frequencies of neural stimulation were adjusted so that the steady-state increase in the heart rate evoked by cardiac sympathetic stimulation alone equaled the steady-state decrease in heart rate induced by vagal stimulation alone. In this experiment, the heart rate increased by about 80 beats/min during sympathetic stimulation at a frequency of 4 Hz, and the heart rate decreased by about 80 beats/min during vagal stimulation at 8 Hz. However, during concurrent sympathetic and vagal stimulation at these respective frequencies (sympathetic stimulation at 4 Hz, vagal stimulation at 8 Hz), the heart rate decreased by about 80 beats/min. Thus the effects of combined vagal and sympathetic stimulation did not differ perceptibly from the effects of vagal stimulation alone; that is, the sympathetic effects were scarcely detectable during combined stimulation. The mechanisms responsible for this overwhelming vagal predominance are discussed later.

Cerebral centers regulate autonomic control

A number of higher cerebral centers help regulate cardiac rate, rhythm, and contractile strength (see also Chapter 10). The excitation of specific nuclei in the **thalamus** or **hypothalamus** alters the heart rate. Hypothalamic centers are also involved in the circulatory responses to fluctuations in environmental temperature. Experimentally induced temperature changes in the an-

terior hypothalamus markedly affect heart rate and peripheral resistance (as described in the section on hypothalamic functions in Chapter 9). Stimuli applied to the H₂ fields of Forel in the **diencephalon** elicit cardiovascular responses that resemble those observed during muscular exercise. In the **cerebral cortex** the centers that influence cardiac function are located mostly in the frontal and temporal lobes; motor, premotor, and orbital cortices; insula; and cingulate gyrus.

Reflex control

The baroreceptors integrate cardiac function with arterial blood pressure

Acute changes in blood pressure reflexly alter heart rate. Such changes in heart rate are mediated mainly by the pressure receptors **(baroreceptors)** located in the carotid sinuses and aortic arch (see also Chapter 23). An example of the heart rate changes elicited by vasodilator and vasoconstrictor medications in a group of conscious, chronically instrumented monkeys is shown in Figure 19-4. As the arterial blood pressure was elevated from about 50 to about 150 mm Hg, the heart rate decreased progressively. Changes in blood pressure above and below this range had little additional effect on heart rate.

Moderate deviations in blood pressure from the normal level are usually accomplished by reciprocal changes in sympathetic and parasympathetic activity. For example, a moderate reduction in blood pressure evokes a rise in heart rate, and this change in rate is mediated usually by a concomitant increase in sympathetic activity and a decrease in vagal activity. Sudden large changes in blood pressure, however, are usually accompanied by activity in only one autonomic division. When the arterial blood pressure is markedly reduced, the sympathetic nerves become very active, and the vagus nerves are virtually quiescent. When the

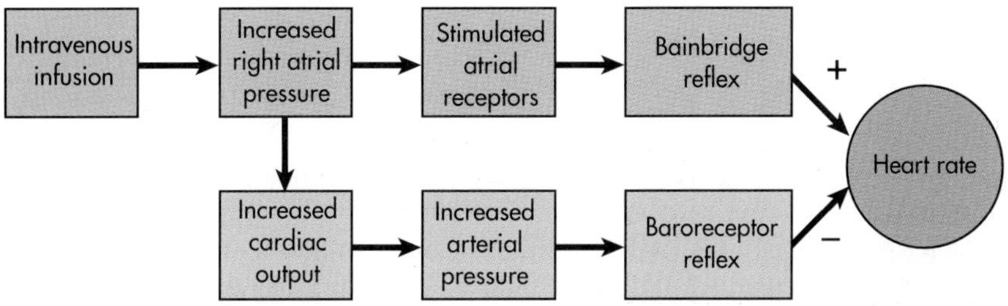

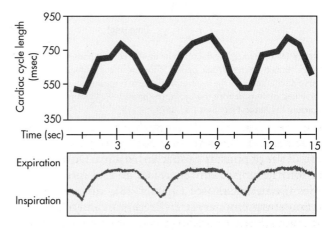

Figure 19-5 Intravenous infusions of blood or electrolyte solutions tend to increase heart rate via the Bainbridge reflex and to decrease heart rate via the baroreceptor reflex. The change in heart rate induced by such infusions is the result of these two opposing reflex actions.

arterial pressure is markedly elevated, the sympathetic nerves become quiescent, and the vagus nerves are hyperactive.

Sensory receptors in the atria regulate cardiac and renal function

In 1915, the British physiologist Francis Bainbridge reported that infusions of blood or saline solution increased the heart rate regardless of whether the infusions raised the arterial blood pressure. Cardiac acceleration was observed when central venous pressure rose enough to distend the right side of the heart, and the effect was abolished by cutting both vagi. Bainbridge postulated that increased cardiac filling raised the heart rate reflexly and that the afferent impulses were conducted by the vagi.

Many investigators have confirmed that the heart rate may accelerate in response to the intravenous administration of fluid. However, the magnitude and direction of the response depend on a number of factors, especially the prevailing heart rate. When the heart rate is relatively slow, intravenous infusions usually accelerate the heart. When the heart rate is more rapid, however, infusions usually slow the heart. Acute increases in blood volume not only evoke the Bainbridge reflex but also activate other reflexes (notably the baroreceptor reflex) that tend to change heart rate in the opposite direction (Figure 19-5). The change in heart rate induced by an intravenous infusion is therefore the result of these antagonistic reflex effects.

Sensory receptors that influence heart rate exist in both atria. The receptors are located principally in the venoatrial junctions. Distention of these receptors sends impulses centrally in the vagi. The efferent impulses are carried by sympathetic and parasympathetic fibers to the SA node. The stimulation of the atrial receptors also increases urine flow. A reduction in renal sympathetic nerve activity might be partially responsible for this diuresis. However, the principal mechanisms appear to be a neurally mediated reduction in the secretion of **vasopressin (antidiuretic hormone)** by the posterior pituitary gland (see Chapter 44) and the release of another peptide, **atrial natriuretic peptide,** which is released from the atrial tissues in response to atrial contraction and stretch (see Chapter 37).

Figure 19-6 Respiratory sinus arrhythmia in a resting, awake dog. The length of the cardiac cycle increases during expiration and decreases during inspiration. *(Redrawn from Warner MR et al: Am J Physiol 251:H1134, 1986.)*

Respiration regulates cardiac rhythm

The length of the cardiac cycle often fluctuates rhythmically depending on the frequency of respiration. Such fluctuations are detectable in most resting adults, and they are more pronounced in children. Typically the cycle length decreases during inspiration and increases during expiration (Figure 19-6).

Recordings of action potentials from the autonomic nerves to the heart in animals reveal that neural activity increases in the sympathetic nerve fibers during inspiration but increases in the vagal fibers during expiration (Figure 19-7). The acetylcholine released at the vagal endings quickly alters the firing of the pacemaker cells in the SA node, and the acetylcholine is also removed very rapidly. Therefore periodic bursts of vagal activity can cause the heart rate to vary rhythmically. Conversely, the norepinephrine released at the sympathetic endings affects the pacemaker cells more gradually than acetylcholine, and norepinephrine is also removed from the cardiac tissues more slowly than acetylcholine. Thus the effects of rhythmic variations in sympathetic activity on heart rate are damped out. Hence THE RHYTHMIC CHANGES IN HEART RATE ASSOCIATED WITH RESPIRATION ARE ASCRIBABLE ALMOST ENTIRELY TO THE OSCILLATIONS IN VAGAL ACTIVITY. Respiratory sinus arrhythmia is exaggerated when vagal tone is enhanced.

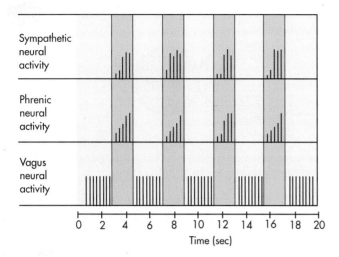

Figure 19-7 Respiratory fluctuations in efferent sympathetic and vagal neural activity in the cardiac nerves of an anesthetized dog. The phrenic nerve discharges mark the inspiratory phase of respiration, whereas the intervening periods denote the expiratory phase. *(Redrawn from Kollai M, Koizumi K: J Auton Nerv Syst 1:33, 1979.)*

Reflex and central factors both contribute to the genesis of the respiratory cardiac arrhythmia. During inspiration, the lung volume increases, and the intrathoracic pressure decreases (see Chapter 28). Lung distention stimulates pulmonary stretch receptors and tends to increase the heart rate reflexly. The reduction in intrathoracic pressure during inspiration increases venous return to the right side of the heart (see Figure 24-12). The resulting distention of the right atrium elicits the Bainbridge reflex (Figure 19-5). After the time delay required for the increased systemic venous return to reach the left side of the heart, the left ventricular stroke volume increases and thereby raises systemic arterial blood pressure. This in turn reduces the heart rate reflexly through baroreceptor stimulation (Figure 19-4).

The respiratory center in the medulla oblongata directly influences the nearby cardiac autonomic centers. This influence has been established in anesthetized animals that have been placed on heart-lung machines. In such preparations, the chest is open, the lungs are collapsed, and the arterial blood pressure and central venous pressure do not fluctuate rhythmically. Nevertheless, respiratory movements of the rib cage and diaphragm demonstrate that the medullary respiratory center is still active. Cyclic heart rate changes accompany the respiratory movements. These rhythmic changes in heart rate are almost certainly induced by a direct interaction between the respiratory and cardiac centers in the medulla.

Arterial chemoreceptors affect cardiac function

The cardiac response to peripheral chemoreceptor stimulation (see Chapter 23) merits special consideration because it illustrates the complexity that may be introduced when one stimulus simultaneously excites two organ systems. In intact animals, stimulation of the carotid chemoreceptors consistently increases ventila-

tory rate and depth (see Chapter 31) but usually has little effect on heart rate. The small, directional changes in heart rate are related to the enhancement of pulmonary ventilation. When chemoreceptor stimulation augments respiration only slightly, the heart rate usually decreases; when the increment in pulmonary ventilation is more pronounced, the heart rate usually increases.

The cardiac response to peripheral chemoreceptor stimulation is the result of primary and secondary reflex mechanisms (Figure 19-8). THE PRIMARY REFLEX EFFECT OF CAROTID CHEMORECEPTOR EXCITATION IS TO STIMULATE THE MEDULLARY VAGAL CENTERS AND THEREBY INHIBIT THE AUTOMATICITY OF THE SA NODE; this primary effect becomes evident when the usual respiratory response is absent. THE SECONDARY REFLEX EFFECTS OF RESPIRATORY EXCITATION TEND TO INHIBIT THE MEDULLARY VAGAL CENTERS AND THEREBY INCREASE HEART RATE. Therefore the respiratory effects of chemoreceptor stimulation tend to mask the primary inhibitory effects that chemoreceptor stimulation exerts on the SA node (Figure 19-8).

A dramatic example of the primary inhibitory influence of chemoreceptor stimulation on heart rate in a human is displayed in Figure 19-9. This electrocardiogram was recorded from a quadriplegic patient who was unable to breathe naturally because of a severe injury to his cervical spinal cord; he required tracheal intubation and artificial respiration. When the tracheal catheter was disconnected briefly to permit removal of excess tracheal secretions, the patient developed marked bradycardia within seconds. The bradycardia reflects the primary inhibitory effects of the chemoreceptor stimulation on heart rate evoked by the hypoxia (diminished arterial O_2 tension [PaO_2]) and hypercapnia (increased arterial CO_2 tension [$PaCO_2$]) that resulted by the patient's inability to breathe (Figure 19-8). The primary inhibitory effects were not opposed by the blood gas changes and pulmonary stretch effects that ordinarily prevail in patients who can breathe normally. The bradycardia could be prevented temporarily in this patient by injecting the muscarinic receptor antagonist **atropine,** and the onset of the bradycardia could be delayed substantially by mechanically hyperventilating the patient's lungs before disconnecting the tracheal cannula.

Sensory receptors in the ventricles regulate cardiac function

Sensory receptors located near the ventricular endocardium initiate reflex effects similar to those elicited by the arterial baroreceptors. Excitation of these endocardial receptors diminishes the heart rate and peripheral vascular resistance. The receptors discharge in a pattern that parallels the changes in ventricular pressure. Impulses that originate in these receptors are transmitted to the medulla oblongata via the vagus nerves.

Other sensory receptors have been identified in the epi-

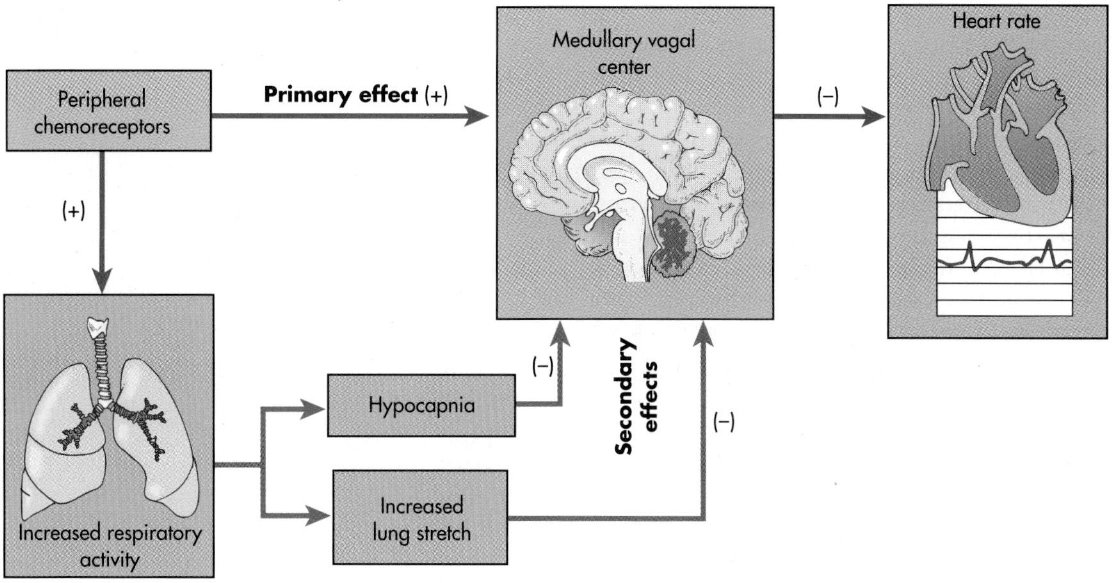

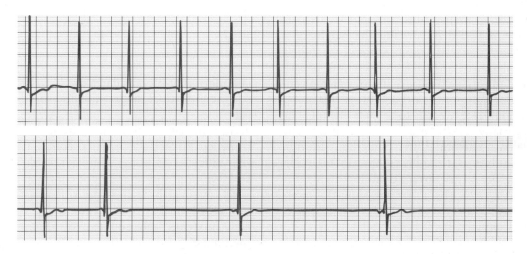

Figure 19-8 The primary effect of arterial chemoreceptor stimulation on heart rate is to excite the cardiac vagal center in the medulla and thus decrease the heart rate. Chemoreceptor stimulation also excites the respiratory center in the medulla. The consequent hypocapnia and increases in lung inflation tend to inhibit the medullary vagal center. Thus the overall heart rate response is the result of these opposing influences.

Figure 19-9 Electrocardiogram of a 30-year-old man who could not breathe spontaneously and required tracheal intubation and artificial respiration because of injury to his cervical spine. The two strips are continuous. When his tracheal catheter was temporarily disconnected from the respirator (at the beginning of the top strip), his heart rate quickly decreased from 65 beats/min to about 20 beats/min. *(Redrawn from Berke JL, Levy MN: Eur Surg Res 9:75, 1977.)*

cardial regions of the ventricles. These receptors discharge in patterns unrelated to the changes in ventricular pressure. These ventricular receptors are excited by various mechanical and chemical stimuli, but their physiological functions are unclear.

Regulation of Myocardial Performance

Intrinsic and extrinsic factors regulate myocardial performance

Just as the heart can initiate its own beat in the absence of any nervous or hormonal control, so also can the myocardium adapt to changing hemodynamic conditions via mechanisms intrinsic to cardiac muscle itself. Experiments

on animals with denervated hearts as well as observations in humans with cardiac transplants reveal that this organ adjusts remarkably well to various types of stress, even in the absence of any cardiac innervation. For example, racing greyhounds with denervated hearts performed almost as well as those with intact innervation. The maximum running speed in the denervated animals was only 5% less than it was before cardiac denervation. In these dogs, the fourfold increase in cardiac output that occurred when they ran was achieved principally by an increase in stroke volume. In normal dogs the increase in cardiac output with exercise is accompanied by a proportionate increase in heart rate; stroke volume does not change much (see also Chapter 26). The cardiac adaptation in the denervated animals was not achieved entirely by intrinsic mechanisms, however; circulating catecholamines contributed significantly. When the β-adrenergic receptors, were blocked by propranolol in greyhounds with denervated hearts, their racing performance was severely impaired.

The principal intrinsic cardiac adaptation involves changes in the resting length of the myocardial fibers. This adaptation is designated **Starling's law of the heart,** or the **Frank-Starling mechanism.** The mechanical and structural bases for this mechanism have been explained in Chapters 12 and 18. However, certain other intrinsic mechanisms that do not depend on changes in resting length also help regulate myocardial performance.

Myocardial fiber length regulates myocardial contraction

In 1895, German physiologist Otto Frank described the response of the isolated frog heart to alterations in the stretching force **(preload)** on the myocardial fibers just before contraction. He observed that as preload was increased, the heart responded with a more forceful contraction. About 20 years later, English physiologist Ernest Starling described the intrinsic response of the canine heart to changes in right atrial and aortic pressure in the isolated heart-lung preparation.

In the heart-lung preparation, the right ventricular filling pressure is varied by altering the height of a reservoir connected to the right atrium; the filling pressure just before ventricular contraction constitutes the preload for the myocardial fibers in the ventricular wall. The right ventricle then pumps this blood through the pulmonary vessels to the left atrium. The lungs are artificially ventilated. Blood is pumped by the left ventricle into the aortic arch and then through some external tubing back to the right atrial reservoir. A resistance device in the external tubing allows the investigator to control the aortic pressure; this pressure constitutes the **afterload** for left ventricular ejection (see also Chapter 18).

One of Starling's recordings of the changes in ventricular volume evoked by a sudden increase in right atrial pressure is shown in Figure 19-10. Aortic pressure in this experiment was permitted to increase only slightly when right atrial pressure (preload) was increased. In the top tracing in Figure 19-10, an increase in ventricular volume is registered as a downward deflection; hence the upper border of the tracing represents the systolic ventricular volume, the lower border indicates the diastolic ventricular volume, and the width of the tracing reflects the stroke volume (i.e., the volume of blood ejected by a ventricle during each heartbeat).

For several beats after the rise in preload, the ventricular volume progressively increases. This indicates that a disparity exists between ventricular inflow during diastole and ventricular outflow during systole; that is, during a given systole, the volume of blood expelled by the ventricles is not as great as the volume that entered them during the preceding diastole. This progressive accumulation of blood dilates the ventricles and lengthens the individual myocardial fibers in the walls of the ventricles.

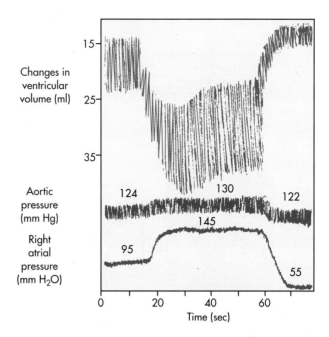

Figure 19-10 Changes in ventricular volume in a canine heart-lung preparation when right atrial pressure was suddenly increased from 95 to 145 mm H_2O and subsequently lowered to 55 mm H_2O. The increase in ventricular volume is registered as a downward shift in the volume tracing. *(Redrawn from Patterson SW, Piper H, Starling EH: J Physiol [Lond] 48:465, 1914.)*

The increased diastolic volume and fiber length somehow facilitate ventricular contraction and enable the ventricles to pump a greater stroke volume. Diastolic volume and fiber length continue to increase on successive heartbeats in response to a sustained increase in preload until at equilibrium, the cardiac output exactly matches the augmented filling volume. The mechanism by which increased fiber length enhances the stroke volume depends in part on a change in the number of interacting cross-bridges between the thick and thin filaments. More important, changes in the length of myocardial fibers substantially alter the sensitivity of the contractile proteins to calcium. An optimum fiber length exists, however, beyond which contraction is impaired (see Chapters 12 and 18). Therefore excessively high preloads may depress rather than enhance the pumping capacity of the ventricles by overstretching the myocardial fibers.

Pronounced changes in preload occur most commonly as a consequence of changes in blood volume. For example, the acute loss of blood **(hemorrhage)** is accompanied by reduced pressure in the great central veins; hence the cardiac filling pressure (preload) is also diminished. Even though blood loss also usually leads to a concomitant reduction in arterial blood pressure (afterload), the influence of preload on cardiac output usually predominates over the influence of afterload, and cardiac output usually decreases in response to hemorrhage (see also Chapters 24 and 26). Large blood transfusions, on the other hand, increase the cardiac filling pressure and therefore increase cardiac output.

Changes in diastolic fiber length also permit the isolated heart to compensate for increased afterload. In Starling's experiments on the heart-lung preparation, arterial pressure (afterload) was abruptly raised while ventricular filling pressure (preload) was held constant. Initially, the increased afterload diminished the ventricular stroke volume. Because venous return to the right atrium was held constant in these experiments, the volume of blood in the ventricles progressively increased for the next several heartbeats. Consequently, the lengths of the ventricular myocardial fibers increased. This change in end-diastolic fiber length finally enabled the ventricles to pump a stroke volume equal to the control stroke volume despite the greater ventricular afterload.

When cardiac compensation involves ventricular dilation, the force required by each myocardial fiber to generate a given intraventricular systolic pressure must be appreciably greater than that developed by the fibers in a ventricle of normal size. The relationship among the ventricular volume, intraventricular pressure, and force that prevails in the ventricular myocardial fibers resembles the relationship for cylindrical tubes (**Laplace's law** [see Chapter 22]) in that for a constant internal pressure, the intramural force (wall tension) varies directly with the radius (see Figure 22-2). Consequently, to attain any given intraventricular pressure, the myocardial fibers in a dilated heart must develop considerably more force than the fibers in a normal-sized heart; therefore these fibers require considerably more O_2 to perform a given amount of external work than those in a normal-sized heart (see also Chapter 25).

The most common clinical condition characterized by a chronic increase in afterload is **essential hypertension,** which is a sustained increase in arterial blood pressure of unknown cause. The principal hemodynamic change responsible for the elevated blood pressure is a generalized arteriolar vasoconstriction. The heart adapts initially to this increased afterload by an increase in diastolic ventricular volume, as previously explained. Ultimately, however, the mass of ventricular muscle cells also increases; that is, the heart **hypertrophies.** This constitutes an additional mechanism by which the heart adapts to a sustained increase in afterload.

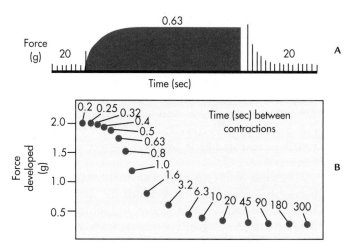

Figure 19-11 **A,** Changes in force development in an isolated papillary muscle from a cat as the interval between contractions was changed from 20 seconds to 0.63 second and then back to 20 seconds. **B,** Steady-state forces developed at the indicated intervals (in seconds). *(Redrawn from Koch-Weser J, Blinks JR: Pharmacol Rev 15:601, 1963.)*

The Frank-Starling mechanism is ideally suited for matching the cardiac output to the venous return and for ensuring that the amount of blood pumped by one ventricle over a substantial series of heartbeats equals the amount of blood pumped by the other ventricle over that same series of beats. Any sudden, excessive output by one ventricle soon results in a greater venous return to the other ventricle. The consequent increase in diastolic fiber length in this other ventricle stimulates increased output by the second ventricle to a value that approaches the output of its mate. For this reason, IT IS THE FRANK-STARLING MECHANISM THAT MAINTAINS A PRECISE BALANCE OVER TIME BETWEEN THE OUTPUTS OF THE RIGHT AND LEFT VENTRICLES. Because the two ventricles are arranged in series in a closed circuit, even a small, maintained imbalance in the outputs of the two ventricles would be catastrophic because the blood volume in one of the vascular systems (systemic or pulmonic) would progressively increase and the blood volume of the other vascular system would progressively diminish.

Contraction frequency alters myocardial contraction
The effects of contraction frequency on the force developed in an isometrically contracting cat papillary muscle are shown in Figure 19-11, *A.* Initially the strip of cardiac muscle was stimulated to contract only once every 20 seconds. When the pacing cycle length was decreased to once every 0.63 second, the developed force increased progressively over the next several beats. This progressive increase in developed force induced by a change in contraction frequency is known as the **staircase,** or **Treppe, phenomenon.** At the new steady state, the developed force was more than five times greater than it was at the longer pacing cycle length. A return to the longer cycle length had the opposite influence on developed force.

The effect of the pacing cycle length on the steady-state level of developed force is shown in Figure 19-11, *B,* for a wide range of cycle lengths. As the cycle length was diminished from 300 seconds down to about 10 seconds, developed force increased only slightly. However, as the cycle length was reduced further, to a value of about 0.5 second, the developed force increased sharply. Further reduction of the cycle length to 0.2 second had little additional effect on developed force.

The progressive rise in developed force as the interval between contractions was suddenly decreased (e.g., from 20 seconds to 0.63 second in Figure 19-11, *A*) is mediated by a gradual rise in the intracellular Ca^{++} content. Ca^{++} enters the cell during each action potential plateau (see Chapter 17). Hence when the time between contractions is reduced (i.e., when the contraction frequency is increased), the Ca^{++} influx per minute increases. As the contraction frequency increases, the action potential plateau shortens (see Figure 17-6), and therefore less Ca^{++} enters the myocardial cell per contraction. However, the fractional increment in the number of beats per minute exceeds the fractional decrement in the Ca^{++} influx per beat. Therefore the intracellular Ca^{++} content rises when the contraction frequency is raised, and hence the contractile force is augmented, as shown in Figure 19-11.

Neural and humoral factors regulate myocardial contraction

Although the heart possesses effective intrinsic mechanisms of adaptation, various extrinsic mechanisms are also important in regulating myocardial contractility. Under many natural conditions the extrinsic mechanisms dominate the intrinsic mechanisms. The extrinsic regulatory factors may be subdivided into nervous and humoral components.

Autonomic nerves regulate myocardial contraction

SYMPATHETIC INFLUENCES. Sympathetic neural activity enhances atrial and ventricular contractility. The density of the sympathetic innervation of the atria and SA and AV nodes is about three times that of the ventricles.

The alterations in ventricular contraction evoked by electrical stimulation of the cardiac sympathetic nerves in an anesthetized dog are shown in Figure 19-12. In this experiment, the heart and lungs were functionally isolated from the rest of the body, and the heart rate was maintained constant by electrical pacing of the right atrium. All venous return to the heart was interrupted, and the coronary arteries were perfused with oxygenated blood at a constant arterial pressure by a heart-lung perfusion apparatus similar to that used clinically for open-heart operations. This perfusion apparatus was also used to maintain adequate perfusion of the entire systemic circulation.

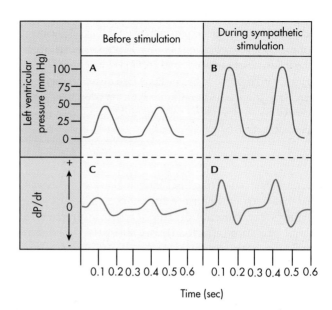

Figure 19-12 In an isovolumic preparation of a canine left ventricle, the left ventricular pressure and rate of change of left ventricular pressure, recorded under control conditions, are shown in **A** and **C,** respectively. Stimulation of the cardiac sympathetic nerves increases the peak left ventricular pressure **(B)** and the maximum rise-and-fall rates of intraventricular pressure (dP/dt) **(D).** (*Unpublished tracing from experiments of Levy MN et al:* Circ Res 19:5, 1966.)

To determine the effects of sympathetic neural activity on cardiac performance, a balloon was inserted into the left ventricle, and enough saline was instilled into the balloon to fill the entire chamber. Because saline is virtually incompressible, the ventricular contractions were isovolumic. When the cardiac sympathetic nerves were stimulated in this preparation, the peak ventricular pressure (Figure 19-12, *B*) and the maximum rate of pressure rise (dP/dt) during systole (Figure 19-12, *D*) were markedly increased. Also, the rate of ventricular relaxation (as indicated by the minimum value of dP/dt) was increased (Figure 19-12, *D*).

Sympathetic stimulation not only enhances the mechanical contraction of the heart but also facilitates ventricular filling. For example, in an experiment (Figure 19-13) on an intact, anesthetized dog not placed on heart-lung bypass, the animal's heart was paced at a constant rate. Stimulation of the cardiac sympathetic nerves increased aortic blood pressure substantially (Figure 19-13, *B*) and increased the stroke volume (not shown). Concurrently, the sympathetic stimulation shortened ventricular systole (Figure 19-13, *D*) and diminished left ventricular pressure during diastole (Figure 19-13, *D*); both of these responses facilitate ventricular filling. The reason for the sympathetically induced reduction in the ventricular diastolic pressure (i.e., preload) is explained in Chapter 24.

The overall effect of increased cardiac sympathoadrenal activity on ventricular performance in intact animals can best be appreciated in terms of families of **ventricular function curves** (see also Chapter 24). Such curves depict the changes in left ventricular perfor-

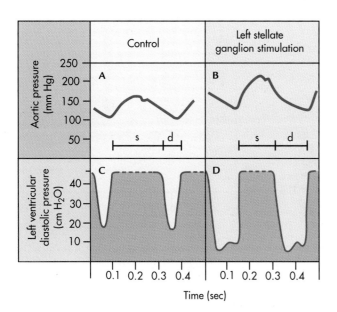

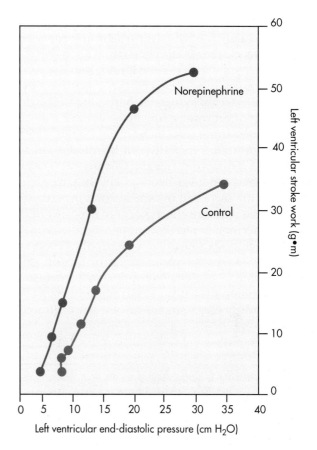

Figure 19-13 Stimulation of the cardiac sympathetic nerves (left stellate ganglion) of an anesthetized dog increases aortic pressure (**A** and **B**) but decreases left ventricular diastolic pressure (**C** and **D**). Note also the abridgment of systole *(s)*, which allows more time in diastole *(d)* for ventricular filling (**D**); the heart was paced at a constant rate. In **C** and **D**, the pen excursion cannot exceed 45 mm Hg *(dashed horizontal lines)*; actual peak ventricular pressures during systole can be estimated from **A** and **B**. *(Redrawn from Mitchell JH, Linden RJ, Sarnoff SJ: Circ Res 8:1100, 1960.)*

Figure 19-14 During a constant infusion of norepinephrine in an anesthetized dog, the left ventricle accomplishes more stroke work than it does under controlled conditions. This effect of norepinephrine is reflected by a leftward shift of the ventricular function curve. *(Redrawn from Sarnoff SJ et al: Circ Res 8:1108, 1960.)*

mance as a function of the end-diastolic pressure (preload) in the ventricle. In the experiment shown in Figure 19-14, **stroke work** (the product of stroke volume and mean aortic pressure) was used as the index of performance. When sympathoadrenal activity was increased by the infusion of norepinephrine, the ventricle was able to accomplish more stroke work at any given level of ventricular end-diastolic pressure; that is, the ventricular function curves are shifted to the left (Figure 19-14).

SYMPATHOADRENAL ACTIVITY ENHANCES MYOCARDIAL PERFORMANCE MAINLY BY FACILITATING THE INFLUX OF Ca^{++} INTO MYOCYTES. The adrenergic agonists norepinephrine and epinephrine interact with β-adrenergic receptors in the cardiac cell membranes. This interaction activates **adenylyl cyclase,** which raises the intracellular levels of **cyclic AMP** (see also Chapters 5, 18, and 47).

PARASYMPATHETIC INFLUENCES. The vagus nerves strongly inhibit the SA node, atrial myocardium, and AV conduction tissue. These parasympathetic nerves also depress the ventricular myocardium, but the effects are less pronounced. In the total heart bypass preparation (such as that used to derive Figure 19-12), vagal stimulation decreases the peak left ventricular pressure and the maximum rates (dP/dt) of pressure development and pressure decline. The effects are opposite to those elicited by sympathetic stimulation (see Figure 19-12).

The effects of increased vagal activity on the ventricular myocardium are achieved largely by antagonizing the facilitatory effects of any concurrent sympathetic activity. This antagonism takes place at two levels. At the level of the autonomic nerve endings in the heart,

the acetylcholine released from vagal endings inhibits the release of norepinephrine from nearby sympathetic endings. At the level of the cardiac cell membranes, the rise in intracellular cyclic AMP that would ordinarily be produced in response to a given quantity of neurally released norepinephrine is attenuated by the acetylcholine released from nearby vagal endings.

These antagonistic interactions between the sympathetic and vagal effects on the ventricular myocardium also take place in other cardiac structures, such as the SA node. For example, in the experiment shown in Figure 19-3, sympathetic stimulation alone at a frequency of 4 Hz substantially increased heart rate. However, during combined sympathetic and vagal stimulation, the vagal influence was so predominant that the heart rate response to combined stimulation did not differ perceptibly from the effects of vagal stimulation alone.

Chemical constituents of the blood regulate myocardial contraction

HORMONES. Various hormones influence cardiac function. The principal hormone secreted by the adrenal medulla is **epinephrine,** although a small quantity of norepinephrine is also released (see Chapter 47). The rate of catecholamine secretion by the adrenal medulla is regulated by essentially the same mechanisms that control the activity of the sympathetic nervous system, and the effects of those catecholamines on the heart are qualitatively similar to those released from the sympathetic nerve endings. However, the concentrations of circulating catecholamines rarely rise high enough to appreciably affect cardiac function.

Numerous studies on intact animals and humans have demonstrated that **thyroid hormones** enhance myocardial contractility (see also Chapter 45). The rates of Ca^{++} uptake and ATP hydrolysis by the sarcoplasmic reticulum are increased in experimental hyperthyroidism, and the opposite effects occur in hypothyroidism. Thyroid hormones increase protein synthesis in the heart, which leads to cardiac hypertrophy. These hormones also affect the composition of myosin isoenzymes in cardiac muscle. They principally increase the concentrations of isoenzymes with the greatest ATPase activity and thereby enhance myocardial contractility substantially.

> Cardiac activity is sluggish in patients with inadequate thyroid function **(hypothyroidism);** that is, the heart rate is slow, and cardiac output is diminished. The converse is true in patients with overactive thyroid glands **(hyperthyroidism).** Characteristically, such patients exhibit tachycardia, high cardiac output, palpitations, and arrhythmias.

Insulin enhances myocardial contractility in several mammals. The effect of insulin is evident even when hypoglycemia is prevented by glucose infusions and when the β-adrenergic receptors are blocked. In fact, the insulin-induced enhancement of contractility is potentiated by β-adrenergic receptor blockade. The improved contractility cannot be explained satisfactorily by the concomitant increase of glucose transport into the myocardial cells.

Glucagon has potent positive inotropic and chronotropic effects on the heart. The endogenous hormone is probably not involved in the normal regulation of the cardiovascular system, but it has been used pharmacologically to treat various cardiac conditions. The effects of glucagon on the heart closely resemble those of the catecholamines, and some of the metabolic effects are similar.

BLOOD GASES.   Changes in the PaO_2 of the blood perfusing the brain and the peripheral chemoreceptors affect the heart through nervous mechanisms, as described earlier in this chapter. These indirect effects of hypoxia are usually prepotent. Moderate degrees of hypoxia characteristically increase the heart rate, cardiac output, and myocardial contractility by increasing sympathetic nervous activity. These changes are largely abolished by β-adrenergic receptor blockade. The PaO_2

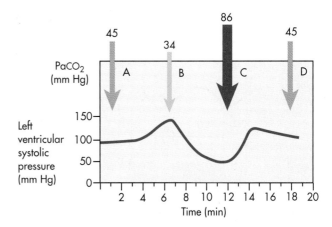

Figure 19-15   A decrease in the $PaCO_2$ from 45 to 34 mm Hg increases left ventricular systolic pressure (arrow B) in an isovolumic canine left ventricle. A subsequent rise in the $PaCO_2$ to 86 mm Hg has the reverse effect. When the $PaCO_2$ is returned to the control level (45 mm Hg), the left ventricular systolic pressure returns to its original value. *(Derived from experiments by Ng ML et al: Am J Physiol 213:115, 1967.)*

of blood perfusing the myocardium also directly influences myocardial performance. The effect of hypoxia is biphasic; moderate degrees are stimulatory, and more severe degrees are depressant.

Changes in the $PaCO_2$ may also directly and indirectly affect the myocardium. The indirect, neurally mediated effects produced by increased $PaCO_2$ are similar to those evoked by a decrease in PaO_2. The direct effects on myocardial performance elicited by changes in $PaCO_2$ in the coronary arterial blood are illustrated in Figure 19-15. In this experiment on an isolated left ventricle, the control $PaCO_2$ was 45 mm Hg (arrow A). Decreasing the $PaCO_2$ to 34 mm Hg (arrow B) was stimulatory, whereas increasing the $PaCO_2$ to 86 mm Hg (arrow C) was depressant. In intact animals, systemic increases in the $PaCO_2$ activates the sympathoadrenal system, and this change tends to compensate for the direct depressant effect of the increased $PaCO_2$ on the heart.

Neither the $PaCO_2$ nor the blood pH is a primary determinant of myocardial behavior; the induced change in intracellular pH is the critical factor. The reduced intracellular pH diminishes the influx of Ca^{++} into the cell via the Ca^{++} channels and the Na^+-Ca^{++} exchanger, and it decreases the amount of Ca^{++} released from the sarcoplasmic reticulum in response to excitation of the myocyte. Intracellular acidosis also directly affects the myofilaments. When they are exposed to a given concentration of Ca^{++}, the myofibrils develop less force as the prevailing intracellular pH decreases.

Figure 19-16 shows the relationship between the changes in contractile performance and intracellular pH when perfusion is halted in an isolated, perfused rabbit heart. When flow ceased, the left ventricular pressure diminished rapidly until the contraction virtually ceased. These changes were accompanied by a

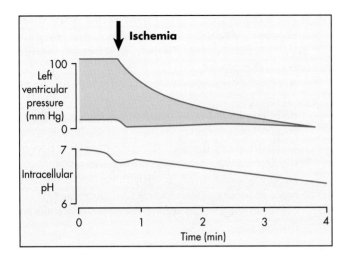

Figure 19-16 Effect of ischemia on left ventricular pressure and intracellular pH in an isolated, perfused rabbit heart. *(Redrawn from Mohabir R et al:* Circ Res *69:1525, 1991.)*

progressive reduction in intracellular pH from a control value of 7.0 to a value of about 6.3 after 4 minutes of ischemia.

In patients with coronary artery disease, a narrowed region of a major coronary artery may suddenly become occluded by a blood clot; this is the most common cause of a "heart attack." The consequent inadequate blood flow **(myocardial ischemia)** to the myocardial tissue leads to progressive impairment of the contractile function of the deprived myocardial cells. This impaired contractility is mediated by a combination of extracellular and intracellular changes in the blood gases and in the pH of the ischemic region. These changes include reductions in P_{O_2} and pH and increases in P_{CO_2}.

SUMMARY

- Cardiac function is regulated by various intrinsic and extrinsic mechanisms.
- The heart rate is regulated mainly by the autonomic nervous system. Sympathetic activity increases and parasympathetic (vagal) activity decreases heart rate.
- The baroreceptor, chemoreceptor, pulmonary inflation, atrial receptor (Bainbridge), and ventricular receptor reflexes all regulate heart rate.
- The principal intrinsic mechanisms that regulate myocardial contraction are the Frank-Starling and rate-related mechanisms.
- The autonomic nervous system regulates myocardial performance mainly by varying the Ca^{++} conductance of the cell membrane via the adenylyl cyclase system.

- Various hormones, including epinephrine, adrenocortical steroids, thyroid hormones, insulin, and glucagon, regulate myocardial performance.
- Changes in the blood concentrations of O_2, CO_2, and H^+ alter cardiac function directly and reflexly.

BIBLIOGRAPHY

Armour JA, Ardell JL, eds: *Neurocardiology,* New York, 1994, Oxford University Press.

Dampney RAL: Functional organization of central pathways regulating the cardiovascular system, *Physiol Rev* 74:323, 1994.

Fozzard HA et al, eds: *Heart and cardiovascular system: scientific foundations,* ed 2, New York, 1991, Raven.

Garfein OB, ed: *Current concepts in cardiovascular physiology,* San Diego, 1990, Academic.

Hainsworth R: Reflexes from the heart, *Physiol Rev* 71:617, 1991.

Hartzell HC: Regulation of cardiac ion channels by catecholamines, acetylcholine, and second messenger systems, *Prog Biophys Mol Biol* 52:165, 1988.

Levy MN: Autonomic interactions in cardiac control, *Ann NY Acad Sci* 601:209, 1990.

Levy MN, Schwartz PJ, eds: *Vagal control of the heart: experimental basis and clinical implications,* Armonk, NY, 1993, Futura.

Marshall JM: Peripheral chemoreceptors and cardiovascular regulation, *Physiol Rev* 74:543, 1994.

Polikar R: Thyroid and the heart, *Circulation* 87:1435, 1993.

Shepherd JT, Vatner SF, eds: *Nervous control of the heart,* Amsterdam, 1996, Harwood Academic.

Sperelakis N, ed: *Physiology and pathophysiology of the heart,* ed 2, Boston, 1995, Kluwer Academic.

Spyer KM: Central nervous mechanisms contributing to cardiovascular control, *J Physiol (Lond)* 474:1, 1994.

Walley KR, Ford LE, Wood LDH : Effects of hypoxia and hypercapnia on the force-velocity relation of rabbit myocardium, *Circ Res* 69:1616, 1991.

Zucker IH, Gilmore JP: *Reflex control of the circulation,* Boca Raton, Fla, 1990, CRC.

CASE STUDY

Case 19-1

A 48-year-old woman was susceptible to occasional, usually brief, episodes of lightheadedness. She noticed that her heart rate was very rapid during these episodes, and that the lightheadedness disappeared when her heart rate returned to normal. Her physician noted no significant abnormalities during physical examination but obtained a 24-hour recording of the patient's electrocardiogram. On reviewing this recording, the physician detected a 7-minute period during which the patient's heart rate increased abruptly from a resting value of about 75 beats/min to a steady level of about 145 beats/min. At the end of the 7 minutes of tachycardia, the heart rate decreased abruptly and attained the resting value again of about 75 beats/min within 1 minute. The patient's problem was diagnosed as paroxysmal supraventricular tachycardia, which is a sudden, pronounced increase in heart rate; this problem is mediated usually by a reentry circuit in the AV junction. During a subsequent visit to her physician, the paroxysmal tachycardia appeared spontaneously. The doctor was able to terminate the tachycardia promptly by carotid sinus massage (i.e., massaging the patient's neck just below the angles of the jaw in the region of the bifurcations of the common carotid arteries). The physician noted that the patient's arterial blood pressure during the tachycardia was 95/75 mm Hg during the tachycardia and that it returned to a value of 130/85 mm Hg (the patient's usual resting blood pressure) soon after termination of the tachycardia.

1. **What would cause a reduction in the patient's mean arterial pressure during the paroxysmal tachycardia?**
   A. A reflex decrease in myocardial contractility
   B. A reflex increase in cardiac cycle duration
   C. A reflex decrease in AV conduction velocity
   D. A reflex increase in norepinephrine release from the cardiac sympathetic nerves
   E. A reflex decrease in calcium conductance of myocytes during the action potential plateau

2. **What would cause a sudden, substantial increase in efferent vagal activity (induced by carotid sinus massage, for example)?**
   A. Strengthening of the contraction of atrial myocytes
   B. Strengthening of the stimulatory action of any concurrent sympathetic activity
   C. Increase in the speed of impulse conduction in the ventricular Purkinje fibers
   D. Decrease in the heart rate within one or two cardiac cycles
   E. Shortening of the AV conduction time

3. **When the patient was in a normal sinus rhythm, what would administration of a medication that antagonizes the muscarinic cholinergic receptors do?**
   A. Abolish or dampen any rhythmic changes in heart rate that occur at the patient's respiratory frequency
   B. Weaken the contractions of the atrial myocytes
   C. Delay AV conduction
   D. Decrease the action potential duration in atrial myocytes
   E. Hyperpolarize the atrial myocytes during the resting phase (phase 4) of the action potential

4. **If the patient had a prominent respiratory sinus arrhythmia when she was not afflicted by the paroxysmal tachycardia, which functional change would take place?**
   A. Efferent vagal activity would decrease during inspiration.
   B. Efferent cardiac sympathetic activity would decrease during inspiration.
   C. The slope of the slow diastolic depolarization of the SA cells would decrease during inspiration.
   D. The respiratory sinus arrhythmia would become more pronounced in response to hemorrhage.
   E. Propranolol would abolish the respiratory sinus arrhythmia.

5. **Why does the heart rate response to vagal activity disappear rapidly when neural activity in the vagus nerves suddenly ceases?**
   A. The cardiac cells gradually become more responsive to acetylcholine.
   B. The vagus nerve endings rapidly take up the released acetylcholine.
   C. The cardiac myocytes rapidly take up the released acetylcholine.
   D. The acetylcholine in the nerve endings is rapidly depleted.
   E. The abundant acetylcholinesterase rapidly degrades the released acetylcholine.

CHAPTER 20

Hemodynamics

- Define the relationship between the velocity of blood flow and cross-sectional area of the vascular bed.
- Describe the factors that govern the relationship between blood flow and pressure gradient.
- Distinguish between resistances in series and resistances in parallel.
- Compare laminar and turbulent flow.
- Describe the influence of the particulates in blood on blood flow.

The electrical and mechanical characteristics of the heart have been described in the preceding chapters. The generation of the signal that initiates the cardiac contraction has been described, the processes involved in excitation-contraction coupling have been explained, and the factors that regulate the cardiac contraction have been identified. This chapter begins to describe the physical factors that regulate blood flow through the various vascular beds. Subsequent chapters describe how the behavior of the blood vessels is regulated.

Various Physical Factors Govern Blood Flow

The fluid mechanics of the circulatory system are very complicated and therefore difficult to analyze precisely. The heart is an intermittent pump, and its behavior is regulated by many physical and chemical factors. The blood vessels are branched, distensible conduits of continuously varying dimensions. The blood is a suspension mainly of erythrocytes but also leukocytes, platelets, and lipid globules, all dispersed in the plasma, which is a colloidal solution of proteins. Despite this complexity, however, an understanding of the relevant, elementary principles of fluid mechanics provides considerable insight into the physical behavior of the vascular system. Certain basic principles are expounded in this chapter in an attempt to illuminate the interrelationships among vascular geometry, blood velocity, blood flow, and blood pressure.

Velocity of the Bloodstream

The relationship between the velocity of the bloodstream and the dimensions of the vascular bed is illustrated by the set of conduits in Figure 20-1; **velocity (v)** refers to the displacement of a particle of the blood per unit time. Consider that the conduit is rigid and that it has a wide section (area $A_1 = 5$ cm^2) and a narrow section (area $A_2 = 1$ cm^2). Also, let an incompressible fluid enter the wide end of the tube at a flow of 5 cm^3/sec (Q_1); **flow (Q)** refers to the volume of fluid that passes a given cross section of the conduit per unit time. Then the velocity (v_1) of a fluid particle as it passes cross section A_1 would be:

$$v_1 = Q_1/A_1 = 1 \text{ cm/sec} \qquad \text{20-1}$$

Thus a particle of fluid advances a distance (ΔL_1) of 1 cm each second (Figure 20-1). When the fluid enters the narrow section of the tube, the volume (Q_2) of fluid that passes cross section A_2 each second must equal the volume (Q_1) that had passed cross section A_1 each second; that is, $Q_2 = Q_1$. The velocity in the narrow section (v_2) would be:

$$v_2 = Q_2/A_2 = 5 \text{ cm/sec} \qquad \text{20-2}$$

Thus each particle of fluid must move past section A_2 five times faster than past section A_1. By the law of conservation of mass:

$$Q_1 = Q_2 \qquad \text{20-3}$$

From Equations 20-1 to 20-3 therefore:

$$v_1/v_2 = A_2/A_1 \qquad \text{20-4}$$

Hence when the caliber of a tube varies with the axial location along the tube, the fluid velocities at these axial sites are inversely proportional to the corresponding cross-sectional areas. This relationship also holds true for more complex hydraulic systems, such as the circulatory system, which is composed of numerous conduits of different calibers and aligned both in series and in parallel.

Note that in Figure 15-3 the velocity decreases progressively as the blood flows through the aorta, its primary and secondary branches, the arterioles, and finally the capillaries. As the blood then passes through the

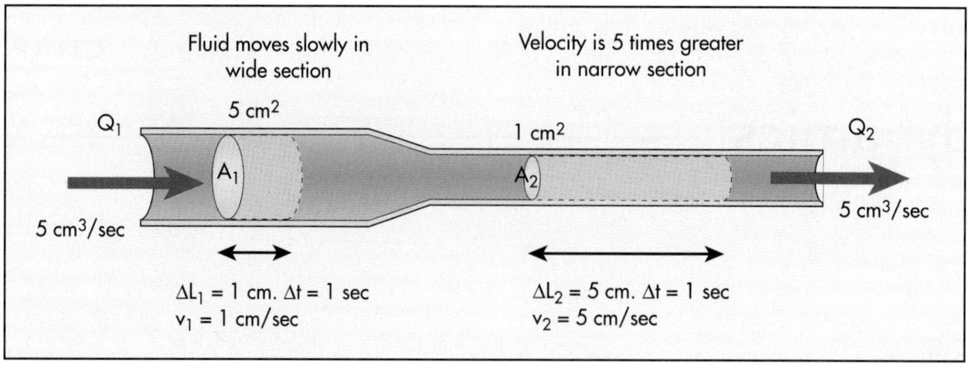

Figure 20-1 In a conduit that contains a wide segment and a narrow segment, the fluid velocities in the two segments are inversely proportional to the cross-sectional areas of the segments.

venules and continues centrally through the intermediate veins toward the venae cavae, the velocity increases progressively again. The velocities in the various serial sections of the circulatory system are inversely proportional to the total cross-sectional areas of the respective sections. The total cross-sectional area of all the parallel systemic capillaries greatly exceeds the total cross-sectional area of any other serial section of the systemic vascular bed (see Figure 15-3). Hence the velocity of the bloodstream in the capillaries is much less than that in any other vascular segment. ᴛʜᴇ ᴠᴇʀʏ sʟᴏᴡ ᴍᴏᴠᴇᴍᴇɴᴛ ᴏғ ᴛʜᴇ ʙʟᴏᴏᴅ ᴛʜʀᴏᴜɢʜ ᴛʜᴇ ᴄᴀᴘɪʟʟᴀʀɪᴇs ᴀʟʟᴏᴡs ᴀᴍᴘʟᴇ ᴛɪᴍᴇ ғᴏʀ ᴛʜᴇ ᴇxᴄʜᴀɴɢᴇ ᴏғ ᴍᴀᴛᴇʀɪᴀʟs ʙᴇᴛᴡᴇᴇɴ ᴛʜᴇ ᴛɪssᴜᴇs ᴀɴᴅ ʙʟᴏᴏᴅ.

The Relationship Between Blood Flow and Pressure Depends on the Characteristics of the Blood and Conduits

The most useful equation that defines the relationships among the various physical factors that govern pressure and flow in hydraulic systems (including the circulatory system) was derived by the French physician Jean Poiseuille over a century ago. This equation, known as **Poiseuille's law,** applies to the flow of fluids through cylindrical tubes, but it applies precisely only under restricted conditions. The equation applies specifically to the steady, laminar flow of newtonian fluids. The term **steady flow** signifies the absence of variations of flow in time. **Laminar flow** is the type of motion in which the fluid moves as a series of infinitesimally thin layers, with each layer moving at a velocity different from that of its neighboring layers (see Figure 20-7). A **newtonian fluid** has certain critical physical properties that are described later. A newtonian fluid is essentially a homogeneous fluid, such as an electrolyte solution.

Flow is proportional to pressure difference

Pressure is a salient determinant of flow. The pressure (P) in dynes/cm^2, at a distance (h) in centimeters below the surface of a liquid:

$$P = h\rho g \qquad\qquad \textbf{20-5}$$

where ρ is the density of the liquid in grams per cubic centimeter, and g is the acceleration of gravity in centimeters per second squared. For convenience, however, pressure is frequently expressed in terms of the height of a column of the liquid above an arbitrary reference level.

Consider the tube that connects reservoirs R_1 and R_2 in Figure 20-2. Let reservoir R_1 be filled with liquid to height h_1 and reservoir R_2 be empty (Figure 20-2, A). The outflow pressure, P_o, is therefore equal to the atmospheric pressure, which is designated as the *zero*, or *reference, level*. The inflow pressure, P_i, is then equal to the same reference level plus the height, h_1, of the column of liquid in reservoir R_1. Under these conditions, let the flow, Q, through the tube be 5 ml/sec.

If reservoir R_1 is filled to twice the height h_2, and reservoir R_2 is again empty (Figure 20-2, B), the flow will be twice as great (i.e., 10 ml/sec) as it is in Figure 20-2, A. Thus with reservoir R_2 empty, flow through the tube will be directly proportional to the inflow pressure, P_i.

If reservoir R_2 is allowed to fill to height h_1 and the fluid level in R_1 is maintained at h_2 (Figure 20-2, C), the flow will again become 5 ml/sec. If the fluid level in reservoir R_2 attains the same height as in reservoir R_1, flow will cease; that is, Q = zero (Figure 20-2, D). ᴛʜᴜs ғʟᴏᴡ ɪs ᴅɪʀᴇᴄᴛʟʏ ᴘʀᴏᴘᴏʀᴛɪᴏɴᴀʟ ᴛᴏ ᴛʜᴇ ᴅɪғғᴇʀᴇɴᴄᴇ ʙᴇᴛᴡᴇᴇɴ ᴛʜᴇ ɪɴ-ғʟᴏᴡ ᴀɴᴅ ᴏᴜᴛғʟᴏᴡ ᴘʀᴇssᴜʀᴇs:

$$Q \propto P_i - P_o \qquad\qquad \textbf{20-6}$$

Blood flow through specific vascular beds is affected by the difference between the inflow (arterial) and outflow (venous) pressures that prevail for that vascular bed. Such pressure differences may be affected substantially by gravitational forces and by the competence of the venous valves, as explained in Chapter 24.

Blood flow through the legs and feet may be entirely different when a person is standing than when recumbent. In a standing person, the arterial blood pressure in the legs is considerably higher than the arterial blood pressure in

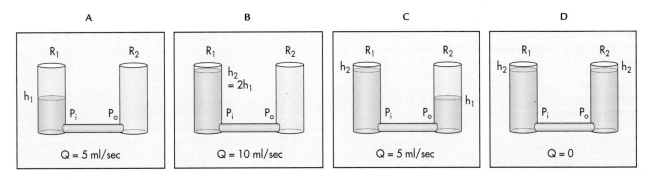

Figure 20-2 The flow *(Q)* of fluid through a tube connecting two reservoirs *(R₁ and R₂)*, is proportional to the difference between the pressure at the inflow end *(Pᵢ)* and the pressure at the outflow end *(Pₒ)* of the tube. **A,** When R_2 is empty, fluid flows from R_1 to R_2 at a rate proportional to the pressure in R_1. **B,** When the fluid level in R_1 is increased twofold, the flow increases proportionately. **C,** Flow from R_1 to R_2 is proportional to the difference between the pressures in R_1 and R_2. **D,** When the pressure in R_2 rises until it is equal to the pressure in R_1, flow ceases.

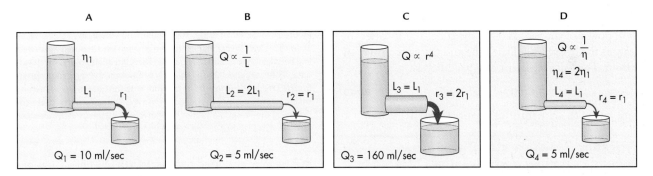

Figure 20-3 The flow *(Q)* of fluid through a tube is inversely proportional to the length *(L)* and the viscosity *(η)* and is directly proportional to the fourth power of the radius *(r)*. **A,** Reference condition: for a given pressure, length, radius, and viscosity, let the flow Q_1 equal 10 ml/sec. **B,** If the tube length doubles, flow decreases by half. **C,** If the tube radius doubles, flow increases sixteenfold. **D,** If viscosity doubles, flow decreases by half.

the thorax; this difference, of course, depends on the person's height. In a person with normal venous valves, the venous blood pressure in the legs and feet may be only slightly higher than the atmospheric pressure (see also Chapters 24 and 25). However, in a patient with **varicose veins** (abnormally dilated veins) in the legs, the venous valves are incompetent. Therefore the blood pressure in the varicose veins in the legs of a standing person may be elevated by the same amount as the arterial blood pressure in the legs. Thus the arteriovenous pressure difference and the blood flow in the legs are substantially greater in a standing person with normal venous valves than in one with varicose veins.

Blood flow depends on tube dimensions

For any given pressure difference between the two ends of a tube, the flow depends on the dimensions of the tube. If the length of the tube in Figure 20-3, *A,* is L and the radius is r_1, the flow Q_1 is observed to be 10 ml/sec.

The tube connected to the reservoir in Figure 20-3, *B,* has the same radius as that in Figure 20-3, *A,* but is twice as long. Under these conditions the flow Q_2 is found to be 5 ml/sec, or only half as great as Q_1. Conversely, for a tube half as long as L_1, the flow would be twice as great as Q_1. In

other words, flow is inversely proportional to the length of the tube:

$$Q \propto 1/L \qquad \textbf{20-7}$$

The length L_3 of the tube connected to the reservoir in Figure 20-3, *C,* is the same as L_1, but the radius r_3 is twice as great as r_1. Under these conditions, the flow Q_3 increases to a value of 160 ml/sec, which is 16 times greater than Q_1. The precise measurements of Poiseuille revealed that flow varies directly as the fourth power of the radius (just as in the previous example):

$$Q \propto r^4 \qquad \textbf{20-8}$$

Blood flow depends on blood viscosity

Finally, for a given pressure difference across a cylindrical tube of given dimensions, the flow is affected by the nature of the fluid itself. This flow-determining property of fluids is termed **viscosity (η).** Suppose that the fluid level in the reservoir in Figure 20-3, *D,* equals that in Figure 20-3, *A,* and that the tubes connected to the bottoms of both reservoirs are identical. However, if viscosity $η_4$ is twice viscosity $η_1$ in Figure 20-3, *D,* then flow Q_4 is only half the flow Q_1:

$$Q \propto 1/η \qquad \textbf{20-9}$$

For most homogeneous liquids, such as water itself or true solutions in water, this inverse proportionality prevails during laminar flow. Such fluids are said to be **newtonian.** For heterogeneous liquids, notably suspensions such as blood, this precise inverse proportionality does not apply. Such fluids are said to be **nonnewtonian.**

Poiseuille's law defines the effects of pressure, tube dimension, and viscosity on blood flow

Poiseuille's law takes into account the various factors that influence the flow of a fluid through a tube; the law applies under restricted conditions. Poiseuille's law states that for the steady, laminar flow of a newtonian fluid through a cylindrical tube, the flow (Q) varies directly as the difference between the inflow and outflow pressures $(P_i - P_o)$ and the fourth power of the radius (r) of the tube, and it varies inversely as the length (L) of the tube and the viscosity (η) of the fluid. The full statement of Poiseuille's is:

$$Q = \pi(P_i - P_o)r^4/8\eta L \qquad \textbf{20-10}$$

where $\pi/8$ is the constant of proportionality.

Hydraulic Resistance to Blood Flow Depends on Flow and Pressure Difference

In electrical theory, **resistance (R)** is defined as the ratio of voltage drop (E) to electrical current flow (I). By analogy, **hydraulic resistance (R)** may be defined as the ratio of pressure drop $(P_i - P_o)$ to fluid flow (Q). For the steady, laminar flow of a newtonian fluid through a cylindrical tube, the physical components of hydraulic resistance may be identified by rearranging Poiseuille's law to yield the hydraulic resistance equation, as follows:

$$R = (P_i - P_o)/Q = 8\eta L/\pi r^4 \qquad \textbf{20-11}$$

Thus when Poiseuille's law applies, the resistance to flow depends only on the dimensions (L and r) of the tube and on the viscosity (η) of the fluid.

THE PRINCIPAL DETERMINANT OF THE RESISTANCE TO BLOOD FLOW THROUGH ANY INDIVIDUAL VESSEL WITHIN THE CIRCULATORY SYSTEM IS ITS CALIBER because resistance varies inversely as the fourth power of the radius. The resistance to flow through small blood vessels in the cat mesentery has been measured, and the resistance per unit length of vessel (R/L) is plotted against the vessel diameter in Figure 20-4. The resistance is highest in the individual capillaries (diameter, 7 μm), and it diminishes as the vessels increase in diameter (or radius) on the arterial and venous sides of the capillaries. The values of R/L were found to be virtually proportional to the fourth power of the diameter for the larger vessels on both sides of the capillaries.

The small arteries and arterioles possess a thick coat of circularly arranged smooth muscle fibers; the lumen

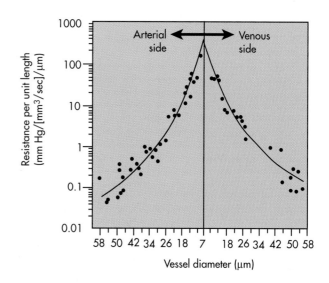

Figure 20-4 Resistance per unit length of individual small blood vessels in cat mesentery. The capillaries (diameter, 7 μm) are denoted by the vertical line between the red and blue panels. The solid circles represent the actual data. The two curves through the data represent the regression equations for the arteriole and venule data. Note that for both types of vessels, the calculated resistance per unit length is inversely proportional to the fourth power of the vessel diameter. *(Redrawn from Lipowsky HH, Kovalcheck S, Zweifach BW: Circ Res 43:738, 1978.)*

radius may be varied because of these fibers. Changes in vascular resistance are induced mainly by nervous and humoral factors that alter the contractile state of the arteriolar smooth muscle cells. The control of vascular resistance is described in Chapter 23.

In severe **arteriosclerosis,** a lipid deposit in the intima of a major artery forms a plaque that may protrude into the lumen and severely narrow it. In this event, the major resistance to flow in the vascular bed supplied by the diseased artery may reside in the large artery itself rather than in the small arteries and arterioles of the vascular bed. Such occlusive lesions in important large arteries, such as the coronary arteries, are often treated using balloon dilation (**angioplasty**) or a **surgical bypass procedure.**

Blood vessels are aligned in series and in parallel

In the cardiovascular system the various types of vessels listed along the horizontal axis in Figure 15-3 lie in **series** with one another. In vessels aligned in series, a red blood cell travels sequentially from one vessel in the series to the next and then on to the next, as illustrated in Figure 20-5. Furthermore, the individual members within each category of vessels are ordinarily arranged in **parallel** with one another (Figure 15-4). In a parallel arrangement, a red blood cell that arrives at the junction of a number of parallel vessels would have the immediate option of traveling

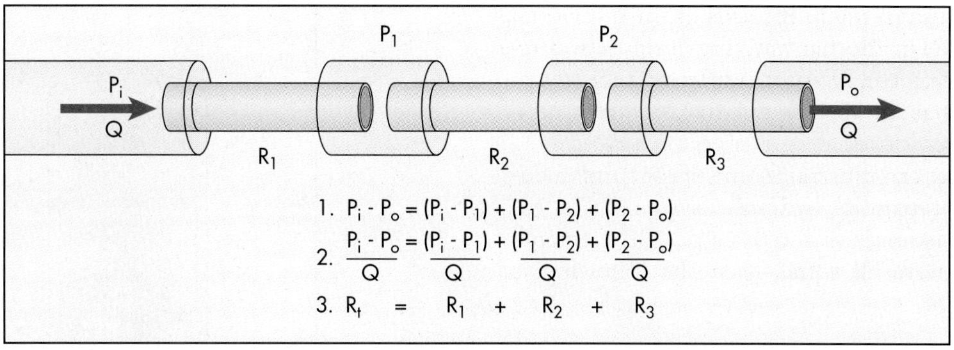

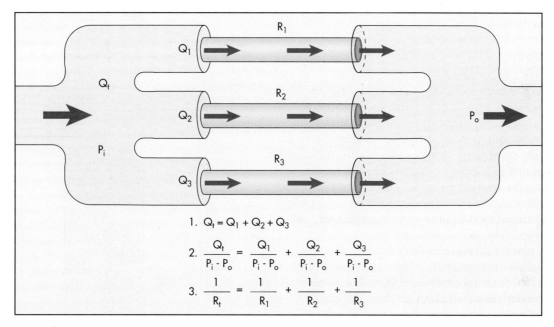

Figure 20-5 For resistances arranged in series (R_1, R_2, R_3), the total resistance (R_t) equals the sum of the individual resistances.

Figure 20-6 For resistances arranged in parallel (R_1, R_2, R_3), the reciprocal of the total resistance (R_t) equals the sum of the reciprocals of the individual resistances.

through just one of these parallel channels, as illustrated in Figure 20-6. The capillaries throughout the lungs are in parallel with one another, and similarly the capillaries throughout the systemic circulation are almost all in parallel with one another. Notable exceptions are the capillaries in the renal vasculature (wherein the peritubular capillaries are in series with the glomerular capillaries) and those in the splanchnic vasculature (wherein the hepatic capillaries are in series with the intestinal capillaries). Formulae for the total hydraulic resistance of conduits arranged in series and in parallel can be derived in the same manner as for electrical resistances.

Three hydraulic resistances (R_1, R_2, and R_3) are aligned in series in Figure 20-5. The pressure drop across the entire system (i.e., the difference between inflow pressure [P_i] and outflow pressure [P_o]) consists of the sum of the pressure drops across each of the individual resistances (Figure 20-5 and Equation 20-1). Under steady-state conditions, the flow (Q) through any given cross section must equal the

flow through any other cross section. When each component in Equation 20-1 is divided by Q (Equation 20-2), it becomes evident from the definition of resistance (i.e., R = [P_i − P_o]/Q) that the total resistance (R_t) of the entire system of resistances in series equals the sum of the individual resistances, as follows:

$$R_t = R_1 + R_2 + R_3 \qquad \textbf{20-12}$$

For resistances in parallel (Figure 20-6), all tubes have the same inflow pressures and the same outflow pressures. The total flow (Q_t) through the system equals the sum of the flows through the individual parallel elements (Figure 20-6 and Equation 20-1). Because the pressure difference (P_i − P_o) is identical for all parallel elements, each term in Equation 20-1 may be divided by that pressure difference to yield Equation 20-2 (Figure 20-6). From the definition of resistance, Equation 20-3 may be derived from Equation 20-2. Equation 20-3 (Figure 20-6) states that the reciprocal of the total resistance

(R_t) equals the sum of the reciprocals of the individual resistances. Stated in another way, if hydraulic **conductance** is defined as the reciprocal of resistance, it becomes evident that FOR TUBES IN PARALLEL, THE TOTAL CONDUCTANCE IS THE SUM OF THE INDIVIDUAL CONDUCTANCES.

A few examples can illustrate some of the fundamental properties of parallel hydraulic systems. For example, if the resistances of the three parallel elements in Figure 20-6 were all equal, then the following is established:

$$R_1 = R_2 = R_3 \qquad \textbf{20-13}$$

Therefore from Equation 20-3 in Figure 20-6 the following is derived:

$$1/R_t = 3/R_1 \qquad \textbf{20-14}$$

and:

$$R_t = R_1/3 \qquad \textbf{20-15}$$

Thus the total resistance is less than any of the individual resistances. Furthermore, for any parallel arrangement, the total resistance must be less than that of any of the individual parallel tubes. For example, consider a system in which a very-high-resistance tube is added in parallel to a low-resistance tube. The total resistance must be less than that of the low-resistance component by itself because the high-resistance component affords an additional pathway, or conductance, for fluid flow.

Similarly, the total resistance across a set of parallel tubes diminishes as the number of tubes increases. This explains why the resistance through the total array of arterioles is greater than that through the total array of capillaries in the systemic circulation, even though the caliber of the individual capillaries is substantially less than that of the individual arterioles. The number of parallel capillaries far exceeds the number of parallel arterioles; this is documented in Figure 15-3 by the much greater cross-sectional area of the capillary bed than of the arteriolar bed. The much greater number of systemic capillaries than of systemic arterioles accounts for the lower resistance to flow through the total array of capillaries than through the total array of arterioles.

Blood Flow May Be Laminar or Turbulent

Under certain conditions, the flow of a fluid in a cylindrical tube will be **laminar,** as illustrated in Figure 20-7. The thin layer of fluid in contact with the inner lining of the tube adheres to the lining and hence is motionless. The thin layer of fluid just central to this external lamina must shear against this motionless layer. Therefore this more central layer moves slowly but with a finite velocity. Similarly, the next more central layer travels still faster. The longitudinal velocity profile is a parabola. The velocity of the fluid adjacent to the wall is zero, whereas the velocity at the center of the stream is

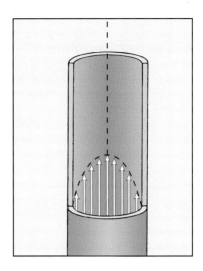

Figure 20-7 In laminar flow, all elements of the fluid move in streamlines parallel to the axis of the tube; no fluid moves in a radial or circumferential direction.

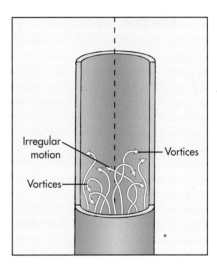

Figure 20-8 In turbulent flow, various elements of the fluid move irregularly in axial, radial, and circumferential directions.

maximum. The maximum velocity of the central component is twice the mean velocity of flow across the entire cross section of the tube. In laminar flow, fluid elements remain in one lamina, or streamline, as the fluid progresses longitudinally along the tube. Flow occurs only in an axial direction (i.e., parallel to the axis of the tube). Particles of fluid do not move in either a radial or a circumferential direction.

Irregular motions of the fluid elements may develop in the flow of fluid through a tube; this irregular flow is called **turbulent flow** (Figure 20-8). Under such conditions, fluid elements do not remain confined to definite laminae, but rapid radial and circumferential mixing occurs, and vortices may develop. More pressure is required to force a given flow of fluid through the same tube when the flow is turbulent than when it is laminar. In turbulent flow the pressure drop is approximately proportional to the square of the flow, whereas in laminar flow, the pressure drop is proportional to the first power of the flow. HENCE TO PRODUCE A GIVEN FLOW, A PUMP SUCH AS THE HEART MUST DO CONSIDERABLY MORE WORK IF TURBULENCE DEVELOPS.

Whether the flow through a tube is turbulent or laminar may be predicted by computing a dimensionless number called **Reynolds' number (N_R),** which is defined as follows:

$$N_R = \rho D \bar{v} / \eta \qquad \text{20-16}$$

where:

ρ = Fluid density
D = Tube diameter
$\bar{v}$ = Mean velocity over the cross section of the tube
η = Fluid viscosity

When N_R is less than 2000, the flow is usually laminar, and when it is more than 3000, turbulence usually prevails. Various flow conditions may develop in the transition range of N_R between 2000 and 3000. Because flow tends to be laminar at low N_R and turbulent at high N_R, Equation 20-16 indicates that large diameters, high velocities, and low viscosities predispose to the development of turbulence.

In addition to these factors, abrupt variations in tube dimensions or irregularities in the tube walls may produce turbulence. Turbulence is usually accompanied by vibrations of the fluid and surrounding structures. Some of these vibrations within the cardiovascular system are in the auditory frequency range, and they may be detected as **murmurs.**

The factors that predispose to turbulence may account for some of the **cardiac murmurs** heard clinically. In certain disorders of the cardiac valves, the valves are **stenotic** (narrowed). As the blood passes through such valves, the flow becomes turbulent, and a cardiac murmur can be detected with the stethoscope. In severe anemia, **functional cardiac murmurs** (murmurs not caused by structural abnormalities) are often detectable. Such murmurs are caused by the high flow velocities that usually prevail in severely anemic patients and by the reduced viscosity of the blood (because of the low red blood cell count).

Blood Is a Nonnewtonian Fluid

The viscosity of a newtonian fluid, such as water, may be determined by measuring the flow that prevails at a given pressure difference through a cylindrical tube of known length and radius. As long as the flow is laminar, the viscosity may be computed by substituting these values into Poiseuille's equation. If the flow is laminar, the calculated viscosity of a given newtonian fluid at a specified temperature will be constant, regardless of the tube

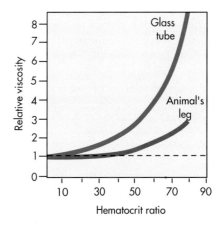

Figure 20-9 The viscosity of whole blood, relative to that of plasma, increases progressively as the hematocrit ratio rises. For any given hematocrit ratio the apparent viscosity of blood is less when measured in a biological viscometer (such as the tissues of an anesthetized animal *[red line]*) than in a glass capillary tube with a lumen diameter of 1 mm *(blue line).* (Redrawn from Levy MN, Share L: Circ Res 1:247, 1953.)

dimensions and flows. However, for a nonnewtonian fluid, the viscosity calculated from Poiseuille's equation may vary considerably when different tube dimensions and flows are used. Therefore regarding the rheological (flow-related) properties of a suspension such as blood, the term *viscosity* does not have a unique meaning. The term **apparent viscosity** is frequently applied to the value of viscosity obtained for nonnewtonian fluids, such as blood, under the particular conditions of measurement.

Rheologically, blood is a suspension, principally of erythrocytes in a relatively homogeneous liquid, the blood plasma. For this reason the apparent viscosity of blood varies as a function of the **hematocrit ratio** (ratio of erythrocyte volume to whole blood volume). In Figure 20-9 the upper curve represents the ratio of the apparent viscosity of whole blood to that of blood plasma over a range of hematocrit ratios up to 80%. The data were derived from measurements of flow through a glass tube 1 mm in internal diameter. The viscosity of plasma is 1.2 to 1.3 times that of water.

When the apparent viscosity of blood with a normal hematocrit ratio of 45% is measured with a glass-tube viscometer (upper curve of Figure 20-9), the apparent viscosity of the blood is about 2½ times that of plasma. In severe anemia, blood viscosity is low. With increasing hematocrit ratios the slope of this curve increases progressively; it is especially steep at the high range of hematocrit ratios. If the hematocrit ratio rises to about 70%, which it may in patients with **polycythemia vera** (abnormally high erythrocyte counts), the apparent viscosity may increase considerably more than twofold (Figure 20-9), and the vascular resistance to blood flow increases proportionally. The effect of such a change on peripheral vascular resistance may be appreciated when it is recognized that in patients with severe **essential hypertension** (the most common cause of a chronic elevation of arterial blood pressure), the total peripheral resistance (ratio of the systemic arteriovenous pressure difference to the cardiac output) rarely increases more than twofold.

For any given hematocrit ratio the apparent viscosity of blood depends on the dimensions of the tube used to estimate the viscosity. Figure 20-10 demonstrates that the apparent viscosity of blood is not appreciably affected by changes in tube diameter when the diameters exceed 0.3 mm, but the apparent viscosity does diminish progressively as the tube diameter is decreased to values below this level. The major resistance to blood flow in vascular beds normally resides in the very small arteries and arterioles, which have diameters substantially smaller than 0.3 mm. Thus these small vessels would be the principal determinants of the apparent viscosity of the blood flowing through living tissues.

The tendency for such small tubes to diminish the apparent viscosity of the blood, as shown in Figure 20-10, explains why the apparent viscosity is less when a biological tissue is used as a viscometer (lower curve of Figure 20-9) than when a glass tube with a lumen diameter of 1 mm is used as a viscometer (upper curve of Figure 20-9). The influence of tube diameter on apparent viscosity is explained in part by the difference in the actual composition of the blood as it flows from large tubes into small tubes. The composition changes because in the small tubes the red blood cells tend to accumulate in the faster axial stream, whereas the plasma is mainly consigned to the slower marginal layers of the bloodstream; the differences in velocity

with radial location in the tube are shown in Figure 20-7. Because red blood cells traverse the tube more quickly than plasma, the hematocrit ratio of the blood in the capillary tube is actually less than the hematocrit ratio of the blood in the reservoir to which the tube is connected (Figure 20-11).

The apparent viscosity of blood diminishes as the shear rate is increased (Figure 20-12), a phenomenon called **shear thinning.** The **shear rate** is the rate at which one layer of fluid moves with respect to the adjacent layers; the shear rate varies directly with the flow. The greater tendency of erythrocytes to accumulate in the axial laminae at higher flow rates is partly responsible for the nonnewtonian behavior of blood. However, a more important factor is that at very slow rates of shear, the suspended cells tend to aggregate, and this tendency increases viscosity. This tendency diminishes as the velocity of flow is increased.

The deformability of the erythrocytes is also a factor in shear thinning, especially when the hematocrit ratio is high. The mean diameter of human red blood cells is

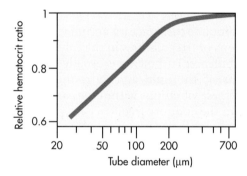

Figure 20-11 "Relative hematocrit ratio" of blood flowing from a feed reservoir through capillary tubes of various calibers as a function of the tube diameter. The relative hematocrit ratio is the ratio of the hematocrit of the blood in the outlet tube to that of the blood in the feed reservoir. *(Redrawn from Barbee JH, Cokelet GR: Microvasc Res 3:6, 1971.)*

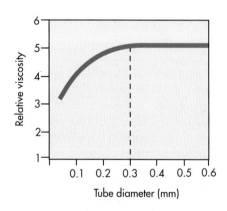

Figure 20-10 The viscosity of blood relative to that of water increases as a function of tube diameter up to a diameter of about 0.3 mm. *(Redrawn from Fahraeus R, Lindqvist T: Am J Physiol 96:562, 1931.)*

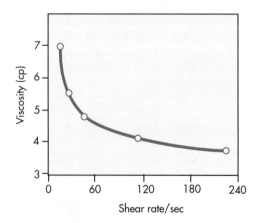

Figure 20-12 The viscosity (in centipoises) of blood as a function of the shear rate, which is the ratio of the velocity of one layer of fluid to that of the adjacent layers. The shear rate is directionally related to the flow. *(Redrawn from Amin TM, Sirs JA: Q J Exp Physiol 70:37, 1985.)*

about 7 μm; yet these cells can pass through openings with a diameter of only 3 μm. As blood that is densely packed with erythrocytes flows at progressively greater rates, the erythrocytes become more deformable. The greater deformability diminishes the apparent viscosity of the blood.

> The flexibility of human erythrocytes is enhanced when the concentration of fibrinogen in the plasma is elevated. Conversely, erythrocytes are misshapen and inflexible in patients with **sickle cell anemia.** This disorder often causes serious disturbances of regional blood flow.

SUMMARY

- The vascular system is composed of two major subdivisions, the systemic and pulmonary circulations, that are in series with one another.
- Each subdivision comprises a number of types of vessels (e.g., arteries, arterioles, capillaries) that are aligned in series with one another. In general, most vessels of a given type (e.g., capillaries) are arranged in parallel with one another.
- The mean velocity of the bloodstream in a given type of vessel is directly proportional to the total blood flow through all the vessels of that type, and it is inversely proportional to the cross-sectional area of all the parallel vessels of that type.
- When blood flow is steady and laminar in vessels larger than arterioles, the flow is proportional to the difference between the inflow and outflow pressures and to the fourth power of the radius, and it is inversely proportional to the length of the vessel and to the viscosity of the fluid (Poiseuille's law).
- For resistances aligned in series, the total resistance equals the sum of the individual resistances.
- For resistances aligned in parallel, the reciprocal of the total resistance equals the sum of the reciprocals of the individual resistances.
- Flow tends to become turbulent when flow velocity is high, fluid viscosity is low, tube diameter is large, and the lumen of the vessel is very irregular.
- Blood flow is nonnewtonian in very small vessels; that is, Poiseuille's law is not applicable.
- The apparent viscosity of the blood diminishes as shear rate (flow) increases and tube dimension decreases.

BIBLIOGRAPHY

Alonso C et al: Transient rheological behavior of blood in low-shear tube flow: velocity profiles and effective viscosity, *Am J Physiol* 268:H25, 1995.

Badeer HS, Hicks JW: Hemodynamics of vascular "waterfall": is the analogy justified? *Resp Physiol* 87:205, 1992.

Cokelet GR, Goldsmith HL: Decreased hydrodynamic resistance in the two-phase flow of blood through small vertical tubes at low flow rates, *Circ Res* 68:1, 1991.

Hoeks APG et al: Noninvasive determination of shear-rate distribution across the arterial wall, *Hypertension* 26:26, 1995.

Jonsson V et al: Significance of plasma skimming and plasma volume expansion, *J Appl Physiol* 72:2047, 1992.

Klanchar M, Tarbell JM, Wang DM: In vitro study of the influence of radial wall motion on wall shear stress in an elastic tube model of the aorta, *Circ Res* 66:1624, 1990.

Lee RT, Kamm RD: Vascular mechanics for the cardiologist, *J Am Coll Cardiol* 23:1289, 1994.

Lowe GDO: *Clinical blood rheology*, vol 1, Boca Raton, Fla, 1988, CRC.

Maeda N, Shiga T: Velocity of O_2 transfer and erythrocyte rheology, *News Physiol Sci* 9:22, 1994.

Pries AR, Secomb TW, Gaetgens P: Design principles of vascular beds, *Circ Res* 77:1017, 1995.

Pries AR et al: Resistance to blood flow in microvessels in vivo, *Circ Res* 75:904, 1994.

Reinhart WH et al: Influence of endothelial surface on flow velocity in vitro, *Am J Physiol* 265:H523, 1993.

Secomb TW: Flow-dependent rheological properties of blood in capillaries, *Microvasc Res* 34:46, 1987.

Sutera SP et al: Vascular flow resistance in rabbit hearts: "apparent viscosity" of RBC suspensions, *Microvasc Res* 36:305, 1988.

White KC et al: Hemodynamics and wall shear rate in the abdominal aorta of dogs: effects of vasoactive agents, *Circ Res* 75:637, 1994.

CASE STUDY

Case 20-1

A 70-year-old man reported to his physician that he experienced severe pain in his right leg when he walked briskly and that the pain disappeared soon after he discontinued walking. His physician referred him to a vascular surgeon, who performed several hemodynamic tests. Angiography showed that the patient had a large arteriosclerotic plaque about 3 cm distal to the origin of the right femoral artery; the left femoral artery appeared to be normal. The mean arterial pressure in the resting patient's left femoral artery was 100 mm Hg, and the blood flow in this artery was 500 ml/min. The mean arterial pressure in the resting patient's right femoral artery proximal to the plaque was 100 mm Hg, and just distal to the plaque, it was 80 mm Hg. The blood flow in this artery was 300 ml/min. The mean venous pressure was 10 mm Hg in the left and right femoral veins.

1. **What is the resistance to blood flow in the vascular bed perfused by the right femoral artery?**
   - **A.** 0.03 mm Hg/ml/min
   - **B.** 0.30 mm Hg/ml/min
   - **C.** 3.00 mm Hg/ml/min
   - **D.** 3.33 mm Hg/ml/min
   - **E.** 33.3 mm Hg/ml/min

2. What is the resistance to blood flow (R_t) in the combined vascular beds perfused by both femoral arteries?
    A. 0.48 mm Hg/ml/min
    B. 0.84 mm Hg/ml/min
    C. 1.10 mm Hg/ml/min
    D. 0.11 mm Hg/ml/min
    E. 11.1 mm Hg/ml/min

3. What is the resistance to flow imposed by the arteriosclerotic plaque in the right femoral artery?
    A. 0.066 mm Hg/ml/min
    B. 0.660 mm Hg/ml/min
    C. 0.15 mm Hg/ml/min
    D. 1.50 mm Hg/ml/min
    E. 15.0 mm Hg/ml/min

CHAPTER 21

Arterial System

OBJECTIVES

- Explain how the pulsatile blood flow in the large arteries is converted into a steady flow in the capillaries.
- Explain the factors that determine the mean, systolic, and diastolic arterial pressures and the arterial pulse pressure.
- Describe the common procedure for measuring the arterial blood pressure in humans.

Preceding chapters described how the heart operates to provide the pumping action required to distribute blood to the peripheral tissues. Chapter 20 presents some of the elementary physical principles that provide some quantitative insight into the relationships between pressure, flow, and vascular dimensions. This chapter describes the operation of the large distributing arteries, which serve as conduits between the heart and the microcirculation, where the exchange of nutrients and waste products take place.

Arteries Serve as Hydraulic Filters

The principal function of the systemic and pulmonary arterial systems is to distribute blood to the capillary beds throughout the body. The arterioles, which are the terminal components of the arterial system, regulate the distribution of blood to the capillary beds. The aorta and pulmonary artery and their major branches constitute a system of conduits between the heart and the arterioles. These conduits have a substantial volume, and in normal individuals, they are very compliant.

Because the normal arteries are so compliant and the arterioles present such a high resistance to blood flow, the arterial system constitutes a **hydraulic filter,** so called because THE ARTERIAL SYSTEM CONVERTS THE INTERMITTENT FLOW GENERATED BY THE HEART TO A VIRTUALLY STEADY FLOW THROUGH THE CAPILLARIES (Figure 21-1). The entire ventricular stroke volume is discharged into the arterial system during ventricular systole, which occupies approximately one third of the cardiac cycle duration. In fact, most of the stroke volume is pumped during the rapid ejection phase of ventricular systole (see Figure 18-8), which constitutes about half of total systole. Part of the energy released by the cardiac contraction is ki-

netic energy; it is dissipated as forward capillary flow during ventricular systole. The remainder is stored as potential energy in that much of the stroke volume is retained by the distensible arteries during systole (Figure 21-1, *A*). During diastole, the elastic recoil of the arterial walls converts this potential energy into capillary blood flow, and this flow continues through the capillaries at a fairly steady rate throughout diastole (Figure 21-1, *B*).

In a patient with severe **arteriosclerosis** (the arterial walls are rigid), capillary flow is more pulsatile than normal. Ventricular ejection leads to an appreciable increase in capillary flow during ventricular systole, and flow virtually ceases during diastole. Similarly, the hydraulic filter is less effective in people with abnormally large stroke volumes than in normal people. For example, in patients with **aortic valve regurgitation** (a leaky aortic valve), the volume of blood ejected during systole is usually greater than the normal stroke volume because much of the ejected volume leaks back into the left ventricle through the incompetent valve during diastole. Such a supernormal stroke volume induces a pulsatile flow in all the systemic capillaries. In such patients, a **capillary pulse** can be perceived in the patient's nail beds during physical examination. Application of a slight force at the distal tip of a fingernail blanches the adjacent region of the nail. In patients with aortic regurgitation, the margin between the pink and blanched regions of the nail bed is perceptibly pulsatile with each heartbeat.

Arteries Are Compliant Tubes

The elastic properties of the arterial wall may be appreciated by first considering the static pressure-volume relationship for the aorta. For one study (Figure 21-2), aortae were obtained at autopsy from people of different ages. All aortic branches were tied, and successive volumes of liquid were injected into this closed elastic system, just as a liquid might be introduced into a balloon. After each increment of volume was injected, the internal pressure in the aorta was measured (Table 21-1).

In Figure 21-2 the curve that relates pressure to volume for the youngest age group (20 to 24 years) is sig-

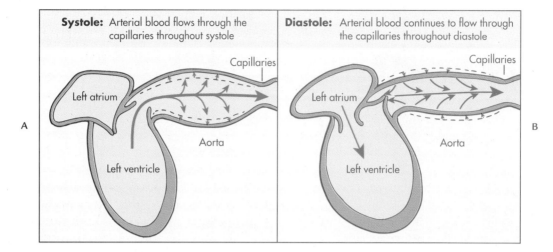

Figure 21-1 A, When the arteries are normally compliant, a substantial fraction of the stroke volume is stored in the arteries during ventricular systole; the arterial walls are stretched. **B,** During ventricular diastole the previously stretched arteries recoil. The volume of blood displaced by the recoil ensures continuous capillary flow throughout diastole.

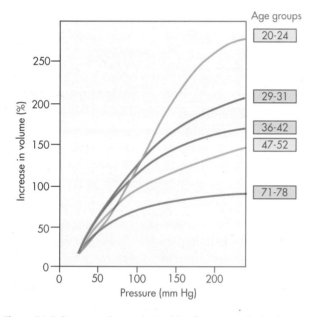

Figure 21-2 Pressure-volume relationships for aortae obtained at autopsy from humans in different age groups (denoted by the numbers at the right end of each curve). *(Redrawn from Hallock P, Benson IC: J Clin Invest 16:595, 1937.)*

Table 21-1	Glossary of Symbols
Symbol	**Meaning**
Capacitance (C)	
C_a	Arterial compliance
C_v	Venous compliance
Flow (Q)	
Q_h	Cardiac output
Q_r	Peripheral runoff
Pressure (P)	
$\overline{P}_a$	Mean arterial pressure
P_a	Arterial pressure
P_d	Diastolic arterial pressure
P_{ra}	Right atrial pressure
P_s	Systolic arterial pressure
P_v	Venous pressure
Resistance (R)	
R_t	Total systemic resistance
Volume (V)	
V_a	Arterial volume
V_h	Volume pumped by the heart
V_r	Runoff volume
V_v	Venous volume

moidal. The curve is approximately linear over most of its extent, but the slope ($\Delta V_a/\Delta P_a$) decreases at the upper and lower ends. At any given point, the slope represents the **arterial compliance (C_a):**

$$C_a = \Delta V_a/\Delta P_a \qquad \text{21-1}$$

Figure 21-2 reveals that in normal young people, C_a is least at very high and very low pressures and is greatest over the normal range of pressure variations. These compliance changes resemble the familiar changes encountered in inflating a balloon. Introducing air into the balloon requires more effort (i.e., the balloon is less compliant) at the beginning of inflation and again at near-maximum volume, just before rupture. At intermediate volumes, however, the balloon is easier to inflate; that is, its compliance is greater.

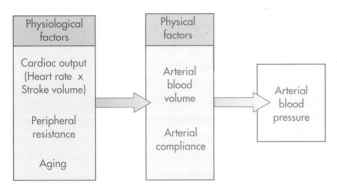

Figure 21-3 Physiological and physical factors that determine arterial blood pressure.

> Figure 21-2 shows that the aortic pressure-volume curves become displaced downward and that the slopes diminish as a function of advancing age; thus compliance decreases with age. Diminished compliance is a manifestation of the progressive increase in the collagen and decrease in the elastin contents of arterial walls. The heart cannot eject a given stroke volume as readily into a rigid arterial system as it can into a more compliant system.

Determinants of Arterial Blood Pressure

The arterial blood pressure is routinely measured when a physician examines a patient, and this measurement provides valuable information about the patient's cardiovascular status. The factors that determine the arterial blood pressure cannot be evaluated precisely. Therefore this chapter takes a simplified approach in an attempt to understand the principal determinants of arterial blood pressure.

The determinants of arterial blood pressure are arbitrarily subdivided into physical and physiological components (Figure 21-3). For simplicity, the arterial system is assumed to be a static, elastic system, much like a tubular balloon. The only two **physical factors** considered are the **blood volume** within the arterial system and the elastic characteristics **(compliance)** of the system, just as the pressure in a balloon depends on the volume of fluid (air or liquid) in the balloon and the compliance of the balloon. The **physiological factors** to be considered are **cardiac output** (the product of **heart rate** and **stroke volume**), **peripheral resistance,** and **aging.** Such physiological factors operate through one or both of the physical factors.

The mean arterial pressure is determined by cardiac output and peripheral resistance

THE MEAN ARTERIAL PRESSURE $(\overline{P}_a)$ IS THE BLOOD PRESSURE IN THE ARTERIES AVERAGED OVER TIME. It may be precisely determined by inserting a needle directly into a peripheral artery and recording the arterial blood pressure with a transducer. The $\overline{P}_a$ can be determined from the arterial blood pressure tracing by dividing the area under the tracing by the elapsed time interval, as shown in Figure 21-4. In the absence of a precise intraarterial pressure tracing, however, the $\overline{P}_a$ usually can be estimated satisfactorily from the measured values of the **systolic pressure (P_s)** and the **diastolic pressure (P_d)** obtained indirectly using a sphygmomanometer (described later). The value of the $\overline{P}_a$ can be estimated by using the following formula:

$$\overline{P}_a \approx P_d + (P_s - P_d)/3 \qquad \textbf{21-2}$$

The physical factors (Figure 21-3) that determine the level of the arterial pressure $(\overline{P}_a)$ can be estimated from a rearrangement of Equation 21-1:

$$\Delta P_a = \Delta V_a/C_a \qquad \textbf{21-3}$$

Thus ANY CHANGE IN P_a VARIES DIRECTLY WITH A CHANGE IN ARTERIAL BLOOD VOLUME (V_a) AND INVERSELY WITH A CHANGE IN C_a.

Many physiological factors regulate the P_a. These factors operate through the physical factors, namely V_a and C_a (Equation 21-3).

Any temporal change in the volume (dV_a/dt) of blood in the arteries depends on the balance between the rate at which the heart pumps blood into the arteries **(cardiac output [Q_h])** and the rate at which the blood flows out of the arteries **(peripheral runoff [Q_r])** through the arterioles and capillaries and into the veins, as follows:

$$dV_a/dt = Q_h - Q_r \qquad \textbf{21-4}$$

This equation is an expression of the **law of conservation of mass.** The equation states that ANY CHANGE IN V_A SIMPLY REFLECTS THE DIFFERENCE IN THE RATES AT WHICH BLOOD ENTERS AND LEAVES THE ARTERIAL SYSTEM. If arterial inflow (Q_h) exceeds the runoff (Q_r), then the arterial volume (V_a) increases, the arterial walls distend, and pressure rises. The converse happens when Q_r exceeds Q_h. Finally, if Q_h equals Q_r, $\overline{P}_a$ remains constant.

Cardiac output is the blood flow into the arterial system
How an alteration in Q_h changes $\overline{P}_a$ can be appreciated by considering some simple examples. Under control conditions, let Q_h be 5 L/min and $\overline{P}_a$ be 100 mm Hg (Figure 21-5, *A*). Under steady-state conditions, $Q_h = Q_r$. The **total peripheral resistance (R_t)** is the resistance to blood flow in the systemic vascular bed:

$$R_t = (\overline{P}_a - \overline{P}_{ra})/Q_r \qquad \textbf{21-5}$$

where $\overline{P}_{ra}$ is the mean right atrial pressure. Because $\overline{P}_{ra}$ is usually close to zero, the following occurs:

$$R_t \approx \overline{P}_a/Q_r \qquad \textbf{21-6}$$

Therefore in the example shown in Figure 21-5, *A*, R_t is 100/5 mm Hg, or 20 mm Hg/L/min.

Now suppose Q_h suddenly increases to 10 L/min (Figure 21-5, *B*) so that Q_h exceeds Q_r. In the first one or

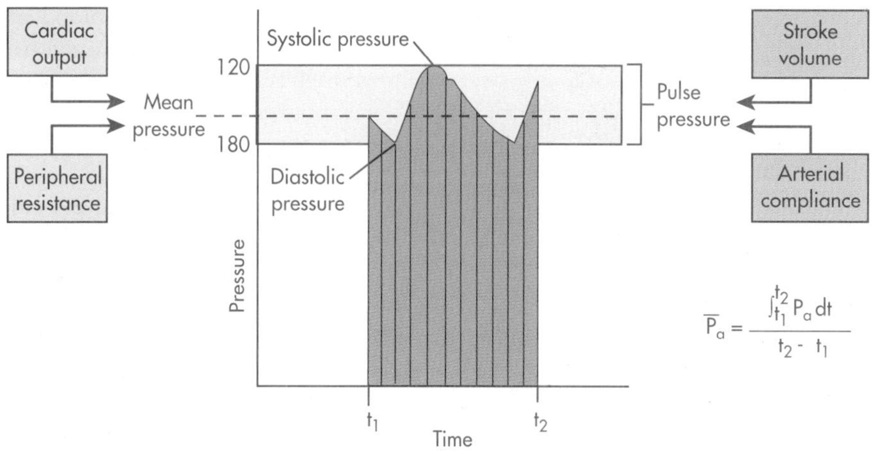

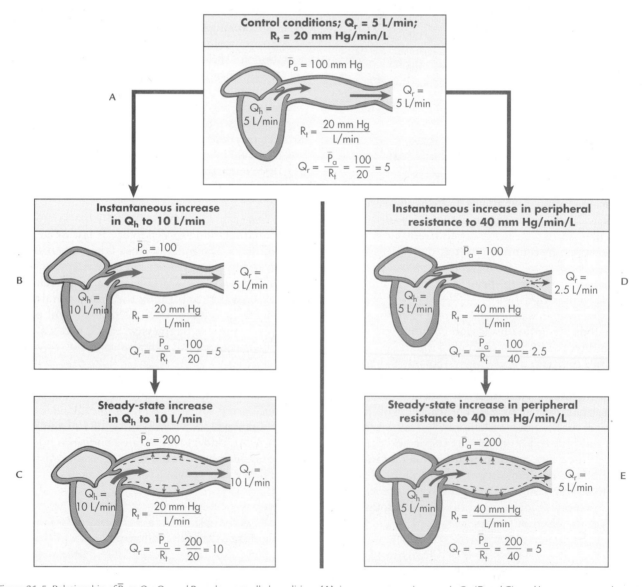

Figure 21-4 Arterial P_s, P_d, pulse pressure, and mean pressure and the factors that determine them.

Figure 21-5 Relationship of $\overline{P}_a$ to Q_h, Q_r, and R_t under controlled conditions **(A)**, in response to an increase in Q_h **(B** and **C)**, and in response to an increase in R_t **(D** and **E)**.

two heartbeats, however, the increment in blood volume in the arteries is negligible, and $\overline{P}_a$ is unchanged. Because Q_r from the arteries depends on $\overline{P}_a$ and R_t, Q_r also does not change appreciably at first. Therefore Q_h, now 10 L/min, exceeds Q_r, still only 5 L/min. Hence V_a progressively increases.

The increase in V_a raises the arterial blood pressure. In this example of a sudden increase in Q_h, blood continues to accumulate in the arteries until the pressure rises high enough to force through the peripheral resistance a runoff, Q_r, that equals the elevated Q_h (Figure 21-5, *C*). If Equation 21-6 is solved for Q_r:

$$Q_r = \overline{P}_a/R_t \qquad \textbf{21-7}$$

This equation makes it evident that Q_r does not attain a value of 10 L/min until the $\overline{P}_a$ reaches 200 mm Hg, provided that R_t remains constant at 20 mm Hg/L/min. Thus $\overline{P}_a$ DEPENDS ONLY ON Q_h AND PERIPHERAL RESISTANCE. C_a does not affect the level that $\overline{P}_a$ attains in response to a change in Q_h or peripheral resistance; the compliance affects only the rate at which the new equilibrium value of $\overline{P}_a$ is attained.

Peripheral resistance regulates the flow out of the arterial system

Similar reasoning may now be applied to explain the changes in $\overline{P}_a$ that accompany alterations in R_t. Suppose the control conditions are identical to the control conditions of the preceding example (Figure 21-5, *A*). If R_t suddenly increases to 40 mm Hg/L/min, from the control value of 20 mm Hg/L/min (Figure 21-5, *D*), over the duration of the first one or two heartbeats, the $\overline{P}_a$ is virtually unchanged because sufficient time has not passed to allow V_a to change substantially. Although $\overline{P}_a$ is still virtually equal to 100 mm Hg, the Q_r suddenly decreases to 2.5 L/min when R_t is increased to 40 mm Hg/L/min. If the Q_h remains constant at 5 L/min, Q_h will exceed Q_r, and thus V_a will increase. Consequently, $\overline{P}_a$ rises and continues to rise until it reaches 200 mm Hg (Figure 21-5, *E*). At this pressure level (Q_r = 200/40 mm Hg = 5 L/min), which equals the Q_h, $\overline{P}_a$ then remains at the new equilibrium level of 200 mm Hg as long as Q_h and R_t do not change.

These findings therefore confirm that $\overline{P}_a$ depends only on Q_h and R_t (Figure 21-4). It is immaterial whether the change in Q_h is accomplished by an alteration in heart rate, stroke volume, or both. Because Q_h equals heart rate multiplied by stroke volume, any change in heart rate that is balanced by an inverse change in stroke volume does not alter Q_h, and therefore $\overline{P}_a$ is not affected.

Arterial pulse pressure is the amplitude of the arterial pressure fluctuation

The arterial pulse pressure for a given heartbeat equals the difference between **P_s** and **P_d** for that heartbeat; P_s and P_d

are the maximum and minimum values, respectively, of the P_a during that heartbeat (Figure 21-4). ARTERIAL PULSE PRESSURE IS DETERMINED BY STROKE VOLUME AND C_a (Figure 21-4).

Stroke volume determines the arterial volume fluctuation

The effect of a change in stroke volume on pulse pressure may be analyzed more clearly under conditions in which C_a remains constant. C_a is constant over any linear region of a pressure-volume curve (Figure 21-2). If the V_a is plotted along the vertical axis and P_a is plotted along the horizontal axis, the slope of the pressure-volume curve (dV_a/dP_a) is by definition the C_a.

The effect of a change in stroke volume on arterial pulse pressure can be appreciated by considering a healthy person who initially has a heart rate of 100 beats/min, a stroke volume of 50 ml, and an R_t of 20 mm Hg/L/min. Because Q_h equals heart rate multiplied by stroke volume, this person's Q_h is 5 L/min. As shown in Figure 21-5, *A*, this person would have a $\overline{P}_a$ of 100 mm Hg. The P_s of course exceeds 100 mm Hg, and the P_d is less than 100 mm Hg. Suppose P_s and P_d for this person is 120 and 90 mm Hg, respectively; the values for $\overline{P}_a$, P_s, and P_d satisfy Equation 21-2. The average normal P_d is about 80 mm Hg; the value of 90 mm Hg is used here only to simplify certain computations.

Several hemodynamic events take place just before and during the rapid ejection phase of systole of a normal heartbeat (see Chapter 18). Throughout the ventricular diastole of the preceding heartbeat and during the brief period of isovolumic contraction, the heart had pumped no blood into the arteries, but blood had flowed out of the arteries and through the resistance vessels continuously. Hence V_a had been declining, and consequently $\overline{P}_a$ had been falling continuously throughout these nonejection phases of the cardiac cycle. In a person whose P_d was 90 mm Hg, this minimum pressure would have been attained at the end of the isovolumic contraction phase of systole (see Figure 18-8).

Under steady-state conditions, the volume of blood that flows out of the arteries and flows through the peripheral resistance vessels during each cardiac cycle equals the stroke volume. In healthy people, most of the stroke volume is ejected during the rapid ejection phase of ventricular systole (see Figure 18-8). If a person has a stroke volume of 50 ml and 80% of that volume is expelled during rapid ejection (i.e., $Q_h = 0.80 \times 50 = 40$ ml, as illustrated in Figure 21-6, *A*), the fractional volume flowing out of the arteries during rapid ejection is approximately equal to the fraction of the cardiac cycle duration occupied by the rapid ejection phase. Assume that during the rapid ejection phase, 16% of the stroke volume exits the arteries through the peripheral resistance; that is, the Q_r during rapid ejection is 0.16×50 ml, or 8 ml (Figure 21-6, *A*).

Hence the **volume increment** (ΔV_a) that prevails in the arteries during the rapid ejection phase of the cardiac cycle equals the quantity of blood ($Q_h = 40$ ml)

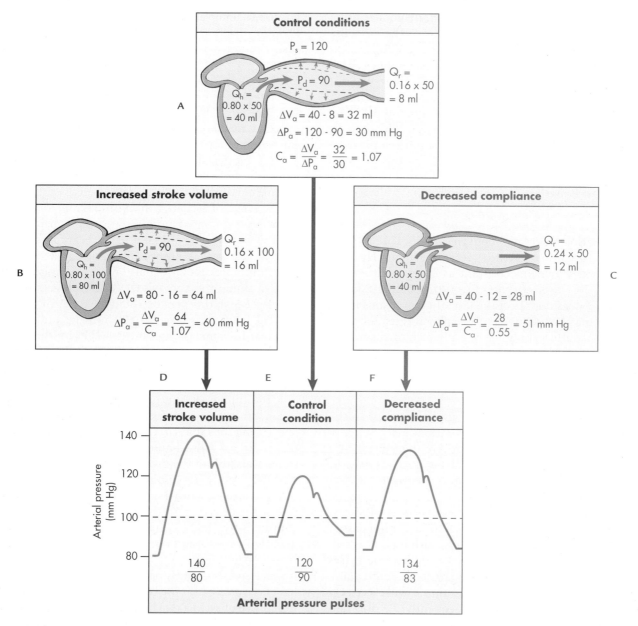

Figure 21-6 Effects of an increase in stroke volume and a decrease in C_a on the arterial pulse pressure. The heart pumps a volume (Q_h) of 40 ml of blood into the arterial system with each heartbeat during rapid ejection **(A)**. Concomitantly, a volume (Q_r) of 8 ml runs out of the arteries through the peripheral resistance. The heart now pumps 80 ml with each beat into the arteries during rapid ejection, and 16 ml runs out of the arteries during the same period **(B)**. The heart still pumps 80% of the stroke volume (50 ml) during the rapid ejection phase despite a decreased C_a (0.55 ml/mm Hg) **(C)**. Under conditions that do not alter the $\overline{P}_a$, an increase in stroke volume **(D)** or a decrease in C_a **(F)** causes the arterial pulse pressure to exceed the control value **(E)** of the arterial pulse pressure.

pumped into the aorta during this phase of the cardiac cycle minus the quantity of blood (Q_r = 8 ml) that has exited through the peripheral resistance vessels during this same period; that is, the ΔV_a equals 32 ml (Figure 21-6, *A*). In this hypothetical subject, the ΔV_a causes P_a to rise from the diastolic level of 90 mm Hg to the systolic level of 120 mm Hg (Figure 21-6). In other words, the ΔV_a of 32 ml produces a pressure increment (ΔP_a) of 30 mm Hg; this pressure increment is by definition the **pulse pressure** (Figure 21-4).

Thus the magnitude of the pulse pressure (ΔP_a) is determined simply by the values of ΔV_a and C_a.

The relationship is evident from a rearrangement of Equation 21-1:

$$\Delta P_a = \Delta V_a / C_a \qquad \textbf{21-8}$$

The pulse pressure equals the V_a increment during the rapid ejection phase of ventricular systole divided by C_a. In the previous example, C_a was equal to $\Delta V_a / \Delta P_a$ = 32/30 mm Hg, or 1.07 ml/mm Hg (Figure 21-6, *A*).

Suppose that the cardiovascular status changes such that the heart rate decreases to 50 beats/min, the stroke volume increases to 100 ml (Figure 21-6, *B*), but the peripheral resistance (20 mm Hg/L/min) and C_a (1.07

ml/mm Hg) remain unchanged. Because Q_h (heart rate × stroke volume) still equals 5 L/min and the peripheral resistance is also unchanged, the $\overline{P}_a$ remains at 100 mm Hg (see Equation 21-6).

To determine the new pulse pressure, assume that the fraction of the stroke volume (100 ml) expelled during rapid ejection is still 80%; that is, Q_h = 0.80 × 100 ml, or 80 ml (Figure 21-6, *B*). Suppose again that 16% of the stroke volume exits the arterial system through the peripheral resistance during rapid ejection. Hence Q_r during rapid ejection is 0.16 × 100 ml, or 16 ml. Thus the ΔV_a during rapid ejection is 80 − 16 ml, or 64 ml.

A ΔV_a of 64 ml in an arterial system with a compliance of 1.07 ml/mm Hg produces a pressure increment (i.e., a pulse pressure) of 60 mm Hg (Figure 21-6, *B*), which is twice the pulse pressure that prevailed under control conditions (Figure 21-6, *A*). If the relationships among the mean pressure, P_s, and P_d satisfy Equation 21-2, this person's P_s and P_d would equal 140 and 80 mm Hg, respectively. Hence if Q_h, peripheral resistance, and C_a remain constant, an increase in stroke volume would raise P_s and lower P_d but would not affect the mean pressure ($\overline{P}_a$) (Figure 21-6, *D*).

Arterial pulse pressure provides valuable clues about a patient's stroke volume, provided that the C_a is essentially normal. Patients who have severe **congestive heart failure** or who have had a severe **hemorrhage** are likely to have very small arterial pulse pressures because their stroke volumes are abnormally small. Conversely, individuals with large stroke volumes are likely to have above-average arterial pulse pressures. For example, well-trained athletes at rest tend to have low heart rates. Thus the prolonged ventricular filling times induce the ventricles to pump more blood per heartbeat. Consequently, the pulse pressures of such athletes tend to be higher than average. Similarly, in patients with **aortic valve regurgitation,** blood leaks back into the left ventricle from the aorta during diastole. This backflow into the ventricle diminishes the aortic P_d and increases the blood volume in the left ventricle during diastole. The augmented ventricular filling volume increases the stroke volume during systole. Characteristically, a patient with aortic valve regurgitation has a low arterial P_d, an elevated arterial P_s, and consequently a greatly increased arterial pulse pressure.

Arterial compliance affects arterial pressure fluctuation
A change in C_a affects the pulse pressure (Figure 21-6, *C*). Assume that heart rate, stroke volume, and peripheral resistance are all the same as in the control condition (Figure 21-6, *A*). However, the arteries are about half as compliant as before (i.e., C_a = 0.55 ml/mm Hg). Because the Q_h and peripheral resistance are the same as in the two preceding examples (Figure 21-6, *A* and *B*), the $\overline{P}_a$ still is 100 mm Hg (Figure 21-6, *F*).

Even though the C_a is much less than the control value, the heart can still pump 80% of the stroke volume during rapid ejection (i.e., Q_h = 40 ml). Because the less compliant arteries accommodate a smaller increment in volume during rapid ejection, the fraction (24%) of the stroke volume that will run out of the arteries during the rapid ejection period (Q_r = 12 ml) will exceed the fraction (16%) that runs out of the arteries in the same period (Q_r = 8 ml) under control conditions. In arteries whose compliance is only 0.55 ml/mm Hg, the V_a increment (V_a = 40 − 12 = 28 ml) produces a pressure increment (pulse pressure) of 51 mm Hg (Figure 21-6, *C*). If the relationships among P_s, P_d, and mean pressure satisfy Equation 21-2, P_s and P_d will be approximately 134 and 83 mm Hg, respectively (Figure 21-6, *F*). Thus when C_a is diminished, P_s will exceed the control P_s, P_d will be lower than the control P_d, and the pulse pressure will be substantially greater than the control pulse pressure (Figure 21-6, *E*).

The C_a of old people in general (Figure 21-2) and of young people with substantial **arteriosclerosis** (hardening of the arteries) is low, and this condition is reflected by the pulse pressures in such individuals. The P_s tends to be abnormally high (so-called **systolic hypertension**), but the P_d tends to be less than average (80 mm Hg) for normal young people.

The characteristic changes in arterial blood pressure in patients with **essential hypertension** (the most common form of chronic hypertension in humans) are a moderate increase in P_d and a substantially greater increase in P_s. Thus the $\overline{P}_a$ and the arterial pulse pressure are augmented. The $\overline{P}_a$ is elevated because the R_t is increased; the reasons for this increase remain to be established. The principal reason for the increase in arterial pulse pressure is that the arteries become less compliant when stretched by the elevated arterial blood pressure. The reduced compliance is reflected by the decrease in the slope of the pressure-volume curve when P_a is elevated (Figure 21-2).

Blood Pressure Measurement in Humans

Needles or catheters may be introduced into peripheral arteries of patients in the cardiac catheterization laboratories or intensive care units of hospitals. Arterial blood pressure can then be measured directly using electronic pressure transducers. Ordinarily, however, blood pressure is estimated indirectly using a **sphygmomanometer.** This instrument consists of a sturdy cuff and an inflatable bag. The cuff is wrapped around the arm above the elbow, and the inflatable bag, which lies between the cuff and the skin, is positioned over the brachial artery. When the patient's blood pressure is measured, a rubber squeeze bulb is used to raise the pressure in the bag to a value in excess of the patient's arterial P_s.

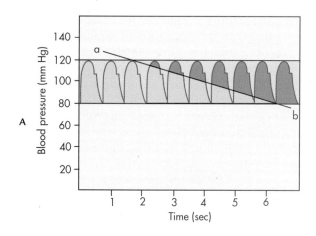

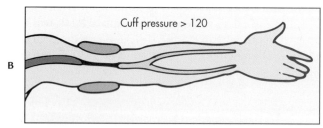

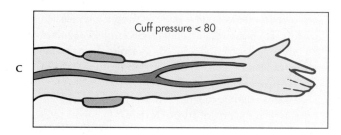

Figure 21-7 Measurement of arterial blood pressure with a sphygmomanometer. **A,** If the patient's arterial blood pressure is 120/80 mm Hg, the pressure *(oblique line)* in a cuff around the patient's arm is allowed to fall from over 120 mm Hg (point a) to below 80 mm Hg (point b) in about 6 seconds. **B,** When the cuff pressure exceeds 120 mm Hg, no blood passes through the arterial segment under the cuff, and no sounds can be detected using a stethoscope bell placed on the arm distal to the cuff. **C,** When the cuff pressure falls below 80 mm Hg, arterial flow through the region surrounded by the cuff is continuous, and no sounds are audible. When the cuff pressure is between 120 and 80 mm Hg, spurts of blood traverse the artery segment under the cuff during each heartbeat, and Korotkoff sounds are heard through the stethoscope.

The elevated pressure in the cuff occludes the brachial artery. Air is then slowly released from the bag using a needle valve in the inflation bulb.

The health care worker listens with a stethoscope applied to the skin in the antecubital space over the brachial artery. While the pressure in the bag exceeds the P_s, the brachial artery is occluded and no sounds are heard (Figure 21-7, *B*). When the inflation pressure falls just below the arterial P_s (upper horizontal line in Figure 21-7, *A*), small spurts of blood pass through the artery each time the P_a exceeds the cuff pressure, and they create turbulence. Consequently, slight tapping sounds (called **Korotkoff sounds**) are heard with each heartbeat. The pressure at which the first sound is detected

represents the **P_s**. As the inflation pressure continues to fall, more blood escapes per beat under the cuff, and the sounds become louder. As the inflation pressure approaches the P_d (lower horizontal line in Figure 21-7, *A*), the Korotkoff sounds become muffled. As the inflation pressure falls just below the minimum pressure in the artery, the sounds disappear; this indicates the **P_d** (Figure 21-7, *C*).

Korotkoff sounds are generated by the impact of the spurt of blood that passes under the cuff and meets the static column of blood beyond the cuff. The impact creates turbulence and generates audible vibrations. Once the inflation pressure is less than the P_d, flow is continuous in the brachial artery, and sounds are no longer heard.

SUMMARY

- The arteries not only conduct blood from the heart to the capillaries but also store some of the ejected blood during each cardiac systole. Consequently, flow can continue through the capillaries throughout cardiac diastole.
- The aging process diminishes the compliance of the arteries.
- The less compliant the arteries, the more work the heart must do to pump a given Q_h.
- The $\overline{P}_a$ varies directly with the Q_h and R_t.
- The arterial pulse pressure varies directly with the stroke volume but inversely with C_a.
- When blood pressure is measured using a sphygmomanometer, the P_s is signaled by a tapping sound that originates in the artery distal to the cuff as the cuff pressure falls below the peak P_a, and the P_d is manifested by the disappearance of the sound as the cuff pressure falls below the minimum P_a.

BIBLIOGRAPHY

Armentano RL et al: Arterial wall mechanics in conscious dogs, *Circ Res* 76:468, 1995.

Burattini R, Campbell KB: Effective distributed compliance of the canine descending aorta estimated by modified T-tube model, *Am J Physiol* 264:H1997, 1993.

Folkow B, Svanborg A: Physiology of cardiovascular aging, *Physiol Rev* 73:725, 1993.

Frasch HF, Kresh JY, Noordergraaf A: Two-port analysis of microcirculation: an extension of Windkessel, *Am J Physiol* 270:H376, 1996.

Fung YC: *Biodynamics: circulation*, Heidelberg, Germany, 1984, Springer-Verlag.

Kelly RP, Tunin R, Kass DA: Effects of reduced aortic compliance on cardiac efficiency and contractile function of in situ canine left ventricle, *Circ Res* 71:490, 1992.

Laskey WK et al: Estimation of total systemic arterial compliance in humans, *J Appl Physiol* 69:112, 1990.

Lee RT, Kamm RD: Vascular mechanics for the cardiologist, *J Am Coll Cardiol* 23:1289, 1994.

Mulvany MJ, Aalkjaer C: Structure and function of small arteries, *Physiol Rev* 70:921, 1990.

O'Rourke M, Kelly R, Avolio A: *Arterial pulse,* Baltimore, 1992, Williams & Wilkins.

Piene H: Pulmonary arterial impedance and right ventricular function, *Physiol Rev* 66:606, 1986.

Stergiopolis N, Meister J-J, Westerhof N: Determinants of stroke volume and systolic and diastolic aortic pressure, *Am J Physiol* 270:H2050, 1996.

Van Gorp AD et al: Technique to assess aortic distensibility and compliance in anesthetized and awake rats, *Am J Physiol* 270:H780, 1996.

▷ CASE STUDY

Case 21-1

A 33-year-old man complained about chest pain on exertion. He was referred to a cardiologist, who performed a number of studies, including right- and left-sided cardiac catheterization for hemodynamic information and coronary angiography to image the status of the coronary arteries. Among the data obtained during these studies were the findings that the patients pulmonary artery and aortic pressures were as follows:

Pressure	Pulmonary Artery (mm Hg)	Aorta (mm Hg)
Systolic	30	120
Diastolic	15	80
Pulse	15	40
Mean	20	93

The hemodynamic and angiographic studies disclosed no serious abnormalities. The patient's physicians recommended certain changes in lifestyle and diet, and the patient continued to do well for about 20 years, when the patient's systemic arterial blood pressure was found to be 190/100 mm Hg and his $\overline{P}_a$ was estimated to be 130 mm Hg. These and other findings led his physicians to the diagnosis of essential hypertension.

1. **Why was the patient's aortic $\overline{P}_a$ (93 mm Hg) much higher than his pulmonary $\overline{P}_a$ (20 mm Hg) at the time of the initial examination?**

   A. His systemic vascular resistance is much greater than his pulmonary vascular resistance.

   B. His aortic compliance is much greater than his pulmonary compliance.

   C. His left ventricular stroke volume is much greater than his right ventricular stroke volume.

   D. The total cross-sectional area of his pulmonary capillary bed is much greater than the total cross-sectional area of his systemic capillary bed.

   E. The duration of the rapid ejection phase of the left ventricle exceeds the duration of the rapid ejection phase of the right ventricle.

2. **When the patient became hypertensive, his arterial pulse pressure (90 mm Hg) increased to a value higher than his pulse pressure (40 mm Hg) before the hypertension. Why?**

   A. His systemic vascular resistance is less than it was before he became hypertensive.

   B. The duration of the reduced ejection phase of the left ventricle decreases as the arterial blood pressure rises.

   C. His C_a was diminished in part because of the hypertension per se and in part because of the effects of aging.

   D. The total cross-sectional area of the systemic capillary bed increases substantially in hypertensive subjects.

   E. His aortic compliance became greater than his pulmonary C_a.

CHAPTER 22

Microcirculation and Lymphatics

OBJECTIVES

- Describe the regulation of regional blood flow by the arterioles.
- Enumerate the physical and chemical factors affecting the microvessels.
- Explain the roles of diffusion, filtration, and pinocytosis in transcapillary exchange.
- Describe the balance between hydrostatic and osmotic forces under normal and abnormal conditions.
- Describe the lymphatic circulation.

The entire circulatory system is geared to supply the body tissues with blood in amounts commensurate with their requirements for O_2 and nutrients and to remove CO_2 and other waste products for excretion by the lungs and kidneys. The exchange of gases, water, and solutes between the vascular and interstitial fluid compartments occurs mainly across the capillaries, which consist of a single layer of endothelial cells. The arterioles, capillaries, and venules constitute the microcirculation, and blood flow through the microcirculation is regulated by the arterioles, also known as the **resistance vessels** (see Chapter 20). The large arteries serve solely as blood conduits, whereas the veins serve as storage or **capacitance vessels** as well as blood conduits.

Functional Anatomy

Arterioles are the stopcocks of the circulation

The arterioles, which range in diameter from about 5 to 100 µm, have a thick smooth muscle layer, a thin adventitial layer, and an endothelial lining (see Figure 15-1). The arterioles give rise directly to the **capillaries** (diameter, 5 to 10 µm) or in some tissues to **metarterioles** (diameter, 10 to 20 µm), which then give rise to capillaries (Figure 22-1). The metarterioles can serve either as thoroughfares to the venules, bypassing the capillary bed, or as conduits for supplying the capillary bed. There are often cross-connections from arteriole to arteriole and from venule to venule as well as in the capillary network. Arterioles that give rise directly

to capillaries regulate flow through their cognate capillaries via constriction or dilation. The capillaries form an interconnecting network of tubes of different lengths; the average length is 0.5 to 1 mm.

The diameter of the resistance vessels is determined by the balance between the contractile force of the vascular smooth muscle and the distending force produced by the intraluminal pressure. The greater the contractile activity of the vascular smooth muscle of an arteriole, the smaller its diameter. At times, the small arterioles may be completely occluded, partly because of infolding of the endothelium (Figure 22-2). With a reduction in the intravascular pressure, vessel diameter decreases, as does tension in the vessel wall (Laplace's law [see Figure 22-4]). When perfusion pressure is progressively reduced, a point is reached at which a segment of the vessel is occluded and blood flow ceases even though a positive pressure gradient from the afferent to the efferent end of the vessel may still exist. The transmural pressure at which flow ceases has been referred to as the **critical closing pressure.**

Capillaries permit the exchange of solutes, water, and gases

Capillary distribution varies from tissue to tissue. In metabolically active tissues such as cardiac and skeletal muscle and glandular structures, capillaries are numerous, whereas less active tissues such as subcutaneous tissue and cartilage have few capillaries. Also, not all capillaries have the same diameter. Because some capillaries have diameters smaller than those of erythrocytes, the red cells must become temporarily deformed to pass through these capillaries. Normal red cells are flexible and readily change their shape to conform to that of the small capillaries (see Chapter 20).

Blood flow in the capillaries is not uniform and depends chiefly on the contractile state of the arterioles. The average velocity of blood flow in the capillaries is 1 mm/sec; however, it can quickly vary from zero to several millimeters per second in the same vessel. The capillary blood flow may vary randomly, or it may oscillate rhythmically at different frequencies as determined by contraction and relaxation (**vasomotion**) of the precapillary vessels. This vasomotion is partly an intrinsic contractile behavior of the vascular smooth muscle. Furthermore, changes in **transmural pressure** (intravascular pressure minus extravascular pressure) affect the contractile state of the precapillary vessels. An increase in the transmural pressure, whether produced by an increase in venous pressure or by the dilation of arterioles, elicits contraction of the terminal arterioles at the points of origin of the capillaries. Conversely, a decrease in the transmural pressure elicits precapillary vessel relaxation. In addition, humoral and neural factors affect vasomotion.

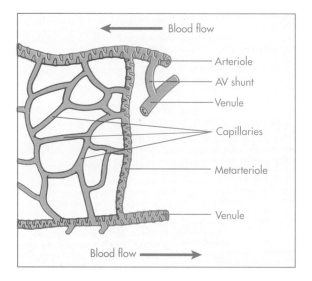

Figure 22-1 Microcirculation. The circular structures on the arteriole and venule represent smooth muscle fibers, and the branching solid lines represent sympathetic nerve fibers. The arrows indicate the direction of blood flow. *AV,* Arteriovenous.

Although reduced transmural pressure relaxes the terminal arterioles, blood flow through the capillaries cannot increase if the reduced intravascular pressure is caused by severe constriction of the parent arterioles or metarterioles. Large arterioles and metarterioles also exhibit vasomotion. However, contraction of these vessels usually does not occlude the lumen and arrest blood flow, whereas contraction of the terminal arterioles may arrest blood flow. Because blood flow through the capillaries provides for the exchange of gases and solutes between blood and tissue, such flow has been termed **nutritional flow,** whereas blood flow that bypasses the capillaries in traveling from the arterial to the venous side of the circulation has been termed **nonnutritional,** or **shunt, flow** (Figure 22-1). In some areas of the body (e.g., fingertips), true arteriovenous shunts exist (see Chapter 25). In many tissues such as muscle, however, evidence of anatomical shunts is lacking.

The true capillaries are devoid of smooth muscle and are therefore incapable of active constriction. Nevertheless, the endothelial cells that form the capillary wall contain actin and myosin and can alter their shape in response to certain chemical stimuli. However, such changes in endothelial cell shape do not regulate blood flow through the capillaries. CHANGES IN CAPILLARY DIAMETER ARE PASSIVE AND ARE CAUSED BY ALTERATIONS IN PRECAPILLARY AND POSTCAPILLARY RESISTANCE.

For many years it was believed that endothelial cells were inert and merely served as barriers to blood cells and large molecules such as plasma proteins. However, it is now known that the endothelium can synthesize substances that affect the contractile state of the arterioles (Figure 22-

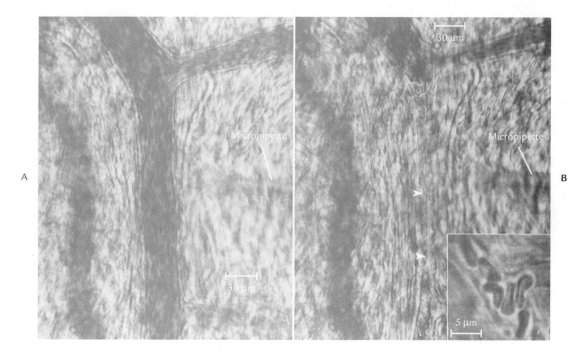

Figure 22-2 Arterioles of a hamster cheek pouch. **A,** Before the microinjection of norepinephrine. **B,** After the injection. Note the complete closure of the arteriole between the arrows and the narrowing of a branch arteriole at the upper right. *Inset,* Capillary with red cells during a period of complete closure of the feeding arteriole. *(Courtesy David N. Damon.)*

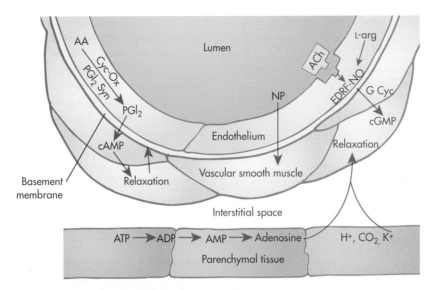

Figure 22-3 Arteriole illustrating endothelium- and nonendothelium-mediated vasodilation. Prostacyclin *(PGI₂)* is formed from arachidonic acid *(AA)* by the action of cyclooxygenase *(Cyc-Ox)* and prostacyclin synthetase *(PGI₂ Syn)* in the endothelium and elicits relaxation of the adjacent vascular smooth muscle via increases in cyclic AMP *(cAMP)*. Stimulation of the endothelial cells with acetylcholine *(ACh)* or other agents (see text) results in the formation and release of an EDRF (NO). The EDRF stimulates guanylyl cyclase *(G Cyc)* to increase cyclic GMP *(cGMP)* in the vascular smooth muscle to produce relaxation. The vasodilator agent nitroprusside *(NP)* acts directly on the vascular smooth muscle. Substances such as adenosine, H⁺, CO₂, and K⁺ can arise in the parenchymal tissue and elicit vasodilation by direct action on the vascular smooth muscle. *L-arg,* L-Arginine.

3). One such vasodilator is **endothelium-derived relaxing factor (EDRF),** which has been shown to be the gas **nitric oxide (NO).** The discoverers of NO were awarded the 1998 Nobel Prize for Medicine and Physiology. NO is formed and released in response to stimulation of the endothelium by various agents (e.g., acetylcholine, ATP, serotonin, bradykinin, histamine, substance P). **Prostacyclin** is another vasodilator that is synthesized by endothelial cells. However, the major function of prostacyclin is to inhibit platelet adherence to the endothelium and platelet aggregation, and thereby it aids in the prevention of intravascular thrombosis (see Chapter 16). A vasoconstrictor substance, **endothelin,** has also been isolated from endothelial cells.

Because of their narrow lumens, the thin-walled capillaries can withstand high internal pressures without bursting. This can be explained in terms of Laplace's law, as follows:

$$T = Pr \qquad\qquad 22\text{-}1$$

where:

  T = Tension in the vessel wall (dynes/cm)
  P = Transmural pressure (dynes/cm²)
  r = Radius of the vessel (cm)

Wall tension is the force per unit length tangential to the vessel wall. This force opposes the distending force (Pr) that tends to pull apart a theoretical longitudinal slit in the vessel (Figure 22-4). Transmural pressure is essentially equal to intraluminal pressure because extravascular pressure is usually negligible.

At normal aortic (100 mm Hg) and capillary (25 mm Hg) pressures, the wall tension of the aorta is about 12,000 times greater than that of the capillary (100 mm Hg × radius of 1.5 cm for the aorta versus 25 mm Hg ×

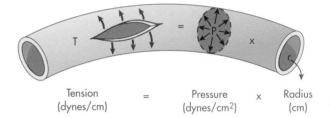

| Tension (dynes/cm) | = | Pressure (dynes/cm²) | × | Radius (cm) |

Figure 22-4 Diagram of a small blood vessel illustrating Laplace's law (T = Pr), in which force tends to pull apart a theoretical longitudinal slit in the vessel. *P,* Intraluminal pressure; *r,* Radius of the vessel; *T,* Wall tension as the force per unit length tangential to the vessel wall.

radius of 5 × 10⁻⁴ cm for the capillary). In a person standing quietly, capillary pressure in the feet may reach 100 mm Hg (see Chapter 24). Under such conditions, capillary wall tension increases to a value that is only one three thousandth that of the wall tension in the aorta at the same internal pressure.

According to Laplace's equation, wall tension increases as vessels dilate, even when internal pressure remains constant. Such is the case in **aneurysm** (local widening) **of the aorta,** in which wall tension may become high enough to rupture the vessel.

Capillary pores

The permeability of the capillary endothelial membrane is not the same in all body tissues. For example, the liver capillaries are very permeable, and albumin escapes at a much greater rate than from the less permeable muscle

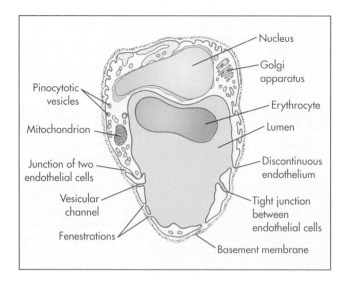

Figure 22-5 Sketch of an electron micrograph, showing a composite capillary in cross section.

capillaries. Also, permeability is not uniform along the whole capillary; the venous ends are more permeable than the arterial ends, and permeability is greatest in the venules. The greater permeability at the venous end of the capillaries and in the venules is caused by the greater number of **pores (clefts).** In most tissues the clefts are sparse and occupy only about 0.02% of the capillary surface area (Figure 22-5). In the brain, clefts are absent in the capillaries, and a **blood-brain barrier** to many small molecules exists.

In addition to clefts, some of the more porous capillaries (e.g., in the kidney and intestine) contain fenestrations 20 to 100 nm wide, whereas other capillaries (e.g., in the liver) have a discontinuous endothelium. The fenestrations appear to be sealed by a thin diaphragm, but they are quite permeable to large molecules. In contrast, only small molecules can pass through the intercellular clefts of the endothelium.

Transcapillary Exchange

Solvents and solutes move across the capillary endothelial wall via three processes: diffusion, filtration, and pinocytosis.

Diffusion is the most important means for solute transfer across the capillary endothelium

Normally only about 0.06 ml of water per minute moves back and forth across the capillary wall per 100 g of tissue as a result of filtration and absorption. In contrast, 300 ml of water per minute per 100 g of tissue moves by diffusion, a 5000-fold difference (see Chapter 1). Only about 2% of the plasma passing through the capillaries is filtered. In contrast, the rate that water diffuses back and forth across the endothelium is 40 times greater than the rate at which it is delivered to the capillaries via blood flow. The trans-

capillary exchange of solutes is also governed by diffusion. Thus DIFFUSION IS THE KEY FACTOR IN THE EXCHANGE OF GASES, SUBSTRATES, AND WASTE PRODUCTS BETWEEN THE CAPILLARIES AND THE TISSUE CELLS. However, the net transfer of fluid across the capillary endothelium is primarily attributable to filtration and absorption.

Lipid-insoluble substances

For small molecules such as water, NaCl, urea, and glucose, the capillary pores do not restrict diffusion. Diffusion proceeds so rapidly that the mean concentration gradient across the capillary endothelium is extremely small. Water passes through the capillary pores between endothelial cells. As the size of lipid-insoluble molecules increases, diffusion through muscle capillaries becomes progressively more restricted. The diffusion of molecules with molecular weights (MWs) greater than 60,000 becomes minimal. With small molecules the only limitations to net movement across the capillary wall is the rate at which blood flow transports the molecules to the capillary; transport is said to be **flow limited.**

When transport across the capillary is flow limited, a small-molecule solute (e.g., an inert tracer) diffuses from the blood near the origin of the capillary from the cognate arteriole into the interstitial fluid and parenchymal cells (Figure 22-6). A somewhat larger molecule moves farther along the capillary before its concentration in the blood becomes insignificant, and a still larger molecule cannot pass at all through the capillary pores (Figure 22-6, *A*). An increase in blood flow velocity extends the detectable concentration of small molecules farther down the capillary and increases the capillary diffusion capacity.

With large molecules, diffusion across the capillaries is the factor that limits exchange **(diffusion limited).** In other words, capillary permeability to a large-molecule solute limits the transport of the solute across the capillary wall (Figure 22-6, *A*).

> Under normal conditions, the diffusion of small lipid-insoluble molecules is so rapid that the exchange of such molecules between blood and tissue is never a problem. Such an exchange can become limited when the distances between capillaries and tissue cells are great (e.g., when capillary density is very low or tissue edema is extensive) [Figure 22-6, *B*].

Lipid-soluble molecules

In contrast to the movement of lipid-insoluble molecules, the movement of lipid-soluble molecules across the capillary wall is not limited to capillary pores because such molecules can pass directly through the lipid membranes of the entire capillary endothelium. Consequently, lipid-soluble molecules move very rapidly between blood and tissue. Lipid solubility (oil-to-

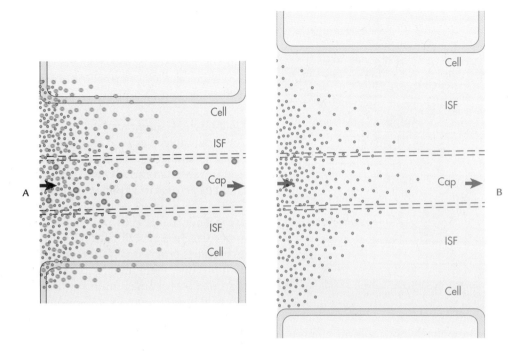

Figure 22-6 Flow- and diffusion-limited transport from capillaries *(Cap)* to tissue. **A,** Flow-limited transport. The smallest water-soluble inert tracer particles *(red dots)* reach negligible concentrations after passing only a short distance down the capillary. Larger particles with similar properties *(blue dots)* travel farther along the capillary before reaching insignificant intracapillary concentrations. Both substances cross the interstitial fluid *(ISF)* and reach the parenchymal tissue. Because of their size, more of the smaller particles are taken up by the tissue cells. The largest particles *(purple dots)* cannot penetrate the capillary pores and thus do not escape from the capillary lumen except by pinocytotic vesicle transport. An increase in the volume of blood flow or an increase in capillary density increases tissue supply for the diffusible solutes. Note that capillary permeability is greater at the venous end of the capillary (also in the venule, not shown) because of the larger number of pores in this region. **B,** Diffusion-limited transport. When the distance between the capillaries and the parenchymal tissue is large as a result of edema or low capillary density, diffusion becomes a limiting factor in the transport of solutes from capillary to tissue, even at high rates of capillary blood flow.

water partition coefficient) is a good index of the ease of transfer of lipid molecules through the capillary endothelium.

O_2 and CO_2 are both lipid soluble and readily pass through the endothelial cells. Calculations based on (1) the diffusion coefficient for O_2, (2) capillary density and diffusion distances, (3) blood flow, and (4) tissue O_2 consumption indicate that the O_2 supply of normal tissue at rest and during activity is not limited by diffusion or by the number of open capillaries.

Measurements of the O_2 tension and O_2 saturation of hemoglobin in the microvessels indicate that in many tissues, the blood O_2 content at the entrance of the capillaries has already decreased to about 80% of that in the aorta. This reduction occurs as a result of the diffusion of O_2 from the arterioles. Furthermore, CO_2 loading and the resulting intravascular shifts in the oxyhemoglobin dissociation curve (see Chapter 30) occur in the precapillary vessels. These findings indicate that O_2 and CO_2 pass directly between adjacent arterioles, venules, and possibly arteries and veins (countercurrent exchange [see Chapter 36]). This exchange of gas represents a diffusional shunt of gas around the capillaries; at low blood flow rates, it may limit the supply of O_2 to the tissue.

Capillary filtration is regulated by the hydrostatic and osmotic forces across the endothelium

The direction and the magnitude of the movement of water across the capillary wall are determined by the algebraic sum of the hydrostatic and osmotic pressures that exist across the membrane. An increase in the intracapillary hydrostatic pressure favors the movement of fluid from the vessel to the interstitial space. Conversely, an increase in the concentration of osmotically active particles within the vessels favors the movement of fluid into the vessels from the interstitial space.

Hydrostatic forces

The hydrostatic pressure (blood pressure) within the capillaries is not constant; it depends on the arterial pressure, the venous pressure, and the precapillary (arterioles) and postcapillary (venules and small veins) resistances. A rise in the arterial or venous pressure increases capillary hydrostatic pressure (P_c), whereas a reduction in either has the opposite effect. An increase in arteriolar resistance reduces capillary pressure, whereas an increase in venous resistance raises capillary pressure.

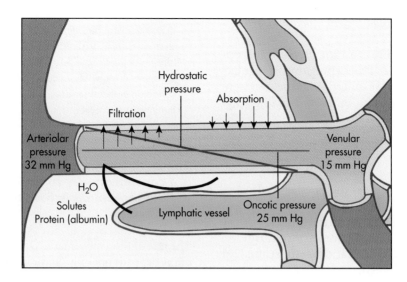

Figure 22-7 Factors responsible for filtration and absorption across the capillary wall and for the formation of lymph.

CAPILLARY HYDROSTATIC PRESSURE IS THE PRINCIPAL FORCE IN CAPILLARY FILTRATION, and the pressure varies from tissue to tissue and even within the same tissue. Average values, which were obtained from many direct measurements in human skin, are about 32 mm Hg at the arterial end of the capillaries and about 15 mm Hg at the venous end of the capillaries at the level of the heart (Figure 22-7). When an individual stands, the hydrostatic pressure in the capillaries of the lower extremities are higher and that of capillaries in the head are lower than when the individual is recumbent.

Tissue pressure, or more specifically **interstitial fluid pressure** (P_i), outside the capillaries, opposes capillary filtration. Hydrostatic pressure minus interstitial fluid pressure ($P_c - P_i$) constitutes the driving force for filtration. In the absence of edema, the P_i is essentially zero.

Osmotic forces

THE KEY FACTOR THAT RESTRAINS FLUID LOSS FROM THE CAPILLARIES IS THE OSMOTIC PRESSURE OF THE PLASMA PROTEINS, USUALLY TERMED THE **COLLOID OSMOTIC PRESSURE** OR **ONCOTIC PRESSURE** (π_p) (see Chapter 1). The total osmotic pressure of plasma is about 6000 mm Hg, whereas the oncotic pressure is only about 25 mm Hg. However, this small oncotic pressure is important in fluid exchange across the capillary wall because the plasma proteins are essentially confined to the intravascular space. The electrolytes that are mainly responsible for the total osmotic pressure of plasma are practically equal in concentration on both sides of the capillary endothelium. The relative permeability of solute to that of water influences the actual magnitude of the osmotic pressure.

The **reflection coefficient** is the relative impediment to the passage of a substance through the capillary membrane. The reflection coefficient of water is zero and that of albumin (to which the endothelium is almost impermeable) is 1. Filterable solutes have reflection coefficients between zero and 1.

Of the plasma proteins, albumin preponderates in determining oncotic pressure. The average albumin molecule (MW, 69,000) is approximately half the size of the average globulin molecule (MW, 150,000), and it is present in a greater concentration than the globulins (4.0 versus 3.0 g/dl of plasma). Albumin also exerts a greater osmotic force than can be accounted for solely on the basis of the number of molecules dissolved in the plasma. Therefore albumin cannot be completely replaced by inert substances of the same molecular size, (e.g., dextran). This additional osmotic force becomes disproportionately greater at high concentrations of albumin (as in plasma), and it is weak to absent in dilute solutions of albumin (as in interstitial fluid).

One reason for the behavior of albumin is its negative charge at a normal blood pH. The negatively charged albumin attracts and retains cations (principally Na^+) in the vascular compartment (the Gibbs-Donnan effect [see Chapter 2]). Furthermore, albumin binds a small number of Cl^- ions, which increases its negative charge and thus its ability to retain more Na^+ inside the capillaries. The small increase in the electrolyte concentration of plasma over that of interstitial fluid produced by the negatively charged albumin enhances its osmotic force to that of an ideal solution containing the same concentration of a solute with an MW of 37,000.

Small amounts of albumin escape from the capillaries and enter the interstitial fluid. This albumin exerts a very small osmotic force (0.1 to 5 mm Hg) because its concentration is low in the interstitial fluid, and at low concentrations, the osmotic force of albumin becomes simply a function of the number of albumin molecules per unit volume of interstitial fluid; the additional osmotic force caused by albumin's negative charge is absent.

Balance of hydrostatic and osmotic forces: Starling's hypothesis

The relationship between hydrostatic pressure and oncotic pressure and the role of these pressures in regulating fluid passage across the capillary endothelium were expounded by Ernest Starling in 1896. Starling's hypothesis is expressed by the following equation:

$$Q_f = k[(P_c + \pi_i) - (P_i + \pi_p)] \qquad \textbf{22-2}$$

where:

   Q_f = Fluid movement across the capillary wall
   k = Filtration constant for the capillary membrane
   P_c = Capillary hydrostatic pressure (mm Hg)
   π_i = Interstitial fluid oncotic pressure (mm Hg)
   P_i = Interstitial fluid hydrostatic pressure (mm Hg)
   π_p = Plasma oncotic pressure (mm Hg)

Net filtration occurs when the algebraic sum of the hydrostatic and osmotic pressures across the capillaries is positive, and net absorption occurs when the sum is negative.

Classically, filtration was thought to occur at the arterial end of the capillary and absorption at its venous end because of the gradient of hydrostatic pressure along the capillary. This is true for the idealized capillary, as depicted in Figure 22-7. However, in some vascular beds (e.g., the renal glomerulus), hydrostatic pressure in the capillary is high enough to result in filtration along the entire length of the capillary. In other vascular beds (e.g., in the intestinal mucosa), the hydrostatic and oncotic forces are such that absorption occurs along the whole capillary.

In the normal steady state, arterial pressure, venous pressure, postcapillary resistance, interstitial fluid hydrostatic and oncotic pressures, and plasma oncotic pressure remain relatively constant, and changes in precapillary resistance determine the movement of fluid across the capillary wall. Because water moves so quickly across the capillary endothelium, the hydrostatic and osmotic forces are nearly in equilibrium along the entire capillary. Thus filtration and absorption normally occur with very small imbalances of pressure across the capillary wall. Only about 2% of the plasma flowing through the vascular system is filtered, and of this, about 85% is absorbed in the capillaries and venules. The remainder returns to the vascular system in the lymph, along with the albumin that escapes from the capillaries.

In the lungs the mean capillary hydrostatic pressure is only about 8 mm Hg. Because the plasma oncotic pressure is 25 mm Hg and interstitial fluid oncotic pressure is approximately 15 mm Hg, the net force slightly favors reabsorption. Pulmonary lymph is formed, however, and it consists of fluid that is osmotically drawn out of the capillaries by the small amount of plasma protein that escapes through the capillary endothelium.

In pathological conditions such as **left ventricular failure** or **mitral valve stenosis,** the pulmonary capillary hydrostatic pressure may exceed plasma oncotic pressure. When this occurs, **pulmonary edema,** a condition that can seriously interfere with gas exchange in the lungs, may occur.

The capillary filtration coefficient is a convenient way to estimate the rate of fluid movement across the capillary endothelium

The rate of fluid movement (Q_f) across the capillary membrane depends not only on the algebraic sum of the hydrostatic and osmotic pressures (ΔP) across the endothelium but also on the area (A_m) of the capillary wall available for filtration, the distance (Δx) across the capillary wall (i.e., the thickness), the viscosity (η) of the filtrate, and the filtration constant (k) of the membrane, as follows:

$$Q_f = \frac{kA_m\Delta P}{\eta\Delta x} \qquad \textbf{22-3}$$

Because the thickness and area of the capillary wall and the viscosity of the filtrate are relatively constant for a given preparation, they can be incorporated with the filtration constant (k_t) in a total filtration constant, which is expressed per unit weight of tissue. Hence the equation can be simplified to the following:

$$Q_f = k_t\Delta P \qquad \textbf{22-4}$$

where k_t is the total capillary filtration coefficient and the units for Q_f are milliliters per minute per 100 g of tissue.

In any given tissue the filtration coefficient per unit area of capillary surface, and thus capillary permeability, is changed neither by physiological conditions such as arteriolar dilation and capillary distention nor by adverse conditions such as hypoxia, hypercapnia, and acidosis.

Capillary injury (e.g., toxins, severe burns) increases capillary permeability greatly (as indicated by an increased filtration coefficient), and significant amounts of fluid and protein leak out of the capillaries into the interstitial space. One of the important therapeutic measures used in the treatment of extensive **burns** is the replacement of lost fluid and plasma proteins.

Disturbances in hydrostatic-osmotic balance

Modest changes in arterial pressure per se may have little effect on filtration because the change may be countered by adjustments of the precapillary resistance vessels (autoregulation [see Chapter 23]).

In a condition such as **hemorrhage,** in which arterial and venous pressures are severely reduced, the capillary hydrostatic pressure falls. Furthermore, the low arterial blood pressure in hemorrhage decreases blood flow (and thus O_2 supply) to the tissues; therefore vasodilator metabolites accumulate and relax the arterioles. The reduced transmural pressure also induces precapillary vessel relaxation. Consequently, absorption predominates over filtration and thereby constitutes one of the body's compensatory mechanisms for restoring blood volume (see also Chapter 26).

An increase in venous pressure, as occurs in the feet when a person changes from the lying to the standing position, elevates capillary pressure and enhances filtration (see Chapter 24). However, the increase in transmural pressure causes precapillary vessel closure (myogenic mechanism [see Chapter 23]); therefore the capillary filtration coefficient decreases. This reduction in the capillary surface available for filtration protects against the extravasation of large amounts of fluid into the interstitial space.

The elevation of venous pressure (e.g., in **pregnancy** or **congestive heart failure,** combined with standing) enhances filtration beyond the capacity of the lymphatic system in the legs to remove the capillary filtrate from the interstitial space. **Edema** of the ankles and lower legs results.

The protein concentration in plasma may also change in pathological states. Thus it may alter the osmotic force and movement of fluid across the capillary membrane.

The plasma protein concentration is increased in **dehydration** (e.g., from water deprivation, prolonged sweating, severe vomiting, or diarrhea), and water moves by osmotic forces from the tissues to the vascular compartment. In contrast, the plasma protein concentration is reduced in **nephrosis** (a renal disease in which protein is lost in the urine), and edema may occur. When capillaries are injured, as in burns, protein along with fluid escapes from the plasma into the interstitial space and increases the oncotic pressure of the interstitial fluid. This greater osmotic force outside the capillaries causes additional fluid loss from the vascular system and may lead to severe intravascular **hypovolemia.**

Pinocytosis enables large molecules to cross the capillary endothelium

Some transfer of substances across the capillary wall can occur in tiny vesicles; this process is called **pinocytosis.** The pinocytotic vesicles, formed by pinching off a section of the surface membrane, can take up substances on one side of the capillary endothelial cell, move by thermal kinetic energy across the cell, and deposit their contents at the other side of the endothelial cell. The amount of material that can be transported in this way is much less than that moved by diffusion. However, pinocytosis may move large (30 nm) lipid-insoluble molecules between the blood and interstitial fluid. The number of pinocytotic vesicles in the endothelium varies with the tissue (muscle > lung > brain) and increases from the arterial to the venous end of the capillary.

The Lymphatics Return Fluid and Solutes that Escape from the Capillaries to the Circulating Blood

The terminal lymphatic vessels consist of a widely distributed closed-end network of highly permeable lymph capillaries that resemble blood capillaries in appearance. However, they generally lack tight junctions between endothelial cells, and they possess fine filaments that anchor them to the surrounding connective tissue. During skeletal muscle contraction, these fine strands may distort the lymphatic vessel and open spaces between the endothelial cells. This distortion permits protein, large particles, and cells in the interstitial fluid to enter the lymphatic capillaries.

The blood capillary filtrate and the protein and cells that have passed from the intravascular compartment to the interstitial fluid compartment are returned to the circulation by virtue of tissue pressure. This process is facilitated by intermittent skeletal muscle contractions, contractions of the lymphatic vessels, and an extensive system of one-way valves. The lymph flows through thin-walled vessels of progressively larger diameter and finally enters the right and left subclavian veins at their junctions with the respective internal jugular veins. Only cartilage, bone, epithelium, and tissues of the central nervous system are devoid of lymphatic vessels.

The volume of fluid that flows through the lymphatic system in 24 hours is about equal to an animal's total plasma volume. The protein returned by the lymphatics to the blood in a day is about one fourth to one half of the circulating plasma proteins. Lymphatic return is the only means whereby protein (mainly albumin) leaving the vascular compartment can be returned to the blood because back diffusion into the capillaries is negligible against the large albumin concentration gradient. If the protein was not removed from the interstitial spaces by the lymph vessels, it would accumulate in the interstitial fluid and act as an oncotic force to draw fluid from the blood capillaries to the interstitial spaces and produce edema.

> In addition to returning fluid and protein to the vascular bed, the lymphatic system filters the lymph at the lymph nodes and removes foreign particles such as bacteria. Thus the lymphatic system is an important component of the body's defense against bacterial invasion.

The largest lymphatic vessel, the thoracic duct, drains the lower extremities, returns protein lost through the permeable liver capillaries, and carries substances (principally fat in the form of chylomicrons) that are absorbed from the gastrointestinal tract to the circulating blood.

Lymph flow varies considerably; it is almost nil in resting skeletal muscle but increases during exercise in proportion to the degree of muscular activity. Lymph flow is increased by any mechanism that enhances the rate of blood capillary filtration; such mechanisms include increased capillary pressure, increased capillary permeability, and decreased plasma oncotic pressure.

> If the volume of interstitial fluid exceeds the drainage capacity of the lymphatics or if the lymphatic vessels become blocked, such as in **elephantiasis** (caused by **filariasis,** a worm infestation), interstitial fluid accumulates (edema), chiefly in the more compliant tissue (e.g., subcutaneous tissue).

SUMMARY

- Blood flow through the capillaries is regulated chiefly by contraction and relaxation of the arterioles (resistance vessels).
- The capillaries, which consist of a single layer of endothelial cells, can withstand high transmural pressure by virtue of their small diameter. According to Laplace's law, wall tension equals the transmural pressure multiplied by the radius of capillary ($T = Pr$).
- The endothelium is the source of EDRF (shown to be NO) and of prostacyclin, which relax vascular smooth muscles.
- The movement of water and small solutes between the vascular and interstitial fluid compartments occurs through capillary pores mainly by diffusion but also by filtration and absorption.
- Because the rate of diffusion is about 40 times greater than the blood flow in the tissue, the exchange of

small lipid-insoluble molecules is flow limited. The larger the molecules, the slower the diffusion until the lipid-insoluble molecules become diffusion limited. Molecules larger than about 60,000 MW are essentially confined to the vascular compartment.
- Lipid-soluble substances such as CO_2 and O_2 pass directly through the lipid membranes of the capillary endothelial cells, and the ease of transfer is directly proportional to the degree of lipid solubility of the substance.
- Capillary filtration and absorption are described by Starling's equation: $Q_f = k[(P_c + \pi_i) - (P_i + \pi_p)]$. Net filtration occurs when the algebraic sum of $(P_c + \pi_i)$ and $(P_i + \pi_p)$ is positive, and net absorption occurs when it is negative.
- By a process called pinocytosis, large molecules can move across the capillary wall in vesicles formed from the lipid membrane of the capillaries.
- Fluid and protein that have escaped from the blood capillaries enter the lymphatic capillaries and are transported via the lymphatic system back to the blood vascular compartment.

BIBLIOGRAPHY

Aukland K: Why don't our feet swell in upright position? *News Physiol Sci* 9:214, 1994.

Aukland K, Reed RK: Interstitial-lymphatic mechanisms in the control of extracellular fluid volume, *Physiol Rev* 73:1, 1993.

Bert JL, Pearce RH: The interstitium and microvascular exchange. In Renkin EM, Michel CC, eds: *Handbook of physiology,* section 2, *The cardiovascular system,* vol 4, parts 1 and 2, *Microcirculation,* Bethesda, Md, 1984, American Physiological Society.

Crone C, Levitt DG: Capillary permeability to small solutes. In Renkin EM, Michel CC, eds: *Handbook of physiology,* section 2, *The cardiovascular system,* vol 4, parts 1 and 2, *Microcirculation,* Bethesda, Md, 1984, American Physiological Society.

Curry FRE: Regulation of water and solute exchange in microvessel endothelium: studies in single perfused capillaries, *Microcirculation* 1:11, 1994.

Feng Q, Hedner T: Endothelium-derived relaxing factor (EDRF) and nitric oxide. II. Physiology, pharmacology, and pathophysiological implications, *Clin Physiol* 10:503, 1990.

Luscher TF, Vanhoutte PM: *The endothelium: modulator of cardiovascular function,* Boca Raton, Fla, 1990, CRC.

Michel CC: Fluid movements through capillary walls In Renkin EM, Michel CC, eds: *Handbook of physiology,* section 2, *The cardiovascular system,* vol 4, parts 1 and 2, *Microcirculation,* Bethesda, Md, 1984, American Physiological Society.

Pries AR et al: Resistance to blood flow in microvessels in vivo, *Circ Res* 75:904, 1994.

Renkin EM: Control of microcirculation and blood-tissue exchange. In Renkin EM, Michel CC, eds: *Handbook of physiology,* section 2, *The cardiovascular system,* vol 4, parts 1 and 2, *Microcirculation,* Bethesda, Md, 1984, American Physiological Society.

Rippe B, Haraldsson B: Transport of macromolecules across microvascular walls: the two-pore theory, *Physiol Rev* 74:163, 1994.

Rosell S: Neuronal control of microvessels, *Ann Rev Physiol* 42:359, 1980.

Welsh DG, Segal SS: Endothelial and smooth muscle cell conduction in arterioles controlling blood flow, *Am J Physiol* 274:H178, 1998.

Xia J, Duling BR: Patterns of excitation-contraction coupling in arterioles: dependence on time and concentration, *Am J Physiol* 274:H323, 1998.

CASE STUDIES

Case 22-1

A 45-year-old man with a long history of alcoholism (average 1 L/day of whiskey) was admitted to the hospital as an emergency because he vomited blood and fainted. In the past few months, he noted progressive anorexia, fatigue, jaundice, generalized itching, and abdominal swelling. Physical examination revealed a semicomatose man with pallor, jaundice, and ascites. The blood pressure was 90/40 mm Hg, the heart rate was 100 beats/min, and the hematocrit was 35%. Liver function tests indicated severe liver damage. The diagnosis was advanced cirrhosis of the liver. Immediate treatment was transfusion with 3 units of blood. The following pressures were noted before the transfusion:

Mesenteric capillary hydrostatic pressure (estimated)	44 mm Hg
Plasma oncotic pressure	23 mm Hg
Pressure in peritoneal cavity	8 mm Hg
Peritoneal fluid oncotic pressure	2 mm Hg

1. Which transcapillary pressure was responsible for the ascites?
   A. 11 mm Hg
   B. 21 mm Hg
   C. 8 mm Hg
   D. 15 mm Hg
   E. 13 mm Hg

2. After lost blood was replaced by transfusion, how was this condition treated?
   A. Dialysis
   B. High-fat diet
   C. Portacaval shunt
   D. Cholecystectomy
   E. Erythromycin

3. Which substance is mainly responsible for the oncotic pressure of the patient's plasma?
   A. Na^+
   B. Albumin
   C. Cl^-
   D. Globulin
   E. K^+

Case 22-2

A 25-year-old man suffered third-degree burns over the upper three fourths of his body in a fire in his home. Several hours elapsed before he reached the hospital. On admission, he was in a shocklike state. His heart rate was 110 beats/min, his blood pressure was 90/70 mm Hg, and his hematocrit was 55%. Blood analysis revealed an Na^+ level of 145 mEq/L, a K^+ level of 4 mEq/L, a Cl^- level of 105 mEq/L, and an albumin level of 3.5 g/dl.

1. The *most* effective treatment is an intravenous infusion of which fluid?
   A. Saline
   B. Whole blood
   C. 5% glucose
   D. Dextran
   E. Plasma

2. After several months of treatment with extensive artificial skin grafts, the patient was able to walk and resume an almost normal life. However, after prolonged standing, he noted slight ankle swelling but no ecchymoses in his feet. Why did the capillaries in his feet not rupture when he stood?
   A. Arterioles reflexly constrict and prevent exposure of the capillaries to high pressure.
   B. The tissue pressure rises and opposes an increase in the capillary pressure.
   C. The total capillary cross-sectional area is large enough to distribute the pressure and thereby compensate for the high intracapillary pressure.
   D. The capillary diameter is so small that the capillary wall tension is low.
   E. Capillaries constrict via a myogenic mechanism.

CHAPTER 23

Peripheral Circulation and Its Control

- Indicate the intrinsic and extrinsic (neural and humoral) factors that regulate peripheral blood flow.
- Explain the autoregulation of blood flow and the myogenic mechanism for local adjustments of blood flow.
- Explain the metabolic regulation of blood flow.
- Explain the role of the sympathetic nerves in blood flow regulation.
- Describe vascular reflexes in the control of blood flow.
- Describe the role of humoral agents in the regulation of blood flow.

The function of the heart and large blood vessels is to pump and carry blood to the tissues of the body, but the distribution of blood to the regions of the body where it is needed and away from where it is not needed rests with the small arteries and arterioles. THE REGULATION OF PERIPHERAL BLOOD FLOW IS ESSENTIALLY UNDER DUAL CONTROL: CENTRALLY BY THE NERVOUS SYSTEM AND LOCALLY IN THE TISSUES BY THE CONDITIONS IN THE IMMEDIATE VICINITY OF THE BLOOD VESSELS. The relative importance of the central and local control mechanisms is not the same in all tissues. In some areas of the body, such as the skin and the splanchnic regions, neural regulation of blood flow predominates, whereas in others, such as the heart and the brain, local factors are dominant.

The small arteries and arterioles that regulate blood flow throughout the body are called the **resistance vessels.** These vessels offer the greatest resistance to the flow of blood pumped to the tissues by the heart and thereby are important in the maintenance of arterial blood pressure. Smooth muscle fibers are the main component of the walls of the resistance vessels (see Figure 15-1). Therefore the vessel lumen can be varied from complete obliteration (by strong contraction of the smooth muscle with infolding of the endothelial lining) to maximal dilation (by full relaxation of the smooth muscle). At any given time, some resistance vessels are closed by partial contraction **(tone)** of the arteriolar smooth muscle. If all the resistance vessels in the body dilated simultaneously, the blood pressure would fall precipitously.

Contraction and Relaxation of Arteriolar Vascular Smooth Muscle Regulate Peripheral Blood Flow

Vascular smooth muscle controls total peripheral resistance and arterial and venous tone. The smooth muscle cells are small, mononucleate, and spindle shaped. They are generally arranged in several helical or circular layers around the larger vessels and in a thick circular layer around the arterioles (see Chapter 14). Passive stretching of the microvessels caused by an increase in intravascular pressure decreases vascular resistance, whereas a decrease in intravascular pressure increases vascular resistance via the recoil of the stretched vascular muscle.

Intrinsic or Local Control of Peripheral Blood Flow

Autoregulation and the myogenic mechanism tend to keep blood flow constant in the face of changes in perfusion pressure

Blood flow is adjusted to the existing metabolic activity in certain tissues. Furthermore, at constant levels of tissue metabolism, imposed changes in the perfusion pressure are met with vascular resistance changes that maintain a constant blood flow. This mechanism, which is illustrated in Figure 23-1, is commonly referred to as the **autoregulation of blood flow.** In the skeletal muscle preparation from which these data were gathered, the muscle was completely isolated from the rest of the animal and was in a resting state. The pressure was abruptly increased or decreased from a control pressure of 100 mm Hg. The blood flows observed immediately after the change in perfusion pressure are represented by the black curve. Maintenance of the pressure at each new level was followed within 60 seconds by a return of flow to or toward the control level; the red curve represents those steady-state flows. Over the pressure range of 20 to 120 mm Hg, the steady-state flow is relatively constant. Calculation of resistance (pressure/flow) across the vascular bed during steady-state conditions indicates that when the perfusion pressure was elevated, the resistance

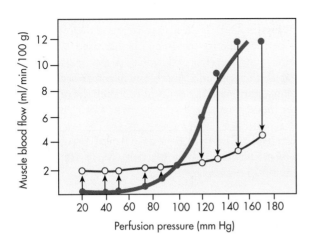

Figure 23-1 Pressure-flow relationship in the skeletal muscle vascular bed of the dog. The closed circles *(blue line)* represent the flows obtained immediately after abrupt changes in perfusion pressure from the control level (point where lines cross). The open circles *(red line)* represent the steady-state flows obtained at the new perfusion pressure. *(Redrawn from Jones RD, Berne RM: Circ Res 14:126, 1964.)*

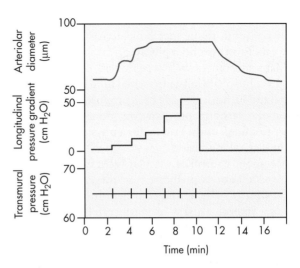

Figure 23-2 Flow-induced vasodilation in an isolated cardiac arteriole perfused at constant transmural pressure. The flow rate was increased by raising a reservoir connected to the proximal end of the cannulated arteriole. The transmural pressure *(bottom line)* was held constant by lowering a reservoir connected to the distal end of the arteriole by the same amount as the proximal reservoir was raised. The longitudinal pressure gradient *(center line)* was elevated in steps by raising the proximal reservoir and lowering the distal reservoir. The flow rate (not shown) was increased proportionately to the increase in the longitudinal pressure gradient (driving pressure). The arteriolar diameter *(top line)* increased with the rise in driving pressure. *(Redrawn from Kuo L, Davis MJ, Chilian WM, Am J Physiol 259:H1063, 1990.)*

vessels constricted, whereas when it was reduced, they dilated.

The mechanism that appears to be responsible for this constancy of blood flow in the presence of an altered perfusion pressure is called the **myogenic mechanism.** AC-CORDING TO THE MYOGENIC MECHANISM, THE VASCULAR SMOOTH MUSCLE CONTRACTS IN RESPONSE TO STRETCH AND RELAXES WITH A REDUCTION IN STRETCH. An abrupt increase in perfusion pressure initially distends the blood vessels. This passive vascular distention is followed by contraction of the smooth muscles of the resistance vessels and a return of blood flow to the previous control level.

Because blood pressure is reflexly maintained at a fairly constant level under normal conditions, the operation of a myogenic mechanism would be expected to be minimal. However, when a person changes from a lying to a standing position, a large increase in transmural pressure occurs in the vessels of the lower extremities. The precapillary vessels constrict in response to this imposed stretch. The constriction diminishes capillary filtration until the increase in plasma oncotic pressure and the increase in interstitial fluid pressure balance the elevated capillary hydrostatic pressure associated with the vertical position (see Chapters 22 and 24).

> If arteriolar resistance did not increase with standing, the hydrostatic pressure in the lower parts of the legs would reach such high levels that large volumes of fluid would pass from the capillaries into the interstitial fluid compartment and produce **edema.** In a patient with elevated venous pressure, as in **heart failure,** the additional hydrostatic pressure in the standing position produces edema of the feet, ankles, and lower legs.

The endothelium actively regulates blood flow

In isolated coronary arterioles perfused at constant transmural pressure, rapid blood flow elicits vasodilation (Figure 23-2). The vasodilation is caused by **endothelium-derived relaxing factor (nitric oxide),** which is released by the endothelial cells in response to the shear stress that the rapid flow exerts on the vascular endothelium. Removal of the endothelium from the arterioles abolishes this dilator response to enhanced flow velocity.

Tissue metabolic activity is the main factor in the local regulation of blood flow

According to metabolic hypothesis, BLOOD FLOW IS GOV-ERNED BY THE METABOLIC ACTIVITY OF THE TISSUE. ANY INTERVEN-TION THAT IMPEDES O_2 SUPPLY TO THE TISSUE RELEASES VASODILA-TOR METABOLITES FROM THE TISSUE. When the metabolic rate of the tissue increases or the O_2 delivery to the tissue decreases, more vasodilator substance is formed, and blood flow increases. If perfusion pressure is constant, a decrease in metabolic activity will decrease the concentration of the vasodilator in the tissue and thereby increase precapillary resistance. Similarly, if metabolic activity is constant, an increase in perfusion pressure and consequently in blood flow will decrease the tissue concentration of the vasodilator agent (metabolite washout) and increase precapillary resistance. An attractive feature of the metabolic hypothesis is that in most tissues, blood flow closely parallels metabolic activity. Thus even when blood pressure is kept fairly constant, tissue metabolic activity and blood flow may vary together under physiological conditions.

Many substances such as lactic acid, CO_2, H^+, Na^+, inorganic phosphate ions, interstitial fluid osmolarity, adenosine, and nitric oxide have been proposed as mediators of metabolic vasodilation. However, none of these agents alone fulfills all of the criteria for a physiological vasodilator in skeletal muscle.

Metabolic control of vascular resistance by the release of a vasodilator is predicated on the existence of **basal tone,** which is the partial contraction (tonic activity) of vascular smooth muscle. In contrast to basal tone in skeletal muscle, basal tone in vascular smooth muscle is independent of the nervous system, and the factor responsible is not known. It could be related to the muscles, a vasoconstrictor substance in the blood, or both.

If arterial inflow to a vascular bed is stopped for a few seconds to several minutes, blood flow immediately after the release of the occlusion exceeds the flow before the occlusion, and it returns only gradually to the control level. This increase in blood flow **(reactive hyperemia)** is illustrated in Figure 23-3, in which blood flow to the leg was stopped by clamping the femoral artery for 15, 30, and 60 seconds. Release of the 60-second occlusion resulted in a peak blood flow that was 70% greater than the control flow, and the flow returned to the control level within about 110 seconds.

When this same experiment is done in humans by inflating a blood pressure cuff on the upper arm, dilation of the resistance vessels of the hand and forearm is evident as a bright red skin color and a fullness of the veins, which occur immediately after the cuff is released. Within limits,

the peak flow and particularly the duration of the reactive hyperemia are proportional to the duration of the occlusion (Figure 23-3). If the arm is exercised during the occlusion period, reactive hyperemia is increased. These observations and the close relationship that exists between metabolic activity and blood flow in the unoccluded limb are consonant with the concept of metabolic regulation of tissue blood flow.

Extrinsic Control of Peripheral Blood Flow Is Mediated Mainly by the Sympathetic Nervous System

Impulses in regions of the medulla descend in the sympathetic nerves to increase vascular resistance

Several regions in the medulla oblongata influence cardiovascular activity (see Chapter 19). Some of the effects of stimulation of the dorsal lateral medulla are vasoconstriction, cardiac acceleration, and enhanced myocardial contractility. Caudal and ventromedial to the pressor region in the medulla is a zone that decreases blood pressure on stimulation. This **depressor area** exerts its effect by the direct inhibition of spinal neurons and by the inhibition of the medullary **pressor region.** These areas do not constitute an anatomical center because no discrete group of cells is discernible. However, these cells do constitute a physiological center in that stimulation of the pressor region produces the responses mentioned previously.

From the vasoconstrictor regions, fibers descend in the spinal cord and synapse at different levels of the thoracolumbar region (T1 to L2 or L3). Fibers from the intermediolateral gray matter of the cord emerge with the ventral roots but leave the motor fibers to join the paravertebral sympathetic chains through the white communicating branches (see Chapter 10). These preganglionic white (myelinated) fibers may pass up or down the sympathetic chains to synapse in the various ganglia within the chains or in certain outlying ganglia. Postganglionic gray branches (unmyelinated) then join the corresponding segmental spinal nerves and accompany them to the periphery to innervate the arteries and veins. Postganglionic sympathetic fibers from the various ganglia join the large arteries and accompany them as an investing network of fibers to the resistance (arterioles) and capacitance (veins) vessels.

The vasoconstrictor regions are tonically active. Reflexes or humoral stimuli that enhance this activity increase the frequency of impulses reaching the terminal branches of the vessels. A constrictor neurohumor (norepinephrine) is released from the postganglionic nerve endings and constricts (α-adrenergic effect) the resistance vessels. Inhibition of the vasoconstrictor area diminishes the frequency of impulses in the efferent fibers, and this effect results in vasodilation. In this manner, NEURAL REGULATION OF THE PERIPHERAL CIRCULATION IS ACCOMPLISHED MAINLY BY ALTERING THE NUMBER OF IMPULSES PASSING DOWN THE VASOCON-

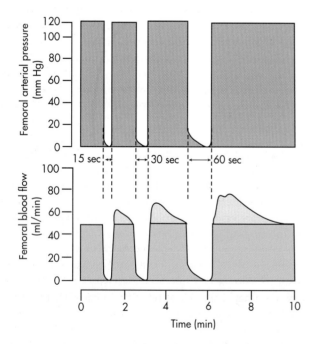

Figure 23-3 Reactive hyperemia in the hind limb of a dog after 15-, 30-, and 60-second occlusions of the femoral artery. *(From Berne RM: Unpublished observations.)*

STRICTOR FIBERS OF THE SYMPATHETIC NERVES TO THE BLOOD VESSELS. The tonic activity of the vasomotor regions may vary rhythmically, which is manifested as oscillations of arterial pressure. Some oscillations occur at the frequency of respiration **(Traube-Hering waves)** and are caused by an increase in sympathetic impulses to the resistance vessels during inspiration. Other oscillations **(Mayer waves)** occur at a lower frequency than that of respiration.

An increase in sympathetic nerve activity constricts resistance and capacitance vessels

The vasoconstrictor fibers of the sympathetic nervous system supply the arteries, arterioles, and veins, but the neural influence on the large vessels is far less important functionally than it is on the microcirculation. Capacitance vessels (veins) are more responsive to sympathetic nerve stimulation than resistance vessels; they are maximally constricted at a lower frequency of stimulation than resistance vessels. However, capacitance vessels do not respond to vasodilator metabolites. Norepinephrine is the neurotransmitter released at the sympathetic nerve terminals at the blood vessels. Many other factors, such as circulating hormones and particularly locally released substances, modify the liberation of norepinephrine from the nerve terminals.

At basal vascular tone, approximately one third of the blood volume in a tissue can be mobilized from the capacitance vessels on stimulation of the sympathetic nerves at physiological frequencies. Because basal tone is very low in capacitance vessels, only small increases in tissue blood volume are obtained with maximum doses of the potent vasodilator acetylcholine. Hence at basal tone the tissue blood volume is close to maximum. In exercise, activation of the sympathetic nerve fibers constricts veins and thus augments central venous pressure and hence the cardiac filling pressure.

In **arterial hypotension,** such as that induced by hemorrhage, the capacitance vessels constrict and thereby aid in overcoming the associated decrease in central venous pressure. In addition, the resistance vessels constrict in **hemorrhagic shock** and thereby assist in the restoration of arterial pressure (see Chapter 26). Furthermore, extravascular fluid is mobilized by a greater reabsorption of fluid from the tissues into the capillaries in response to the lowered capillary hydrostatic pressure caused by the lower arterial pressure.

Parasympathetic neural influence is apparent only in blood vessels in the cranial and sacral regions

The efferent fibers of the cranial division of the parasympathetic nervous system supply the blood vessels of the head and viscera, whereas fibers of the sacral division supply the blood vessels of the genitalia, bladder, and large bowel. Skeletal muscle and skin do not receive parasympathetic innervation. Because only a small proportion of the resistance vessels of the body receives parasympathetic fibers, the effect of these cholinergic fibers on total vascular resistance is small.

Epinephrine and norepinephrine are the chief humoral factors that affect vascular resistance

Epinephrine and norepinephrine exert a profound effect on the peripheral blood vessels. In skeletal muscle, epinephrine in low concentrations dilates resistance vessels (β-adrenergic effect) and in high concentrations constricts them (α-adrenergic effect). However, in skin, only vasoconstriction occurs with epinephrine. In contrast, norepinephrine elicits vasoconstriction in all vascular beds. When stimulated, the adrenal gland releases mainly epinephrine but also some norepinephrine into the systemic circulation (see Chapter 47). Under physiological conditions, however, the effect of catecholamine release from the adrenal medulla is much less important than the effect of norepinephrine release from the sympathetic nerves.

Vascular reflexes are responsible for rapid adjustments of blood pressure

Areas of the medulla oblongata that mediate sympathetic and vagal effects are under the influence of neural impulses (arising in the baroreceptors, chemoreceptors, hypothalamus, cerebral cortex, and skin) and of local CO_2 and O_2 concentrations.

Baroreceptors
The **baroreceptors** (or **pressoreceptors**) are stretch receptors located in the **carotid sinuses** (slightly widened areas of the internal carotid arteries at their points of origin from the common carotid arteries [Figure 23-4]) and in the **aortic arch.** Impulses arising in the carotid sinus travel up afferent fibers in the **carotid sinus nerve,** which is a branch of the glossopharyngeal nerve. Impulses arising in the baroreceptors of the aortic arch reach the medulla via afferent fibers in the vagus nerves. These fibers from both sets of baroreceptors travel to the **nucleus of the tractus solitarius (NTS)** in the medulla. The NTS is the site of central projection of the chemoreceptors and baroreceptors. Its stimulation inhibits sympathetic nerve impulses to the peripheral blood vessels and produces vasodilation **(depressor effect),** whereas experimental destruction of the NTS produces vasoconstriction **(pressor effect).**

THE BARORECEPTOR NERVE TERMINALS IN THE WALLS OF THE CAROTID SINUS AND AORTIC ARCH RESPOND TO THE VASCULAR STRETCH AND DEFORMATION INDUCED BY ARTERIAL PRESSURE. The frequency of firing is enhanced by an increase in blood pressure and diminished by a reduction in blood pressure. An increase in the impulse frequency inhibits the medullary vasoconstrictor regions and results in peripheral vasodilation and a lowering of blood pressure.

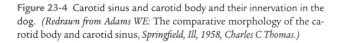

Figure 23-4 Carotid sinus and carotid body and their innervation in the dog. *(Redrawn from Adams WE: The comparative morphology of the carotid body and carotid sinus, Springfield, Ill, 1958, Charles C Thomas.)*

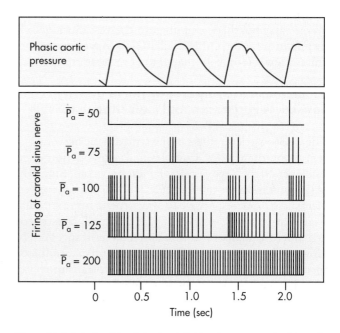

Figure 23-5 Relationship of phasic aortic blood pressure to the firing of a single afferent nerve fiber from the carotid sinus at different levels of mean arterial pressure $(\overline{P}_a)$.

Contributing to a lowering of the blood pressure is bradycardia caused by stimulation of the vagal nuclei in the medulla. The carotid sinus baroreceptors are more sensitive to pressure change than the aortic baroreceptors. However, when the blood pressure changes are pulsatile, the two sets of baroreceptors respond similarly.

The carotid sinus with the sinus nerve intact can be isolated from the rest of the circulation and can be artificially perfused. Under these conditions, changes in the pressure within the carotid sinus elicit reciprocal changes in the blood pressure of the experimental animal. The receptors in the walls of the carotid sinus show some adaptation, and therefore they are more responsive to constantly changing pressures than to sustained constant pressures; this is illustrated in Figure 23-5. At normal levels of blood pressure a barrage of impulses from a single fiber of the carotid sinus nerve is initiated in early systole by the pressure rise; only a few spikes are observed during late systole and early diastole (Figure 23-5). At lower pressures, these phasic changes are even more evident, but the overall frequency of discharge is reduced. The blood pressure threshold for eliciting sinus nerve impulses is about 50 mm Hg, and a maximum level of sustained firing is reached at approximately 200 mm Hg.

Because the baroreceptors do adapt, their response is greater to a large than to a small pulse pressure. This is illustrated in Figure 23-6, which shows the effects of damping pulsations in the carotid sinus on the fre-

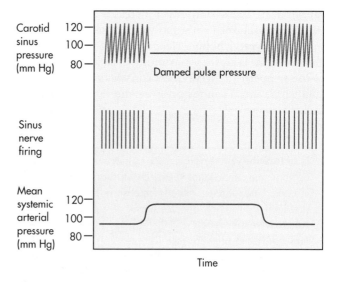

Figure 23-6 Effect of reducing pulse pressure in the vascularly isolated perfused carotid sinuses *(top)* on impulses recorded from a fiber of a sinus nerve *(middle)* and on the mean systemic arterial pressure *(bottom)*. The mean pressure in the carotid sinuses *(red line, top)* is constant when pulse pressure is damped.

quency of firing in a sinus nerve fiber and on the systematic arterial pressure. When the pulse pressure in the carotid sinuses is reduced but mean pressure remains constant, the frequency of the neural impulses recorded from a sinus nerve fiber decreases, and the systemic arterial pressure increases. Restoration of the pulse pressure in the carotid sinus returns the frequency of sinus nerve discharge and systemic arterial pressure to control levels (Figure 23-6).

The resistance increases that occur in the peripheral vascular beds in response to reduced pressure in the carotid sinus vary from one vascular bed to another and thereby redistribute blood flow. For example, the resistance changes elicited in the dog by altering the carotid sinus pressure are greatest in the femoral vessels, less in the renal vessels, and least in the mesenteric and celiac vessels.

> The sensitivity of the carotid sinus reflex can be altered. For example, in **hypertension**, when the carotid sinus becomes stiffer and less deformable as a result of the high intraarterial pressure, baroreceptor sensitivity decreases. In some individuals the carotid sinus is overly sensitive to pressure; tight collars or other forms of external pressure over the region of the carotid sinus may elicit **hypotension** and **fainting**.

THE BARORECEPTORS PLAY A KEY ROLE IN SHORT-TERM ADJUSTMENTS OF BLOOD PRESSURE WHEN THE CHANGES IN BLOOD VOLUME, CARDIAC OUTPUT, AND PERIPHERAL RESISTANCE ARE RELATIVELY ABRUPT (AS IN EXERCISE). HOWEVER, LONG-TERM CONTROL OF BLOOD PRESSURE (I.E., OVER DAYS OR WEEKS) IS DETERMINED MAINLY BY THE INDIVIDUAL'S FLUID BALANCE, NAMELY THE BALANCE BETWEEN FLUID INTAKE AND OUTPUT. When peripheral resistance is constant, an increased blood volume raises blood pressure by augmenting cardiac output (see Chapter 24). BY FAR, THE MOST IMPORTANT ORGAN IN CONTROL OF BODY FLUID VOLUME AND THUS BLOOD PRESSURE IS THE KIDNEY. With overhydration the excess fluid is excreted, whereas with dehydration, urine output is reduced.

Cardiopulmonary baroreceptors

In addition to the carotid sinus and aortic baroreceptors, cardiopulmonary receptors also exist; both types of receptors are necessary for the full expression of blood pressure regulation. The cardiopulmonary receptors initiate reflexes via vagal and sympathetic afferent and efferent nerves. These reflexes are tonically active, and they can alter peripheral resistance in response to changes in intracardiac, venous, and pulmonary vascular pressures.

Peripheral chemoreceptors are stimulated by decreases in arterial blood O_2 tension and increases in arterial blood CO_2 tension

The **peripheral chemoreceptors** consist of the carotid body (at the bifurcation of the carotid artery) and several small, highly vascular bodies in the regions of the aortic arch. THE CHEMORECEPTORS ARE SENSITIVE TO CHANGES IN ARTERIAL BLOOD O_2 TENSION (Pa_{O_2}), CO_2 TENSION (Pa_{CO_2}), AND pH.

Although they are concerned mainly with the regulation of respiration (see Chapter 31), the peripheral chemoreceptors reflexly influence the circulatory system to a minor degree.

A reduction in Pa_{O_2} stimulates the chemoreceptors. The resulting increase in the frequency of impulses in the afferent nerve fibers from the carotid and aortic bodies stimulates the vasoconstrictor regions; this action increases tone in the resistance and capacitance vessels. The reflex vascular effect induced by an increased Pa_{CO_2} and by a reduced pH is much less than the direct effect of **hypercapnia** (an elevated Pa_{CO_2}) and of H^+ on the vasomotor regions in the medulla. When hypoxia and hypercapnia coexist **(asphyxia)**, the stimulation of the chemoreceptors is greater than the sum of the two blood gas stimuli when they act independently. Simultaneous stimulation of the chemoreceptors and reduction of arterial pressure (reduced stimulation of the baroreceptors) enhance the vasoconstrictor response of the peripheral vessels. However, when both the baroreceptors and chemoreceptors are stimulated together (e.g., high carotid sinus pressure and low Pa_{O_2}), the cardiovascular effects of the baroreceptors predominate.

> Chemoreceptors with sympathetic afferent fibers exist in the heart. These cardiac chemoreceptors are activated by myocardial ischemia, and they transmit the precordial pain **(angina pectoris)** associated with an inadequate blood supply to the myocardium.

Hypothalamus

Optimal function of the cardiovascular reflexes requires the integrity of pontine and hypothalamic structures. Furthermore, these structures are responsible for behavioral and emotional control of the cardiovascular system. Stimulation of the anterior hypothalamus decreases blood pressure and heart rate, whereas stimulation of the posterolateral region increases blood pressure and heart rate. The hypothalamus also contains a temperature-regulating center that affects the skin vessels. Cooling of the skin or the blood perfusing the hypothalamus results in constriction of the skin vessels and heat conservation, whereas warm stimuli have the opposite effects.

Cerebrum

The cerebral cortex can also affect the blood flow distribution in the body. Stimulation of the motor and premotor areas can affect blood pressure; usually a pressor response is obtained. However, vasodilation and hypotensive responses may be evoked (e.g., blushing, fainting) in response to an emotional stimulus.

Skin and viscera

Painful stimuli can elicit either an increase or a decrease in blood pressure depending on the magnitude and location of the stimulus. Distention of the viscera often decreases blood pressure, whereas painful stimuli on the body surface usually raise blood pressure.

Pulmonary reflexes

Inflation of the lungs reflexly dilates systemic resistance vessels and decreases arterial blood pressure. Conversely, collapse of the lungs causes the constriction of systemic vessels. Afferent fibers that mediate this reflex are carried in the vagus nerves. Stimulation of the pulmonary stretch receptors inhibits the vasomotor areas. The magnitude of the depressor response to lung inflation is directly related to the degree of inflation and to the existing level of vasoconstrictor tone; the greater the vascular tone, the greater the hypotension produced by lung inflation.

Chemosensitive regions of the medulla

Increases in Pa_{CO_2} stimulate the medullary vasoconstrictor regions and thereby increase peripheral resistance. Reduction in Pa_{CO_2} below normal levels (as with hyperventilation) decreases the tonic activity in these areas and thus decreases peripheral resistance. The chemosensitive regions are also affected by changes in pH. A lowering of blood pH stimulates and a rise in blood pH inhibit these areas.

Changes in Pa_{O_2} usually have little direct effect on the vasomotor region in the medulla. The reflex effect of hypoxia is mediated mainly by the carotid and aortic chemoreceptors. A moderate reduction of Pa_{O_2} stimulates the vasomotor region, but severe reduction depresses vasomotor activity, just as a very low Pa_{O_2} depress other areas of the brain.

> **Cerebral ischemia,** such as that which can occur with an expanding **intracranial tumor,** results in severe peripheral vasoconstriction. The stimulation is probably caused by a local accumulation of CO_2 and a reduction of O_2 in certain regions of the brain. With prolonged severe ischemia, extreme depression of cerebral function eventually supervenes, and the blood pressure falls.

Balance Between Intrinsic and Extrinsic Factors in the Regulation of Peripheral Blood Flow

Dual control of the peripheral vessels by intrinsic and extrinsic mechanisms constitutes a complex system of vascular regulation. This system enables the body to direct blood flow to areas where the need is greater and to divert it away from areas where the need is less. In some tissues the relative potency of extrinsic and intrinsic mechanisms is constant. However, in other tissues the ratio is changeable depending on that tissue's

state of activity. In the brain and heart, which are vital structures with very limited tolerance for a reduced blood supply, intrinsic flow-regulating mechanisms are dominant.

> Massive discharge of the medullary vasoconstrictor region (which might occur in response to a severe, acute hemorrhage) has negligible effects on the cerebral and cardiac resistance vessels, but it greatly constricts the skin, renal, and splanchnic blood vessels.

In the skin, extrinsic vascular control is dominant. Not only do the cutaneous vessels participate strongly in a general vasoconstrictor discharge, but they also respond selectively through the hypothalamic pathways that subserve body temperature regulation. However, intrinsic control can be demonstrated by local changes of skin temperature that can modify or override the central influence on the resistance and capacitance vessels.

In skeletal muscle the changing balance between extrinsic and intrinsic mechanisms can be clearly seen. In resting skeletal muscle, neural control (vasoconstrictor tone) is dominant. This can be demonstrated by the large increment in blood flow that occurs immediately after the sympathetic nerves to the muscle are cut. Just before and at the start of running, blood flow increases

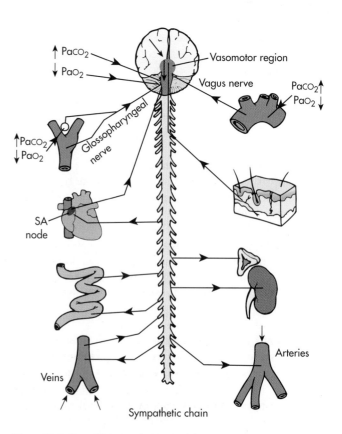

Figure 23-7 Neural input and output of the vasomotor region. *SA node,* Sinoatrial node.

in the leg muscles. After the onset of exercise, the intrinsic flow-regulating mechanism assumes control. Because of the local increase in metabolites, vasodilation occurs in the active muscles. Vasoconstriction occurs in the inactive muscles and other tissues as a manifestation of the general sympathetic discharge associated with exercise. However, the constrictor impulses that reach the resistance vessels of the active muscles are overridden by the local metabolic effect, which dilates the vessels. Operation of this dual-control mechanism thus provides more blood where it is required and shunts it away from the inactive areas.

Similar effects may be achieved by a general increase in Pa_{CO_2}. Normally the hyperventilation associated with exercise keeps the Pa_{CO_2} at normal levels. However, if the Pa_{CO_2} increases during exercise, generalized vasoconstriction occurs because of the stimulation of the medullary vasoconstrictor region by CO_2. In the active muscles, where the CO_2 concentration is highest, the smooth muscle of the arterioles relaxes in response to the high Pa_{CO_2} concentration locally. Factors that affect and that are affected by the medullary vasomotor region are summarized in Figure 23-7.

SUMMARY

- The arterioles, often referred to as the *resistance vessels,* are important in the regulation of blood flow through their cognate capillaries. Smooth muscle, which constitutes a major fraction of the wall of the arterioles, contracts and relaxes in response to neural and humoral stimuli.
- Most tissues show autoregulation of blood flow, a phenomenon characterized by a relatively constant blood flow in the face of a substantial change in perfusion pressure. A logical explanation of autoregulation is the myogenic mechanism, by which an increase in transmural pressure elicits a direct contractile response of the vascular smooth muscle, whereas a decrease in transmural pressure directly elicits relaxation.
- The striking parallelism between tissue blood flow and tissue O_2 consumption indicates that blood flow is regulated largely by a metabolic mechanism. A decrease in the O_2 supply/demand ratio of a tissue releases one or more vasodilator metabolites that dilate arterioles and thereby enhance the O_2 supply.
- Neural regulation of blood flow is accomplished mainly by the sympathetic nervous system. Sympathetic nerves to blood vessels are tonically active; inhibition of the vasoconstrictor center in the medulla reduces peripheral vascular resistance. Stimulation of the sympathetic nerves constricts resistance and capacitance vessels.
- In the organs and tissues supplied by the cranial and sacral divisions of the parasympathetic nervous system, blood vessels are under parasympathetic (as well as sympathetic) control. Parasympathetic activity usually induces vasodilation, but the effect is ordinarily weak.
- The baroreceptors (or pressoreceptors) in the internal carotid arteries and aorta are tonically active and regulate blood pressure on a moment-to-moment basis. Stretch of these receptors caused by an increase in arterial pressure reflexly inhibits the vasoconstrictor center in the medulla and induces vasodilation, whereas a decrease in arterial pressure disinhibits the vasoconstrictor center and induces vasoconstriction.
- The carotid baroreceptors predominate over those in the aorta, and both respond more vigorously to pulsatile pressure (stretch) than to steady (nonpulsatile) pressures.
- Baroreceptors are also present in the cardiac chambers and large pulmonary vessels (cardiopulmonary baroreceptors); they have less influence on blood pressure than arterial baroreceptors, but they participate in blood volume regulation.
- Peripheral chemoreceptors in the carotid bodies and aortic arch and central chemoreceptors in the medulla oblongata are stimulated by a decrease in Pa_{O_2} and by an increase in Pa_{CO_2}. Stimulation of these chemoreceptors generally increases the rate and depth of respiration but also produces peripheral vasoconstriction.
- Peripheral vascular resistance and hence blood pressure can be affected by stimuli arising in the skin, viscera, lungs, and brain.
- The combined effect of neural and local metabolic factors is to distribute blood to active tissues and divert it from inactive tissues. In vital structures such as the heart and brain and in contracting skeletal muscle, metabolic factors predominate over neural factors.

BIBLIOGRAPHY

Berg BR, Cohen KD, Sarelius IH: Direct coupling between blood flow and metabolism at the capillary level in striated muscle, *Am J Physiol* 272:H2693, 1997.

Cowley AW Jr: Long-term control of blood pressure, *Physiol Rev* 72:231, 1992.

Doyle MP, Duling BR: Acetylcholine induces conducted vasodilation by nitric oxide–dependent and –independent mechanisms, *Am J Physiol* 272:H1364, 1997.

Hainsworth R: Reflexes from the heart, *Physiol Rev* 71:617, 1991.

Hickner RC et al: Role of nitric oxide in skeletal muscle blood flow at rest and during dynamic exercise in humans, *Am J Physiol* 273:H405, 1997.

Kuo L, Davis JJ, Chilian WM: Endothelium-dependent flow-induced dilation of isolated coronary arterioles, *Am J Physiol* 259:H1063, 1990.

Marshall JM: Peripheral chemoreceptors and cardiovascular regulation, *Physiol Rev* 74:543, 1994.

Persson PB: Modulation of cardiovascular control mechanisms and their interaction, *Physiol Rev* 76:193, 1996.

Persson PB, Kirchheim HR, eds: *Baroreceptor reflexes,* Berlin, 1991, Springer-Verlag.

Porter VA et al: Frequency modulation of Ca^{2+} sparks is involved in regulation of arterial diameter by cyclic nucleotides, *Am J Physiol* 274:C1346, 1998.

Shepard JT: Cardiac mechanoreceptors. In Fozzard HA et al, eds: *The heart and cardiovascular system: scientific foundations,* ed 2, Philadelphia, 1991, Raven.

Shoemaker JK et al: Contributions of acetylcholine and nitric oxide to forearm blood flow at exercise onset and recovery, *Am J Physiol* 273:H2388, 1997.

Zucker IH, Gilmore JP, eds: *Reflex control of the circulation,* Boca Raton, Fla, 1991, CRC.

▷ CASE STUDIES

Case 23-1

A 40-year-old man goes to see his physician because of pain in the calves of both legs when he walks moderate distances; the pain is especially noticeable when he walks uphill or when he climbs stairs. The onset of the pain was insidious and has progressively increased in frequency and severity. He has had no other symptoms. He has a normal diet, has two cocktails before dinner, and has smoked two packs of cigarettes per day for the past 22 years. The results of the physical examination were essentially normal except for the absence of pulses in the dorsalis pedis and posterior tibial arteries in both legs. Arteriography revealed a narrowing of the major arteries of both lower legs. He was diagnosed as having **thromboangiitis obliterans,** a severe progressive obstructive disease of large arteries.

1. **What do the arterioles in the lower legs show at rest?**
   A. Myogenic constriction
   B. Metabolic dilation
   C. Autoregulation
   D. Myogenic dilation
   E. Metabolic constriction

2. **What will the physician probably recommend?**
   A. Stopping smoking
   B. A vasodilator medication
   C. Bilateral sympathectomy of the lower extremities
   D. Application of heat to the lower legs three or four times a day
   E. A vasoconstrictor medication

Case 23-2

A 72-year-old man was admitted to the hospital for repeated brief episodes of loss of consciousness.

1. **Which of the following diagnoses should *not* be considered?**
   A. Carotid sinus hypersensitivity
   B. Complete heart block
   C. Orthostatic hypotension
   D. Atrial or ventricular tachycardia
   E. Diabetic coma

2. **The electrocardiogram indicated supraventricular (atrial) tachycardia (SVT) as the cause of his syncope, a rare complication of SVT. Which of the following would *not* be prescribed for treatment of this arrhythmia?**
   A. Intravenous adenosine
   B. Valsalva's maneuver
   C. Digitalis
   D. Carotid sinus massage
   E. Electrical ablation of the atrial ectopic focus

CHAPTER 24

Control of Cardiac Output: Coupling of the Heart and Blood Vessels

- Describe the principal determinants of cardiac output.
- Describe the principal determinants of cardiac preload and afterload.
- Explain the mechanical coupling between the heart and blood vessels.
- Explain the effects of gravity on venous function.

The first few chapters in this part of the book deal with the operation of the heart, which is the energy source responsible for pumping blood to all the tissues of the body. The next several chapters deal with the operation and control of the various types of blood vessels that serve as the conduits for blood delivery to the tissues. The purpose of this chapter is to describe and explain the principal interactions between the cardiac and vascular components of the cardiovascular system. Not only does the heart determine how much blood is pumped through the blood vessels, but also the blood vessels concurrently influence the quantity of blood that the heart pumps to the tissues.

Critical Cardiac and Vascular Factors Regulate Cardiac Output

FOUR MAJOR FACTORS CONTROL CARDIAC OUTPUT (Q_h): HEART RATE, MYOCARDIAL CONTRACTILITY, PRELOAD, AND AFTERLOAD (Figure 24-1). Heart rate and myocardial contractility are strictly **cardiac factors.** They are intrinsic characteristics of the cardiac tissues, although they are modulated by various neural and humoral mechanisms. As explained in Chapter 18, **preload** is the stretching force that acts on cardiac muscle before contraction, whereas **afterload** is the force that opposes cardiac muscle shortening. The preload and afterload depend on the characteristics of both the heart and the vascular system. NOT ONLY ARE PRELOAD AND AFTERLOAD IMPORTANT DETERMINANTS OF Q_h, BUT THESE FEATURES ARE ALSO DETERMINED BY Q_h. Hence preload and afterload may be designated as **coupling**

factors (Figure 24-1) because they constitute a functional coupling between the heart and blood vessels.

The heart pumps blood around the vascular system, which is a closed circuit. The rate at which the blood is pumped around the circuit (i.e., Q_h) is an important determinant of preload and afterload. Concomitantly, the physical characteristics of the blood vessels determine preload and afterload. Hence these coupling factors regulate the quantity of blood that the heart pumps around the circuit per unit time. Understanding the regulation of Q_h thus requires an appreciation of the nature of the coupling between the heart and vascular system.

Graphs that relate Q_h to preload are used to analyze some of the critical interactions between the heart and blood vessels. This graphical analysis involves two independent functional relationships between Q_h and preload. In this analysis, attention is directed to the right ventricular preload, which is the pressure in the right atrium and thoracic venae cavae; this pressure is often called the **central venous pressure (P_v).**

The curve that defines the dependence of Q_h on preload is called the **cardiac function curve.** It expresses the well-known Frank-Starling relationship (see Chapters 18 and 19). The cardiac function curve is a characteristic of the heart itself; classically, it was studied in hearts completely isolated from the rest of the circulatory system. Over the normal range of Q_h and P_v, this curve indicates that a rise in P_v leads to an increase in Q_h; that is, Q_h ORDINARILY VARIES DIRECTLY WITH P_v.

The other functional relationship between P_v and Q_h is defined by a second curve. THIS CURVE, THE **VASCULAR FUNCTION CURVE,** DEPICTS HOW Q_H AFFECTS P_V. This relationship depends on certain critical characteristics of the vascular system, namely peripheral resistance, arterial (C_a) and venous (C_v) compliances, and blood volume. The vascular function curve is entirely independent of the characteristics of the heart; it applies even if the heart is replaced by a mechanical pump. The vascular function curve indicates that if the Q_h is increased, the P_v decreases; that is, P_v VARIES INVERSELY WITH Q_h.

Thus the cardiac function curve indicates that Q_h ordinarily varies directly with P_v, whereas the vascular function curve indicates that P_v varies inversely with Q_h. These assertions might seem contradictory, but as the following discussion indicates, this is not the case.

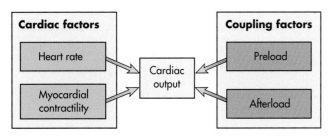

Figure 24-1 Determinants of cardiac output (Q_h).

Cardiac Output Affects Central Venous Pressure

The vascular function curve defines the changes in P_v generated by changes in Q_h. Therefore in this relationship, P_v is the dependent variable (or response), and Q_h is the independent variable (or stimulus).

The simplified schema of the circulation in Figure 24-2 helps elucidate how the Q_h determines the level of the P_v. The essential components of the cardiovascular system have been lumped into four elements. The right and left sides of the heart and the pulmonary vascular bed are considered simply to be a pump-oxygenator, much as that used during open-heart surgery. In Figure 24-2, the energy source is simply called a *pump*. The high-resistance microcirculation is designated as the peripheral resistance. Finally, the entire compliance of

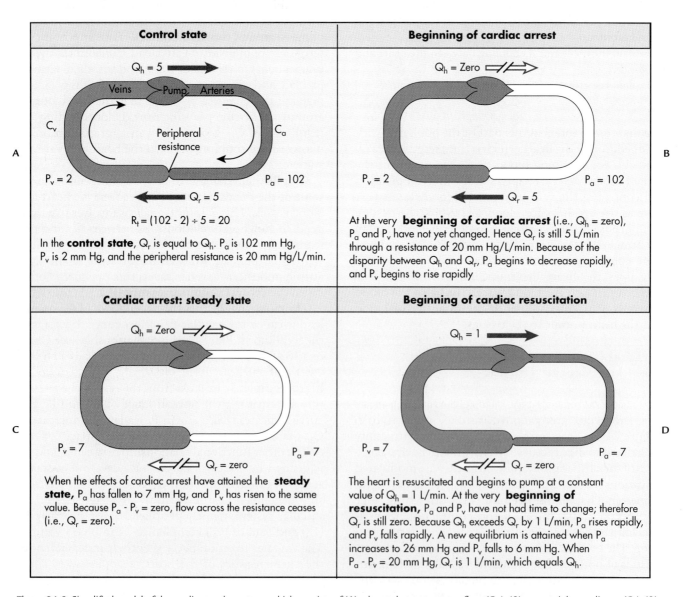

Figure 24-2 Simplified model of the cardiovascular system, which consists of (1) a heart that generates a flow (Q_h), (2) an arterial compliance (C_a), (3) a total peripheral resistance (R_t), (4) a flow through that resistance (Q_t), and (5) a venous compliance (C_v). Q_r, Flow through the peripheral resistance.

the system is subdivided into the following components: total C_a and total C_v (see Table 21-1). As defined in Chapter 21, compliance is the increment of volume (ΔV) accommodated per unit change of pressure (ΔP), as follows:

$$C \equiv \Delta V/\Delta P \qquad \text{24-1}$$

C_v normally is about 20 times greater than C_a. In the following example, the ratio of C_v to C_a is set at 19:1 to simplify certain calculations. Thus if it were necessary to add x ml of blood to the arterial system to increase the arterial pressure (P_a) by 1 mm Hg, then it would be necessary to add $19x$ ml of blood to the venous system to raise P_v by the same amount.

Figure 24-2 illustrates very simply why P_v varies inversely with Q_h. In this example, the model is endowed with characteristics that resemble those of a normal, resting adult (Figure 24-2, *A*). Suppose Q_h is 5 L/min, P_a is 102 mm Hg, and P_v is 2 mm Hg. The total peripheral resistance (R_t) is the ratio of pressure difference $(P_a - P_v)$ to flow (runoff) (Q_r) through the peripheral resistance. At equilibrium, Q_r equals Q_h. Hence R_t equals 100/5 mm Hg, or 20 mm Hg/L/min. From heartbeat to heartbeat, the volume of blood in the arteries (V_a) and the volume of blood in the veins (V_v) remain constant because the volume of blood transferred from the veins to the arteries each minute by the heart (Q_h) equals the volume of blood that flows each minute from the arteries through the resistance vessels and into the veins (Q_r).

The initiation of cardiac arrest in this model (Figure 24-2, *B*) helps explain why the relationship between Q_h and P_v is inverse in the vascular function curves. At the very moment that the heart ceases, V_a and V_v have not had time to change appreciably. The P_a and P_v depend on V_a and V_v, respectively. Therefore these pressures are identical to the respective pressures in Figure 24-2, *A* (i.e., $P_a = 102$ mm Hg, $P_v = 2$ mm Hg). The arteriovenous pressure gradient of 100 mm Hg forces a flow of 5 L/min through the peripheral resistance of 20 mm Hg/L/min. Thus although Q_h now equals zero, the flow (Q_r) through the microcirculation equals 5 L/min (Figure 24-2, *B*). In other words, AT THE VERY BEGINNING OF CARDIAC ARREST, THE POTENTIAL ENERGY STORED IN THE ARTERIES BY THE PREVIOUS CONTRACTIONS OF THE HEART CAUSES BLOOD TO BE TRANSFERRED FROM ARTERIES TO VEINS CONTINUOUSLY, INITIALLY AT THE NORMAL CONTROL RATE, EVEN THOUGH THE HEART CAN NO LONGER TRANSFER BLOOD FROM THE VEINS BACK INTO THE ARTERIES.

After the initiation of cardiac arrest, blood continues to flow from the systemic arteries to the systemic veins as long as P_a exceeds P_v (Figure 24-2, *B*). Therefore V_a progressively decreases, and V_v progressively increases. Because the vessels are elastic structures, P_a progressively falls, and P_v progressively rises. This process continues until P_a and P_v become equal (Figure 24-2, *C*). Once this condition is reached, the flow (Q_r) from ar-

teries to veins through the resistance vessels is zero, as is the Q_h.

At zero flow equilibrium (Figure 24-2, *C*), P_a and P_v depend on the relative compliances of these vessels. Had the C_a and C_v been equal, the decline in P_a would have been equal to the rise in P_v because the decrement in V_a equals the increment in V_v (principle of conservation of mass). P_a and P_v would have both attained the average of P_a plus P_v in Figure 24-2, *A* and *B*; that is, $P_a = P_v = (102$ mm Hg + 2 mm Hg)/2 = 52 mm Hg.

In actual subjects, however, veins are much more compliant than arteries; the ratio is approximately equal to the ratio $(C_v : C_a = 19)$ assumed for the model. Hence the transfer of blood from arteries to veins at equilibrium would induce a fall in P_a 19 times greater than the concomitant rise in P_v. As Figure 24-2, *C*, shows, P_v increases by 5 mm Hg (to an equilibrium value of 7 mm Hg), whereas P_a falls by $19 \times 5 = 95$ mm Hg (to an equilibrium value of 7 mm Hg). This equilibrium pressure that exists in the absence of flow is referred to as the **mean circulatory pressure (static pressure) (P_{mc})**. The pressure in the static system reflects the total volume of blood in the system and the overall compliance of the system.

Two important points on the vascular function curve have already been derived, as shown in Figure 24-3. One point represents the normal status (depicted in Figure 24-2, *A*). Under control conditions, when Q_h was 5 L/min, P_v was 2 mm Hg. When flow stopped $(Q_h =$ zero), P_v became 7 mm Hg at equilibrium; this pressure is the P_{mc}. This point is the Y-axis intercept in Figure 24-3.

The inverse relationship between P_v and Q_h simply expresses the fact that when Q_h is suddenly decreased, the rate (Q_r) at which blood flows from arteries to the veins through the resistance vessels is temporarily greater than the rate (Q_h) at which the heart pumps it

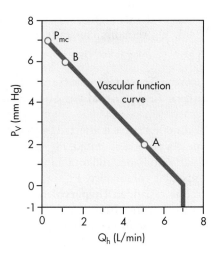

Figure 24-3 Changes in P_v produced by changes in Q_h. P_{mc} is the equilibrium pressure throughout the cardiovascular system when $Q_h =$ zero. Points B and A represent P_v when $Q_h = 1$ and 5 L/min, respectively.

from the veins back into the arteries. During that transient period, a net volume of blood is translocated from the arteries to veins; hence P_a falls, and P_v rises.

In the circulation model shown in Figure 24-2, *D,* when the heart has been resuscitated after a period of cardiac arrest, it immediately begins to generate a Q_h of 1 L/min. Instantaneously, virtually no blood has yet been transferred from the veins to the arteries; therefore the arteriovenous pressure gradient is zero (Figure 24-2, *D*). Consequently, blood does not flow at first from the arteries through the capillaries and into the veins; that is, Q_r = zero. When pumping resumes, blood is being transferred from the veins to the arteries at the rate of 1 L/min; P_v begins to fall, and P_a begins to rise. Because of the difference in compliances, P_a rises 19 times more rapidly than P_v falls.

The resulting arteriovenous pressure gradient causes blood to flow through the resistance vessels. If the pump maintains a constant output of 1 L/min, the P_a will continue to rise, and the P_v will continue to fall until the pressure gradient becomes 20 mm Hg. It forces a flow of 1 L/min through a resistance of 20 mm Hg/L/min. This gradient is achieved by a rise of 19 mm Hg (to 26 mm Hg) in P_a and a fall of 1 mm Hg (to 6 mm Hg) in P_v. This equilibrium value of P_v = 6 mm Hg for a Q_h of 1 L/min appears as point B in Figure 24-3. It reflects a net transfer of blood from the venous to the arterial side of the circuit and a consequent reduction of the P_v.

The vascular function curve shows that as Q_h is increased, P_v is diminished. The reduction of P_v that can be achieved by an increase in Q_h is limited, however. At some critical maximum value of Q_h, sufficient fluid is translocated from the venous to the arterial side of the circuit to reduce the P_v below the ambient pressure (i.e., the intrathoracic pressure). In a system of very distensible vessels, such as the venous system, the vessels are collapsed by the greater external pressure. This venous collapse constitutes an impediment to venous return to the heart. Hence it limits the maximum value of Q_h regardless of the strength of the pump. Note that in Figure 24-3, Q_h remains constant as P_v decreases below zero.

Blood volume affects the relationship between cardiac output and central venous pressure

The vascular function curve is affected by changes in total blood volume. As previously stated, P_{mc} depends only on overall vascular compliance and total blood volume. Thus for a given vascular compliance, P_{mc} increases when the blood volume is expanded **(hypervolemia),** and it decreases when the blood volume is diminished **(hypovolemia).** In the three vascular function curves shown in Figure 24-4, for example, either blood was transfused into the static system (Q_h = zero) until P_{mc} reached 9 mm Hg at equilibrium *(top curve),* or it was withdrawn from the static system until P_{mc} reached 5 mm Hg at equilibrium *(bottom curve).* P_{mc} is the Y-axis intercept in Figure 24-4.

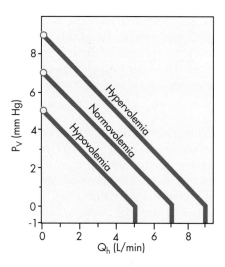

Figure 24-4 Effects of increased blood volume (hypervolemia) and decreased blood volume (hypovolemia) on the vascular function curve.

The various vascular function curves in Figure 24-4 are all parallel to one another. To understand why the curves are parallel, consider the example of hypervolemia *(top curve),* in which P_{mc} had been raised to 9 mm Hg. When the system is static, P_a and P_v would both be 9 mm Hg. If Q_h were then suddenly increased to 1 L/min (as in Figure 24-2, *D*) and if the peripheral resistance were still 20 mm Hg/L/min, an arteriovenous pressure gradient of 20 mm Hg would still be necessary for 1 L/min to flow through the resistance vessels. This does not differ from the example for normovolemia. Assuming the same ratio of C_v to C_a of 19:1, the pressure gradient would be achieved by a decline of 1 mm Hg in P_v and a rise of 19 mm Hg in P_a.

Therefore a change in Q_h from 0 to 1 L/min would evoke the same reduction in P_v irrespective of the total blood volume as long as the C_v:C_a ratio and the peripheral resistance remain constant. The slope of the vascular function curve is by definition the change in P_v per unit change in Q_h. Because the change in P_v induced by a unit change in Q_h is not affected by the blood volume, the vascular function curves that represent different blood volumes are parallel to one another, as shown in Figure 24-4.

Figure 24-4 also shows that the Q_h at which P_v becomes zero varies directly with the blood volume. Therefore the maximum value that Q_h can attain becomes progressively more limited as the total blood volume is reduced. However, the pressure at which the veins collapse (sharp change in slope of the vascular function curve) is not altered appreciably by changes in blood volume. This pressure depends only on the ambient pressure. When P_v falls below the ambient pressure, the veins collapse, and venous return to the heart is thereby limited.

Peripheral resistance affects the relationship between cardiac output and central venous pressure

The modifications of the vascular function curve that are associated with changes in R_t are shown in Figure 24-5. The arterioles contain only about 3% of the total

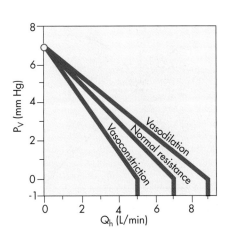

Figure 24-5 Effects of arteriolar vasodilation and vasoconstriction on the vascular function curve.

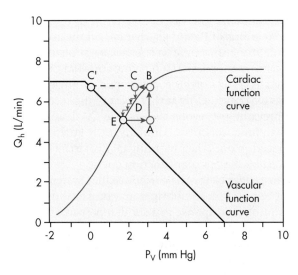

Figure 24-6 Typical vascular and cardiac function curves plotted on the same coordinate axes. The coordinates of the equilibrium point, at the intersection of the two curves, represent the stable values of Q_h and P_v at which the system tends to operate. Any perturbation (such as when P_v is suddenly increased to point A) initiates a sequence of changes in Q_h and P_v such that these variables gradually approach their equilibrium values.

blood volume. Hence changes in the contractile state of these vessels do not significantly alter P_{mc}. Thus the vascular function curves that represent various peripheral resistances converge at a common point (P_{mc}) on the P_v axis.

For any given Q_h, the P_v decreases as the peripheral resistance is increased (Figure 24-5). The principal reason for this relationship is that for a given Q_h, an increase in peripheral resistance redistributes the blood volume such that a greater fraction of the blood resides in the arteries (Figure 21-5), and consequently a lesser fraction resides in the veins. This reduction in V_v would be attended by a proportionate fall in P_v.

Increases in peripheral resistance are associated with a clockwise rotation of the vascular function curves about a common intercept on the P_v axis because an increase in peripheral resistance tends to decrease P_v without affecting P_{mc} (Figure 24-5). Conversely, arteriolar vasodilation is associated with a counterclockwise rotation. A higher maximum Q_h is attainable when the arterioles are dilated than when they are normal or constricted (Figure 24-5).

The Heart and Blood Vessels Interact with Each Other

The P_v constitutes the filling pressure (essentially, the preload) for the right ventricle. In accordance with the Frank-Starling mechanism (see Chapters 18 and 19), P_v is a cardinal determinant of the Q_h. Ordinarily, Q_h varies directly with P_v; that is, OVER A WIDE RANGE OF VENOUS PRESSURES, A RISE IN P_v INCREASES Q_h. In the discussion to follow, graphs of Q_h as a function of P_v are called **cardiac function curves.** Alterations in myocardial contractility are represented by shifts in these curves.

Appreciation of the coupling between the heart and blood vessels requires an examination of the interrelationship of the cardiac function and vascular function curves (Figure 24-6). Both curves reflect the relationship between Q_h and P_v. As stated in the preceding paragraph, THE CARDIAC FUNCTION CURVE EXPRESSES HOW Q_h VARIES IN RESPONSE TO A CHANGE IN P_v. Hence Q_h is the **dependent variable** (or response), and P_v is the **independent variable** (or stimulus). By convention, the dependent variable is scaled along the Y axis and the independent variable is scaled along the X axis. Note that in Figure 24-6, the assignment of X and Y axes is conventional for the cardiac function curve.

THE VASCULAR FUNCTION CURVE, CONVERSELY, REFLECTS HOW P_v IS AFFECTED BY A CHANGE IN Q_h. For the vascular function curve, P_v is the dependent variable (or response), and Q_h is the independent variable (or stimulus). By convention, P_v should be scaled along the Y axis and Q_h along the X axis. Note that this convention was observed for the vascular function curves displayed in Figures 24-3 to 24-5.

However, so that the vascular function curve can be included on the same set of coordinate axes with the cardiac function curve, as in Figure 24-6, the plotting convention for one of these curves must be violated. In this case, the convention for the vascular function curve has been arbitrarily violated. NOTE THAT THE VASCULAR FUNCTION CURVE IN FIGURE 24-6 REFLECTS HOW P_v (SCALED ALONG THE X AXIS) VARIES IN RESPONSE TO A CHANGE OF Q_h (SCALED ALONG THE Y AXIS).

Simultaneous examination of the two curves, one that characterizes cardiac function and the other that characterizes vascular function, provides some insight about the coupling between the heart and vessels. Theoretically the heart can operate at all combinations of P_v and Q_h that fall on the appropriate cardiac function curve. Similarly, the vascular system can operate at all combinations of P_v and Q_h that fall on the appropriate vascular function curve. AT EQUILIBRIUM, THEREFORE THE EN-TIRE CARDIOVASCULAR SYSTEM (I.E., THE COMBINATION OF HEART AND VESSELS) MUST OPERATE AT THE POINT OF INTERSECTION OF THESE TWO CURVES. Only at this point of intersection does the prevailing P_v evoke the specific Q_h defined by the cardiac function curve. Similarly, only at this point of intersection does the prevailing Q_h evoke the specific P_v defined by the vascular function curve.

The tendency for the cardiovascular system to operate about such an equilibrium may best be illustrated by examining its response to a sudden perturbation. Consider the changes elicited by a sudden rise in P_v from the equilibrium point to point A in Figure 24-6. Such a change in P_v might be induced during ventricular systole by the rapid injection of a given volume of blood on the venous side of the circuit accompanied by the rapid withdrawal of an equal volume from the arterial side; the total blood volume would remain constant.

As defined by the cardiac function curve in Figure 24-6, this elevated P_v would increase Q_h (from points A to B) during the very next ventricular systole. The increased Q_h would in turn result in the net transfer of blood from the venous to the arterial side of the circuit, with a consequent reduction in P_v. In one heartbeat, this reduction would be small (from points B to C) because the heart would transfer only a small fraction of the total V_v over to the arterial side. Because of this reduction in P_v, the Q_h during the very next beat would diminish (from points C to D) by an amount dictated by the cardiac function curve. Because point D is still above the intersection point, the heart pumps blood from the veins to the arteries at a rate greater than the blood flows across the peripheral resistance from arteries to veins. Because the venoarterial transport exceeds the arteriovenous transport, P_v continues to fall. This process continues in ever-diminishing steps until the point of intersection (point E) is reached. Only one specific combination of Q_h and P_v (denoted by the coordinates of the point of intersection) simultaneously satisfies the conditions defined by the cardiac and vascular function curves.

Changes in myocardial contractility are reflected by shifts in the cardiac function curves

Graphs of cardiac and vascular function curves help explain the effects of alterations in ventricular contractility. **Contractility** refers to an alteration in myocardial performance based on processes (such as a change in responsiveness to intracellular Ca^{++}) that involve the contractile proteins. Semantically, the term specifically excludes any effects imposed by a change in preload or afterload, even if those changes are mediated by an altered responsiveness to Ca^{++}.

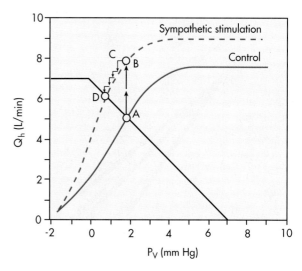

Figure 24-7 When myocardial contractility is enhanced (e.g., by cardiac sympathetic nerve stimulation), the equilibrium values of Q_h and P_v shift from the intersection (point A) of the vascular function curve with the control cardiac function curve to the intersection (point D) of the same vascular function curve with the cardiac function curve that represents the effects of cardiac sympathetic nerve stimulation.

In Figure 24-7, the lower cardiac function curve represents the control state of contractility, whereas the upper curve reflects an enhanced state of contractility. This pair of hypothetical cardiac function curves is analogous to the experimentally derived pair of ventricular function curves shown in Figure 19-14. The change in contractility reflected by the two hypothetical cardiac function curves might be achieved experimentally by selective stimulation of the sympathetic nerves only to the heart. Such selective stimulation would not directly affect the vasculature, so only one vascular function curve need be included in Figure 24-7.

During the control state, the equilibrium values for Q_h and P_v in Figure 24-7 are designated by point A. At the beginning of cardiac sympathetic nerve stimulation (assuming the effects to be instantaneous and constant), the combination of the prevailing level of P_v and the enhanced contractility would abruptly raise Q_h to point B. However, this high Q_h would increase the net transfer of blood from the venous to the arterial side of the circuit; consequently P_v begins to fall (to point C). Q_h continues to fall until it reaches a new equilibrium (point D), which is located at the intersection of the vascular function curve with the new cardiac function curve. The new equilibrium (point D) lies above and to the left of the control equilibrium (point A). This shift reveals that sympathetic stimulation increases Q_h despite the diminution of the ventricular filling pressure (i.e., P_v). Such a change accurately describes the true response. In the experiment shown in Figure 24-8, stimulation of the left stellate ganglion in an anesthetized dog increased Q_h but decreased the right and left atrial pressures.

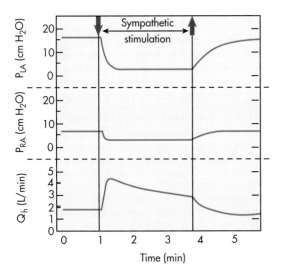

Figure 24-8 During electrical stimulation of the cardiac sympathetic nerves in an anesthetized dog, Q_h increased while pressures in the left atrium (P_{LA}) and right atrium (P_{RA}) diminished. *(Redrawn from Sarnoff SJ et al: Circ Res 8:1108, 1960.)*

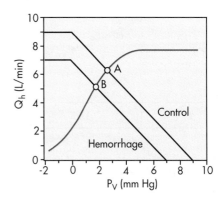

Figure 24-9 Hemorrhage is reflected by a shift of the vascular function curve to the left. Therefore the equilibrium values of Q_h and P_v are both decreased, as denoted by the translocation of the equilibrium from points A to B.

Similar changes occur in patients with **congestive heart failure** when they are treated with medications that improve myocardial contractility, such as digitalis. Classically, patients with congestive heart failure had a high P_v and an abnormally low Q_h. Medications that exert a **positive inotropic effect** (i.e., that enhance contractility) raise the Q_h and decrease the P_v. When such observations were first made, they were interpreted to be incompatible with Starling's law. Now it is recognized that this important physiological principle is more faithfully represented by a family of cardiac function curves and that changes in contractility are reflected by shifts from one component curve to another.

Changes in blood volume mainly affect the vascular function curve

Changes in blood volume do not directly affect the cardiac function curve, but they do influence the vascular function curve in the manner shown in Figure 24-4. For a clear understanding of the circulatory alterations evoked by a given change in blood volume, the appropriate cardiac function curve must be plotted along with the vascular function curves that represent the control and altered vascular states, as shown in Figure 24-9.

The parallel shift in the vascular function curve in Figure 24-9 reflects the response to **acute hemorrhage.** Equilibrium (point B), which denotes the values for Q_h and P_v immediately after sudden hemorrhage, lies below and to the left of control equilibrium (point A). Thus a pure, sudden reduction in blood volume decreases both Q_h and P_v.

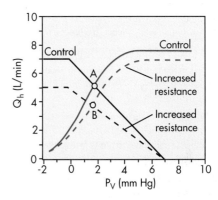

Figure 24-10 An increase in peripheral resistance is reflected by downward shifts of the cardiac and vascular function curves. At equilibrium, Q_h is less (point B) when the peripheral resistance is high than when it is normal (point A).

Changes in peripheral resistance affect cardiac output relatively more than central venous pressure

Predictions concerning the effects of changes in peripheral resistance on Q_h and P_v are complex because changes in peripheral resistance are associated with shifts in both the cardiac and vascular function curves (Figure 24-10). In the vascular function curves plotted in Figure 24-5, vasoconstriction was accompanied by a clockwise rotation of the vascular function curve. The axes are reversed in Figure 24-10, however, and therefore vasoconstriction is associated with a counterclockwise rotation of the vascular function curve depicted in this figure. Hence for any given value of P_v, Q_h is diminished by vasoconstriction. The cardiac function curve is also shifted downward because at any given cardiac filling pressure (P_v), the heart pumps less blood

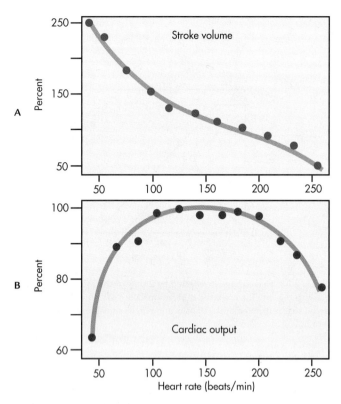

A

B

Figure 24-11 Changes in stroke volume **(A)** and in cardiac output **(B)** induced by changes in the rate of atrial pacing in an anesthetized dog. *(Redrawn from Kumada M, Azuma T, Matsuda K:* Jpn J Physiol *17:538, 1967.)*

when the peripheral resistance is increased; an increase in peripheral resistance characteristically raises the P_a (the afterload). Because both curves are displaced downward by vasoconstriction, the new equilibrium (point B) falls below control (point, A).

Changes in Heart Rate Have Variable Effects on Cardiac Output

Q_h IS THE PRODUCT OF STROKE VOLUME AND HEART RATE. Analysis of the effects of changes in heart rate on Q_h is complicated because a change in heart rate alters the other factors (namely the preload, afterload, and contractility) that determine stroke volume (Figure 24-1). For example, an increase in the heart rate decreases the duration of diastole. Hence the time available for ventricular filling is abridged, and preload is reduced. If the proposed increase in heart rate did alter Q_h, P_a (afterload) would change. Finally, an increase in heart rate would augment the net influx of Ca^{++} into the cardiac myocytes, and this would enhance myocardial contractility (see Figure 19-15).

Many investigators have varied heart rate by artificial pacing in experiments on animals and in humans. The effects on Q_h qualitatively resemble the experimental results shown in Figure 24-11. In that experiment, as the

atrial pacing frequency was gradually increased in an anesthetized dog, the stroke volume progressively diminished (Figure 24-11, *A*). Presumably, the reduction in stroke volume was induced by the decreased time for ventricular filling. However, the change in Q_h evoked by a change in heart rate was influenced markedly by the actual level of the heart rate. In this experiment, for example, as the pacing frequency was raised within the range of 50 to 100 beats/min, an increase in heart rate increased the Q_h. Presumably, at these lower frequencies, the decrement in stroke volume *(SV)* evoked by a given increase in heart rate *(HR)* was proportionately less than the increment in heart rate itself. Stated mathematically, the equation $Q_h = SV \times HR$ signifies that if an increment in heart rate exceeds the consequent decrement in stroke volume, then the consequent value of Q_h will exceed the initial value of Q_h.

Over the frequency range from about 100 to 200 beats/min, however, Q_h in these experiments (Figure 24-11, *B*) was not affected appreciably by changes in pacing frequency. Hence as the pacing frequency was increased, the decrease in stroke volume was proportional to the increase in heart rate. Finally, at excessively high pacing frequencies (>200 beats/min), increments in heart rate diminished Q_h. Therefore the induced decrement in stroke volume must have exceeded the applied increment in heart rate over this high pacing frequency range. Although the relationship of Q_h to heart rate is characteristically that of an inverted **U**, the relationship varies quantitatively among subjects and among physiological states in any given subject.

The characteristic relationship between Q_h and heart rate explains the urgent need for the treatment of patients who have excessively slow or excessively fast heart rates. Profound **bradycardias** (slow rates) may occur as the result of a very slow sinus rhythm in patients with **sick sinus syndrome** or as the result of a slow **idioventricular rhythm** in patients with **complete atrioventricular block.** In either rhythm disturbance, the capacity of the ventricles to fill during a prolonged diastole is limited (often by the noncompliant pericardium). These rhythm disturbances often require the installation of an artificial pacemaker.

Excessively high heart rates in patients with **supraventricular** or **ventricular tachycardias** may also require emergency treatment. The Q_h may be critically low because of the diminished filling time. Reversion of the tachycardia to a more normal rhythm may be accomplished pharmacologically or in emergencies, by delivering a strong electrical current across the thorax or directly to the heart through an implanted device.

Ancillary Factors Also Regulate Cardiac Output

In the previous discussion, the interrelationship between P_v and Q_h has been oversimplified because the effects elicited by changes in just one factor were explained. However, because many feedback-control mechanisms regulate the cardiovascular system, an isolated change in a single variable rarely occurs. A change in blood volume, for example, reflexly alters cardiac function, peripheral resistance, and venomotor tone. Furthermore, several auxiliary factors also contribute to the regulation of Q_h. Among these, some serve as additional energy sources to help the heart pump blood around the body.

Gravity affects cardiac output

Soldiers standing at attention for long periods, particularly in hot weather, may faint because the Q_h decreases substantially. Under such conditions, gravity impedes venous return from the dependent regions of the body, but it also promotes flow on the arterial side of the same circuit. Therefore in the dependent regions of the body, the vascular system behaves much like a U-shaped tube, where the effects of gravity in the descending limb (arteries) and ascending limbs (veins) of the tube neutralize each other. Such neutralization does not take place in the vessels above the level of the heart because the pressure in the veins at some level above the heart might fall below the ambient pressure, thus collapsing these veins.

The compliance of the blood vessels accounts for the gravitational effects on Q_h. When a person stands, the blood vessels below the level of the heart are distended by the gravitational forces that act on the columns of blood in the vessels. The distention is more prominent on the venous than on the arterial side of the circuit because C_v is much higher than C_a (as explained earlier). Such venous distention is readily observed on the backs of the hands when the arms are allowed to hang below the level of the heart. The hemodynamic effects of distention of the veins **(venous pooling)** below the heart level resemble those caused by the loss of an equivalent volume of blood from the body. When a person shifts from a supine position to a relaxed standing position, 300 to 800 ml of blood may be pooled in the legs. This may reduce Q_h by about 2 L/min.

The compensatory adjustments to the erect position are similar to the adjustments to blood loss. For example, venous pooling and other gravitational effects tend to lower the pressure in the regions of the arterial baroreceptors. The resulting diminution in baroreceptor excitation reflexly speeds the heart, strengthens cardiac contraction, and constricts arterioles and veins (see Chapters 19 and 23). The baroreceptor reflex has a greater effect on the resistance vessels (arterioles) than on the capacitance vessels (veins). On hot days, the compensatory vasomotor reactions are less efficacious, and the absence of muscular activity exaggerates the pooling effects of gravity, as explained later.

> Many of the vasodilator medications used to treat **essential hypertension** and other circulatory disorders also interfere with the reflex adaptation to standing. Similarly, astronauts exposed to weightlessness lose their adaptations after a few days, and they experience difficulties when they first return to a normal gravitational field. When individuals with impaired reflex adaptations stand, their blood pressures may fall dramatically. This response is called **orthostatic hypotension,** which may cause lightheadedness or fainting.

Muscular activity and venous valves constitute an auxiliary blood pump

When a relaxed individual stands, the pressure in the veins below the heart rises. P_v in the legs increases gradually and does not reach equilibrium until almost 1 minute after the subject stands. The slowness of the rise in P_v is attributable to the **venous valves,** which permit flow only toward the heart. When a person stands, the valves prevent blood in the veins from actually falling toward the feet. Hence the column of venous blood is supported at numerous levels by these valves; temporarily the venous column consists of many separate segments. However, blood continues to enter the column from many venules and small tributary veins, and pressure continues to rise. As soon as the pressure in one segment exceeds that in the segment just above it, the valve between the two segments is forced open. Ultimately, all the valves in the dependent veins are open, and the column is continuous.

Precise measurement reveals that the final level of P_v in the feet of an individual during quiet standing is only slightly greater than that in a static column of blood extending from the right atrium to the feet. When the person begins to walk or run, the P_v in the legs and feet decreases appreciably. Because of the intermittent venous compression produced by the contracting muscles and because of the presence of the venous valves, blood is forced from the veins toward the heart (see Figure 25-2). Hence MUSCULAR CONTRACTION LOWERS THE P_v IN THE LEGS AND SERVES AS AN AUXILIARY BLOOD PUMP. Furthermore, muscular activity prevents venous pooling and lowers capillary hydrostatic pressure and thereby reduces the tendency for edema fluid to collect in the feet during standing. This mechanism operates very effectively in normal people in that not much motion is required for appreciable auxiliary pumping to occur. Thus if a standing person shifts weight periodically, the pressure in the foot veins is considerably less than the pressure that prevails if he or she remains absolutely still.

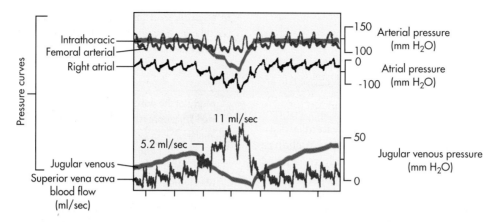

Figure 24-12 In an anesthetized dog, intrathoracic, right atrial, and jugular venous pressures decrease, and flow in the superior vena cava increases (from 5.2 to 11 ml/sec) during inspiration. *(Redrawn from Brecher GA: Venous return, New York, 1956, Grune & Stratton.)*

This auxiliary pumping mechanism is not very effective in people with **varicose veins** in the legs. The valves in such veins do not operate properly; therefore when the leg muscles contract, the blood in the leg veins can be forced in the retrograde as well as in the antegrade direction. Thus when such an individual stands or walks, the P_v in the ankles and feet is excessively high. The consequent high capillary pressure leads to the accumulation of extracellular fluid (**edema**) in the ankles and feet.

Respiration alters venous return

The normal, periodic activity of the respiratory muscles causes rhythmic variations in vena caval flow, and it constitutes an auxiliary pump to promote venous return of blood to the heart. Coughing, straining at stool, and other activities that require the respiratory muscles may affect Q_h substantially.

The changes in blood flow in the superior vena cava during the respiratory cycle of an anesthetized dog are shown in Figure 24-12. During respiration, the changes in intrathoracic pressure are transmitted to the lumina of the thoracic blood vessels. The reduction in P_v during inspiration increases the pressure gradient between the extrathoracic and intrathoracic veins. The consequent acceleration of venous return to the right atrium is displayed in Figure 24-12 as an increase in superior vena caval blood flow from 5.2 ml/sec during expiration to 11 ml/sec during inspiration.

During expiration, flow into the central veins decelerates. However, the mean rate of venous return during normal respiration exceeds the venous flow that occurs in the temporary absence of respiration. Hence normal inspiration facilitates venous return more than normal expiration impedes it. This facilitation is partly attributable to the valves in the veins of the extremities and neck. These valves prevent any reversal of flow during expiration. Thus the re-

spiratory muscles and venous valves also constitute an auxiliary pump for venous return.

SUMMARY

- Two important relationships between Q_h and P_v prevail in the cardiovascular system. One applies to the heart and the other to the vascular system.
- With respect to the heart, Q_h varies directly with P_v (preload) over a wide range of P_v. This relationship is represented by the cardiac function curve, and it expresses the Frank-Starling mechanism.
- With respect to the vascular system, P_v varies inversely with Q_h. This relationship is represented by the vascular function curve, and it reflects the fact that an increase in Q_h, for example, augments total blood volume in the arteries and hence decreases blood volume in the veins.
- The principal mechanisms that govern the cardiac function curve are the changes in contractility and afterload.
- The principal factors that govern the vascular function curve are C_a and C_v, peripheral vascular resistance, and total blood volume.
- The equilibrium values of Q_h and P_v that prevail under a given set of physiological conditions are determined by the intersection of the cardiac and vascular function curves.
- At very low and very high heart rates, the heart cannot pump an adequate Q_h.
- Gravity influences Q_h because the veins are very compliant, and substantial quantities of blood tend to pool in the veins of the dependent portions of the body.
- Respiration changes the pressure gradient between the intrathoracic and extrathoracic veins and hence alters venous return.

BIBLIOGRAPHY

Aukland K: Why don't our feet swell in the upright position? *News Physiol Sci* 9:214, 1994.

Geddes LA, Wessale JL: Cardiac output, stroke volume, and pacing rate: a review of the literature and a proposed technique for selection of the optimum pacing rate for an exercise responsive pacemaker, *J Cardiovasc Electrophysiol* 2:408, 1991.

Hainsworth R: The importance of vascular capacitance in cardiovascular control, *News Physiol Sci* 5:250, 1990.

Lacolley PJ et al: Microgravity and orthostatic intolerance: carotid hemodynamics and peripheral responses, *Am J Physiol* 264:H588, 1993.

Rothe CF: Mean circulatory filling pressure: its meaning and measurement, *J Appl Physiol* 74:499, 1993.

Rothe CF, Gaddis ML: Autoregulation of cardiac output by passive elastic characteristics of the vascular capacitance system, *Circulation* 81:360, 1990.

Sagawa K et al: *Cardiac contraction and the pressure-volume relationship,* New York, 1988, Oxford University Press.

Seymour RS, Hargens AR, Pedley TJ: The heart works against gravity, *Am J Physiol* 265:R715, 1993.

Sheriff DD et al: Dependence of cardiac filling pressure on cardiac output during rest and dynamic exercise in dogs, *Am J Physiol* 265:H316, 1993.

Smith JJ, ed: *Circulatory response to the upright posture,* Boca Raton, Fla, 1990, CRC.

Stick, C, Jaeger H, Witzleb E: Measurements of volume changes and venous pressure in the human lower leg during walking and running, *J Appl Physiol* 72:2063, 1992.

Tyberg JV: Venous modulation of ventricular preload, *Am Heart J* 123:1098, 1992.

Yin FCP, ed: *Ventricular/vascular coupling,* New York, 1987, Springer-Verlag.

▷ CASE STUDY

Case 24-1

A 44-year-old woman had been extremely ill with severe coronary artery disease, and she underwent cardiac transplantation. She recovered very well, and 1 month after surgery her cardiovascular function was normal even though her new heart was entirely denervated. About 3 months after surgery, she developed a duodenal ulcer, which suddenly began to bleed. The patient was estimated to have lost about 600 ml of blood in 1 hour. Her physician treated her with diet and antibiotics, and her ulcer was cured in about 2 weeks. The patient appeared to be healthy for about 3 years but then gradually lost some of her strength and energy. Her physician determined that the cardiac transplant was slowly being rejected. Her physician began to treat her with a new medication that substantially and specifically increased myocardial contractility. Occasionally, the patient experienced brief periods of tachycardia with a rate of about 250 beats/min; the electrocardiogram indicated that the tachycardia originated in the atrioventricular junction.

1. **How would acute blood loss from the duodenal ulcer affect the patient?**
    A. Decrease P_v and increase Q_h
    B. Increase P_v and decrease P_a
    C. Decrease P_v and decrease Q_h
    D. Increase P_a and decrease Q_h
    E. Decrease P_v and increase aortic pulse pressure

2. **What would the administration of a medication that acts specifically to improve myocardial contractility do?**
    A. Decrease P_v and increase Q_h
    B. Decrease P_v and decrease P_a
    C. Increase P_v and increase aortic pulse pressure
    D. Decrease P_v and decrease Q_h
    E. Increase P_v and increase C_a

3. **Strapping the patient to a tilt-table and tilting her to the vertical, head-up position would do what?**
    A. Increase the pressure in a foot vein and increase P_v
    B. Decrease the pressure in a foot vein and decrease Q_h
    C. Decrease P_v and increase P_a
    D. Decrease the pressure in a foot vein and decrease the arterial pulse pressure
    E. Increase the pressure in a foot vein and decrease Q_h

4. **When the patient was experiencing tachycardia, what critical hemodynamic changes would be expected?**
    A. Increase in P_a and increase in P_v
    B. Decrease in stroke volume and decrease in Q_h
    C. Increase in stroke volume and increase in aortic compliance
    D. Increase in P_v and increase in Q_h
    E. Decrease in P_v and increase in arterial pulse pressure

CHAPTER 25

Special Circulations

- Describe the regulation of cutaneous blood flow and the role of the skin in maintaining a constant body temperature.
- Indicate the relative importance of the local and neural factors in adjustments of muscle blood flow at rest and during exercise.
- Explain the physical, neural, and chemical factors that affect coronary blood flow.
- Describe the regulation of cerebral blood flow.
- Relate the intestinal and hepatic components of the splanchnic circulation.
- Explain the changes in the fetal circulation that occur at birth.

Previous chapters on the circulatory system described how the heart and vessels provide the tissues of the body with O_2 and nutrients and remove CO_2 and waste products. Because the circulations of the various organs of the body differ to some degree with respect to their function and regulation, it is necessary to include this chapter on special circulations, which discusses the regulatory mechanisms in the cutaneous, muscular, coronary, cerebral, splanchnic, and fetal circulations. The circulations of the kidneys and lungs are described in the renal and pulmonary sections of this text.

Cutaneous Circulation

The O_2 and nutrient requirements of the skin are relatively small. The supply of these essential materials is not the chief governing factor in the regulation of cutaneous blood flow, in contrast to the regulation in most other body tissues. THE PRIMARY FUNCTION OF THE CUTANEOUS CIRCULATION IS MAINTENANCE OF A CONSTANT BODY TEMPERATURE. Consequently, blood flow to the skin fluctuates widely depending on the need for loss or conservation of body heat. The mechanisms responsible for alterations in skin blood flow are activated mainly by changes in ambient and internal body temperatures.

Skin blood flow is regulated mainly by the sympathetic nervous system

Essentially the following types of resistance vessels are present in skin: **arterioles** and **arteriovenous (AV) anastomoses.** The arterioles are similar to those found elsewhere in the body. AV anastomoses shunt blood from the arterioles to the venules and venous plexuses; thus they bypass the capillary bed (Figure 25-1). AV anastomoses are found mainly in the fingertips, palms, toes, soles of the feet, ears, nose, and lips. AV anastomoses differ morphologically from the arterioles in that they are either short and straight vessels or long and coiled vessels, about 20 to 40 μm in lumen diameter. They have thick muscular walls and are richly supplied with nerve fibers. These vessels are almost exclusively under sympathetic neural control, and they dilate maximally when their nerve supply is interrupted. Conversely, reflex stimulation of the sympathetic fibers to these vessels may constrict them to the point that the vascular lumen is completely obliterated. Although AV anastomoses do not exhibit basal tone (tonic activity of the vascular smooth muscle independent of innervation), they are highly sensitive to vasoconstrictor agents such as epinephrine and norepinephrine. Furthermore, AV anastomoses are not under metabolic control, and they fail to show reactive hyperemia or autoregulation of blood flow. Thus the regulation of blood flow through these anastomotic channels is governed mainly by temperature receptors or by higher centers of the central nervous system.

THE BULK OF THE SKIN RESISTANCE VESSELS EXHIBIT SOME BASAL TONE. VASCULAR RESISTANCE IN THE SKIN IS UNDER DUAL CONTROL OF THE SYMPATHETIC NERVOUS SYSTEM AND LOCAL REGULATORY FACTORS in much the same manner as other vascular beds. IN THE SKIN, HOWEVER, NEURAL CONTROL IS MORE IMPORTANT THAN LOCAL FACTORS. The stimulation of sympathetic nerve fibers to skin blood vessels (i.e., arteries, veins, arterioles) induces vasoconstriction, and severance of the sympathetic nerves induces vasodilation. After chronic denervation of the cutaneous blood vessels, the degree of tone that existed before denervation is gradually regained over several weeks. This is accomplished by an enhanced basal tone that compensates for the degree of tone previously contributed by sympathetic nerve fiber activity. Epinephrine and norepinephrine elicit only vasoconstriction in cutaneous vessels.

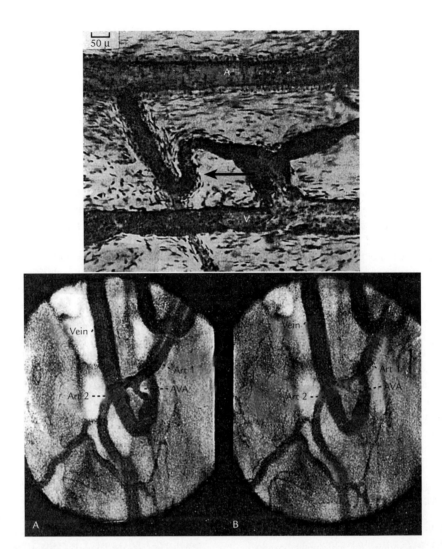

Figure 25-1 *Top,* AV anastomosis in a human ear injected with Berlin blue. The walls of the AV anastomoses in the fingertips are thicker and more cellular. *A,* Artery; *V,* vein; *arrow,* AV anastomosis. *Bottom,* Two frames from a motion-picture record of the same relatively large AV anastomosis *(AVA)* in a stable rabbit ear chamber installed 3½ months previously. On the left *(A),* the AV anastomosis is dilated; on the right *(B),* it is contracted. On this day the lumen measured 51 μm dilated and 5 μm contracted at its narrowest point. Arrows indicate the direction of blood flow. *Art,* Artery. *(Top from Pritchard MML, Daniel PM: J Anatomy 90:309, 1956. Bottom from Clark ER, Clark EL: Am J Anat 54:229, 1934.)*

Parasympathetic vasodilator nerve fibers do not supply the cutaneous blood vessels. However, stimulation of the sweat glands, which are innervated by cholinergic fibers of the sympathetic nervous system, results in dilation of the skin resistance vessels. Sweat contains an enzyme that acts on a protein moiety in the tissue fluid to release bradykinin, a polypeptide with vasodilator properties. Bradykinin formed in the tissue can act locally to dilate the arterioles and increase blood flow to the skin.

The skin vessels of certain body regions, particularly the head, neck, shoulders, and upper chest, are under the influence of the higher centers of the central nervous system. For example, blushing (e.g., that caused by embarrassment or anger) is attributable to the inhibition of sympathetic nerve fibers to the face, whereas blanching (e.g., that caused by fear or anxiety) is attributable to the stimulation of the sympathetic nerve fibers to the face.

In contrast to AV anastomoses in the skin, the cutaneous resistance vessels show autoregulation of blood flow and reactive hyperemia. If the arterial inflow to a limb is stopped by briefly inflating a blood pressure cuff, the skin reddens greatly below the point of vascular occlusion when the cuff is deflated. This increased cutaneous blood flow **(reactive hyperemia)** is also manifested by distention of the superficial veins in the erythematous extremity.

Under normal conditions, ambient temperature is the main factor in the regulation of skin blood flow

The primary function of the skin is to preserve the internal milieu and protect it from adverse changes in the environment, and the ambient temperature is one of the most important external variables with which the body must contend. Therefore it is not surprising that the vasculature of the skin is chiefly influenced by environmental temperature. Exposure to cold elicits a generalized cutaneous vaso-constriction that is most pronounced in the hands and feet. This response is chiefly mediated by the nervous system because arrest of the circulation to the hand caused by inflation of a pressure cuff and then immersion of that hand in cold water results in vasoconstriction in the skin of the other extremities that have been exposed only to room temperature. When circulation to the chilled hand is not occluded, the reflex vasoconstriction is caused partly by the cooled blood returning to the general circulation and stimulating the temperature-regulating center in the anterior hypothalamus. Direct application of cold to this region of the brain produces cutaneous vasoconstriction.

The skin vessels of the cooled hand also respond directly to cold. Moderate cooling or exposure of the hand to severe cold (up to 15° C) for brief periods constricts the resistance and capacitance vessels, including AV anastomoses. However, prolonged exposure of the hand to severe cold has a secondary vasodilator effect. Prompt vasoconstriction and severe pain are elicited by immersion of the hand in water near 0° C, but these reactions are soon followed by dilation of the skin vessels, reddening of the immersed part, and alleviation of the pain. With continued immersion of the hand, alternating periods of constriction and dilation occur, but the skin temperature rarely drops as low as it did during the initial vasoconstriction. Prolonged severe cold damages the tissue.

> The rosy faces of people outdoors in the cold are examples of cold vasodilation. However, blood flow through the skin of the face may be very low despite the flushed appearance. The redness of the slowly flowing blood is largely the result of the reduced O_2 uptake by the cold skin and the change in the affinity of hemoglobin for O_2 as reflected by the cold-induced shift to the left of the oxyhemoglobin dissociation curve (see Chapter 30).

Direct application of heat produces not only local vasodilation of resistance and capacitance vessels and AV anastomoses but also reflex dilation in other parts of the body. The local effect is independent of the vascular nerve supply, whereas the reflex vasodilation is a combination of anterior hypothalamic stimulation by the returning warmed blood and stimulation of receptors in the heated part.

The proximity of the major arteries and veins to each other permits considerable heat exchange (**countercurrent**) between the artery and vein. Cold blood that flows in veins from a cooled hand toward the heart takes up heat from adjacent arteries; this warms the venous blood and cools the arterial blood. Heat exchange occurs in the opposite direction when the extremity is exposed to heat. Thus heat conservation is enhanced during exposure of the extremities to cold, and heat gain is minimized during exposure of the extremities to warmth.

> In patients with **Raynaud's disease,** exposure to cold or emotional stimuli may initiate ischemic attacks in the extremities (especially the fingers). The response is characterized by blanching followed by cyanosis and then redness. The attacks are often associated with numbness, tingling, pain, and burning sensations.

In light skin the color is a function of the amount of blood in the skin and subcutaneous tissue and the O_2 content of that blood

The color of the skin is determined in large part by pigment, but in all but very dark skin, the pallor or ruddiness depends on the color and amount of blood in the skin. With little blood in the venous plexus the skin appears pale, whereas with larger quantities of blood in the venous plexus, the skin has more color. Whether this color is bright red, blue, or some intermediate shade is determined by the degree of oxygenation of blood in the subcutaneous vessels. For example, a combination of vasoconstriction and reduced hemoglobin can make the skin an ashen gray, whereas a combination of venous engorgement and reduced hemoglobin can make it dark purple. Skin color provides little information about the rate of cutaneous blood flow. Rapid blood flow and pale skin may coexist when the AV anastomoses are open, and slow blood flow and red skin may coexist when the extremity is exposed to cold.

Skeletal Muscle Circulation

Blood flow to skeletal muscle varies directly with the contractile activity of the tissue and the type of muscle. Blood flow and capillary density in red (slow-twitch, high-oxidative) muscle are greater than in white (fast-twitch, low oxidative) muscle. In resting muscle the arterioles exhibit asynchronous intermittent contractions and relaxations. Thus at any given moment, a large percentage of the capillary bed is not perfused. Consequently the total blood flow through quiescent skeletal muscle is low (1.4 to 4.5 ml/min/100 g). During exercise, the resistance vessels relax, and the muscle blood flow may increase many-fold (≤15 to 20 times the resting level); the magnitude of the increase depends largely on the severity of the exercise.

Control of muscle circulation is achieved by neural and local factors

The relative contribution of neural and local factors is dictated by muscle activity. IN SUBJECTS AT REST, NEURAL AND MYOGENIC REGULATIONS ARE PREDOMINANT, WHEREAS DURING EXERCISE, METABOLIC CONTROL SUPERVENES. As with all tissues, physical factors such as arterial pressure, tissue pressure, and blood viscosity influence blood flow to muscle. However, another physical factor plays a role during exercise: the squeezing effect of the active muscle on the vessels (see also Chapter 24). With intermittent contractions, inflow is restricted and venous outflow enhanced during each brief contraction. The presence of the venous valves prevents the backflow of blood in the veins between contractions, and thus the valves aid in the forward propulsion of blood (Figure 25-2). With strong sustained contractions, the vascular bed can be compressed to the point at which blood flow ceases temporarily.

Basal tone and sympathetic nerve activity to muscle vessels regulate blood flow in resting subjects

Although the resistance vessels of muscle have a high basal tone, they also display a tone attributable to continuous low-frequency activity in the sympathetic vasoconstrictor nerve fibers. The tonic activity of the sympathetic nerves is greatly influenced by the baroreceptor reflex. An increase in carotid sinus pressure dilates the vascular bed of the muscle, and a decrease elicits vasoconstriction. Because muscle is the major body component on the basis of mass and thereby represents the largest vascular bed, the reflex participation of resistance vessels in the muscles is important in maintaining a constant arterial blood pressure.

Metabolic activity is the main factor in regulating muscle blood flow during exercise

It already has been stressed that neural regulation of muscle blood flow is superseded by metabolic regulation (see Chapter 23) when the muscle changes from the resting to the contracting state. However, local control also occurs in innervated resting skeletal muscle when the vasomotor nerves are not active. Thus autoregulation can be observed in innervated as well as in denervated muscle. In both conditions, autoregulation is characterized by a low venous blood O_2 saturation.

Coronary Circulation

Coronary blood flow is under the influence of physical, neural, and metabolic factors

The main force responsible for perfusion of the myocardium is aortic pressure, which is generated by the heart itself. Changes in aortic pressure generally shift coronary blood flow in the same direction. However, alterations of cardiac work, which are produced by increased or decreased aortic pressure, have a considerable effect on coronary resistance. Increased metabolic activity of the heart decreases coronary resistance, whereas a reduction in cardiac metabolism increases coronary resistance. Under normal conditions, blood pressure is kept within relatively narrow limits by the baroreceptor reflex. Therefore CHANGES IN CORONARY BLOOD FLOW ARE CAUSED PRIMARILY BY CALIBER CHANGES OF THE CORONARY RESISTANCE VESSELS IN RESPONSE TO THE METABOLIC DEMANDS OF THE HEART. When the rate of myocardial metabolism is unchanged and coronary perfusion pressure is raised or lowered, coronary blood flow remains relatively constant (**autoregulation of blood flow**).

In addition to providing the head of pressure to drive blood through the coronary vessels, the heart also influences its own blood supply by the squeezing effect of the contracting myocardium on the blood vessels that course through it (**extravascular compression** or **extracoronary resistance**). This force is so great during early ventricular systole that blood flow in a large coronary artery supplying the left ventricle is briefly reversed. Left coronary inflow is maximal in early diastole, when the ventricles have relaxed and extravascular compression of the coronary vessels is virtually absent. This flow pattern is seen in the phasic coronary flow curve for the left coronary artery (Figure 25-3). After an initial reversal in early systole, left coronary blood flow parallels the aortic pressure until early diastole, when it rises abruptly. It then declines slowly as aortic pressure falls during the remainder of diastole.

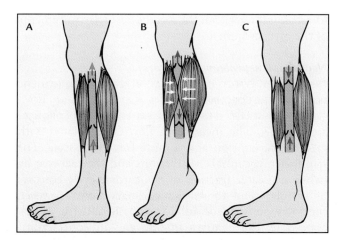

Figure 25-2 Action of the muscle pump in venous return from the legs. **A,** Standing at rest. The venous valves are open, and blood flows upward toward the heart by virtue of the pressure generated by the heart, which is transmitted through the capillaries to the veins from the arterial side of the vascular system (vis a tergo). **B,** Contraction of the muscle compresses the vein so that the increased pressure in the vein drives blood toward the thorax through the upper valve and closes the lower valve in the uncompressed segment of the vein just below the point of muscular compression. **C,** Immediately after muscle relaxation, the pressure in the previously compressed venous segment falls, and the reversed pressure gradient causes the upper valve to close. The valve below the previously compressed segment opens because the pressure below it exceeds that above it, and the segment fills with blood from the foot. As blood flow continues from the foot, the pressure in the previously compressed segment rises. When it exceeds the pressure above the upper valve, this valve opens, and continuous flow occurs as in **A.**

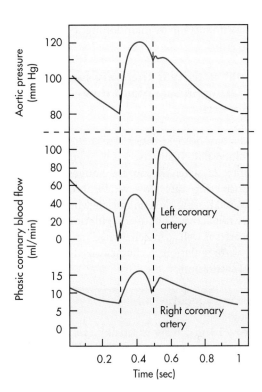

Figure 25-3 Comparison of phasic coronary blood flow in the left and right coronary arteries.

The minimum extravascular resistance and absence of left ventricular work during diastole are used to advantage clinically to improve myocardial perfusion in patients with damaged myocardium and low blood pressure. The method is called **counterpulsation,** and it consists of the insertion of an inflatable balloon into the thoracic aorta through a femoral artery. The balloon is inflated during ventricular diastole and deflated during systole. This procedure enhances coronary blood flow during diastole by raising diastolic pressure at a time when coronary extravascular resistance is lowest. Furthermore, it reduces cardiac energy requirements by lowering aortic pressure (afterload) during ventricular ejection.

Left ventricular myocardial pressure (pressure within the wall of the left ventricle) is greatest near the endocardium and lowest near the epicardium. However, under normal conditions, this pressure gradient does not impair endocardial blood flow because a greater blood flow to the endocardium during diastole compensates for the greater blood flow to the epicardium during systole. In fact, blood flow is slightly higher in the endocardium than in the epicardium under normal conditions. Because extravascular compression is greatest at the endocardial surface of the ventricle, the equality of epicardial and endocardial blood flow must mean that the tone of the endocardial resistance vessels is less than that of the epicardial vessels.

Under abnormal conditions, when diastolic pressure in the coronary arteries is low, such as in **severe hypotension, partial coronary artery occlusion,** or **severe aortic stenosis,** blood flow to the endocardial regions is more severely impaired than that to the epicardial regions of the ventricle. For this reason, myocardial damage after occlusion of the anterior descending branch of the left coronary artery is usually greatest in the inner wall of the left ventricle.

Flow in the right coronary artery shows a similar pattern (Figure 25-3), but because of the lower pressure developed by the thin right ventricle during systole, blood flow does not reverse in early systole. Systolic blood flow in the right coronary artery constitutes a much greater proportion of total coronary inflow than it does in the left coronary artery.

Tachycardia and bradycardia have dual effects on coronary flow. A change in heart rate is accomplished chiefly by shortening or lengthening diastole. During tachycardia, the proportion of time the heart spends in systole (when the vessels are compressed and flow is restricted) increases. However, this mechanical reduction in mean coronary flow is overridden by the coronary dilation associated with the increased metabolic activity of the more rapidly beating heart. During bradycardia the opposite is true; restriction of coronary inflow is less (diastole is longer), but the metabolic (O_2) requirements of the myocardium are also less.

Neural and neurohumoral factors

THE PRIMARY EFFECT OF STIMULATION OF THE SYMPATHETIC NERVES TO THE CORONARY VESSELS IS VASOCONSTRICTION. HOWEVER, THE OBSERVED EFFECT IS A GREAT INCREASE IN CORONARY BLOOD FLOW. The increase in flow is associated with cardiac acceleration and a more forceful systole. The stronger myocardial contractions and the tachycardia (when a greater fraction of the cardiac cycle consists of systole) tend to restrict coronary flow. However, the increase in myocardial metabolic activity, as evidenced by the changes in rate and in contractility, tends to dilate the coronary resistance vessels. The increase in coronary blood flow elicited by cardiac sympathetic nerve stimulation is the algebraic sum of these factors.

Metabolic factors

One of the most striking characteristics of the coronary circulation is the close parallelism between the level of myocardial metabolic activity and the magnitude of the coronary blood flow. This relationship is also found in the denervated heart. The link between cardiac metabolic rate and coronary blood flow remains unsettled. However, it appears that A DECREASE IN THE RATIO OF O_2 SUPPLY TO O_2 DEMAND (whether produced by a reduction in

O_2 supply or by an increment in O_2 demand) RELEASES A VASODILATOR SUBSTANCE FROM THE MYOCARDIUM INTO THE INTERSTITIAL FLUID, WHERE THE SUBSTANCE CAN RELAX THE CORONARY RESISTANCE VESSELS.

As diagrammed in Figure 25-4, a decrease in arterial blood O_2 content, a decrease in coronary blood flow, or an increase in metabolic rate decreases the O_2 supply/demand ratio. This causes the release of a vasodilator substance such as adenosine, which dilates the arterioles and thereby adjusts the O_2 supply to the O_2 demand. A decreased O_2 demand would reduce the amount of vasodilator substance released and permit greater expression of basal tone.

Numerous agents, generally referred to as **metabolites,** have been suggested as mediators of the vasodilation evoked by increased cardiac work. Among the substances implicated are CO_2, O_2 (reduced O_2 tension [Po_2]), H^+ (lactic acid), K^+, nitric oxide, and adenosine. Of these agents, adenosine comes closest to satisfying the criteria for the physiological mediator. Accumulation of vasoactive metabolites may also be responsible for reactive hyperemia in the heart because the duration of coronary flow after the release of the briefly occluded vessel is, within certain limits, proportional to the duration of the period of occlusion.

Cardiac O_2 consumption is determined by the kind of work done by the heart

The volume of O_2 consumed by the heart is determined by the amount and type of activity the heart performs. Under basal conditions, myocardial O_2 consumption is about 8 to 10 ml/min/100 g of heart. It can increase severalfold with exercise and decrease moderately under conditions such as hypotension and hypothermia. The cardiac venous blood normally has a low O_2 content (about 5ml/dl), and the myocardium can therefore receive little additional O_2 by further O_2 extraction from the coronary blood.

Left ventricular work per beat **(stroke work)** is approximately equal to the product of the stroke volume and the mean aortic pressure against which blood is ejected by the left ventricle. At resting levels of cardiac output, the kinetic energy component is negligible (see Chapter 20). However, at high cardiac outputs, as in strenuous exercise, the kinetic component can account for up to 50% of total cardiac work. One can simultaneously halve the aortic pressure and double the cardiac output, or vice versa, and still arrive at the same value for cardiac work. However, the O_2 requirements are greater for any given increment of cardiac work when it is achieved by a rise in pressure than when it is achieved by an increase in stroke volume. Pumping an increase in cardiac output at a constant aortic pressure **(volume work)** is accomplished with a small increase in left ventricular O_2 consumption. Conversely, pumping against an increased arterial pressure at a constant cardiac output **(pressure work)** is accompanied by a large increment in myocardial O_2 consumption.

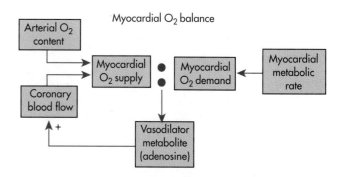

Figure 25-4 An imbalance in the O_2 supply/demand ratio alters coronary blood flow by changing the rate of release of a vasodilator metabolite (adenosine) from the cardiomyocytes. A decrease in the ratio elicits an increase in vasodilator release, whereas an increase in the ratio has the opposite effect.

> The greater energy demand of pressure work over volume work is clinically important. For example, in **aortic stenosis** (a narrowed aortic valve), left ventricular O_2 consumption is increased because of the high intraventricular pressure developed during systole to overcome the resistance of the stenotic valve, whereas coronary perfusion pressure is normal or reduced because of the pressure drop across the narrowed orifice of the diseased aortic valve. The result is a greater O_2 need by the myocardium in the face of a reduced O_2 supply. This can produce **angina pectoris** (chest pain) and eventually left ventricular failure.

Coronary collateral vessels develop in response to the impairment of coronary blood flow

In the normal human heart, there are virtually no functional intercoronary channels, and an abrupt occlusion of a coronary artery or one of its branches leads to **ischemic necrosis** (tissue death caused by inadequate blood flow) and eventual fibrosis of the areas of myocardium supplies by the occluded vessel.

> If a coronary artery narrows slowly over a period of weeks, months, or years, as often occurs in **coronary atherosclerosis,** collateral vessels develop, and they may furnish sufficient blood to the ischemic myocardium to prevent or reduce the extent of myocardial injury if a major coronary artery is occluded abruptly.

Collateral vessels develop between branches of occluded and nonoccluded arteries. They originate from preexisting small vessels that undergo proliferative changes of the endothelium and smooth muscle, possi-

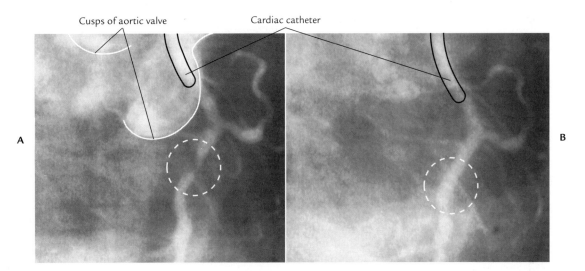

Figure 25-5 A, Angiogram (intracoronary radiopaque dye) of a person with marked narrowing of the circumflex branch of the left coronary artery *(circle)*. Reflux of dye into the root of the aorta outlines two of the aortic valve cusps. **B,** Same segment of the coronary artery after angioplasty. *(Courtesy Dr. Eric R. Powers.)*

bly in response to wall stress and chemical agents released by the ischemic tissue.

> When disease causes discrete occlusions or severe narrowing in coronary arteries (lumen diameters as small as 1 mm), the lesions can be bypassed with an artery or vein graft, or the narrow segment can be dilated by inserting a balloon-tipped catheter into the diseased vessel via a peripheral artery and inflating the balloon. Distention of the vessel by balloon inflation **(angioplasty)** can produce a lasting dilation of a narrowed coronary artery (Figure 25-5).

Cerebral Circulation

Blood reaches the brain through the internal carotid and vertebral arteries. The latter join to form the basilar artery, which in conjunction with branches of the internal carotid arteries, forms the **circle of Willis.** A unique feature of the cerebral circulation is that it all lies within a rigid structure, the cranium. Because intracranial contents are incompressible, any increase in arterial inflow, such as that occurring with arteriolar dilation, must be associated with a comparable increase in venous outflow. The volume of blood and extravascular fluid can vary considerably in most tissues. In brain the volume of blood and extravascular fluid is relatively constant; change in either of these fluid volumes must be accompanied by a reciprocal change in the other. In contrast to most other organs, the total cerebral blood flow is held within a relatively narrow range; in humans, it averages 55 ml/min/100 g of brain.

Local factors predominate over neural factors in the regulation of cerebral blood flow

Of the various body tissues, the brain is the least tolerant of ischemia. Interruption of cerebral blood flow for as little as 5 seconds results in loss of consciousness. Ischemia lasting just a few minutes results in irreversible tissue damage. Fortunately, regulation of the cerebral circulation is mainly under the direction of the brain itself. Local regulatory mechanisms and reflexes that originate in the brain tend to maintain cerebral circulation relatively constant. This constancy prevails even in the presence of adverse extrinsic effects such as sympathetic vasomotor nerve activity, circulating humoral vasoactive agents, and changes in arterial blood pressure. Under certain conditions the brain also regulates its blood flow by initiating changes in systemic blood pressure.

> The elevation of intracranial pressure, such as that which may occur with a brain tumor, results in an increased systemic blood pressure. This response, called **Cushing's phenomenon,** is apparently caused by ischemic stimulation of vasomotor regions of the medulla. It aids in maintaining cerebral blood flow in the face of elevated intracranial pressure.

Neural factors

The cerebral vessels are innervated by the cervical sympathetic nerve fibers that accompany the internal carotid and vertebral arteries into the cranial cavity. Relative to the control of other vascular beds, the sympathetic control of the cerebral vessels is weak, and the

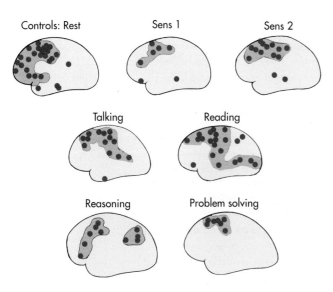

Controls: Rest   Sens 1   Sens 2

Talking   Reading

Reasoning   Problem solving

Figure 25-6 Effects of different stimuli on the regional blood flow in the contralateral human cerebral cortex. *Sens 1,* Low-intensity electrical stimulation of the hand; *Sens 2,* high-intensity electrical stimulation of the hand (pain). *(Redrawn from Ingvar DG: Brain Res 107:181, 1976.)*

contractile state of the cerebrovascular smooth muscle depends mainly on local metabolic factors. There are no known sympathetic vasodilator nerves to the cerebral vessels. However, the vessels do receive parasympathetic fibers from the facial nerve, and stimulation of these fibers produces slight vasodilation.

Local factors

GENERALLY, TOTAL CEREBRAL BLOOD FLOW IS CONSTANT. HOWEVER, REGIONAL CORTICAL BLOOD FLOW IS ASSOCIATED WITH REGIONAL NEURAL ACTIVITY. For example, movement of one hand results in increased blood flow only in the hand area of the contralateral sensorimotor and premotor cortex. Also, talking, reading, and other stimuli to the cerebral center are associated with increased blood flow in the appropriate regions of the cortex (Figure 25-6). The mediator of the link between cerebral activity and blood flow has not been established, but nitric oxide and adenosine may be involved.

The cerebral vessels are very sensitive to CO_2 tension. Increases in arterial blood CO_2 tension (Pa_{CO_2}) elicit marked cerebral vasodilation; inhalation of 7% CO_2 results in a twofold increment in cerebral blood flow. By the same token, decreases in Pa_{CO_2}, which may be elicited by hyperventilation, decrease the cerebral blood flow. CO_2 changes arteriolar resistance by altering the perivascular pH and probably the intracellular pH of the vascular smooth muscle. By independently changing the Pa_{CO_2} and bicarbonate concentration, it has been demonstrated that pial vessel diameter (and presumably blood flow) and pH are inversely related, regardless of the level of the Pa_{CO_2}.

The cerebral circulation shows reactive hyperemia and excellent autoregulation between pressures of about 60 and 160 mm Hg. Mean arterial pressures less than 60 mm Hg result in reduced cerebral blood flow and syncope, whereas mean pressures greater than 160 mm Hg may increase the permeability of the blood-brain barrier and cause cerebral edema.

Splanchnic Circulation

The splanchnic circulation consists of the blood supply to the gastrointestinal tract, liver, spleen, and pancreas. The most noteworthy feature of the splanchnic circulation is that two large capillary beds are partly in series with each other. The small splanchnic arterial branches supply the capillary beds in the gastrointestinal tract, spleen, and pancreas. From these capillary beds the venous blood ultimately flows into the portal vein, which normally provides most of the blood supply to the liver. However, the hepatic artery also supplies blood to the liver.

Intestinal circulation

Neural regulation

Neural control of the mesenteric circulation is almost exclusively sympathetic. Increased sympathetic activity constricts the mesenteric arterioles and capacitance vessels. These responses are mediated by α-receptors, which are prepotent in the mesenteric circulation; however, β-receptors are also present. Infusion of a β-receptor agonist such as isoproterenol causes vasodilation.

Autoregulation

Autoregulation in the intestinal circulation is not as well developed as it is in certain other vascular beds, such as those in the brain and kidney. The principal mechanism responsible for autoregulation is metabolic, although a myogenic mechanism probably also participates.

Functional hyperemia

Food ingestion increases intestinal blood flow. The secretion of the gastrointestinal hormones gastrin and cholecystokinin augments intestinal blood flow. The absorption of food also increases intestinal blood flow; the principal mediators of mesenteric hyperemia are glucose and fatty acids.

Hepatic circulation

Regulation of flow

Blood flow in the portal venous and hepatic arterial systems varies reciprocally. When blood flow is curtailed in one system, the flow increases in the other. However, the resultant increase in flow in one system usually does not fully compensate for the initiating reduction in flow in the other.

The portal venous system does not autoregulate. As the portal venous pressure and flow are raised, resistance either remains constant or decreases. However, the hepatic arterial system does autoregulate.

The sympathetic nerves constrict the presinusoidal resistance vessels in the portal venous and hepatic arterial systems. However, neural effects on the capacitance vessels are more important. The effects are mediated mainly by α-receptors.

Capacitance vessels

The liver contains about 15% of the total blood volume of the body. Under appropriate conditions, such as in response to hemorrhage, about half of the hepatic blood volume can be rapidly expelled. Thus the liver constitutes an important blood reservoir in humans. In certain species, notably the dog, the spleen also may serve as an effective blood reservoir. It does not play an important role in humans, however.

Extensive fibrosis of the liver, such as that which occurs in **hepatic cirrhosis,** increases hepatic vascular resistance, which raises portal venous pressure substantially. The consequent increase in the capillary pressure throughout the splanchnic circulation leads to extensive fluid transudation (**ascites**) into the peritoneal cavity.

Fetal Circulation

The fetal circulation supplies the tissues with O_2 and nutrients from the placenta and bypasses the fetal lungs

The circulation of the fetus differs from that of the postnatal infant. The fetal lungs are functionally inactive, and the fetus depends completely on the placenta for O_2 and nutrients. Oxygenated fetal blood from the placenta passes through the umbilical vein to the liver. Approximately half passes through the liver, and the remainder bypasses the

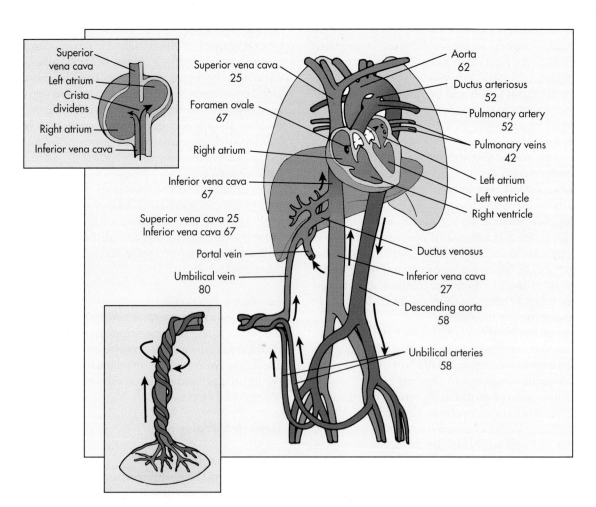

Figure 25-7 Fetal circulation. The numbers represent the percentage of O_2 saturation of blood flowing in the indicated blood vessel. *Upper inset,* Direction of flow of a major portion of the inferior vena caval blood through the foramen ovale to the left atrium. *Bottom inset,* Umbilical vessels and placenta. *(Data for O_2 saturations from Dawes GS et al:* J Physiol *126:563, 1954.)*

liver to the inferior vena cava through the **ductus venosus** (Figure 25-7). In the inferior vena cava, blood from the ductus venosus joins blood returning from the lower trunk and extremities, and this combined stream is in turn joined by blood from the liver through the hepatic veins.

The streams of blood tend to maintain their identity in the inferior vena cava, but they are divided into two streams of unequal size by the edge of the interatrial septum **(crista dividens).** The larger stream, which is mainly blood from the umbilical vein, is shunted to the left atrium through the **foramen ovale,** which lies between the inferior vena cava and the left atrium (Figure 25-7, *upper inset*). The other stream passes into the right atrium, where it is joined by superior vena caval blood returning from the upper parts of the body and by blood from the myocardium.

In contrast to the adult, in whom the right and left ventricles pump in series, the ventricles in the fetus operate essentially in parallel. Because of the large pulmonary resistance, only one tenth of the right ventricular output goes through the lungs. The remainder passes through the **ductus arteriosus** from the pulmonary artery to the aorta at a point distal to the origins of the arteries to the head and upper extremities. Blood flows from the pulmonary artery to the aorta because the pulmonary artery resistance is high and the diameter of the ductus arteriosus is as large as the descending aorta.

The large volume of blood coming through the foramen ovale into the left atrium is joined by blood returning from the lungs, and it is pumped out by the left ventricle into the aorta. Most of the blood in the ascending aorta goes to the head, upper thorax, and arms, and the remainder joins blood from the ductus arteriosus and supplies the rest of the body and the placenta. The amount of blood pumped by the left ventricle is about half of that pumped by the right ventricle. The major fraction of the blood that passes down the descending aorta comes from the ductus arteriosus and right ventricle and flows by way of the two umbilical arteries to the placenta.

Figure 25-7 indicates the O_2 saturations of blood at various points of the fetal circulation. Fetal blood leaving the placenta is 80% saturated, but the saturation of blood passing through the foramen ovale is reduced to 67% because it mixes with desaturated blood returning from the lower part of the body and the liver. The addition of the desaturated blood from the lungs reduces the O_2 saturation of left ventricular blood to 62%, which is the level of saturation of blood reaching the head and upper extremities.

Blood in the right ventricle, a mixture of desaturated superior vena caval blood, coronary venous blood, and inferior vena caval blood, is only 52% saturated with O_2. When the major portion of this blood traverses the ductus arteriosus and joins that pumped out by the left ventricle, the resulting O_2 saturation of blood traveling to the lower part of the body and back to the placenta is 58%. Thus the tissues that receive blood of the highest O_2 saturation are the liver, heart, and upper parts of the body, including the head.

At the placenta the chorionic villi dip into the maternal sinuses, and O_2, CO_2, nutrients, and metabolic waste products exchange across the membranes. The barrier to exchange is large, and the equilibrium of Po_2 between the two circulations is not reached at normal rates of blood flow. Therefore the Po_2 of the fetal blood leaving the placenta is low. If fetal hemoglobin did not have a greater affinity for O_2 than adult hemoglobin, the fetus would not receive an adequate O_2 supply. The fetal oxyhemoglobin dissociation curve is shifted to the left. Therefore at equal O_2 pressures, fetal blood carries significantly more O_2 than maternal blood.

In early fetal life the high cardiac glycogen levels that prevail may protect the heart from acute periods of hypoxia. The glycogen levels gradually decrease to adult levels by term.

At birth, several changes occur in the circulatory system

The umbilical vessels have thick muscular walls that are very reactive to trauma, tension, sympathomimetic amines, bradykinin, angiotensin, and changes in Po_2. In animals in which the umbilical cord is not tied, hemorrhage of the newborn is prevented because these large vessels constrict in response to one or more of the stimuli just listed. Closure of the umbilical vessels increases total peripheral resistance and blood pressure. When blood flow through the umbilical vein ceases, the ductus venosus, a thick-walled vessel with a muscular sphincter, closes. The factor initiating closure of the ductus venosus is still unknown.

The asphyxia that starts with constriction or clamping of the umbilical vessels, plus the cooling of the body, activates the respiratory center of the newborn. After the lungs fill with air, pulmonary vascular resistance decreases to about one tenth of the value that existed before lung expansion. This resistance change is not caused by the presence of O_2 in the lungs because the change is just as great if the lungs are filled with nitrogen.

Left atrial pressure is raised above that in the inferior vena cava and right atrium (1) by the decrease in pulmonary resistance with the resulting large flow of blood through the lungs to the left atrium, (2) by the reduction of flow to the right atrium caused by occlusion of the umbilical vein, and (3) by the increased resistance to left ventricular output produced by occlusion of the umbilical arteries. This reversal of the pressure gradient across the atria abruptly closes the valve over the foramen ovale, and the septal leaflets fuse over several days.

With the decrease in pulmonary vascular resistance, the pressure in the pulmonary artery falls to about half its previous level (≈ 35 mm Hg). This change in pressure, coupled with a slight increase in aortic pressure, reverses the flow of blood through the ductus arteriosus. However, within several minutes the large ductus arteriosus begins to constrict, producing turbulent flow, which manifests as a murmur in the newborn. Constriction of the ductus arteriosus is progressive and usually is complete within 1 to 2 days after birth. Closure of the ductus arteriosus appears to be initiated by the high Pa_{O_2} of the arterial blood passing through it; pulmonary ventilation with O_2 closes the ductus, whereas ventilation with air low in O_2 opens this shunt vessel. Whether O_2 acts directly on the ductus or mediates the release of a vasoconstrictor substance is unknown.

At birth the walls of the two ventricles are about equally thick, or the right ventricle is slightly thicker. Also, in the newborn, the pulmonary arterioles are thick, which is partly responsible for the high pulmonary vascular resistance of the fetus. After birth, the thickness of the walls of the right ventricle diminishes, as does the muscle layer of the pulmonary arterioles; the left ventricular walls become thicker. These changes are progressive for several weeks after birth.

> The **ductus arteriosus** occasionally fails to close after birth. This constitutes a common congenital cardiac abnormality that is amenable to surgical correction.

SUMMARY

- Most of the resistance vessels in the skin are under the dual control of the sympathetic nervous system and local vasodilator metabolites, but the AV anastomoses found in the skin of the hands, feet, and face are solely under neural control.
- The main function of skin blood vessels is to aid in the regulation of body temperature either by constricting, which conserves heat, or by dilating, which loses heat.
- Skin blood vessels dilate directly and reflexly in response to heat and constrict directly and reflexly in response to cold.
- Skeletal muscle blood flow is regulated centrally by the sympathetic nerves and locally by the release of vasodilator metabolites.
- Neural regulation of blood flow in resting subjects is paramount, but metabolic regulation prevails during muscle contractions.
- The physical factors that influence coronary blood flow are the viscosity of the blood, frictional resistance of the vessel walls, aortic pressure, and extravascular compression of the vessels within the walls of the left ventricle.
- Left coronary blood flow is restricted during ventricular systole as a result of extravascular compression, and it is greatest during diastole, when the intramyocardial vessels are not compressed.
- Neural regulation of coronary blood flow is much less important than metabolic regulation. Activation of the cardiac sympathetic nerves directly constricts the

coronary resistance vessels. However, the enhanced myocardial metabolism caused by the associated increase in heart rate and contractile force produces vasodilation, which overrides the direct constrictor effect of sympathetic nerve stimulation. Stimulation of the cardiac branches of the vagus nerves slightly dilates the coronary arterioles.

- The metabolic activity of the heart parallels the coronary blood flow. A decrease in O_2 supply or an increase in O_2 demand apparently releases a vasodilator that decreases coronary resistance.
- In response to the gradual occlusion of a coronary artery, collateral vessels develop from adjacent unoccluded arteries, and they supply blood to the compromised myocardium distal to the point of occlusion.
- Cerebral blood flow is regulated predominantly by metabolic factors, especially CO_2, K^+, and adenosine.
- Increased regional cerebral activity produced by stimuli such as touch, pain, hand motion, talking, reading, reasoning, and problem solving are associated with enhanced blood flow in the activated areas of the cerebral cortex.
- The microcirculation in the intestinal villi constitutes a countercurrent exchange system for O_2. This places the villi in jeopardy in states of low blood flow.
- The splanchnic resistance and capacitance vessels are very responsive to changes in sympathetic neural activity.
- The liver receives about 25% of the cardiac output; about three fourths of this comes via the portal vein and about one fourth via the hepatic artery.
- When blood flow is diminished in either the portal or the hepatic system, flow in the other system usually increases but not proportionately.
- The liver tends to maintain a constant O_2 consumption, in part because its mechanism for extracting O_2 from the blood is so efficient.
- The liver normally contains about 15% of the total blood volume. It serves as an important blood reservoir for the body.
- In the fetus a large percentage of the right atrial blood passes through the foramen ovale to the left atrium, and a large percentage of the pulmonary artery blood passes through the ductus arteriosus to the aorta.
- At birth, the umbilical vessels, ductus venosus, and ductus arteriosus close by contraction of their muscle layers.
- The reduction in the pulmonary vascular resistance caused by lung inflation is the main factor that reverses the pressure gradient between the atria, thereby closing the foramen ovale.

BIBLIOGRAPHY

Belardinelli L, Linden J, Berne RM: The cardiac effects of adenosine, *Prog Cardiovasc Dis* 32:73, 1989.

Faber JJ, Thornburg KL: *Placental physiology,* New York, 1983, Raven.

Faraci FM, Heistad DD: Regulation of the cerebral circulation: role of endothelium and potassium channels, *Physiol Rev* 78:53, 1998.

Fozzard HA et al, eds: *The heart and cardiovascular system,* ed 2, New York, 1991, Raven.

Greenway CV, Lautt WW: Hepatic circulation. In Schultz SG, ed: *Handbook of physiology,* section 6, *The gastrointestinal system,* vol 1, *Motility and circulation,* Bethesda, 1989, American Physiological Society.

Guissani DA et al: Dynamics of cardiovascular responses to repeated partial umbilical cord compression in late-gestation sheep fetus, *Am J Physiol* 273(5 Pt 2):H2351, 1997.

Hudetz AG, Shen H, Kampine JP: Nitric oxide from neuronal NOS plays critical role in cerebral capillary flow response to hypoxia, *Am J Physiol* 274:H982, 1998.

Ishibashi Y et al: ATP-sensitive K$^+$ channels, adenosine, and nitric oxide–mediated mechanisms account for coronary vasodilation during exercise, *Circ Res* 82:346, 1998.

Lautt WW, Legare DJ: Passive autoregulation of portal venous pressure: distensible hepatic resistance, *Am J Physiol* 263:G702, 1992.

Miller FJ, Dellsperger KC, Gutterman DD: Myogenic constriction of human coronary arterioles, *Am J Physiol* 273:H257, 1997.

Olsson RA, Bunger R, Spaan JAE: Coronary circulation. In Fozzard HA et al, eds: *The heart and cardiovascular system,* ed 2, New York, 1991, Raven.

Phillis JW, ed: *The regulation of cerebral blood flow,* Boca Raton, Fla, 1993, CRC.

Rådegran G, Saltin B: Muscle flow at onset of dynamic exercise in humans, *Am J Physiol* 274:H314, 1998.

Schaper W et al: Collateral circulation. In Fozzard HA et al, eds: *The heart and cardiovascular system,* ed 2, New York, 1991, Raven.

CASE STUDIES

Case 25-1

A 70-year-old man with a long history of angina pectoris has been treated successfully with nitroglycerin. He entered the hospital because of short episodes of lightheadedness and occasional loss of consciousness. The results of the physical examination were unremarkable, except for a pulse rate of 35 beats/min. His blood pressure was 130/50 mm Hg. The electrocardiogram showed an atrial rate of 72 beats/min and a ventricular rate of 35 beats/min, with complete disassociation of the P and R waves. The chest x-ray film showed a moderately enlarged heart. The diagnosis was coronary artery disease with complete (third-degree) heart block. A pacemaker was inserted, and the patient was discharged from the hospital.

1. What did the severe bradycardia produce?
   A. Myogenic constriction of the coronary vessels
   B. Metabolic dilation of the coronary vessels
   C. Reflex dilation of the coronary vessels
   D. A decrease and an increase in coronary resistance
   E. Reversal of the endocardial to epicardial blood flow ratio

2. Within 2 to 3 months after leaving the hospital the patient experienced more frequent and more severe bouts of angina pectoris, and he was admitted to the hospital for study. An angiogram showed advanced coronary artery disease with almost complete occlusion of the three main coronary arteries. He was then scheduled for coronary bypass surgery. During the operation, the surgeon electrically stimulated the right and left stellate ganglia. What did this stimulation cause?
   A. No change in coronary blood flow
   B. An increase in ventricular rate and a decrease in atrial rate
   C. A decrease in ventricular rate and an increase in atrial rate
   D. Sustained coronary dilation in one of the partially occluded vessels
   E. Sustained coronary constriction in one of the partially occluded vessels

3. Shortly after bypass surgery the reactivity of his coronary vessels was tested by intracoronary administration (via a catheter) of several vasoactive agents. Which of the following substances elicited an increase in coronary resistance?
   A. Nitroglycerin
   B. Endothelin
   C. Prostacyclin
   D. Adenosine
   E. Acetylcholine

4. Despite the coronary bypass surgery the patient's cardiac function progressively deteriorated. He became severely short of breath (dyspneic) and developed intractable cardiac failure. A suitable donor was found, and he had a heart transplant. After cardiac transplant, which of the following is true?
   A. Coronary blood flow increases with vagus nerve stimulation.
   B. Coronary blood flow decreases with sympathetic nerve stimulation.
   C. Heart rate increases with inspiration.
   D. Heart rate decreases with inspiration.
   E. Stroke volume increases with exercise.

Case 25-2

A 53-year-old man has consumed substantial amounts of alcohol over the past 3 decades. For the past 2 or 3 years, he has noticed that his belt size has progressively increased and that his abdomen was distended. His physician was able to evoke a fluid wave across the abdomen when he tapped the patient's abdomen. His doctor made the diagnosis of hepatic cirrhosis, which is associated with extensive fibrosis of the liver.

1. What is the reason for the large accumulation of fluid in the patient's abdomen?

   A. The hydrostatic pressure in the splanchnic capillaries was abnormally high.

   B. The hydrostatic pressure in the hepatic artery was abnormally high.

   C. The hydrostatic pressure in the hepatic veins exceeded that in the portal vein.

   D. The hydrostatic pressure in the hepatic veins exceeded that in the splenic vein.

   E. The hepatic vascular resistance was subnormal.

CHAPTER 26

Interplay of Central and Peripheral Factors in Control of the Circulation

OBJECTIVES

- Describe the sequence of cardiovascular events during exercise.
- Describe how most cardiovascular functions are integrated in exercise.
- Explain the effects of blood loss on the cardiovascular system.
- Explain the various compensatory mechanisms that protect against hemorrhagic shock.
- Explain the various decompensatory mechanisms that intensify the effects of blood loss.

The primary function of the circulatory system is to deliver the supplies needed for tissue metabolism and growth and to remove the products of metabolism. Explaining how the heart and blood vessels serve this function requires a morphological and functional analysis of the system and a discussion of how the component parts contribute to maintain adequate tissue perfusion under different physiological conditions.

Once the functions of the various components are understood, it is essential that their interrelationships in the overall role of the circulatory system be considered. Tissue perfusion depends on arterial pressure and local vascular resistance, and arterial pressure in turn depends on cardiac output and total peripheral resistance (TPR). Arterial pressure is maintained within a relatively narrow range in the healthy individual, a feat accomplished by reciprocal changes in cardiac output and TPR. However, cardiac output and TPR are each influenced by a number of factors, and it is the interplay among these factors that determines the level of these two variables. The autonomic nervous system and the baroreceptors play the key role in regulating blood pressure. However, from the long-range point of view, control of fluid balance by the kidney, adrenal cortex, and central nervous system is crucial in maintaining a constant blood volume.

In a well-regulated system, one way to study the extent and sensitivity of the regulatory mechanism is to disturb the system and observe how it restores the preexisting steady state. Disturbances in the form of physical exercise and hemorrhage are used in this chapter to illustrate the effects of the factors that regulate the circulatory system.

Exercise

Cardiovascular adjustments in exercise represent an integration of neural and local chemical factors. The neural factors consist of central command, reflexes originating in the contracting muscle, and the baroreceptor reflex. **Central command** is the cerebrocortical activation of the sympathetic nervous system that produces cardiac acceleration, increased myocardial contractile force, and peripheral vasoconstriction. Reflexes can be activated via stimulation of intramuscular mechanoreceptors (stretch, tension) and chemoreceptors (products of metabolism) in response to muscle contraction. Impulses from these receptors travel centrally via small myelinated (group III) and unmyelinated (group IV) afferent nerve fibers. The central connections of this reflex are unknown, but the efferent limb consists of the sympathetic nerve fibers to the heart and peripheral blood vessels. The baroreceptor reflex is described in Chapters 19 and 23, and the local factors that influence skeletal muscle blood flow (metabolic vasodilators) are described in Chapters 23 and 25.

Exercise activates the autonomic nervous system

The concerted inhibition of parasympathetic control areas and activation of sympathetic control areas in the medulla oblongata increase the heart rate and myocardial contractility. The tachycardia and enhanced contractility increase cardiac output.

Total peripheral resistance is decreased in whole body exercise

At the same time that the sympathetic nervous system stimulates the heart, it also changes vascular resistance in the periphery. In the skin, kidneys, splanchnic regions, and inactive muscle, sympathetic-mediated vasoconstriction increases vascular resistance, which diverts blood away from these areas. This increased resistance in the vascular beds of inactive tissues persists throughout exercise.

As cardiac output and blood flow to active muscles increase with the progressive increase in the intensity of exercise, blood flow to the splanchnic and renal vasculatures decreases. Blood flow to the myocardium increases, whereas that to the brain is unchanged. Skin blood flow initially decreases during exercise and then increases as body temperature rises with the length and intensity of exercise. Skin blood flow finally decreases when the skin vessels constrict as the total body O_2 consumption nears maximum.

THE MAJOR CIRCULATORY ADJUSTMENT TO PROLONGED EXERCISE INVOLVES THE VASCULATURE OF THE ACTIVE MUSCLES. The local formation of vasoactive metabolites markedly dilates the resistance vessels; this dilation progresses as the intensity of exercise is raised. The local accumulation of metabolites relaxes the terminal arterioles. Blood flow through the muscle may increase to 15 to 20 times above the resting level. This metabolic vasodilation of the precapillary vessels in active muscles occurs very soon after the onset of exercise, and the decrease in TPR enables the heart to pump more blood more efficiently at a lesser load (less pressure work [see Chapter 25]) than if TPR were unchanged.

Only a small number of the capillaries are perfused in resting muscle, whereas in actively contracting muscle, all or nearly all of the capillaries contain flowing blood (**capillary recruitment**). The surface available for the exchange of gases, water, and solutes increases many-fold. Furthermore, the hydrostatic pressure in the capillaries is increased because of the relaxation of the resistance vessels. Hence there is a net movement of water and solutes into the muscle tissue. Tissue pressure rises and remains elevated during exercise as fluid continues to move out of the capillaries and is carried away by the lymphatic system. Lymph flow is increased as a result of the rise in capillary hydrostatic pressure and the massaging effect of the contracting muscles on the valve-containing lymphatic vessels.

The contracting muscle avidly extracts O_2 from the perfusing blood (increased arteriovenous-O_2 difference [Figure 26-1]), and the release of O_2 from the blood is facilitated by the nature of oxyhemoglobin dissociation (see Chapter 30). The reduction in pH caused by the high concentration of CO_2 and the formation of lactic acid, and the increase in temperature in the contracting muscle diminish the affinity of hemoglobin for O_2, as reflected by a shift in the oxyhemoglobin dissociation curve to the right. At any given partial pressure of O_2, less O_2 is held by the he-

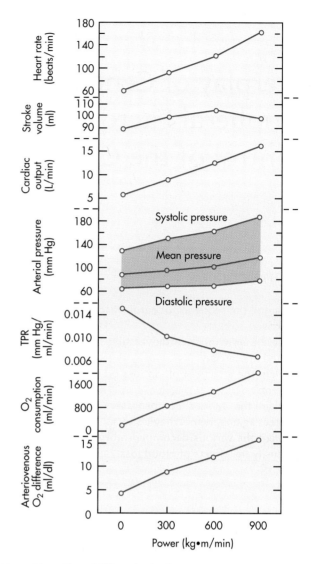

Figure 26-1 Effect of different levels of exercise on several cardiovascular variables. *(Data from Carlsten A, Grimby G: The circulatory response to muscular exercise in man, Springfield, Ill, 1966, Charles C Thomas.)*

moglobin in the red cells; consequently, O_2 removal from the blood is more effective. O_2 consumption may increase as much as sixtyfold with only a fifteenfold increase in muscle blood flow. However, the partial pressure of arterial O_2 and arterial CO_2 are normal during exercise. Muscle myoglobin serves as a limited O_2 store in exercise and can release bound O_2 at very low partial pressures. It also facilitates O_2 transport from the capillaries to the mitochondria by serving as an O_2 carrier.

Heart rate, cardiac output, and venous return increase with exercise

The enhanced sympathetic drive and the reduced parasympathetic inhibition of the sinoatrial node continue during exercise; consequently, tachycardia persists. If the workload is moderate and constant, the heart rate reaches a certain level and remains there throughout exercise. However, if the workload increases, the heart rate increases concomitantly until a plateau at about 180 beats/min is reached in severe exercise (Figure 26-1). In contrast to the large increase in heart rate, the increase in stroke volume is only about 10% to 35% (Figure 26-1), the larger values occurring in trained individuals. In very well-trained distance runners, whose cardiac outputs can reach six to seven times the resting level, stroke volume reaches about twice the resting value.

If the baroreceptors are denervated in animals, the cardiac output and heart rate responses to exercise are more sluggish than in animals with normally innervated baroreceptors. However, in the absence of autonomic innervation of the heart, such as that which occurs experimentally after total cardiac denervation, exercise still elicits an increment in cardiac output comparable to that observed in normal animals, but then it is associated with an elevated stroke volume.

In addition to the contribution made by sympathetically mediated constriction of the capacitance vessels in both exercising and nonexercising parts of the body, venous return to the heart is aided by the working skeletal muscles and the muscles of respiration (see also Chapters 24 and 25). The intermittently contracting muscles compress the vessels that course through them. The valves in the compressed veins permit blood flow only toward the right atrium. (The valves prevent backflow.) The flow of venous blood to the heart is also aided by the increase in the pressure gradient developed by the more negative intrathoracic pressure produced by deeper and more frequent respirations.

In a healthy resting person an increase in heart rate does not usually increase cardiac output appreciably (see Chapter 24). However, in whole body exercise, the enhanced venous return caused by a decreased TPR (Figure 26-1) in concert with the skeletal muscle pump (see Figure 25-2) is associated mainly with an increase in heart rate. If the heart rate cannot increase normally in response to exercise (e.g., in a patient with complete atrioventricular block), the patient's ability to exercise will be severely limited. HENCE AN INCREASE IN HEART RATE IS NECESSARY TO ENABLE THE REDUCED TPR AND SKELETAL MUSCLE PUMP TO APPROPRIATELY AUGMENT CARDIAC OUTPUT DURING EXERCISE.

In humans, little evidence exists that blood reservoirs contribute much to the circulating blood volume, with the exception of the skin, lungs, and liver. In fact, blood volume is usually reduced slightly during exercise, as evidenced by a rise in the hematocrit ratio, because of water loss externally through sweating and enhanced ventilation and through fluid movement into the contracting muscle. The fluid loss from the vascular compartment into the interstitium of contracting muscle reaches a plateau as interstitial fluid pressure rises and opposes the increased hydrostatic pressure in the capillaries of the active muscle. The fluid loss is partially offset by the movement of fluid from the splanchnic regions and inactive muscle into the bloodstream. This influx of fluid occurs as a result of a decrease

in the hydrostatic pressure in the capillaries of these tissues and an increase in the plasma osmolarity because of movement of osmotically active particles into the blood from the contracting muscle. In addition, reduced urine formation by the kidneys helps conserve body water.

In light to moderate exercise, blood returning to the heart is so rapidly pumped through the lungs and out into the aorta that the central venous pressure (diastolic filling pressure) increases only slightly. In fact, CHEST X-RAY FILMS OF INDIVIDUALS AT REST AND AT EXERCISE REVEAL A DECREASE IN HEART SIZE DURING EXERCISE, which is in harmony with the observations of a constant ventricular diastolic volume. However, in maximal or near-maximal exercise, right atrial pressure and end-diastolic ventricular volume increase. Thus the Frank-Starling mechanism contributes to the enhanced stroke volume in vigorous exercise.

Arterial pressure increases with exercise

If exercise involves a large proportion of the body musculature, such as in running or swimming, the reduction in total vascular resistance can be considerable (Figure 26-1). Nevertheless, arterial pressure starts to rise with the onset of exercise, and the increase in blood pressure roughly parallels the severity of the exercise performed (Figure 26-1). Therefore the increase in the inactive tissues by the sympathetic nervous system (and to some extent by the release of catecholamines from the adrenal medulla) is important for maintaining normal or increased blood pressure; sympathectomy or drug-induced block of the adrenergic sympathetic nerve fibers results in a decreased arterial pressure **(hypotension)** during exercise.

Sympathetic-mediated vasoconstriction also occurs in active muscle when additional muscles are activated after about half the total skeletal musculature is contracting. In experiments in which one leg is working at maximal levels and then the other leg starts to work, blood flow decreases in the first working leg. Furthermore, blood levels of norepinephrine rise significantly in exercise, and most of it comes from sympathetic nerves in the active muscles.

As body temperature rises during exercise, the skin vessels dilate in response to the thermal stimulation of the heat-regulating center in the hypothalamus, and TPR decreases further. This would decrease blood pressure were it not for the increasing cardiac output and constriction of arterioles in the renal, splanchnic, and other tissues.

In general, the mean arterial pressure rises during exercise as a result of the increased cardiac output. However, the effect of enhanced cardiac output is offset by the overall decrease in TPR, so the increase in mean blood pressure is relatively small (Figure 26-1). Vasoconstriction in the inactive vascular beds contributes to the maintenance of a normal arterial blood pressure for adequate perfusion of the active tissues. The actual pressure attained represents a balance between the cardiac output and TPR. Systolic pressure usually increases more than diastolic pressure, which results in an increased pulse pressure (Figure 26-1). The larger pulse pressure is primarily attributable to a greater stroke volume and to a lesser degree to a more rapid ejection of blood by the left ventricle, with less peripheral run-off during the brief ventricular ejection period.

In exercise taken to the point of exhaustion, the compensatory mechanisms begin to fail. The heart rate attains a maximum level of about 180 beats/min, and stroke volume reaches a plateau and often decreases, resulting in a fall in blood pressure. Dehydration occurs. Sympathetic vasoconstrictor activity supersedes the vasodilator influence on the cutaneous vessels, and its effect on the capacitance vessels produces a slight increase in effective blood volume. However, cutaneous vasoconstriction also decreases the rate of heat loss. Body temperature is normally elevated, and the reduction in heat loss through cutaneous vasoconstriction can, under these conditions, lead to very high body temperatures with associated feelings of acute distress (**heat exhaustion** or **heat stroke**). The tissue and blood pH decrease as a result of increased lactic acid and CO_2 production. The reduced pH is probably the key determinant of the maximal amount of exercise an individual can tolerate because of muscle pain and the subjective feeling of exhaustion.

A summary of the neural and local effects of exercise on the cardiovascular system is presented in Figure 26-2.

When exercise stops, the heart rate and cardiac output abruptly decrease

The TPR remains low for some time after exercise ends, presumably because of the accumulation of vasodilator metabolites in the muscles during the exercise. As a result of the reduced cardiac output and persistence of vasodilation in the muscles, arterial pressure may fall briefly below preexercise levels. Blood pressure is then stabilized at normal levels by the baroreceptor reflexes.

Inadequate O_2 supply limits exercise performance

The two main forces that could limit skeletal muscle performance are the rate of O_2 use by the muscles and the O_2 supply to the muscles. Muscle O_2 use is probably not critical because when maximum O_2 consumption (Vo_{2max}) is reached during exercise of a large percentage of the body muscle mass, the recruitment of additional muscles does not produce a further increase in O_2 consumption. If muscle O_2 use were limiting, the recruitment of more contracting muscle would use additional O_2 to meet the enhanced O_2 requirements and would thereby increase total body O_2 consumption. Therefore O_2 supply to the ac-

tive muscles must be inadequate. The limitation of O_2 supply could be caused by inadequate oxygenation of blood in the lungs or by the limitation of the supply of O_2-laden blood to the muscles. Failure of the lungs to fully oxygenate blood can be excluded because even with the most strenuous exercise in subjects at sea level, arterial blood is fully saturated with O_2. Therefore O_2 delivery (blood flow) to the active muscles appears to be the limiting factor in muscle performance.

This limitation in muscle performance translates into the inability of the heart to increase its output beyond a certain level. Cardiac output equals heart rate multiplied by stroke volume, and heart rate reaches maximum levels before Vo_{2max} is reached. Hence stroke volume must be the limiting factor. However, blood pressure provides the energy for skeletal muscle perfusion, and blood pressure depends on TPR as well as on cardiac output. During intense exercise at peak Vo_{2max} and peak cardiac output, blood pressure falls as more muscle vascular beds dilate in response to locally released vasodilator metabolites if some

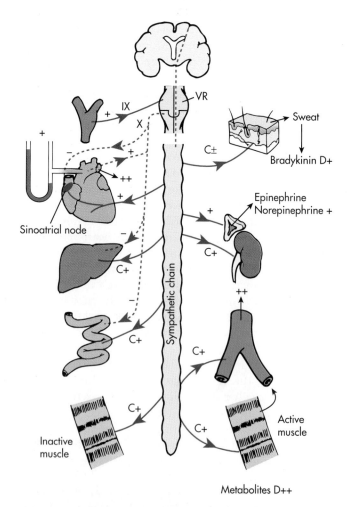

Figure 26-2 Cardiovascular adjustments in exercise. *C,* Vasoconstrictor activity; *D,* vasodilator activity; *IX,* glossopharyngeal nerve; *VR,* vasomotor region; *X,* vagus nerve; +, increased activity, −, decreased activity.

centrally mediated vasoconstriction (via the baroreceptor reflex) does not occur in the resistance vessels of the active muscles. Hence the adjustment of resistance in the active muscles appears to be an important factor in the limitation of whole-body exercise (e.g., swimming, running). However, THE MAJOR FACTOR IS THE PUMPING CAPACITY OF THE HEART. When the exercise involves only a small group of muscles (e.g., those of the hand), the cardiovascular system is not taxed, and the limiting factor, although unknown, lies within the muscle.

Physical training and conditioning increase peak O_2 consumption

The response of the cardiovascular system to regular exercise is to increase its capacity to deliver O_2 to the active muscles and improve the ability of the muscle to use O_2. The Vo_{2max} is quite reproducible in a given individual, and it varies with the level of physical conditioning. Training progressively increases the Vo_{2max}, which reaches a plateau at the highest level of conditioning. Highly "trained" athletes have a lower resting heart rate, greater stroke volume, and lower TPR than they had before training or after deconditioning (becoming sedentary). The low resting heart rate is caused by a higher vagal tone and a lower sympathetic tone. With exercise, the maximum heart rate of the trained individual is the same as that in "untrained" persons, but it is attained at a higher level of exercise. The trained person also exhibits a low vascular resistance that is inherent in the muscle. For example, if an individual exercises one leg regularly over an extended period and does not exercise the other leg, the vascular resistance is lower and the Vo_{2max} is higher in the trained leg than in the untrained leg. Also, the well-trained athlete has a lower resting sympathetic outflow to the viscera than a sedentary counterpart.

Physical conditioning is also associated with greater extraction of O_2 from the blood (greater arteriovenous-O_2 difference) by the muscles. With long-term training, capillary density in skeletal muscle increases, as do the concentrations of oxidative enzymes in the mitochondria. Also, the levels of ATPase, myoglobin, and enzymes involved in lipid metabolism appear to increase with physical conditioning.

Endurance training such as running or swimming increases left ventricular volume without increasing left ventricular wall thickness. In contrast, strength exercises such as weight lifting increase left ventricular wall thickness **(hypertrophy)** but have little effect on ventricular volume. However, this increase in wall thickness is small relative to that observed in **chronic hypertension,** in which the elevation of afterload persists because of the high TPR.

Hemorrhage

In an individual who has lost a large quantity of blood, the arterial systolic, diastolic, and pulse pressures are reduced, and the arterial pulse is rapid and feeble. The skin is pale, moist, and slightly **cyanotic** (blue). The cutaneous veins are collapsed and fill slowly when compressed centrally. Respiration is rapid, but the depth of respiration may be shallow or deep.

Arterial blood pressure declines when blood is lost

The changes in mean arterial pressure evoked by acute hemorrhage in animals are illustrated in Figure 26-3. If an animal is bled rapidly to bring the mean arterial pressure to 50 mm Hg, the arterial pressure tends to rise spontaneously toward control over the subsequent 20 to 30 minutes. In some animals (curve A in Figure 26-3), this trend continues, and normal pressures are regained within a few hours. These animals tend to survive even if their shed blood is not returned to them. In other animals (curve B in Figure 26-3), the pressure begins to decline after the initial rise and continues to fall at an accelerating rate until death ensues. If blood is transfused early in the phase of declining arterial pressure, the animals usually survive. However, at some point later in this phase of declining pressure, the deterioration becomes irreversible.

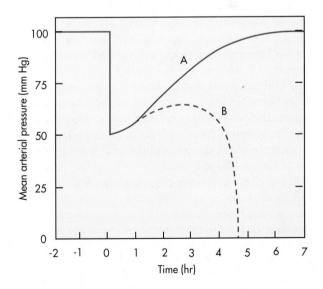

Figure 26-3 Changes in mean arterial pressure after rapid hemorrhage. At time zero, the animal is bled rapidly to a mean arterial pressure of 50 mm Hg. The arterial pressure tends to return toward normal at first. In some animals *(curve A),* the pressure continues to improve until the normal pressure is attained even though none of the shed blood has been transfused back into the animal. In other animals *(curve B),* after a temporary period of apparent improvement, the arterial blood pressure begins to decline and falls at a steeper and steeper rate until death ensues.

When the arterial blood pressure fails to return to normal, the state is known as **hemorrhagic shock.** This state usually has a lethal outcome regardless of whether the animal already in shock receives a transfusion of its own shed blood or a transfusion of a larger quantity of matched blood from a donor.

Compensatory mechanisms protect against blood loss

The prominent tendency for arterial blood pressure to rise toward normal levels immediately after acute blood loss (Figure 26-3) indicates that potent compensatory mechanisms must be invoked. Any mechanism that acts to restore normal levels of arterial blood pressure in response to blood loss may be designated as a **negative-feedback mechanism.** The term *negative* is applied because the direction of the induced change in pressure is opposite to that of the initiating change. The following negative-feedback mechanisms are evoked by hemorrhage:

1. Baroreceptor reflexes
2. Chemoreceptor reflexes
3. Cerebral ischemia responses
4. Reabsorption of tissue fluids into the plasma compartment
5. Release of endogenous vasoconstrictor substances
6. Renal conservation of salt and water

Baroreceptor reflexes minimize arterial pressure declines

The reductions in the mean arterial and pulse pressures during hemorrhage decrease the excitation of the baroreceptors in the carotid sinuses and aortic arch (see Chapter 23). Several cardiovascular responses are thus evoked reflexly, all of which act to restore the normal arterial blood pressure. Unloading of the arterial baroreceptors decreases vagal tone and augments sympathetic tone, and both of these changes in efferent neural activity increase the heart rate and enhance myocardial contractility (see Chapter 19).

Generalized arteriolar vasoconstriction is the principal mechanism that is invoked by the diminished baroreceptor stimulation and that protects the subject from a critical reduction in arterial blood pressure in response to hemorrhage. Although arteriolar vasoconstriction is widespread throughout the systemic vascular bed, it is by no means uniform. Hemorrhage-induced vasoconstriction is most severe in the skin, skeletal muscle, and splanchnic vascular beds.

In the early states of mild to moderate hemorrhage, the changes in renal resistance are usually slight. The tendency for increased sympathetic activity to constrict the renal vessels is counteracted by autoregulatory mechanisms (see Chapter 33). In response to more prolonged and more severe hemorrhage, however, renal va-

soconstriction becomes intense. The reductions in renal circulation are most severe in the outer layers of the renal cortex; the inner zones of the cortex and outer zones of the medulla are spared.

If renal vasoconstriction persists too long, it is harmful. Frequently, patients who have lost substantial amounts of blood survive the acute hypotensive period, only to die several days later from **kidney failure** resulting from renal ischemia.

Reflexly induced arteriolar vasoconstriction tends to be slight or absent in the cerebral and coronary circulations. In many instances the cerebral and coronary vascular resistances are diminished. Thus the reduced cardiac output is redistributed to favor flow through the brain and heart, which are certainly among the most crucial of the body's organs.

The increased sympathetic discharge also evokes a generalized venoconstriction, which has the same hemodynamic consequences as a transfusion of blood (see Chapter 24). Sympathetic activation constricts certain blood reservoirs. This constriction provides an autotransfusion of blood into the circulating bloodstream. In the dog, considerable quantities of blood are mobilized by contraction of the spleen. In humans, the spleen is not an important blood reservoir. Instead, constriction of the cutaneous and hepatic vasculatures in response to blood loss contributes blood volume to the circulating bloodstream. Therefore these regional structures act as blood reservoirs.

Severe cutaneous vasoconstriction accounts for the characteristic pale, cold skin of patients suffering from blood loss. Warming the skin of such patients improves their appearance considerably, much to the satisfaction of well-meaning individuals who might render first aid. However, it also inactivates an effective, natural compensatory mechanism to the patient's possible detriment.

Chemoreceptor reflexes help sustain arterial blood pressure

Hemorrhage-induced reductions in arterial pressure below about 60 mm Hg do not evoke any additional responses through the baroreceptor reflexes because this pressure level constitutes the threshold for baroreceptor stimulation (see Chapter 23). However, low arterial pressure may lead to arterial chemoreceptor stimulation because the resulting inadequate blood flow to the aortic and carotid bodies diminishes the partial pressure of O_2 in the chemoreceptor tissues. Chemoreceptor excitation augments the prevailing vasoconstriction evoked by the baroreceptor reflexes. Also, the

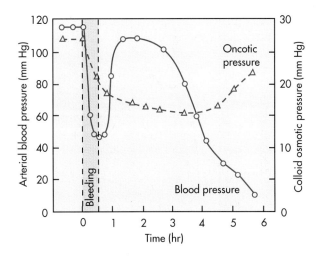

Figure 26-4 Changes in arterial blood pressure *(circles)* and plasma colloid osmotic pressure *(triangles)* in response to the withdrawal of 45% of the estimated blood volume over a 30-minute period, beginning at time zero, in a group of anesthetized cats. *(Redrawn from Zweifach BW: Anesthesiology 41:157, 1974.)*

respiratory stimulation induced by chemoreceptor excitation assists venous return by the auxiliary pumping mechanism described in Chapter 24.

Cerebral ischemia helps sustain arterial blood pressure

When hemorrhage lowers the arterial blood pressure below about 40 mm Hg, the resulting cerebral ischemia activates the sympathetic nervous system. The resulting sympathetic nervous discharge is intense; it is several times greater than the maximal activity that occurs when the baroreceptors cease to be stimulated. Therefore the vasoconstriction and facilitation of myocardial contractility evoked by cerebral ischemia may be pronounced. When cerebral ischemia is severe, the vagal centers also become activated. The resulting bradycardia may aggravate the hypotension that initiated the cerebral ischemia.

The reabsorption of tissue fluids helps restore plasma volume

The arterial hypotension, arteriolar constriction, and reduced central venous pressure induced by hemorrhage lower the hydrostatic pressure in the capillaries. Consequently, the balance of forces across the capillary endothelium promotes the net reabsorption of interstitial fluid into the vascular compartment. The rapidity of this response in an experiment on anesthetized cats is displayed in Figure 26-4. In this experiment, 45% of the estimated blood volume was removed over a 30-minute period. The mean arterial blood pressure declined rapidly to about 45 mm Hg during the hemorrhage. When bleeding was terminated, the arterial pressure rose rapidly but only temporarily to near the control level. About 2½ hours after cessation of the hemorrhage, the arterial pressure began to fall, and it declined progressively until the animals died. The time

course of this response to hemorrhage resembles that of curve B in Figure 26-3.

Associated with these changes in arterial blood pressure, the plasma colloid osmotic pressure declines markedly during bleeding and continues to decrease more gradually for several hours (Figure 26-4). The reduction in the colloid osmotic pressure reflects the dilution of the blood by tissue fluids. Considerable quantities of fluid may be drawn into the circulation during hemorrhage. Approximately 1 L/hr of fluid might be autoinfused from the interstitial fluid into the circulatory system of an average individual after acute blood loss.

Considerable quantities of fluid also may be slowly shifted from the intracellular to the extracellular spaces. This fluid exchange is probably mediated by the secretion of cortisol from the adrenal cortex in response to hemorrhage.

Endogenous vasoconstrictors help maintain arterial blood pressure

Catecholamines (epinephrine and norepinephrine) are released from the adrenal medulla and postganglionic sympathetic nerve endings in response to acute blood loss (see Chapter 47). The concentrations of epinephrine and norepinephrine increase substantially in the arterial blood within the first minute of hemorrhage and remain elevated (up to 50 times normal) throughout hemorrhage. Retransfusion of the shed blood reduces the blood catecholamine levels to normal.

Vasopressin, a potent vasoconstrictor, is actively secreted by the posterior pituitary gland in response to hemorrhage (see Chapter 44). Removal of about 20% of the blood volume in animals increases vasopressin secretion about fortyfold. The sensory receptors responsible for the augmented release are the sinoaortic baroreceptors and the stretch receptors in the left atrium.

Diminished renal perfusion during hemorrhagic hypotension leads to the secretion of **renin** from the juxtaglomerular apparatus (see Chapters 37 and 46). Consequently, the concentration of renin in the peripheral blood rises as a function of the volume of shed blood. Renin is an enzyme that acts on the plasma protein **angiotensinogen** to form **angiotensin,** which is a very powerful vasoconstrictor.

The kidneys conserve water during hemorrhage

The diminution in arterial blood pressure induced by the loss of blood decreases the glomerular filtration rate and thus curtails the excretion of water and electrolytes (see Chapter 37). During hemorrhage, fluid and electrolytes are also conserved by the kidneys in response to the release of various hormones, including vasopressin and renin, as noted in the preceding section. The peptide angiotensin, which is formed by the action of renin, accelerates the release of aldosterone from the adrenal cortex. Aldosterone in turn stimulates Na$^+$ reabsorption by the renal tubules, and water accompanies the Na$^+$ that is actively reabsorbed (see Chapters 36 and 37).

Decompensatory mechanisms intensify the effects of hemorrhage

In contrast to the negative-feedback mechanisms just described, latent **positive-feedback mechanisms** are also invoked by hemorrhage. Such mechanisms exaggerate the primary changes initiated by the blood loss. Specifically, positive-feedback mechanisms aggravate the hypotension induced by blood loss and tend to initiate vicious cycles that may be fatal. The operation of positive-feedback mechanisms is manifested in the accelerating and eventually lethal decline in blood pressure reflected by curve B of Figure 26-3.

Whether a positive-feedback mechanism leads to a vicious cycle depends on the **gain** of that mechanism; the gain is the ratio of the secondary change evoked by a given feedback mechanism to the primary change itself. A gain greater than 1 induces a vicious cycle; a gain less than 1 does not. For example, consider a positive-feedback mechanism with a gain of 2. If an intervention such as the rapid loss of a specific volume of blood causes the mean arterial blood pressure to decrease quickly by 10 mm Hg, a positive-feedback mechanism (with a gain of 2) subsequently evokes a secondary pressure reduction of 20 mm Hg. This secondary change in turn causes a further decrement of 40 mm Hg; that is, each change induces a subsequent change of twice the magnitude. Hence mean arterial pressure declines at an ever-increasing rate until death, as depicted by curve B in Figure 26-3.

A positive-feedback mechanism with a gain less than 1 also amplifies the effect of any initiating intervention, but it probably does not generate a vicious cycle. For example, if a primary intervention suddenly decreases the arterial blood pressure by 10 mm Hg, a positive-feedback mechanism with a gain of 0.5 initiates a secondary, additional pressure decline of 5 mm Hg. This, in turn, provokes a decrease of 2.5 mm Hg. The process continues in ever-diminishing steps, and the arterial blood pressure approaches some equilibrium value asymptotically. Some of the important positive-feedback mechanisms invoked in response to hemorrhage include cardiac failure, acidosis, inadequate cerebral blood flow, aberration of blood clotting, and depression of the reticuloendothelial system (RES).

Cardiac failure exaggerates the effects of hemorrhage

Whether cardiac failure plays a significant role in the progression of hemorrhagic shock is controversial. All investigators agree that the heart fails terminally, but the importance of cardiac failure during earlier stages of hemorrhagic hypotension remains to be established. Rightward shifts in ventricular function curves (Figure 26-5) constitute experimental evidence of a progressive

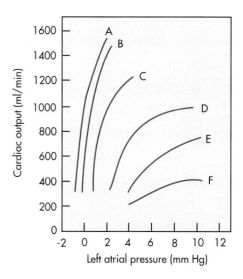

Figure 26-5 Left ventricular function curves in an anesthetized dog during hemorrhagic shock. Curve A represents the control curve. Curves B through F represent the curves at 117, 247, 280, 295, and 310 minutes, respectively, after the initial hemorrhage. *(Redrawn from Crowell JW, Guyton AC: Am J Physiol 203:248, 1962.)*

depression of myocardial contractility during a sustained reduction in blood volume.

The hypotension induced by hemorrhage reduces the coronary blood flow, which tends to depress ventricular function. The consequent reduction in cardiac output leads to a further decline in arterial pressure, a classic example of a positive-feedback mechanism. Furthermore, the reduced tissue blood flow leads to a local accumulation of vasodilator metabolites, which decreases TPR and therefore intensifies the decline in arterial pressure.

Acidosis exaggerates the effects of blood loss

Inadequate blood flow during hemorrhage affects the metabolism of all cells in the body. The resulting stagnant anoxia accelerates the production of lactic acid and other acid metabolites by the tissues. Furthermore, impaired kidney function prevents adequate excretion of the excess H$^+$, and generalized metabolic acidosis ensues (Figure 26-6). The depressant effect of the metabolic acidosis on the heart further reduces tissue perfusion and thus aggravates the acidosis. The reactivity of the heart and arterioles to neurally released and circulating catecholamines is diminished by the acidosis, which intensifies the hypotension.

Central nervous system depression impairs the response to hemorrhage

The arterial hypotension associated with hemorrhagic shock reduces cerebral blood flow. Moderate degrees of cerebral ischemia evoke a pronounced sympathetic nervous stimulation of the heart, arterioles, and veins. Hence moderate cerebral ischemia mobilizes various salutary negative-feedback mechanisms, as previously explained. When hypotension is severe, however, the

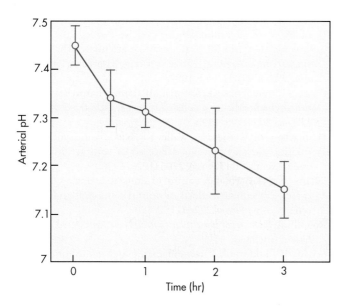

Figure 26-6 Reduction in arterial blood pH (mean plus or minus standard deviation) in 11 anesthetized dogs whose blood pressure had been held at 35 mm Hg by arterial bleeding into a reservoir, beginning at time zero. *(Redrawn from Markov AK et al: Circ Shock 8:9, 1981.)*

cardiovascular centers in the brainstem are depressed because the reduction in blood flow to the brain is so pronounced. The resulting curtailment of sympathetic neural activity then exaggerates the diminution of cardiac output and TPR. The consequent decline in mean arterial pressure intensifies the inadequate cerebral perfusion.

Various endogenous **opioids,** such as **enkephalins** and **β-endorphin,** may be released into the brain substance or into the circulation in response to the same stresses that provoke circulatory shock. Enkephalins exist along with catecholamines in secretory granules in the adrenal medulla, and they are released together in response to stress (see Chapter 47). Similar stimuli release β-endorphin from the anterior pituitary gland (see Chapter 44). These opioids depress the centers in the brainstem that mediate some of the compensatory autonomic adaptations to blood loss and other shock-provoking stresses. Conversely, the opioid antagonist **naloxone** improves cardiovascular function and survival in various forms of shock.

Aberrations of blood clotting intensify the effects of hemorrhage

THE ALTERATIONS OF BLOOD CLOTTING AFTER HEMORRHAGE ARE TYPICALLY BIPHASIC; AN INITIAL PHASE OF HYPERCOAGULABILITY IS FOLLOWED BY A SECONDARY PHASE OF HYPOCOAGULABILITY AND FIBRINOLYSIS (see Chapter 15). In the initial phase, intravascular clots, or **thrombi,** develop within a few minutes of the onset of severe hemorrhage, and coagulation may be extensive throughout the microcirculation.

Thromboxane A$_2$, which is released from various ischemic tissues, aggregates platelets. The trapped platelets release more thromboxane A$_2$, which then

traps additional platelets. This positive-feedback response intensifies the clotting process. The mortality rate from certain standard shock-provoking procedures has been reduced considerably by the administration of anticoagulants such as **heparin.**

In the later stages of hemorrhagic hypotension, the clotting time is prolonged, and fibrinolysis is prominent. Hemorrhage into the intestinal lumen is common after several hours of hemorrhagic hypotension in various species of animals. Blood loss into the intestinal lumen, of course, aggravates the hemodynamic effects of the original hemorrhage.

Blood loss depresses the reticuloendothelial system

Hemorrhage curtails the phagocytic activity of the RES. Consequently, the antibacterial and antitoxic defense mechanisms of the body are impaired. **Endotoxins** from the normal bacterial flora of the intestine constantly enter the circulation. Ordinarily they are inactivated by the RES, principally in the liver. When the RES is depressed, however, these endotoxins invade the general circulation.

ENDOTOXINS TEND TO LOWER ARTERIAL BLOOD PRESSURE BY AUGMENTING THE SYNTHESIS OF NITRIC OXIDE SYNTHASE, MAINLY IN THE VASCULAR SMOOTH MUSCLE. The nitric oxide generated by the activity of this enzyme is a potent vasodilator, and therefore it intensifies the hypotension caused by the blood loss.

Positive and negative-feedback mechanisms interact

Hemorrhage alters a multitude of circulatory and metabolic activities. As previously stated, some of these alterations constitute compensatory or decompensatory feedback systems. Some of those systems possess a high gain; others, a low gain. Furthermore, the gain of any specific system usually varies with the severity of the hemorrhage. For example, when the loss of blood is minimal, the mean arterial pressure is usually within the normal range, and the gain of the baroreceptor reflexes is high. When hemorrhage is more severe, the mean arterial pressure may be below about 60 mm Hg (i.e., below the threshold for the baroreceptors), and therefore further reductions have no additional influence via the baroreceptor reflexes. Hence below this critical pressure the baroreceptor reflex gain is near zero.

When blood loss is minor, the gains of the negative-feedback mechanisms are usually high, whereas those of the positive-feedback mechanisms are usually low. The converse is true when hemorrhage is more severe. In a specific, complex pathophysiological state, such as severe blood loss, the generation of a vicious cycle depends on whether the overall gain of the various compensatory and decompensatory systems exceeds 1. The development of a vicious cycle is, of course, more likely when blood losses are severe. Therefore to avert a vicious cycle in a subject who has suffered a severe hemorrhage, the subject must be treated quickly and intensively, mainly by blood replacement, before the process becomes irreversible.

Summary

- In anticipation of exercise the vagus nerve impulses to the heart are inhibited, and the sympathetic nervous system is activated by central command. The result is an increase in heart rate, myocardial contractile force, and regional vascular resistance.
- With exercise, vascular resistance increases in the skin, kidneys, splanchnic regions, and inactive muscles and decreases in active muscles.
- During exercise, the increase in cardiac output is accomplished mainly by the increase in heart rate. Stroke volume increases only slightly.
- During exercise, TPR decreases, O_2 consumption and blood O_2 extraction increase, and systolic and mean blood pressures increase slightly.
- As body temperature rises during exercise, the skin blood vessels dilate. However, when the heart rate becomes maximal during severe exercise, the skin vessels constrict. This increases the effective blood volume but causes greater increases in body temperature and a feeling of exhaustion.
- The limiting factor in exercise performance is the delivery of blood to the active muscles.
- Acute blood loss induces the following hemodynamic changes: tachycardia, hypotension, generalized arteriolar vasoconstriction, and generalized venoconstriction.
- Acute blood loss invokes various negative-feedback (compensatory) mechanisms such as baroreceptor and chemoreceptor reflexes, responses to moderate cerebral ischemia, reabsorption of tissue fluids, release of endogenous vasoconstrictors, and renal conservation of water and electrolytes.
- Acute blood loss also invokes various positive-feedback (decompensatory) mechanisms such as cardiac failure, acidosis, central nervous system depression, aberrations of blood coagulation, and depression of the RES.
- The outcome of acute blood loss depends on the gains of the various feedback mechanisms and the interactions between the positive and negative-feedback mechanisms.

BIBLIOGRAPHY

Astiz ME, Rackow EC, Weil MH: Pathophysiology and treatment of circulatory shock, *Crit Care Clin* 9:183, 1993.

Blomqvist CG, Saltin B: Cardiovascular adaptations to physical training, *Ann Rev Physiol* 15:169, 1983.

Cameron JD, Dart AM: Exercise training increases total systemic arterial compliance in humans, *Am J Physiol* 266:H693, 1994.

Cheng K-P, Igarashi Y, Little WC: Mechanism of augmented rate of left ventricular filling during exercise, *Circ Res* 70:9, 1992.

Collins HL, DiCarlo SE: Daily exercise attenuates the sympathetic component of the atrial baroreflex control of heart rate, *Am J Physiol* 273:H2613, 1997.

Geerdes BP, Frederick KL, Brunner MJ: Carotid baroreflex control during hemorrhage in conscious and anesthetized dogs, *Am J Physiol* 265:R195, 1993.

Herbertson MJ, Werner HA, Walley KR: Nitric oxide synthase inhibition partially prevents decreased LV contractility during endotoxemia, *Am J Physiol* 270:H1979, 1996.

Iellamo F et al: Baroreflex control of sinus node during dynamic exercise in humans: effects of central command and muscle reflexes, *Am J Physiol* 272:H1157, 1997.

Rowell LB: *Human cardiovascular control,* New York, 1993, Oxford University Press.

Schadt JC, Ludbrook J: Hemodynamic and neurohumoral responses to acute hypovolemia in conscious mammals, *Am J Physiol* 260:H305, 1991.

Sheriff DD et al: Dependence of cardiac filling pressure on cardiac output during rest and dynamic exercise in dogs, *Am J Physiol* 265:H316, 1993.

Szabo C: Alterations in nitric oxide production in various forms of circulatory shock, *New Horizons* 3:2, 1995.

Vissing SF, Scherrer U, Victor RG: Stimulation of skin sympathetic nerve discharge by central command: differential control of sympathetic outflow to skin and skeletal muscle during static exercise, *Circ Res* 69:229, 1991.

Yao Y-M et al: Significance of NO in hemorrhage-induced hemodynamic alterations, organ injury, and mortality in rats, *Am J Physiol* 270:H1616, 1996.

Case Studies

Case 26-1

A 23-year-old male track star decided to enter the Boston Marathon. He had run only in short-distance events, up to 10 km, before entry in the marathon. At the 15-mile mark, he was leading the race, but he was soon passed by one of his competitors. This inspired him to make a strong effort to retake the lead, but he was unable to increase his speed. At the 20-mile mark, he began to feel faint; within the next mile he became sick to his stomach and somewhat disoriented, and he finally staggered and fell to the ground, exhausted.

1. **When the runner was at the 17-mile mark, what limited him from achieving his goal of retaking the lead?**
   A. His leg muscles were unable to use more O_2.
   B. His respiratory system was unable to saturate the arterial blood with O_2.
   C. He had inadequate vasoconstriction in the splanchnic regions and inactive muscles.
   D. His stroke volume became inadequate.
   E. His arteriovenous-O_2 difference was decreased.

2. At the time of his collapse, which of the following did *not* occur?

 A. His body temperature fell.

 B. His heart rate reached a maximum level.

 C. His skin blood vessels constricted.

 D. His blood pH decreased.

 E. His blood pressure decreased.

Case 26-2

A 47-year-old woman had an acute episode of severe abdominal pain, and she suddenly vomited a large amount of bloody material. Her husband called for an ambulance to take her to the hospital. The emergency department physician learned that the patient had frequent, severe episodes of upper abdominal pain over the past 6 weeks. Physical examination revealed that the patient's skin was very pale and cold, her heart rate was 110 beats/min, and her blood pressure was 85/65 mm Hg. Examination of the patient's blood revealed that the hematocrit ratio (i.e., the ratio of red cell volume to whole blood volume) was 40%. The physician made the tentative diagnosis of a bleeding peptic ulcer.

1. Why was the patient's skin pale and cold?

 A. The arterial baroreceptors reflexly induced the parasympathetic nerves to the skin to release acetylcholine.

 B. The arterial chemoreceptors reflexly induced the parasympathetic nerves to the skin to release vasoactive intestinal peptide.

 C. The arterial chemoreceptors reflexly induced the parasympathetic nerves to the skin to release neuropeptide Y.

 D. The arterial baroreceptors reflexly induced the sympathetic nerves to the skin to release nitric oxide.

 E. The arterial baroreceptors reflexly induced the sympathetic nerves to the skin to release norepinephrine.

2. What does the patient's arterial blood pressure of 85/65 mm Hg indicate?

 A. The patient's left ventricle was producing an abnormally low cardiac output and low stroke volume.

 B. The patient's left ventricle was pumping more blood than was her right ventricle.

 C. The patient's left ventricle was producing an abnormally low cardiac output but a normal stroke volume.

 D. The patient's left ventricle was producing a normal cardiac output and an abnormally low stroke volume.

 E. The patient's left ventricle was pumping less blood than her right ventricle.

3. If the patient's bleeding had stopped before she arrived at the hospital, which of the following changes would be expected in the blood 1 hour after the patient arrived at the hospital?

 A. The individual red blood cells would be larger than normal.

 B. The hematocrit ratio would be reduced.

 C. The lymphocyte count would be abnormally high.

 D. The plasma albumin concentration would be increased.

 E. The plasma globulin concentration would be increased.

RESPIRATORY SYSTEM

V

Mario Castro

CHAPTER 27

Overview of the Respiratory System

OBJECTIVES

- Explain the role of the respiratory system in normal body physiology.
- Describe the function of the lung in the distribution of inspired air and gas exchange.
- Describe O_2 and CO_2 transport and tissue gas exchange.
- Examine the important factors in the control of breathing.
- Compare the relationship of the various structures of the respiratory system to their function.

There are two essential physiological functions necessary to life: breathing and circulation of blood. A person may live for several days without liver, kidney, or higher brain function. However, without breathing or circulation for about 5 minutes, lack of oxygenated blood to all the body's cells is usually fatal. This chapter provides an overview of the respiratory system, including the relationship of the lung structures to their function, and sets the groundwork for the subsequent chapters on the respiratory system. Abbreviations for the respiratory system are listed in Table 27-1.

Necessity of Respiration

The lung's primary role is to distribute air and blood flow for gas exchange

Breathing is an automatic, rhythmic, and centrally regulated mechanical process by which contraction of the skeletal muscles of the diaphragm and rib cage move gas in and out of the airways and alveoli. Respiration includes breathing, but it also includes the circulation of blood to and from the tissue capillaries so that O_2 can reach every cell and be used to oxidize metabolites and produce useful energy. CO_2, the spent fuel of cellular respiration, is carried away by venous blood to the lungs for exhalation (see Chapters 22 and 23). THE PRINCIPAL FUNCTION OF THE LUNGS IS TO PROVIDE ADEQUATE DISTRIBUTION OF INSPIRED AIR AND PULMONARY BLOOD FLOW such that the exchange of O_2 and CO_2

between the gas in the alveoli and the pulmonary capillary blood is accomplished with a minimal expenditure of energy.

Ventilation and perfusion to the lung need to be matched

Ventilation ($\dot{V}$) is measured as the frequency of breathing multiplied by the volume of each breath **(tidal volume).** Ventilation maintains the normal concentrations of O_2 and CO_2 in the alveolar gas and maintains the normal O_2 and CO_2 partial pressures in the blood flowing from the capillaries by the process of **diffusive gas exchange. Perfusion** ($\dot{Q}$) refers to pulmonary blood flow, which equals the heart rate multiplied by the right ventricular stroke volume.

VENTILATION AND PERFUSION ARE NORMALLY MATCHED IN THE LUNG SO THAT GAS EXCHANGE (VENTILATION) NEARLY MATCHES THE PULMONARY ARTERIAL BLOOD FLOW (PERFUSION). Ideally, the ventilation/perfusion ratio ($\dot{V}/\dot{Q}$) is identical in all parts of the lungs. The difference between the O_2 and CO_2 partial pressures in the expired gas and the systemic arterial blood is useful in determining the efficiency of overall lung function. The normal ventilation and perfusion matching process in the lungs with respect to the partial pressures of O_2 and CO_2 in gas and blood is depicted in Fig. 27-1.

The following extreme example illustrates the importance of ventilation and perfusion matching. A 2-year-old child is brought to the hospital emergency room because he inhaled a peanut into the main bronchus of the left lung and ventilation of that lung was blocked. The child was born with a very narrow right pulmonary artery; therefore nearly all pulmonary blood flow goes to the left lung. This congenital defect did not seriously bother the child before he aspirated the peanut, but now it threatens his life. All of the fresh air goes to the right lung, but nearly all of the lung's blood flow goes to the left lung. Hence little useful gas exchange occurs.

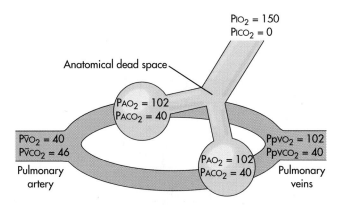

Figure 27-1 Model of the normal ventilation/perfusion process. The normal matching of ventilation to perfusion is simplified by showing only two parallel lung units, which are arranged vertically so that the reader will not automatically think of right and left lungs. Each unit receives equal quantities of fresh air (V̇) and blood flow (Q̇) for its size. The numbers indicate normal human adult resting values in millimeters of mercury (mm Hg) for the gas partial pressures *(P)* in inspired air *(I)*, alveolar gas *(A)*, and mixed venous *(v̄)* blood arriving at the capillaries from the right ventricle via the pulmonary artery. *pv,* Pulmonary venous.

Blood Gas Transport and Tissue Gas Exchange

Oxygenated blood leaves the lungs via the pulmonary veins and is pumped by the left ventricle through the systemic arteries to the capillaries, where it supplies cells in the tissues. Metabolism by these cells produces CO_2, which is transported away from the respiring cells via the systemic veins to the lungs for elimination.

Hemoglobin is essential for O_2 transport

Hemoglobin in red blood cells is able to combine rapidly and reversibly with O_2 to dramatically increase the solubility of O_2 in blood. The normal **oxyhemoglobin equilibrium curve** (see Figure 30-2) shows the relationship between the partial pressure of O_2 in blood and the amount bound to normal hemoglobin (O_2 percent saturation). The normal blood hemoglobin concentration of 150 g/L accounts for the normal arterial blood O_2 concentration of 200 ml/L of O_2 at an arterial O_2 partial pressure of 100 mm Hg. Only about 25% of the O_2 bound to hemoglobin is exchanged between the blood and systemic tissues during each circulation; that is, the arterial-venous O_2 difference is 50 ml/L.

The cardiac output in a resting human adult is about 5 L/min (see Chapter 18). During strenuous exercise, cardiac output is unlikely to increase to more than three times the resting level. Because O_2 consumption by the body during steady-state exercise may increase sixfold from the resting value (from 250 to 1500 ml/min of O_2), the extraction of O_2 from arterial blood must double. (That is, 50% extraction from arterial blood = 100 ml/L, and 100 ml/L (cardiac output of 15 L/min = O_2 delivery to the tissues of 1500 ml/min of O_2). Highly trained athletes can increase their exercise

Table 27-1	Abbreviations for the Respiratory System
Abbreviation	**Meaning**
Ca_{O_2}	Arterial O_2 content
$C\bar{v}_{O_2}$	Mixed venous O_2 content
f	Frequency
Fe^{++}	Ferrous iron (reduced state)
Fe^{+++}	Ferric iron
FEV_1	Forced expiratory volume in 1 second
Fi_{O_2}	Fraction of inspired O_2
FRC	Functional residual capacity
Hb	Hemoglobin
HbO_2	Oxyhemoglobin
HCO_3^-	Bicarbonate
H_2CO_3	Carbonic acid
MbO_2	Oxymyoglobin
N_2	Nitrogen
$NaHCO_3$	Sodium bicarbonate
NH_3	Ammonia
NHCOO	Carbamino group
NO	Nitric oxide
P_B	Barometric pressure
Pa_{CO_2}	Arterial blood CO_2 tension
Pa_{O_2}	Arterial blood O_2 tension
PA_{O_2}	Alveolar O_2 tension
P_{CO_2}	Partial pressure of CO_2 (in gas or liquid [does not specify arterial or venous])
$\bar{P}la$	Mean left atrial pressure
P_{O_2}	Partial pressure of O_2 (in gas or liquid [does not specify arterial or venous])
$\bar{P}pa$	Mean pulmonary artery pressure
Ppl	Pleural pressure
Ppv_{O_2}	Pulmonary vein blood O_2 tension
Pt_{O_2}	Tissue O_2 tension
Pv_{O_2}	Pulmonary artery blood O_2 tension (mixed venous blood O_2 tension)
PVR	Pulmonary vascular resistance
Q̇	Perfusion
RDS	Respiratory distress syndrome
RQ	Respiratory quotient
RV	Residual volume
S_{O_2}	Relative amount of O_2 to hemoglobin (saturation)
TLC	Total lung capacity
V̇	Ventilation
VC	Vital capacity
V_{DS}	Physiological dead space
$\dot{V}_{O_2}$	O_2 consumption
V̇/Q̇	Ventilation/perfusion ratio
V_T	Tidal volume

cardiac output or O_2 consumption to more than twice the values of an untrained person (see also Chapter 26).

Gas exchange depends on diffusion

Diffusion is the passive thermodynamic flow of molecules between regions with different partial pressures (see Chapters 1 and 22). The diffusion of gas (primarily O_2 and CO_2) must occur between alveolar gas and blood in the pulmonary capillaries and between blood in the systemic capillaries and the mitochondria of the cells in the tissue.

CO_2 is transported from tissue to the lungs mainly in solution and as sodium bicarbonate. Fortunately, CO_2 dissolves in water much better than O_2. Even more important, CO_2 reacts with water to form carbonic acid, which dissociates to release the bicarbonate ion (HCO_3^-), the principal constituent of blood CO_2 transport.

Control of Breathing

Inspiration is active breathing, and expiration is passive breathing

Inspiration is the active phase of breathing. It is initiated by neural impulses from the respiratory control centers in the brainstem (medulla and pons) (Figure 27-2). These neural impulses stimulate the diaphragm and intercostal muscles to contract. The muscle contraction causes the thoracic cavity to expand, which lowers the pressure in the pleural space surrounding the lungs. As the pressure falls, the distensible lungs expand passively, which causes the pressure in the alveoli (terminal air spaces) to decrease. As the alveolar pressure decreases, air flows along the airways into the alveoli until alveolar pressure equals the pressure (usually atmospheric pressure) at the airway opening. During **expiration,** which occurs passively via elastic recoil of the lungs, the process is reversed. Pleural and alveolar pressures rise, and gas flows out of the lung. Normal breathing at rest is completely automatic and uses little energy.

Breathing is automatically regulated by a variety of strategically placed sensors (Figure 27-2). **Mechanoreceptors** located within the chest wall and lungs monitor muscular effort and the rate of lung volume change. **Chemoreceptors** (for CO_2 and O_2) located at the bifurcation of the carotid artery in the neck and in the aortic arch sense arterial blood oxygenation, and chemoreceptors near the ventrolateral surface of the brainstem (medulla) sense CO_2 tension within the brain tissue. Breathing is also susceptible to conscious (volitional) control from higher brain centers (cerebral cortex).

Structure-Function Relationships

In adults, the lung weight represents about 1.5% of body weight (1 kg in a 70-kg adult); lung tissue accounts for 60%, and blood accounts for the remain-

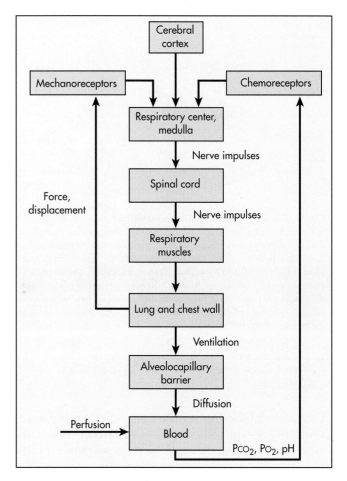

Figure 27-2 Diagram showing overall regulation of breathing. The respiratory center neurons, dispersed into several groups in the medulla, show spontaneous cyclic activity but are strongly influenced by stimuli descending from the cerebral cortex (volitional control) and from two sensory loops, mechanoreceptors and chemoreceptors (automatic control). P_{CO_2}, Partial pressure of carbon dioxide; P_{O_2}, partial pressure of oxygen.

der. Figure 27-3 is a light microscopic photograph of a thin slice of an expanded normal lung. The lung volume is occupied mainly by the alveolar spaces, and only a small fraction of the volume is accounted for by the alveolar tissue between the alveoli (**interstitium**). Figure 27-4 is an electron micrograph of several alveoli. The average distance between alveolar gas and red blood cells in the capillaries is 1.5 μm. This short diffusion pathway permits rapid and efficient gas exchange across the normal alveolar-capillary interface.

In the human lung the vast number of alveoli constitute a total internal surface area of some 70 m^2 when the lung is at **functional residual capacity** (i.e., volume of gas in the lung at the end of a normal expiration). This area is necessary for distributing the pulmonary blood flow (right ventricular output) into a thin stream, one red blood cell thick, so that the time spent by each erythrocyte flowing along the capillaries is sufficient to permit the equilibration of O_2 and CO_2 between blood and alveolar gas.

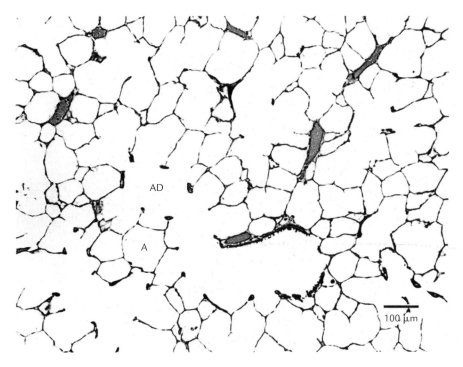

Figure 27-3 Low-magnification section of a normal, well-inflated lung. The larger central openings are the alveolar ducts *(AD)*, the final branches of the airways. Surrounding each duct are the anatomical alveoli *(A)*. *(Courtesy KH Albertine, University of Utah.)*

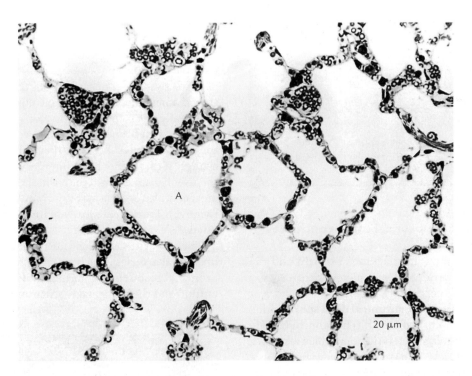

Figure 27-4 Low-magnification electron microscopic view of a very thin section of lung tissue. The lung was at low volume when it was fixed, which permits numerous alveolar walls to be seen. The bulk of the alveolar walls is capillaries, the other tissue being reduced to optimize O_2 diffusion from the alveoli *(A)*, to the erythrocytes *(black objects)* in the capillaries. *(Courtesy KH Albertine, University of Utah.)*

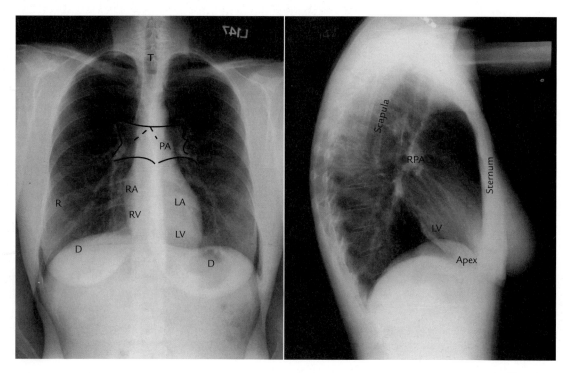

Figure 27-5 Normal posteroanterior *(left)* and lateral *(right)* chest roentgenograms taken at the end of a deep inspiration. The chest wall (ribs *[R]* and diaphragm *[D]*) can be seen. The lungs fill all of the thoracic cavity, except for the heart and mediastinum (which contains the trachea *[T]* dividing into the right and left mainstem bronchi *[inverted V-shaped dashed line]*). Some of the larger distributing pulmonary vessels in the lung can be seen because they contain blood, in contrast to the air-filled lung. Normally, no detail of the alveolar structures can be seen. Outlined are the main pulmonary artery *(PA)* and the left atrium *(LA)*, into which the pulmonary veins empty. *RPA,* Right pulmonary artery; *LV,* left ventricle.

> What is seen in a normal chest x-ray film is mainly the larger airways (bronchi) and blood in the arteries and veins (Figure 27-5). Because lung roentgenograms are usually obtained after a maximal inspiration, the alveolar walls and capillaries are too thin to affect the penetration of the x rays. That makes it easier for the radiologist to see changes in the air or in the spaces between alveoli.

The airways include bronchi and bronchioles

The conducting airways (cartilaginous **bronchi** and the larger membranous **bronchioles**) do not participate in gas exchange. Thus their portion of each breath is wasted ventilation and constitute the **anatomical dead space,** which is about 30% of each normal breath. The bronchi (Figure 27-6) are lined with columnar epithelium, which rests on a layer of smooth muscle. The epithelium contains a large number of ciliated cells, whose rhythmic beating in a thin liquid layer on the surface effectively transports secreted mucus and inhaled particles out of the lung via the trachea. The bronchi decrease in diameter and length with each successive branching, and the cartilaginous support gradually disappears until it is absent in tubes smaller than about 1 mm in diameter.

The bronchioles (Figure 27-7) are the continuation of the bronchi. They constitute all of the airways smaller than 1 mm in diameter, contain no cartilage, and are lined with a simple cuboidal epithelium. The bronchioles are embedded directly in the connective tissue framework of the lung; their diameter depends on lung volume.

Distally, the bronchioles develop outpouchings: the alveoli. The first bronchioles with alveoli are called **respiratory bronchioles** because they participate in gas exchange. With further branchings, the number and size of the alveoli increase until the walls of the bronchioles are almost completely replaced by the mouths of the alveoli (Figure 27-6). These final airway branches are called **alveolar ducts.**

The airways receive their nutritive blood supply via the **bronchial arteries,** which are small branches of the aorta. Bronchial blood flow is normally about 1% of the cardiac output, and the bronchial vascular resistance is high.

> **Asthma** is a large-airway disease characterized by inflammation (predominantly lymphocytes and eosinophils) in the large airway's submucosa and reversible constriction of the bronchial tubes **(bronchospasm)** (see Chapter 28). **Respiratory bronchiolitis** is a small-airway disease most often caused by viruses in early life. **Emphysema** is a lung disease in which the alveolar walls or alveoli are destroyed or fragmented, forming large air spaces that are ineffective in oxygenating or removing CO_2 from the blood. Emphysema occurs most often in cigarette smokers.

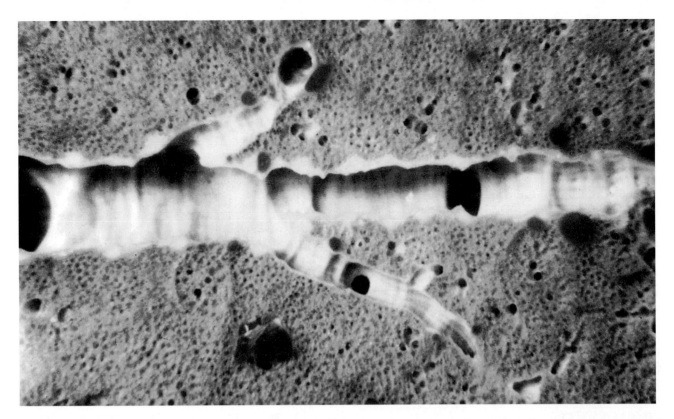

Figure 27-6 Cartilaginous bronchi cut in longitudinal section in a block of frozen lung. There are frequent irregular branchings in all directions, with each daughter bronchus smaller than the parent bronchus. The gas in the bronchi represents wasted ventilation (anatomical dead space). The design of the airway keeps the anatomical dead space as small as possible, commensurate with keeping airflow resistance as low as possible. *(From Staub NC: Basic respiratory physiology, New York, 1991, Churchill Livingstone.)*

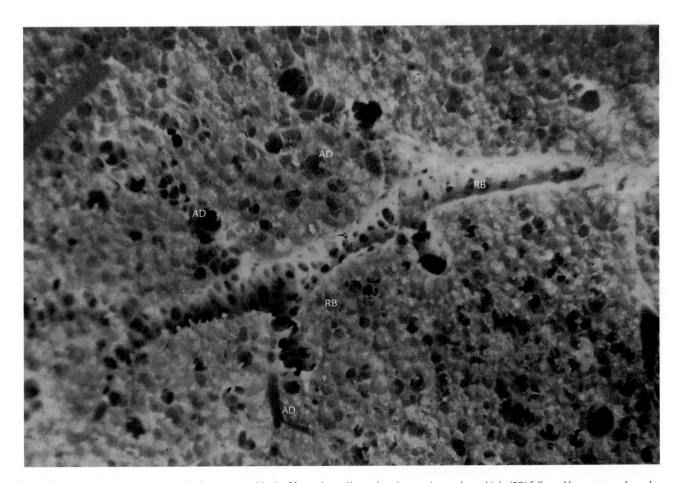

Figure 27-7 Bronchioles cut in longitudinal section in a block of frozen lung. Shown here is a respiratory bronchiole *(RB)* followed by numerous branches. Also shown are the alveolar ducts *(AD)* evolving from numerous small alveoli. The alveolar ducts are seen mainly as right-angle branches above and below the row of respiratory bronchioles. *(From Staub NC: Basic respiratory physiology, New York, 1991, Churchill Livingstone.)*

The airways are controlled by the autonomic nervous system

The airways are innervated by both the motor and sensory nerves of the sympathetic and parasympathetic branches of the autonomic nervous system. These nerves regulate breathing, airway caliber, glandular secretion, and bronchial activity. For example, when airway smooth muscle contracts (usually from activity in the parasympathetic nerves), the bronchial lumen is narrowed.

Sensory fibers are located beneath and within the intercellular junctions of the epithelial cells. There are two main types of large airway receptors: those sensitive to physical distortion (stretch) and those sensitive to chemical substances (irritants). All along the airways are small, nonmyelinated, slowly conducting C fibers. These fibers are abundant, and they can be stimulated by various chemical mediators, which can elicit certain pulmonary-cardiac reflex responses. Control of breathing, including the sensory and motor nerves of the airways, is discussed in more detail in Chapter 31.

Pulmonary Circulation

Lung perfusion usually matches ventilation

The pulmonary artery accompanies and branches with the airways (Figure 27-8). Thus a **ventilation/perfusion matching** relationship is established. In contrast, the pulmonary veins do not follow the airways. The pulmonary veins are situated within the interlobular loose connective tissue septa and receive blood from many lung units. These veins connect with the left atrium. Pulmonary arteries and veins are thin walled and elastic, and they contain nearly 10% (500 ml) of the total body blood volume. Although the pulmonary circulation normally has a low pressure and low resistance, the smaller arteries (<500 μm in diameter) are muscular and can actively regulate their diameters and alter resistance to blood flow.

> In the fetus, the pulmonary vessels are constricted; therefore only a small fraction of right ventricular output flows through the lungs (see Chapters 25 and 30). Pulmonary vascular resistance is high. At the onset of air breathing, the vessels dilate, and vascular resistance falls. In a small number of babies, a congenital opening in the septum between the right and left ventricles persists **(ventricular septal defect),** so some of the left ventricular blood at high pressure flows into the right ventricle. This results in abnormally high pressures and flow in the pulmonary arteries, which respond by constricting; **pulmonary hypertension** eventually develops. If the defect can be corrected early, the long-term effects on the pulmonary vessels can be prevented or reversed.

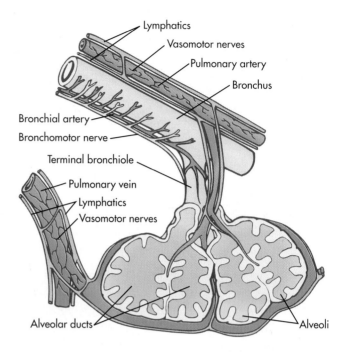

Figure 27-8 Model of normal lung structure-function relationships, showing the correct anatomical relation between the pulmonary artery and the airways. The veins have no relationship to the airways. Two physiological lung units are represented by the two respiratory bronchioles *(RB)*. Note that the small pulmonary arterial (resistance) vessels are surrounded by the alveolar gas of the unit they perfuse (see Chapter 30).

The motor nerve supply to the arterial and venous smooth muscle of the pulmonary vessels is through the sympathetic branch of the autonomic nervous system. In contrast to the systemic circulation, the normal pulmonary circulation shows little evidence of active external regulation (see Chapter 30). The extensive sensory innervation, located in the adventitia (outer connective tissue layer) of the blood vessels, can be stimulated by vascular pressure changes (stretch) and various chemical substances.

Capillary blood volume is equal to right ventricular stroke volume

The pulmonary capillaries form an extensive interdigitating network that is continuous over several alveoli. When the capillaries are well filled with blood, about 75% of the surface area of the alveolar wall overlies red cells (Figure 27-4). In a resting human, the effective volume of blood in the pulmonary capillaries is about 70 ml, although the maximum capillary volume of the human adult lung is about 200 ml. Capillary volume can be increased by opening closed or compressed capillary segments. This regularly occurs during exercise as cardiac output increases. The capillaries can also be distended as the internal pressure rises (see Chapter 30). Capillary blood volume at any instant is about equal to the stroke volume of the right ventricle. This means that the average erythrocyte remains in the capillaries a sufficient time (0.8 second) for the diffusive exchange of O_2 and CO_2 to reach equilibrium across the thin alveolar-capillary barrier.

Physiological Lung Unit

The **physiological (functional) lung unit** is the largest lung unit (usually the respiratory bronchiole) in which the partial pressures of O_2 and CO_2 are each uniform. The physiological unit is much larger than any anatomical alveolus. The human adult lung has 60,000 of these units. Each contains 5000 anatomical alveoli and 250 alveolar ducts. Figure 27-8 shows the relationships among the various structural elements of the lung.

SUMMARY

- The main function of the lung is to bring fresh air into close contact with blood flowing in the pulmonary capillaries so that the exchange of O_2 and CO_2 by passive diffusion can take place efficiently.
- Ventilation is the volume of each breath multiplied by the frequency of breathing. Perfusion (pulmonary blood flow) is the heart rate multiplied by the right ventricular stroke volume.
- Ventilation and perfusion are normally well matched so that O_2 transport from the outside air to the systemic arterial blood is nearly optimal.
- Hemoglobin within red blood cells vastly increases the ability of blood to transport O_2.
- CO_2 is transported from the tissue capillaries back to the lung, mainly as bicarbonate ion in plasma.
- The passive diffusion of O_2 is normally not a rate-limiting step either at the alveolar-capillary barrier or at the systemic capillary–tissue barrier, but it can become limiting in very stressful conditions or severe lung disease.
- Inspiration is the active phase of breathing; the muscles of the chest wall, mainly the diaphragm, contract and lower the pressure in the lung's alveoli so that air can flow into the lungs.
- Breathing is controlled from the respiratory center in the medulla (brainstem) via sensory information from mechanoreceptors that monitor chest wall motion and lung volume and via chemoreceptors that detect the CO_2 and O_2 partial pressures in brain interstitial fluid and systemic arterial blood, respectively.
- Two types of airways are the bronchi (cartilaginous) and the bronchioles. The alveolar ducts (final branches of the bronchioles), together with the alveoli, form the gas-exchange part of the lung.
- One pulmonary artery branch accompanies each airway and branches with it. To maximize the rate of O_2

and CO_2 diffusional exchange with the pulmonary blood flow, the lung has the most extensive capillary network of any organ; this network occupies about 75% of the alveolar surface area.
- Erythrocytes remain in the capillaries long enough for gas exchange to reach equilibrium, even during strenuous exercise.
- Groups of alveolar ducts and their alveoli, together with their supplying arteries, are combined into small functional lung units. These physiological lung units are arranged in parallel, thus ensuring the efficient distribution of inspired air and mixed venous blood.

BIBLIOGRAPHY

Konig MF, Lucocq JM, Weibel ER: Demonstration of pulmonary vascular perfusion by electron and light microscopy, *J Appl Physiol* 75:1877, 1993.

Staub NC, Albertine KH: The structure of the lung relative to its principal function. In Murray JF, Nadel JA, eds: *Textbook of respiratory medicine*, ed 2, Philadelphia, 1994, WB Saunders.

Taylor CR et al: Matching structures and functions in the respiratory system. In Wood SC, ed: *Comparative pulmonary physiology: current contents*, New York, 1989, Marcel Dekker.

Tyler WS, Julian MD: Gross and subgross anatomy of lungs, pleura, connective tissue septa, distal airways and structural units. In Parent RA, ed: *Comparative biology of the normal lung*, Boca Raton, Fla, 1991, CRC.

▷ CASE STUDIES

Case 27-1

A 75-year-old man is seen for evaluation of shortness of breath for the past 10 years. He has smoked two packs of cigarettes a day for 50 years. On examination, he has a barrel chest and is using his accessory respiratory muscles. On auscultation, he has markedly decreased breath sounds bilaterally. Chest radiography demonstrates enlarged lungs (hyperinflation) with flattening of the diaphragm. Pulmonary function tests demonstrate decreased expiratory flows (forced expiratory volume in 1 second is 35% of predicted), increased lung volume (total lung capacity is 140% of predicted), and increased residual volume (150% predicted).

1. **An arterial blood gas sample (a specimen of arterial blood that provides a direct measurement of the partial pressure of O_2 [Pa_{O_2}] and CO_2 [Pa_{CO_2}] is obtained. The patient probably has emphysema. What effect would this patient's emphysema have on the arterial blood gas?**

   A. The Pa_{O_2} would be reduced.
   B. The Pa_{CO_2} would be increased.
   C. The Pa_{CO_2} would be decreased.
   D. The arterial pH would be reduced.
   E. The effect on the arterial blood gas is unpredictable.

2. Which of the following could *not* be an effect of increased lung volumes (hyperinflation)?
   A. The diaphragm would be flattened on chest radiography because of the enlarged lung volumes.
   B. The maximum inspiratory pressure would be increased.
   C. The diaphragmatic muscle fiber's length-force relationship would not be optimal.
   D. The primary inspiratory muscle in this patient is the diaphragm.
   E. The scalene and sternocleidomastoid muscles can function as accessory inspiratory muscles.

Case 27-2

A 50-year-old man with a history of alcohol intoxication is minimally responsive when he comes to the emergency department. He had also aspirated stomach contents into his lungs. Examination demonstrates decreased breath sounds over the right upper lung and no evidence of heart murmurs. The chest x-ray film demonstrates pneumonia involving the right upper lung. Analysis of arterial blood gas (obtained at sea level) reveals the following values:

pH	7.46
Pao_2	50 mm Hg
$Paco_2$	34 mm Hg
Hemoglobin	15 g/dl

1. Which of the following is the *least* likely explanation for his hypoxemia (low Pao_2)?
   A. Ventilation/perfusion mismatch
   B. Right to left intrapulmonary shunt
   C. Diffusion barrier to gas transfer
   D. Hypoventilation
   E. Bronchial obstruction

2. To further evaluate the cause of hypoxemia in this patient, the physician decides to calculate the alveolar to arterial O_2 gradient. Which of the following statements is *false* regarding gas gradients in the lung?
   A. The alveolar to arterial CO_2 gradient in the lung is usually zero.
   B. The alveolar to arterial O_2 gradient in the lung is usually less than 15 mm Hg.
   C. The alveolar to arterial O_2 gradient will help the physician determine whether the hypoxemia is due to the aspiration pneumonia (diffusion abnormal) or the alcohol intoxication (hypoventilation).
   D. The alveolar to arterial carbon monoxide gradient is usually greater than 50 mm Hg.
   E. The physician needs to know the barometric pressure to calculate the alveolar O_2 concentration.

CHAPTER 28

Mechanical Aspects
of Breathing

OBJECTIVES

- Describe the components of ventilation and lung volumes.
- Explain alveolar ventilation and the gas equations.
- Explain the breathing pump.
- Analyze pulmonary pressure-volume relationships.
- Explain the effect of surfactant on lung compliance.
- Analyze airway resistance in normal and abnormal lungs.

This chapter discusses the basic concepts of ventilation, which are crucial to understanding the respiratory system and subsequent chapters. The measurements of airflow, lung volumes, compliance, and resistance are used every day by physicians to understand whether the respiratory system is functioning normally. This chapter covers these concepts in detail and further elaborates on how they are affected in disease states.

Components of Ventilation

The main purpose of ventilation is to maintain an optimal composition of alveolar gas

Ventilation raises the alveolar O_2 tension (P_{AO_2}) above that of mixed venous blood, as shown in Figure 27-1. O_2 molecules then diffuse along their partial pressure gradient into the pulmonary capillary blood and increase the oxyhemoglobin (HbO_2) concentration. Ventilation lowers the alveolar CO_2 tension (P_{ACO_2}) below that in mixed venous blood. CO_2 molecules then diffuse along their partial pressure gradient into the alveolar gas and reduce the CO_2 concentration in pulmonary capillary blood.

When the demand for O_2 is increased, as in exercise, the partial pressure of O_2 (P_{O_2}) of venous blood decreases, and the partial pressure of CO_2 (P_{CO_2}) increases. Ventilation must be increased in a regulated manner to maintain the P_{O_2} and P_{CO_2} at normal levels in arterial blood.

The measurement of lung volumes is essential

A good understanding of lung volumes and mechanics is essential for understanding pulmonary physiology. Figure 28-1 demonstrates the various lung volumes and capacities that are routinely measured in pulmonary function testing. The volume of gas moved during normal quiet breathing is the **tidal volume (V_T),** usually about 0.5 L. The **functional residual capacity (FRC)** is the volume of gas that remains in the lung at the end of a passive expiration; normally, it is 2 to 2.4 L (40% of maximum lung volume) in adults. The **total lung capacity (TLC)** is the maximum lung volume (5 to 6 L in normal adults) that can be achieved voluntarily. If a person inspires to the TLC and then breathes out as much as possible, he or she can decrease lung volume below FRC to the **residual volume (RV),** which is normally 1 to 1.2 L. The volume of air moved between the TLC and RV is the **vital capacity** (VC); normally, it amounts to 4 to 5 L in adults. The VC is the largest possible breath that can be inspired or expired.

Alveolar ventilation is always less than minute ventilation

Minute ventilation is the total volume of air entering or leaving the lungs each minute. It is measured with an electronic flowmeter **(pneumotachograph)** to mathematically integrate the airflow at the mouth, as shown in Figure 28-2.

Alveolar ventilation ($\dot{V}_A$) is the volume of air that enters the alveoli each minute. $\dot{V}_A$ is always less than total ventilation; how much less depends on the anatomical dead space and the V_T. Inspired air in the conducting airways (mouth to terminal bronchioles) that does not participate in gas exchange is called the **anatomical dead space.** It normally measures about 0.15 L (2 ml/kg of body weight) in adults:

$$\dot{V}_A = V_T \times f \qquad \textbf{28-1}$$

$\dot{V}_A$ equals the breathing frequency (f) (e.g., 12 breaths/min at rest) multiplied by the difference between V_T (0.5 L) and the anatomical dead space (0.15 L). In the normal resting adult, $\dot{V}_A$ is $12 \times (0.5 - 0.15) = 4.2$ L/min.

Physiological dead space is the sum of anatomical and alveolar dead spaces

Alveolar dead space is the volume of gas in an alveolus with little or no perfusion. An extreme example, the blockage of a pulmonary artery branch by an embolus, is illustrated in Figure 28-3. The $\dot{V}_A$ to the portion of the lung with the obstructed blood flow is wasted because it

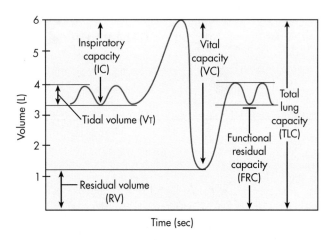

Figure 28-1 Real-time tracing of lung volume changes during two normal tidal breaths (*V*t), after which the subject made a maximal inspiration to total lung capacity (*TLC*) then an expiration to the residual volume (*RV*). (The volume exhaled between the total lung capacity and the residual volume is the vital capacity [*VC*].) The tracing ends with two more tidal breaths. The inspiratory capacity (*IC*) is the volume between the end expiration of a tidal breath and the total lung capacity. The functional residual capacity (*FRC*) is the volume of gas that remains in the lung after passive expiration. The left-hand Y axis shows the average volumes of each of these measurements. Note that normal tidal breathing is near the middle of the total lung capacity.

does not participate in gas exchange. **Physiological dead space** ($VDS_{physiol}$) is normally 30% of the V_T; that is, $VDS_{physiol}/V_T$ is normally 0.15 or less.

A common cause of dyspnea, or shortness of breath, is increased ventilatory demand caused by an increased $VDS_{physiol}$; that is, $VDS_{physiol}/V_T = 0.50$ or greater. For example, a patient with severe **emphysema** has an increased anatomical dead space, which is the air located in the conducting airways and destroyed alveoli and that does not participate in gas exchange. A patient with a pulmonary embolus has increased alveolar dead space because ventilated alveoli are not being perfused. The increased $VDS_{physiol}$ in a patient with emphysema or pulmonary embolus results in marked dyspnea.

The arterial O_2 tension controls alveolar ventilation

It is not the O_2 supply to the alveoli but the partial pressure of CO_2 in arterial blood ($PaCO_2$) that is sensed by the brainstem respiratory center and that regulates $\dot{V}A$ (see Chapter 31). The **alveolar ventilation equation** describes the exact relationship between $\dot{V}A$ and $PaCO_2$ for any given rate of CO_2 production ($\dot{V}CO_2$).

$$\dot{V}A \times PaCO_2 = \dot{V}CO_2 \times K \qquad \textbf{28-2}$$

$\dot{V}A$ is given in liters per minute, $PaCO_2$ in millimeters of mercury, and $\dot{V}CO_2$ in milliliters per minute (see Chapter 41). Usually, the unit conversion constant (*K*) is 0.863 mm Hg × L/ml. When ventilation rises, $PaCO_2$ decreases; when it falls, $PaCO_2$ increases.

The adequacy of $\dot{V}A$ is measured in terms of $PaCO_2$. When ventilation is normal, the $PaCO_2$ equals about 40 mm Hg. **Hyperventilation** (overventilation) means that $\dot{V}A$ is excessive for metabolic needs; the $PaCO_2$ is less than 35 mm Hg. Hyperventilation may occur in response to hypoxia or anxiety. **Hypoventilation** (underventilation) means that $\dot{V}A$ is too low for metabolic needs; $PaCO_2$ is more than 45 mm Hg. The most common cause of hypoventilation is respiratory failure (e.g., that caused by severe lung disease or nervous system depression).

The alveolar-arterial O_2 gradient is usually less than 10 mm Hg

If the $PaCO_2$ is known, the effective PAO_2 can be calculated using the **alveolar gas equation:**

$$PAO_2 = PIO_2 - PaCO_2 [FIO_2 + (1 - FIO_2)/R] \qquad \textbf{28-3}$$

The alveolar gas equation assumes that $PaCO_2$ is equivalent to $PACO_2$. The **partial pressure of inspired O_2 (PIO_2)** is calculated by subtracting the partial pressure of water, 47 mm Hg, from the barometric pressure (**PB**) (the absolute atmospheric pressure at sea level is 760 mm Hg) and multiplying the result by the fraction of air that is O_2 (**FIO_2**). For example, at a PB of 730 mm Hg and with room air ($FIO_2 = 21\%$), the $PIO_2 = (730 - 47) \times 0.21 = 143$ mm Hg.

The respiratory exchange ratio (R) is calculated by dividing the CO_2 by the O_2 consumption; normally, it is 0.8 (see Chapter 30). Therefore in this same example, $PAO_2 = 143 - 40 [0.21 + (1 - 0.21/0.8)] = 143 - 40(1.1975) = 95.1$ mm Hg. The difference between PAO_2 and PaO_2 ($PAO_2 - PaO_2$ gradient) is normally less than 10 mm Hg. A $PAO_2 - PaO_2$ gradient greater than 20 mm Hg indicates that gas exchange is abnormal (see Chapter 30).

When the $PaCO_2$ rises (hypoventilation), the PAO_2 must decrease, and when the $PaCO_2$ falls (hyperventilation), the PAO_2 must increase because the total pressure of all alveolar gases cannot exceed the PB. Ideally, when the $PaCO_2$ is 40 mm Hg, the PAO_2 is 100 mm Hg in subjects at sea level (see Figure 27-1).

The Breathing Pump

The diaphragm is the main muscle of the breathing pump

The diaphragm is responsible for approximately 75% of inspiration during quiet breathing. It is a dome-shaped structure that separates the thoracic and abdominal cavities (Figures 27-5 and 28-4). The diaphragm receives its blood supply from intercostal arteries, and its venous blood flows into the inferior vena cava. It is innervated by the two phrenic nerves, which arise at the third to fifth cervical segments of the spinal cord and then pass caudally in the mediastinum to the right and left halves of the diaphragm (Figure 28-4, *A*).

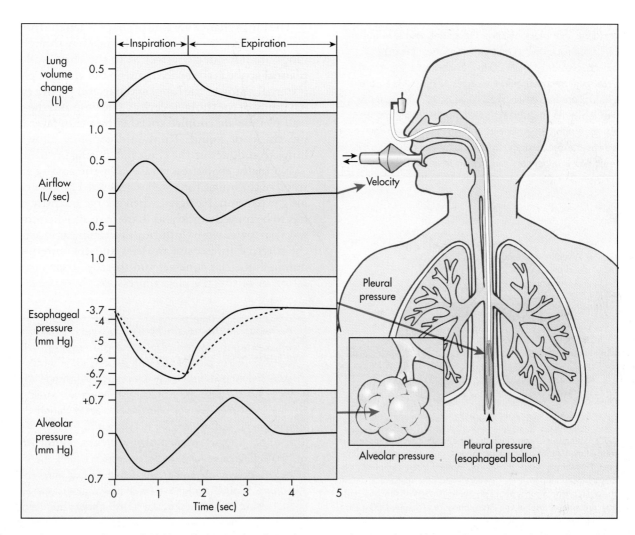

Figure 28-2 Dynamics of a normal tidal breath, showing the relationships among changes in lung volume, airflow, esophageal (pleural) pressure, and alveolar pressure. In modern pulmonary physiology, flow is measured at the mouth using a device called a pneumotachograph. The flow signal is integrated (added up over time) to generate the lung volume change. Pleural pressure is approximated by pressure in the intrathoracic portion of the esophagus, measured with a long flaccid balloon. The duration of the breath is 5 seconds (frequency = 12 breaths/min). Inspiration lasts 2 seconds. The curve for pleural pressure includes the pressure required to change volume *(dashed line)* plus the pressure needed to generate airflow; total pressure is the solid line.

When the diaphragm contracts, it displaces the abdominal contents caudally (downward in upright subjects) or ventrally (outward). At its attachments to the lower ribs, the contracting diaphragm rotates the ribs toward the horizontal plane (Figure 28-4, *B*). In erect subjects, the rib motion toward the horizontal plane (inspiration) increases the cross-sectional area of the thoracic cavity ("pail-handle effect"). Rib motion away from the horizontal plane (expiration) has the opposite effect.

Obstructive airways disease (e.g., emphysema, asthma) involves obstruction of airflow out of the lungs. Processes that impede airflow out of the lungs trap the air in the lungs and overinflate them. The thoracic cage may become more barrel shaped, and the diaphragm may flatten. This causes the diaphragm to maintain a flattened configuration even during expiration; hence diaphragmatic movement is impaired (Figure 28-4). The length-force relationship of the muscle fibers in the diaphragm is not optimal (see Chapter 12). This impairment of the diaphragmatic pail-handle effect may be a primary cause of shortness of breath in patients with obstructive lung disease.

The inspiratory muscles of the rib cage are the **external intercostals;** the expiratory muscles are the **internal intercostals.** The rib cage muscles are supplied by intercostal arteries and veins and are innervated by intercostal motor and sensory nerves. Some of the muscles of the neck **(sternocleidomastoids** and the **scalenes)** are called **accessory muscles** of breathing because when they contract, they pull up on the upper ribs and assist inspiration. These accessory muscles are activated in exercise or when inspiratory airflow is limited, as in respiratory failure.

In accidents that block or sever the spinal cord low in the neck, diaphragmatic breathing continues because the phrenic nerves arise (from C3 to C5) above the injury site. The rib cage and abdominal muscles of course are paralyzed, as are all other skeletal muscles whose motor nerves leave the spinal cord caudal to the injury site. Because expiration is passive and the primary inspiratory muscle is the diaphragm, quadriplegic patients with the phrenic nerve intact can breathe on their own.

The lungs change volume or shape when the thoracic cavity changes its volume or shape, even though the lungs are not directly attached to the chest wall. The **pleural space** is the space between the **visceral pleura** (external lining of the lung) and **parietal pleura** (internal lining of the thoracic cavity). The lung and the chest wall pleurae are coupled together by a thin layer ($\approx$20 μm thick) of liquid. The liquid coupling allows the lungs to slide across the chest wall during breathing.

Normally, expiration is caused by the passive elastic recoil of the lungs; the recoil is generated by inspiratory lung expansion. However, when a large quantity of air has to be moved quickly, as in exercise, or when the airways narrow excessively during expiration, as in asthma, the internal intercostal muscles and the anterior abdominal muscles contract and thereby accelerate expiration by raising the pleural pressure.

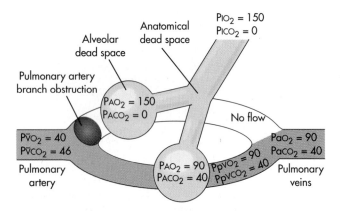

Figure 28-3 Wasted ventilation includes the anatomical dead space plus any portion of the VA that does not exchange O_2 or CO_2 with the pulmonary blood. This simple sketch shows a pulmonary artery completely obstructed by a blood clot. However, in most subjects the anatomical definition of the wasted ventilation is not easily made. $PaCO_2$, Pressure of arterial CO_2; PaO_2, pressure of arterial O_2; $PICO_2$, pressure of inspired CO_2; PIO_2, pressure of inspired O_2; $P\bar{v}O_2$, mixed venous O_2 content; $PpvCO_2$, pressure of pulmonary venous CO_2; $PpvO_2$, pressure of pulmonary venous O_2; $P\bar{v}CO_2$, mixed venous CO_2 content.

An important characteristic of the rib cage is its stiffness, which prevents any inward (paradoxical) movement of the thoracic wall as pleural pressure becomes more subatmospheric during inspiration. In newborns, the rib cage is not very stiff because the ribs consist mainly of cartilage. Therefore when pleural pressure decreases during diaphragmatic contraction, the rib portion of the chest wall retracts. In the **respiratory distress syndrome (RDS)** (immature lungs in the premature infant), this can be a serious problem because the lungs are stiffer than normal. In adults, trauma to the chest wall that causes several ribs to break can produce a **flail chest.** This can induce respiratory failure as a result of the lung affected by the flail chest.

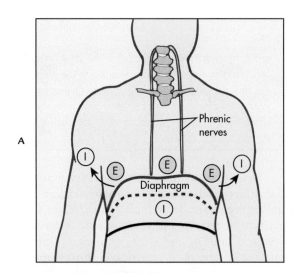

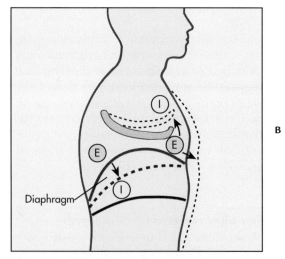

Figure 28-4 A, Front view in an upright human, showing the descent of the diaphragm and the flaring of the lower ribs caused by the contraction of the diaphragm at its rib attachments during inspiration (*I*) (*dashed line*). The phrenic motor nerves to the diaphragm are also shown from their origin in the neck. *E,* Expiration (*blue line*). **B,** Lateral view, showing the outward bulge of the abdominal wall as the contracting diaphragm shortens and moves caudally. The limited rotatory motion (pail-handle action) permitted for the rib cage is also shown. In severe emphysema, the diaphragm excursion is limited even in expiration, resulting in a flattened diaphragm (*purple line*). (**B** *redrawn from Staub NC:* Basic respiratory physiology, *New York, 1991, Churchill Livingstone.*)

The Breathing Cycle

Airflow requires a pressure difference

Airflow can be achieved by generating a difference between ambient pressure (atmosphere) and alveolar pressure (PA). Thus during inspiration, PA is subatmospheric, whereas it is higher than PB during expiration. The changes in PA during airflow are generated by changes in the pleural pressure. Thus translung pressure (PL) during inspiration is slightly greater and during expiration, is slightly less than is necessary to sustain the lung volume changes, as shown in the pleural pressure curve in Figure 28-2.

Compliance is a measure of the pressure-volume relationship

COMPLIANCE OF THE LUNG OR CHEST WALL, SINGLY OR TOGETHER, REFERS TO THE EASE WITH WHICH EITHER OR BOTH CAN BE DISTENDED. The standard procedure for measuring compliance in humans is to determine the pressure-volume relationship during a passive expiration (no-breathing muscle activity) from TLC. If the respiratory system deflates slowly, the PA is essentially equal to the PB, and pleural pressure is nearly the same as the pressure in the esophagus, which can be measured with a swallowed thin-walled balloon attached via a plastic tube to a pressure-sensing device (Figure 28-2).

Compliance is the slope ($\Delta V/\Delta P$) of the straight line joining any two points on the deflation of the pressure-volume curve (see also Chapter 21). For the respiratory system, there are three different compliance curves: lung, chest wall, and combined (Figure 28-5). **Lung compliance** is the change in lung volume divided by the change in PL: $\Delta V/\Delta PL$. **Chest wall compliance** is the change in lung volume divided by the change in trans–chest wall pressure: $\Delta V/\Delta PCW$. *Respiratory system compliance* is the change in lung volume divided by the change in trans–respiratory system pressure: $\Delta V/\Delta PRS$.

Lung and chest wall compliances may be affected by disease

In **emphysema,** the alveoli in the lungs are destroyed or fragmented. The alveoli form large air spaces that are ineffective in oxygenating or removing CO_2 from the blood. The breakdown of alveolar tissues also results in loss of lung elasticity (decreased recoil, increased compliance). During exhalation, the lungs do not recoil inward in a normal fashion. Small changes in transpulmonary pressure evoke large changes in lung volume (blue line in Figure 28-6). This leads to air trapping and hyperinflation of the lungs. Hyperinflation in turn leads to configurational changes in the chest wall and flattening of the diaphragm. Hence patients with emphysema have abnormal lung tissue and disadvantageous conformational changes in the diaphragm. Their work of breathing may be much greater than that in a healthy individual. In **asthma** (yellow line in Figure 28-6), because the alveolar tissue is preserved, lung compliance is much closer to normal. In **restrictive lung disease (pulmonary fibrosis),** the lungs have increased stiffness (low compliance), and therefore large changes in transpulmonary pressure evoke only small changes in lung volume (purple line in Figure 28-6).

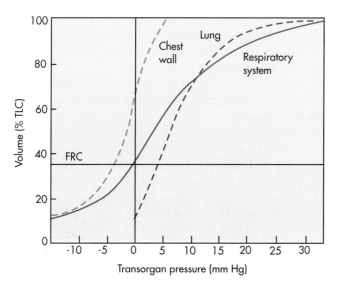

Figure 28-5 Distensibilities (compliances) of the lungs and chest wall and their sum, the respiratory system. These are passive, static pressure-volume curves. From below the FRC up to about 75% of the TLC, lung compliance is high, fairly linear, and parallel to that of the chest wall. The lungs become stiffer near the TLC as the noncompliant collagen fibers of the lung become taut. Over the normal range of breathing, the respiratory system curve has a lower slope (lower compliance) than either the lungs or the chest wall. At FRC, the lung and chest wall recoil pressures are equal and opposite.

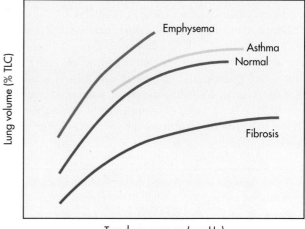

Figure 28-6 Compliance (distensibility) curves representing lungs with various chronic diseases See text.

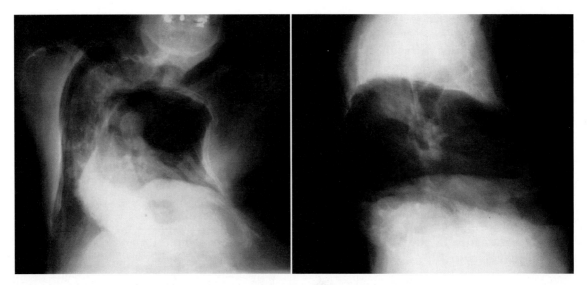

Figure 28-7 Chest wall compliance is affected by diseases such as kyphoscoliosis. This chest x-ray film demonstrates the severe chest wall deformity caused by kyphoscoliosis as a result of restriction of all vital organs in the chest, including the lungs. This deformity causes decreased chest wall compliance, reduced effective expansion of the rib cage, and decreased diaphragmatic movement, resulting in markedly decreased lung volumes (restrictive lung disease). *Left,* Posteroanterior. *Right,* Lateral.

Changes in chest wall compliance are less common than changes in lung compliance. In **kyphoscoliosis** (a distorted spinal column), the rib cage cannot move normally. (Compare the x-ray film in Figure 28-7 with the one in Figure 27-7.) Hence in **restrictive lung disease,** lung volume is reduced, as is the chest wall compliance. When the abdominal pressure is elevated, the chest wall compliance is also decreased because the abdomen interferes with the descent of the diaphragm.

The chest wall's outward recoil tendency balances the lung's inward recoil

At normal end-expiration (FRC), the PRS must be zero because the system is at rest. This stable normal condition is caused by a balance between the inward recoil (collapsing tendency) of the lung and the outward recoil (expanding tendency) of the chest wall. The PL at FRC is +3.7 mm Hg. This inward recoil of the lung exactly balances the outward recoil of the chest wall (the PCW at FRC is −3.7 mm Hg). These recoil forces indicate that the lungs are above their unstressed volume (the volume at which PL is zero) and that the chest wall is below its resting volume (the volume at which PCW is zero). This important relationship is shown in Figure 28-5 (compare the pressures along the line labeled FRC).

When the chest wall is opened during thoracic surgery, air enters the pleural space because the pleural pressure is less than the PB. The lungs tend to collapse, whereas the thoracic cavity gets larger. The condition is called a **pneumothorax** (air in the thoracic cavity outside the lung) (compare Figure 28-8 to the normal chest x-ray film

in Figure 27-7). A traumatic or spontaneous pneumothorax may be life threatening because ventilation is inadequate and the increased intrathoracic pressure (tension pneumothorax) compromises venous return to the heart.

When lung volume exceeds the FRC by about 25% of the TLC (normally FRC = 1 to 1.5 L), the PCW is zero (Figure 28-5); hence pleural pressure must be equal to PB on the body surface. The total pressure across the respiratory system equals the translung pressure: PRS = PL. The compliance lines of the lung and respiratory system cross (Figure 28-5).

Surfactant diminishes surface tension in the lungs

The alveoli are lined by a thin film of liquid. At the interface between the liquid and the alveolar gas, strong intermolecular forces in the liquid tend to cause the lining area to shrink; that is, the alveoli tend to get smaller. These forces contribute more to the elastic recoil of the lung than the lung tissue components (elastic and collagen fibers). The effects of surface forces on lung compliance become evident when the pressure-volume curves of air- and saline-filled lungs are compared.

Ventilating the lung with saline eliminates the air-liquid interface and abolishes the surface forces without affecting lung tissue. At any given volume, the transpulmonary pressure of the liquid-inflated lung is less than that of the air-inflated lung. In the air-inflated lung, compliance is less during inflation than during deflation, as indicated by the higher pressure required at any given volume (Figure 28-9).

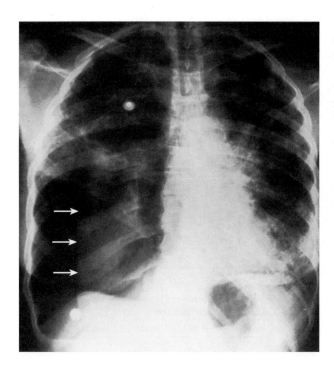

Figure 28-8 Chest x-ray film demonstrating a large pneumothorax affecting the right lung *(arrows)*. Pneumothoraces are often caused by trauma penetrating the chest wall or pleural surface or spontaneously caused by cysts or blebs in the lung rupturing on the pleural surface. Because the pleural pressure is subatmospheric, it causes air entry and collapse of the underlying lung.

THE MOST IMPORTANT COMPONENT OF THE LIQUID FILM THAT LINES THE ALVEOLAR WALLS IS **SURFACTANT.** Surfactant is produced by type 2 pneumocytes, and its major constituent is **dipalmitoyl phosphatidylcholine,** a phospholipid with detergent properties. Surfactant is special because it allows alveolar surface tension to vary with lung volume. Alveolar surface tension rises as the lung is inflated toward TLC. That is why the inflation limb of the pressure-volume curve in Figure 28-10 is displaced to the right (higher pressure at any volume). As deflation begins, alveolar surface tension decreases rapidly, which is why the deflation limb of the pressure-volume curve of the air-filled lung moves to the left; less PL is needed during deflation to maintain a given volume than during inflation. By reducing surface tension during deflation, surfactant promotes stability among the alveoli, which anatomically are of different sizes. Thus the smaller alveoli do not collapse **(atelectasis)** at end-expiration (FRC).

Alveolar surface tension contributes to translung pressure

The Laplace equation (see Chapter 22) relates transmural pressure to the wall tension and radius of a cylindrical blood vessel: $P_{tm} = T/r$. The Laplace equation also applies to the alveoli because in the air-filled lung, wall tension is almost entirely surface tension, as illustrated in Figure 28-10. The component of PL caused by surface tension (st) is $P_{L_{st}} = 2T/r$.

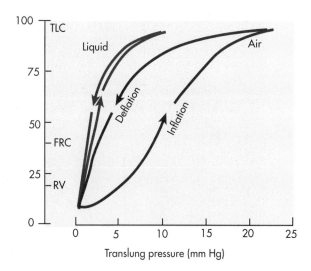

Figure 28-9 Pressure-volume loops of a normal human lung for the liquid- and air-filled states. Conventionally, each loop begins and ends at a PL equal to zero (minimum lung volume). The blue lines show the liquid-filled lung. The curve is steep, and the inflation and deflation lines are nearly the same. TLC is achieved at a PL of 11 mm Hg. The air-filled pressure-volume curve is indicated by the red lines. The inflation limb is displaced far to the right of the curve of the liquid-filled lung, whereas the deflation limb is closer to it. This means that the pressure-volume curve of the lung depends on something that is different between inflation and deflation: alveolar surface tension.

At end-inspiration, the surface tension in all the expanding, interconnected alveoli is about the same. As deflation begins, PL decreases rapidly because surface tension falls. The low surface tension is important for maintaining alveolar stability as lung volume decreases toward FRC.

In RDS, a leading cause of morbidity and mortality in babies with immature lungs, the key defect is failure of type 2 alveolar epithelial cells to secrete adequate quantities of surfactant. The lungs are more difficult to inflate, but the main problem is that during deflation, the alveoli collapse because surface tension does not fall. The deflation limb of the pressure-volume curve is similar to the inflation limb. Thus each lung inflation is like the first breath of air after birth, when the liquid-filled lungs must be inflated with air. The increased work required to inflate the lungs contributes to respiratory fatigue and failure. Recently, surfactant replacement therapy has made a significant impact in improving ventilation and decreasing the mortality rate in immature babies.

The airways can regulate airway resistance

The submucosal smooth muscle bands that encircle the airways can change the caliber of the bronchi and bronchioles independently of lung volume or PL. This capability allows the individual airways to alter their resistance to airflow. In the normal lung, airway smooth muscle tone is continuously modulated by airway reflexes.

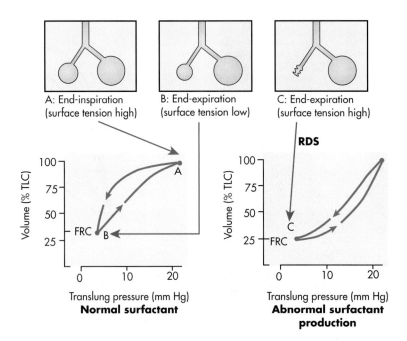

Figure 28-10 Effect of alveolar surface tension. **A,** At the end of a normal inspiration the surface tension in the lung's alveoli is essentially uniform and high. **B,** Surface tension decreases rapidly as the lung volume starts to decrease. The decrease is greater in the more rapidly deflating alveoli. Consequently, all alveoli deflate relatively uniformly in proportion to their volumes. This maintains even the smallest alveoli inflated at FRC and makes the next lung inflation much less work. **C,** If there is a deficiency in surfactant production or secretion by the type 2 alveolar epithelial cells (RDS of immature babies), surface tension remains high throughout the breathing cycle. The inflation curve is shifted to the right. (That is, more work required to inflate the lungs.) The deflation limb follows the inflation limb. The smaller alveoli collapse to minimal volume; even the large ones are smaller. The FRC is lower.

Stimulation of the vagus nerves, which are the motor nerves to the airway smooth muscles, increases airway resistance (RAW). Stimulation of pulmonary sympathetic nerves inhibits airway constriction.

Asthma is characterized by: (1) airflow obstruction that is reversible (although not completely in some patients) either spontaneously or with treatment, (2) chronic inflammatory disorder of the airways, and (3) increased airway responsiveness or sensitivity to a variety of stimuli such as allergens, histamine, exercise, and cold air. These substances cause contraction of the smooth muscle around the airways, swelling of the lining of the airways, and increased mucous secretion. The overall result of these responses is narrowing of the cross-sectional area of the airways and plugging of the airways with mucus. In asthma, the lung compliance is normal (as opposed to emphysema or pulmonary fibrosis), although the FRC may be increased (yellow line in Figure 28-6). The main symptoms that the patient experiences are wheezing, shortness of breath, and cough (which may be productive of thick mucous plugs). If the lung becomes markedly hyperinflated, the diaphragm will become flattened and will work inefficiently. **Bronchodilator drugs** stimulate the sympathetic nerves or inhibit the parasympathetic nerves and dilate the airways.

Airway resistance is determined by the driving pressure and the airflow

Airway resistance equals driving pressure divided by flow: $RAW = \Delta P/\dot{V}$, where ΔP is the difference between the pressure at the open mouth (P_B) and in the alveoli (P_A). During tidal inspiration, the average difference between P_{ao} and P_A is about 0.4 mm Hg, and the average airflow rate is 0.25 L/sec. Thus $RAW = 0.4/0.25 = 1.6$ mm Hg/L/sec. Therefore the average P_A is higher than the P_B by about 0.4 mm Hg, and the average airflow velocity is 0.2 L/sec (expiration is slower than inspiration). Thus $RAW = 0.4/0.2 = 2.0$ mm Hg/L/sec, which is slightly greater than that during inspiration.

From the trachea to the alveolar ducts, the total cross-sectional area of the airways progressively increases. Thus the velocity of airflow diminishes rapidly. In the trachea and main bronchi, airflow is turbulent (noisy), and it accounts for 80% of the total resistance to airflow (see also Chapter 20). Turbulence is why one can hear breath sounds with a stethoscope. At the low-airflow velocities in the small airways, flow is laminar and silent.

Breathing is time dependent
Breathing is a dynamic event that depends on time. Some of the dynamic events associated with normal breathing are depicted in Figure 28-2. Inspiration lasts about 2.0 seconds and expiration about 3.0 seconds

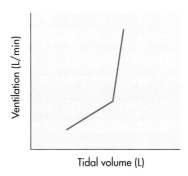

Figure 28-11 Relationship between ventilation and tidal volume. Ventilation is increased voluntarily or in response to a stimulus in an awake person in two phases. See text.

(breathing frequency = 12 breaths/min). One can increase minute ventilation either by increasing the V_T of each breath or by increasing the breathing frequency (see Chapter 31). Based on the earlier equation for ventilation, one can take time dependency into account:

$$V = V_T \times f = [V_T/T_I] \times [T_I/T_{tot}] \qquad \textbf{28-4}$$

Minute ventilation depends on the average inspiratory flow rate (V_T/T_I) and the timing of inspiration in the respiratory cycle (T_I/T_{tot}); T_I is the inspiratory time, and T_{tot} is the total duration of the respiratory cycle. The relationship of V_T to ventilation is expressed in Figure 28-11. In the first phase, ventilation increases in a linear fashion with V_T until approximately half of the VC is reached. Then higher levels of ventilation are brought about by increases in respiratory frequency (f) with little or no change in V_T. Breathing at this higher frequency is inefficient (wasted ventilation is higher), and it requires more energy.

Breathing affects airway dimensions

The bronchi are passively affected by P_L because they are not directly attached to the lung and are distensible and collapsible. During inspiration, as pleural pressure becomes more negative, the bronchi and bronchioles dilate slightly as a result of increased transmural pressure. During expiration, the pleural pressure rises, and the bronchi are compressed, which increases the R_{AW}. The bronchioles are not compressed as long as lung volume does not change much.

During forced expiration, the pleural pressure may exceed the pressure within the bronchi and thus tends to compress them. The site of the bronchial compression is usually in the mainstream bronchi because these airways are less well supported by their cartilaginous plates. Coughing is the best example of forced expiration; it compresses the posterior membranous portion of the trachea and narrows the tracheal diameter. Airflow at the point of compression is high and turbulent (coughing makes noise); both effects help expel irritants from the upper airways.

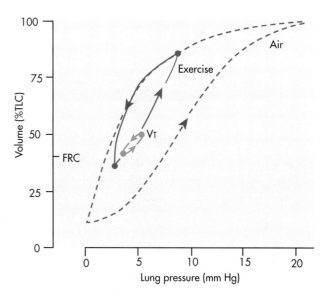

Figure 28-12 Dynamic pressure-volume loops of the lung: resting V_T (*green loop*) and during exercise (*red loop*). The maximum air-filled lung pressure-volume loop (*purple line*) from Figure 28-9 is also shown. The dynamic compliance of the tidal breath (slope of the line connecting end-inspiration with end-expiration) is less than that of the lung during exercise.

Dynamic lung compliance is less than static lung compliance

During normal tidal breathing, the pressure-volume loop is much different from the static pressure-volume loop shown in Figure 28-9 because neither volume nor P_L change much, as shown in Figure 28-12. The small tidal breathing loop is located approximately in the center of the static pressure-volume loop.

The slope of the line that joins the points of no flow (end-expiration and end-inspiration) is used to calculate the **dynamic lung compliance.** In Figure 28-12, the tidal pressure-volume loop is tilted toward the X axis slightly more than either the inflation or deflation limb of the static loop at the same lung volumes. Thus dynamic lung compliance is less than static lung compliance; this difference is attributed to the fact that alveolar surface tension is higher during normal tidal breathing because the lung volume changes are slight (0.5 L).

During exercise (the red loop in Figure 28-12), the slope of the dynamic compliance line becomes steeper. This indicates that the lung is more distensible because the larger V_T stretches the alveolar walls and recruits more surfactant, which lowers surface tension.

Maximal expiratory airflow is displayed by the flow-volume curve

One of the most useful pulmonary function tests it the **flow-volume curve,** which is derived by simultaneously measuring the flow at the mouth (obtained with a pneu-

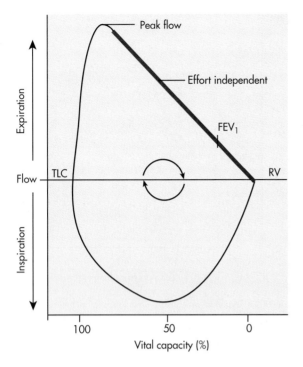

Figure 28-13 Flow-volume loop, the modern way to assess the dynamics of breathing. The small loop in the center represents normal tidal breathing. The large loop represents a maximal forced (as fast as possible) inspiration from RV to TLC, followed by a maximal forced expiration back to RV (forced vital capacity maneuver). The most important information is contained in the expiratory curve; the red portion of this curve is independent of effort. The effort-independent flow velocity is a function of airway collapsibility (dynamic compression). Also shown are the peak expiratory flow rate, the maximal flow that can be achieved with expiration, and the forced expiratory volume in 1 second (*FEV₁*).

motachograph [see Figure 28-2]) and the lung volume (obtained by integrating the flow signal). Figure 28-13 shows the flow-volume curves for tidal breathing and for a forced vital capacity.

THE MOST IMPORTANT ASPECT OF THE FORCED FLOW-VC LOOP IS THE EXPIRATORY PORTION. This portion shows the **maximal expiratory flow** that can be achieved at any given lung volume, no matter how much effort is expended. Contracting the powerful anterior abdominal muscles and the intercostal muscles (active expiration) generates a high flow velocity when lung volume is at or near TLC. Expiratory flow resistance increases as the velocity increases. The velocity decreases rapidly (approximately linearly) as volume decreases but not because of decreasing effort. Once the linear portion of the expiratory flow-volume curve has been reached, it is effort independent; that is, no matter how hard he or she tries, a person cannot exceed the maximal expiratory flow at the given volume. Additional increases in effort to raise the driving pressure diminishes the increases in expiratory flow. The high pleural pressure during this maneuver causes dynamic compression of the airways, which limits flow progressively as lung volume decreases. Patients with emphysema or asthma generate less

flow during maximal expiration (airflow limitation) because of dynamic airway compression.

> Pulmonary function tests often measure expiratory airflow using **forced vital capacity (FVC)** and **forced expiratory volume in 1 second (FEV₁)** (Figure 28-13). The FVC refers to the maximal amount of air one can move in a breathing maneuver from TLC to RV. The FEV₁ is the maximal amount of air that can be expired in 1 second. Patients with emphysema or asthma have a reduced FEV₁ as they experience more airway collapse during expiration at lower lung volumes. Patients with restrictive lung disease have a symmetrically reduced FEV₁ and FVC (normal FEV₁/FVC ratio) as their lung disease restricts their lung capacity without affecting airflow.

The work of breathing is mainly expended during inspiration

THE WORK (ENERGY COST) OF BREATHING IS ACCOMPLISHED PRIMARILY BY THE INSPIRATORY MUSCLES. The work of breathing is low under normal conditions (about 1% to 2% of the total resting O_2 consumption); therefore the respiratory muscles have a large metabolic reserve. However, in patients with severe emphysema, the diaphragm and other chest wall muscles become fatigued because of the high work requirements.

Most of the work used to expand the chest wall and lungs during inspiration is stored as elastic energy, which is used to restore the system to FRC during expiration. In fact, expiration could not occur passively without the potential energy stored during inspiration. However, the work expended to cause airflow is wasted (unrecoverable frictional heat). During expiration, the potential energy stored in the expanded lung pulls the chest wall back to its FRC position and overcomes the expiratory RAW.

SUMMARY

- The FRC is the volume of gas in the lungs at end-expiration. TLC is the maximum lung volume that can be achieved.
- The alveolar ventilation equation states that $\dot{V}A$ multiplied by PAO_2 is a constant at any given level of aerobic metabolism.
- The main muscle of the chest wall is the diaphragm, but the intercostal muscles aid expansion, especially during exercise.
- Coordinated muscle contraction in the chest wall enlarges the thoracic cavity during inspiration, and the lungs expand passively in all directions to fill the cavity.

- At end-expiration the lungs tend to recoil to a smaller volume, whereas the chest wall tends to recoil in the opposite direction toward a larger volume because the chest wall is normally under compression, except at very high volumes. FRC is the condition that occurs when these opposite recoil tendencies are equal.
- The lungs and chest wall must move together. The total compliance of the respiratory system is less than either component alone.
- Lung compliance (distensibility) during inflation is less than its compliance during deflation because of the variable air-liquid surface tension in the alveoli. The reason for the variable surface tension is a special detergent (surfactant) secreted by type 2 alveolar epithelial cells; surfactant's chief component is dipalmitoyl phosphatidylcholine.
- Lung compliance is determined from the slope of the pressure-volume curve during a passive slow deflation from the TLC.
- Because of the resistance to airflow, the P_A is either slightly above or slightly below the P_B (ambient pressure), except at points of no airflow (i.e., end-inspiration and end-expiration).
- An important physical factor that affects R_{AW} is the transmural pressure across the bronchi, whose walls are distensible and collapsible. In a forced expiratory maneuver, the pleural pressure may rise above the large airway pressure and dynamically compress the airways and thereby limit expiratory flow velocity.
- The work of breathing at rest is small. In various lung or chest wall diseases, work may be increased to such an extent that respiratory failure occurs.

BIBLIOGRAPHY

Altose MD: Pulmonary mechanics. In Fishman AP et al, eds: *Pulmonary diseases and disorders,* ed 3, New York, 1998, McGraw-Hill.

Bates DV, Macklem PT, Christie RV: *Respiratory function in disease,* ed 2, Philadelphia, 1971, WB Saunders.

Crystal RG, West JB: *The lung: scientific foundations,* 1991, Raven.

D'Angelo E, Agostoni E: Statics of the chest wall. In Roussos C, ed: *The thorax,* ed 2, New York, 1995, Marcel Dekker.

Derenne JPH, Macklem PT, Roussos CH: The respiratory muscles. I. Mechanics, control and pathophysiology, *Am Rev Respir Dis* 118:581, 1978.

DeTroyer A, Farkas G: Linkage between parasternals and external intercostals during resting breathing, *J Appl Physiol* 69:509, 1990.

Fishman AP et al: *Handbook of physiology,* Baltimore, 1986, Williams & Wilkins.

Similowski T et al: Contractile properties of the human diaphragm during chronic hyperinflation, *N Engl J Med* 325:917, 1991.

Van Gould IMG, Tatenberg JJ, Robertson B: The pulmonary surfactant system: biochemical aspects and functional significance, *Physiol Rev* 68:374, 1988.

Ward ME, Ward JW, Macklem PT: Analysis of chest wall motion using a two compartment rib cage model, *J Appl Physiol* 72:1338, 1992.

CASE STUDIES

Case 28-1

A 30-year-old anxious woman is admitted to the hospital for evaluation of shortness of breath and chest pain. She is at sea level ($P_B = 760$ mm Hg) and is breathing room air (21% O_2). On examination, her respiratory rate is 30 breaths/min, her V_T is 600 ml, and her anatomical dead space is 200 ml. The results of an arterial blood sample follow:

pH	7.47
Pa_{O_2}	60 mm Hg
Oxygen saturation	90%
Pa_{CO_2}	30 mm Hg

1. What is the $\dot{V}_A$ in this patient?
- **A.** 4 L/min
- **B.** 6 L/min
- **C.** 8 L/min
- **D.** 10 L/min
- **E.** 12 L/min

2. What would the expected $\dot{V}_{CO_2}$ be in this patient? (The unit conversion constant [K] is 0.863 mm Hg × L/ml.)
- **A.** 180 ml/min
- **B.** 310 ml/min
- **C.** 900 ml/min
- **D.** 1520 ml/min
- **E.** 2300 ml/min

3. It is suspected that the patient may have had a blood clot in a branch of the pulmonary artery (pulmonary embolus). Her physician wants to know whether she is hypoxemic. Therefore the $P_{A_{O_2}} - Pa_{O_2}$ gradient is calculated. Which is the correct $P_{A_{O_2}} - Pa_{O_2}$ gradient?
- **A.** 54 mm Hg
- **B.** 22 mm Hg
- **C.** 42 mm Hg
- **D.** 4 mm Hg
- **E.** 15 mm Hg

Case 28-2

A 60-year-old man is admitted to the intensive care unit for shortness of breath caused by exacerbation of emphysema. He previously smoked two packs of cigarettes per day for 40 years. His respiratory rate is 40 breaths/min, and he uses accessory muscles to breathe. His physician decides to place him on mechanical ventilation and temporarily paralyze him with medications. The ventilator is set for 12 breaths/min with a V_T of 1000 ml. The ventilator measures airway pressure at the end of each delivered V_T (at a point of no airflow); at this point, the airway pressures is 25 cm H_2O. The ventilator then allows him to passively exhale, and the airway pressure returns to zero (P_B).

1. **What is the compliance of his respiratory system?**
   A. 5 ml/cm H_2O
   B. 100 ml/cm H_2O
   C. 20 ml/cm H_2O
   D. 40 ml/cm H_2O
   E. 55 ml/cm H_2O

2. **On further examination, the physician notes that the patient has bilateral wheezes when she listens to his chest. His R_{AW} is measured. The peak airway pressure is 35 cm H_2O, and airflow is 1 L/sec. The physician occludes the airway at the point of peak airway pressure (end-inspiration), and it measures 25 cm H_2O. What is the total R_{AW} (including the endotracheal tube)?**
   A. 2 cm H_2O/L/sec
   B. 5 cm H_2O/L/sec
   C. 8 cm H_2O/L/sec
   D. 20 cm H_2O/L/sec
   E. 25 cm H_2O/L/sec

Pulmonary and Bronchial Circulations and the Distribution of Ventilation and Perfusion

■ Describe the normal pulmonary and bronchial circulation of the lung.

■ Describe the regulation of the pulmonary circulation by active and passive mechanisms.

■ Analyze the distribution of ventilation and perfusion in the normal lung and their relationship.

This chapter discusses the pulmonary and bronchial circulation and its relationship to ventilation (see also Chapter 28). The work of pumping all the cardiac output through the lungs is less than 10% of that required for systemic circulation. The difference is attributed to the enormous parallel array of pulmonary resistance arteries that are normally dilated so that pulmonary vascular resistance (PVR) is very low. Under appropriate conditions the pulmonary vascular bed exerts considerable vasomotor control so that blood flow to the myriad lung units supplied by the small resistance arteries matches the ventilation of those units (ventilation/perfusion matching) and thereby maintains the arterial O_2 tension (PaO_2) and arterial CO_2 tension ($PaCO_2$) near their ideal levels. Flow in the normal pulmonary circulation is regulated by potent local mechanisms, of which alveolar O_2 tension (PAO_2) is the most important.

Pulmonary Circulation

The pulmonary circulation is ideal for gas exchange

The pulmonary circulation is a large network of capillaries in the alveolar walls (70 m^2 or 40 times the body surface area). In resting adults, it contains about 75 ml of blood spread out in this vast array, generally one red cell thick. During exercise, the capillary blood volume increases and approaches the maximum anatomical capillary volume,

which is about 200 ml. The average thickness of the alveolocapillary wall is less than 1 μm, which helps optimize O_2 diffusion between the alveolar gas and the hemoglobin in the red blood cells, as shown in Figure 27-4. One of the principal design features of the lung is to allow erythrocytes to remain in the capillaries long enough to ensure equilibration between alveolar gas and blood; that is, the diffusive exchange of O_2 and CO_2 is not rate limiting, except under extreme conditions.

> Because airplanes routinely fly at altitudes above 30,000 feet (barometric pressure [PB] ≤ 230 mm Hg), the airlines must pressurize the cabins to about 7000 feet (PB = 600 mm Hg) so that the passengers and flight crew do not lose consciousness because of inadequate O_2 **(hypoxemia).** In spite of the pressurized cabin, people with severe chronic lung disease may require additional O_2 during flights.

The blood volume of the lung (main pulmonary artery to left atrium) in a normal adult is about 500 ml, which is about 10% of the total circulating blood volume. The relatively large volume serves as a reservoir (buffer) for filling of the left atrium. During normal breathing, as pleural pressure falls during inspiration (see Chapter 28), venous return into the right ventricle rises, whereas the stroke volume of the left ventricle is reduced. During expiration, the opposite occurs.

> **Mechanical ventilation** refers to the use of a machine that inflates the lungs by delivering positive pressure at the nose and mouth or through a tube in the trachea. During mechanical ventilation, pressure is often applied at the end of expiration (positive end-expiratory pressure) to keep the alveoli open and improve oxygenation. However, this can also result in increased intrathoracic pressure, which may cause low blood pressure (hypotension) by impeding venous return to the right side of the heart.

The lung has its own metabolic needs. Although the alveolar wall tissue can get all of the nutrients it requires from the pulmonary circulation and O_2 from the alveolar gas, the large conduit or support structures (i.e., bronchi, arteries, veins, pleura, and interlobular connective tissue) cannot. Thus these structures receive a systemic blood supply, consisting of small bronchial arteries, which branch from the aorta or intercostal arteries.

The pulmonary circulation is a low-pressure, high-flow system

The normal pressures in the human pulmonary and systemic circulations are depicted in Figure 29-1. The data are for a resting adult lying supine. The mean pressure in the pulmonary artery ($\overline{Ppa}$) is about one seventh that in the aorta. Mean left atrial pressure ($\overline{Pla}$) is usually about 5 mm Hg higher than mean right atrial pressure. The transpulmonary pressure is equal to the pressure difference from the pulmonary artery to the left atrium ($\overline{Ppa} - \overline{Pla}$). PVR is equal to the transpulmonary pressure divided by flow. Therefore at the normal resting cardiac output (Q) of 5 L/min, PVR = $(\overline{Ppa} - \overline{Pla})/Q = (14 - 8)/5 = 1.2$ mm Hg/(L/min). A comprehensive view of pulmonary hemodynamics under a given set of conditions can be obtained by measuring the changes in transpulmonary pressure ($\overline{Ppa} - \overline{Pla}$) as cardiac output varies. The resulting graphs are called **pressure-flow curves.** A normal curve is shown in Figure 29-2.

PVR is represented on a pressure-flow curve by the slope of the line drawn from the origin of the graph to a specified point on the curve, not by the slope of the curve itself. The most important aspect of the pressure-flow curve is its nonlinear shape. The curve bends toward the flow axis as flow increases (Figure 29-2), meaning that PVR DECREASES AS FLOW INCREASES BECAUSE OF THE PASSIVE DISTENSIBILITY OF THE RESISTANCE VESSELS.

> When someone with lung cancer has half a lung removed, the PVR at rest may be only modestly elevated because the pulmonary vascular bed of the remaining lung can take up the doubled flow via the recruitment of more alveolar wall capillaries. However, when the patient tries to exercise, much less vascular recruitment is available. Hence $\overline{Ppa}$ rises during exercise and limits exercise ability.

The pulmonary circulation varies with the location of the vessels

Only the alveolar wall capillaries and the smallest venules and arterioles are functionally in the lung because only these vessels are exposed on their external surfaces to the total pressure of the alveolar gas. These vessels are usually called **alveolar vessels.** The outer surfaces of all other ar-

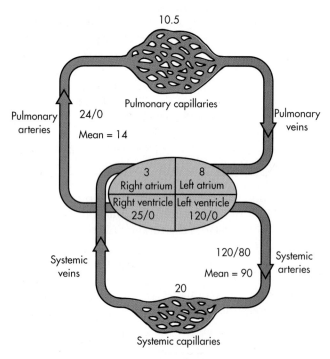

Figure 29-1 Phasic or mean pressure distribution within the systemic and pulmonary circulations in a normal, resting human adult lying in the dorsal recumbent position. (All pressures are shown in millimeters of mercury [mm Hg]). The driving pressure in the systemic circuit ($\overline{Pa} - \overline{Pra}$) is 90 − 3 = 87 mm Hg compared with the driving pressure in the pulmonary circuit ($\overline{Ppa} - \overline{Pla}$): 14 − 8 = 6 mm Hg. Cardiac output must be the same in both circuits in the steady state because the circuits are in series. Therefore the resistance to flow through the lungs is less than 10% that of the rest of the body. Furthermore, the pressures in the left heart chambers are higher than those in the right side of the heart. Thus any congenital openings between the right and left sides favor left-to-right flow.

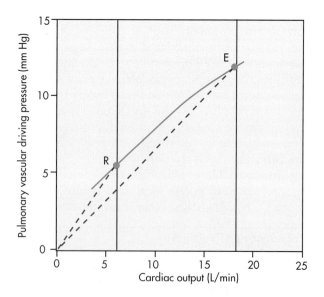

Figure 29-2 Representative pressure-flow curve that might be obtained in the pulmonary circulation of a dorsally recumbent (supine) normal human. The slopes of the dashed red lines from the origin to the two points on the curve represent the PVR ($\Delta P/\Delta Q$). The key feature is that the pressure-flow line *(green line)* bends toward the abscissa (flow) as flow rises, meaning that resistance decreases because of the recruitment of capillaries and the passive distention of resistance vessels. *E,* Submaximal steady-state exercise; *R,* resting condition.

teries and veins are exposed to pleural pressure (subatmospheric) because the conduit vessels are not attached directly to the lung connective tissue structure (see Chapter 27). These vessels are usually called **extraalveolar vessels.** The importance of the distinctions of these vessels is discussed in the section on lung zones.

The lung is wrapped around the extraalveolar vessels and the conducting blood vessels, and the bronchi can be easily separated from the lung tissue using liquid (as in **pulmonary edema**) or air (as in **interstitial** or **subcutaneous emphysema**). This anatomical arrangement is important to the thoracic surgeon, who must separate the lung tissue from the main conduit vessels before removing a portion of a lung lobe. If these vessels cannot be separated from the lung tissue, the entire lobe has to be removed, even if only a small portion is cancerous.

BECAUSE ALL OF THE PULMONARY VESSELS, INCLUDING THE RESISTANCE VESSELS, ARE RELATIVELY THIN-WALLED SOFT TUBES, THEIR DIAMETERS ARE SENSITIVE TO THE DISTENDING PRESSURE (I.E., THE DIFFERENCE BETWEEN THE PRESSURES INSIDE AND OUTSIDE OF EACH VESSEL). The pressure outside the alveolar vessels is the alveolar gas pressure, which is ordinarily the atmospheric pressure. The pressure outside the extraalveolar vessels, however, is below the alveolar pressure; the outside pressure is similar to the pleural pressure. (-3.7 mm Hg at functional residual capacity [FRC]).

In normal breathing, when the lung expands and pleural pressure falls, the pressure outside the extraalveolar vessels decreases. This enlarges the extraalveolar vessels during inspiration and thereby increases pulmonary blood volume. On the other hand, alveolar pressure does not vary much with breathing.

Mechanical ventilation applies positive pressure in the airways and raises alveolar pressure. Unfortunately, this compresses the capillaries. The PVR is increased, but if there is lung disease, the pressure effect may not be uniformly distributed. This nonuniformity may markedly affect the matching of perfusion to ventilation and disturb not only the work of the right ventricle but also the systemic arterial O_2 concentration.

Pulmonary blood flow is affected by gravity

Gravity affects venous return (cardiac output) and the distribution of systemic blood volume (see Chapters 23 and 24). A systemic arterial pressure of 120/80 mm Hg refers to pressure at the level of the heart when the subject is in the dorsal recumbent (supine) position (Figure 29-1). Luminal pressure rises in both arteries and veins by 0.7 mm Hg for each centimeter below the heart and falls by a comparable amount above the heart.

THE EFFECTS OF GRAVITY ARE GREATER IN THE PULMONARY CIRCULATION THAN IN THE SYSTEMIC CIRCULATION BECAUSE THE VASCULAR PRESSURES ARE MUCH LOWER. Furthermore, the heart is about halfway up the lung in the upright human posture (see Figure 27-3). At FRC (normal lung volume at end-expiration), the bottom of the lung is about 12 cm below the lung hilum (level of the left atrium). Although the higher pressure toward the bottom of the lung does not change the driving pressure along the vessels, it does change the transmural distending pressure, which tends to decrease the resistance to flow. Flow is greater toward the bottom of the lung. The opposite effect occurs for the 12 cm of lung above the heart level. When the lung is at FRC, the mean pulmonary arterial pressure at the top is 5 mm Hg, and the pulmonary venous (outflow) pressure is -1 mm Hg (i.e., less than alveolar [atmospheric] pressure). When the pressure inside a distensible vessel is less than the pressure outside, the vessel is compressed and thereby increases resistance to flow at the point of compression. The pressure differences resulting from gravity affect the distribution of blood flow up and down the lung, as illustrated in Figure 29-3.

There are three **lung zones** depending on the relationship among pulmonary arterial, venous, and alveolar pressures. In **zone 1,** there is no blood flow because pulmonary arterial pressure is lower than alveolar pressure (capillaries compressed). In **zone 3,** flow is high because all vessels are distended. In **zone 2,** the alveolar pressure exceeds the venous outflow pressure, so the capillaries or venules exposed to alveolar pressure are compressed at the outflow end of the alveolar compartment (Figure 29-3). Although all three zones can exist in the human lung, pulmonary arterial pressure is normally high enough so that the zone 1 condition of no flow does not occur. Also, the condition described for zone 2 is limited to the top of the lung because the $\overline{P}$la is normally well above alveolar pressure.

Mechanical ventilation is often used in patients with diseased lungs. If the pressure that inflates the lungs is too high, some of the lung may be put into zone 1, where there is no blood flow. In fact, the healthiest part of the lung may be most affected; thus blood flow may be shifted to the more diseased parts of the lung. Hence the ventilator may make ventilation/perfusion mismatching worse instead of better.

Venous admixture reduces the efficiency of gas exchange

Venous blood that returns to the lungs and does not pass by air-filled alveoli leads to **venous admixture** because the venous blood mixes with oxygenated blood from the lung. Venous admixture always lowers the systemic Pa_{O_2} and he-

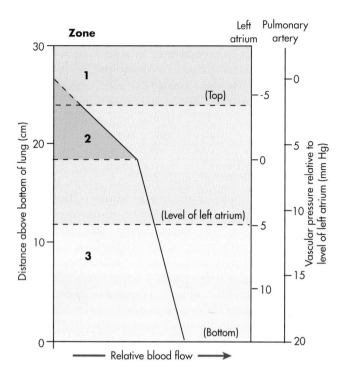

Figure 29-3 Distribution of flow in the normal upright human lung at rest. At FRC, the top **(zone 1)** of the lung is at 24 cm (left-hand ordinate) above the bottom. At the level of the left atrium **(zone 2)**, the $\bar{P}la$ and $\bar{P}pa$ are 5 and 11 mm Hg, respectively, as shown on the two parallel scales along the right-hand ordinate. Note that these pressures are each about 3 mm Hg less than in the supine resting individual (see Figure 29-1). This is the result of gravity affecting the whole body in the upright posture. Most of the lung is in **zone 3** because the $\bar{P}la$ does not fall below zero until some 18 cm above the bottom. In zone 3, although the driving pressure is constant, flow (abscissa shows relative flow only) continues to increase toward the bottom of the lung because of the passive distention of vessels by the increasing vascular pressure. Zone 2 occurs in the upper 6 cm. In zone 2, flow is regulated by alveolar pressure compressing the outflow from the alveolar microvessels. Near the top, the alveolar wall capillaries may even be completely compressed if the arterial pressure falls below the alveolar pressure (zone 1).

moglobin saturation. Venous admixture includes anatomical shunts and blood from mismatched ventilation/perfusion lung units. A small amount of venous admixture is normal. This can be less than 1% of the cardiac output normally, but in some diseases the percentage may be much higher. In the normal fetus, nearly all of the cardiac output bypasses the lungs. Some blood flows through a hole **(foramen ovale)** in the septum between the atria, but most of the blood flows through a vessel **(ductus arteriosus)** that connects the pulmonary artery to the ascending aorta (see Chapter 25). After birth, as the blood is oxygenated by the lungs and the PVR falls toward the low adult levels, these fetal shunts quickly close.

> After birth, normally the $\bar{P}la$ is higher than right atrial pressure, and aortic pressure is higher than $\bar{P}pa$ (Figure 29-1). Even if the foramen ovale or the ductus arteriosus

remains open after birth, blood flow is from **left to right,** so systemic arterial blood is normally oxygenated. In a few uncommon anomalies (abnormal developmental anatomy) blood flows in the other direction, causing **cyanotic heart disease** ("blue babies," who have low O_2 saturation of the hemoglobin in their arterial blood).

When a left-to-right shunt exists, the pulmonary blood flow exceeds systemic blood flow, and the left ventricular stroke volume exceeds the right ventricular volume by the amount of blood that flows through the shunt. Venous admixture represents a stream of blood being pumped around the body without delivering any O_2 or picking up any CO_2. Therefore venous admixture reduces the efficiency of blood gas exchange. Venous admixture is the blood flow equivalent of wasted ventilation. Wasted ventilation results in an infinitely great ventilation/perfusion ratio ($\dot{V}/\dot{Q} = \infty$).

> Venous admixture occurs commonly in pulmonary diseases because ventilation is diminished more than perfusion in many lung units. Low ventilation/perfusion units effectively shunt some of the blood around the alveolar gas (wasted blood flow). On the other hand, high ventilation/perfusion units cause only wasted ventilation but not venous admixture.

The lung is leaky

All capillaries throughout the body are leaky in varying degrees to the liquid, electrolytes, and proteins of blood plasma (see Chapter 22). Net outward filtration continues throughout life, and most of the filtrate is returned to the circulation as lymph by the lymphatic system. The lung is no exception. The hydrostatic pressure that favors liquid filtration from the microvessels is higher near the bottom of the lung than near the top. The accumulation of excess extracellular liquid in the lung **(pulmonary edema)** may be life threatening because it may cause serious ventilation/perfusion mismatching and interfere with diffusion (see Chapter 30). Alveoli full of liquid cannot be adequately ventilated.

> In patients with **congestive heart failure,** the $\bar{P}la$ is elevated, and edema fluid tends to accumulate, especially in the lower half of the lung. Reduced breath sounds or bubbling **rales** (noises in the small airways) are audible near the lung bases. The chest roentgenogram shows greater density (more fluid) toward the bottom of the lung. Patients with left ventricular failure often complain that they must sit up **(orthopnea)** in bed to sleep. When the patient lies flat, pulmonary vascular pressures rise, and

fluid filtration increases throughout the lung; these problems cause a feeling of suffocation. The accumulating edema fluid in the alveoli interferes with O_2 exchange and causes systemic arterial O_2 desaturation.

The pulmonary circulation is predominantly passive

During exercise, cardiac output can increase at least three-fold in most humans. As mentioned earlier, this increase is accommodated by the pulmonary circulation without an equivalent rise in the pulmonary vascular driving pressure because of the recruitment and distention of microvessels. For example, during exercise, the volume of blood in the pulmonary capillaries may more than double, so the resistance to blood flow in the capillaries decreases substantially.

In pulmonary hypertension the work required of the right side of the heart to pump blood through the pulmonary vessels increases. The right side of the heart may begin to fail, and the blood may become poorly oxygenated. The initial complaint may be exertional shortness of breath, which then progresses to resting shortness of breath and hypoxemia. **Primary pulmonary hypertension** (i.e., high pressure in the pulmonary arteries of unknown cause) may strike young women and may progress rapidly. **Secondary pulmonary hypertension** may be caused by massive destruction of alveolar wall capillaries. Such destruction may occur in advanced chronic obstructive lung disease, in interstitial lung disease, in inflammation of pulmonary blood vessels (vasculitis), or after multiple chronic pulmonary emboli. Surgical resection of more than about 60% of the total lung mass leads to pulmonary hypertension, even when the patient is at rest.

The pulmonary circulation can be actively regulated by the nervous system

Although the passive effects of pressure on the distensible pulmonary bed are generally predominant, active regulation occurs under various physiological and pathological conditions. The smooth muscle associated with the small muscular pulmonary arteries, arterioles, and veins is adequate to substantially alter the PVR. The smooth muscle may hypertrophy remarkably in pathological conditions.

The pulmonary vascular bed is innervated by **parasympathetic (cholinergic) nerves** (the vagus nerves) and by **sympathetic (adrenergic) nerves.** However, external autonomic stimulation does not greatly affect vascular resistance, but it seems chiefly to modulate lung vascular distensibility (compliance). Efferent vagal stimulation releases acetylcholine, which acts via endothelial cell receptors to release nitric oxide (NO), which increases vascular compliance. It also relaxes the resistance vessels, but the effect is normally minimal because the vessels are already relaxed.

When humans and other mammals go to high altitude, pharmacological blockade of the release of NO tends to increase the PVR. This response indicates that NO production is increased at high altitude. This, however, is probably a local effect, not an autonomic reflex, because the carotid chemoreceptors are stimulated by hypoxemia, and this tends to constrict the PVR vessels (see Chapter 31).

Sympathetic nerves are the main motor nerves to pulmonary vascular smooth muscle. Baroreceptor stimulation may dilate pulmonary resistance vessels, most likely because of the withdrawal of sympathetic tone. The sympathetic nerves release norepinephrine, which acts principally via α-adrenergic receptors on the smooth muscle cells to increase their tone and thereby increase vascular resistance and reduce vascular distensibility. The main circulating catecholamine, however, is epinephrine, which stimulates β-adrenergic receptors on the smooth muscle cells to relax them.

The alveolar O_2 level is the most important regulator of the pulmonary vasculature

A number of naturally occurring substances affect the vasomotor tone of pulmonary arterial or venous vessels. Some of these substances are normally **constrictors.** The more important of these include thromboxane A_2, α-adrenergic catecholamines, several arachidonic acid metabolites, neuropeptides, endothelin, and increased Pa_{CO_2}. Other substances, such as increased PA_{O_2}, α-adrenergic catecholamines, prostacyclin, and NO, are normally **dilators.** THE CRUCIAL FACTOR THAT USUALLY GOVERNS MINUTE-TO-MINUTE REGULATION OF THE PULMONARY CIRCULATION IS THE PA_{O_2}. This factor is critical because the small muscular pulmonary arteries are surrounded by the alveolar gas of the terminal respiratory units they subserve. Ordinarily, the PA_{O_2} is about 100 mm Hg.

The response of pulmonary vascular smooth muscle to a low PA_{O_2} differs from that of the systemic circulation. In the lung, a low PA_{O_2} **constricts** nearby arterioles, whereas in the systemic circulation, the PA_{O_2} **relaxes** the resistance vessels. In the lung a low PA_{O_2} appears to act directly on the vascular smooth muscle cells. The intracellular sensing mechanism that mediates smooth muscle contraction is unknown, but it may involve a protein kinase, cyclic GMP (see Chapter 5). As the PA_{O_2} falls in any region of the lung, the adjacent arterioles constrict. This decreases local blood flow and shifts it to other regions of the lung. Because alveolar hypoxia usually results from inadequate ventilation, the local hypoxic vasoconstriction reduces perfusion. Hence the $\dot{V}/\dot{Q}$ is restored toward normal; this is an efficient self-control mechanism. On the other hand, a global reduction in PA_{O_2}, such as that which occurs at high altitude, causes all of the resistance vessels to constrict and thereby raises PVR. The PVR in people traveling or living at altitudes above 10,000 feet may be more than twice normal.

As previously stated, a sustained elevation in the $\overline{P}pa$ may occur in some disease states and may be mediated by two interdependent physiological and pathological mechanisms: persistent vasoconstriction and vascular structural remodeling. Unfortunately, this combination of effects on the pulmonary circulation imposes a burden that cannot be overcome by normal adaptive mechanisms.

An important clinical test for assessing the possible reversibility of a pulmonary hypoxic response is to have the subject breathe 100% O_2. This should reverse any hypoxic component of pulmonary hypertension. Recently, however, potent pulmonary vasodilators have begun to supplant the O_2 test; these include prostacyclin, calcium channel antagonists, and NO.

The most important of the vasoconstrictors is probably **thromboxane A_2,** a product of arachidonic acid metabolism. Many cells, including leukocytes, macrophages, platelets, and possibly endothelial cells, can produce and release thromboxane. Thromboxane A_2 is one of the most powerful constrictors of vascular and airway smooth muscle, but it acts mainly locally because it is rapidly inactivated. **Prostacyclin** (prostaglandin I_2), another product of arachidonic acid metabolism, is a potent vasodilator and has an antiaggregatory influence on platelets (see Chapter 16). Vascular endothelial cells and smooth muscle cells produce prostacyclin locally, especially at the site of vessel injury.

Bronchial Circulation

The bronchial circulation provides separate nourishment to the lung

The bronchial arteries supply water and nutrients to the airways down to and including the terminal bronchioles. They also nourish the pulmonary arteries and veins, pleura, and interlobular septa. The pressure in the main bronchial arteries is essentially the same as in the aorta; hence the driving pressure is high. Although bronchial blood flow is normally less than 1% of cardiac output, it is adequate for the portion of the lung tissue it serves. About half of the bronchial blood flow returns to the right side of the heart via the bronchial veins. The remainder flows through small bronchopulmonary anastomoses (<100 μm in diameter) into the pulmonary veins and thereby contributes to the small, normal venous admixture (right-to-left shunt).

In certain inflammatory diseases of the airways (i.e., **bronchitis, bronchiectasis, bronchogenic carcinoma**), the bronchial circulation expands dramatically and may contribute as much as 10% to 20% to the venous admixture. This explains why patients with these diseases may often cough up blood (**hemoptysis**).

The bronchial circulation warms and humidifies the inspired air, especially when the inspired air bypasses the nose, as in mouth-breathing during exercise. The inhaled air is completely warmed and humidified in the upper airways, and this process prevents any evaporation from the alveolar surfaces.

The ventilation/perfusion ratio is not uniformly distributed in the lung

In the ideal lung the $\dot{V}/\dot{Q}$ is uniform at about 0.8. This value yields the normal PaO_2 of 100 mm Hg and $PaCO_2$ of 40 mm Hg, as shown in Figure 29-4. However, neither ventilation nor blood flow is uniformly distributed in the real lung, even in a healthy adult. In patients with cardiopulmonary disease, the most common cause of systemic arterial hypoxemia is uneven matching of alveolar ventilation to alveolar blood flow (ventilation/perfusion mismatching).

Ventilation/perfusion mismatching is generally expressed in terms of its effect on the alveolar-arterial difference in the partial pressure of O_2 ($PAO_2 - PaO_2$ gradient) (see Equation 28-2). Note that in the ideal lung, the PAO_2 does not differ from the PaO_2 (Figure 29-4). The two

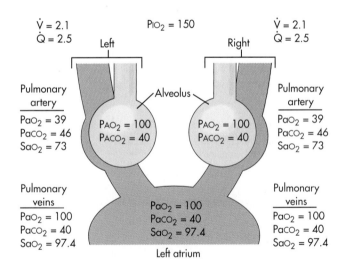

Figure 29-4 Two-compartment schema showing the effect of uniform alveolar $\dot{V}/\dot{Q}$s of 0.84 on the partial pressure of oxygen (*PO₂*) and partial pressure of carbon dioxide (*PCO₂*) in millimeters of mercury (mm Hg) and the O_2 saturation (*SO₂*) in percentages (%) of the pulmonary venous blood that leaves each compartment and mixes in the left atrium (systemic arterial blood). Each lung receives half the total ventilation (in liters per minute [L/min]) so that the left atrial blood has the same O_2 saturation, 97.4%, as the outflowing blood from each lung. *PACO₂, Partial pressure of alveolar carbon dioxide; PIO₂, partial pressure of inspired O_2; SaO₂, arterial oxygen saturation.*

extreme examples of ventilation/perfusion mismatching are **wasted ventilation ($\dot{V}/\dot{Q} = \infty$)** and **venous admixture ($\dot{V}/\dot{Q}$ = zero).** Between totally wasted ventilation and totally venous admixture lie all possible values for $\dot{V}/\dot{Q}$. The average $\dot{V}/\dot{Q}$ is about 0.8, but the ventilation/perfusion distribution throughout the normal lung is not homogeneous. Some lung units are overventilated, and some are underventilated.

The distribution of $\dot{V}/\dot{Q}$ in a normal adult is illustrated in Figure 29-5. The average ratio in this individual is 0.84, as shown by the thin vertical line. The Y axis shows the ventilation or perfusion in liters per minute. The range of $\dot{V}/\dot{Q}$ (derived by dividing each ventilation value by its associated perfusion value) is shown on the X axis; the scale is logarithmic to encompass the wide range of such ratios. In conclusion, THE NORMAL LUNG FUNCTIONS EXCEEDINGLY WELL, EVEN THOUGH GRAVITY CAUSES AN UNEVEN LUNG EXPANSION AND AN UNEVEN DISTRIBUTION OF BLOOD FLOW (see Chapter 28).

The distribution of ventilation depends on transpulmonary pressure and volume

The end-expiratory volume (FRC) of the alveoli toward the bottom of the lung is less than that for the alveoli toward the top (Figure 29-6). This is because in a lung expanded to FRC, the transpulmonary pressure in a given region of the lung increases as a function of the vertical distance of that region from the base of the lung. However, as long as the compliance (slope of the pressure-volume line in Figure 29-6) is constant, the inspired air goes proportionally to all alveoli; that is, each alveolus (terminal lung unit) receives air in proportion to its volume. Thus maldistribution of ventilation in different lung regions is rarely a problem in a healthy young person.

The regional maldistribution of ventilation can be increased by temporarily reducing end-expiratory lung vol-

ume to residual volume or by inspiring to total lung capacity. Both of these effects depend entirely on the shape of the pressure-volume curve (Figure 29-6). Increased regional maldistribution is a normal part of the aging process because the lung as a whole becomes more distensible (increased compliance).

Local maldistribution of ventilation is probably more important than regional maldistribution in the normal adult. Resistance of the small airways and compliance measurements among terminal respiratory units (alveoli) vary substantially on both functional and anatomical grounds. THE RATE OF FILLING AND EMPTYING OF A LUNG UNIT DEPENDS ON ITS TIME CONSTANT: THE PRODUCT OF RESISTANCE AND COMPLIANCE ($R \times C$).

Figures 29-7 shows how three different units inflate during a normal 2-second inspiration. One unit is normal, one has twice the airway resistance of the others, and one has a reduced compliance. At the normal breathing rate of 12 breaths/min, the inspiratory time is about 2 seconds, which may not be long enough for every functional lung unit to achieve a new steady state. The normal unit and the low-compliance unit both attain new steady states, although the volume of the stiff (low-compliance) unit is reduced. The unit with increased resistance fills to only 80%

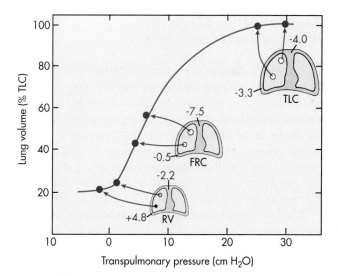

Figure 29-6 Regional distribution of lung volume at end-expiration. Because of the gradually more subatmospheric pleural pressure (greater translung distending pressure [X axis]) from the bottom to the top of the lung, the end-expiratory volume is less in individual lung units near the bottom **(FRC).** As long as the various lung ventilation units are on the nearly linear part of the lung pressure-volume (compliance) curve, each unit is ventilated during normal tidal breathing in proportion to its volume so that the regional distribution range of ventilation is fairly narrow. However, if end-expiratory lung volume falls below FRC (e.g., to **residual volume [RV]**), some lower ventilation units are compressed. During the next tidal breath, they are less well ventilated because their compliance is less. If a maximal inspiration is taken to **total lung capacity (TLC),** all ventilation units are fully expanded uniformly despite pleural surface pressure differences down the lung. At residual volume and FRC, pleural pressure gradients *(red numbers)* cause the upper regions of lung to be more expanded than lower regions.

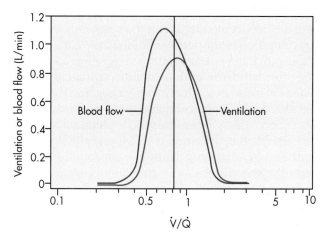

Figure 29-5 Normal ventilation *(blue line)* and blood flow (perfusion) *(red line)* distribution curves in an adult. On the X axis is the $\dot{V}/\dot{Q}$ distribution, shown on a logarithmic scale ranging from 0.1 to 10. The overall lung normal value of 0.84 in this man is shown by the vertical line. The Y axis gives the absolute value of ventilation or blood flow for each $\dot{V}/\dot{Q}$.

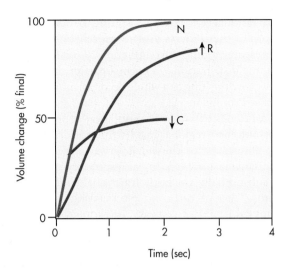

Figure 29-7 Three examples of local variation of ventilation among lung units caused by differences in airway resistance (R) or compliance (C). The normal unit (N) reaches 97% of its equilibrium volume during a 2-second normal inspiration. The unit with increased resistance fills slowly, reaching only 80% of its equilibrium volume in the 2 seconds available; it is underventilated relative to its FRC volume. The unit with decreased compliance fills as fast as the normal unit, but because it is stiffer, it is also underventilated.

of its steady-state volume. If inspiration is prolonged, the high-resistance unit will eventually fill.

The distribution of perfusion is gravity dependent

As previously discussed, gravity affects the regional distribution of blood flow in the lung via its effect on the transmural distending pressure of the blood vessels and on the relative arterial, venous, and alveolar pressures (Figure 29-3). In the range of normal breathing at rest, the gravitational effects on the blood flow distribution over the height of the lung may not be very large. Most of the lung behaves as if it were in zone 3, where flow changes do occur but not as dramatically as in zone 2 (Figure 29-3).

The local distribution of blood flow among alveoli may be very uneven based on two factors. The first is anatomical; that is, the diameter and length of the vessels to each functional unit determine the resistance to flow, according to Poiseuille's equation (see Chapter 20). Local uneven flow is not affected by large changes in total lung blood flow. The second factor is the P_{AO_2}, which alters local vasomotor tone and thereby affects the vascular resistance within the various lung units. Normally, the vasoconstrictor effect of hypoxia is insignificant; the inhalation of 100% O_2 changes the PVR only slightly.

Ventilation/perfusion mismatching alters arterial oxygenation

In healthy young adults, right-to-left shunts (i.e., bronchopulmonary anastomotic flow, intracardiac venous leakage through thebesian veins) account for only 1% to 2% of

cardiac output, and ventilation/perfusion mismatching accounts for some 4% to 5%. Thus the normal systemic P_{aO_2} in humans is about 90 mm Hg compared with a P_{AO_2} of 100 mm Hg, which gives a $P_{AO_2} - P_{aO_2}$ gradient of about 10 mm Hg. In a subject breathing room air, a $P_{AO_2} - P_{aO_2}$ gradient less than 20 mm Hg, is considered normal. However, if a patient breathes 100% O_2, the percentage of venous admixture is roughly 1% for every difference of 20 mm Hg. For example, if the P_{AO_2} is 550 mm Hg but the P_{aO_2} is 150 mm Hg, the $P_{AO_2} - P_{aO_2}$ gradient is 400 mm Hg, and the venous admixture is 20%. In healthy resting adults the average alveolar ventilation is 4.2 L/min, and the average pulmonary blood flow is about 5.0 L/min. Thus the $\dot{V}/\dot{Q}$ normally is about 0.84 (Figure 29-5). In Figure 29-4, half the alveolar ventilation and half the blood flow go to each lung. Thus the $\dot{V}/\dot{Q}$ of each lung is also 0.84, and the pulmonary venous blood leaving each lung has the same O_2 saturation: 97.5%. When the two streams join in the left atrium, the O_2 saturation remains at 97.5%.

Pulmonary emboli are blood clots that lodge in the pulmonary arteries. These clots arise from the systemic veins or the right heart chambers. Pulmonary emboli can cause shortness of breath, pleurisy, cough, hemoptysis, tachycardia, and a fall in blood oxygenation levels. Pulmonary emboli cause ventilation/perfusion mismatching by restricting the blood supply to alveoli that are still being ventilated. This results in a high $\dot{V}/\dot{Q}$ and hypoxemia. Figure 29-8, A, demonstrates a normal perfusion scan in which blood flow is symmetrically and homogenously distributed. Figure 29-8, B, demonstrates an abnormal perfusion scan, with absent perfusion to the right and left lower lobes (caused by pulmonary emboli).

Figure 29-9 shows that the right lung is overventilated but has a normal blood flow. Thus the $\dot{V}/\dot{Q}$ is high, and the P_{aO_2} is increased. This, however, only raises the O_2 saturation in the outflowing blood to 98.0% because the hemoglobin is nearly saturated (see Figure 30-2). On the other hand, the left lung is underventilated but has a normal blood flow. Thus its $\dot{V}/\dot{Q}$ is low, and the P_{aO_2} is decreased, which reduces the saturation of the outflowing blood to 89%. When the venous blood mixes in the left atrium, the saturation is 93.5%, and the P_{aO_2} is 68 mm Hg. Ventilation/perfusion mismatching also affects the systemic P_{aCO_2} (Figure 29-9). However, compensation is usually effective, so the P_{aCO_2} is only slightly above normal.

When the trachea is intubated for general anesthesia, care must be taken to properly position the endotracheal tube. Infrequently, the endotracheal tube may selectively

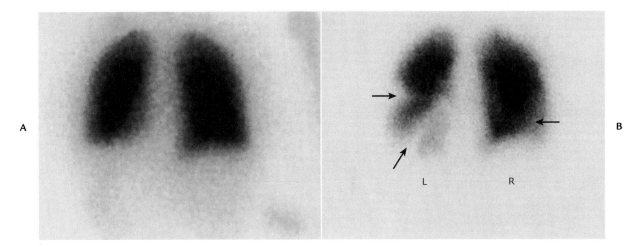

Figure 29-8 A, Normal perfusion scan (performed by intravenous injection of a radioactive tracer) demonstrates normal blood flow distribution in all lobes of the lung. **B,** Abnormal perfusion scan demonstrates diminished blood flow to the right and left lower lobes as a result of occluding pulmonary emboli *(arrows).* The ventilation/perfusion mismatching explains this patient's hypoxemia.

go down the right mainstem bronchus, causing overventilation and increased airway pressures in the right lung and resulting in a high $\dot{V}/\dot{Q}$. The left lung will be underventilated, although it will still receive normal flow, resulting in a low $\dot{V}/\dot{Q}$ and a decreased O_2 saturation. The absence of breath sounds and ventilation to the left lung should promptly alert the anesthesiologist to this complication before the O_2 saturation drops to dangerously low levels.

The most important compensatory mechanism for ventilation/perfusion mismatching is hypoxic vasoconstriction

A number of compensatory mechanisms come into play to alleviate partial ventilation/perfusion mismatching. Initially, these mechanisms may involve increasing the overall ventilation because the $Paco_2$ is increased. However, increasing total ventilation is only a stopgap measure because much of the increased ventilation goes to the lung that is already overventilated. Local regulatory factors are much more important. As already mentioned, HYPOXIC VASOCONSTRICTION (IN HYPOVENTILATED UNITS) IS THE SINGLE MOST EFFECTIVE MECHANISM FOR SHIFTING FLOW AWAY FROM UNDERVENTILATED UNITS, as Figure 29-10 demonstrates. Likewise, when ventilation is wasted (hyperventilated unit), the local $Paco_2$ falls. This change lowers the H^+ concentration (raises pH) in and around the associated airway smooth muscle. The fall in the H^+ concentration increases the local airway resistance and shifts ventilation to units with a higher $\dot{V}/\dot{Q}$ (Figures 29-6 and 29-10). If blood flow is sufficiently reduced to a lung unit, the local alveolar cell metabolism (notably, surfactant production) may be decreased. The increase in the air-liquid interfacial tension reduces the unit's compliance, and its FRC volume decreases (Figure 29-7).

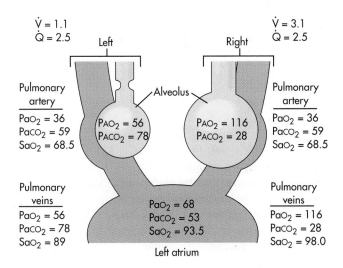

Figure 29-9 Two-compartment schema showing the effect of uneven alveolar $\dot{V}/\dot{Q}$ on the partial pressure of oxygen *(Po$_2$)* and partial pressure of carbon dioxide *(Pco$_2$)* in millimeters of mercury (mm Hg) and the O_2 saturation *(So$_2$)* in percentages (%) of the pulmonary venous blood leaving each compartment and after mixing in the left atrium (systemic arterial blood). The right lung receives 3.1 instead of 2 L/min ventilation in the ideal lung (see Figure 29-4), but it still receives half of the normal blood flow, 2.5 L/min. Its $\dot{V}/\dot{Q}$ is 3.1/2.5 = 1.2; it is clearly overventilated. Its Pco_2, which must be calculated using the alveolar ventilation equation (Equation 28-2), is 28 mm Hg: hyperventilation, by definition. Its Po_2 is increased to 116 mm Hg. However, O_2 saturation of the outflowing venous blood is only slightly increased: to 98.0%. The left lung, of course, is underventilated by 1.1 L/min but still receives half of the total blood flow. Its $\dot{V}/\dot{Q}$ is 1.1/2.5 = 0.44. Its Pco_2, calculated using the alveolar ventilation equation, is 78 mm Hg: hypoventilation, by definition. Its Po_2 is decreased to 56 mm Hg, which gives an O_2 saturation equal to 89% in the outflowing venous blood. When the two bloodstreams mix in the left atrium, the resultant systemic arterial blood is hypoxemic (arterial O_2 saturation *[Sao$_2$]* = 93.5%, Pao_2 = 68 mm Hg). Clearly, the hyperventilated lung compartment cannot compensate for the hypoventilated compartment because of the markedly alinear shape of the oxyhemoglobin equilibrium curve (see Figure 30-2). Note that the $Paco_2$ is increased in this uncompensated example. *Paco$_2$,* Partial pressure of alveolar carbon dioxide.

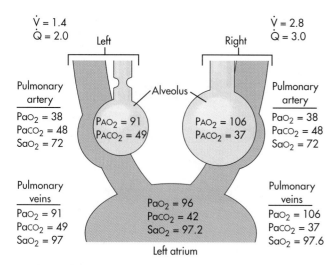

$\dot{V} = 1.4$
$\dot{Q} = 2.0$

Left

Right

$\dot{V} = 2.8$
$\dot{Q} = 3.0$

Pulmonary
artery

$PaO_2 = 38$
$PaCO_2 = 48$
$SaO_2 = 72$

Alveolus

$PAO_2 = 91$
$PACO_2 = 49$

$PAO_2 = 106$
$PACO_2 = 37$

Pulmonary
artery

$PaO_2 = 38$
$PaCO_2 = 48$
$SaO_2 = 72$

Pulmonary
veins

$PaO_2 = 91$
$PaCO_2 = 49$
$SaO_2 = 97$

$PaO_2 = 96$
$PaCO_2 = 42$
$SaO_2 = 97.2$

Pulmonary
veins

$PaO_2 = 106$
$PaCO_2 = 37$
$SaO_2 = 97.6$

Left atrium

Figure 29-10 Two-compartment schema showing the marked improvement of the systemic arterial blood gas levels after modest local compensatory mechanisms have occurred. Hypoxic vasoconstriction has occurred in the left lung compartment, shifting the blood flow of 0.5 L/min to the right, overventilated lung. Increased airway resistance in the right lung has shifted a blood flow of 0.3 L/min to the left lung. These shifts bring the $\dot{V}/\dot{Q}$ of the left and right lungs to 0.7 and 0.94, respectively. The compensation brings the systemic arterial blood gases to near normal. The partial pressure of oxygen (PO_2) and partial pressure of carbon dioxide (PCO_2) are in millimeters of mercury (mm Hg), and the O_2 saturation (SO_2) is in percentages (%). $PACO_2$, Partial pressure of alveolar carbon dioxide; SaO_2, arterial oxygen saturation.

SUMMARY

- The pulmonary vascular resistance (PVR) is normally much less than systemic vascular resistance.
- Blood flowing from the systemic veins to the systemic arteries without being fully oxygenated (right-to-left shunt) decreases the systemic PaO_2 and O_2 concentration.
- In left-to-right shunts, pulmonary blood flow is increased, but the systemic arterial O_2 concentration is normal.
- The distribution of pulmonary blood flow is sensitive to gravity over the height of the air-filled lung. Gravity leads to three flow conditions. In zone 1, there is no flow. In zone 2, flow is regulated by the compression of microvessels at the outflow from the alveolar walls. In zone 3, flow depends on the driving pressure, vascular geometry, and smooth muscle tone.
- The normal passive regulation of pulmonary blood flow distribution predominates, but active regulation may become very important.
- The main regulator of flow distribution is the PAO_2; a decrease in the PAO_2 (alveolar hypoxia) leads to a local increase in vascular resistance.
- The bronchial circulation nourishes the walls of the airways and blood vessels; it warms and humidifies incoming air.

- The $\dot{V}/\dot{Q}$ among normal functional lung units is not uniform and may deviate markedly from normal in disease states. The limiting ratios are wasted ventilation $(\dot{V}/\dot{Q} = \infty)$ and venous admixture $(\dot{V}/\dot{Q} = \text{zero})$.
- Ventilation is distributed nonuniformly in the lung on regional (gravitational) and local (nongravitational) bases.
- Blood flow is also distributed nonuniformly in the lung on regional and local bases.
- The overall effect of ventilation/perfusion distribution can be judged by determining the $PAO_2 - PAO_2$ gradient, which is normally 10 to 15 mm Hg.

BIBLIOGRAPHY

Deffebach ME, Widdicombe J: The bronchial circulation. In Crystal RG et al, eds: *The lung: scientific foundations,* vol 1, New York, 1991, Raven.

Glenny RW et al: Gravity is minor determinant of pulmonary blood flow distribution, *J Appl Physiol* 71:620, 1991.

Hakim TS, Dean GW, Lisbona R: Effect of body posture on spatial distribution of pulmonary blood flow, *J Appl Physiol* 64:1160, 1988.

Pearl RG: The pulmonary circulation, *Curr Opin Anesthesiol* 5:848, 1992.

Wagner PD: Ventilation/perfusion matching during exercise, *Chest* 101:192S, 1992.

Wagner PD: Ventilation, pulmonary blood flow, and ventilation/perfusion relationships. In Fishman AP et al, eds: *Pulmonary diseases and disorders,* ed 3, New York, 1998, McGraw-Hill.

West JB: *Ventilation/blood flow and gas exchange,* Oxford, England, 1990, Blackwell Scientific.

CASE STUDIES

Case 29-1

A 65-year-old man, previously a heavy smoker, has hemoptysis, cough, weight loss, and shortness of breath. A chest x-ray film demonstrates a left lung mass. He subsequently undergoes a left pneumonectomy (removal of the entire left lung). He recovers and undergoes a second evaluation.

1. **What is the result if cardiac output is unchanged?**
   A. The patient would have significant elevations in the $\overline{P}pa$ because of loss of capillary beds.
   B. The patient would have a significant elevation in the $\overline{P}pa$ and PVR because of the loss of capillary beds and the effects of surgery.
   C. The patient would have a transient increase in the $\overline{P}pa$ and PVR in the postoperative period, and then these values would return to normal.
   D. The patient would be hypoxemic and have pulmonary hypertension caused by reflexive pulmonary vasoconstriction.
   E. The patient would be hypoxemic and hypercarbic as a result of poor ventilation.

2. How would the current ventilation/perfusion relationship in this patient be best described?

    A. Low ventilation/perfusion units in the left side as a result of persistent circulation to that side with absent ventilation

    B. Little effect on ventilation/perfusion balance as a result of equal increases in ventilation and perfusion to the right lung

    C. A decrease in arterial oxygenation as a result of loss of the capillary bed but no change in arterial CO_2 levels

    D. High ventilation/perfusion units in the right lung as a result of increase in ventilation with little ability to increase pulmonary circulation

    E. Low ventilation/perfusion units in the right lung as a result of increased perfusion to the right lung

Case 29-2

A 30-year-old woman faints when running up an incline, but otherwise she has been in good health. On physical examination, her physician notes a loud second pulmonary valve heart sound. Because of this, a pulmonary artery catheterization is performed, and the following values are recorded:

$\bar{P}pa$	74/29 mm Hg (mean, 45 mm Hg)
Right atrial pressure	19/18 mm Hg (mean, 16 mm Hg)
Right ventricular pressure	74/13 mm Hg (mean, 17 mm Hg)
Pulmonary artery occlusion pressure	15 mm Hg
Cardiac output	3.0 L/min

A pulmonary angiogram demonstrates no evidence of pulmonary emboli.

1. What is the calculated PVR in this patient?

    A. 10 mm Hg/L × min

    B. 6 mm Hg/L × min

    C. 16 mm Hg/L × min

    D. 20 mm Hg/L × min

    E. 25 mm Hg/L × min

2. Which of the following responses to chemical substances is *not* true?

    A. The inhalation of NO would cause vasodilation.

    B. The inhalation of 100% O_2 may reverse hypoxia-induced pulmonary vasoconstriction.

    C. The administration of calcium channel blockers may lower the $\bar{P}pa$ and cardiac output.

    D. The administration of prostacyclin (prostaglandin I_2) may cause vasodilation.

    E. The administration of leukotriene D_4 would cause vasodilation and bronchodilation.

CHAPTER 30

Transport of O_2 and CO_2 Between the Lungs and Body Cells

- Describe the mechanisms of O_2 and CO_2 transport.
- Analyze the hemoglobin-O_2 equilibrium curve.
- Describe respiratory gas diffusion.

This chapter introduces the key concepts of respiratory gas exchange and transport, which are essential to understanding the interaction of multiple organ systems covered in other sections of this book. All organ systems depend on O_2 delivery to varying degrees. Failure of gas exchange is a common abnormality in medicine and has critical implications to the body systems as a whole. Respiratory gas exchange occurs both at the alveolar-capillary level in the lung and the capillary-tissue level systemically (Figure 30-1). One of the primary functions of the cardiovascular system is to transport O_2 from the lungs to all the systemic capillaries and to transport CO_2 from the systemic capillaries back to the lungs. O_2 is transported for metabolic purposes only in the systemic arterial blood from the lungs to the tissue capillaries. CO_2 is transported for metabolic purposes only in the systemic venous blood from the tissue capillaries to the lungs.

O_2 Transport

O_2 is transported primarily by hemoglobin

As briefly outlined in Chapter 27, ALMOST ALL OF THE O_2 TRANSPORTED IN THE SYSTEMIC ARTERIAL BLOOD IS CHEMICALLY BOUND TO HEMOGLOBIN. Normal human hemoglobin (**hemoglobin A**) (molecular weight, 16,400) consists of four O_2-binding heme molecules (iron-containing porphyrin rings), each attached to a polypeptide chain (see also Chapter 16). Normally, the concentration of hemoglobin in blood is about 15.0 g/dl. Each gram of hemoglobin can combine with about 1.34 ml of O_2. Thus the hemoglobin in 1 L of blood can combine with approximately 200 ml of O_2 (100% hemoglobin saturation). The O_2 content in

blood equals both dissolved O_2 and O_2 bound to hemoglobin. The normal O_2 content of 1 L of mixed venous blood is 150 ml of O_2 (75% hemoglobin saturation).

The amount of O_2 bound to hemoglobin is described two ways: the actual concentration in milliliters per liter of blood (**O_2 content**) and the relative percentage of the maximum amount that can be bound (**O_2 capacity**). The relative amount is called the **oxygen saturation (So_2);** for example, the So_2 is 50% when partial pressure of oxygen (Po_2) is 26 mm Hg, as Figure 30-2 shows. The normal So_2 of systemic arterial blood (Sao_2) is 97.5% when its Po_2 (Pao_2) is 100 mm Hg, and the normal So_2 of systemic mixed venous (pulmonary arterial) blood ($S\bar{v}o_2$) is 75% when its Po_2 ($P\bar{v}o_2$) is 40 mm Hg.

The oxyhemoglobin relationship maximizes O_2 uptake and release

THE BINDING OF O_2 TO HEMOGLOBIN IS DIRECTLY DEPENDENT ON THE Po_2 IN A RELATIONSHIP CALLED THE **OXYHEMOGLOBIN (HbO_2) EQUILIBRIUM CURVE.** The normal HbO_2 curve for human adult systemic arterial blood is shown in Figure 30-2. There are three important physiological properties of the chemical binding between hemoglobin and O_2:

1. Hemoglobin combines reversibly with O_2. The O_2-bound form is called **oxyhemoglobin,** and the deoxygenated form is called **hemoglobin.**
2. Molecular O_2 rapidly reacts with hemoglobin. This fast reaction is critical for O_2 transport because blood remains in the pulmonary and systemic capillaries less than 1 second (see Chapters 27 and 29).
3. Heme group interaction affects the shape of the HbO_2 equilibrium curve. This **S** shape of the curve is caused by a change in the configuration of the hemoglobin molecule after the iron in three of a molecule's heme groups binds O_2. The shape change reflects the alterations in hemoglobin's affinity for O_2 as partial pressure is varied. Functionally, the shape of the curve shows that the

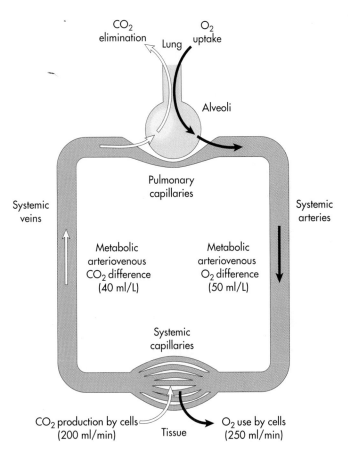

Figure 30-1 O_2 and CO_2 transport in the blood. O_2 is carried from the pulmonary capillaries to the systemic capillaries by the systemic arteries. CO_2 is carried from the systemic capillaries to the pulmonary capillaries by the systemic veins.

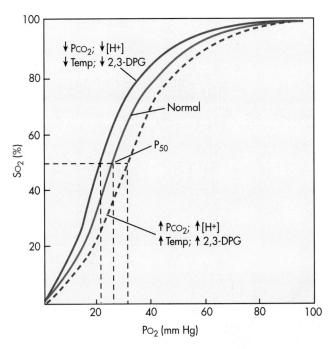

Figure 30-2 The position of the hemoglobin-O_2 equilibrium curve is shifted to the right *(dashed purple line)* when any of the four physiological factors shown—partial pressure of CO_2 *[Pco_2]*; [H^+]; temperature; 2,3-diphosphoglycerate *[2,3-DPG]*—is increased. A shift to the right decreases the ability of hemoglobin to bind O_2 (decreased O_2 affinity). A shift to the left *(solid red line)* signifies a decrease in one or more of the four physiological factors and represents an increased O_2 affinity for hemoglobin. P_{50}, Po_2 at 50% hemoglobin saturation.

The oxyhemoglobin equilibrium curve is modified by physiological factors

The normal conditions in the HbO_2 equilibrium curve for human adults (Figure 30-2) are:

H^+ concentration [H^+]	40 nmol/L (pH, 7.40)
Carbon dioxide tension (Pco_2)	40 mm Hg
Temperature	37° C
2,3-Diphosphoglycerate (2,3-DPG) concentration	15 μmol/g of hemoglobin

When any of these four physiological factors increases, the affinity of hemoglobin for O_2 decreases. It is customary to describe changes in hemoglobin affinity in terms of the Po_2 at 50% hemoglobin saturation (P_{50}). The P_{50} increases (decreased affinity) when any of the factors increases (shift to the right of the dashed purple curve in Figure 30-2). Conversely, when the concentration of any of the physiological factors decreases, the affinity of hemoglobin for O_2 increases and the P_{50} decreases. The entire HbO_2 equilibrium curve is shifted proportionally to the left (solid red curve in Figure 30-2).

The effect of [H^+] is caused by a greater affinity of hydrogen for hemoglobin than for HbO_2. CO_2, which forms carbonic acid in plasma, has its principal effect by

quantity of O_2 taken up in the lungs is maximized even at lower-than-normal alveolar O_2 tension and that the quantity released in the systemic capillaries is substantial at a relatively high Po_2.

Individuals with **anemia** have lower-than-normal blood hemoglobin contents; for example, in anemia associated with **chronic renal failure** the circulating hemoglobin concentration may be 50 g/L because of inadequate renal output of the hormone **erythropoietin.** Erythropoietin regulates the number of erythrocytes and the concentration of hemoglobin. In patients with chronic renal failure, each liter of blood has only one third the normal O_2-carrying capacity, even though the hemoglobin may be normally saturated in systemic arterial blood. Such patients may complain only of tiredness or the inability to do much exercise. When the patient is treated properly with recombinant human erythropoietin, the blood O_2 capacity may improve dramatically. Improving the O_2-carrying capacity of the blood is very important in the treatment of anemia, whatever the cause may be.

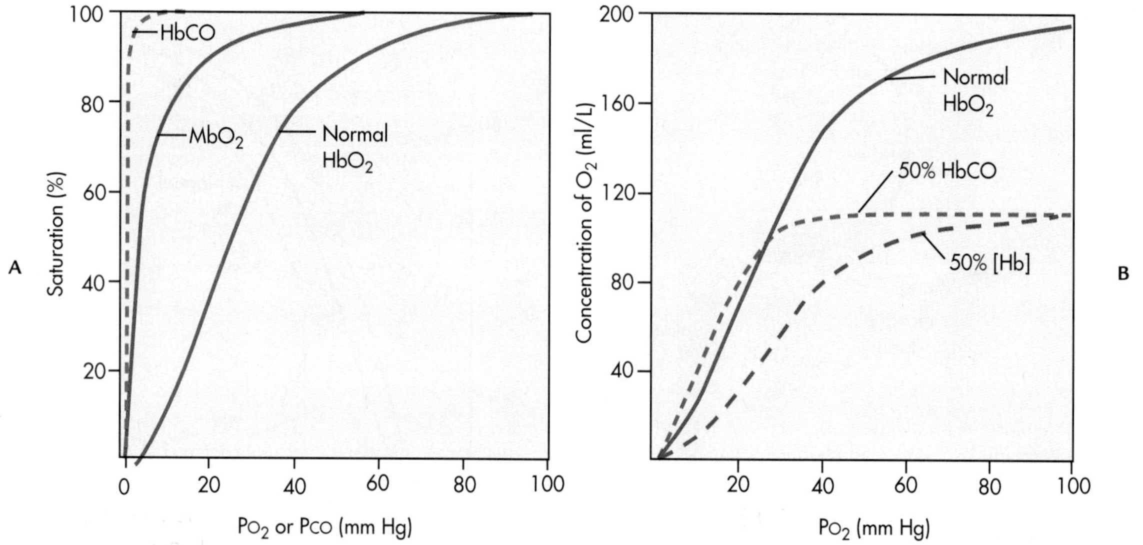

Figure 30-3 Comparison among the saturation curves of hemoglobin *(red line)*, carbon monoxide *(blue line)*, and MbO_2 (the skeletal muscle O_2 storage protein) *(purple line)* for O_2. **A,** The P_{50} of MbO_2 is less than 5 mm Hg, which is similar to the normal intracellular Po_2 of muscle. **B,** The full effect of the damage caused by the carbon monoxide to O_2 transport is seen when the concentration of O_2 in blood is plotted versus the Po_2. This panel compares normal blood *(red line)* with blood with half the normal hemoglobin concentration *[Hb]* (anemia) *(purple line)* and with blood with 50% carboxyhemoglobin *(HbCO) (blue line)*. The dramatic change in the shape of the HbO_2 equilibrium curve in CO poisoning can be seen by the shift in the mixed venous point if the arteriovenous difference in Po_2 remains at 50 ml/L. *Pco,* Partial pressure of carbon monoxide.

increasing the $[H^+]$. The shift in the position of the HbO_2 equilibrium curve, caused by a change in the Pco_2, is called the **Bohr effect.** The compound 2,3-DPG is present in erythrocytes in a higher concentration than in other cells because mature red blood cells, having no mitochondria, respire by anaerobic metabolism (glycolysis), which produces 2,3-DPG as a side reaction. 2,3-DPG binds to hemoglobin more strongly than to HbO_2, and this binding reduces the affinity of hemoglobin for O_2. Increases in 2,3-DPG occur in chronic hypoxemia (decreased Pao_2) and decreased blood $[H^+]$, whereas 2,3-DPG levels decrease in blood stored for transfusions.

> One of the factors that favors O_2 diffusion across the placenta to the developing fetus is that fetal hemoglobin produced in utero is not affected by 2,3-DPG; therefore fetal HbO_2 has a slightly greater affinity for O_2 than maternal HbO_2. Furthermore, the hemoglobin concentration in fetal blood is high (≤ 200 g/L). Thus the fetus's arterial blood has nearly the same O_2 concentration as that of the mother, even though the fetus's arterial Po_2 is less than 40 mm Hg.

Myoglobin stores O_2 in the skeletal muscles

If the hemoglobin molecule were separated into its four globin chains, each with one heme group, the result would be a molecule very much like **oxymyoglobin (MbO_2),** which is the O_2-binding heme protein (molecular weight, 16,500) in skeletal muscle cells. The important physiological features of the MbO_2 equilibrium curve are that it lies far to the left of the HbO_2 equilibrium curve and that it has a hyperbolic shape (purple line in Figure 30-3, *A*). Because each MbO_2 molecule has only one heme group, there cannot be any molecular interaction. Also, because of the low Po_2 at which MbO_2 binds O_2, MbO_2 is unsuited for O_2 transport. However, MbO_2 IS USEFUL FOR STORING O_2 TEMPORARILY IN SKELETAL MUSCLE CELLS, WHERE THE Po_2 IS NORMALLY LOW AND IN THE RANGE OVER WHICH MbO_2 IS ONLY PARTLY SATURATED. The P_{50} of MbO_2 is less than 5 mm Hg.

Carbon monoxide and nitric oxide have high affinities for O_2

Carbon monoxide (CO) is an odorless and colorless gas that has 240 times the affinity for hemoglobin than O_2. Figure 30-3, *B*, also shows the equilibrium curve for pathological **carboxyhemoglobin.** CO associates readily with hemoglobin but does not dissociate appreciably unless its partial pressure is less than 1.0 mm Hg. CO binding to hemoglobin is competitive with that to O_2, so CO binding reduces the O_2-carrying capacity of hemoglobin and O_2 delivery to the tissues. Therefore **CO poisoning** is a more serious problem than an equivalent reduction of hemoglobin O_2 capacity caused by anemia (Figure 30-3, *B*). Carboxyhemoglobin has a hyperbolic equilibrium curve that is shifted much farther to the left than the equilibrium curve of an equivalent hemoglobin-deficiency anemia (50% decrease in O_2 capacity). The Pao_2 level may be entirely normal in CO poisoning. **Nitric oxide (NO)** (see Chapters 23 and 29) binds to hemoglobin 200,000 times more strongly than O$_2$ and 1000 times more strongly than CO. NO is strictly a local hormone, active only at its site of production, because any NO that diffuses into the blood is rapidly and irreversibly bound by hemoglobin.

The oxidation of hemoglobin interferes with O$_2$ transport

Hemoglobin binds O$_2$ only when the iron atoms in the porphyrin rings are in the ferrous (Fe^{++}, reduced) state. One of the developmental advantages of having hemoglobin packaged within erythrocytes is that several reducing systems are present that keep hemoglobin functional. Certain chemicals (nitrates and sulfates) and drugs can oxidize the iron to the inactive ferric (Fe^{+++}) form and cause **methemoglobinemia.**

Dissolved O$_2$ contributes minimally to O$_2$ transport

Unlike CO$_2$, O$_2$ has a low physical solubility in water or whole blood, so normally, one can disregard the contribution of dissolved O$_2$ to O$_2$ transport. However, when a person breathes 100% O$_2$, the high Po$_2$ (up to 675 mm Hg at sea level: (barometric pressure minus water pressure and alveolar Pco$_2$) permits about 20 ml/L of O$_2$ to be carried in physical solution, nearly 40% of the normal arteriovenous difference in Po$_2$ in a resting individual. Dissolved O$_2$ represents 0.0031 ml for every millimeter of mercury of O$_2$ tension in 100 ml of blood. Under such conditions, the dissolved O$_2$ participates substantially in blood O$_2$ transport.

O$_2$ reserves are short term

For the body as a whole, the tissue Po$_2$ is low, and O$_2$ is poorly soluble in water. Some O$_2$ is stored in the alveoli of the lung. When the lung is at an functional residual capacity of 2.4 L and the Pao$_2$ is 100 mm Hg, there is approximately 500 ml of O$_2$ available for about 1 to 2 minutes of basal O$_2$ consumption. The circulating blood volume (about 5 L) contains 150 ml of O$_2$ per liter of blood. This quantity of O$_2$ can provide another 3 minutes of O$_2$ consumption, provided that all of it can be used. Finally, in skeletal and cardiac muscle, O$_2$ is stored in combination with MbO$_2$. However, the content of MbO$_2$ is low, only about 4 mg/g in cardiac ventricular muscle; this amount of MbO$_2$ can supply O$_2$ for 3 to 4 seconds when the basal O$_2$ consumption of the heart is normal. The MbO$_2$ concentration in skeletal muscle is less than that in the heart; the total O$_2$ stored as MbO$_2$ in skeletal muscle is less than 10 ml. This small amount of O$_2$ is useful during brief muscle contractions, when the blood flow is temporarily stopped or slowed. Overall, the O$_2$ in the body is sufficient to provide about 5 minutes of basal O$_2$ consumption.

> Victims of severe cold exposure may have a low body temperature and no detectable evidence of heartbeat or breathing for as long as 1 hour and still recover. The reason they may recover without permanent brain damage is the result of the low body temperature, which drastically reduces the O$_2$ demand by the brain and other tissues. In fact, before the advent of heart-lung bypass machines, surgeons used whole-body hypothermia to reduce O$_2$ consumption so that they could stop the heart for several minutes to do a quick surgical repair of cardiac lesions.

O$_2$ use increases with exercise

In individuals at rest, the uptake of O$_2$ (O$_2$ consumption) is estimated by determining the difference between the amount of inspired O$_2$ and the amount of expired O$_2$. From the Fick equation (see Chapter 18):

$$\dot{V}o_2 = Q(Cao_2 - C\bar{v}o_2)$$

where:

$\dot{V}o_2$ = Oxygen consumption
Q = Cardiac output in liters per minute
Cao_2 = O$_2$ content of arterial blood
$C\bar{v}o_2$ = O$_2$ content of mixed venous blood

Because the normal arterial O$_2$ content is 200 ml of O$_2$ per liter of blood, the cardiac output is 5 L/min, and the mixed venous blood content is 150 ml/L of O$_2$, the normal O$_2$ consumption 5 L/min × (200 − 150) = 250 ml/min of O$_2$. During maximal steady-state exercise, O$_2$ consumption can rise to 10 times the basal level. Well-trained athletes often have O$_2$ consumption levels greater than 3 L/min. When steady-state exercise is maximal, the cardiac output may reach 15 to 20 L/min, 70% of which goes to the exercising muscle. The total body arteriovenous concentration difference increases to about 100 ml/L of O$_2$ blood during maximal exercise. It is uncommon for steady-state S$\bar{v}o_2$ to fall below 50% (P$\bar{v}o_2$ = 29 mm Hg), although the O$_2$ saturation of venous blood from individual organs may do so (see also Chapter 26).

Respiratory Gas Diffusion in the Body

CO$_2$ diffuses twice as fast as O$_2$ across the alveolar-capillary barrier

The diffusion of O$_2$ or CO$_2$ across the alveolar-capillary barrier is favored by a large surface area, a short distance to travel from a region of high concentration to lower concentration, a large partial pressure difference, and a high diffusivity (small molecular size and high solubility in water). Diffusion is a fast, efficient process over short distances, but it can be seriously rate limiting when the distance exceeds several micrometers (see Chapter 1). Although O$_2$ is a smaller molecule than CO$_2$, CO$_2$ is much more soluble

Lung

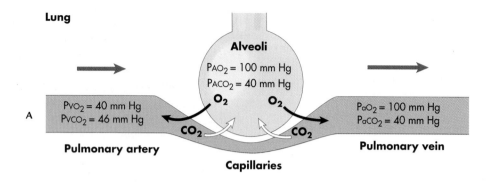

Tissue

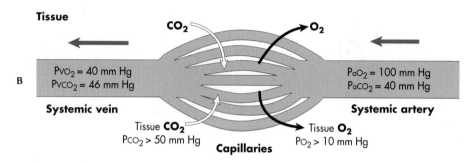

Figure 30-4 The respiratory gases O_2 and CO_2 generally diffuse in opposite directions, each along its partial pressure gradient. The diffusion streams are completely independent of each other. $PaCO_2$, Partial pressure of arterial blood oxygen; $PACO_2$, partial pressure of alveolar carbon dioxide; PAO_2, partial pressure of alveolar oxygen; $P\bar{v}CO_2$, partial pressure of mixed venous blood oxygen. **A,** Pulmonary capillaries. **B,** Systemic capillaries.

THAN O_2 IN WATER, AND CO_2 DIFFUSES ABOUT TWICE AS RAPIDLY AS O_2 ACROSS THE ALVEOLAR-CAPILLARY BARRIER. The initial partial pressure difference between CO_2 in mixed venous blood and alveolar gas is normally about 6 mm Hg, and that for O_2 is 60 mm Hg. Despite this difference in partial pressure, the **diffusivity** (diffusion coefficient multiplied by solubility) of CO_2 is much greater than that of O_2. The respiratory gases (i.e., O_2, CO_2, N_2) or anesthetic gases (i.e., ether, nitrous oxide) diffuse along their partial pressure gradients (from a region of higher to a region of lower partial pressure) independently of the movements of any other gases. Thus O_2 and CO_2 diffuse in opposite directions in the lungs and systemic capillaries, as illustrated in Figure 30-4. Some of the adaptations of the lungs for enhancing the diffusion of O_2 and CO_2 are to provide an ample alveolocapillary surface area and to provide a very thin barrier (see Chapter 27). Furthermore, the relatively large capillary blood volume in the lung (75 ml in resting men) allows blood to remain in the exchange vessels long enough (one heartbeat) for complete equilibration.

The diffusion of O_2 to tissue mitochondria is improved by capillary recruitment

Sufficient O_2 is moved from the capillary blood to the mitochondria of the tissue cells throughout the body (so that tissue respiration is aerobic) by maximizing the transit time in the systemic capillaries and minimizing the dis-tance between the capillaries and mitochondria. However, because all body organs, except the lung, are solid (mostly water), the distance from the capillaries to the mitochondria is much longer in those tissues than in the lung. Arterial blood enters the systemic capillaries at a P_{O_2} of 100 mm Hg. However, Figure 30-2 reveals that the P_{O_2} of the capillary blood must fall to below 80 mm Hg before any significant quantity of O_2 dissociates from hemoglobin. Thus the mean capillary P_{O_2} of 55 mm Hg is closer to the P_{O_2} of end-capillary blood ($P\bar{v}_{O_2}$ = 40 mm Hg) than to that of arterial blood.

As in the lungs, the driving force for O_2 diffusion depends directly on the difference between the P_{O_2} in capillary blood and the P_{O_2} in most distant mitochondria. Fortunately, mitochondria can perform oxidative metabolism at a tissue O_2 tension as low as 1 to 2 mm Hg. In the steady state, all mitochondria normally receive adequate amounts of O_2. A reasonable estimate of the mean resting tissue O_2 tension is about 10 mm Hg, which in skeletal muscle means that the O_2-storage protein MbO_2 is about 75% saturated (Figure 30-3, *A*). In the left ventricular myocardium, which requires a large O_2 supply per unit mass, the capillaries are about 25 μm apart, the width of one left ventricular muscle fiber (see Chapter 25). Thus from each capillary, O_2 must diffuse outward within a tissue cylinder radius of about 13 μm. Although that distance seems short, it is 10 times greater than that across the alveolocapillary barrier in the lung. In brain cortex, the capillaries are about 40 μm apart, and in resting skeletal muscle, they are about 80 μm apart. THE BODY'S MOST EFFECTIVE MECHANISM FOR IMPROVING O_2 DELIVERY TO TISSUE CELLS IS TO DECREASE THE DIFFUSION PATH LENGTH BY RECRUITING MORE FUNCTIONAL CAPILLARIES. This process also increases the capillary surface area across which O_2 diffuses. In skeletal muscle the functional capillary density increases threefold during heavy exercise (see Chapters 23 and 26).

There are five clinical causes of low PO_2 (hypoxemia): hypoxia, hypoventilation, ventilation/perfusion mismatching, right-to-left shunt, and diffusion abnormality. **Hypoxia** refers to a reduced inspired O_2 concentration, which may occur at high altitudes or because of a reduced O_2-carrying capacity (as a result of anemia or CO poisoning). **Hypoventilation** produces hypoxia because of inadequate ventilation (see Equation 28-3). Areas of the lung with low ventilation/perfusion ratios (**ventilation/perfusion mismatching**) may produce hypoxemia (see Chapter 29). **Right-to-left shunts** may occur with congenital abnormalities such as atrial septal defect, in which blood is being shunted from the right atrium to the left atrium without being oxygenated in the pulmonary circulation. The sum of anatomical shunts and the shuntlike effect of lung units with low ventilation/perfusion ratios is called **venous admixture**. Last, **diffusion problems** across the alveolar-capillary barrier may produce hypoxemia. The diffusion of O_2 from the alveolus to the capillary may be impaired by **interstitial fibrosis (pulmonary fibrosis)** or **edema** (congestive heart failure).

CO₂ Transport

The respiratory quotient is determined by the ratio of CO₂ production to O₂ consumption

Metabolic CO_2 transport is solely a function of systemic venous blood, just as metabolic O_2 transport is solely a function of systemic arterial blood (Figure 30-1). Under basal steady-state conditions, humans exhale 80 molecules of CO_2 for every 100 molecules of O_2 taken up from the alveoli into the pulmonary capillary blood. This ratio is called the **respiratory exchange ratio.** It is calculated by dividing the CO_2 production by the O_2 consumption. This ratio is normally 80/100, or 0.8.

In the steady state the respiratory exchange ratio is the same as the **respiratory quotient:** the latter applies to the respiratory events at the mitochondria (aerobic oxidation). The respiratory exchange ratio can vary from 0.7 (lipid metabolism) to 1.0 (carbohydrate metabolism); amino acids yield an intermediate value (0.85) (see Chapter 41). Lipid is the major fuel under basal conditions because the respiratory exchange ratio is about 0.8.

During exercise, athletes can increase cardiac output twofold and increase O_2 consumption tenfold. With progressively higher workloads, the O_2 supply becomes inadequate, and anaerobic metabolism begins. As the body tissues become more acidic (because of the formation of lactic acid and other acids), the body stores of carbonic acid (mainly as bicarbonate [HCO_3^-]) are converted to CO_2 gas and are exhaled. Therefore carbon dioxide production starts to outpace O_2 consumption (**anaerobic** or **ventilatory threshold**). The anaerobic threshold is the highest O_2 uptake during exercise above which sustained lactic acidosis occurs. The respiratory exchange ratio often reaches levels of 1.0 to 1.2 during heavy exercise or anaerobic metabolism. In disease states, O_2 consumption may be decreased as a result of inadequate cardiac output (e.g., congestive heart failure) or inadequate ventilation (e.g., emphysema).

CO₂ is transported mainly by bicarbonate in the blood

IN CONTRAST TO HEMOGLOBIN AND ITS REVERSIBLE BINDING OF O_2, NO SINGLE EFFICIENT CO_2-TRANSPORT MOLECULE EXISTS IN BLOOD. HOWEVER, THREE MECHANISMS ACHIEVE CO_2 TRANSPORT: DISSOLVED CO_2, CARBAMINOHEMOGLOBIN COMPOUNDS, AND SODIUM BICARBONATE, as shown in Figure 30-5. Because CO_2 is 20 times more soluble in blood than O_2, about 10% of systemic venous CO_2 transport occurs by physical solution, even though the normal difference in the arteriovenous PCO_2 is only 6 mm Hg. Carbaminohemoglobin is CO_2 bound to the amine side groups (NH_2) available on the amino acids in hemoglobin, and it accounts for about 30% of the normal venous CO_2 transport. CO_2 diffuses into red blood cells and reacts with hemoglobin-NH_2 to form carbaminohemoglobin, which dissociates into $NHCOO^-$ and H^+ (Figure 30-5).

Sodium bicarbonate is the principal form by which CO_2 is carried in blood. As CO_2 is formed and diffuses into capillary blood, it reacts with water to form carbonic acid, which in turn instantly dissociates to form H^+ and HCO_3^-:

$$CO_2 + H_2O \xleftrightarrow{CA} H_2CO_3 \leftrightarrow H^+ + HCO_3^- \qquad \textbf{30-1}$$

where CA is carbonic anhydrase. However, the formation of carbonic acid proceeds relatively slowly, with a half-time of many seconds. This process is too slow because each unit of blood passes through capillaries in about 1 second and arrives at the lungs within 30 seconds. Circulation time (one trip around the body) averages 60 seconds. The enzyme **carbonic anhydrase** is present in red blood cells (and many other body cells) but not present in plasma. Carbonic anhydrase catalyzes the reaction shown in Equation 30-1; it speeds up the reaction more than 10,000-fold in either direction depending on the PCO_2 and HCO_3^-. Thus the HCO_3^- concentration rises or falls more rapidly in erythrocytes than in the plasma in the capillaries.

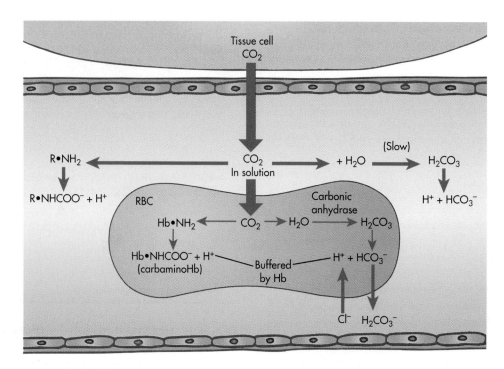

Figure 30-5 CO_2 transport in blood and a red blood cell *(RBC)*. As CO_2 diffuses into capillary blood from the peripheral tissues, it may slowly react with water to form carbonic acid or with the amine side groups of plasma proteins to form carbamino compounds. However, the majority of CO_2 diffuses into the red cell, where it rapidly forms carbonic acid, a reaction catalyzed by carbonic anhydrase. The HCO_3^- ions formed by this reaction are transported out of the red cell and exchanged with Cl^- (Cl^- shift). As hemoglobin *(Hb)* loses its O_2, it becomes more able to bind CO_2 to its NH_2 side groups to form carbaminohemoglobin compounds. In addition, hemoglobin is a weaker acid when deoxygenated, which facilitates the buffering of H^+ ions released during CO_2 hydration.

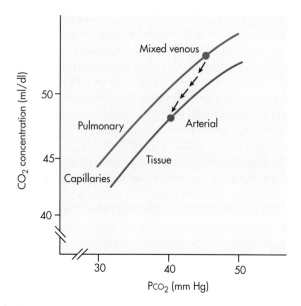

Figure 30-6 CO_2 equilibrium curves for normal systemic arterial and mixed venous blood. In the pulmonary capillaries, as the P_{O_2} of the blood increases, the $[H^+]$ of the red cells tends to rise. (HbO_2 is a stronger acid than hemoglobin.) Thus CO_2 is liberated from carbamino compounds and from HCO_3^- (leftward shift of the CO_2 equilibrium curve). Conversely, in the tissue capillaries, as the P_{O_2} of the blood decreases, the erythrocyte cytoplasm becomes less acidic, and more CO_2 can be carried by the blood (rightward shift of the CO_2 equilibrium curve). Therefore oxygenated blood carries less CO_2 for the same P_{CO_2} (Haldane effect).

The red blood cell membrane is very permeable to HCO_3^- and other anions. Hence HCO_3^- diffuses rapidly between the erythrocyte and plasma along its concentration gradient. As with other mammalian cell membranes, the red cell membrane is not very permeable to cations (i.e., Na^+, K^+, H^+). However, the laws of physical chemistry require electrical neutrality in the bulk phase of solutions. To achieve this, Cl^-, the main plasma anion, diffuses along its concentration gradient and counterbalances the flux of HCO_3^-. This exchange of Cl^- for HCO_3^- in tissue or pulmonary capillaries is called the **Cl^- shift.**

The CO_2 equilibrium curve for venous blood is shifted to the left

As a result of the three mechanisms for CO_2 transport previously described, the CO_2 concentration in whole blood varies with the P_{CO_2}, but here the analogy to the HbO_2 equilibrium curve completely breaks down. Over the range of P_{CO_2} found in life, the CO_2 equilibrium curve is essentially a straight line (Figure 30-6). The CO_2 equilibrium curve of systemic venous blood at a P_{O_2} of 40 mm Hg is shifted to the left of that for systemic arterial blood at a P_{O_2} of 100 mm Hg. This relationship improves O_2 dissociation in capillaries (the Bohr effect). This CO_2 equilibrium curve shift increases the transport of CO_2 in systemic venous blood and is referred to as the **Haldane effect.** The Haldane effect is attributed to the fact that deoxygenated hemoglobin is a weaker acid than HbO_2.

The regulation of CO_2 is essential to acid-base balance

The role of P_{CO_2} and its associated products (carbonic acid and HCO_3^-) as part of the various H^+ buffer systems of the body is covered more fully in the renal section (see Chapter 39). The alveolar ventilation equation (see Chapter 28) describes how the body's P_{CO_2} regulates or is regulated by breathing. When the systemic arterial blood $[H^+]$ rises, as it does in **metabolic acidosis** (see Chapter 39), the body's P_{CO_2} also rises. This response stimulates the brain to increase alveolar ventilation, which acts to return P_{CO_2} toward normal. On the other hand, if alveolar ventilation is impaired, as in **respiratory insufficiency** (advanced emphysema is the most common cause), alveolar P_{CO_2} rises and increases the body's P_{CO_2}, which characterizes **respiratory acidosis.** The increase in ventilation that occurs during exercise results in decreased alveolar P_{CO_2}. This decreases the body's $[H^+]$; this condition is called **respiratory alkalosis.** Likewise, the loss of body acids, such as during prolonged vomiting, leads to **metabolic alkalosis.** This decreases alveolar ventilation, which raises body P_{CO_2} and HCO_3^- concentration. Thus there are four distinct abnormalities of acid-base balance, two caused mainly by changes in breathing and P_{CO_2} (respiratory acidosis and alkalosis) and two in which secondary, compensatory changes in breathing and P_{CO_2} occur (metabolic acidosis and alkalosis).

S UMMARY

- O_2 is transported from the lungs to the systemic capillaries in arterial blood, whereas CO_2 formed by aerobic metabolism is transported from the systemic tissues to the lungs in venous blood.
- Hemoglobin quickly and reversibly binds with O_2. The O_2 capacity of normal human blood is 200 ml/L of O_2 (absolute concentration) or 100% saturation (relative concentration).
- The nature of the association between O_2 and hemoglobin, as defined by the HbO_2 equilibrium curve, is well suited for the loading of O_2 in the lungs and for its unloading in systemic tissue capillaries.
- Normal physiological factors that affect the association between hemoglobin and O_2 are $[H^+]$, P_{CO_2}, temperature, and the concentration of 2,3-DPG in erythrocytes. Increases in any of these factors are reflected by a shift in the position of the HbO_2 curve to the right, which denotes a decrease in the affinity of hemoglobin for O_2.
- O_2 affinity decreases as blood passes through the systemic capillaries because the P_{CO_2} and $[H^+]$ in the capillary blood increase. This reduced affinity increases the unloading of O_2 in the systemic capillaries; the reverse change occurs in the lung and favors O_2 uptake.
- The shape of the HbO_2 equilibrium curve indicates that in the systemic capillaries, hemoglobin releases large quantities of O_2 as the P_{O_2} falls below 70 mm Hg.
- The association between O_2 and hemoglobin is affected by CO, which has an affinity for hemoglobin more than 200 times greater than O_2. Even in very low concentrations, CO combines avidly with hemoglobin, interferes with O_2 binding, and destroys heme group interactions.
- The diffusion of O_2 between body compartments depends on the P_{O_2} difference. The principal diffusion limitation for O_2 is from the systemic capillaries through several micrometers of interstitial fluid to the mitochondria of the respiring cells.
- The number of actively perfused capillaries is an important mechanism for increasing O_2 diffusion to skeletal muscle cells during muscle activity.
- CO_2 is produced by aerobic metabolism in mitochondria. The CO_2 diffuses into systemic capillary blood and is transported to the lungs, where it diffuses into alveolar gas and is exhaled.
- CO_2 is transported in blood via a combination of three mechanisms: physical solution, carbaminohemoglobin, and the principal transport molecule, HCO_3^-.
- CO_2 slowly combines chemically with water to produce carbonic acid. In erythrocytes the enzyme carbonic anhydrase catalyzes this reaction.
- Once formed, carbonic acid dissociates instantly into H^+ and HCO_3^-. The H^+ is removed by combining chemically with the enormous amount of hemoglobin within the red cells. The HCO_3^- diffuses out of the red cells in exchange for Cl^- (Cl^- shift).
- There are four deviations of acid-base balance from normal. Respiratory acidosis and alkalosis are caused primarily by changes in breathing and P_{CO_2}, and metabolic acidosis and alkalosis are caused by changes in the blood $[H^+]$ with compensatory changes in breathing and the P_{CO_2}.

BIBLIOGRAPHY

Bidami A: Analysis of abnormalities of capillary CO_2 exchange in vivo, *J Appl Physiol* 70:1686, 1991.

Fencl V, Leith DE: Stewart's quantitative acid-base chemistry: applications in biology and medicine, *Respir Physiol* 91:1, 1993.

Heidelberger E, Reeves RB: O_2 transfer kinetics in a whole blood unicellular thin layer, *J Appl Physiol* 68:1854, 1990.

Hlastala MP, Swenson ER: Blood-gas transport. In Fishman AP et al, eds: *Pulmonary diseases and disorders*, ed 3, New York, 1998, McGraw-Hill.

Jennings DB: The physiochemistry of $[H^+]$ and respiratory control: roles of P_{CO_2}, strong ions, and their hormonal regulators, *Can J Physiol Pharmacol* 72:1499, 1994.

Reeves RB, Park HK: CO uptake kinetics of red cells and CO diffusing capacity, *Respir Physiol* 88:1, 1992.

Rose B: *Clinical physiology of acid-base and electrolyte disorders,* ed 4, New York, 1994, McGraw-Hill.

Swenson ER et al: In vivo quantification of carbonic anhydrase and band 3 protein contributions to pulmonary gas exchange, *J Appl Physiol* 74:838, 1993.

Wasserman K et al: *Principles of exercise testing and interpretation,* ed 2, Philadelphia, 1994, Lea & Febiger.

Weibel ER et al: Morphometric model for pulmonary diffusing capacity. I. Membrane diffusing capacity, *Respir Physiol* 93:125, 1993.

CASE STUDIES

Case 31-1

A 20-year-old man is rescued from a fire and brought to the emergency department. His vital signs (i.e., heart rate, blood pressure, respiratory rate) are stable, and he has evidence of smoke inhalation. The results of an arterial blood test demonstrates the following values while the subject is breathing 100% O_2:

Arterial P_{O_2}	190 mm Hg
Arterial P_{CO_2}	36 mm Hg
pH	7.47
Sa_{O_2}	60%
Carboxyhemoglobin value	40%
Barometric pressure	738 mm Hg

1. **Which of the following is a true statement about the effect of smoke inhalation on this patient's O_2 transport?**

    A. O_2 delivery would not be affected because the Pa_{O_2} is normal.

    B. The HbO_2 equilibrium curve would be shifted downward and to the left.

    C. The O_2 saturation is reduced; therefore carboxyhemoglobin delivers some O_2 to the tissue.

    D. The increase in pH accounts for a rightward shift of the HbO_2 equilibrium curve.

    E. O_2 content will be normal or above normal because the Pa_{O_2} is 190 mm Hg.

2. **When this patient is breathing 100% O_2, what is the alveolar-arterial O_2 pressure gradient?**

    A. 500 mm Hg

    B. 300 mm Hg

    C. 200 mm Hg

    D. 100 mm Hg

    E. 10 mm Hg

Case 30-2

A 70-year-old woman has a history of chronic anemia. She is admitted to the intensive care unit for the treatment of shock resulting from a urinary tract infection that spread to her bloodstream. She is on a mechanical ventilator (inspired O_2, 60%), and a pulmonary artery catheter is in place. Physical examination reveals that she is febrile (39° C) and has a low blood pressure (90/60 mm Hg). The following information is obtained:

Arterial blood gas levels	
$\quad Pa_{O_2}$	60 mm Hg
$\quad Pa_{CO_2}$	35 mm Hg
$\quad$ pH	7.27
$\quad Sa_{O_2}$	92%
$\quad$ Hemoglobin value	7 g/dl
Cardiac output	8 L/min
Mixed venous O_2 pressure	40 mm Hg
Pulmonary artery pressure	40/20 mm Hg
$S\bar{v}_{O_2}$	73%

1. **What is the arterial O_2 content?**

    A. 150 ml/L

    B. 127 ml/L

    C. 53 ml/L

    D. 88 ml/L

    E. 208 ml/L

2. **What is the O_2 consumption?**

    A. 144 ml/min

    B. 320 ml/min

    C. 40 ml/min

    D. 660 ml/min

    E. 200 ml/min

3. **Which treatment would have the greatest effect on O_2 transport?**

    A. Transfusion of three units of red blood cells (increased hemoglobin to 10 g/dl)

    B. Increase in cardiac output by administering inotropic medications to 10 L/min

    C. Increase in inspired O_2 concentration to 100%

    D. Placement of compression trousers on the lower extremity to increase venous return

    E. Administration of antibiotics to treat the bloodstream infection

CHAPTER 31

Control of Breathing

OBJECTIVES

- Explain the factors that control breathing.
- Describe the neural and chemical regulation of breathing.
- Analyze the effects of sleep and high altitude on the control of breathing.
- Describe the effects of failure of the control of breathing.

As discussed in previous chapters, the primary function of respiration is to supply O_2 and remove CO_2. For the respiratory system to perform this function, it must be tightly controlled. This chapter discusses the neural and chemical controls of respiration that are so fundamental to life. Furthermore, special alterations that occur in this system during respiratory failure, sleep, and acclimatization to altitude are discussed.

Central Organization of Breathing

Breathing is controlled mainly at the brainstem level

Two patterns are involved in the control of breathing: metabolic and volitional. **Metabolic,** or automatic, breathing is the basic pattern, and it is concerned with the regulation of the partial pressure of arterial CO_2 (Pa_{CO_2}) through the modulation of alveolar ventilation. Metabolic breathing is state dependent. For example, during slow-wave sleep, the respiratory drive is diminished, and minute ventilation is reduced by 1 or 2 L/min, resulting in an increased partial pressure of alveolar CO_2 (Pa_{CO_2}). DURING METABOLIC BREATHING, BOTH THE RATE (FREQUENCY) AND THE DEPTH OF BREATHING (TIDAL VOLUME), WHICH DETERMINE MINUTE VENTILATION, ARE REGULATED SO THAT THE Pa_{CO_2} AND Pa_{CO_2} ARE MAINTAINED CLOSE TO 40 MM Hg, as established by the alveolar ventilation equation (see Equation 28-2). Although the Pa_{CO_2}-sensitive mechanism is the main controller, it can be overridden in systemic arterial hypoxemia (e.g., during acclimatization to high altitude) by a controller sensitive to the partial pressure of arterial O_2 (Pa_{O_2}).

The **metabolic controller** (respiratory neuronal groups in Figure 31-1) resides within the brainstem. Formerly, the neurons responsible for inspiration and expiration were believed to be located in specific brainstem cen-

ters, but now the organization is known to be much looser. Surrounding and interdigitating throughout the brainstem is a loose network of interneurons known as the **reticular activating system** that influences the brainstem controller by affecting the state of alertness (wakefulness) of the brain. Hence breathing is regulated somewhat differently during sleep than wakefulness.

Knowledge regarding the neural basis for **volitional** control is limited. This control is known to involve the thalamus (primitive integrating system) and the cerebral cortex (higher integrating system). These areas are required to coordinate breathing in relation to the many complex but volitional motor activities involving the lungs and chest walls. Several pathways carry the rostrally located (anterior) cortical and thalamic neuronal axons caudally to the pontine and medullary controllers. Some volitional activities include talking, singing, suckling, swallowing, coughing, sneezing, defecation, parturition, and responses to anxiety and fear. Volitional control of ventilation allows ventilation to be altered but within limits; for example, breath-holding has its limits. Like the metabolic controller, volitional control can modify the rate and depth of breathing (see Chapter 28).

> Defining the brain centers involved in breathing is one area in which patients with neurological disorders have provided important insights. For example, after **head trauma** that damages the pons, a patient may breathe with inspiratory breath-holds that last many seconds, followed by brief exhalations; this pattern is called **apneustic breathing.**

Respiration is controlled by two areas in the brainstem

Two regions in the brainstem contain the intrinsic breathing controllers: the **medullary respiratory areas** and the **pontine respiratory group (PRG).** The precise anatomical and functional organization of the respiratory medullary neurons is still under investigation. The current schema, in which regional groups of mixed respiratory neurons (dorsal, ventral, and pontine) exhibit phasic discharges locked to either the inspiratory or expiratory phase of the respiratory cycle is depicted in Figure 31-1. Note also that the cranial nerves to the face, mouth, throat, and lungs, which must be coordinated in metabolic and volitional breathing activities, are close to the respiratory neuron groups.

The medullary respiratory areas include the **dorsal respiratory group (DRG)** and **ventral respiratory group (VRG)** of neurons. The DRG acts as the initial processing station for afferent feedback from the airways, lungs, and peripheral chemoreceptors. The DRG also provides excitatory inspiratory stimuli to the phrenic motor neurons. The VRG contains axons to cranial motor neurons and bulbospinal axons to the phrenic and intercostal respiratory motor neurons that exhibit respiratory cycle rhythmicity. Transection of the **PRG (pneumotaxic center)** with vagotomy results in **apneustic breathing,** which is characterized by long inspiratory phases (transection level 2 of Figure 31-2). The function of the PRG in respiration is unclear, but it may be involved in the change from inspiration to expiration and vice versa.

The respiratory motor neurons that traverse the spinal cord along the ventral horn can be influenced at many levels. Excitation and inhibition of the respiratory muscles (i.e., diaphragm, intercostal and abdominal muscles) involve segmental interneuronal networks. For example, inhibition of the antagonist muscles takes place through interneurons that travel between the motor neurons of the inspiratory and expiratory muscles. Stretch of the intercostal muscles or electrical stimulation of sensory input into T9 to T12 excites the intercostal and phrenic motor neurons to enlarge the thoracic cavity. In contrast, stimuli to segments T1 to T8 inhibit phrenic motor neuron activity and terminate inspiration. Spinal reflexes are important because they augment muscle force when the resistance to breathing is increased or lung compliance is decreased.

Normal people cannot breathe and swallow simultaneously without gagging or coughing. However, a newborn can. A baby is born with a large flexible epiglottis to direct incoming milk laterally into the oropharynx, down

---

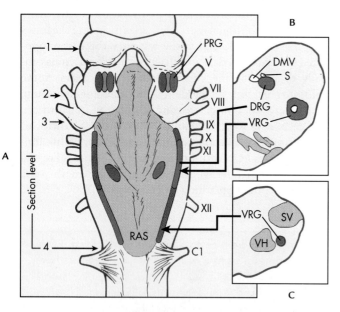

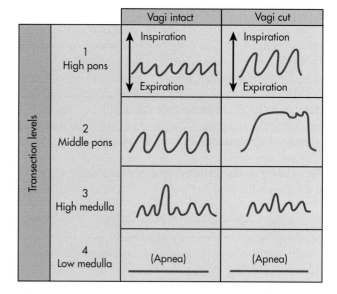

Figure 31-1 Brainstem (dorsal view) **(A)** and cross sections **(B and C)** at the midmedulla and caudal medulla, respectively, illustrating locations of the dorsal *(DRG)*, ventral *(VRG)*, and pontine *(PRG)* respiratory neuron groups (the metabolic controllers of breathing). The colors roughly indicate the locations of neurons that fire during inspiration *(red)*, expiration *(blue)*, or both *(yellow)*. The reticular activating system *(RAS)* surrounds and interdigitates with the various neuronal groups. The roman numerals (right side of **A**) show the corresponding cranial nerves, some of which have both sensory and motor divisions. The arabic numerals (left side of **A**) show the classic levels of brainstem transections *(1 to 4)*, which helped early physiologists to localize the respiratory neuron groups. Breathing patterns caused by successive ablations from rostral to caudal are shown in Figure 31-2. *C1,* First cervical nerve; *DMV,* dorsal motor nucleus of the vagus; *S,* nucleus of the tractus solitarius; *SV,* spinal trigeminal nucleus; *VH,* ventral horn.

Figure 31-2 Different patterns of breathing produced by successive transections of the brainstem in anesthetized animals. These patterns may also occur in humans with selected brainstem lesions. The four levels of transection correspond to the numbers in Figure 31-1, *A*. The importance of the sensory division of the vagus nerve, carrying information about the state of lung inflation, is shown by contrasting the intact to the cut columns. For transection level 1, there is no effect on the basic breathing pattern, showing that the main controller lies caudal. Furthermore, it eliminates all volitional (conscious) changes in breathing (not shown here). When vagal sensory input is eliminated, breathing slows, and tidal volume increases. Skipping down to transection level 4, breathing stops completely, showing that the main controller lies rostral. For transection level 2, as long as sensory input from the vagus nerve continues, ablation of the PRG has only a moderate slowing effect on breathing, with tidal volume increased to maintain alveolar ventilation at approximately normal. After vagotomy, apneustic breathing (deep inspiration held for many seconds) appears. For transection level 3, irregular, gasping breathing develops, which is not affected by cutting the vagus nerves. Clearly, medullary controllers are sufficient to sustain life but are not adequate for providing normal modulation of breathing.

and around the glottis. Also the breathing interrupter reflexes that are activated when swallowing begins in an older child and adult are absent in a baby. The ability to breathe and swallow simultaneously is lost at about 1 year of age.

Respiratory rhythm is regulated by the inhibition of tonic inspiratory impulses

An explanation for rhythmic breathing has been formulated into an operational model of brainstem mechanisms that generate the breathing rhythm (Figure 31-3). The system is represented by three neuron pools that are responsible for different phases of breathing. Signals (increased CO_2 tension [PCO_2] or decreased O_2 tension [PO_2]) from the central and peripheral chemoreceptors reinforce activity in inspiratory neurons that are tonically active (pool A in Figure 31-3); these neurons are located in both the DRG and VRG. Some of these neurons send axons to the phrenic nerve and intercostal muscle neurons in the spinal cord and increase their activity. Stimulation via this pathway causes inspiration.

The central inspiratory activity stimulates neurons in pool B (Figure 31-3). These neurons are also reinforced by impulses from the lung stretch receptors. As the lung expands, the stretch receptor signals become stronger. Some of the pool B neurons project anteriorly to stimulate pool C (PRG). The pool C neurons send inhibitory impulses to the inspiratory neurons in the dorsal medulla until the impulse activity in these inspiratory neurons is extinguished and inspiration ends and expiration begins. This scheme of breathing pattern generation—tonic inspiratory activity, which is inhibited only when sufficient inhibitory sig-

nals are received—is an attractive model because no spontaneous cyclic breathing rhythm is postulated and none has been found. The scheme also integrates the effects of CO_2 and O_2 (chemoreceptor activity) and other reflex stimuli into various normal and abnormal breathing patterns.

Chemoreceptor Control of Breathing

Respiration is controlled by both central and peripheral chemoreceptors

Two main types of chemoreceptors (central and peripheral) are involved in the control of breathing. By far the more important ones are located in the central nervous system at or near the ventrolateral surface of the medulla and between the origins of the seventh and tenth cranial nerves (Figure 31-4). The main **peripheral chemoreceptors** are the **carotid bodies,** which are located at the bifurcation of the common carotid arteries (see Chapter 23). Chemoreceptors are also located in the aortic arch (**aortic bodies),** but these are less studied and appear to be of minimal importance.

In awake, resting humans the **central chemoreceptors** account for about 90% of the CO_2-induced increases in ventilation. The relationship between PCO_2 and ventilation is linear (Figure 31-5). In normal individuals the average ventilatory response to inspired CO_2 is about 2.5 L/min, but the response varies among individuals of different body sizes and ages. THE MEDULLARY CHEMORECEPTOR CELLS RESPOND TO CHANGES IN THE H^+ CONCENTRATION

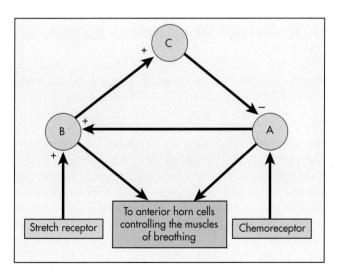

Figure 31-3 Basic wiring of the brainstem ventilatory controller. The signs on the main outputs *(arrows)* of the neuron pools indicate excitatory *(+)* or inhibitory *(−)*. The pools are named A, B, and C.

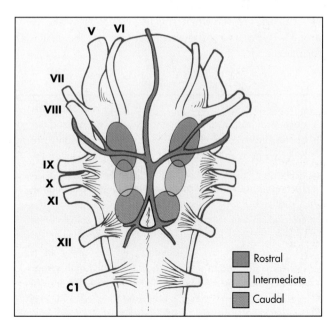

Figure 31-4 Ventral view of the brainstem, showing the locations of the central chemoreceptors. The chemosensitive cells are believed to lie just beneath the surface of the medulla. Hence they are affected by the H^+ concentration in brain interstitial and cerebrospinal fluids. *C1,* First cervical nerve.

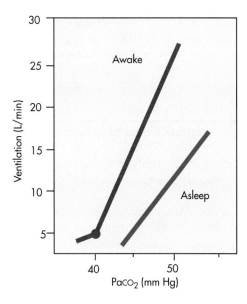

Figure 31-5 CO_2-ventilation response curve. Ventilation is sensitive to $PaCO_2$, as shown by the red line (awake). The normal operating point is 5 L/min at 40 mm Hg (large dot). In the awake (alert) state, ventilation becomes insensitive to a decrease in CO_2 below 40 mm Hg. When the reticular activating system is turned off, as during sleep (blue line), the CO_2 intercept is increased (shifted to the right), and the slope is decreased (decreased sensitivity).

OF THE INTERSTITIAL FLUID IN THE SURROUNDING BRAINSTEM AND NEARBY CEREBROSPINAL FLUID. Because CO_2 is very soluble in lipid and water, it easily crosses the blood-brain barrier and rapidly equilibrates with brain fluids. Conversely, increases in arterial blood acidity evoke much slower responses because H^+ does not readily cross the blood-brain barrier or the cell membranes. The effects of CO_2 are greater when the individual is awake (Figure 31-5) because of greater activity in the reticular formation.

One cause of respiratory failure is acute narcotic overdose with respiratory depressants such as benzodiazepines and alcohol. The effects of these depressants are reflected by a shift to the right in the CO_2-ventilation response curve and a reduction of the slope (Figure 31-5). This results in a new set point such that alveolar ventilation is reduced, $PaCO_2$ is increased, and PaO_2 is slightly decreased. In this setting, it is often helpful to calculate the alveolar-arterial PO_2 gradient to determine whether the decrease in arterial oxygenation is due solely to a decrease in alveolar ventilation or whether another reason accounts for the hypoxemia. If the alveolar-arterial gradient is normal, the gas-exchange abnormality is caused only by the respiratory depressant. If the gradient is increased, other reasons, such as ventilation/perfusion mismatching or diffusion abnormality from aspiration, must be evaluated (see Chapter 30).

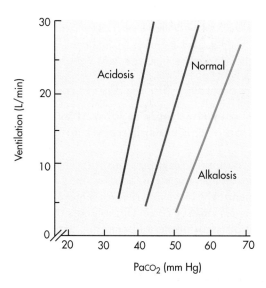

Figure 31-6 Effect of the H^+ concentration on CO_2 ventilatory response. In chronic metabolic acidosis, ventilatory sensitivity to CO_2 is increased, resulting in greater levels of ventilation than in normal or alkalotic states. *(Redrawn from Fencl V et al: J Appl Physiol 27:67, 1969.)*

Increases in $PaCO_2$ cause marked cerebral vasodilation, which is an important phenomenon to consider in patients with cerebral edema. The increased cerebral blood flow washes CO_2 from the tissues, reducing the ventilatory drive stimulated by CO_2 via the central chemoreceptors. Finally, an increased H^+ concentration in the peripheral blood stimulates the peripheral chemoreceptors. This increase in ventilatory drive then decreases the $PaCO_2$. Furthermore, in chronic acid-base disorders, metabolic acidosis increases the ventilatory sensitivity to $PaCO_2$ (red line in Figure 31-6) and metabolic alkalosis (green line in Figure 31-6) decreases the ventilatory sensitivity.

O_2 affects respiration differently than CO_2

UNLIKE THE EFFECT OF CO_2 ON VENTILATION, THE EFFECT OF A REDUCED PaO_2 ON BREATHING IS SMALL UNTIL THE PaO_2 FALLS TO 70 MM Hg. Below this level, ventilation increases in a hyperbolic fashion (Figure 31-7). The oxyhemoglobin equilibrium curve (see Figure 30-2) shows that the arterial O_2 saturation does not decrease much until the PaO_2 falls below 70 mm Hg (saturation = 94%). Therefore when the PaO_2 decreases to about 55 mm Hg, ventilation increases markedly. This stimulation is explained in part by increases in peripheral chemoreceptor activity. Low PaO_2 levels (hypoxemia) reduce K^+ channel activity in type I cells (glomus cells) in the carotid body. This results in depolarization of the type I cells, Ca^{++} influx, neurotransmitter release, and stimulation of adjacent carotid body sensory nerve terminals. Hypoxemia also affects the body's ventilatory response to CO_2. THE SENSITIVITY OF CO_2-INDUCED VENTILATION IS ENHANCED BY HYP-

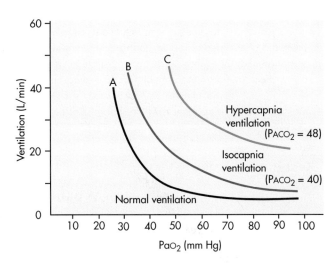

Figure 31-7 O_2-ventilation dose-response curve. *Black curve:* Ventilation is not sensitive to the PaO_2 until the tension falls below about 70 mm Hg. The normal ventilation response to decreased inspired O_2 causes the $PaCO_2$ to decrease, which opposes the hypoxic drive. *Red curve:* When the $PaCO_2$ is maintained at 40 mm Hg (isocapnic ventilation) by adding CO_2 to the inspired air, the ventilatory response begins at a higher PO_2. *Green curve:* When the $PaCO_2$ is increased (hypercarbia: $PaCO_2 = 48$ mm Hg), the ventilatory response occurs at an even higher PaO_2.

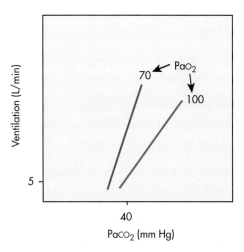

Figure 31-8 Effect of O_2 and CO_2 ventilatory response. The normal ventilatory response to CO_2 is enhanced by hypoxia; both the threshold (extrapolated X-intercept) and the sensitivity (slope of response line) are affected.

OXIA (Figure 31-8). In hyperoxia (blue line in Figure 31-8), the response of the central chemoreceptors to CO_2 is blunted.

Patients with chronic respiratory acidosis and hypercapnia who complain of air hunger or dyspnea are sometimes inadvertently given high doses of O_2. This improves the PaO_2 levels but may also contribute to respiratory failure. The higher PaO_2 blunts the patient's ventilatory response to high CO_2 levels, and they may develop CO_2 narcosis. The treatment is to remove or decrease the O_2 supply so that PaO_2 levels fall back to a range that will stimulate ventilation. In some situations, patients require mechanical ventilation until their gas exchange is back to baseline values.

Hypoxic ventilatory response is affected by CO_2 levels

The increase in ventilation induced by hypoxemia decreases the $PaCO_2$. This decrease then blunts stimulation from both the central and the peripheral chemoreceptors. Thus when a person's sensitivity to low inspired O_2 is tested, the difference between tests in which the $PaCO_2$ is maintained constant, and tests in which it is allowed to change can be distinguished. The ventilatory response to hypoxia when $PaCO_2$ is controlled at 40 mm Hg and when it is not controlled is depicted by the red line in Figure 31-7 **(isocapnia ventilation).**

Mechanical Control of Breathing

Sensory receptors in the lung provide feedback to control respiration

The three types of lung sensory receptors follow:
1. **Stretch receptors** (slowly adapting and rapidly adapting), which are located within the smooth muscle layer of the extrapulmonary airways
2. **Irritant receptors** (a type of rapidly adapting stretch receptor), which are located adjacent to the epithelial cells of the nasal cavity, pharynx, and larynx and in the bronchi
3. **C fibers** (unmyelinated), which are situated in the lung interstitium and alveolar walls

The afferent nerve fibers of all these receptors travel to the brain in the vagus nerves (cranial nerve X), and they enter the medulla adjacent to the respiratory nerve pools.

Lung stretch receptors, both slowly and rapidly adapting, are myelinated sensory nerve receptors that send impulses up the vagus nerves to the ventral medullary motor group (Figure 31-1). The slowly adapting stretch receptors are thought to be located among airway smooth muscle cells in intrathoracic and extrathoracic airways, and they are stimulated predominantly by increases in lung volume. These receptors adapt slowly to steady lung inflation. They send impulses rostrally to the PRG (pneumotaxic center), which then sends inhibitory impulses to the dorsal medullary motor group to turn off the inspiratory neurons and promote expiration **(Hering-Breuer reflex).**

Irritant receptors are a type of rapidly adapting receptor; that is, with sustained lung inflation, these nerves stop sending impulses up the vagus nerve after the initial burst of activity. These receptors are thought to be located among airway epithelial cells in the large airways. They respond to chemical stimuli such as noxious exogenous agents (e.g., cigarette smoke, sulfur dioxide, ammonia) and endogenous agents (e.g., histamine, leukotriene C_4, bradykinin) or to mechanical stimuli (e.g., particulate matter impinging on the bronchial epithelium). Irritant receptor stimulation constricts the airways and promotes rapid, shallow breathing. One likely effect of this response is to limit penetration of harmful substances deep into the lung and thereby prevent injury of the gas-exchanging surfaces. Apparently, the irritant receptors also contribute to the initiation of the periodic sighs that occur during normal breathing. These sighs expand the alveolar surface area and replenish surface-active molecules (see Chapter 28).

The unmyelinated **C fibers** are located within the bronchi and in the lung parenchyma adjacent to the pulmonary capillaries. These fibers are excited by mechanical distortion of the lung's connective tissue structure, such as that caused by fluid accumulation (edema), or by exogenous or endogenous chemicals, including capsaicin (the active irritant in pepper), histamine, bradykinin, and serotonin. Activation of the C fibers initially causes expiratory apnea, hypotension, and bradycardia, but these are quickly followed by rapid, shallow breathing. Furthermore, activation of the C fibers can produce bronchoconstriction and mucous secretion. C fibers may play a role in a variety of pulmonary pathological conditions such as pulmonary edema, pulmonary embolism, and asthma.

Chest wall receptors also help control respiration

There are various sensory nerve receptors (joint, tendon, and muscle spindles, as in other skeletal muscles) in the chest wall. **Joint receptors** are stimulated by the movement of the ribs relative to the vertebrae and the sternum. **Golgi tendon organs** are located in the intercostal muscles and diaphragm at the point of insertion of the muscle fiber into its tendon. The Golgi tendon organs monitor the force of muscle contraction and act to inhibit inspiration (and perhaps prevent the muscle from being overloaded). **Muscle spindles** are abundant in the intercostal and abdominal wall muscles but scarce in the diaphragm. The spindles help coordinate breathing during changes in posture and speech, and they stabilize the rib cage when breathing is impeded by increases in airway resistance or decreases in lung compliance.

Dyspnea is a feeling of not getting enough air to breathe. Often, this occurs in patients with underlying cardiopul-

monary disease. However, in some situations, people may complain of dyspnea at rest or during mild exercise. The sensation of dyspnea may be disproportionate to the level of cardiopulmonary impairment. On the other hand, healthy people who exercise to exhaustion, such as a marathon runner, experience severe shortness of breath.

Respiratory Failure

As lung disease progresses, it eventually reaches a stage at which alveolar ventilation is inadequate. This condition, called **respiratory failure,** means that ventilation cannot keep up with O_2 demand and CO_2 production. The alveolar ventilation equation (see Equation 28-2) indicates that $Paco_2$, $Paco_2$, and tissue Pco_2 rise during respiratory failure. This results in a respiratory and metabolic acidosis (as lactic acid and carbonic acid accumulate). Acutely, this may occur during maximal strenuous exercise. More often, it occurs in the setting of chronic respiratory failure, such as with emphysema or restrictive lung disease. In these conditions, alveolar ventilation is diminished, so gas exchange is inadequate, and $Paco_2$ is increased. Over time, the compensatory mechanisms lead to the near normalization of arterial pH despite increased levels of $Paco_2$ (see Chapters 30 and 39).

Sleep

SLEEP CONSISTS OF TWO MAIN STAGES: NON–RAPID EYE MOVEMENT (NON-REM) AND REM (DEEP SLEEP DURING WHICH DREAMING OCCURS [see also Chapter 11]). Non-REM sleep is characterized by high-voltage, low-frequency brain wave activity, and it consists of four stages of progressively deeper sleep (slow-wave sleep). REM sleep is characterized by low-voltage, high-frequency brain wave activity, rapid eye movements, and the absence of tonic muscle activity.

Sleep stages affect respiration

During slow-wave sleep, minute ventilation usually decreases. Hence the Pao_2 decreases, and the $Paco_2$ increases. The CO_2 response curve is shifted to the right (blue line in Figure 31-5). However, the ventilatory response to hypoxia, but not to hypercapnia, is maintained in slow-wave sleep.

REM sleep (dreaming) is divided into phasic and tonic substages. In tonic REM sleep, breathing is regular, but tidal volume may decrease progressively because the ventilatory responses to inspired CO_2 are less pronounced than in non-REM sleep (first stage). External stimuli and changes in blood gas tensions are less effective in producing arousal than they are in slow-wave sleep. Phasic REM sleep is associated with irregular breathing patterns be-

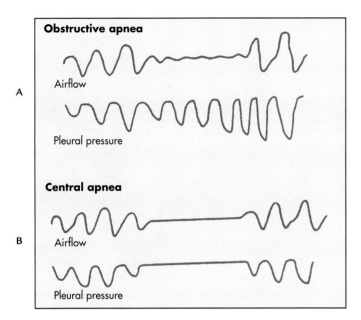

Figure 31-9 Types of sleep apnea. **A,** In obstructive sleep apnea, pleural pressure swings are augmented, indicating that airflow resistance is very high because of blockage of the oropharynx by the soft palate or tongue. **B,** Central apnea is characterized by no attempt to breathe, as demonstrated by no change in pleural pressure. O_2 desaturation is seen in both types of sleep apnea.

cause the activity of the higher brain centers modulates medullary respiratory neuronal activity.

Obstructive sleep apnea disrupts sleep

Sleep apneas are classified into three categories: obstructive, central, and mixed (Figure 31-9). **Obstructive sleep apnea** is a common sleep disorder; it affects 2% of women and 4% of men. When a person is awake, the muscles of the tongue and throat are tonically active, and they maintain a patent oropharynx. Activity of the skeletal muscle decreases during sleep; the oropharyngeal muscles are almost completely relaxed. Furthermore, the soft palate and uvula may be drawn dorsally (especially when a person sleeps in the supine position) because of the slight negative pressure in the upper airways during inspiratory airflow. This process is frequently manifested by snoring, and it indicates a partial obstruction of the oropharynx. In obstructive sleep apnea, occlusion of the oropharynx becomes complete, and airflow ceases despite continued activation of the inspiratory muscle. As shown in Figure 31-9, *A,* the hallmark of this malady is that pleural pressure cycles but there is no airflow. The apnea may last for many seconds, and the arterial O_2 saturation may fall below 75% ($Pa_{O_2} \leq 40$ mm Hg). The pleural pressure swings increase as the Pa_{CO_2} rises. Obstructive apnea occurs in all stages of sleep, but it is more common in slow-wave sleep. It ends as a result of activation of the arousal response evoked by chemical and mechanical stimuli. Often, this arousal proceeds to a

lighter stage of sleep and thereby activates the upper airway muscles and opens the upper airway. These arousals can occur frequently (in some patients, more than 100 times per hour) and thus profoundly disrupt the quality of sleep.

> **Obstructive sleep apnea** has a number of important clinical implications. It is the leading cause of excessive daytime sleepiness and probably leads to a significant number of motor vehicle accidents each year. It contributes to the development of high blood pressure, pulmonary hypertension, right-sided heart failure, chronic respiratory failure, cardiac arrhythmias during sleep, and possibly sudden death.

Respiratory drive is abnormal in central sleep apnea

Central sleep apnea is characterized by a cessation of all breathing efforts as a result of transient decreases in respiratory drive. As shown in Figure 31-9, *B,* the hallmark of central sleep apnea is no attempt to breathe. In addition to no airflow, pleural pressure does not change. **Periodic breathing,** a type of central apnea, is characterized by the regular waxing and waning of ventilation as a result of fluctuations in the central respiratory drive. Central sleep apnea includes a number of disorders with three potential abnormalities of respiratory control:

1. Defect in the respiratory control system (such as in the chronic alveolar hypoventilation syndrome) or respiratory neuromuscular apparatus
2. Transient fluctuations in respiratory drive (see later examples)
3. Reflex inhibition of central respiratory drive (such as that induced by aspiration)

Cheyne-Stokes respiration, a type of periodic breathing, is characterized by cycles of hypopneas (decreased breathing effort associated with reduced airflow) or apneas alternating with hyperpnea (hyperventilation). This breathing pattern, during which the systemic Pa_{CO_2} and Pa_{O_2} fluctuate markedly, may appear in healthy individuals in the transition from wakefulness to sleep. While the subject is awake, a threshold for P_{CO_2} to drive ventilation is set. During transition to sleep, the Pa_{CO_2} level is below the new threshold value for sleep. During this time, a period of hypopnea or apnea may occur until the Pa_{CO_2} drifts up to the critical threshold level.

Another potential explanation for Cheyne-Stokes breathing is related to delays in information transfer, during which the transit time of respiratory stimulants around the circulation is prolonged. Ordinarily, changes in Pa_{CO_2} are sensed by the central chemoreceptors within several seconds. In severe congestive heart failure, in which cardiac output may be only half of nor-

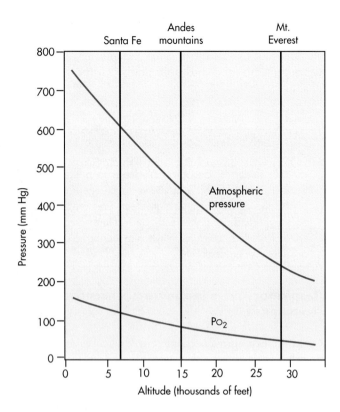

Figure 31-10 The barometric pressure and P_{O_2} fall exponentially as a person ascends to high altitude. Vertical lines show some locations relative to human ability to live at altitude. Santa Fe, New Mexico, at 7000 feet (barometric pressure = 585 mm Hg, P_{O_2} = 118 mm Hg), is the highest large U.S. city. The highest permanent human community is in the Andes mountains at about 15,000 feet (barometric pressure = 430 mm Hg, P_{O_2} = 90 mm Hg). The top of Mt. Everest is at 29,000 feet (barometric pressure = 235 mm Hg, P_{O_2} = 49 mm Hg).

mal, the time required for the blood to circulate from the lungs to the central chemoreceptors is prolonged. Therefore the controller "hunts" for an appropriate level of response; that is, the controller increases and decreases ventilation as it seeks a level that will maintain the Pa_{CO_2} in the normal range.

Biot's breathing is another form of central apnea; it is characterized by periods of normal breathing interrupted suddenly by periods of apnea. This breathing pattern occurs in patients with central nervous system diseases (e.g., meningitis). The mechanism for this pattern is unclear.

Acclimatization to Altitude

Barometric pressure and inspired P_{O_2} decrease with increasing altitude (Figure 31-10); the relationship is approximately exponential. As a person ascends to higher altitudes, the resulting systemic arterial hypoxemia elicits a variety of compensatory responses. Some of these occur quickly, whereas others develop gradually during prolonged exposure (weeks). The initial hyperventilation that occurs at high altitude is caused by stimula-

tion of the peripheral chemoreceptors, particularly the carotid bodies. The increase in ventilation reduces the Pa_{CO_2} and H^+ concentration. These changes decrease the excitation of central chemoreceptors and thus act as a negative-feedback mechanism (opposing the hypoxia-induced hyperventilation). After a person has spent a few days at high altitude, ventilation increases further until breathing achieves a new steady state. Acclimatization occurs in part via the following mechanisms:

1. The renal excretion of Na^+ reduces the plasma bicarbonate concentration, which raises the blood H^+ concentration toward normal (decreases pH to near normal).

2. At the same time, the bicarbonate concentration is decreased in brain interstitial fluid, probably by an active metabolic process that moves Na^+ from the brain interstitial fluid into the blood.

3. A small amount of anaerobic metabolism may occur in the hypoxic brain and allow the lactate anions in the brain to replace bicarbonate ions.

Another important acclimatization response is reflected by a leftward shift of the ventilatory response to CO_2 and a steepening of the slope of the response curve (increased sensitivity) caused by the interaction with a reduced Pa_{O_2} (Figure 31-8). Consequently, the threshold for central breathing stimulation occurs at a lower P_{CO_2}. Overall, the acclimatization process decreases the negative feedback that opposes the carotid chemoreceptor–induced drive to increase ventilation; hence the rate and depth of breathing increase.

Exposure to high altitude also increases the circulating hemoglobin concentration as more erythropoietin is manufactured and secreted by the hypoxic kidney cells. The concentration of 2,3-diphosphoglycerate also rises in the red blood cells and decreases the affinity of hemoglobin for O_2 (rightward shift of the curve). The P_{O_2} at 50% hemoglobin saturation is increased, and the higher P_{O_2} improves the unloading of O_2 in the systemic capillaries (see Chapter 30). Occasionally, the tolerance of high altitude disappears and serious symptoms, such as ventilatory depression, severe **polycythemia** (hematocrit may rise above 60%), high-altitude pulmonary edema, and high-altitude cerebral edema, develop. This intolerance to altitude **(chronic mountain sickness)** is relieved by the descent to a lower altitude or by the administration of O_2. People who have suffered from chronic mountain sickness should never go to high altitude again.

SUMMARY

- There are two main components to the regulation of breathing. Metabolic (automatic) control is concerned with delivering O_2 and maintaining normal levels of Pa_{CO_2}. Volitional control is related to coordinated activities during which breathing may be temporarily suspended or altered.

- The respiratory control system consists of a central controller (driver) located in the brainstem (medulla and pons), an effector (the muscles of the chest wall, especially the diaphragm), and various sensory receptors, which report the results of the intended action back to the central controller.

- The brainstem controller contains a tonically active inspiratory neuron pool that receives input from a variety of sensors. As lung volume increases, the summed sensory input from various receptors inhibits inspiratory activity.

- The cortex, thalamus, and hypothalamus alter volitional breathing by temporarily overriding the brainstem pattern generator.

- The sensory components of breathing control include central chemoreceptors (near the surface of the medulla), peripheral chemoreceptors (carotid bodies), and proprioceptors (lung stretch, irritant, and C-fiber receptors; muscle spindles; and Golgi tendon and joint organs).

- The medullary receptors are sensitive to the P_{CO_2} in the brain and cerebrospinal fluid.

- The carotid body chemoreceptors are sensitive mainly to a substantially reduced Pa_{O_2}.

- Irritant receptors in the nose and large airways protect the delicate alveolar surfaces from inhaled water, particles, and chemical vapors.

- C-fiber receptors in the lung interstitium are stimulated by distortion of the alveolar walls.

- Sleep is a complex phenomenon that consists of non-REM and REM sleep. Sensitivities to CO_2 and O_2 are both diminished, and the reticular activating system is depressed.

- The immediate hyperventilation that occurs at high altitude is caused by stimulation of the peripheral chemoreceptors via a lower Pa_{O_2}.

- The chronic adjustments to hypoxia are achieved by the restoration of the pH in the brain interstitium and cerebrospinal fluid.

BIBLIOGRAPHY

Berger AJ: Control of breathing. In Murray J, Nadel J, eds: *Textbook of respiratory medicine,* ed 2, Philadelphia, 1994, WB Saunders.

Coleridge JCG, Coleridge HMG: Afferent vagal C fibre innervation of the lung and airways and its functional significance, *Rev Physiol Biochem Pharmacol* 99:1, 1984.

Lydic R: State-dependent aspects of regulatory physiology, *FASEB J* 1:6, 1987.

Phillipson EA: Sleep disorders. In Murray J, Nadel J, eds: *Textbook of respiratory medicine,* ed 2, Philadelphia, 1994, WB Saunders.

Schiaefke ME: Central chemosensitivity: a respiratory drive, *Rev Physiol Biochem Pharmacol* 90:171, 1981.

von Euler C: On the central pattern generator for the basic breathing rhythmicity, *J Appl Physiol* 55:1647, 1983.

von Euler C, Lagercrantz H, eds: *Neurobiology of the control of breathing,* New York, 1987, Raven.

▷ **C**ASE **S**TUDIES

Case 31-1

A young, previously healthy man was in a motor vehicle accident and fractured his cervical vertebrae, which resulted in spinal transection at C2. When he arrived at the hospital, he was alert and oriented. The results of a physical examination revealed a blood pressure of 90/60 mm Hg. His respiratory rate was 26 breaths/min, but his pattern of breathing was abnormal. He demonstrated paradoxical breathing (outward movement of his abdominal muscles with inspiration).

1. **Which one of the following structures of respiratory control has been affected by this injury?**
   A. Middle pons
   B. Medulla
   C. Reticular activating system
   D. Phrenic nerve
   E. DRG

2. **Which one of the following effects on breathing would *not* be noted in this patient?**
   A. Periods of apneic episodes during sleep
   B. A reduced vital capacity
   C. Mild hypercapnia and hypoxemia
   D. Lack of diaphragmatic movement noted on examination
   E. A reduced maximal inspiratory pressure indicative of inspiratory muscle weakness

Case 31-2

An obese 56-year-old woman complains of fatigue, sleepiness, and morning headaches. She admits to sleep disruption, and her husband states that she is a loud snorer. She states that she no longer drives long distances because she is afraid she will fall asleep at the wheel. In addition, over the past month, she has noticed swelling in her legs. On physical examination, she weighs 320 pounds and is 5 feet, 4 inches tall. Her respiratory rate is 22 breaths/min and regular. Her oropharynx is narrow, and her uvula is elongated. The results of the remainder of her examination are normal, except for mild pitting edema of the lower extremities. When she breathes room air, her arterial blood gas levels are Pa_{O_2}, 58 mm Hg; Pa_{CO_2}, 67 mm Hg; pH, 7.35; and saturation of arterial O_2, 86%. Her hemoglobin concentration is 14 g/dl.

1. **The physician suspects that the patient has obstructive sleep apnea, and an overnight polysomnogram is ordered. Which one of the following**

findings on the polysomnogram would the physician *not* expect to find?

A. Absence of airflow for periods up to 60 seconds and decreased O_2 saturation

B. Absence of airflow for periods up to 60 seconds despite abdominal and chest wall movement

C. Absence of abdominal and chest wall contraction associated with an arousal

D. Decreased airflow (>50% reduction) associated with episodes of O_2 desaturation

E. Decreased airflow (>50% reduction) associated with abdominal and chest wall movements

2. **While awaiting the performance of the polysomnogram, the patient develops shortness of breath and is transferred to the emergency department. She is treated with O_2 (6 L/min) and a nebulized bronchodilator and is observed for 1 hour. She is now a little sleepy. The following arterial blood gas levels are now obtained: Pa_{O_2}, 88 mm Hg; Pa_{CO_2}, 71 mm Hg; pH, 7.33; and saturation of arterial O_2, 92%. What is the most likely explanation for the change in the arterial blood gas levels?**

A. The administration of a nebulized bronchodilator improved the gas exchange in the dead space.

B. Increased levels of CO_2 resulted in responses reflected by a downward shift of the O_2-ventilatory response curve and an enhanced sensitivity to O_2, thereby explaining the increased Pa_{O_2}.

C. Increased levels of O_2 stimulated mainly the peripheral chemoreceptors.

D. The development of acidosis resulted in responses reflected by a rightward shift of the CO_2-ventilatory response curve and a decreased sensitivity to CO_2.

E. The increased levels of O_2 resulting in responses reflected by a rightward shift of the CO_2-ventilatory response curve cause decreased sensitivity to CO_2 and a worsening of the hypercapnia.

GASTROINTESTINAL SYSTEM

VI

Howard C. Kutchai

CHAPTER 32

Motility of the Gastrointestinal Tract

OBJECTIVES

- Describe the characteristics and functions of the layers of the wall of the gastrointestinal tract.
- Explain the neural control of gastrointestinal functions.
- Describe the function of slow waves.
- Describe the swallowing reflex.
- Explain the control of gastric emptying.
- Describe the contractile behavior of the small intestine.
- Describe the motility of the colon and the defecation reflex.

The gastrointestinal system consists of the gastrointestinal tract and certain associated glandular organs producing secretions that function in the gastrointestinal tract. The major functions of the gastrointestinal system are to digest foodstuffs and absorb nutrient molecules into the bloodstream. The activities by which the gastrointestinal system carries out these functions may be subdivided into motility (discussed in this chapter), secretion (see Chapter 33), and digestion and absorption (see Chapter 34). **Motility** refers to gastrointestinal movements that mix and circulate the gastrointestinal contents and propel them along the length of the tract.

The Wall of the Gastrointestinal Tract Has a Layered Structure

The structure of the gastrointestinal tract varies greatly from region to region, but common features exist in the overall organization of the tissue. Figure 32-1 depicts the general layered structure of the gastrointestinal tract wall.

The **mucosa** consists of the epithelium, the lamina propria, and the muscularis mucosae. The **epithelium** is a single layer of specialized cells that lines the lumen of the gastrointestinal tract. The nature of the epithelium varies greatly from one part of the digestive tract to another. The **lamina propria** consists largely of loose connective tissue containing collagen and elastin fibrils. It is rich in several types of glands and contains lymph nodules and capillaries. The **muscularis mucosae** is the thin, innermost layer of intestinal smooth muscle. Contractions of the muscularis mucosae throw the mucosa into folds and ridges.

The **submucosa** consists largely of loose connective tissue with collagen and elastin fibrils. In some regions, submucosal glands are present. The larger nerve trunks and blood vessels of the intestinal wall travel in the submucosa.

The **muscularis externa** typically consists of two substantial layers of smooth muscle cells: an inner circular layer and an outer longitudinal layer. Contractions of the muscularis externa mix and circulate the contents of the lumen and propel them along the gastrointestinal tract.

The wall of the gastrointestinal tract contains many neurons. A dense network of nerve cells in the submucosa is the **submucosal plexus (Meissner's plexus).** The prominent **myenteric plexus (Auerbach's plexus)** is located between the circular and longitudinal smooth muscle layers. The submucosal and myenteric plexuses, together with the other neurons of the gastrointestinal tract, constitute the **intramural plexuses** or the **enteric nervous system,** which helps integrate the motor and secretory activities of the gastrointestinal system. If the sympathetic and parasympathetic nerves to the gut are cut, many motor and secretory activities continue because these processes are controlled by the enteric nervous system.

The **serosa,** or **adventitia,** is the outermost layer. It consists mainly of connective tissue covered with a layer of squamous mesothelial cells.

The Functions of the Gastrointestinal Tract Are Regulated by Hormones, Paracrine Agonists, and Nerves

Hormones are produced by endocrine cells and released into the blood to reach their target cells via the circulation. Paracrine agonists are released by cells in the vicinity of the target cells and reach the target cells by diffusion. Regulation may be classified as **endocrine, paracrine,** or **neurocrine** depending on the cell type that produces the regulatory substance and the

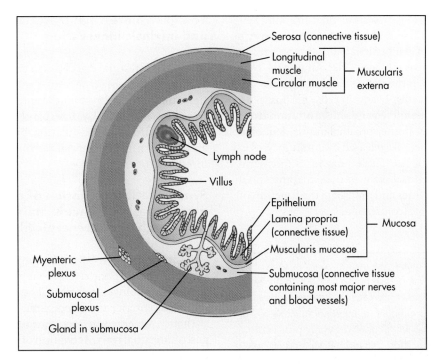

Figure 32-1 General organization of the layers of the gastrointestinal tract.

substance's route of delivery to the target cell (see Chapter 5).

MUCH HORMONAL AND NEURAL REGULATION IS INTRINSIC TO THE GASTROINTESTINAL TRACT. That is, the cells that regulate and the cells that respond reside in the gastrointestinal tract. However, gastrointestinal functions are also controlled by hormones released by cells outside the gastrointestinal tract and by neurons whose cells bodies lie outside the gastrointestinal tract. The overlapping layers of intrinsic and extrinsic hormonal and neural control allow for the subtle and precise control of gastrointestinal functions.

Hormones and paracrine mediators influence gastrointestinal functions

Endocrine cells in the mucosa or submucosa of the stomach and intestine and in the pancreas produce an array of hormones (Table 32-1). Some of these act on secretory cells located in the wall of the gastrointestinal tract, in the pancreas, or in the liver to alter the rate or the composition of their secretions (see Chapter 33). Other hormones act on smooth muscle cells in particular segments of the gastrointestinal tract, on gastrointestinal sphincters, or on the musculature of the gallbladder (see Chapter 33).

Paracrine substances also regulate the secretory and motor functions of the gastrointestinal tract. For example, histamine released from cells in the wall of the stomach is a key physiological agonist of HCl secretion by gastric parietal cells.

Other paracrine agonists are released by cells of the **gastrointestinal immune system.** The mass of cells with im-

Table 32-1	Gastrointestinal Hormones
Location of Endocrine Cells that Produce Hormone	**Hormone**
Stomach	Gastrin
	Somatostatin
Duodenum or jejunum	Secretin
	Cholecystokinin
	Motilin
	Gastric inhibitory peptide
	Somatostatin
Pancreatic islets	Insulin
	Glucagon
	Pancreatic polypeptide
	Somatostatin
Ileum or colon	Enteroglucagon
	Peptide YY
	Neurotensin
	Somatostatin

Gastrin, cholecystokinin, secretin, gastric inhibitory peptide, and motilin have physiological roles in the gastrointestinal system. The physiological roles of the other listed hormones remain to be explained.

mune function in the gastrointestinal tract is approximately equal to the combined mass of immunocytes in the rest of the body. The gastrointestinal immune system secretes antibodies in response to certain food antigens and mounts an immunological defense against many pathogenic microorganisms.

The components of the gastrointestinal immune system include cells in mesenteric lymph nodes, **Peyer's patches** in the wall of the intestine, and immunocytes in the mucosa and submucosa (Figure 32-2). Among the cells with immune function in the mucosa and submucosa are intraepithelial lymphocytes, B and T cells, plasma cells, mast cells, macrophages, and eosinophils. **Inflammatory mediators** such as histamine, prostaglandins, leukotrienes, cytokines, and others are released by immunocytes in the mucosa and submucosa. These substances diffuse to secretory and smooth muscle cells in the gastrointestinal tract to affect their activities and modulate the function of certain neurons in the gastrointestinal tract.

> The gastrointestinal immune system is involved in several troublesome gastrointestinal diseases, one of which is **celiac disease,** also known as **gluten enteropathy.** Patients with this disease mount an intestinal immune response against a component of gluten, a major protein of wheat. Celiac disease is characterized by clubbing of the villi of the small intestine, causing the absorptive surface area to be dramatically reduced. Malabsorption of carbohydrates, proteins, and lipids may occur. The majority of cases of celiac disease can be managed with a diet free of gluten.

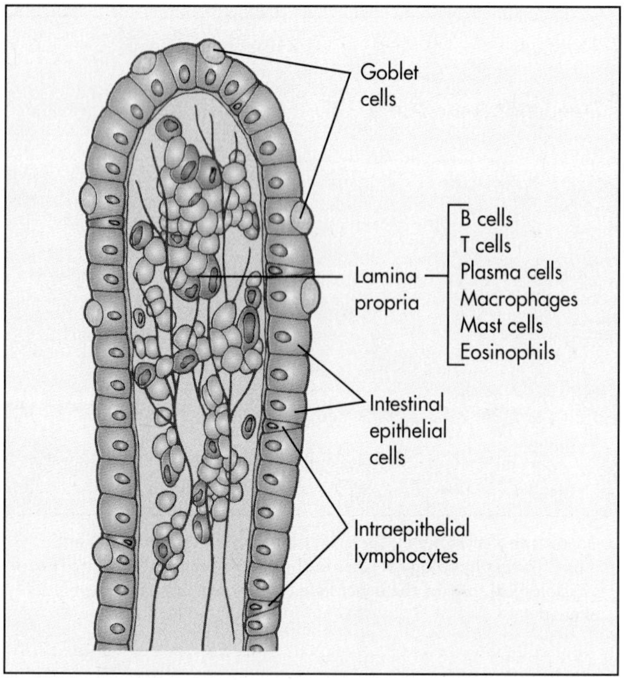

The gastrointestinal tract has both autonomic and intrinsic innervation

The gastrointestinal tract is innervated by the sympathetic and parasympathetic nervous systems (extrinsic innervation) and by the neurons of the enteric nervous system (intrinsic innervation). The interplay between local control by enteric neurons and regulation by the parasympathetic and sympathetic systems allows for fine control of gastrointestinal functions.

Sympathetic innervation of the gastrointestinal tract is mainly via postganglionic adrenergic fibers

Postganglionic sympathetic fibers, whose cell bodies are in prevertebral and paravertebral ganglia (Figure 32-3), innervate the gastrointestinal tract. The celiac, superior and inferior mesenteric, and hypogastric plexuses provide sympathetic innervation to various segments of the gastrointestinal tract. Activation of the sympathetic nerves usually inhibits the motor and secretory activities of the gastrointestinal system. MOST OF THE SYMPATHETIC FIBERS DO NOT DIRECTLY INNERVATE STRUCTURES IN THE GASTROINTESTINAL TRACT BUT RATHER TERMINATE ON NEURONS IN THE INTRAMURAL PLEXUSES. Some vasoconstrictor sympathetic fibers directly innervate the blood vessels of the gastrointestinal tract.

Figure 32-2 Small intestinal villus, showing intraepithelial lymphocytes and various immunocytes in the lamina propria. *(Redrawn from Kagnoff MF. In Sleisenger MH, Fordtran JS, eds:* Gastrointestinal disease, *ed 5, Philadelphia, 1993, WB Saunders.)*

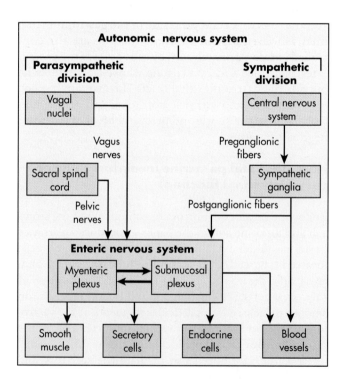

Figure 32-3 Major features of the autonomic innervation of the gastrointestinal tract. In most cases the autonomic nerves influence the functions of the gastrointestinal tract by modulating the activities of the neurons of the enteric nervous system. *(Redrawn from Costa M, Furness JB:* Br Med Bull *38:247, 1982.)*

Other sympathetic fibers innervate glandular structures in the wall of the gut.

Stimulation of sympathetic input to the gastrointestinal tract inhibits motor activity of the muscularis externa but stimulates contraction of the muscularis mucosae and certain sphincters. The sympathetic nerves do not directly inhibit contractions of the muscularis because few sympathetic nerve endings lie in the muscularis externa. Rather, the sympathetic nerves influence neural circuits in the enteric nervous system, and these circuits provide input to the smooth muscle cells. The sympathetic nerves may reinforce this effect by reducing blood flow to the muscularis externa. Other fibers that travel with the sympathetic nerves may be cholinergic; still others release neurotransmitters that remain to be identified.

Parasympathetic innervation of most of the gastrointestinal tract is via branches of the vagus nerves

Parasympathetic innervation of the gastrointestinal tract down to the level of the transverse colon is provided by branches of the vagus nerves (Figure 32-3). The remainder of the colon, the rectum, and the anus receive parasympathetic fibers from the pelvic nerves. These parasympathetic fibers are preganglionic and predominantly cholinergic. Other fibers that travel in the vagus and its branches release other transmitters, some of which have not been identified. The parasympathetic fibers terminate predominantly on the ganglion cells in the intramural plexuses. The ganglion cells then directly innervate the smooth muscle and secretory cells of the gastrointestinal tract. Excitation of parasympathetic nerves usually stimulates the motor and secretory activities of the gastrointestinal tract.

The enteric nervous system can coordinate many of the activities of the gastrointestinal tract in the absence of extrinsic innervation

The myenteric and submucosal plexuses are the most well-defined plexuses in the wall of the gastrointestinal tract (Figure 32-4). The plexuses are networks of nerve fibers and ganglion cell bodies. Interneurons in the plexuses connect afferent sensory fibers with efferent neurons to smooth muscle and secretory cells to form reflex arcs that are wholly within the gastrointestinal tract wall. Consequently the myenteric and submucosal plexuses can coordinate activity in the absence of extrinsic innervation of the gastrointestinal tract. Axons of plexus neurons innervate gland cells in the mucosa and submucosa, smooth muscle cells in the muscularis externa and muscularis mucosae, and intramural endocrine and exocrine cells.

Reflex control of the gastrointestinal tract occurs via local and central reflex pathways

AFFERENT FIBERS IN THE GASTROINTESTINAL TRACT PROVIDE THE AFFERENT LIMBS OF BOTH LOCAL AND CENTRAL REFLEX ARCS (Figure 32-5). **Chemoreceptor** and **mechanoreceptor** endings are present in the mucosa and muscularis externa. The cell bodies of many of these sensory receptors are located in the myenteric and submucosal plexuses. The axons of some of these receptor cells synapse with other cells in the

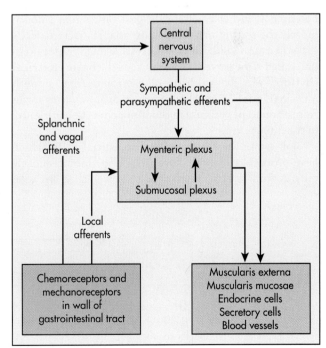

Figure 32-5 Local and central reflex pathways in the gastrointestinal system.

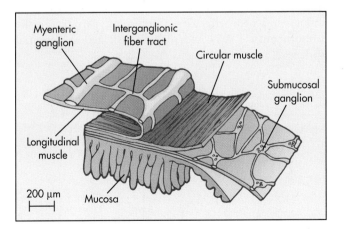

Figure 32-4 Enteric neurons of the submucosal and myenteric plexuses in the wall of the gastrointestinal tract. The plexuses consist of ganglia interconnected by fiber tracts. *(Redrawn from Wood JD. In Johnson RL, ed: Physiology of the gastrointestinal tract, ed 2, New York, 1987, Raven.)*

plexuses to mediate local reflex activity. Other sensory receptors send their axons back to the central nervous system. The complex afferent and efferent innervation of the gastrointestinal tract allows for fine control of secretory and motor activities.

Gastrointestinal Smooth Muscle Cells Have Unique Mechanical and Electrophysiological Properties

The general properties of smooth muscle are discussed in Chapter 14. The smooth muscle cells of the gastrointestinal tract are long (about 500 μm) and slender (5 to 20 μm across). They are arranged in bundles that are separated and defined by connective tissues.

Oscillations of the resting membrane potential of gastrointestinal smooth muscle are called slow waves

The resting membrane potential of gastrointestinal smooth muscle is typically smaller than that of skeletal muscle. The resting membrane potential of gastrointestinal smooth muscle cells ranges from approximately -40 to -80 mV. The electrogenic Na^+,K^+ pump (see Chapter 2) contributes significantly to the resting membrane potential in smooth muscle. In guinea pig taenia coli, for example, about one third of the resting membrane potential results from the electrogenicity of Na^+,K^+-ATPase.

In most other excitable tissues the resting membrane potential is rather constant. In gastrointestinal smooth muscle the resting membrane potential characteristically varies in time. Oscillations of the resting membrane potential, called **slow waves** (also known as the **basic electrical rhythm**), are characteristic of gastrointestinal smooth muscle (Figure 32-6). The frequency of slow waves varies from about 3 per minute in the stomach to 12 per minute in the duodenum.

Slow waves are generated by **interstitial cells,** which have properties of both fibroblasts and smooth muscle cells. A thin layer of interstitial cells is located between the longitudinal and circular layers of muscularis externa. Processes of the interstitial cells form gap junctions with longitudinal and circular smooth muscle cells. These gap junctions enable the slow waves to be conducted rapidly to both muscle layers. Because the smooth muscle cells of both longitudinal and circular layers are well coupled electrically, the slow wave spreads throughout the smooth muscle of each segment of the gastrointestinal tract.

The amplitude and, to a lesser extent, the frequency of the slow waves can be modulated by the activity of intrinsic and extrinsic nerves and by circulating hormones. In general, sympathetic nerve activity decreases the amplitude of the slow waves or abolishes them, whereas stimulation of parasympathetic nerves increases the size of the slow waves. IF THE PEAK OF THE SLOW WAVE IS ABOVE THRESHOLD FOR THE CELLS TO FIRE ACTION POTENTIALS, ONE OR MORE ACTION POTENTIALS MAY BE TRIGGERED DURING THE PEAK OF THE SLOW WAVE (Figure 32-6).

Ca^{++} enters smooth muscle cells during action potentials that may occur on the crests of the slow waves

Action potentials in gastrointestinal smooth muscle are more prolonged (10 to 20 msec) than those of skeletal muscle and have little or no overshoot. The rising phase of the action potential is caused by ion flow through channels that conduct both Ca^{++} and Na^+ and that are relatively slow to open. Ca^{++} that enters the cell during the action potential helps initiate contraction.

When the membrane potential of gastrointestinal smooth muscle reaches threshold, typically near the peak of a slow wave, a train of action potentials (1 to 10 per second) occurs (Figure 32-6). The extent of depolarization of the cells and the frequency of action potentials are enhanced by certain hormones and compounds liberated from excitatory nerve endings. Inhibitory hormones and neuroeffector substances hyperpolarize the smooth muscle cells and may abolish action potential spikes.

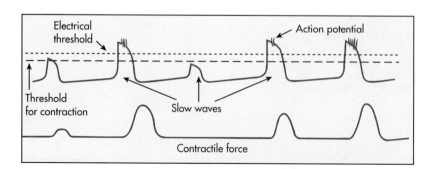

Figure 32-6 Contraction of small intestinal smooth muscle occurs when the depolarization caused by the slow wave exceeds a threshold for contraction. When depolarization of a slow wave exceeds the electrical threshold, a burst of action potentials occurs. Action potentials elicit much stronger contractions than occur in the absence of action potentials.

Action potentials greatly increase the force of contractions of gastrointestinal smooth muscle cells

In the example shown in Figure 32-6 the slow waves without action potentials elicit weak contractions of the smooth muscle layers. Much stronger contractions are evoked by the action potentials intermittently triggered near the peaks of the slow waves. THE GREATER THE NUMBER OF ACTION POTENTIALS OCCURRING AT THE PEAK OF A SLOW WAVE, THE MORE INTENSE THE CONTRACTION OF THE SMOOTH MUSCLE. Because smooth muscle cells contract rather slowly (about one tenth as fast as skeletal muscle), the individual contractions caused by each action potential in a burst are not visible as distinct twitches; rather, they sum temporally to produce a smoothly increasing level of tension (Figure 32-6).

Between bursts of action potentials the tension developed by gastrointestinal smooth muscle falls but not to zero. This nonzero resting, or baseline, tension developed by the smooth muscle is called **tone.** The tone of gastrointestinal smooth muscle is altered by neuroeffectors, hormones, and drugs.

Gastrointestinal smooth muscle cells are electrically coupled to their neighbors

Neighboring cells are said to be well coupled electrically if a perturbation of the membrane potential of one cell spreads rapidly and with little decrement to the other cell. The smooth muscle cells of the circular layer are better coupled than those of the longitudinal layer. The cells of the circular layer are joined by frequent gap junctions that allow the spread of electrical current from one cell to another (see also Chapter 4).

The Enteric Nervous System Functions as a Semiautonomous "Enteric Brain"

Typically, the enteric nervous system directly controls the patterns of muscular and secretory activities, but contraction and secretion are also regulated more indirectly by the autonomic nervous system. The neurons of the intramural plexuses send axons to the smooth muscle layers, and each axon may branch extensively to innervate many smooth muscle cells. Neuromuscular interactions in the gastrointestinal tract do not involve true neuromuscular junctions with specialization of the postjunctional membrane, as occurs at neuromuscular junctions in skeletal muscle. The circular smooth muscle layer of the muscularis externa is heavily innervated by excitatory and inhibitory motor nerve terminals closely associated with the plasma membranes of the smooth muscle cells. Longitudinal smooth muscle cells are much less richly innervated by the neurons of the intrinsic plexuses than the cells of the circular layer, and the neuromuscular contacts are not so intimate.

The enteric nervous system of the large and small intestines alone contains about 10^8 neurons, about as many neurons as in the spinal cord. Figure 32-4 depicts the myenteric and submucosal plexuses and their locations in the wall of the intestine. Both plexuses consist of ganglia that are interconnected by tracts of fine, unmyelinated nerve fibers. The neurons in the ganglia include sensory neurons, with their sensory endings in the wall of the gastrointestinal tract. These sensory endings respond to mechanical deformation, particular chemical stimuli, and temperature. Some of the neurons in the enteric ganglia are effector neurons that send axons to smooth muscle cells of the circular or longitudinal layers, secretory cells of the gastrointestinal tract, or gastrointestinal blood vessels. Many of the neurons in the enteric ganglia are interneurons that are part of the network of neurons integrating the sensory input to the ganglia and formulating the output of the effector neurons.

A large number of neuromodulatory substances are present in enteric neurons. Most of the neuromodulatory substances that function in the central nervous system (see Chapter 4) are also present in the gastrointestinal tract. Box 32-1 lists some of the neuroactive substances present in the gastrointestinal tract.

Many neurons in myenteric ganglia are motor neurons that excite or inhibit the smooth muscle cells of the muscularis externa

Excitatory motor neurons release **acetylcholine** onto muscarinic receptors on the smooth muscle cells; they also release **substance P.** Inhibitory motor neurons release **vasoactive intestinal polypeptide (VIP)** and **nitric oxide.**

Box 32-1   Substances Established or Proposed as Neurotransmitters and Neuromodulators in the Enteric Nervous System

Acetylcholine
Adenosine triphosphate
γ-Aminobutyric acid
Calcitonin gene–related peptide
Cholecystokinin
Dynorphin and dynorphin-related peptides
Enkephalin and enkephalin-related peptides
Galanin
Gastrin-releasing peptide (mammalian bombesin)
Neuropeptide Y
Nitric oxide
Norepinephrine
Serotonin (5-hydroxytryptamine)
Somatostatin
Tachykinins (substance P, neurokinin A, neuropeptide K, neuropeptide Y)
Vasoactive intestinal peptide (and peptide histidine isoleucine)

out one third of neurons in myenteric ganglia are sensory. Other myenteric neurons project to neurons in submucous ganglia. Most myenteric interneurons release acetylcholine onto nicotinic receptors on motor neurons or on other interneurons.

Many neurons in submucous ganglia regulate secretion via glandular, endocrine, and epithelial cells

Stimulatory secretomotor neurons release acetylcholine and VIP onto gland cells or epithelial cells. The numerous sensory neurons in submucous ganglia respond to chemical stimuli or mechanical deformation of the mucosa, and they are the afferent limbs of secretomotor reflexes. Submucous interneurons release acetylcholine onto other neurons in submucous ganglia or project to myenteric ganglia. Submucous ganglia also contain vasodilator neurons that release acetylcholine, VIP, or both products onto submucous blood vessels. There are apparently no inhibitory secretomotor neurons in the enteric nervous system.

The component cells of intrinsic reflexes are all located in the walls of the gastrointestinal tract

Numerous intrinsic reflexes control the motor and secretory activities of each segment of the gastrointestinal tract. A well-characterized intrinsic reflex is shown in Figure 32-7. LOCALIZED MECHANICAL OR CHEMICAL STIMULATION OF THE INTESTINAL MUCOSA ELICITS CONTRACTION ABOVE (ORAL TO) AND RELAXATION BELOW (ANAL TO) THE POINT OF STIMULATION.

Chewing Is Frequently a Reflex Behavior

Chewing can be carried out voluntarily, but it is more frequently a reflex behavior. Chewing lubricates food by mixing it with salivary mucus, mixes starch-containing food with salivary amylase, and subdivides food so that it can be mixed more readily with the digestive secretions of the stomach and duodenum.

Swallowing Is Accomplished via a Complex Reflex

Swallowing can be initiated voluntarily, but thereafter it is almost entirely under reflex control. THE SWALLOWING REFLEX IS A RIGIDLY ORDERED SEQUENCE OF EVENTS THAT PROPELS FOOD FROM THE MOUTH TO THE STOMACH. During swallowing, respiration is reflexly inhibited, thereby preventing the entrance of food into the trachea. The afferent limb of the swallowing reflex begins with touch receptors, most notably those near the opening of the pharynx. Sensory impulses from these receptors are transmitted to certain areas in the medulla. The central integrating areas for swallowing lie in the medulla and lower pons; these areas are collectively called the **swallowing cen-**

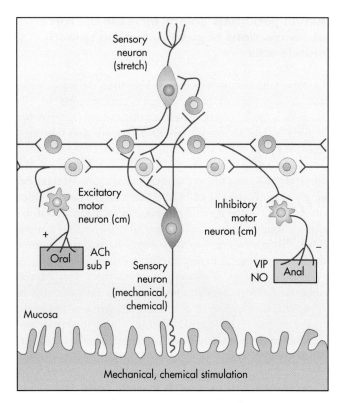

Figure 32-7 Localized mechanical or chemical stimulation of the intestinal mucosa typically elicits contraction above and relaxation below the point of stimulation. This figure depicts the enteric neuronal circuitry responsible for this reflex behavior. In the center are two sensory neurons: a stretch-sensitive neuron in the muscle layer *(pink cytoplasm)* and a mechanosensitive or chemosensitive neuron *(blue cytoplasm)* with its receptive ending in the mucosa. Stimulation of either sensory neuron results in activation of ascending (oral) excitatory pathways and descending (anal) pathways to circular muscle *(cm)*. *ACh*, Acetylcholine; *NO*, nitric oxide; *sub P*, substance P. *(Courtesy Dr Terence K Smith.)*

ter. Motor impulses travel from the swallowing center to the musculature of the pharynx and upper esophagus via various cranial nerves and to the remainder of the esophagus via vagal motor neurons.

The oral phase of swallowing is voluntary

The **oral phase** of swallowing is initiated when the tip of the tongue separates a bolus of food from the mass in the mouth. The bolus to be swallowed is moved upward and backward in the mouth by pressing first the tip of the tongue and later the more posterior portions of the tongue against the hard palate. This forces the bolus into the pharynx, where the bolus stimulates the tactile receptors that initiate the swallowing reflex.

The pharyngeal phase of swallowing propels food from the pharynx into the esophagus

The **pharyngeal phase** of swallowing involves the following sequence of events, which occur in less than 1 second:
1. The soft palate is pulled upward, and the palatopharyngeal folds move inward toward one an-

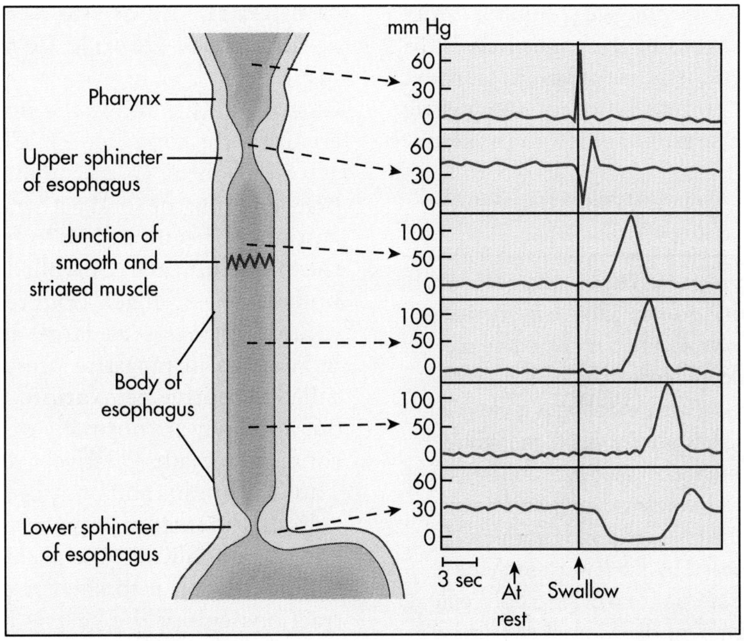

Figure 32-8 Pressures in the pharynx, esophagus, and esophageal sphincters during swallowing. Note the reflex relaxation of the upper and lower esophageal sphincters and the timing of the relaxation. *(Redrawn from Christensen JL. In Christensen JL, Wingate DL, eds: A guide to gastrointestinal motility, Bristol, England, 1983, John Wright & Sons.)*

other. This prevents the reflux of food into the nasopharynx and provides a narrow passage through which food moves into the pharynx.

2. The vocal cords are pulled together. The larynx is moved forward and upward against the epiglottis. These actions prevent food from entering the trachea and help open the upper esophageal sphincter.
3. The upper esophageal sphincter relaxes to receive the bolus of food (Figure 32-8). Then the pharyngeal superior constrictor muscles contract strongly to force the bolus deeply into the pharynx.
4. A **peristaltic wave** is initiated with contraction of the pharyngeal superior constrictor muscles, and the wave moves toward the esophagus (Figure 32-8). This forces the bolus of food through the relaxed **upper esophageal sphincter.**

DURING THE PHARYNGEAL STAGE OF SWALLOWING, RESPIRATION IS REFLEXLY INHIBITED.

The esophageal phase of swallowing involves the body of the esophagus and both esophageal sphincters

The **esophageal phase** of swallowing is controlled mainly by the swallowing center. After the bolus of food passes the upper esophageal sphincter, the sphincter reflexly constricts. A peristaltic wave then begins just below the upper esophageal sphincter and traverses the entire esophagus in less than 10 seconds (Figure 32-8). This initial wave, called **primary peristalsis,** is controlled by the swallowing center. The peristaltic wave travels down the esophagus at 3 to

5 cm/sec. THE **LOWER ESOPHAGEAL SPHINCTER** RELAXES EARLY IN THE ESOPHAGEAL PHASE AND REMAINS RELAXED UNTIL FOOD IS DRIVEN THROUGH IT BY THE ESOPHAGEAL PERISTALTIC WAVE (Figure 32-8).

If primary peristalsis is insufficient to clear the esophagus of food, distention of the esophagus initiates another peristaltic wave, called **secondary peristalsis,** which begins above the site of distention and moves downward. Input from esophageal sensory fibers to the central and enteric nervous systems modulates esophageal peristalsis.

The Esophagus Moves Food from the Pharynx to the Stomach

In the upper third of the esophagus, both the inner circular and the outer longitudinal muscle layers are striated. In the lower third, the muscle layers are composed entirely of smooth muscle cells. In the middle third, skeletal and smooth muscles coexist, with a gradient from all skeletal muscle above to all smooth muscle below. The esophageal musculature, both striated and smooth, is innervated mainly by branches of the vagus nerve. Somatic motor fibers of the vagus nerves form motor endplates on striated muscle fibers. Visceral motor nerves are preganglionic parasympathetic fibers that synapse primarily on the nerve cells of the myenteric plexus. Neurons of the myenteric plexus directly innervate the smooth muscle cells of the esophagus and communicate with one another.

The upper and lower esophageal sphincters prevent the entry of air and gastric contents, respectively, into the esophagus. The lower esophageal sphincter opens when a wave of esophageal peristalsis begins (Figure 32-

8). The opening of the lower esophageal sphincter is mediated by impulses in branches of the vagus nerves. In the absence of esophageal peristalsis the sphincter must remain tightly closed to prevent reflux of the gastric contents, which would cause esophagitis and the sensation of heartburn.

In individuals with **incompetence of the lower esophageal sphincter,** gastric juice can **reflux** (move back up) into the lower esophagus and cause erosion of the esophageal mucosa. Reflux can be a problem because the pressure in the thoracic esophagus is close to intrathoracic pressure, which is usually less than intraabdominal pressure. The difference between intraabdominal and intrathoracic pressures increases during each inspiration (see Chapter 28). The reflux of gastric contents up into the esophagus is opposed by the lower esophageal sphincter. In addition, because the crura of the diaphragm wrap around the esophagus at the level of the lower esophageal sphincter, contraction of the diaphragm increases the pressure in the lower esophageal sphincter with each inspiration. Weakness of the diaphragm or **hiatal hernia** can exacerbate incompetence of the lower esophageal sphincter.

The lower esophageal sphincter is controlled by nerves and hormones

The resting pressure in the lower esophageal sphincter is about 30 mm Hg. The tonic contraction of the circular musculature of the sphincter is regulated by nerves, both intrinsic and extrinsic, and by hormones and neuromodulators. A significant fraction of basal tone in this sphincter is mediated by vagal cholinergic nerves. Stimulation of sympathetic nerves to the sphincter also causes the lower esophageal sphincter to contract.

Vagal inhibitory fibers relax the lower esophageal sphincter. The intrinsic and extrinsic innervation of the lower esophageal sphincter is both excitatory and inhibitory. A major component of the sphincter's relaxation that occurs in response to primary peristalsis in the esophagus is mediated by noncholinergic vagal fibers inhibitory to the circular muscle of the lower esophageal sphincter.

In some individuals the sphincter fails to relax sufficiently during swallowing, so food may not be able to enter the stomach. This condition is known as **achalasia.** Therapy for achalasia may involve mechanically dilating or surgically weakening the lower esophageal sphincter or administering drugs that inhibit the tone of the lower esophageal sphincter. Individuals with **diffuse esophageal spasm** have prolonged and painful contraction of the lower part of the esophagus instead of the normal esophageal peristaltic wave after swallowing.

Contractions of the Stomach Mix and Propel Gastric Contents

Gastric motility allows the stomach (1) to serve as a reservoir for the large volume of food that may be ingested at a single meal, (2) to fragment food into smaller particles and mix the food with gastric secretions so that digestion can begin, and (3) to empty gastric contents into the duodenum at a controlled rate. The **fundus** and the **body** of the stomach (Figure 32-9) can accommodate volume increases as large as 1.5 L without a great increase in intragastric pressure; the phenomenon is called **receptive relaxation.** Contractions of the fundus and body are normally weak, so much of the gastric contents remains relatively unmixed for long periods. Thus the fundus and body of the stomach serve as reservoirs. In the antrum, however, contractions are vigorous and thoroughly mix antral chyme with gastric juice and subdivide food into smaller particles. The antral contractions empty the gastric contents in small squirts into the duodenal bulb. The rate of gastric emptying is adjusted by several mechanisms so that chyme is not delivered to the duodenum too rapidly. The physiological mechanisms that underlie this behavior are discussed later.

The structure and extrinsic innervation of the stomach

The basic structure of the gastric wall follows the scheme presented in Figure 32-1. The circular muscle layer of muscularis externa is more prominent than the longitudinal layer. The muscularis externa of the fundus and body is relatively thin, but that of the antrum is considerably thicker, and the thickness increases toward the pylorus.

The stomach is richly innervated by extrinsic nerves and by the neurons of the enteric nervous system. Axons from the cells of the intramural plexuses innervate the smooth muscle and secretory cells.

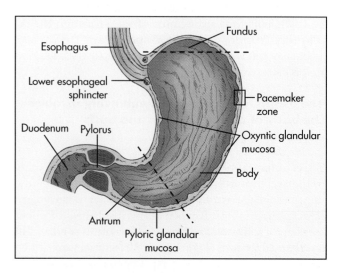

Figure 32-9 Major anatomical subdivisions of the stomach.

Parasympathetic innervation is by the vagus nerves, and sympathetic innervation is from the celiac plexus. In general, parasympathetic nerves stimulate gastric smooth muscle motility and gastric secretions, whereas sympathetic activity inhibits these functions. Numerous sensory afferent fibers leave the stomach in the vagus nerves, and some travel with sympathetic nerves. Other fibers are the afferent links of intrinsic reflex arcs via the intramural plexuses of the stomach. Some of these afferent fibers relay information about intragastric pressure, gastric distention, intragastric pH, or pain.

The body and fundus relax in response to gastric filling

When a wave of esophageal peristalsis begins, the lower esophageal sphincter reflexly relaxes. This is followed by receptive relaxation of the fundus and body of the stomach. The stomach also relaxes if it is directly filled with gas or liquid. The nerve fibers in the vagi are a major efferent pathway for reflex relaxation of the stomach. The vagal fibers that mediate this response release VIP as their transmitter.

> Before effective drugs for blocking gastric acid secretion were available, it was common to treat duodenal ulcers by cutting the vagus nerves to the stomach (vagotomy) to diminish the rate of gastric acid secretion. This procedure also eliminated the efferent pathway of the receptive relaxation reflex so that in response to ingestion of a meal, intragastric pressure increases to a much greater level than normal. The accelerated emptying of gastric contents that results is known as the **dumping syndrome.** Gastric contents are emptied into the small intestine faster than they can be processed; thus these patients may have chronic diarrhea.

The rate of emptying of gastric contents depends on their physical properties

The muscle layers in the fundus and body are thin; weak contractions characterize these parts of the stomach. As a result, the contents of the fundus and the body tend to form layers based on the density of the contents. Gastric contents may remain unmixed for as long as an hour after eating. Fats tend to form an oily layer on top of the other gastric contents. Consequently, fats are emptied later than other gastric contents. Liquids can flow around the mass of food contained in the body of the stomach and are emptied more rapidly into the duodenum (Figure 32-10). Large or indigestible particles are retained in the stomach for a longer period.

Gastric contractions, with a frequency of about three per minute, usually begin in the middle of the body of the stomach and travel toward the pylorus. The contractions increase in force and velocity as they approach the gas-

troduodenal junction. As a result, the major mixing activity occurs in the antrum, the contents of which are mixed rapidly and thoroughly with gastric secretions.

The pattern of gastric contractions after eating differs from that during fasting

After an individual eats, regular contractions of the antrum occur at a rate of about three per minute. As discussed later, the rate of gastric emptying is regulated by feedback mechanisms that diminish the force of antral contractions.

IN A FASTED ANIMAL THE PATTERN OF ANTRAL CONTRACTIONS IS DIFFERENT. The antrum is quiescent for 75 to 90 minutes; then a brief period (5 to 10 minutes) of intense electrical and motor activity occurs. This activity is characterized by strong contractions of the antrum and a relaxed pylorus. During this period, even large chunks of material that remain from the previous meal are emptied from the stomach. The period of intense contractions is followed by another 75 to 90 minutes of quiescence. This cycle of contractions in the stomach is part of a pattern of contractile activity that periodically sweeps from the stomach to the terminal ileum during fasting. This cyclic contractile activity is known as the **migrating myoelectric complex** (MMC) and is discussed later.

Slow waves and action potentials elicit gastric contractions

The gastric peristaltic waves occur at the frequency of the gastric slow waves that are generated by a **pacemaker zone** (Figure 32-9) near the middle of the body of the stomach. These waves are conducted toward the pylorus. In humans the frequency of slow waves is about three per minute.

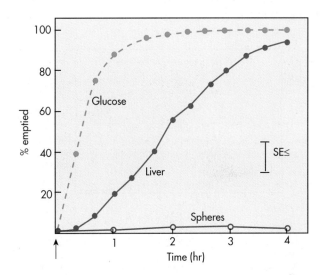

Figure 32-10 Rates of emptying of different meals from a dog's stomach. A solution (400 ml of 1% glucose *[green line]*) is emptied faster than a digestible solid (50 g of cubed liver *[blue line]*). The indigestible solid (40 7-mm plastic spheres *[red line]*) remains in the stomach under these conditions. *SE,* Standard error. *(Redrawn from Hinder RA, Kelly KA: Am J Physiol 233:E335, 1977.)*

The gastric slow wave is triphasic (Figure 32-11). Its shape resembles that of action potentials in cardiac muscle. However, the gastric slow wave lasts about 10 times longer than the cardiac action potential, and it does not overshoot. Gastric smooth muscle contracts when depolarization during the slow wave exceeds threshold for contraction (Figure 32-11). The greater the extent of depolarization and the longer the cell remains depolarized above the threshold, the greater the force of contraction. In the gastric antrum, action potential spikes may occur during the plateau phase; when action potentials occur, the resulting contraction is much stronger than in the absence of action potentials (Figure 32-6). Acetylcholine and the hormone **gastrin** stimulate gastric contractility by increasing the amplitude and duration of the plateau phase of the gastric slow wave. Norepinephrine has the opposite effect.

The passage of gastric contents through the pylorus is highly regulated

The pylorus separates the gastric antrum from the duodenal bulb, the first part of the **duodenum.** The pylorus functions as a sphincter. The circular smooth muscle of the pylorus forms two ringlike thickenings followed by a connective tissue ring that separates the pylorus from the duodenum.

The duodenum has a basic electrical rhythm of 10 to 12 slow waves per minute compared with the 3 per minute of the stomach. The duodenal bulb is influenced by the basic electrical rhythms of both the stomach and the postbulbar duodenum. Thus the duodenal bulb contracts somewhat irregularly. However, the antrum and duodenum are coordinated; when the antrum contracts, the duodenal bulb relaxes. The essential functions of the gastroduodenal junction are to (1) allow the carefully regulated emptying of gastric contents at a rate consistent

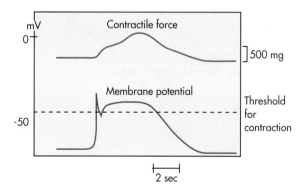

Figure 32-11 Relationship between the contraction of the smooth muscle of a dog's stomach *(upper tracing)* and an intracellularly recorded slow wave *(lower tracing).* Contraction occurs when the depolarizing phase of the slow wave exceeds the threshold for contraction, even though there are no action potential spikes on the plateau of the slow wave. When action potentials occur, a much stronger contraction is elicited. *(Redrawn from Szurszewski J. In Johnson LR, eds: Physiology of the gastrointestinal tract, New York, 1981, Raven.)*

with the ability of the duodenum to process the chyme and (2) prevent regurgitation of duodenal contents back into the stomach.

> The gastric mucosa is highly resistant to acid, but it may be damaged by bile. The duodenal mucosa has the opposite properties. Thus too-rapid gastric emptying may lead to **duodenal ulcers,** whereas regurgitation of duodenal contents may contribute to **gastric ulcers.**

The pylorus is densely innervated by both vagal and sympathetic nerve fibers. Sympathetic fibers increase the constriction of the sphincter. Vagal fibers are either excitatory or inhibitory to pyloric smooth muscle. Excitatory cholinergic vagal fibers stimulate constriction of the sphincter. Inhibitory vagal fibers release another transmitter, probably VIP, that relaxes the sphincter. The hormones cholecystokinin, gastrin, gastric inhibitory peptide, and secretin all elicit constriction of the pyloric sphincter.

Gastric emptying is regulated in response to the nature of duodenal contents

The duodenal and jejunal mucosa have receptors that sense acidity, osmotic pressure, certain fats, and amino acids and peptides (Figure 32-12). The presence of fatty acids or monoglycerides (products of fat digestion) in the duodenum dramatically decreases the rate of gastric emptying. The chyme that leaves the stomach is usually hypertonic, and it becomes more hypertonic because of the action of the digestive enzymes in the duodenum. Gastric emptying is retarded by hypertonic solutions in the duodenum, a duodenal pH below 3.5, and the presence of amino acids and peptides in the duodenum. The results of these mechanisms are:

1. Fat is not emptied into the duodenum at a rate greater than that at which it can be emulsified by the bile acids and lecithin of the bile.
2. Acid is not dumped into the duodenum more rapidly than it can be neutralized by pancreatic and duodenal secretions and other mechanisms.
3. The rates at which the other components of chyme are presented to the small intestine do not exceed the rate at which the small intestine can process those components.

Neural and hormonal mechanisms elicited by duodenal contents slow gastric emptying. In response to the acid in the duodenum, the force of gastric contractions promptly decreases, and duodenal motility increases. This response has neural and hormonal components. The presence of acid in the duodenum releases **secretin,** which diminishes the rate of gastric emptying by inhibiting antral contractions and stimulating contraction of the pyloric sphincter (Figure 32-12).

The presence of fat digestion products in the duodenum and jejunum decreases the rate of gastric emptying. This response results mainly from the release of **cholecystokinin** from the duodenum and jejunum. Cholecystokinin decreases the rate of gastric emptying. The presence of fatty acids in the duodenum and jejunum releases another hormone, **gastric inhibitory peptide,** that also decreases the rate of gastric emptying. Hyperosmotic solutions in the duodenum and jejunum slow the rate of gastric emptying. This response has both neural and hormonal components. Hypertonic solutions in the duodenum release an unidentified hormone that diminishes the rate of gastric emptying.

Peptides and amino acids release **gastrin** from **G cells** located in the antrum of the stomach and the duodenum. Gastrin increases the strength of antral contractions and increases constriction of the pyloric sphincter; the net effect probably diminishes the rate of gastric emptying.

> In some patients with **duodenal ulcers** the underlying physiological malfunction may be diminished effectiveness of the mechanisms by which hormones released from the duodenum decrease the rates of gastric emptying and gastric acid secretion. In normal individuals, experimental instillation of acid into the duodenum via a nasogastric tube dramatically decreases the rate and force of contractions of the gastric antrum. In some patients with duodenal ulcers, this response to acid in the duodenum is markedly diminished.

Vomiting Is the Expulsion of Gastric (and Sometimes Duodenal) Contents from the Gastrointestinal Tract via the Mouth

Vomiting often is preceded by a feeling of nausea, a rapid or irregular heartbeat, dizziness, sweating, pallor, and dilation of the pupils. It is usually preceded by **retching,** in which gastric contents are forced up into the esophagus but do not enter the pharynx.

Vomiting is a reflex behavior controlled and coordinated by a **vomiting center** in the medulla oblongata. Many areas in the body have receptors that provide afferent input to the vomiting center. Distention of the stomach and duodenum is a strong stimulus that elicits vomiting. Tickling the back of the throat, painful injury to the genitourinary system, dizziness, and certain other stimuli can bring about vomiting.

> Certain chemicals, called **emetics,** can elicit vomiting. Some emetics do this by stimulating receptors in the stomach or more often in the duodenum. The widely used emetic **ipecac** stimulates duodenal receptors. Certain other emetics (e.g., **apomorphine**) act at the level of the central nervous system on receptors in the floor of the fourth ventricle, in an area known as the **chemoreceptor trigger zone.** The chemoreceptor trigger zone lies on the blood side of the blood-brain barrier and thus can be reached by most blood-borne substances.

When the vomiting reflex is activated, the sequence of events is the same regardless of the stimulus that ini-

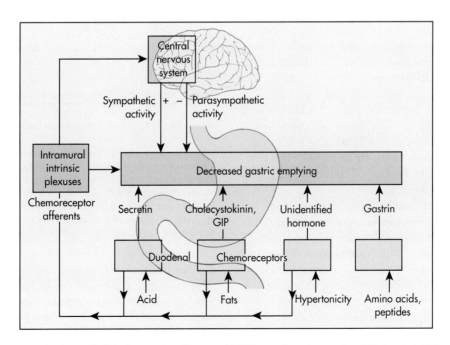

Figure 32-12 Duodenal stimuli elicit the neural and hormonal inhibition of gastric emptying. *GIP,* Gastric inhibitory peptide.

tiates the reflex. Early events include a wave of **reverse peristalsis** that sweeps from the middle of the small intestine to the duodenum. The pyloric sphincter and the stomach relax to receive the intestinal contents. Then a forced inspiration occurs against a closed glottis. This decreases intrathoracic pressure, whereas the lowering of the diaphragm increases intraabdominal pressure. Then a forceful contraction of abdominal muscles sharply elevates intraabdominal pressure and drives gastric contents into the esophagus. The lower esophageal sphincter relaxes reflexly to receive gastric contents, and the pylorus and antrum contract reflexly. When a person retches, the upper esophageal sphincter remains closed, which prevents vomiting. When the respiratory and abdominal muscles relax, the esophagus is emptied by secondary peristalsis into the stomach. Often a series of stronger and stronger retches precedes vomiting.

When a person vomits, the rapid propulsion of gastric contents into the esophagus is accompanied by a reflex relaxation of the upper esophageal sphincter. **Vomitus** is projected into the pharynx and mouth. Entry of vomitus into the trachea is prevented by approximation of the vocal chords, closure of the glottis, and inhibition of respiration.

The Motility of the Small Intestine Mixes and Propels Intestinal Contents

The small intestine accounts for about three fourths of the length of the human gastrointestinal tract. The small intestine is about 5 m long, and chyme typically takes 2 to 4 hours to traverse it. The first 5% or so of the small intestine is the duodenum, which has no mesentery and can be distinguished from the rest of the small intestine histologically. The remaining small intestine is divided into the jejunum and the ileum. The **jejunum** is more proximal and occupies about 40% of the length of the small bowel. The **ileum** is the distal part of the small intestine and accounts for its remaining length.

The small intestine, particularly the duodenum and the jejunum, is the site of most digestion and absorption. The movements of the small intestine mix chyme with digestive secretions, bring fresh chyme into contact with the absorptive surface of the microvilli, and propel chyme toward the colon.

The most frequent type of movement of the small intestine is termed **segmentation.** Segmentation (Figure 32-13) is characterized by closely spaced contractions of the circular muscle layer. The contractions divide the small intestine into small, neighboring segments. In rhythmic segmentation the sites of the circular contractions alternate so that a given segment of gut contracts and then relaxes. Segmentation effectively mixes chyme with digestive secretions and brings fresh chyme into contact with the mucosal surface.

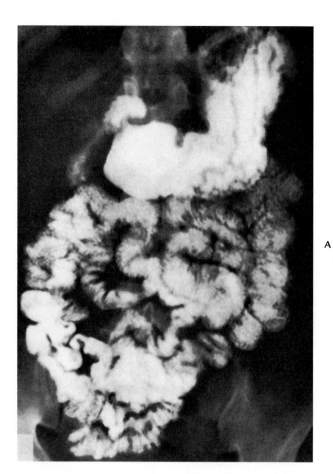

A

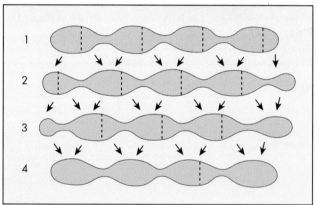

B

Figure 32-13 A, X-ray view showing the stomach and small intestine filled with barium contrast medium in a normal individual. Note that segmentation of the small intestine divides its contents into ovoid segments. **B,** Sequence of segmental contractions in a portion of a cat's small intestine. Lines 1 through 4 indicate successive patterns in time. The dotted lines indicate where contractions will occur next. The arrows show the direction of chyme movement.   (*A from Gardner EM et al: Anatomy: a regional study of human structure, ed 4, Philadelphia, 1975, WB Saunders. B redrawn from Cannon WB: Am J Physiol 6:251, 1902.*)

Peristalsis is the progressive contraction of successive sections of circular smooth muscle. The contractions move along the gastrointestinal tract in an orthograde direction. Peristaltic waves occur in the small intestine, but they usually involve only a short length of intestine.

Slow waves and action potentials determine the frequency and force of intestinal contractions

Regular slow waves occur all along the small intestine. The frequency is highest (11 to 13 per minute in humans) in the duodenum and declines along the length of the small bowel (to a minimum of 8 or 9 per minute in humans in the terminal part of the ileum). The slow waves may be accompanied by bursts of action potential spikes. When action potentials occur, they elicit much stronger contractions of the smooth muscle that cause the major mixing and propulsive movements of the small intestine (Figure 32-6). Action potential bursts are localized to short segments of the intestine, and they elicit the highly localized contractions of the circular smooth muscle that cause segmentation.

The basic electrical rhythm of the small intestine is independent of extrinsic innervation. The frequency of the action potential spike bursts that elicit strong contractions depends on the excitability of the smooth muscle cells of the small intestine. The excitability is influenced by circulating hormones, the autonomic nervous system, and enteric neurons. Excitability is enhanced by parasympathetic nerves and is inhibited by sympathetic nerves, both acting via the intramural plexuses. Even though much of the direct control of intestinal motility resides in the intramural plexuses, the parasympathetic and sympathetic innervation of the small intestine modulates contractile activity. The extrinsic neural circuits are essential for certain long-range intestinal reflexes, which are discussed later.

Contractions of the duodenum, jejunum, and ileum mix the contents with digestive secretions

Contractions of the duodenal bulb mix chyme with pancreatic and biliary secretions, and they propel the chyme along the duodenum. Contractions of the duodenal bulb typically follow contractions of the gastric antrum. This helps prevent regurgitation of duodenal contents into the stomach.

Segmental contractions occur at about 12 per minute in the duodenum, 10 or 11 per minute in the jejunum, and 8 or 9 per minute in the ileum. Segmentation is more effective at mixing intestinal contents than at propelling them. The low rate of propulsion of chyme in the small intestine allows time for digestion and absorption.

The importance of the slow rate of propulsion in the small intestine can be demonstrated by treatment with agents that alter small intestinal motility. For example, the administration of **codeine** and other **opiates** markedly reduces the frequency and volume of stools. This action results from a decrease in small intestinal motility and a consequent increase in the transit time of jejunal contents.

The longer transit time allows more complete absorption of salts and water and certain nutrients in the small intestine so that less than a normal volume enters the colon. **Castor oil,** a potent laxative, contains hydroxy fatty acids that stimulate small intestinal motility and decrease small intestinal transit time. Hence salts and water are delivered to the colon at a rate that overwhelms the ability of the colon to absorb them; this results in diarrhea.

Intestinal reflexes involve the enteric and autonomic nervous systems

When a bolus of material is placed in the small intestine, the intestine typically contracts behind the bolus and relaxes ahead of it (Figure 32-7), a response known as the **law of the intestine.** This response, which is integrated chiefly in the enteric nervous system, propels the bolus in an orthograde direction, similar to a peristaltic wave.

Certain intestinal reflexes can occur along a considerable length of the gastrointestinal tract. These long-range reflexes depend on the function of both intrinsic and extrinsic nerves. Overdistention of one segment of the intestine relaxes the smooth muscle in the rest of the intestine. This response is known as the **intestinointestinal reflex.**

The stomach and terminal part of the ileum interact reflexly. Elevated secretory and motor functions of the stomach increase the motility of the terminal part of the ileum and accelerate the movement of material through the **ileocecal sphincter.** This response is called the **gastroileal reflex.**

The migrating myoelectric complex occurs during fasting

The contractile behavior of the small intestine previously discussed is characteristic of the period after ingestion of a meal. SEVERAL HOURS AFTER PROCESSING OF THE PREVIOUS MEAL, SMALL INTESTINAL MOTILITY FOLLOWS A VERY DIFFERENT PATTERN CHARACTERIZED BY BURSTS OF INTENSE ELECTRICAL AND CONTRACTILE ACTIVITY SEPARATED BY LONGER QUIESCENT PERIODS. This pattern, the **migrating myoelectric complex (MMC),** appears to be propagated from the stomach to the terminal ileum (Figure 32-14). The MMC in the stomach is discussed earlier in this chapter.

The MMC repeats every 75 to 90 minutes in humans (Figure 32-14). About the time that one MMC reaches the distal ileum, the next MMC begins in the stomach. The strongest contractions of the MMC, both in the stomach and the small intestine, are more vigorous and more propulsive than the contractions that occur in a fed individual. These intense contractions sweep the small bowel clean and empty its contents into the colon. Thus the MMC has been termed the housekeeper of the small intestine.

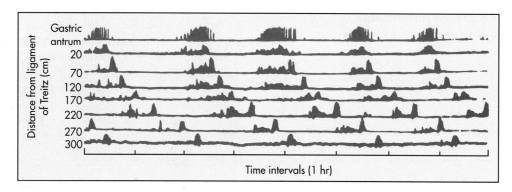

Figure 32-14 Contractile activity during the MMC in the stomach and small intestine of a fasting dog. The ligament of Treitz marks the border between the duodenum and the jejunum. *(From Itoh Z, Sekiguchi T: Scand J Gastroenterol [Suppl] 82:121, 1983.)*

> The MMC inhibits the migration of colonic bacteria into the terminal ileum. Individuals with weak or absent phase 3 contractions may be troubled by bacterial overgrowth in the ileum.

The muscularis mucosae contracts irregularly

Irregular contractions of the muscularis mucosae, on average about three per minute, alter the pattern of ridges and folds of the mucosa, mix the luminal contents, and bring different parts of the mucosal surface into contact with freshly mixed chyme. Irregular contractions of intestinal villi, especially in the jejunum, help empty the central lacteals and increase intestinal lymph flow.

Neural mechanisms regulate the passage of material through the ileocecal sphincter

The **ileocecal sphincter** separates the terminal end of the ileum from the **cecum,** the first part of the colon. Normally the sphincter is closed, but short-range peristalsis in the terminal part of the ileum relaxes the sphincter and allows a small amount of chyme to squirt into the cecum. The ileocecal sphincter normally allows ileal chyme to enter the colon at a slow enough rate that the colon can absorb most of the salts and water of the chyme. The ileocecal sphincter is coordinated primarily by the neurons of the intramural plexuses but is also influenced by autonomic reflexes and hormones.

> ### The Motility of the Colon Facilitates the Absorption of Salts and Water and Permits the Orderly Evacuation of Feces

The colon receives 500 to 1500 ml of chyme per day from the ileum. Most of the salts and water that enter the colon are absorbed; the feces normally contain only about 50 to 100 ml of water each day. Colonic contractions mix the chyme and circulate it across the mucosal surface of the colon. As the chyme becomes semisolid, this mixing resembles a kneading process. The

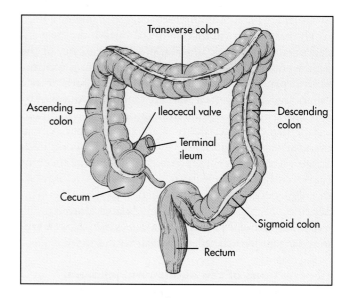

Figure 32-15 Major anatomic subdivisions of the colon.

progress of colonic contents is slow, about 5 to 10 cm/hr at most.

One to three times daily a wave of contraction, called a **mass movement,** occurs. A mass movement resembles a peristaltic wave in which the contracted segments remain contracted for some time. Mass movements push the contents of a significant length of colon in an orthograde direction.

Structure and extrinsic innervation of the colon

The major subdivisions of the large intestine (Figure 32-15) are the cecum, ascending colon, transverse colon, descending colon, sigmoid colon, rectum, and anal canal. The structure of the wall of the large bowel follows the general plan presented earlier in this chapter, but the longitudinal muscle layer of the muscularis externa is concentrated into three bands called the **taenia coli.** In between the taenia coli the longitudinal muscle layer is thin. The longitudinal muscle of the rectum and anal canal is substantial and continuous.

Parasympathetic innervation of the cecum and the ascending and transverse colon is via branches of the vagus nerves; that of the descending and sigmoid colon, rectum, and anal canal is via the pelvic nerves from the sacral spinal cord. The parasympathetic fibers end mainly on neurons of the intramural plexuses.

Sympathetic fibers innervate the proximal part of the large intestine via the superior mesenteric plexus, the distal part of the large intestine via the inferior mesenteric and superior hypogastric plexuses, and the rectum and anal canal via the inferior hypogastric plexus. STIMULATION OF THE SYMPATHETIC NERVES STOPS COLONIC MOVEMENTS. VAGAL STIMULATION CAUSES SEGMENTAL CONTRACTIONS OF THE PROXIMAL PART OF THE COLON. STIMULATION OF THE PELVIC NERVES BRINGS ABOUT EXPULSIVE MOVEMENTS OF THE DISTAL COLON AND SUSTAINED CONTRACTION OF SOME SEGMENTS.

The anal canal usually is kept closed by the internal and external sphincters. The **internal anal sphincter** is a thickening of the circular smooth muscle of the anal canal. The **external anal sphincter** is more distal and consists entirely of striated muscle. The external anal sphincter is innervated by somatic motor fibers via the pudendal nerves, which allow the sphincter to be controlled both reflexly and voluntarily.

The motility of the colon promotes the efficient absorption of water and electrolytes and the orderly evacuation of feces

The motility of the cecum and proximal colon is minimally propulsive. Most contractions of the cecum and proximal part of the large bowel are segmental and are more effective at mixing and circulating the contents than at propelling them. In the proximal colon, "antipropulsive" patterns occur. Reverse peristalsis and segmental propulsion toward the cecum both take place; consequently, chyme is retained in the proximal colon, and the absorption of salts and water is facilitated.

Because the taenia coli are shorter than the circular muscle layer of the colon, the colon is divided into neighboring ovoid segments, called **haustra** (Figure 32-16). Localized segmental contractions of colonic circular muscle, called **haustral contractions,** result in back-and-forth mixing of luminal contents.

Normally the distal part of the colon is filled with semisolid feces via a mass movement. Segmental contractions knead the feces and thereby facilitate absorption of the remaining salts and water. About one to three times daily, mass movements occur and sweep the feces toward the rectum.

Colonic motility is regulated by intrinsic and extrinsic nerves. As in other segments of the gastrointestinal tract, the intramural plexuses control the contractile behavior of the colon, and the extrinsic autonomic nerves to the colon are modulatory. The **defecation reflex,** discussed later, is

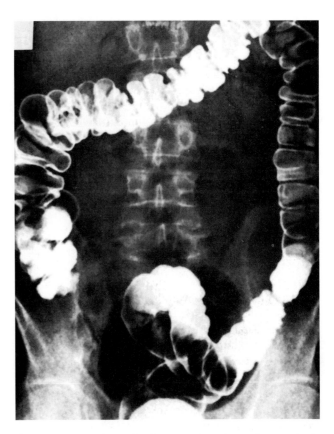

Figure 32-16 X-ray image showing a prominent haustral pattern in the colon of a normal individual. *(From Keats TE: An atlas of normal roentgen variants, ed 2, St Louis, 1979, Mosby.)*

an exception to this rule: It requires the function of the sacral spinal cord via the pelvic nerves.

Colonic smooth muscle has both slow waves and myenteric potential oscillations

Two classes of rhythm-generating cells reside in the colon. Interstitial cells near the inner border of the circular muscle produce regular slow waves with a frequency about six per minute. The slow waves have high amplitude, and their shape resembles that of gastric slow waves. Interstitial cells near the outer border of the circular muscle produce **myenteric potential oscillations,** which are low in amplitude and much higher in frequency than the slow waves.

The circular muscle does not usually fire action potentials. Contractile agonists, such as acetylcholine released from excitatory enteric motor neurons, enhance contractions by increasing the duration of the slow waves. The longer slow waves elicit contractions of the circular muscle.

Longitudinal colonic muscle displays the myenteric potential oscillations. In contrast with the circular smooth muscle, the longitudinal muscle cells fire occasional action potentials at the peaks of the myenteric potential oscillations. The action potentials elicit contraction of the longitudinal muscle. Contractile agonists increase the frequency of action potentials.

Reflex control of colonic motility involves intrinsic and extrinsic neurons

Distention of one part of the colon reflexly relaxes other parts. This **colonocolonic reflex** is mediated by the enteric nervous system and is modulated by the sympathetic fibers that supply the colon. After a meal enters the stomach, the motility of proximal and distal colon and the frequency of mass movements increase reflexly via the **gastrocolic reflex.**

Coordination of the rectum and the anal canal is important in defecation. The rectum is usually empty or nearly so. The rectum is more active than the sigmoid colon in segmental contractions, so the rectal contents tend to move retrogradely into the sigmoid colon. The anal canal is tightly closed by the anal sphincters. Before defecation, the rectum is filled as a result of a mass movement in the sigmoid colon. Filling the rectum brings about reflex relaxation of the internal anal sphincter and reflex constriction of the external anal sphincter and causes the urge to defecate. People who lack functional motor nerves to the external anal sphincter defecate involuntarily when the rectum is filled. The reflex reactions of the sphincters to rectal distention are transient. If defecation is postponed, the sphincters regain their normal tone, and the urge to defecate temporarily subsides.

In **Hirschsprung's disease,** also known as **congenital megacolon,** enteric neurons are congenitally absent from part of the colon. Frequently, only a short length of colon proximal to the internal anal sphincter is involved, but larger segments of the colon may also be affected. In a normal person, filling of the rectum by a mass movement leads to reflex relaxation of the distal rectum and the internal anal sphincter. In the absence of enteric neurons, this reflex relaxation cannot occur. This results in functional obstruction of the distal colon and dilation of the colon above the obstruction.

The integrating center for the defecation reflex is in the sacral spinal cord. When circumstances are appropriate, an individual voluntarily relaxes the external anal sphincter to allow defecation to proceed. Defecation is a complex behavior involving both reflex and voluntary actions. The integrating center for the reflex actions is in the sacral spinal cord and is modulated by higher centers. The principal efferent pathways are cholinergic parasympathetic fibers in the pelvic nerves. The sympathetic nervous system does not play a significant role in normal defecation.

Voluntary actions are important in defecation. The external anal sphincter is voluntarily held in the relaxed state. Intraabdominal pressure is elevated to aid in the expulsion of feces. Evacuation is normally preceded by a deep breath, which moves the diaphragm downward. The glottis is then closed, and contractions of the respiratory muscles on full lungs elevates both the intrathoracic and intraabdominal pressures. Contractions of the muscles of the abdominal wall further increase intraabdominal pressure, which may be as great as 200 cm H_2O. This helps force feces through the relaxed sphincters. The muscles of the pelvic floor are relaxed to allow the floor to drop. This helps straighten the rectum and prevent rectal prolapse.

▪ SUMMARY

- The gastrointestinal tract has a characteristic layered structure consisting of mucosa, submucosa, muscularis externa, and serosa.
- The gastrointestinal tract receives both sympathetic and parasympathetic innervation.
- Contractions of the smooth muscle of the muscularis externa mix and propel the contents of the gastrointestinal tract.
- Gastrointestinal smooth muscle cells are electrically coupled, and their resting membrane potential oscillates with a rhythm characteristic of each segment of the gastrointestinal tract.
- The membrane potential oscillations, called slow waves, control the timing and force of contractions of gastrointestinal smooth muscle.
- The nerve plexuses of the gastrointestinal tract, the enteric nervous system, contain about 10^8 neurons, as many as in the spinal cord. The enteric nervous system contains motor neurons, sensory neurons, and interneurons.
- Enteric sensory neurons function as the afferent arms of enteric reflex arcs by which the enteric nervous system controls most of the motor and secretory activities of the gastrointestinal tract.
- The autonomic nervous system modulates the activities of the enteric nervous system.
- Swallowing is a reflex coordinated by a swallowing center in the medulla and pons.
- Contractions of the stomach mix food with gastric juice and mechanically subdivide the food.
- Hormonal and neural mechanisms initiated by the presence of acid, fats, amino acids, and peptides, as well as hypertonicity in the duodenum, regulate gastric emptying.
- Segmentation is the major contractile activity in the small intestine. Segmental contractions mix and circulate intestinal contents but are not very propulsive.
- In a fasted individual a different pattern of motility, the MMC, occurs. The MMC sweeps the stomach and small intestine clear of any debris left from the previous meal.

- In the proximal colon, antipropulsive contractions predominate, which allows time for the absorption of salts and water. In the transverse and descending colon, haustral contractions mix and knead colonic contents to facilitate the extraction of salts and water.
- Filling the rectum with feces initiates the defecation reflex. The integrating center for the defecation reflex is in the sacral spinal cord.

BIBLIOGRAPHY

Abell TL, Werkman RF: Gastrointestinal motility disorders, *Am Fam Physic* 53:895, 1996.

Diamant NE: Neuromuscular mechanisms of primary peristalsis, *Am J Med* 103(5A):40S, 1997.

Furness JB et al: Roles of peptides in the enteric nervous system, *Trends Neurosci* 15:66, 1992.

Goyal R, Hirano I: The enteric nervous system, *New Engl J Med* 334:1106, 1996.

Jannsens J, ed: *Progress in understanding and management of gastrointestinal motility disorders,* Belgium, 1993, University of Leuven.

Lang IM: Digestive tract motor correlates of vomiting and nausea, *Can J Physiol Pharmacol* 68:242, 1990.

MacDonald IA: Physiological regulation of gastric emptying and glucose absorption, *Diabetic Med* 13(suppl 5):S11, 1996.

Makhlouf GM: Neuromuscular function of the small intestine. In Johnson RL, ed: *Physiology of the gastrointestinal tract,* ed 3, New York, 1994, Raven.

Plant RL: Anatomy and physiology of swallowing, *Otolarygnol Clin North Am* 31:477, 1998.

Pope CE II: The esophagus for the nonesophagologist, *Am J Med* 103(5A):19S, 1997.

Quigley EM: Gastric and small intestinal motility in health and disease, *Gastroenterol Clin North Am* 25:113, 1996.

Sanders KM: Ionic mechanisms of electrical rhythmicity in gastrointestinal smooth muscles, *Annu Rev Physiol* 54:439, 1992.

Sanders KM: A case for interstitial cells of Cajal as pacemakers and mediators of neurotransmission in the gastrointestinal tract, *Gastroenterology* 112:492, 1996.

Smith TK, Bornstein JC, Furness JB: Interactions between reflexes evoked by distention and mucosal stimulation: electrophysiological studies of guinea-pig ileum, *J Autonom Nerv Syst* 34:69, 1991.

Walsh JH, Dockray GJ, eds: *Gut peptides: biochemistry and physiology,* ed 3, New York, 1994, Raven.

▷ CASE STUDIES

Case 32-1

A 42-year-old woman reports difficulty in swallowing solid foods; liquids are less difficult to swallow. Chest pain follows eating, and she frequently regurgitates after eating. When the recumbent patient underwent fluoroscopy after a barium swallow, her lower esophagus was somewhat dilated compared to normal, but her upper esophagus was of normal caliber. Subsequent swallows initiated by the patient showed that the barium was cleared from the esophagus very slowly. The acute administration of amyl nitrite caused the barium to be cleared more rapidly. Manometric studies showed a resting pressure in the lower esophageal sphincter of about 60 mm Hg, with a decrease to about 45 mm Hg after a swallow. The patient was treated with forceful dilation of the lower esophageal sphincter using a pneumatic dilating device. The patient's ability to swallow solid food was dramatically improved after the dilation procedure. Some 15 months after the dilation, the patient returned because swallowing had again become difficult.

1. **Which statement about this patient is true?**
   A. The resting pressure in the lower esophageal sphincter is close to normal.
   B. The pressure in the lower esophageal sphincter is much higher than normal in the relaxed state.
   C. A normal esophageal peristaltic pressure wave would be expected when the patient swallows.
   D. The lower esophageal sphincter pressures do not explain the slowness of the barium clearance from the esophagus.
   E. None of the above.

2. **Which statement about this patient is true?**
   A. The efficacy of amyl nitrite shows that there is no abnormality of the musculature of the lower esophageal sphincter.
   B. The innervation of the lower esophageal sphincter is functioning normally.
   C. Hypertrophy of the lower esophageal sphincter may be present.
   D. The patient suffers from diffuse esophageal spasm.
   E. None of the above.

3. **Which statement about this patient is true?**
   A. The recurrence of her problems 15 months after dilation is unexpected.
   B. Pharmacological therapy is unlikely to help the patient.
   C. Surgical intervention might help alleviate the symptoms.
   D. Repeating the dilation of the lower esophageal sphincter is unlikely to help relieve the symptoms.
   E. None of the above.

Case 32-2

A 5-week-old boy has abdominal distention. His parents report that his bowel movements are infrequent (once every other day, on average) and that he vomits frequently. Digital examination of the baby's rectum reveals that the rectal ampulla is empty; a short squirt of fecal material is expressed when the physician's finger is removed. A lateral x-ray study performed after a barium enema reveals that the distal 7 cm of the rectum has a narrowed lumen and that most of the colon above the narrowed segment is enlarged. When the rectum is distended with a balloon, the internal anal sphincter fails to show the normal transient relaxation. The provisional diagnosis is Hirschsprung's disease.

1. Which statement about this patient is true?

   A. Failure of the internal anal sphincter to relax on rectal distention clinches the diagnosis of Hirschsprung's disease.

   B. The next step should be a full-thickness biopsy of the rectum.

   C. A suction biopsy of the mucosa would not add useful information.

   D. The presence of enlarged nerve trunks in the mucosa would help confirm the diagnosis.

   E. None of the above.

2. Which statement about this patient is true?

   A. The probability that a younger male sibling will have Hirschsprung's disease is 0.25.

   B. The disorder will spontaneously become less severe as the baby grows and develops.

   C. The disorder can be managed with drugs that relax colonic muscle.

   D. The recommended treatment is surgical.

   E. None of the above.

3. What does the recommended surgical treatment of Hirschsprung's disease involve?

   A. Incising the circular muscle of the aganglionic segment of colon to weaken it

   B. Removing most of the colon

   C. Constructing a permanent colostomy

   D. Removing only the aganglionic segment of the colon

   E. None of the above

CHAPTER 33

Gastrointestinal Secretions ———

OBJECTIVES

- Describe the composition of saliva and explain the cellular processes in acinar and duct cells responsible for the secretion of saliva.
- Explain the physiological functions of gastric juice.
- Describe the physiological mechanisms that regulate the secretion of hydrochloric acid in the stomach.
- Explain how mucus and bicarbonate create a "gastric mucosal barrier."
- Explain the physiological functions of pancreatic juice.
- Explain the physiological mechanisms that regulate the secretion of bile.

This chapter deals with the glandular secretion of fluids and compounds that have important functions in the digestive tract. In particular, the secretions of the salivary glands, gastric glands, exocrine pancreas, and liver are considered. The functions of these secretions in digestion are discussed in Chapter 34. In each case the nature of the secretions and their functions in digestion are discussed, and the regulation of the secretory processes is emphasized. These gastrointestinal secretions are elicited by the action of specific neurocrine, endocrine, and paracrine effector substances on the secretory cells (see Chapter 5). A substance that stimulates secretion is called a **secretagogue.**

Saliva Lubricates Food and Begins the Digestion of Starch

In humans the salivary glands produce about 1 L of saliva each day. Saliva lubricates food for greater ease of swallowing and also facilitates speaking.

In people who lack functional salivary glands, **xerostomia** (dry mouth), **dental caries,** and infections of the buccal mucosa are prevalent. Saliva contains **secretory immunoglobulins** (antibodies) directed against microorganisms in the mouth. In the absence of these antibod-

ies, organisms that cause buccal infections and dental caries proliferate. The basic pH of saliva also helps prevent dental caries.

Saliva contains mucins and an α-amylase

Mucins, which are glycoproteins produced by the submaxillary and sublingual glands, lubricate food so that it can be more readily swallowed. The major digestive function of saliva is the action of **salivary amylase** on starch. Salivary amylase is an enzyme with the same specificity as the α-amylase of pancreatic juice; it reduces starch to oligosaccharide molecules. The pH optimum of salivary amylase is about 7, but it is active between a pH of 4 and 11. Amylase action continues in the mass of food in the stomach and is terminated only when the contents of the antrum are mixed with enough gastric acid to lower the pH to less than 4. More than half the starch in a well-chewed meal may be reduced to small oligosaccharides by the action of salivary amylase. However, because of the large capacity of the pancreatic α-amylase to digest starch in the small intestine, starch is well-absorbed even in the absence of salivary amylase.

Secretory endpieces in salivary glands are drained by a system of ducts

In humans the **parotid glands,** the largest salivary glands, are entirely serous. Their watery secretion lacks mucins. The **submaxillary** and **sublingual glands** are mixed mucous and serous glands, and they secrete a more viscous saliva that contains mucins. Many smaller salivary glands are present in the oral cavity. The microscopic structure of a mixed salivary gland is depicted in Figure 33-1. The **serous acinar cells** located in the **secretory endpieces** (also called **acini**) have apical **zymogen granules** that contain salivary amylase and perhaps certain other salivary proteins. **Mucous acinar cells** secrete mucins into the saliva. **Intercalated ducts** drain the acinar fluid into somewhat larger ducts, the **striated ducts,** which empty into still larger **excretory ducts.** A single large duct brings the secretions of each major gland into the mouth.

A **primary secretion** is elaborated in the secretory endpieces. The cells that line the ducts modify the primary secretion.

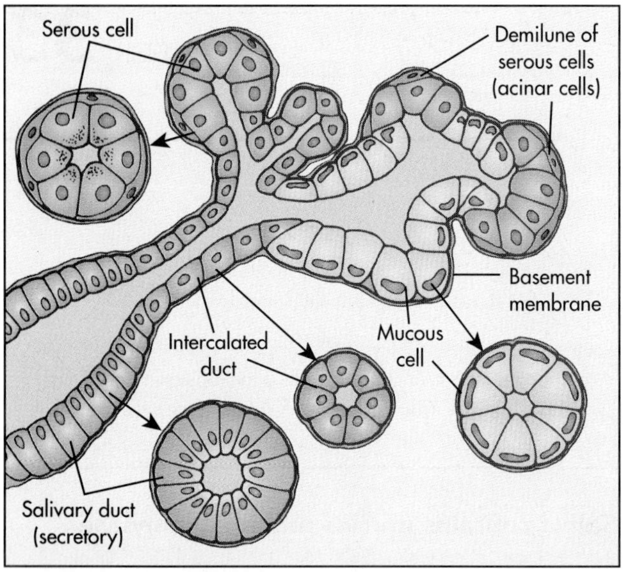

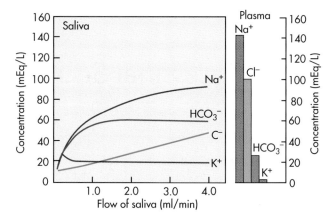

Figure 33-1 Structure of the human submandibular gland as seen with the light microscope. (*Redrawn from Braus H:* Anatomie des Menschen, *Berlin, 1934, Julius Springer.*)

Actively secreting salivary glands have a high metabolic rate and a high blood flow

The salivary glands produce a prodigious flow of saliva. The maximum rate in humans is about 1 ml/min/g of gland; AT THIS RATE THE GLANDS ARE PRODUCING THEIR OWN WEIGHT IN SALIVA EACH MINUTE. Salivary glands have a high rate of metabolism and a high blood flow; both are proportional to the rate of saliva formation. The blood flow to maximally secreting salivary glands is approximately 10 times that of an equal mass of actively contracting skeletal muscle. Stimulation of the parasympathetic nerves to salivary glands increases blood flow via dilation of the vasculature of the glands. **Vasoactive intestinal polypeptide (VIP)** and **acetylcholine** are released from parasympathetic nerve terminals in the salivary glands; both of these compounds contribute to vasodilation during secretory activity.

Both acinar cells and duct cells help determine the composition of saliva

Saliva is hypotonic to plasma

As shown in Figure 33-2, salivary concentrations of Na^+ and Cl^- are less than those of plasma. The greater the secretory flow rate, the higher the tonicity of the saliva; at maximum flow rates the tonicity of saliva in humans is about 70% of that of plasma. The pH of saliva from resting glands is slightly acidic. During active secretion, however, the saliva becomes basic, with the pH near 8. The increase in pH with the secretory flow rate is partly caused by the increase in the salivary bicarbonate (HCO_3^-) concentration.

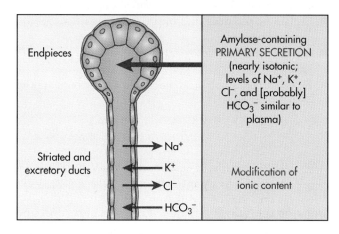

Figure 33-2 Average composition of parotid saliva as a function of salivary flow rate. Saliva is hypotonic to plasma at all flow rates. The bicarbonate (HCO_3^-) level in saliva exceeds that in plasma, except at very low flow rates. (*Redrawn from Thaysen JH et al:* Am J Physiol *178:155, 1954.*)

Figure 33-3 Two-stage model of salivary secretion. The primary secretion, containing salivary amylase, is secreted by the acinar cells. The striated and excretory ducts modify the composition of saliva.

Acinar cells elaborate a primary secretion, which is modified by the duct cells

A two-stage model of salivary secretion (Figure 33-3) postulates the following:

1. The secretory endpieces, perhaps with the participation of intercalated ducts, produce a primary secretion that is isotonic to plasma. The amylase concentration and the rate of fluid secretion vary with the level and type of stimulation. However, the electrolyte composition of the secretion is fairly constant, and the levels of Na^+, K^+, and Cl^- are close to plasma levels.

2. The excretory ducts and probably the striated ducts modify the primary secretion by extracting Na^+ and Cl^- from the saliva and adding K^+ and HCO_3^- to it. The ducts do not add to the volume of saliva.

As saliva flows down the ducts, it becomes progressively more hypotonic. Thus the ducts remove more ions from saliva than they contribute to it. The faster the flow rate of the saliva down the striated and excretory ducts, the closer it is to isotonicity.

In their apical cytoplasm, serous acinar cells have zymogen granules that contain salivary amylase. When the gland is stimulated to secrete, the zymogen granules fuse with the plasma membrane and release their contents into the lumen of an acinus by exocytosis.

Salivary gland functions are regulated principally by parasympathetic nerves

Excitation of either sympathetic or parasympathetic nerves to the salivary glands stimulates salivary secretion, but the effects of the parasympathetic nerves are stronger and last longer. Interruption of the sympathetic nerves causes no major defect in the function of the salivary glands. If the parasympathetic supply is interrupted, however, the salivary glands atrophy. THE ESSENTIAL PHYSIOLOGICAL CONTROL OF SALIVARY SECRETIONS IS VIA THE PARASYMPATHETIC NERVOUS SYSTEM.

Sympathetic fibers to the salivary glands come from the superior cervical ganglion. Preganglionic parasympathetic fibers come via branches of the facial and glossopharyngeal nerves (cranial nerves VII and IX, respectively), and they synapse with postganglionic neurons in or near the salivary glands. The acinar cells and ducts are supplied with parasympathetic nerve endings.

Parasympathetic stimulation increases the synthesis and secretion of salivary amylase and mucins, enhances the transport activities of the ductular epithelium, greatly increases blood flow to the glands, and stimulates glandular metabolism and growth. The increase in salivary secretion that results from stimulation of sympathetic nerves is transient. Sympathetic stimulation constricts blood vessels, with consequent reductions in salivary gland blood flow.

Duct cells are stimulated by acetylcholine and norepinephrine

The ducts of salivary glands respond to both cholinergic and adrenergic agonists by increasing their rates of secretion of K^+ and HCO_3^-.

Acinar cells are stimulated by several neurocrine agonists

Neuroeffector substances that stimulate acinar cell secretions act mainly by elevating intracellular cyclic AMP or by increasing the level of Ca^{++} in the cytosol. Acetylcholine, norepinephrine, substance P, and VIP are released in salivary glands by specific nerve terminals. Each of these neuroeffectors may increase the secretion of salivary amylase and the flow of saliva.

Norepinephrine, acting on β-receptors, and VIP elevate cyclic AMP in acinar cells. In contrast, acetylcholine, substance P, and the activation of α-receptors by norepinephrine increase intracellular Ca^{++}.

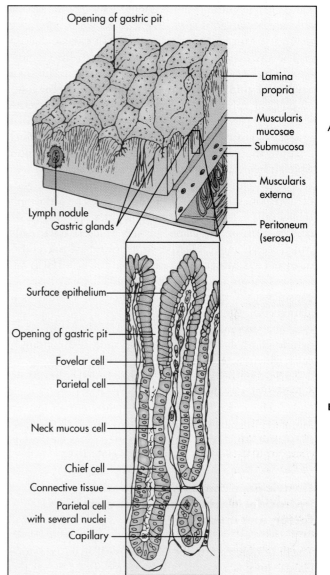

Figure 33-4 Structure of the gastric mucosa. **A,** Reconstruction of part of the gastric wall. **B,** Two gastric glands from a human stomach. *(A redrawn from Braus H:* Anatomie des Menschen, Berlin, 1934, Julius Springer. *B redrawn From Weis L, ed:* Histology: cell and tissue biology, ed 5, New York, 1981, Elsevier.)

Gastric Secretions Begin the Digestion of Proteins and Have Other Important Functions

The wall of the stomach contains exocrine glands and endocrine cells

The surface of the gastric mucosa (Figure 33-4) is covered by columnar **epithelial cells** that secrete mucus and an alkaline fluid that protects the epithelium from mechanical injury and gastric acid. The surface is studded with **gastric pits;** each pit is the opening of a duct into which one or more **gastric glands** empty (Figure 33-4, *A*). THE GASTRIC PITS ARE SO NUMEROUS THAT THEY ACCOUNT FOR A SIGNIFICANT FRACTION OF THE TOTAL SURFACE AREA OF THE GASTRIC MUCOSA.

The gastric mucosa can be divided into three regions based on the structures of the glands present. The small **cardiac glandular region,** which is just below the lower esophageal sphincter, contains mainly mucus-secreting gland cells. The remainder of the gastric mucosa is divided into the **oxyntic** (acid-secreting) **glandular region,** which is above the notch, and the **pyloric glandular region,** which is below the notch (see Figure 32-9).

The structure of a gastric gland from the oxyntic glandular region is illustrated in Figure 33-4, *B.* The surface epithelial cells extend slightly into the duct opening. In the narrow neck of the gland are the **mucous neck cells,** which secrete mucus. Deeper in the gland are **parietal** or **oxyntic cells,** which secrete hydrochloric acid (HCl) and intrinsic factor, and **chief** or **peptic cells,** which secrete pepsinogens. Oxyntic cells are particularly numerous in glands in the fundus.

Mucus-secreting cells predominate in the glands of the pyloric glandular region. Pyloric glands also contain **G cells,** which secrete the hormone **gastrin.**

Surface epithelial cells are exfoliated into the lumen at a considerable rate during normal gastric function. They are replaced by mucous neck cells, which differentiate into columnar epithelial cells and migrate up out of the necks of the glands. The capacity of the stomach to repair damage to its epithelial surface in this way is remarkable.

Gastric juice contains salts, water, hydrochloric acid, pepsins, intrinsic factor, and mucus

The fluid secreted into the stomach is called **gastric juice.** Gastric juice is a mixture of the secretions of the surface epithelial cells and the secretions of gastric glands. Secretion of all these components increases after a meal.

The ionic composition of gastric juice depends on the rate of secretion. The higher the secretory rate, the higher the concentration of hydrogen ion (Figure 33-5). At lower secretory rates, the H^+ concentration diminishes and the Na^+ concentration increases. The K^+ concentration is always higher in gastric juice than in plasma, and consequently, prolonged vomiting may lead to hypokalemia. At all rates of secretion, Cl^- is the major anion of gastric juice. At high rates of secretion, the composition of gastric juice resembles that of an isotonic solution of HCl. Gastric HCl converts pepsinogens to active pepsins (see later section) and provides an acid pH at which pepsins are active.

Basal (unstimulated) rates of gastric acid production typically range from about 1 to 5 mEq/hr in humans. On maximal stimulation, HCl production rises to 6 to 40 mEq/hr. On average, less HCl is secreted in patients with gastric ulcers, but more than normal is secreted in patients with duodenal ulcers. The reasons for this are discussed later.

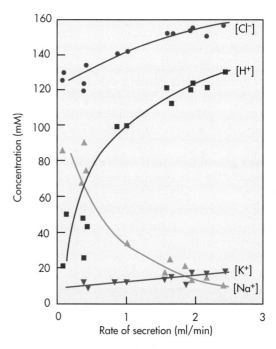

Figure 33-5 Concentrations of ions in gastric juice as a function of the rate of secretion in a normal young person. At low flow rates, gastric juice is hypotonic to plasma. At high flow rates, gastric juice approaches isotonicity and contains predominantly H^+ and Cl^-. *(Modified from Nordgren B: Acta Physiol Scand 58[suppl 202]:1, 1963.)*

> The high acidity of gastric juice kills most ingested microorganisms. Individuals who have low rates of gastric acid secretion, either because they have a disease or they are taking medications that suppress HCl secretion, are more susceptible to infection by ingested pathogens.

Dramatic morphological changes in parietal cells accompany gastric acid secretion

Parietal cells have a distinctive ultrastructure (Figure 33-6) and an elaborate system of branching **secretory canaliculi,** which course through the cytoplasm and are connected by a common outlet to the cells' luminal surface. Microvilli line the surfaces of the canaliculi. The cytoplasm of unstimulated parietal cells contains numerous tubules and vesicles: the **tubulovesicular system.** The membranes of the tubovesicles contain the transport proteins responsible for the secretion of H^+ and Cl^- into the lumen of the gland. When parietal cells are stimulated to secrete HCl (Figure 33-6, *B*), tubulovesicular membranes fuse with the plasma membrane of the secretory canaliculi; this extensive membrane fusion greatly increases the number of HCl pumping sites available at the surface of the secretory canaliculi.

The prime mover in gastric H^+ secretion is a proton-pumping ATPase

At maximal rates of secretion, H^+ is pumped against a concentration gradient that is more than one million to one. Cl^- also enters the gastric lumen against a large

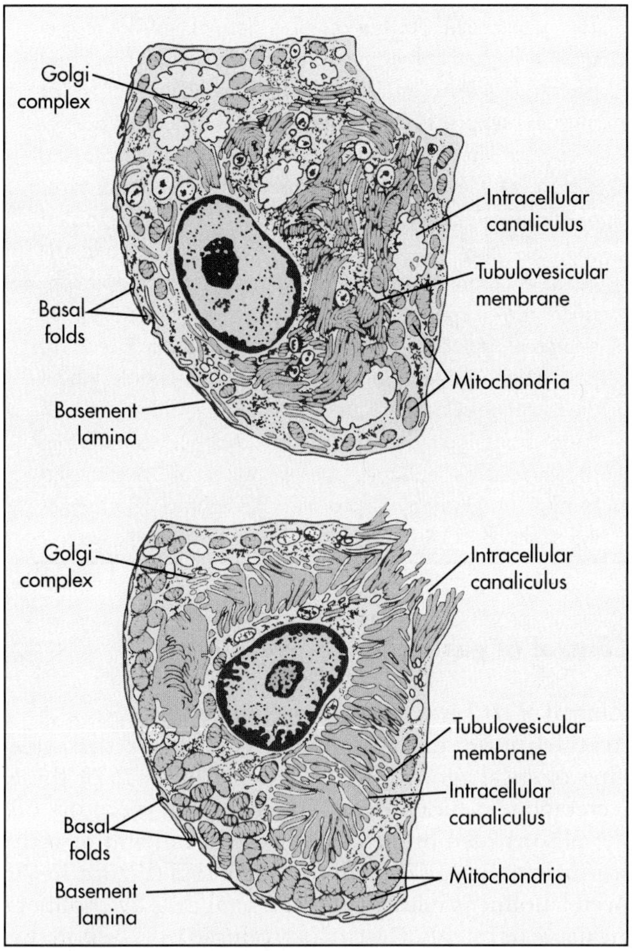

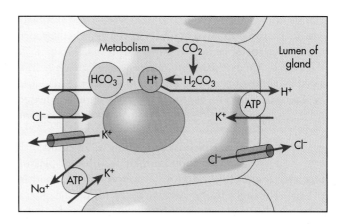

Figure 33-7 Simplified view of the major ionic transport processes involved in the secretion of H^+ and Cl^- by parietal cells. Cl^- enters the cell across the basolateral membrane against an electrochemical gradient. Its entry is powered by the downhill efflux of HCO_3^-. The high level of HCO_3^- in the cytosol is generated by the active extrusion of H^+ across the luminal membrane. Protons are pumped into the secretory canaliculus by H^+,K^+-ATPase. Cl^- enters the canalicular fluid via an electrogenic ion channel.

Figure 33-6 A, Resting parietal cell with a cytoplasm full of tubulovesicles and an internalized intracellular canaliculus. **B,** Acid-secreting parietal cell. The tubulovesicles have fused with the membrane of the intracellular canaliculus, which is now open to the lumen of the gland and is lined with abundant long microvilli. *(Redrawn from Ito S. In Johnson LR, ed:* Physiology of the gastrointestinal tract, *New York, 1981, Raven.)*

electrochemical potential difference. Thus energy is required for the transport of both H^+ and Cl^-.

The apical membrane of the parietal cell (the membrane that lines the secretory canaliculus) contains H^+,K^+-ATPase, which exchanges H^+ for K^+ (Figure 33-7). This ATPase is the primary H^+ pump. Both H^+ and K^+ are pumped against their electrochemical potential gradients.

When H^+ is pumped out of the parietal cell, an excess of HCO_3^- is left behind. HCO_3^- flows down its electrochemical gradient across the basolateral plasma membrane. The protein that mediates HCO_3^- efflux transports Cl^- in the opposite direction. Cl^- moves against its electrochemical potential gradient into the cell, and the energy for the active transport of Cl^- comes from the downhill movement of HCO_3^-.

As a result of the combined action of H^+,K^+-ATPase and the Cl^-–HCO_3^- counter-transporter, Cl^- is concentrated in the cytoplasm of the parietal cell. Cl^- leaves

the parietal cell at the apical membrane via an electrogenic anion channel.

Pepsins begin the digestion of proteins

Pepsins, often collectively called **pepsin,** are a group of proteases secreted by the chief cells of the gastric glands. Pepsins are secreted as inactive proenzymes called **pepsinogens.** The cleavage of acid-labile linkages converts pepsinogens to active pepsins: The lower the pH, the more rapid the conversion. Pepsins also act proteolytically on pepsinogens to form more pepsins.

The pepsins have their highest proteolytic activity at a pH of 3 and below. Pepsins may digest as much as 20% of the protein in a typical meal. When the duodenal contents are neutralized, pepsins are inactivated irreversibly by the neutral pH. Pepsinogens are contained in membrane-bound zymogen granules in the chief cells. The contents of the zymogen granules are released by exocytosis when the chief cells are stimulated to secrete.

Intrinsic factor is required for the normal absorption of vitamin B$_{12}$

Intrinsic factor, a glycoprotein, is secreted by the parietal cells of the stomach. Intrinsic factor is released in response to the same stimuli that evoke the secretion of HCl by parietal cells. THE SECRETION OF INTRINSIC FACTOR IS THE ONLY GASTRIC FUNCTION THAT IS ESSENTIAL FOR HUMAN LIFE.

Mucus and bicarbonate help protect surface epithelial cells

Secretions that contain glycoprotein mucins are viscous and sticky and are collectively termed **mucus.** Mucins are secreted by mucous neck cells in the necks of gastric glands and by the surface epithelial cells of the stomach. Mucus is stored in large granules in the apical cytoplasm of mucous neck cells and surface epithelial cells; it is released by exocytosis. The secretion of mucus is stimulated by some of the same stimuli that enhance acid and pepsinogen secretion, especially via acetylcholine released from parasympathetic nerve endings near the gastric glands.

The surface epithelial cells also secrete watery fluid with Na^+ and Cl^- concentrations similar to those of plasma but with higher K^+ and HCO_3^- concentrations than in plasma. The high HCO_3^- concentration makes the mucus alkaline. Mucus is secreted by the resting mucosa and lines the stomach with a sticky, viscous, alkaline coat. When food is eaten, the rates of secretion of mucus and HCO_3^- increase.

The gastric mucosal barrier requires both mucus and bicarbonate

Mucus forms a gel on the luminal surface of the mucosa. MUCUS AND THE ALKALINE SECRETIONS ENTRAPPED WITHIN IT CONSTITUTE A GASTRIC MUCOSAL BARRIER THAT PREVENTS DAMAGE TO THE MUCOSA FROM GASTRIC CONTENTS (Figure 33-8). Pepsins cleave certain peptide bonds in the mucin molecules and thereby dissolve the gel. The gel must be replenished via the synthesis of new mucin molecules.

The mucous gel layer prevents the HCO_3^--rich secretions of the surface epithelial cells from rapidly mixing with the contents of the gastric lumen. Thus the surface of the epithelial cells can be maintained at a nearly neutral pH despite a luminal pH of about 2. The protection depends on the secretion of both mucus and HCO_3^-; neither mucus alone nor HCO_3^- alone can hold the pH at the epithelial cell surface near neutral.

The gastric mucosal barrier of a normal individual can protect the stomach even when secretion rates of HCl and pepsins are elevated. If the secretion of either HCO_3^- or mucus is suppressed, however, the gastric mucosal barrier is compromised, and the effects of acid and pepsin on the surface of the stomach may produce **gastric ulcers.** α-Adrenergic agonists diminish HCO_3^- secretion. This effect may play a role in the pathogenesis of **stress ulcers:** A chronically elevated level of circulating epinephrine may suppress HCO_3^- secretion sufficiently to decrease protection of the epithelial cell surface. Aspirin and other nonsteroidal antiinflammatory agents inhibit the secretion of both mucus and HCO_3^-; prolonged use of these drugs may damage the mucosal surface. Certain prostaglandins enhance the secretion of mucus and HCO_3^- and thereby help protect the epithelial surface of the stomach.

Control of gastric acid secretion

Control of HCl secretion by the parietal cell

Acetylcholine, histamine, and **gastrin** are the three physiological agonists of HCl secretion. Each of these secretagogues binds to a distinct class of receptors on the plasma membrane of the parietal cell and directly stimulates the parietal cell to secrete HCl (Figure 33-9). Acetylcholine is released near parietal cells by cholinergic nerve terminals. Gastrin is produced by G cells in the mucosa of the gastric antrum and the duodenum and reaches parietal cells via the bloodstream. Histamine, a paracrine agonist, is released from cells in the gastric mucosa and diffuses to the parietal cells.

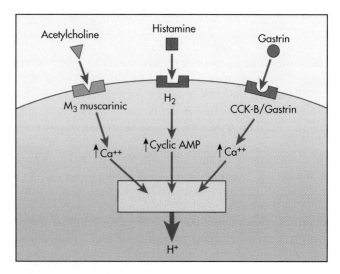

Figure 33-9 Secretagogues that elicit acid secretion from the parietal cells. Acetylcholine binds to M_3 muscarinic receptors. Histamine acts via H_2-histamine receptors *(H_2)*. Gastrin binds to cholecystokinin/gastrin receptors *(CCK-B/Gastrin)*. Acetylcholine and gastrin act to increase levels of cytosolic free Ca^{++}. Histamine increases intracellular levels of cyclic AMP.

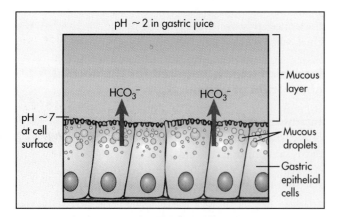

Figure 33-8 The protection provided to the mucosal surface of the stomach by the HCO_3^--containing mucus layer is known as the gastric mucosal barrier. Buffering by the HCO_3^--rich secretions of the surface epithelial cells and the restraint to convective mixing caused by the high viscosity of the mucus layer allow the pH at the cell surface to remain near 7, whereas the pH in the gastric juice in the lumen is 1 to 2.

Cellular mechanisms of parietal cell agonists

The receptors for acetylcholine, gastrin, and histamine on the parietal cell membrane and the intracellular second messengers by which these secretagogues act are shown in Figure 33-9. Histamine is a major physiological mediator of HCl secretion. **Cimetidine,** a specific antagonist of H$_2$ receptors, blocks a large portion of the acid secretion elicited by any known secretagogue. **Enterochromaffin-like** (ECL) **cells,** present in the gastric muscosa, synthesize and store histamine. When stimulated by acetylcholine or gastrin, the ECL cells release histamine, which diffuses to nearby parietal cells to stimulate HCl secretion.

Gastrin is not as potent a direct stimulant of parietal cells as acetylcholine or histamine. The physiological response to elevated levels of gastrin in the blood is greatly attenuated by cimetidine. Thus a major component of the physiological response to gastrin results from the gastrin-stimulated release of histamine.

> The availability of cimetidine and other H$_2$-receptor blockers has revolutionized therapy for duodenal ulcer disease and other disorders related to the hypersecretion of gastric acid. These drugs usually diminish the secretion of HCl dramatically, and they have few side effects. H$_2$-receptor blockers are not as effective in patients with **Zollinger-Ellison syndrome.** Such patients have gastrin-secreting tumors and thus have very high serum levels of gastrin. **Omeprazole** (a specific and irreversible inhibitor of H$^+$,K$^+$-ATPase) is the current drug of choice for treating these patients.

The three phases of gastric acid secretion are the cephalic, gastric, and intestinal phases

When the stomach has been empty for several hours, HCl is secreted at a basal rate, which is approximately 10% of the maximal rate. After a meal, the rate of acid secretion by the stomach increases promptly. There are three phases of increased acid secretion in response to food: the **cephalic phase,** elicited before food reaches the stomach; the **gastric phase,** elicited by the presence of food in the stomach; and the **intestinal phase,** elicited by mechanisms that originate in the duodenum and upper jejunum (Table 33-1).

THE CEPHALIC PHASE OF GASTRIC SECRETION IS NORMALLY ELICITED BY THE SIGHT, SMELL, AND TASTE OF FOOD. Cholinergic vagal fibers and cholinergic neurons of the intramural plexuses evoke cephalic phase secretion. Acetylcholine released from these neurons directly stimulates parietal cells to secrete HCl. Acetylcholine also indirectly stimulates acid secretion by releasing gastrin from G cells in the antrum and duodenum and by releasing histamine from ECL cells in the gastric mucosa.

A low pH in the antrum of the stomach diminishes the amount of HCl secreted during the cephalic phase. In the absence of food in the stomach to buffer the acid secreted, the pH of the antral contents falls rapidly during the cephalic phase. A low pH limits the amount of acid secreted by inhibiting the parietal cells directly and by evoking inhibitory intrinsic neural reflexes.

IN THE GASTRIC PHASE THE PRINCIPAL STIMULI ARE DISTENTION OF THE STOMACH AND THE PRESENCE OF AMINO ACIDS AND PEPTIDES RESULTING FROM THE ACTIONS OF PEPSINS. Most of the acid secreted in response to a meal is secreted during the gastric phase. The secretion of HCl is blocked effectively by bathing of the mucosal surface with a solution having a pH of 2 or less. Once the buffering capacity of the gastric contents is saturated, the gastric pH falls rapidly and inhibits further acid release. In this way the acidity of gastric contents regulates itself.

The presence of amino acids and peptides in the antrum elicits HCl secretion by causing G cells in the antrum to release gastrin. Intact proteins do not have this effect. Other ingested substances that can enhance gastric acid secretion include Ca^{++}, caffeine, and alcohol.

DURING THE INTESTINAL PHASE, GASTRIC SECRETION IS MODULATED BY THE DUODENAL CONTENTS. The presence of chyme in the duodenum causes neural and endocrine responses that first stimulate and later inhibit the secretion of acid by the stomach. Early in gastric emptying, when the pH of gastric chyme is greater than 3, the stimulatory influences predominate. Later, when the

Table 33-1	Major Mechanisms for Stimulation of Gastric Acid Secretion		
Phase	**Stimulus**	**Pathway**	**Stimulus to Parietal Cell**
Cephalic	Chewing, swallowing, etc.	Vagus nerve to:	
		Parietal cells	Acetylcholine
		G cells	Gastrin
Gastric	Gastric distention	Local and vagovagal reflexes to:	
		Parietal cells	Acetylcholine
		G cells	Gastrin
Intestinal	Protein digestion products in duodenum	Intestinal G cells	Gastrin
		Intestinal endocrine cells	Enterooxyntin

Modified from Johnson LR, ed: *Gastrointestinal physiology,* ed 4, St Louis, 1991, Mosby.

buffer capacity of gastric chyme is exhausted and the pH of chyme emptied into the duodenum falls to less than 3, inhibitory influences prevail. Tables 33-1 and 33-2 summarize the major mechanisms that stimulate and inhibit gastric acid secretion.

Gastric secretion is enhanced by distention of the duodenum and by the presence of protein digestion products (peptides and amino acids) in the duodenum. The duodenum and proximal jejunum contain G cells that release gastrin when stimulated by peptides and amino acids.

Several mechanisms that operate during the intestinal phase inhibit gastric secretion (Table 33-2). These mechanisms are evoked by the presence of acid, fat digestion products, and hypertonicity in the duodenum and proximal part of the jejunum.

Acid solutions in the duodenum release the hormone **secretin** into the bloodstream. Secretin inhibits gastric acid by inhibiting the release of gastrin by G cells and by decreasing the response of parietal cells to secretagogues. Acid in the duodenum also inhibits gastric acid secretion via a local nervous reflex. Acid in the duodenal bulb releases another hormone, **bulbogastrone,** which inhibits acid secretion by the parietal cells.

The products of triglyceride digestion in the duodenum and proximal part of the jejunum release two hormones, **gastric inhibitory peptide** and **cholecystokinin** (CCK), that inhibit acid secretion by parietal cells. Hyperosmotic solutions in the duodenum release an uncharacterized hormone that inhibits gastric acid secretion.

> Patients with gastric ulcers frequently have subnormal rates of HCl secretion. This may be counterintuitive. Gastric ulcers may be caused by a failure of the gastric mucosal barrier to prevent a large decrease in pH at the surface of the gastric mucosa. This decrease suppresses HCl secretion. Duodenal ulcer patients, in contrast, often have elevated rates of HCl secretion. In some cases, hypersecretion of HCl is caused by diminished sensitivity of the mechanisms that inhibit gastric HCl secretion. As a result, HCl is emptied into the duodenum more rapidly than H⁺ can be neutralized; this leads to ulceration of the duodenum.

Many of the agents that stimulate the secretion of hydrochloric acid also elicit the secretion of pepsinogens

The release rates of acid by parietal cells and of pepsinogens by chief cells are highly correlated. Acetylcholine is a potent stimulus that causes the chief cells to release pepsinogens. Gastrin also directly stimulates chief cells. Acid in contact with the gastric mucosa stimulates pepsinogen release via a local neural reflex. Secretin and CCK released by the duodenal mucosa stimulate chief cells to secrete pepsinogens.

Helicobacter pylori infection is responsible for nearly all cases of gastric and duodenal ulcers not related to medication

The term **peptic ulcer disease** includes both gastric and duodenal ulcers. Among the mechanisms that may contribute to ulcer formation are infection by *Helicobacter pylori* bacteria, diminished effectiveness of the gastric mucosal barrier, and hypersecretion of acid.

Diminished effectiveness of the gastric mucosal barrier and formation of gastric ulcers may result from long-term treatment with nonsteroidal antiinflammatory agents that diminish the rates of secretion of mucus and HCO_3^-. Hypersecretion of acid may contribute to the formation of duodenal ulcers. In **Zollinger-Ellison's syndrome** a gastrin-secreting tumor results in increased secretion of HCl and the formation of duodenal ulcers.

H. pylori thrives in an acidic environment. These bacte-

Table 33-2	Major Mechanisms for Inhibition of Gastric Acid Secretion			
Region	**Stimulus**	**Mediator**	**Inhibition of Gastrin Release**	**Inhibition of Acid Secretion by Parietal Cell**
Antrum	Acid (pH < 3.0)	None, direct	+	
Duodenum	Acid	Secretin	+	+
		Bulbogastrone	+	+
		Neural reflex		+
Duodenum and jejunum	Hyperosmotic solutions	Unidentified enterogastrone		+
	Fatty acids, monoglycerides	Gastric inhibitory peptide	+	+
		Cholecystokinin		+
		Unidentified enterogastrone		+

Modified from Johnson LR, ed: *Gastrointestinal physiology,* ed 4, St Louis, 1991, Mosby.

ria have high levels of urease, the enzyme that catalyzes the conversion of urea to ammonia and carbon dioxide. Ammonia helps buffer the acid surrounding the bacteria. *H. pylori* colonizes the mucous layer of the stomach and duodenum. It does not invade the mucosa but secretes proteins that evoke both cellular and humoral immune responses. The invasion of the mucosa by macrophages and other immunocytes results in **chronic superficial gastritis,** which frequently leads to ulcer disease.

The stomachs of about 40% of the people in the world are infected with *H. pylori*. Most of these people may have chronic superficial gastritis that causes mild symptoms. In other individuals, *H. pylori* causes more severe gastritis or ulcerations. Chronic severe gastritis caused by *H. pylori* probably predisposes the individual to the development of gastric cancer.

Most duodenal ulcers are associated with *H. pylori* infection of the duodenum. Patients with duodenal ulcers are often hypersecretors of HCl; this may be partly attributed to diminished sensitivity to the inhibition of HCl secretion by secretin released from the duodenum. The resulting decreased pH of the duodenum conduces to infection by acid-loving *H. pylori*.

Antibiotic therapy is part of the recommended treatment of gastric or duodenal ulcer disease in *H. pylori*–infected patients. Usually a drug is also administered to suppress HCl secretion because such suppression renders *H. pylori* more sensitive to antibiotics. Treatment with **omeprazole** or H_2-receptor antagonists, but without antibiotics, diminishes the population of *H. pylori* and promotes the healing of ulcers. But when the administration of blockers of acid secretion is discontinued, *H. pylori* again flourish, and in most cases, ulcers recur.

Pancreatic Secretions Include Enzymes that Digest all the Major Foodstuffs

The human pancreas weighs less than 100 g; yet each day it secretes about 1 L (10 times its mass) of pancreatic juice. The pancreas is unusual in having both endocrine and exocrine secretory functions. The exocrine juice is composed of an **aqueous component** that is rich in HCO_3^- and that helps neutralize duodenal contents and an **enzyme component** that contains enzymes for digesting carbohydrates, proteins, and fats. Pancreatic exocrine secretion is controlled by both neural and hormonal signals elicited mainly by the presence of acid and digestion products in the duodenum. Secretin chiefly elicits secretion of the aqueous component, and CCK stimulates the secretion of pancreatic enzymes.

The structure of the exocrine pancreas resembles that of the salivary glands

Microscopic, blind-ended tubules are surrounded by polygonal acinar cells whose primary function is to secrete the enzyme component of pancreatic juice. The acini are

organized into lobules; the tiny ducts that drain the acini are called **intercalated ducts.** These ducts empty into the somewhat larger **intralobular ducts.** The intralobular ducts of a particular lobule drain into a single **extralobular duct** that empties the lobule into still larger ducts. The larger ducts converge into a main duct that enters the duodenum with the **common bile duct.**

The endocrine cells of the pancreas reside in the **islets of Langerhans.** Although islet cells account for less than 2% of the volume of the pancreas, their hormones are essential in regulating metabolism. **Insulin, glucagon, somatostatin,** and **pancreatic polypeptide** are hormones released from cells of the islets of Langerhans (see Chapter 42).

The pancreas is innervated by branches of the vagus nerve. Vagal fibers synapse with cholinergic neurons that lie within the pancreas and that innervate both acinar and islet cells. Postganglionic sympathetic nerves from the celiac and superior mesenteric plexuses innervate pancreatic blood vessels. Secretion of pancreatic juice is stimulated by parasympathetic activity and inhibited by sympathetic activity.

The aqueous component of pancreatic juice is elaborated mainly by ductular epithelial cells

Na^+ and K^+ concentrations of pancreatic juice are similar to those in plasma. HCO_3^- (at levels well above those in plasma) and Cl^- are the major anions. The HCO_3^- concentration varies from approximately 80 mEq/L at low rates of secretion to about 140 mEq/L at high secretory rates (Figure 33-10). HCO_3^- and Cl^- concentrations vary reciprocally. The aqueous component secreted by the duct cells is slightly hypertonic, and its HCO_3^- concentration is

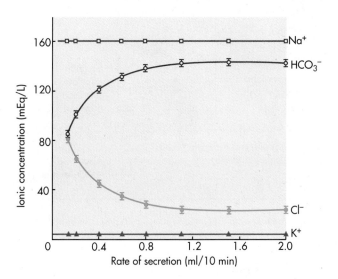

Figure 33-10 Concentrations of the major ions in cat pancreatic juice as functions of the secretory flow rate. At all flow rates the concentration of HCO_3^- in pancreatic juice is well above the plasma level. Secretion was stimulated by the intravenous injection of secretin. *(Redrawn from Case RM, Harper AA, Scratcherd T: J Physiol [Lond] 201:335, 1969.)*

high. As the secretion flows down the ducts, water equilibrates across the epithelium so that the pancreatic juice becomes isotonic with plasma and some HCO_3^- exchanges for Cl^- (Figure 33-11).

Under resting conditions, the aqueous component is produced mainly by the intercalated and other intralobular ducts. When secretion is stimulated by secretin, however, the additional flow comes mostly from the extralobular ducts (Figure 33-11). Secretin is the major physiological stimulus for secretion of the aqueous component.

Acinar cells secrete the enzyme component of pancreatic juice

The secretions of the acinar cells constitute the **enzyme component** of pancreatic juice. The fluid secreted by the acinar cells resembles plasma in its tonicity and in its concentrations of various ions. The enzyme component contains enzymes that are important for the digestion of all the major classes of foodstuffs. If pancreatic enzymes are absent, lipids, proteins, and carbohydrates are malabsorbed.

Proteases of pancreatic juice are secreted in inactive zymogen form. The major pancreatic proteases are **trypsin, chymotrypsin,** and **carboxypeptidase.** They are secreted as trypsinogen, chymotrypsinogen, and procarboxypeptidase, respectively. Trypsinogen is specifically activated by **enteropeptidase** (also called **enterokinase**), which is se-

creted by the duodenal mucosa. Trypsin then activates **trypsinogen, chymotrypsinogen,** and **procarboxypeptidase. Trypsin inhibitor,** a protein present in pancreatic juice, prevents the premature activation of proteolytic enzymes in the pancreatic ducts.

Pancreatic juice contains an **α-amylase** that is secreted in active form. **Pancreatic amylase** cleaves starch molecules into oligosaccharides. Pancreatic juice also contains a number of lipid-digesting enzymes, or **lipases.** Among the major pancreatic lipases are **triacylglycerol hydrolase, cholesterol ester hydrolase,** and **phospholipase A$_2$.**

Cl^- enters the acinar lumen via electrogenic Cl^- channels in the apical plasma membranes of the acinar cells. The primary molecular defect in **cystic fibrosis** is a mutation in the gene that encodes this Cl^- channel; this mutation results in a dramatic reduction of the number of Cl^- channels present in the apical plasma membranes of certain epithelial cells. The decreased transport of Cl^- into the acinar lumen impairs the transport of Na^+ and water. Consequently, in cystic fibrosis, the acini and intercalated ducts of the pancreas and the small airways of the lungs become clogged with mucus. The pancreatic exocrine function of most infants with cystic fibrosis has been irreversibly damaged in utero. For this reason, infants with cystic fibrosis frequently have severe digestive difficulties, especially in the digestion and absorption of fats.

Neural and hormonal stimuli elicit the secretion of pancreatic juice

Stimulation of the vagal branches to the pancreas enhances secretion. The activation of sympathetic fibers inhibits pancreatic secretion, partly by decreasing blood flow to the pancreas. Secretin and CCK, hormones released from the duodenal mucosa, stimulate secretion of the aqueous and enzyme components, respectively. Because the aqueous and enzyme components of pancreatic juice are separately controlled (Figure 33-11), the protein content of the juice varies from less than 1% to as much as 10%.

Gastrin is an angonist during the cephalic phase
Gastrin is released from the mucosa of the gastric antrum in response to vagal impulses, and it stimulates pancreatic secretion during the cephalic phase. Gastrin is a member of the same class of peptides as CCK, but it is much less potent as a pancreatic secretagogue than CCK is. Figure 33-12 shows the agonists that can elicit secretion from pancreatic acinar cells.

Gastric phase pancreatic secretion is elicited by gastrin and neural reflexes
During the gastric phase of secretion, gastrin, which is released in response to gastric distention and the presence of amino acids and peptides in the antrum of the

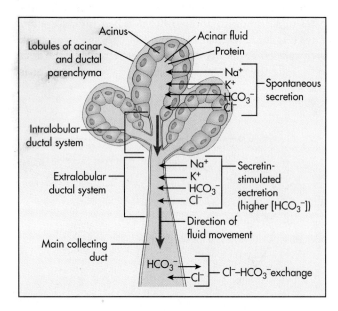

Figure 33-11 Locations of important transport processes involved in the elaboration of pancreatic juice. Acinar fluid is isotonic and resembles plasma in its concentrations of Na^+, K^+, Cl^-, and HCO_3^-. The secretion of acinar fluid and the proteins it contains is stimulated by CCK and acetylcholine. A spontaneous secretion produced by the intralobular ducts has higher concentrations of K^+ and HCO_3^- than plasma. The hormone secretin stimulates water and electrolyte secretion by the cells lining the extralobular ducts. The secretin-stimulated secretion is still richer in HCO_3^- than the spontaneous secretion. *(Modified from Swanson CH, Solomon AK: J Gen Physiol 62:407, 1973.)*

stomach, enhances secretion by the pancreas. In addition, neural reflexes elicited by distention of the stomach evoke pancreatic secretion.

The greatest volume of pancreatic secretion occurs during the intestinal phase

In the intestinal phase of secretion, certain components of the chyme in the duodenum and upper jejunum evoke pancreatic secretion. Acid in the duodenum and upper jejunum elicits the secretion of a large amount of pancreatic juice low in enzyme content. THE HORMONE SECRETIN IS THE MAJOR MEDIATOR OF THIS RESPONSE TO ACID. Secretin is released by certain cells in the mucosa of the duodenum and upper jejunum in response to acid in the lumen, and it directly stimulates the epithelial cells of the pancreatic extralobular ducts to secrete the HCO_3^--rich aqueous component of the pancreatic juice.

The presence of peptides and certain amino acids in the duodenum elicits the secretion of pancreatic juice rich in enzyme components. Fatty acids and monoglycerides in the duodenum also elicit the secretion of protein-rich pancreatic juice. CCK, A HORMONE RELEASED BY PARTICULAR CELLS IN THE DUODENUM AND UPPER JEJUNUM IN RESPONSE TO THESE DIGESTION PRODUCTS, IS THE MOST IMPORTANT PHYSIOLOGICAL MEDIATOR OF THE ENZYME COMPONENT OF PANCREATIC JUICE. CCK potentiates the stimulatory effect of secretin on the ducts. Secretin potentiates the effect of CCK on acinar cells.

Functions of the Liver and Gallbladder

The liver is organized into lobules

Each liver **lobule** is organized around a **central vein** (Figure 33-13). At the periphery of the lobule blood enters the **sinusoids** from branches of the **portal vein** and the **hepatic artery** (see also Chapter 25). In the sinusoids, blood flows toward the center of the lobule between plates of **hepatocytes** one or two cells thick. Because of the large fenestrations between the endothelial cells lining the sinusoids, each hepatocyte is in direct contact with sinusoidal blood. The intimate contact of a large fraction of the hepatocyte surface with blood contributes to the liver's ability to effectively clear the blood of certain classes of compounds. **Biliary canaliculi** lie between adjacent hepatocytes, and the canaliculi drain into bile ducts at the periphery of the lobule.

The metabolic functions of the liver are required for life

The liver is essential in regulating metabolism, synthesizing many proteins and other molecules, storing certain vitamins and iron, degrading certain hormones, and inactivating and excreting many drugs and toxins. It regulates the metabolism of carbohydrates, lipids, and proteins. Liver and skeletal muscle are the two major sites of glycogen storage in the body. When the level of glucose in the blood is high, glycogen is deposited in the liver. When the

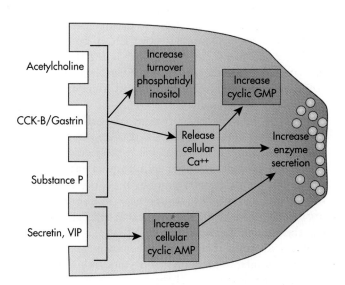

Figure 33-12 Agonists that elicit secretion from pancreatic acinar cells and their second-messenger mechanisms. Acetylcholine, CCK, gastrin, and substance P activate the hydrolysis of inositol lipids, mobilize intracellular Ca^{++}, and increase levels of cyclic GMP. Secretin and VIP activate adenylyl cyclase and thereby increase levels of cyclic AMP.

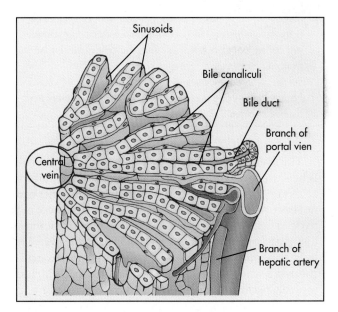

Figure 33-13 Hepatic lobule. A central vein is located in the center of the lobule, with plates of hepatocytes disposed radially. Branches of the portal vein and hepatic artery are located on the periphery of the lobule, and blood from both perfuses the sinusoids. Peripherally located bile ducts drain the bile canaliculi that run between the hepatocytes. *(Modified from Bloom W, Fawcett DW: A textbook of histology, ed 10, Philadelphia, 1975, WB Saunders.)*

blood glucose level is low, glycogen is broken down to glucose **(glycogenolysis),** and the glucose is then released into the blood. In this way the liver helps maintain a relatively constant blood glucose level. The liver is also the major site of **gluconeogenesis,** the conversion of amino acids, lipids, or simple carbohydrates (e.g., lactate) into glucose. Carbohydrate metabolism by the liver is regulated by several hormones (see Chapters 42 and 47).

The liver is also centrally involved in lipid metabolism. As described in Chapter 34, lipids absorbed by the intestine leave the intestine in **chylomicrons** in the lymph. **Lipoprotein lipase** on the endothelial cell surface of blood vessels hydrolyzes some of the triglyceride in the chylomicrons and releases glycerol and fatty acids that are taken up by **adipocytes.** This results in the formation of **chylomicron remnants** rich in cholesterol. Chylomicron remnants are taken up by hepatocytes and degraded. Hepatocytes synthesize and secrete **very-low-density lipoproteins,** which are then converted to the other types of serum lipoproteins. These lipoproteins are the major sources of cholesterol and triglycerides for most other tissues of the body. CHOLESTEROL PRESENT IN BILE REPRESENTS CHOLESTEROL'S ONLY ROUTE OF EXCRETION. Hepatocytes are thus a principal source of cholesterol in the body and the major site of excretion of cholesterol. Thus HEPATOCYTES PLAY AN IMPORTANT ROLE IN THE REGULATION OF SERUM CHOLESTEROL LEVELS (see also Chapter 41).

Because carbohydrate use is impaired in **diabetes mellitus,** β-oxidation of fatty acids provides a major source of energy for the body (see Chapter 42). In the liver the oxidation of fatty acids produces acetoacetate, β-hydroxybutyrate, and acetone. These three compounds are called **ketone bodies.** Ketone bodies are released from hepatocytes and carried via the circulation to other tissues, where they are metabolized. The levels of ketone bodies in the urine and blood can indicate the severity of diabetic acidosis.

The liver is centrally involved in protein metabolism. When proteins are broken down (catabolized), amino acids are deaminated to form ammonia. Ammonia cannot be further metabolized by most tissues and becomes toxic at levels achievable by metabolism. Ammonia is dissipated by conversion to urea, mainly in the liver. The liver also synthesizes all the nonessential amino acids. THE LIVER SYNTHESIZES ALL THE MAJOR PLASMA PROTEINS, including the plasma lipoproteins, albumins, globulins, fibrinogens, and proteins involved in blood clotting.

The liver stores certain substances that are important in metabolism. Next to hemoglobin in red blood cells, the liver is the most important storage site for iron. Also, certain vitamins, most notably A, D, and B_{12}, are stored in the liver. Hepatic storage protects the body from limited dietary deficiencies of these vitamins.

The liver transforms and excretes many hormones, drugs, and toxins. These substances are frequently converted to inactive forms by reactions that occur in hepatocytes. The smooth endoplasmic reticulum of hepatocytes contains systems of enzymes and cofactors that are responsible for the chemical transformations of many substances. Certain other enzymes in the endoplasmic reticulum catalyze the conjugation of many compounds with glucuronic acid, glycine, or glutathione. The transformations that occur in the liver render many compounds more water soluble; thus they are more readily excreted by the kidneys. Some liver metabolites are secreted into the bile.

Bile is secreted by hepatocytes and ductular epithelial cells

The hepatic function most important to the digestive tract is the secretion of **bile.** Bile, which is elaborated by hepatocytes, contains bile acids, cholesterol, lecithins, and bile pigments. These constituents, along with an isotonic fluid that resembles plasma in its electrolyte concentrations, are all synthesized and secreted by hepatocytes into the bile canaliculi. The bile canaliculi merge into ever-larger ducts and finally into a single large bile duct. The epithelial cells that line the bile ducts secrete a watery fluid that is rich in HCO_3^- and that contributes to the volume of bile leaving the liver.

The secretory function of the liver shares important features with that of the exocrine pancreas. In both organs the major parenchymal cell type elaborates a primary secretion containing the substances responsible for the major digestive function of the organ. In both the liver and the pancreas, the primary secretion is isotonic to plasma and contains Na^+, K^+, and Cl^- at close to plasma levels, and the primary secretion is stimulated by CCK. In both the pancreas and the liver the epithelial cells lining the duct systems modify the primary secretion. When stimulated by secretin, the epithelial cells contribute an aqueous secretion with a high HCO_3^- concentration.

Between meals, bile is diverted into the **gallbladder.** THE GALLBLADDER EPITHELIUM EXTRACTS SALTS AND WATER FROM THE STORED BILE, AND THE BILE ACIDS ARE THEREBY CONCENTRATED FIVEFOLD TO TWENTYFOLD. After an individual has eaten, the gallbladder contracts and empties its concentrated bile into the duodenum. The most potent stimulus for emptying the gallbladder is CCK. From 250 to 1500 ml of bile enters the duodenum each day.

Bile acids emulsify lipids and thereby increase the surface area available to lipolytic enzymes. Bile acids then form **mixed micelles** (see Chapter 34) with the products of lipid digestion. Micelles increase the transport of the products of lipid digestion products to the brush border surface; thus they enhance the absorption of lipids by the epithelial cells. Bile acids are actively absorbed, mainly in the terminal ileum. A small fraction of bile acids escapes absorption and is excreted. Bile acids returning to the liver are avidly taken up by hepatocytes and are rapidly resecreted during the course of digestion. The entire bile acid pool is recirculated two or more times in response to a typical meal. The recirculation of the bile acids is known as the **enterohepatic circulation.** Approximately 20% of the bile acid pool is excreted in the feces each day and is replenished by hepatic synthesis of new bile acids. Figure 33-14 summarizes some major aspects of the enterohepatic circulation.

Bile acids lost into the feces are a significant mechanism of cholesterol excretion. Treatment with drugs that inhibit the reabsorption of bile acids in the ileum promotes the synthesis of new bile acids from cholesterol. Such drugs have been used to lower the level of cholesterol in the blood.

The fraction of bile secreted by hepatocytes contains bile acids, phospholipids, cholesterol, and bile pigments

BILE ACIDS ARE THE MAJOR COMPONENT OF BILE. They constitute about 50% of the dry weight of bile. Other important compounds secreted by hepatocytes into the bile include phospholipids, bile pigments, and proteins. Bile acids have a steroid nucleus and are synthesized by the hepatocytes from cholesterol. The major bile acids synthesized by the liver are called **primary bile acids.** These are **cholic acid** (3-hydroxyl groups) and **chenodeoxycholic acid** (2-hydroxyl groups). The presence of the carboxyl and hydroxyl groups make the bile acids more water soluble than the cholesterol from which they are synthesized.

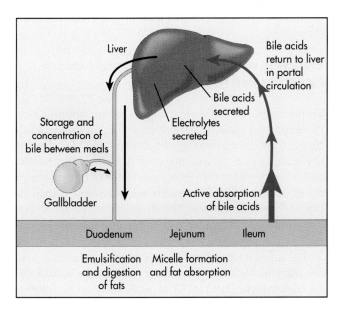

Figure 33-14 Overview of the enterohepatic circulation of bile. Bile is dumped into the duodenum as a result of contractions of the gallbladder. In the small intestine, bile acids first emulsify dietary fat and then form mixed micelles with the products of fat digestion. In the terminal ileum, bile acids are reabsorbed. Bile acids return to the liver in the portal blood; they are avidly taken up by hepatocytes and resecreted into bile.

Bacteria in the digestive tract dehydroxylate bile acids to form **secondary bile acids.** The major secondary bile acids are **deoxycholic acid** (from dehydroxylation of cholic acid) and **lithocholic acid** (from dehydroxylation of chenodeoxycholic acid). Bile contains both primary and secondary bile acids.

Bile acids normally are secreted conjugated with glycine or taurine. In conjugated bile acids the glycine or taurine is linked by a peptide bond between the carboxyl group of an unconjugated bile acid and the amino group of glycine or taurine. At the near-neutral pH of the gastrointestinal tract, conjugated bile acids are more completely ionized and thus more water soluble than unconjugated bile acids. Conjugated bile acids are present almost entirely as salts of various cations (mostly Na^+) and are often called **bile salts.**

The steroid nucleus of bile acids is almost planar. In solution, bile acids have their polar (hydrophilic) substituents—the hydroxyl groups, the carboxyl moiety of glycine or taurine, and the peptide bond—all on one surface of the molecule. This makes the bile acid molecule amphipathic (i.e., having both hydrophilic and hydrophobic domains). Because they are amphipathic, bile acids tend to form molecular aggregates called **micelles** in which the hydrophobic side of the bile acid faces inside and away from water and the hydrophilic surface faces outward and toward the water (see Chapter 34). When the concentration of bile acids exceeds a certain concentration (called the **critical micelle concentration**), bile acid micelles form. Above this concentration, any additional bile acid goes into the micelles exclusively and not into molecular solution. Normally in bile, the bile acid concentration is much greater than the critical micelle concentration.

PHOSPHOLIPIDS IN BILE HELP SOLUBILIZE CHOLESTEROL. Hepatocytes also secrete phospholipids, especially lecithins, into bile. Cholesterol is also secreted into the bile, and this is the major route for cholesterol excretion. Although lecithin and cholesterol are essentially insoluble in water, they dissolve in the bile acid micelles. Lecithin increases the amount of cholesterol that can be solubilized in the micelles.

If more cholesterol is present in the bile than can be solubilized in the micelles, crystals of cholesterol form in the bile. These crystals are important in the formation of **cholesterol gallstones** (the most common gallstones) in the duct system of the liver or more often in the gallbladder.

BILE PIGMENTS ARE END PRODUCTS OF PORPHYRIN CATABOLISM. When senescent red blood cells are degraded in reticuloendothelial cells, the porphyrin moiety of hemoglobin is converted to **bilirubin.** Bilirubin is released into the plasma, where it is bound to albumin. Hepatocytes efficiently remove bilirubin from blood in the sinusoids and conjugate bilirubin with one or two glucuronic acid molecules. Bilirubin glucuronides are secreted into the bile. Bilirubin is yellow and contributes to the yellow color of bile.

The bile duct epithelium elaborates a bicarbonate-rich secretion

The epithelial cells that line the bile ducts contribute an aqueous secretion that accounts for about 50% of the total volume of bile. The secretion of the bile duct epithelium is isotonic with plasma and contains Na^+ and K^+ at levels similar to those of plasma. However, the concentration of HCO_3^- is greater and the concentration of Cl^- is less than in plasma. The secretory activity of the bile duct epithelium is specifically stimulated by secretin.

Bile is concentrated and stored in the gallbladder

Between meals, the tone of the **sphincter of Oddi,** which guards the entrance of the common bile duct into the duodenum, is high. Thus most bile flow is diverted into the gallbladder. The gallbladder is a small organ, having a capacity of 15 to 60 ml (average about 35 ml) in humans. Many times this volume of bile may be secreted by the liver between meals. The gallbladder concentrates the bile by absorbing Na^+, Cl^-, HCO_3^-, and water from the bile, such that the bile acids are concentrated 5 to 20 times. The active transport of Na^+ is the primary active process in the concentrating action of the gallbladder.

Because of its high rate of water absorption, the gallbladder serves as a model for water and electrolyte transport by tight-junctioned epithelia. The **standing osmotic gradient mechanism** for fluid absorption was first proposed for the gallbladder. It was noted that during fluid reabsorption by the gallbladder, the lateral intercellular spaces between the epithelial cells were large and swollen. When fluid transport was blocked, the intercellular spaces almost disappeared. These observations suggested that the intercellular spaces are a major route of fluid flow during absorption.

The primary active transport process in the standing osmotic gradient mechanism is the active transport of Na^+ into the lateral intercellular spaces (Figure 33-15). Na^+,K^+-ATPase molecules are especially concentrated in the basolateral membrane near the mucosal (apical) end of the intercellular channels. Cl^- and HCO_3^- are also transported into the intercellular space, probably because of the electrical potential created by electrogenic Na^+ transport. The high ion concentration near the apical end of the intercellular space causes the fluid there to be hypertonic. This produces an osmotic flow of water from the lumen via adjacent cells into the intercellular space. Water distends the intercellular channels because of increased hydrostatic pressure. As a result of water flow

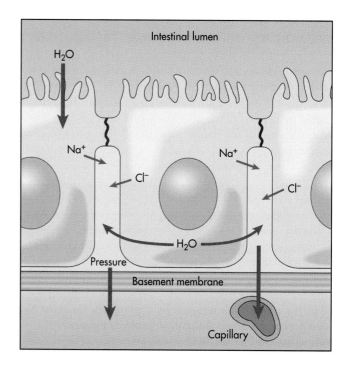

Figure 33-15 Water absorption from the gallbladder via the standing gradient osmotic mechanism. Na^+ is actively pumped into the lateral intercellular spaces; Cl^- follows. Water is drawn by osmosis into the intercellular spaces, elevating the intercellular hydrostatic pressure. Water, Na^+, and Cl^- are filtered across the porous basement membrane and enter the capillaries.

from adjacent cells, the fluid becomes less hypertonic as it flows down the intercellular channel, so the fluid is essentially isotonic when it reaches the serosal (basal) end of the channel. Ions and water move across the basement membrane of the epithelium, and they are carried away by the capillaries.

Emptying of the gallbladder is regulated by nerves and hormones

Emptying of the gallbladder begins several minutes after the start of a meal. Intermittent contractions force bile through the partially relaxed sphincter of Oddi. During the cephalic and gastric phases of digestion, contraction and relaxation of the sphincter are mediated by cholinergic fibers in branches of the vagus nerve and by gastrin released from the stomach. The stimulation of sympathetic nerves to the gallbladder and duodenum inhibits emptying of the gallbladder.

The highest rate of gallbladder emptying occurs during the intestinal phase of digestion; the strongest stimulus for the emptying is CCK. CCK reaches the gallbladder via the circulation and causes strong contractions of the gallbladder and relaxation of the sphincter of Oddi. Substances that mimic the actions of CCK in promoting gallbladder emptying, such as CCK and gastrin, are called **cholecystagogues.** Gastrin has the same sequence of five amino acids at its C-terminus as CCK does; however, gastrin is not nearly as potent a cholecystagogue as CCK. Nevertheless, gastrin helps elicit gallbladder contractions during the cephalic and gastric phases of digestion.

Under normal circumstances the rate of gallbladder emptying is sufficient to keep the concentration of bile acids in the duodenum above the critical micelle concentration.

Bile acids are reabsorbed in the distal ileum and return to the liver in the portal blood

The functions of bile acids in emulsifying dietary lipid and in forming mixed micelles with the products of lipid digestion are discussed in Chapter 34. Normally, by the time chyme reaches the terminal part of the ileum, dietary fat is almost completely absorbed. Bile acids are then absorbed. Transport mechanisms are present in the brush border of the terminal ileum for uptake of both conjugated and unconjugated bile acids. Conjugated bile acids can be taken up against a large concentration gradient. Because bile acids are also lipid soluble, they can also be taken up by simple diffusion. Bacteria in the terminal part of the ileum and colon deconjugate bile acids and also dehydroxylate them to produce secondary bile acids. Both deconjugation and dehydroxylation lessen the polarity of bile acids and thereby enhance their lipid solubility and their absorption by simple diffusion.

Typically, about 0.5 g of bile acids escapes absorption and is excreted in the feces each day. This quantity is 15% to 35% of the total bile acid pool, and normally it is replenished via the synthesis of new bile acids by the liver. Bile acids, whether absorbed by active transport or simple diffusion, are transported away from the intestine in the portal blood, mostly bound to plasma proteins. In the liver, hepatocytes avidly extract the bile acids from the portal blood. IN A SINGLE PASS THROUGH THE LIVER, THE PORTAL BLOOD IS ESSENTIALLY CLEARED OF BILE ACIDS. Bile acids in all forms, primary and secondary, both conjugated and deconjugated, are taken up by the hepatocytes. The hepatocytes reconjugate almost all the deconjugated bile acids and rehydroxylate some of the secondary bile acids. These bile acids are secreted into the bile along with newly synthesized bile acids (Figure 33-14).

Bile acids in blood stimulate hepatocytes to secrete
The rate of return of the bile acids to the liver affects the rate of synthesis and secretion of bile acids. Bile acids in the portal blood stimulate the uptake and resecretion of bile acids by hepatocytes. This is called the **choleretic effect** of bile acids; substances that enhance bile acid secretion are called choleretics. So powerful is the stimulus to resecrete the returning bile acids that the entire pool of bile acids (1.5 to 31.5 g) recirculates twice in response to a typical meal. In response to a meal with a very high fat content, the bile acid pool may recirculate five or more times.

Gallstones have cholesterol or bile pigments as major constituents

Cholesterol is essentially insoluble in water. When bile contains more cholesterol than can be solubilized in the bile acid–lecithin micelles, crystals of cholesterol form in the bile. Such bile is said to be **supersaturated** with cholesterol. The greater the concentration of bile acids and lecithin in bile, the greater the amount of cholesterol that can be contained in the mixed micelles.

> **Bile pigment gallstones** are another major class of gallstones; their major constituent is the calcium salt of unconjugated bilirubin. Conjugated bilirubin is quite soluble and does not form insoluble calcium salts in bile. In liver disease, bile may contain elevated levels of unconjugated bilirubin because hepatocytes are deficient in forming the glucuronides of bilirubin. Individuals with liver disease are more likely to form bile pigment stones.

Electrolytes, Water, and Mucus Are Secreted by Intestinal Mucosa

The mucosa of the intestine, from the duodenum through the rectum, elaborates secretions that contain mucus, electrolytes, and water. The total volume of intestinal secretions is about 1500 ml/day. The mucus in the secretions protects the mucosa from mechanical damage. The nature of the secretions and the mechanisms that control secretion vary in different segments of the intestine.

Duodenal secretions are mostly produced by duodenal glands

The duodenal submucosa contains branching glands that elaborate a secretion rich in mucus. The duodenal epithelial cells also contribute to duodenal secretions, but most of the secretions are produced by the glands. The duodenal secretion contains mucus and an aqueous component that does not differ significantly from plasma in its concentrations of the major ions.

Goblet cells, which lie among the columnar epithelial cells of the small intestine, secrete mucus. During normal digestion, an aqueous secretion is elaborated by the epithelial cells at a rate only slightly less than that of fluid absorption by the small intestine.

The secretions of the colon are smaller in volume but richer in mucus than the secretions of the small intestinal. Mucus is produced by numerous goblet cells in the colonic mucosa. The aqueous component of colonic secretions is rich in K^+ and HCO_3^-. Colonic secretion is stimulated by mechanical irritation of the mucosa and by activation of cholinergic pathways to the colon. The stimulation of sympathetic nerves to the colon decreases the rate of colonic secretion.

Summary

- The epithelial cells that line the gastrointestinal tract and the cells of various glands associated with the gastrointestinal tract produce secretions that contain water, electrolytes, and proteins.
- Gastrointestinal secretion is regulated by intrinsic and extrinsic neurons, hormones, and paracrine mediators.
- Salivary glands produce a hypotonic fluid with HCO_3^- and Na^+ concentrations in excess of plasma levels. Saliva contains an α-amylase that begins the digestion of starch.
- The stomach serves as a reservoir for ingested food and empties gastric contents into the duodenum at a regulated rate. Parietal cells secrete HCl and intrinsic factor into the stomach. Chief cells secrete pepsinogens.
- The regulation of HCl secretion in the stomach involves extrinsic and intrinsic nerves, with acetylcholine as the major stimulatory neurotransmitter. Gastrin, a hormone released by G cells in the gastric antrum and in the duodenum, and histamine, a paracrine agonist released by ECL cells in the stomach, are also important physiological agonists of HCl secretion.
- HCl catalyzes the conversion of pepsinogens to active pepsins. Pepsins convert a significant fraction of ingested protein to oligopeptides.
- Mucus and HCO_3^- secretions form the "gastric mucosal barrier" that protects the epithelial cells of the stomach from the effects of HCl and pepsins.
- The pancreas produces an HCO_3^--rich fluid that contains enzymes essential for the digestion of carbohydrates, proteins, and fats. Pancreatic acinar cells produce the enzyme component of pancreatic juice; the intralobular and extralobular ducts secrete most of the aqueous component (water and electrolytes) of pancreatic juice.
- CCK and secretin are hormones released by cells in the duodenum and jejunum in response to the presence of fat digestion products and acid, respectively. CCK is the major physiological agonist of acinar cell secretion of the enzyme component. Secretin is the major stimulus for secretion of HCO_3^--rich fluid by the extralobular ducts of the pancreas.
- The liver produces and the gallbladder concentrates bile. Bile is an HCO_3^--rich fluid that contains bile acids, bile pigments, lecithin, cholesterol, and numerous other components. Bile acids play a vital role in the digestion and absorption of lipids.
- Hepatocytes are responsible for secreting the organic components of bile. The cells of the bile ducts secrete an HCO_3^--rich fluid. CCK is a major secretagogue for

secretion by the hepatocytes. Secretin stimulates the bile ducts to produce their HCO_3^--rich fluid.
- Bile acids are absorbed in the terminal ileum and return to the liver in the portal vein. Hepatocytes rapidly clear the blood of bile acids and resecrete them. Bile acids in the portal blood are a powerful stimulus that causes the hepatocytes to resecrete bile acids.

BIBLIOGRAPHY

Arias IM et al: *The liver: biology and pathobiology,* ed 3, New York, 1994, Raven.

Blaser MJ: The bacteria behind ulcers, *Sci Am* 274:104, 1996.

Chew CS: Intracellular mechanisms in control of acid secretion. *Curr Opin Gastroenterol* 7:856, 1991.

El-Omer EM et al: *Helicobacter pylori* infection and abnormalities of gastric secretion in patients with duodenal ulcer disease, *Gastroenterology* 109:681,1995.

Gerber JG, Payne NA: The role of gastric secretagogues in regulating gastric histamine release *in vivo, Gastroenterology* 102:403, 1992.

Go VLW et al, eds: *The pancreas: biology, pathobiology, and disease,* ed 2, New York, 1993, Raven.

Johnson LR, ed: *Physiology of the gastrointestinal tract,* ed 3, New York, 1994, Raven.

Rabon EC, Reuben MA: The mechanism and structure of the gastric H,K-ATPase, *Annu Rev Physiol* 52:321, 1990.

Raeder M: The origin and subcellular mechanisms causing pancreatic bicarbonate secretion, *Gastroenterology* 103:1674, 1992.

Raufman J-P: Gastric chief cells: receptors and signal transduction mechanisms, *Gastroenterology* 102:699, 1992.

Shamburek RD, Schubert ML: Control of gastric acid secretion, *Gastroenterol Clin North Am* 21:527, 1992.

Siegers C-P, Watkins JB III, eds: *Biliary excretion of drugs and other chemicals,* New York, 1991, Gustav Fischer Verlag.

Sleisenger M, Fordtran JS, eds: *Gastrointestinal diseases,* ed 5, Philadelphia, 1993, WB Saunders.

Tavoloni N, Berk PD, eds: *Hepatic transport and bile secretion,* New York, 1993, Raven.

Case Studies

Case 33-1

A 25-year-old woman has persistent diarrhea, steatorrhea, and abdominal pain. An upper gastrointestinal radiological series suggests the presence of a duodenal ulcer. The presence of the ulcer is confirmed by endoscopy. The patient's basal rate of secretion of gastric HCl is about 12 mmol/hr (the normal range is 1 to 5 mmol/hr). The patient has an elevated serum gastrin level (1145 pg/ml); the normal range is 50 to 150 pg/ml. After a test meal, the patient's serum gastrin level does not increase significantly. The diagnosis is Zollinger-Ellison syndrome, a disorder in which ectopic cells secrete high levels of gastrin.

1. Which of the following statements is correct?

A. The patient is likely to be secreting elevated levels of pepsinogens.

B. Her duodenal ulcer is due partly to increased pepsin levels and H^+ concentrations in the duodenum.

C. Her steatorrhea may be a consequence of a low duodenal pH.

D. Muscarinic antagonists might partially alleviate the symptoms.

E. All of the above.

2. Which of the following statements is correct?

A. All patients with elevated gastrin levels have high rates of HCl secretion.

B. If the diagnosis is correct, her serum gastrin level should increase after eating.

C. The patient may have an increased number of glands in her gastric fundus.

D. The patient has a high probability of gastric ulcers.

E. None of the above.

3. Which of the following statements is correct?

A. This disorder should be managed only with drugs that suppress HCl secretion.

B. H_2-receptor blockers should be as effective in this woman as in a healthy individual.

C. Sectioning the vagus nerve branches to the fundus and the body would be ineffective.

D. Omeprazole should effectively block HCl secretion in this patient.

E. None of the above.

Case 33-2

A 38-year-old woman complains of pain in the right upper quadrant of her abdomen. The pain usually occurs after eating a heavy meal or a fatty snack. Pain tends to be constant, lasts for about an hour, and is accompanied by nausea. The patient was given 6 g of calcium ipodate (a radiographic contrast agent concentrated in the gallbladder) by mouth over 12 hours, and then x-ray studies of the patient's gallbladder, cystic duct, and common bile duct were performed. Several radiolucent stones (5 to 10 mm in diameter) were detected in the gallbladder, but no stones were found in the cystic or common bile duct. The diagnosis is **cholecystitis** probably caused by gallstones in the gallbladder.

1. Which of the following statements is correct?

A. It is most likely that the patient has cholesterol gallstones.

B. The fact that the stones are radiolucent indicates that significant calcification of the gallstones has not occurred.

C. Ultrasonography would probably confirm the presence of stones in the gallbladder.

D. The absence of calcification favors the use of lithotripsy in this patient.

E. All of the above.

2. Which of the following statements is correct?

A. Cholesterol hypersecretion contributes to the formation of most cholesterol gallstones.

B. Abnormalities of gallbladder motility do not usually influence the formation of cholesterol gallstones.

C. Mucus secretion by gallbladder epithelial cells protects against cholesterol gallstone formation.

D. Treatment with nonsteroidal antiinflammatory drugs would not influence the rate at which cholesterol gallstones form.

E. All of the above.

3. Which of the following statements is correct?

A. If the patient's condition were treated with chenodeoxycholate and ursodeoxycholate, the stones would dissolve in a matter of weeks.

B. This patient is not a good candidate for lithotripsy.

C. Treating this patient with an inhibitor of 3-hydroxy-3-methylglutaryl–coenzyme A reductase is likely to be ineffective.

D. Once the patient's stones are dissolved, additional stones are unlikely to form.

E. None of the above.

CHAPTER 34

Digestion and Absorption

- Describe the digestion and absorption of sucrose, lactose, and branched starch molecules.
- Describe the digestion and absorption of proteins and lipids.
- Explain the transport of water and electrolytes in the small and large intestines.
- Describe the absorption of Ca^{++} and iron.
- Explain the absorption of water-soluble vitamins, especially vitamin B_{12}.

In most instances, nutrients cannot be absorbed by the cells that line the gastrointestinal tract in the forms in which they are ingested. **Digestion** refers to the processes by which ingested molecules are cleaved into smaller ones via reactions catalyzed by enzymes in gastrointestinal secretions (see Chapter 33) or on the luminal surface of the gastrointestinal tract. As a result of digestion, ingested molecules are converted to smaller molecules that can be absorbed from the lumen of the gastrointestinal tract. **Absorption** refers to the processes by which molecules are transported through the epithelial cells that line the gastrointestinal tract and then enter the blood or lymph, draining that region of the gastrointestinal tract.

Digestion and Absorption of Carbohydrates

Carbohydrates are the principal source of calories for most people

Plant starch, **amylopectin,** is the major source of carbohydrate in most human diets. Amylopectin is a high-molecular-weight ($MW > 10^6$), branched polymer of glucose units. A smaller proportion of dietary starch is **amylose,** a lower-molecular-weight ($MW > 10^5$), linear α–1,4-linked polymer of glucose. **Cellulose** is a β–1,4-linked glucose polymer. Intestinal enzymes cannot hydrolyze β-glycosidic links. Thus cellulose and other molecules with β-glycosidic links remain undigested and contribute to **dietary fiber.**

The amount of the animal starch, **glycogen,** that is ingested varies widely among cultures and among individuals within a given culture. **Sucrose** and **lactose** are the principal dietary disaccharides, and **glucose** and **fructose** are the major monosaccharides.

Saliva and pancreatic juice contain α-amylases that begin the digestion of starch

The structure of a branched starch molecule is depicted in Figure 34-1. Starch is a polymer of glucose and consists of chains of glucose units linked by α-1,4 glycosidic bonds. The α-1,4 chains have branch points formed by α-1,6 glycosidic links.

The digestion of starch begins in the mouth with the action of **salivary amylase.** This enzyme catalyzes the hydrolysis of the internal α-1,4 links of starch, but it cannot hydrolyze the α-1,6 branching links. As shown in Figure 34-1, the principal products of the α-amylase digestion of starch are maltose, maltotriose, and branched oligosaccharides known as **α-limit dextrins.** Considerable digestion of starch by the salivary amylase may occur normally, but this enzyme is not required for the normal digestion and absorption of starch. After salivary amylase is inactivated by the low pH of gastric contents, no further processing of carbohydrate occurs in the stomach.

Pancreatic juice contains a highly active α-amylase. The products of starch digestion by the pancreatic enzyme are the same as those for the salivary amylase, but the total amylase activity in pancreatic juice is considerably greater than that in saliva, Within 10 minutes after entering the duodenum, starch is entirely converted to the oligosaccharides shown in Figure 34-1.

The further digestion of these oligosaccharides is accomplished by enzymes that reside in the brush border membrane of the epithelium of the duodenum and jejunum (Figure 34-2). The major brush border oligosaccharidases are (1) **lactase,** which splits lactose into glucose and galactose; (2) **sucrase,** which splits sucrose into glucose and fructose; (3) α-**dextrinase** (also called **isomaltase**), which "debranches" the α-limit dextrins by cleaving the α-1,6 links at the branch points; and (4) **glucoamylase,** which cleaves the terminal α-1,4 glycosidic bonds to break maltooligosaccharides down to glucose units. The activities of these four enzymes are highest in the brush border of the upper jejunum, and they gradually decline through the rest of the small intestine.

Glucose, galactose, and fructose are the only well-absorbed monosaccharides

The duodenum and upper jejunum have the highest capacity for absorbing sugars. The capacities of the lower jejunum and ileum are progressively less. Glucose and galactose are actively taken up across the brush border plasma membrane of epithelial cells through an Na^+-powered, secondary active transport protein called **SGLT1** (Figure 34-3). Glucose and galactose compete for entry. Na^+ and glucose or galactose are transported into the cell by SGLT1, which has two Na^+-binding sites and one sugar-binding site. The presence of Na^+ in the intestinal lumen enhances the absorption of glucose and galactose, and vice versa. The energy released by Na^+ moving down its electrochemical potential gradient is harnessed to transport glucose or galactose into the cell against a concentration gradient of the sugar (see Chapter 1). Glucose and galactose leave the intestinal epithelial cell at the basal and lateral plasma membranes via a facilitated transport protein **(GLUT2)**, and they diffuse into the mucosal capillaries.

Fructose does not compete well for the glucose-galactose transporter. However, fructose is transported almost as rapidly as glucose and galactose and much more rapidly than other monosaccharides. Fructose is taken up across the brush border membrane by a fructose-specific facilitated transporter **(GLUT5)**. Fructose, along with glucose and galactose, crosses the basolateral membrane via GLUT2.

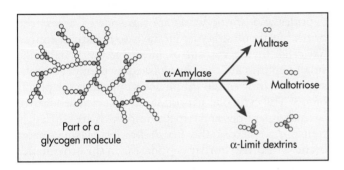

Figure 34-1 Structure of a branched starch molecule and the action of α-amylase. The open gray circles represent glucose monomers. The filled brown circles show glucose units linked by α-1,6 links at the branch points. The α-1,6 links and terminal α-1,4 bonds cannot be cleaved by α-amylase.

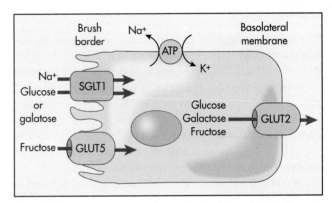

Figure 34-3 Glucose and galactose enter the jejunal epithelial cells against a concentration gradient via SGLT1. The gradient of Na^+ provides the energy for sugar entry. The facilitated transport of fructose across the brush border membrane is mediated by GLUT5. All three monosaccharides leave the cell at the basolateral membrane via facilitated transport by GLUT2.

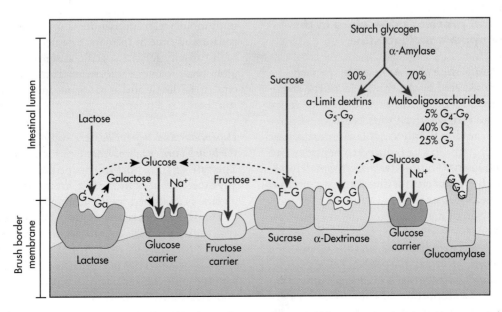

Figure 34-2 Functions of the major brush border oligosaccharidases. Glucose, galactose, and fructose molecules released by enzymatic hydrolysis are then transported into the epithelial cells by specific transport proteins in the brush border membrane. *F,* Fructose; *G,* glucose; *Ga,* galactose. *(Redrawn from Gray GM: N Engl J Med 292:1225, 1975.)*

In individuals with low levels of brush border lactase activity, undigested lactose is passed on to the colon. The colonic bacteria rapidly metabolize the lactose, and the bacteria produce gas and release metabolic products that enhance colonic motility and cause diarrhea. This condition is called **lactose intolerance.** Lactose intolerance in the newborn, **congenital lactose intolerance,** is uncommon. Lactose-intolerant infants are usually fed formula with sucrose as the major source of carbohydrate. In contrast, more than 50% of the world's adults are lactose intolerant. This is genetically determined. Most Asian and African adults are lactose intolerant, but most Northern European adults tolerate lactose.

Digestion and Absorption of Proteins

The amount of dietary protein varies greatly among cultures and among individuals within a culture. In poor societies, it is difficult for adults to obtain the amount of protein (0.5 to 0.7 g/day/kg of body weight) required to balance the normal catabolism of proteins. It is even more difficult for children to receive the relatively greater amounts of protein required to sustain normal growth. In wealthy societies a typical individual ingests protein far in excess of the nutritional requirement.

In normal humans, essentially all ingested protein is digested and absorbed by the time intestinal chyme has reached the middle of the jejunum. Most of the protein in digestive secretions and exfoliated cells is also digested and absorbed. The small amount of protein in the feces is derived principally from colonic bacteria, exfoliated colonic cells, and proteins in mucous secretions of the colon.

The digestion of proteins takes place in the stomach and upper small intestine

Pepsins begin the digestion of proteins in the stomach
Pepsinogens are secreted by the chief cells of the stomach and are converted in an acid environment to active **pepsins.** The extent to which pepsins hydrolyze dietary protein is significant but highly variable. At most, about 15% of dietary protein may be reduced to peptides and amino acids by pepsins. The duodenum and small intestine have such a high capacity for digesting protein that the total absence of pepsins does not impair the digestion and absorption of dietary protein.

The digestion of proteins in the small intestine involves the actions of pancreatic proteases and peptidases
Proteases in pancreatic juice play a major role in protein digestion. The most important of these proteases are **trypsin, chymotrypsin,** and **carboxypeptidase.** Pancreatic juice contains these enzymes in inactive, proenzyme forms. The enzyme **enteropeptidase** (also known as **enterokinase**), secreted by the mucosa of the duodenum and jejunum, converts trypsinogen to active trypsin. Trypsin activates trypsinogen and also converts chymotrypsinogen and procarboxypeptidase to the active enzymes. The pancreatic proteases are very active in the duodenum, and they rapidly convert dietary protein to small peptides. About 50% of ingested protein is digested and absorbed in the duodenum. The brush border of the duodenum and small intestine contains a number of peptidases. These peptidases are integral membrane proteins whose active sites face the intestinal lumen.

The principal products of protein digestion by pancreatic proteases and brush border peptidases are small peptides and single amino acids. The small peptides (mainly dipeptides, tripeptides, and tetrapeptides) are about three or four times more concentrated than the single amino acids. As discussed next, small peptides and amino acids are transported across the brush border plasma membrane into intestinal epithelial cells. In the cytosol of intestinal epithelial cells, small peptides are then hydrolyzed by peptidases; consequently, only single amino acids appear in the portal blood. The cytosolic peptidases are particularly active against dipeptides and tripeptides, which are efficiently transported across the brush border plasma membrane. The brush border peptidases, on the other hand, are active mainly against peptides of four or more amino acids.

The absorption of protein digestion products is accomplished via transporters for amino acids and small peptides

Some intact proteins and large peptides that can trigger immunological responses are absorbed. In ruminants and rodents but not in humans, the neonatal intestine has a high capacity for the specific absorption of the immune globulins present in colostrum. This absorptive process is vital in the development of normal immune competence in ruminants and rodents.

Dipeptides and tripeptides are rapidly transported across the brush border membrane
The rate of transport of dipeptides or tripeptides usually exceeds that of individual amino acids. For example, glycine is absorbed by the human jejunum less rapidly as amino acid than it is as glycylglycine or as glycylglycylglycine. A single membrane transport system with broad specificity is responsible for the absorption of small peptides. The transport system has a high affinity for dipeptides and tripeptides but a very low affinity for peptides of four or more amino acid residues. The transport of dipeptides and tripeptides across the brush border plasma membrane is a secondary active transport

process and is powered by the electrochemical potential difference of H^+ across the membrane.

Brush border and basolateral plasma membranes differ in their amino acid transport proteins

Amino acids are transported across the brush border plasma membrane into the intestinal epithelial cell by certain specific amino acid transport proteins. Some of the transporters depend on the Na^+ gradient, whereas others are independent of Na^+.

> **Hartnup disease** is a rare hereditary disorder in which one of the major neutral amino acid transport proteins is deficient in the brush border of the small intestine and the proximal renal tubule. Individuals with Hartnup disease have elevated urinary levels of certain neutral amino acids. However, such patients are not malnourished because the affected neutral amino acids are absorbed well as components of dipeptides and tripeptides in the upper small intestine.

Intestinal Absorption of Water and Electrolytes

Under normal circumstances, humans absorb almost 99% of the water and ions presented to them in ingested food and gastrointestinal secretions (Figure 34-4). Thus net fluxes of water and ions are normally directed from the lumen of the gut to the blood. In most cases the net fluxes of water and ions are the differences between much larger unidirectional flows from lumen to blood and from blood to lumen.

The gastrointestinal tract absorbs more than 8 L of fluid per day

Typically about 2 L of water is ingested each day, and approximately 7 L/day is contained in gastrointestinal secretions (Figure 34-4). Only about 50 to 150 ml of water per day is lost in the feces.

Very little net absorption occurs in the duodenum, but the chyme is brought to isotonicity in the duodenum. The chyme that is delivered from the stomach is often hypertonic. The action of digestive enzymes creates still more osmotic activity. The epithelium of the duodenum is highly permeable to water and ions, and very large fluxes of water occur from lumen to blood and from blood to lumen. Usually the net flux is from blood to lumen because of the hypertonicity of the chyme. Large net water absorption occurs in the small intestine; the jejunum is more active than the ileum in absorbing water. The net absorption that occurs in the colon is relatively small, approximately 400 ml/day.

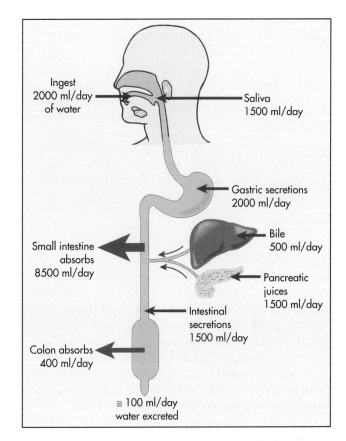

Figure 34-4 Overall fluid balance in the human gastrointestinal tract. Approximately 2 L of water is ingested each day, and 7 L of various secretions enters the gastrointestinal tract. Of this total of 9 L, about 8.5 L is absorbed in the small intestine. Approximately 500 ml is passed on to the colon, which normally absorbs 80% to 90% of the water presented to it.

Na^+ is absorbed along the entire length of the intestine

Net absorption of Na^+ is result of the large unidirectional fluxes of Na^+ from blood to lumen and from lumen to blood. These fluxes are greater in the proximal than in the distal intestine. Na^+ crosses the brush border membrane down an electrochemical gradient, and it is actively extruded from the epithelial cells by Na^+,K^+-ATPase in the basolateral plasma membrane. The contents of the small bowel are normally isotonic to plasma. Luminal contents have about the same Na^+ concentration as plasma, and therefore Na^+ absorption normally occurs in the absence of a significant net concentration gradient.

The net rate of Na^+ absorption is highest in the jejunum. There, Na^+ absorption is enhanced by the presence of glucose, galactose, and neutral amino acids in the lumen. These substances and Na^+ cross the brush border membrane on the same transport proteins. Na^+ moves down its electrochemical potential gradient and provides the energy for moving the sugars (glucose and galactose) and neutral amino acids into the epithelial cells against a concentration gradient. In this way, Na^+ enhances the absorption of sugars and amino acids and vice versa.

> The ability of glucose to enhance the absorption of Na^+, and hence Cl^- and water, is exploited in oral rehydration therapy for **cholera** and other secretory diarrheas. When patients with cholera drink a solution containing glucose, sodium chloride (NaCl), and certain other constituents, the absorption of glucose, salt, and water helps counteract the secretory fluxes of salt and water that characterize this disease.

In the ileum, the net rate of Na^+ absorption is smaller than that in the jejunum. Na^+ absorption is only slightly stimulated by sugars and amino acids because the sugar and amino acid transport proteins are less concentrated in the ileum than in the jejunum. The ileum can absorb Na^+ against a larger electrochemical potential than the jejunum can.

In the colon, Na^+ is normally absorbed against a large electrochemical potential difference. Na^+ concentrations in the luminal contents can be as low as 25 mM, compared with about 120 mM in the plasma.

Cl$^-$ and bicarbonate are absorbed in large amounts in the jejunum, but in the ileum and colon, Cl$^-$ is usually absorbed in exchange for bicarbonate

By the end of the jejunum, most of the bicarbonate (HCO_3^-) of the hepatic and pancreatic secretions has been absorbed. In the ileum, Cl^- is absorbed, but HCO_3^- is normally secreted. If the HCO_3^- concentration in the lumen of the ileum exceeds about 45 mM, the flux from lumen to blood exceeds that from blood to lumen, and net absorption occurs. In the colon, the transport of these ions is similar to that in the ileum: Cl^- is absorbed, and HCO_3^- is usually secreted.

The absorption of water creates a concentration gradient favoring the absorption of K$^+$

As with the other ions, the net movement of K^+ across the intestinal epithelium is the difference between large unidirectional fluxes from lumen to blood and from blood to lumen. In the jejunum and in the ileum, the net flux is from lumen to blood. As the volume of intestinal contents is reduced because of the absorption of water, the increased concentration of K^+ provides a driving force for the movement of K^+ across the intestinal mucosa and into the blood.

In the colon, there is usually a net secretion of K^+. Net secretion occurs when the luminal concentration is less than about 25 mM; if it is greater than 25 mM, net absorption occurs. The secretion of K^+ is powered by the negative luminal electrical potential (about -30 mV) in the colon. Table 34-1 summarizes the transport of Na^+, K^+, Cl^-, and HCO_3^- in the small and large intestines.

> Most absorption of K^+ results from its increased concentration in the lumen. This high concentration is caused by the absorption of water. Significant amounts of K^+ may be lost in diarrhea. If the diarrhea is prolonged, the K^+ level in the extracellular fluid compartment falls. Maintaining normal K^+ levels is important, especially for the heart and other muscles. K^+ imbalance can have life-threatening consequences, such as **cardiac arrhythmias.** Infants with prolonged diarrhea are particularly susceptible to **hypokalemia** (low plasma K^+ levels).

Ion and water transport occurs via paracellular and transcellular routes

The tight junctions between intestinal epithelial cells are leaky; that is, they are somewhat permeable to water and ions. The tight junctions of the duodenum are the least

Table 34-1	Transport of Na^+, K^+, Cl^-, and HCO_3^- in the Large and Small Intestines			
Segment of Intestine	**Na^+**	**K^+**	**Cl^-**	**HCO_3^-**
Jejunum	Actively absorbed; absorption enhanced by sugars, neutral amino acids	Passively absorbed when concentration rises because of absorption of water	Absorbed	Absorbed
Ileum	Actively absorbed	Passively absorbed	Absorbed, some in exchange for HCO_3^-	Secreted, partly in exchange for Cl^-
Colon	Actively absorbed	Net secretion occurs when K^+ concentration in lumen <25 mM	Absorbed, some in exchange for HCO_3^-	Secreted, partly in exchange for Cl^-

tight, and hence they have the highest permeability. Tight junctions in the jejunum are somewhat tighter, those in the ileum are still tighter, and those in the colon are the tightest.

Because the tight junctions are leaky, some fraction of the water and ions that traverse the intestinal epithelium passes between, rather than through, the epithelial cells. Transmucosal movement through the tight junctions and the lateral intracellular spaces is called **paracellular transport.** Passage through the epithelial cells is termed **transcellular transport.**

Because the tight junctions in the duodenum are very leaky, most of the large unidirectional fluxes of water and ions that take place in the duodenum occur via the paracellular pathway. The proportions of water or of a particular ion that pass through the transcellular and paracellular routes are determined by the relative permeabilities of the two pathways for the substance in question. Even in the ileum, where the junctions are much tighter than in the duodenum, the paracellular pathway contributes more to the total ionic conductance of the mucosa than the transcellular pathway does.

The net absorption of water is powered by the absorption of solutes from the intestine

The absorption of water depends on the absorption of nutrients such as sugars and amino acids and on the absorption of ions, principally Na^+ and Cl^-. Water absorption in the small intestine normally occurs in the absence of a significant osmotic pressure difference between the luminal contents and the blood in the intestinal capillaries. A significant fraction of the net water absorption occurs via a mechanism known as **standing gradient osmosis** (see Chapter 33). As shown in Figure 33-15, the active pumping of Na^+ into the lateral intercellular spaces by Na^+,K^+-ATPase drives the absorption of Cl^- and water.

> Any substance that cannot be absorbed in the intestine will, because of its osmotic effect, prevent an isoosmotic equivalent of water from being absorbed. This is the basis for the action of **osmotic laxatives** such as magnesium sulfate (Epsom salt). When a nutrient is malabsorbed, as in **lactose intolerance,** the osmotic effect of unabsorbed nutrient contributes to the diarrhea.

Electrolyte transport in the intestine is regulated by hormones, neurotransmitters, and paracrine substances

Stimulation of sympathetic nerves to the intestine or an elevated plasma level of epinephrine increases the absorption of Na^+, Cl^-, and water. Stimulation of parasympathetic nerves to the gut decreases the net rate of ion and water absorption.

Adrenal cortical hormones stimulate the absorption of electrolytes and water. Aldosterone strongly stimulates the secretion of K^+ and the absorption of Na^+ and water by the colon and to a much lesser extent by the ileum. Aldosterone acts by increasing the number of Na^+ channels in the luminal membrane of the colonic epithelial cells (Figure 34-5, C) and the number of active Na^+,K^+-ATPase molecules in the basolateral membrane. Aldosterone has similar effects on the epithelial cells of the distal tubule of the kidney (see Chapter 37). The enhanced absorption of NaCl and water induced by aldosterone in the colon and kidney is an important mechanism in the body's compensatory response to dehydration. Glucocorticoids also increase the content of Na^+,K^+-ATPase in the basolateral membrane and thereby enhance Na^+ and water absorption and K^+ secretion in the colon.

Ion transport processes vary from one segment of the intestine to another

The ion transport processes that occur in the jejunum, ileum, and colon are summarized in Figure 34-5.

In the jejunum, large amounts of Na^+, Cl^-, bicarbonate, and water are absorbed

Na^+ enters jejunal epithelial cells at the brush border via the nutrient-coupled, Na^+-powered transporters (electrogenic) and via the Na^+/H^+ exchanger. Na^+ is extruded from the cell across the basolateral membrane by Na^+,K^+-ATPase. The absorption of Cl^- and HCO_3^- is powered by (1) the slight luminal electronegativity generated by Na^+ uptake at the brush border and by Na^+,K^+-ATPase and (2) the concentration of luminal ions via the large net absorption of water in the jejunum.

Acidification of the jejunal contents by gastric acid and by the Na^+/H^+ exchanger pushes the bicarbonate/carbonic acid equilibrium toward carbonic acid, which is in equilibrium with carbon dioxide and water. Carbon dioxide is highly diffusible (see Chapter 30) and is readily absorbed across the mucosa and into the blood. Most of the HCO_3^- dumped into the duodenum in bile and pancreatic juice is absorbed by this mechanism.

In the ileum, Cl^- is absorbed in exchange for bicarbonate

In the ileum (Figure 34-5, *B*), the net absorption of Na^+ and Cl^- occurs via mechanisms similar to those in the jejunum. The Na^+-powered nutrient transporters are less numerous than in the jejunum. The net secretion of HCO_3^- in exchange for the absorption of Cl^- occurs via an **anion exchanger** in the brush border membrane. HCO_3^- enters the epithelial cells across the basolateral membrane via Na^+-powered, secondary active transport. The coupled operation of the

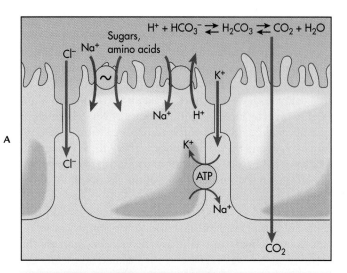

$$H^+ + HCO_3^- \rightleftarrows H_2CO_3 \rightleftarrows CO_2 + H_2O$$

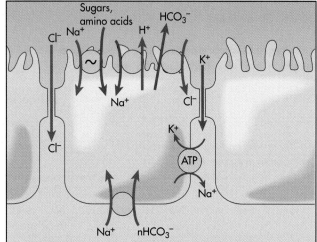

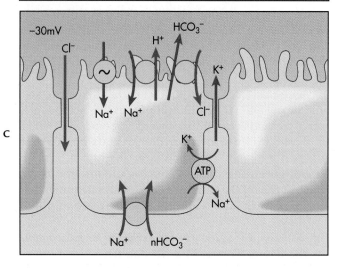

Figure 34-5 Summary of the major ion-transport processes that occur in the jejunum **(A)**, ileum **(B)**, and colon **(C)**.

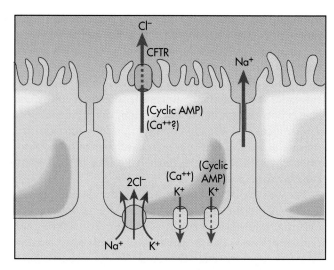

Figure 34-6 Ion transport processes involved in the secretion of Cl^-, Na^+, and water by the epithelial cells in the crypts of Lieberkühn in the small intestine. Cl^- is actively taken up into the cell at the basolateral membrane; this is powered by the Na^+ gradient. Cl^- enters the lumen via an electrogenic channel; the resulting luminal negativity drives the secretion of Na^+, partly via the tight junctions. The secretion of Na^+ and Cl^- results in the osmotic movement of water into the lumen. *CFTR,* Cystic fibrosis transmembrane regulator.

Na^+/H^+ exchanger and the Cl^-/HCO_3^- transporter of the luminal membrane results in the absorption of NaCl and the secretion of carbonic acid (H_2CO_3). In both the jejunum and the ileum, K^+ is concentrated by the absorption of water; the elevated K^+ concentration drives the net absorption of K^+, predominantly via the tight junctions.

In the colon, Na^+ is absorbed across the brush border membrane via an electrogenic Na^+ channel

In the colon, the net absorption of Na^+ and Cl^- and net secretion of HCO_3^- occur via mechanisms similar to those in the ileum. In the colon, however, the entry of Na^+ across the brush border membrane occurs via an electrogenic Na^+ channel. Because the tight junctions of the colon are so tight, electrogenic Na^+ transport produces an electrical potential of about 30 mV (lumen negative) across the mucosa. This potential drives the net secretion of K^+ into the lumen, mostly via the tight junctions. In the distal colon, the active absorption of K^+ and the secretion of H^+ are powered by an H^+,K^+-ATPase that resembles the gastric H^+ pump.

Large secretory fluxes of water and electrolytes occur in each segment of the intestine

The normal net absorption of Na^+, Cl^-, and water is the result of large unidirectional fluxes from lumen to blood and from blood to lumen. Mature intestinal epithelial cells near the tips of the villi are active in the net absorption of Na^+, Cl^-, and water; the processes previously described and shown in Figure 34-5 occur in the cells at the villous tips. The more immature epithelial cells in the crypts of Lieberkühn are net secretors of Na^+, Cl^-, and water (Figure 34-6). Secretion by the crypt cells is a normal physiological function and is subject to physiological regulation.

Cl^- is actively transported into the crypt cell across the basolateral membrane (Figure 34-6); Cl^- is driven into the cell by the electrochemical potential of Na^+ via a transporter known as the $Na^+,K^+,2\,Cl^-$ transporter. Cl^- is secreted into the lumen across the brush border membrane via an **electrogenic Cl^- channel.** Na^+ is secreted along with Cl^- to preserve electroneutrality, and water is secreted because of the osmotic pressure generated by the secretion of Na^+ and Cl^-.

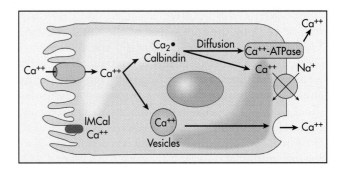

Figure 34-7 Cellular mechanisms involved in Ca^{++} absorption in the small intestine. *IMCal,* Intestinal membrane Ca^{++}-binding protein.

In **secretory diarrheal diseases** such as **cholera,** the secretion of Cl^-, Na^+, and water into the intestinal lumen by the cells in the crypts of Lieberkühn is specifically elevated. Cholera is caused by cholera toxin produced by the bacterium *Vibrio cholerae.* Cholera toxin permanently activates adenylyl cyclase and thereby elevates the level of cyclic AMP in the crypt cells. Cyclic AMP activates the brush border Cl^- channels and thereby enhances the secretion of Cl^- (and therefore also of Na^+ and water). Cholera patients may produce up to 20 L/day of watery stool. Such patients are likely to die unless they are promptly and adequately rehydrated.

The brush border Cl^- channel is the same protein that is defective in **cystic fibrosis (CF).** CF is by far the most common autosomal recessive disorder; about 1 in 20 American adults are CF carriers. CF carriers, who have one normal and one defective copy of the gene for the Cl^- channel, may be less likely to suffer the severe symptoms of cholera than normal individuals. Because cholera and related secretory diarrheas are the major causes of loss of life in children in societies that lack modern sanitation, the resistance of CF carriers to secretory diarrheas may explain the unusual prevalence of this mutation.

Ca^{++} Is Actively Absorbed in All Segments of the Intestine

The duodenum and jejunum are especially active in absorbing Ca^{++}, and they can absorb Ca^{++} against a greater than tenfold concentration gradient. The ability of the intestine to absorb Ca^{++} is regulated. Animals with a Ca^{++}-deficient diet increase their ability to absorb Ca^{++}, but animals receiving high-Ca^{++} diets have less capacity to absorb it. The intestinal absorption of Ca^{++} is stimulated by vitamin D and is slightly stimulated by parathyroid hormone (see Chapter 43).

Ca^{++} moves down its electrochemical potential gradient into intestinal epithelial cells through Ca^{++} channels in the brush border plasma membrane (Figure 34-7). An integral protein of the brush border plasma membrane, called **intestinal membrane Ca^{++}-binding protein** (IMCal), appears to bind Ca^{++} near the inner surface of the brush border membrane.

Ca^{++} is bound to calbindin in the cytosol epithelial cells

The cytosol of the intestinal epithelial cells contains a Ca^{++}-binding protein called **calbindin,** or **CaBP.** In mammals, calbindin has a molecular weight of about 9000 and binds two Ca^{++} with high affinity. The level of calbindin in the epithelial cells correlates well with the capacity to absorb Ca^{++}. Calbindin allows large amounts of Ca^{++} to traverse the cytosol, but it averts concentrations of free Ca^{++} that are high enough to form insoluble salts with intracellular anions. In addition, Ca^{++} traverses the epithelial cell cytosol in membrane-bounded vesicles, with which a fraction of the calbindin is associated.

Ca^{++} is transported across the basolateral membrane by two transport proteins

The basolateral plasma membrane contains two transport proteins that are capable of ejecting Ca^{++} from the cell against its electrochemical potential gradient. Ca^{++}-ATPase uses the energy of ATP to extrude Ca^{++} across the basolateral plasma membrane. A smaller amount of Ca^{++} is transported across the basolateral plasma membrane by an Na^+/Ca^{++} exchanger. The Ca^{++}-containing vesicles are believed to extrude Ca^{++} across the basolateral plasma membrane via exocytosis (Figure 34-7).

Vitamin D enhances Ca^{++} absorption

Vitamin D is essential for development of the normal capacity for Ca^{++} absorption by the intestine. The actions of vitamin D are also discussed in Chapter 43.

In **rickets,** a disease caused by vitamin D deficiency, the absorption rate of Ca^{++} is very low. In children with rickets, the growth of bones is abnormal because of insufficient levels of Ca^{++}. Because of a failure to deposit normal levels of calcium salts in the bone matrix, bones are softer and more flexible than normal. These changes contribute to the characteristic "bowlegged" appearance of children with rickets.

Vitamin D has multiple effects that enhance the absorption of Ca^{++} by the epithelium of the small intestine. Treatment with vitamin D increases the transport of Ca^{++} across the brush border membrane; the mechanism of this effect is unclear. Vitamin D treatment also enhances the transport of Ca^{++} through the cytosol of the intestinal epithelial cell by dramatically increasing the level of calbindin. Vitamin D increases the rate of extrusion of Ca^{++} across the basolateral membrane of intestinal epithelial cells by increasing the level of Ca^{++}-ATPase in the membrane.

Ingested Iron Is Absorbed

A typical adult should ingest approximately 15 to 20 mg of iron daily. Of this amount, only 0.5 to 1 mg is absorbed by normal adult men and 1 to 1.5 mg is absorbed by premenopausal women. Iron depletion (e.g., that caused by hemorrhage) increases the capacity of the intestine to absorb iron. Growing children and pregnant women absorb greater amounts of iron than men.

Iron absorption is limited because iron tends to form insoluble salts with hydroxide, phosphate, HCO$_3^-$, and other anions present in intestinal secretions. Iron also forms insoluble complexes with other substances typically present in food, such as phytate, tannins, and the fiber of cereal grains. These iron complexes are more soluble at a low pH. Therefore the hydrochloric acid (HCl) secreted by the stomach enhances iron absorption, whereas iron absorption is usually low in individuals deficient in HCl secretion.

Vitamin C effectively promotes iron absorption by forming a soluble complex with iron and by reducing Fe^{+++} to Fe^{++}. Iron that is complexed with ascorbate or is in the form of Fe^{++} has less tendency to form insoluble complexes than Fe^{+++} and thus is better absorbed. Individuals who take iron supplements are advised to ingest vitamin C with their iron tablets.

Heme iron is relatively well absorbed

Iron is present in the diet as inorganic iron salts and as part of the heme prosthetic groups of proteins such as hemoglobin, myoglobin, and cytochromes. About 20% of ingested heme iron is absorbed. Proteolytic enzymes release heme groups from proteins in the intestinal lumen. Heme is taken up via facilitated transport by the epithelial cells that line the upper small intestine. In the epithelial cell, iron is split from the heme (Figure 34-8). No intact heme is transported into the portal blood.

The absorption of Fe^{++} involves a transporter and an iron-binding protein

Duodenal epithelial cells are principally responsible for the absorption of nonheme iron. The brush border plasma membrane has transport proteins that bind Fe^{++}

and transport it into the duodenal epithelial cells (Figure 34-8); Fe^{+++} is not transported. In the epithelial cell cytosol, Fe^{++} is bound to an iron-binding protein, which is called **mobilferrin**. Mobilferrin may function analogously to calbindin, namely (1) to receive Fe^{++} from the brush border transporter, (2) to prevent Fe^{++} from forming insoluble complexes with intracellular anions, and (3) to facilitate the diffusion of Fe^{++} through the cytosol.

The basolateral membrane has transferrin receptors. These receptors bind plasma transferrin, and they apparently mediate the transfer of Fe^{++} from mobilferrin in the cytosol to transferrin on the extracellular face of the basolateral membrane. The Fe^{++}-transferrin complex is then released to the extracellular fluid and diffuses into the blood. The transport of Fe^{++} across the basolateral membrane is the rate-limiting step in its absorption; the rate of transport is limited by the number of transferrin receptors present in the basolateral membrane.

Iron absorption is regulated in accordance with the body's need for iron

In chronic iron deficiency or after hemorrhage, the capacity of the duodenum and jejunum to absorb iron is increased. The intestine also protects the body from the consequences of absorbing too much iron. An important mechanism for preventing excess absorption of iron is the almost irreversible binding of iron to ferritin in the intestinal epithelial cell. Iron bound to ferritin is not available for transport into the plasma (Figure 34-9), and it is lost into the intestinal lumen and excreted in the feces when the intestinal epithelial cell is sloughed off. The amount of apoferritin present in the intestinal cells determines how much iron can be trapped in the nonabsorbable pool. The synthesis of apoferritin is stimulated by iron, and this protects against absorption of excessive amounts of iron.

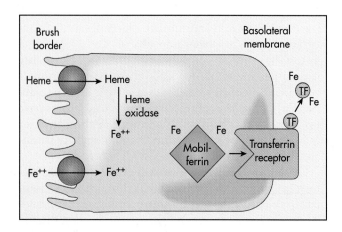

Figure 34-8 Iron absorption by the epithelial cells of the small intestine. In the cytosol of intestinal epithelial cells, iron is bound to mobilferrin. *Tf,* Transferrin.

The capacity of the duodenum and jejunum to absorb iron increases 3 or 4 days after hemorrhage. The intestinal epithelial cells require this time to migrate from their sites of formation in the crypts of Lieberkühn to the tips of the villi, where they enhance absorption. The iron-absorbing capacity of the epithelial cells is programmed when the cells are in the crypts of Lieberkühn. The brush border membranes of the duodenum and jejunum of an iron-deficient animal also have an increased number of receptors for the complex of iron with transferrin and thus absorb the iron-transferrin complex from the lumen more rapidly.

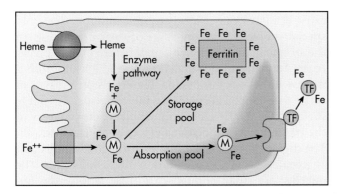

Figure 34-9 In the epithelial cells of the small intestine, there are two pools of iron. One pool is bound to mobilferrin *(M)* in the cytosol and is available for absorption into the blood, where iron is bound to transferrin *(Tf)*. The other pool, iron that becomes bound to ferritin in the epithelial cell, is unavailable for transport across the basolateral membrane; this iron is lost into the lumen when the epithelial cell is sloughed off.

Absorption of Other Ions

Magnesium is absorbed along the entire length of the small intestine. About half the normal dietary intake is absorbed, and the rest is excreted. **Phosphate** is absorbed, in part by active transport, all along the small intestine. **Copper** is absorbed in the jejunum; approximately 50% of the ingested load is absorbed. Copper is secreted in the bile bound to certain bile acids; this copper is lost in the feces.

Transport Proteins Mediate the Absorption of Most Water-Soluble Vitamins

Most water-soluble vitamins can be absorbed by simple diffusion if they are taken in sufficiently high doses. Nevertheless, specific transport mechanisms are important in the normal absorption of most water-soluble vitamins (Table 34-2).

The normal absorption of vitamin B_{12} requires intrinsic factor

A specific active transport process has been implicated in the absorption of vitamin B_{12}. The dietary requirement for this vitamin is fairly close to its maximal absorptive capacity (Table 34-2). Enteric bacteria synthesize B_{12} and other B vitamins, but the colonic epithelium lacks specific mechanisms for their absorption.

Table 34-2 Intestinal Absorption of Vitamins

Vitamin	Species	Site of Absorption	Transport Mechanism	Maximal Absorptive Capacity*	Dietary Requirement*
Ascorbic acid (C)	Humans, guinea pig	Ileum	Active	>5000 mg	<50 mg
Biotin	Hamster	Upper small intestine	Active	?	?
Choline	Guinea pig, hamster	Small intestine	Facilitated	?	?
Folic acid					
Pteroylglutamate	Rat	Jejunum	Facilitated	>1000 µg/dose	100-200 µg
5-Methyltetrahydrofolate	Rat	Jejunum	Diffusion		
Nicotinic acid	Rat	Jejunum	Facilitated	?	10-20 mg
Pantothenic acid		Small intestine	?	?	(?) 10 mg
Pyridoxine (B_6)	Rat, hamster	Small intestine	Diffusion	>50 mg/dose	1-2 mg
Riboflavin (B_{21})	Humans, rat	Jejunum	Facilitated	10-12 mg/dose	1-2 mg
Thiamin (B_1)	Rat	Jejunum	Active	8-14 mg	≈1 mg
Vitamin B_{12}	Humans, rat, hamster	Distal ileum	Active	6-9 µg	3-7 µg

Data from Matthews DM. In Smyth DH, ed: *Intestinal absorption,* vol 4B, *Biomembranes,* London, 1974, Plenum; and Rose RC: *Annu Rev Physiol* 42:157, 1980.
*In humans (per day).

When the intestinal absorption of vitamin B_{12} is impaired, the resulting deficiency retards the maturation of red blood cells and causes **pernicious anemia.** Because of the occurrence of this disorder, much attention has focused on the absorption of vitamin B_{12}. Most patients with pernicious anemia have pronounced atrophy of gastric glands, and their stomachs are defective in secreting HCl and pepsins, as well as intrinsic factor (IF). These individuals have circulating antibodies against parietal cells; the antibodies may cause the destruction of parietal cells.

The liver contains a large store (2 to 5 mg) of vitamin B_{12}. Vitamin B_{12} is normally present in the bile (0.5 to 5 µg daily), but approximately 70% of this is normally reabsorbed. Because only about 0.1% of the store is lost daily, even if absorption totally ceases, the store will last 3 to 6 years.

Events in the stomach and intestine influence the absorption of vitamin B_{12}

Most of the vitamin B_{12} in food is bound to proteins. The low pH in the stomach and the digestion of proteins by pepsins releases free vitamin B_{12}, which is then rapidly bound to a class of glycoproteins known as **R proteins.** R proteins are present in saliva and gastric juice, and they bind vitamin B_{12} tightly over a wide pH range.

IF is a vitamin B_{12}–binding protein secreted by the gastric parietal cells. IF binds vitamin B_{12} with less affinity than the R proteins; thus in the stomach most of the vitamin B_{12} food is bound to R proteins.

Pancreatic proteases degrade the complex between R proteins and vitamin B_{12}, which causes vitamin B_{12} to be released. The free vitamin B_{12} is taken up by IF, which is highly resistant to digestion by pancreatic proteases.

Receptors that bind the intrinsic factor–vitamin B_{12} complex are present on the brush border of the distal ileum

The normal absorption of vitamin B_{12} depends on the presence of IF (Figure 34-10). The brush border plasma membranes of the epithelial cells of the ileum contain receptor proteins that recognize and bind the IF-B_{12} complex. Free IF does not compete for binding, and the receptor does not recognize free vitamin B_{12}. Binding to the receptor is required for normal B_{12} uptake. After being absorbed, vitamin B_{12} appears in the portal blood bound to a protein called **transcobalamin II.**

In the complete absence of IF, approximately 1% to 2% of the vitamin B_{12} ingested is absorbed. If large doses are taken (about 1 mg/day), enough can be absorbed to treat pernicious anemia.

Digestion and Absorption of Lipids

The primary lipids of a normal diet are **triglycerides.** The diet contains smaller amounts of **sterols** (such as cholesterol), **sterol esters,** and **phospholipids.** Because lipids are only slightly soluble in water, they pose special problems at every stage of their processing. In the stomach, lipids tend to separate into an oily phase. In the duodenum and small intestine, lipids are **emulsified** with the aid of bile acids. The emulsion consists of small droplets of lipid coated by bile acids. The large surface area of the emulsion droplets allows access of the water-soluble lipolytic enzymes to their substrates. The digestion products of lipids form small molecular aggregates, known as **micelles,** with the bile acids. The micelles are small enough to diffuse among the microvilli and to allow absorption of the lipids from molecular solution along the entire surface of the intestinal brush border.

Because fats tend to separate into an oily phase, they usually are emptied from the stomach later than the other gastric contents. Fat in the duodenum strongly inhibits gastric emptying. This helps ensure that the fat is not emptied from the stomach more rapidly than it can be accommodated by the duodenal mechanisms that provide for emulsification and digestion.

The digestion of lipids occurs in the stomach and small intestine

Lingual lipase is produced by serous glands in the tongue. **Gastric lipase** is secreted by chief cells. Together, these two lipases constitute **preduodenal lipase.** These enzymes are specific for the hydrolysis of triglycerides. In humans, gastric lipase is more abundant than lingual lipase. The amount of triglyceride hydrolyzed by preduodenal lipases varies considerably among individuals.

Lipases present in pancreatic juice are responsible for the hydrolysis of most dietary lipid. The lipolytic enzymes of the pancreatic juice are water-soluble molecules and thus have access to lipids only at the surfaces of the fat droplets. THE SURFACE AVAILABLE FOR DIGESTION IS INCREASED MANY THOUSAND TIMES BY EMULSIFICATION OF THE LIPIDS. Bile acids themselves are rather poor emulsifying agents. However, with the aid of lecithins, which are present in high concentration in bile, the bile acids emulsify dietary fats.

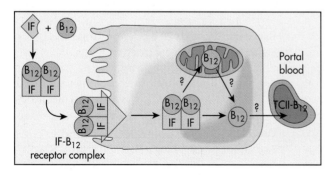

Figure 34-10 Mechanism of absorption of vitamin B_{12} by epithelial cells in the ileum. Vitamin B_{12} in portal blood is bound to transcobalamin II (*TCII*).

Pancreatic juice contains the major lipolytic enzymes responsible for the digestion of lipids

Glycerol ester hydrolase, also called **pancreatic lipase,** cleaves the 1 and 1′ fatty acids preferentially from a triglyceride to produce two free fatty acids and one 2-monoglyceride. **Colipase,** a small protein present in pancreatic juice, is essential for the function of glycerol ester hydrolase. Colipase is required for glycerol ester hydrolase to bind to the surface of the emulsion droplets in the presence of bile acids.

Cholesterol esterase cleaves the ester bond in a cholesterol ester to give one fatty acid and free cholesterol. **Phospholipase A_2** cleaves the ester bond at the 2 position of a glycerophosphatide to yield, in the case of lecithin, one fatty acid and one lysolecithin.

Infants with CF secrete extremely low levels of pancreatic enzymes. This is because the defective Cl^- channels in the apical membranes of pancreatic ductular epithelial cells make the cells unable to secrete Cl^-, Na^+, and water into the acinar lumen. Because little water is secreted, mucus obstructs the small pancreatic ducts, and the pancreatic acinar cells are destroyed. (Obstruction of the bronchioles by mucus is responsible for the pulmonary problems associated with CF.) Because of the deficiency of pancreatic lipases, children with CF have marked difficulties in digesting dietary lipids. Consequently, they may suffer from **steatorrhea** (fatty stool) and malnutrition.

Bile acids form mixed micelles with the products of lipid digestion

Triglycerides are not often good micelle formers, but 2-monoglycerides are effective in forming mixed micelles with bile acids. The micelles are multimolecular aggregates (about 5 nm in diameter) that contain approximately 20 to 30 molecules (Figure 34-11). Bile acids are flat molecules that have a polar face and a nonpolar face. Much of the surface of the micelles is covered with bile acids, with the nonpolar face toward the lipid interior of the micelle and the polar face toward the outside. Hydrophobic molecules, such as long-chain fatty acids, monoglycerides, phospholipids, cholesterol, and fat-soluble vitamins, tend to partition into the micelles.

Bile acids must be present at a certain minimal concentration, called the critical micelle concentration, before micelles form. Bile acids are normally present in the duodenum at greater than the critical micelle concentration.

The absorption of lipid digestion products takes place in the small intestine

The diffusion of mixed micelles through the unstirred layer is the rate-limiting step in the absorption of lipid digestion products

Micelles are important in the absorption of the products of lipid digestion and in the absorption of most other fat-soluble molecules (e.g., fat-soluble vitamins). The micelles diffuse among the microvilli that form the brush border, and this allows the huge surface area of the brush border membrane to participate in lipid absorption (Figure 34-12). The presence of micelles tends to keep the aqueous solution near the brush border plasma membrane saturated with fatty acids, 2-monoglycerides, cholesterol, and other micellar contents.

Because of their high lipid solubility, the fatty acids, 2-monoglycerides, cholesterol, and lysolecithin can diffuse across the brush border membrane. In addition, the brush border plasma membrane contains specific transport proteins that facilitate the transport of particular lipid digestion products. A Na^+-dependent **fatty acid transport protein** enhances the movement of long-chain fatty acids across the brush border plasma membrane. Another transport protein mediates facilitated transport of cholesterol across the brush border plasma membrane.

Because lipids can be taken up across the brush border plasma membrane quite rapidly, the main limitation to the rate of lipid uptake by the epithelial cells of

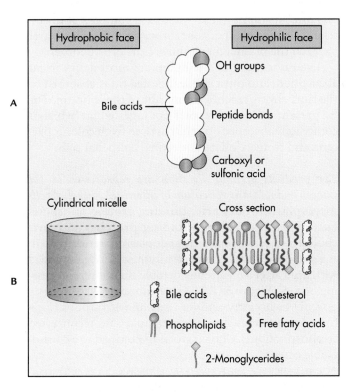

Figure 34-11 Structure of bile acids and micelles. **A,** A bile acid molecule is amphipathic because it has a hydrophobic face and a hydrophilic face. **B,** Model of the structure of a bile acid–lipid mixed micelle, showing the way that bile acids and the major products of lipid digestion pack into the mixed micelle.

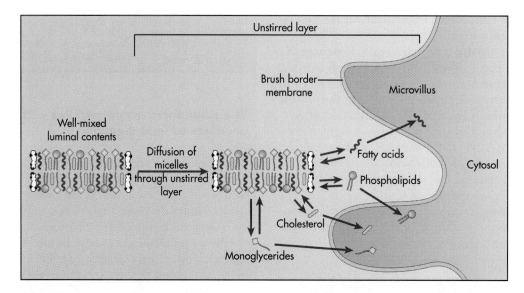

Figure 34-12 Lipid absorption in the small intestine. Mixed micelles of bile acids and lipid digestion products diffuse through the unstirred layer. As lipid digestion products are absorbed from free solution, more lipids partition out of the micelles.

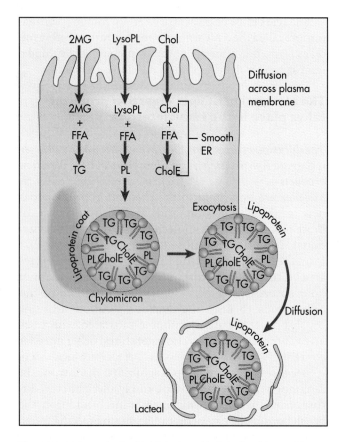

Figure 34-13 Resynthesis of lipids in the epithelial cells of the small intestine, formation of chylomicrons, and subsequent transport of chylomicrons into the lymphatic vessels. *Chol,* Cholesterol; *CholE,* cholesterol ester; *ER,* endoplasmic reticulum; *FFA,* free fatty acid; *lysoPL,* lysophospholipid; *2MG,* 2-monoglyceride; *PL,* phospholipid; *TG,* triglyceride.

the upper small intestine is the diffusion of the mixed micelles through an unstirred layer on the luminal surface of the brush border plasma membrane (Figure 34-12). Partly because of the convoluted surface of the intestinal mucosa, the fluid in immediate contact with the epithelial cell surface is not readily mixed with the bulk of the luminal contents. This fluid forms an effective **unstirred layer** with an effective thickness of 200 to 500 µm. Nutrients in the well-mixed contents of the intestinal lumen must diffuse through the unstirred layer to reach the plasma membrane of the brush border.

The duodenum and jejunum are most active in fat absorption, and most of the ingested fat is absorbed by the time chyme reaches the middle of the jejunum. The fat present in normal stool is not ingested fat (which is completely absorbed), but it is derived from colonic bacteria and from exfoliated intestinal epithelial cells.

The products of lipid digestion are reprocessed in the smooth endoplasmic reticulum of intestinal epithelial cells A **cytoplasmic fatty acid–binding protein** transports fatty acids, and a **sterol-binding protein** transports cholesterol to the smooth endoplasmic reticulum. In the smooth endoplasmic reticulum, which is engorged with lipid after a meal, considerable chemical reprocessing occurs (Figure 34-13). The 2-monoglycerides are re-esterified with fatty acids at the 1 and 1′ carbons to reform triglycerides. Lysophospholipids are reconverted to phospholipids. Cholesterol is reesterified to a considerable extent.

CHYLOMICRONS ARE FORMED FROM THE PRODUCTS OF LIPID DIGESTION. The reprocessed lipids accumulate in the vesicles of the smooth endoplasmic reticulum. Phospholipids cover the external surfaces of these lipid droplets. The lipid droplets, approximately 10 nm in diameter at this point, are known as **chylomicrons.** About

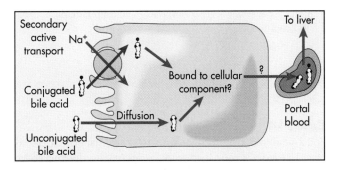

Figure 34-14 Absorption of bile acids by epithelial cells of the terminal ileum. Bile acids are absorbed both by simple diffusion and by Na^+-powered, secondary active transport. Conjugated bile acids are absorbed mainly by active transport; unconjugated bile acids are absorbed chiefly by diffusion.

10% of their surface is covered by β-lipoprotein, some of which is synthesized in the intestinal epithelial cells.

Chylomicrons are ejected from the epithelial cell by exocytosis (Figure 34-13). The chylomicrons leave the cells at the level of the nuclei and enter the lateral intercellular spaces. Chylomicrons are too large to pass through the basement membrane that invests the mucosal capillaries. However, they do enter the lacteals, which have sufficiently large fenestrations for the chylomicrons to pass through. The chylomicrons leave the intestine with the lymph, primarily via the thoracic lymphatic duct, and flow into the venous circulation.

The absorption of bile acids occurs in the terminal ileum
The absorption of dietary lipids is typically complete by the time chyme reaches the middle of the jejunum. In contrast, bile acids are absorbed largely in the terminal part of the ileum. Bile acids cross the brush border plasma membrane via two routes: a Na^+-powered, secondary active transport process and simple diffusion (Figure 34-14). Conjugated bile acids are the principal substrates for active absorption; deconjugated bile acids have less affinity for the transporter. Deconjugation and dehydroxylation make bile acids less polar, and thus they are better absorbed by simple diffusion.

Absorbed bile acids are carried away from the intestine in the portal blood. Hepatocytes avidly extract bile acids, and they essentially clear the bile acids from the blood in a single pass through the liver. Most deconjugated bile acids are reconjugated in the hepatocytes, and some secondary bile acids are rehydroxylated. The reprocessed bile acids, together with newly synthesized bile acids, are secreted into bile (see Chapter 33).

Fat-soluble vitamins are mostly absorbed from mixed micelles

The fat-soluble vitamins (A, D, E, and K) partition into the mixed micelles formed by the bile acids and lipid digestion products. THE PRESENCE OF BILE ACIDS AND LIPID DIGESTION PRODUCTS ENHANCES THE ABSORPTION OF FAT-SOLUBLE VITAMINS.

The fat-soluble vitamins diffuse across the brush border plasma membrane into the intestinal epithelial cell. In the intestinal epithelial cell, the fat-soluble vitamins enter the chylomicrons and leave the intestine in the lymph. In the absence of bile acids, a significant fraction of the ingested load of a fat-soluble vitamin may be absorbed and leave the intestine in the portal blood.

SUMMARY

- The α-amylases of saliva and pancreatic juice cleave branched starch molecules into maltose, maltotriose, and α-limit dextrins. These digestion products are then reduced to glucose molecules by glucoamylase and α-dextrinase on the brush border membrane.
- Sucrase and lactase on the brush border membrane cleave sucrose and lactose into monosaccharides that can be transported into the intestinal epithelial cells.
- Protein digestion begins in the stomach by pepsins. Pancreatic proteases rapidly cleave proteins in the duodenum and jejunum, primarily to oligopeptides. Peptidases on the brush border membrane reduce oligopeptides to single amino acids and to small peptides.
- Amino acids are transported across the brush border membrane via an array of amino acid transporters. Dipeptides and tripeptides are taken up by a brush border peptide transporter with broad specificity.
- A typical human ingests about 2 L of water daily, and about 7 L enters the gastrointestinal tract in various secretions. About 99% of the water presented to the gastrointestinal tract is absorbed.
- The absorption of water is powered by the absorption of nutrients and salts. The greatest quantity of water is absorbed in the small intestine, especially the jejunum. Mature cells at the tips of the villi are active in salt, nutrient, and water absorption. Cells in the crypts of Lieberkühn are net secretors of ions and water.
- Ca^{++} is actively absorbed in the small intestine. Calbindin, a Ca^{++}-binding protein, facilitates the transport of Ca^{++} through the cytosol of the intestinal epithelial cell. Ca^{++} is transported across the basolateral membrane by Ca^{++}-ATPase and the Na^+/Ca^{++} exchange protein.
- Vitamin D stimulates the absorption of Ca^{++} by enhancing the synthesis of calbindin and the absorption of Ca^{++}-ATPase of the basolateral membrane.
- About 5% of inorganic iron ingested is absorbed by the small intestine; approximately 20% of heme iron is absorbed. Inorganic iron is transported across the brush border plasma membrane bound to Fe^{++} receptors. In the epithelial cells, some iron is bound to ferritin and is unavailable for absorption. The capacity to absorb iron increases in response to hemorrhage.

- Most water-soluble vitamins are taken up by specific transporters in the small intestinal brush border plasma membrane.
- Vitamin B_{12} is bound to R proteins in saliva and gastric juice. When R proteins are digested, vitamin B_{12} is bound by IF. Receptors on the ileal brush border membrane bind the IF-B_{12} complex and allow vitamin B_{12} to be taken up into the ileal epithelial cell. Vitamin B_{12} appears in the plasma bound to transcobalamin II.
- Triglycerides are the major dietary lipids. Lipids form droplets in the stomach and are emulsified in the duodenum by bile acids. Emulsification greatly increases the surface area available for the action of lipid-digesting enzymes of pancreatic juice.
- The products of triglyceride digestion, the 2-monoglycerides and fatty acids, form mixed micelles with bile acids. Cholesterol, fat-soluble vitamins, and other lipids partition into the micelles. Mixed micelles are small enough to diffuse among the microvilli and thus greatly enhance the brush border surface area available for lipid absorption.
- In epithelial cells, triglycerides and phospholipids are resynthesized and packaged along with other lipids into chylomicrons. Chylomicrons are coated with apolipoproteins and released at the basolateral membrane via exocytosis. Chylomicrons leave the intestine in the lymphatic vessels and thoracic duct.

BIBLIOGRAPHY

Caspary WF: Physiology and pathophysiology of intestinal absorption, *Am J Clin Nutr* 55:S299, 1992.

Cheeseman CI: Molecular mechanisms involved in regulation of amino acid transport, *Progr Biophys Mol Biol* 55:71, 1991.

Cooke HJ: Neuroimmune signaling in regulation of intestinal transport, *Am J Physiol* 266:G167, 1994.

Eastwood MA: The physiological effect of dietary fiber: an update, *Annu Rev Nutr* 12:19, 1992.

Field M, ed: *Diarrheal diseases*, New York, 1991, Elsevier.

Field M, Frizzell RA, eds: *Handbook of physiology*, section 6, vol 4, Bethesda, Md, 1991, The American Physiological Society.

Gray GM: Starch digestion and absorption in nonruminants, *J Nutr* 122:172, 1992.

Johnson LR, ed: *Physiology of the gastrointestinal tract*, ed 3, New York, 1994, Raven.

Johnson LR, ed: *Gastrointestinal physiology*, ed 5, St Louis, 1996, Mosby.

Matthews DM: *Protein absorption: development and present state of the subject*, New York, 1991, Wiley-Liss.

Sleisenger MH, Fordtran JS, eds: *Gastrointestinal disease*, ed 5, Philadelphia, 1993, WB Saunders.

Thurnhofer H, Hauser H: Uptake of cholesterol by small intestinal brush border membrane is protein mediated, *Biochemistry* 29:2142, 1990.

Turk E et al: Glucose/galactose malabsorption caused by a defect in the Na/glucose cotransporter, *Nature* 350:354, 1991.

Wasserman RH et al: Intestinal calcium transport and calcium extrusion processes at the basolateral membrane, *J Nutr* 122:662, 1992.

Yamada T, ed: *Textbook of gastroenterology*, ed 2, Philadelphia, 1995, JB Lippincott.

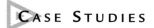 CASE STUDIES

Case 34-1

A 12-year-old boy has a skin rash reminiscent of pellagra. The rash is reported to occur occasionally and to be exacerbated by exposure to the sun. The patient's diet is judged to contain sufficient niacin and calories but is relatively low in protein. The patient is not malnourished. The patient's urine contains most of the neutral amino acids in levels from 5 to 20 times their levels in urine of normal individuals. When the patient is fed a mixture of amino acids, there is only a very small rise (compared to normal individuals) in the plasma levels of the neutral amino acids that are enriched in the patient's urine. The diagnosis is **Hartnup disease.**

1. Which of the following statements is correct?

   A. Many patients with Hartnup disease are malnourished.

   B. The patient would benefit from being given large oral doses of niacin daily.

   C. The patient probably has very low plasma levels of the neutral amino acids.

   D. High urinary levels of neutral amino acids are not expected in Hartnup disease.

   E. None of the above.

2. Which of the following statements is correct?

   A. A diet richer in protein would be expected to benefit this patient.

   B. If the patient were fed a mixture of all 20 amino acids, the plasma levels of many neutral amino acids would not rise as much as they would in a normal individual.

   C. If the patient has multiple siblings, some of them may have a similar disorder.

   D. It would be incorrect to say that this patient has pellagra.

   E. All of the above.

3. Which of the following statements is correct?

   A. The patient would benefit from being fed those amino acids that are in high concentration in his urine.

   B. All the neutral amino acids are expected to be at high levels in the patient's urine.

   C. It is unlikely that one of the patient's parents has Hartnup disease.

   D. After the patient is fed partially hydrolyzed protein, his plasma levels of neutral amino acids will rise much less than in a normal individual.

   E. None of the above.

Case 34-2

A 3-month-old infant is brought to the clinic because she does not seem to be growing at a normal rate and has stools that are bulky, malodorous, and greasy. Examination of a stool smear reveals numerous clear fat droplets. The baby was of normal birth weight, but after the first 3 months of life she fell below the 10th percentile in body weight. A sweat chloride test shows levels of NaCl in her sweat that are twice the normal levels. The diagnosis is **CF.**

1. Which of the following statements is correct?

   A. Digestive difficulties are unexpected in CF.

   B. CF is an uncommon disease.

   C. The baby is less likely to be deficient in pancreatic proteases than in pancreatic lipases.

   D. The baby should be put on a low-fat diet immediately.

   E. None of the above.

2. Which of the following statements is correct?

   A. The baby would benefit from taking pancreatic enzymes in enterically coated microspheres that are resistant to acid but that release enzymes at a pH of 5.5 to 6 with each meal.

   B. The baby would benefit from an inhibitor of gastric acid secretion.

   C. The baby would benefit from the administration of water-soluble forms of fat-soluble vitamins.

   D. The baby might benefit from a formula enriched in medium-chain triglycerides.

   E. All of the above.

3. Which of the following statements is not correct?

   A. The baby is at no increased risk of abnormalities of the endocrine pancreas.

   B. The baby is likely to have decreased levels of some of the brush border carbohydrate-digesting enzymes.

   C. The baby is likely to have high levels of serum trypsinogen.

   D. The baby is unlikely to have edema.

   E. None of the above.

RENAL SYSTEM

VII

Bruce M. Koeppen and Bruce A. Stanton

CHAPTER 35

Elements of Renal Function

- Describe the anatomy of the kidney and lower urinary tract.
- Explain the process of ultrafiltration and the concepts of glomerular filtration rate and renal blood flow.
- Describe the process of micturition.
- Explain why knowledge of the glomerular filtration rate is essential in evaluating the severity and course of kidney disease.
- Describe the concept of autoregulation of the glomerular filtration rate and renal blood flow.
- Explain how hormones and the sympathetic nerves affect the glomerular filtration rate and renal blood flow.

The kidneys are excretory and regulatory organs. By excreting water and solutes, the kidneys rid the body of excess water and waste products. In conjunction with the cardiovascular, endocrine, and nervous systems, the kidneys regulate the volume and composition of the body fluids within a very narrow range despite wide variations in the intake of food and water. Because of the kidneys' homeostatic role, the tissues and cells of the body can carry out their normal functions in a relatively constant environment.

The Kidneys Have Several Major Functions

The kidneys regulate (1) body fluid osmolality and volumes, (2) electrolyte balance, (3) acid-base balance, (4) the excretion of metabolic products and foreign substances, and (5) the production and secretion of hormones. Control of body fluid osmolality is important for the maintenance of normal cell volume in all tissues of the body. Control of body fluid volume is necessary for normal function of the cardiovascular system. The kidneys are also essential in regulating the amount of several important inorganic ions in the body, including Na^+, K^+, Cl^-, bicarbonate (HCO_3^-), hydrogen (H^+), Ca^{++}, and phosphate ($PO_4^=$). The excretion of these electrolytes must be equal to their daily intake to maintain appropriate balance,. If the intake of an electrolyte exceeds its excretion, the amount of this electrolyte in the body increases, and the individual is in positive balance for that electrolyte. Conversely, if excretion of an electrolyte exceeds its intake, its amount in the body decreases, and the individual is in negative balance for that electrolyte. For many electrolytes the kidneys are the sole or primary route for excretion from the body.

Another important function of the kidneys is the regulation of acid-base balance. Many of the metabolic functions of the body are exquisitely sensitive to pH. Thus the pH of the body fluids must be maintained within narrow limits. The pH is maintained by buffers within the body fluids and by the coordinated action of the lungs, liver, and kidneys.

The kidneys excrete a number of the end products of metabolism. These waste products include urea (from amino acids), uric acid (from nucleic acids), creatinine (from muscle creatine), end products of hemoglobin metabolism, and metabolites of hormones. The kidneys eliminate these substances from the body at a rate that matches their production. Thus the kidneys regulate hormone concentrations within the body fluids. The kidneys also represent an important route for the elimination of foreign substances such as drugs, pesticides, and other chemicals from the body.

Finally, the kidneys are important endocrine organs that produce and secrete renin, calcitriol, and erythropoietin. Renin activates the renin-angiotensin-aldosterone system, which helps regulate blood pressure and Na^+ and K^+ balance. **Calcitriol,** a metabolite of vitamin D_3, is necessary for the normal resorption of Ca^{++} by the gastrointestinal tract and for its deposition in bone (see also Chapter 38). In patients with renal disease, the kidneys' ability to produce calcitriol is impaired, and levels of this hormone are reduced. As a result, Ca^{++} resorption by the intestine is decreased. This reduced intestinal Ca^{++} resorption contributes to the bone formation abnormalities seen in patients with chronic renal disease. Another consequence of many kidney diseases is a reduction in erythropoietin production and secretion. Erythropoietin stimulates red blood cell formation by the bone marrow. Decreased erythrocyte production causes the anemia that occurs in chronic renal failure. This chapter reviews the anatomy of the kidneys, glomerular filtration rate (GFR), and renal blood flow (RBF).

Structure and Function Are Closely Linked in the Kidneys

The kidneys lie on the posterior wall of the abdomen behind the peritoneum on either side of the vertebral column. The gross anatomical features of the human kidney are illustrated in Figure 35-1. The medial side of each kidney contains an indentation through which pass the renal artery and vein, nerves, and pelvis. If a kidney were cut in half, two regions would be evident: an outer region called the **cortex** and an inner region called the **medulla.** The cortex and medulla are composed of nephrons, (the functional units of the kidney), blood vessels, lymphatics, and nerves. The medulla in the human kidney is divided into conical masses called the **renal pyramids.** The base of each pyramid originates at the corticomedullary border, and the apex terminates in a **papilla,** which lies within a **minor calyx.** Minor calyces collect urine from each papilla. The numerous minor calyces expand into two or three open-ended pouches, the **major calyces.** The major calyces in turn feed into the **pelvis.** The pelvis represents the upper expanded region of the **ureter,** which carries urine from the pelvis to the urinary bladder.

The blood flow to the two kidneys is equal to about 25% (1.25 L/min) of the cardiac output in resting individuals. However, the kidneys constitute less than 0.5% of total body weight. As illustrated in Figure 35-2 *(left)*, the renal artery branches to progressively form the **interlobar artery,** the **arcuate artery,** the **interlobular artery,** and the **afferent arteriole,** which leads into the **glomerular capillaries** (i.e., glomerulus). The glomerular capillaries come together to form the **efferent arteriole,** which leads into a second capillary network, the peritubular capillaries, which supply blood to the

nephron. The vessels of the venous system run parallel to the arterial vessels and progressively form the interlobular vein, arcuate vein, interlobar vein, and renal vein, which courses beside the ureter.

The functional unit of the kidney is the nephron

Each human kidney contains approximately 1.2 million nephrons, which are hollow tubes composed of a single cell layer. The nephron consists of a renal corpuscle, proximal tubule, loop of Henle, distal tubule, and collecting duct system (Figure 35-1). The renal corpuscle consists of glomerular capillaries and **Bowman's capsule.** The proximal tubule initially forms several coils, followed by a straight piece that descends toward the medulla. The next segment is the loop of **Henle,** which is composed of the straight part of the proximal tubule, descending thin limb, ascending thin limb (only in nephrons with long loops of Henle), and thick ascending limb. Near the end of the thick ascending limb, the nephron passes between the afferent and efferent arterioles of the same nephron. This short segment of the thick ascending limb is called the **macula densa.** The distal tubule begins a short distance beyond the macula densa and extends to the point in the cortex where two or more nephrons join to form a cortical collecting duct. The cortical collecting duct enters the medulla and becomes the outer medullary collecting duct and then the inner medullary collecting duct.

Nephrons may be subdivided into superficial and juxtamedullary types (Figure 35-2). The renal corpuscle of each **superficial nephron** is located in the outer region of the cortex. Its loop of Henle is short, and its efferent arteriole branches into peritubular capillaries that surround the nephron segments of its own and adjacent nephrons. This capillary network conveys oxygen and important nutrients to the nephron segments, delivers substances to the nephron for secretion (i.e., the movement of a substance from the blood into the tubular fluid), and serves as a pathway for the return of resorbed water and solutes to the circulatory system.

The renal corpuscle of each **juxtamedullary nephron** is located in the region of the cortex adjacent to the medulla (Figure 35-2, *right*). In comparison with the superficial nephrons, the juxtamedullary nephrons differ anatomically in two important ways: the loop of Henle is longer and extends deeper into the medulla, and the efferent arteriole forms not only a network of peritubular capillaries but also a series of vascular loops called the **vasa recta.**

As shown in Figure 35-2, the vasa recta descend into the medulla, where they form capillary networks that surround the collecting ducts and ascending limbs of the loop of Henle. The blood returns to the cortex in the ascending vasa recta. Although less than 0.7% of the RBF enters the vasa recta, these vessels subserve important functions, including (1) conveying oxygen and important nutrients to

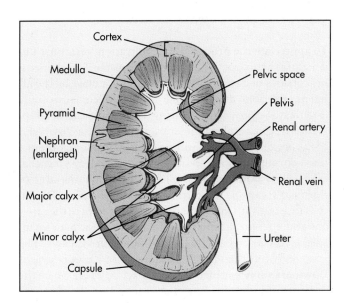

Figure 35-1 Structure of a human kidney, cut open to show the internal structures. *(Modified from Marsh DJ: Renal physiology, New York, 1983, Raven.)*

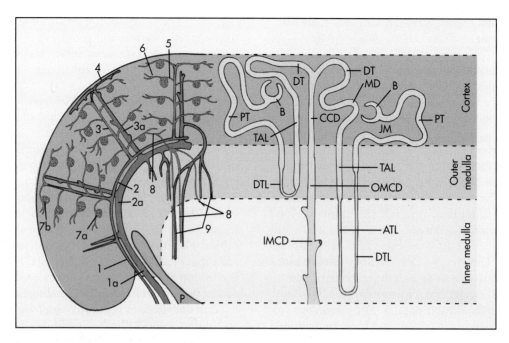

Figure 35-2 *Left,* Organization of the vascular system of the human kidney. *1,* Interlobar arteries; *1a,* interlobar veins; *2,* arcuate arteries; *2a,* arcuate veins; *3,* interlobular arteries; *3a,* interlobular veins; *4,* stellate vein; *5,* afferent arterioles; *6,* efferent arterioles; *7a, 7b,* glomerular capillary networks; *8,* descending vasa recta; *9,* ascending vasa recta. *Right,* Organization of the human nephron. A superficial nephron is illustrated on the left and a juxtamedullary *(JM)* nephron is illustrated on the right. The loop of Henle includes the straight portion of the proximal tubule *(PT),* descending thin limb *(DTL),* ascending thin limb *(ATL),* and thick ascending limb *(TAL). B,* Bowman's capsule; *CCD,* cortical collecting duct; *DT,* distal tubule; *IMCD,* inner medullary collecting duct; *MD,* macula dense; *OMCD,* outer medullary collecting duct; *P,* pelvis. *(Modified from Kriz W, Bankir LA:* Am J Physiol *254:F1, 1988; and Koushanpour E, Kriz W:* Renal physiology: principles, structure, and function, *ed 2, New York, 1986, Springer-Verlag.)*

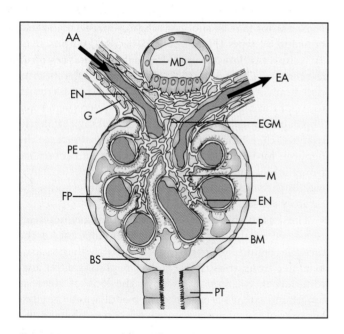

Figure 35-3 Anatomy of the renal corpuscle and juxtaglomerular apparatus. The juxtaglomerular apparatus is composed of the macula densa *(MD)* of the thick ascending limb, extraglomerular mesangial cells *(EGM),* and renin-producing granular cells *(G)* of the afferent arterioles *(AA). BM,* Basement membrane; *BS,* Bowman's space; *EA,* efferent arteriole; *EN,* endothelial cell; *FP,* foot processes of podocyte; *M,* mesangial cells between capillaries; *P,* podocyte cell body (visceral cell layer); *PE,* parietal epithelium; *PT,* proximal tubule cell. *(Modified from Kriz W, Kaissling B. In Seldin DW, Giebisch G, eds:* The kidney: physiology and pathophysiology, *ed 2, New York, 1992, Raven.)*

nephron segments, (2) delivering substances to the nephron for secretion, (3) serving as a pathway for the return of resorbed water and solutes to the circulatory system, and (4) concentrating and diluting the urine.

The first step in urine formation begins with the passive movement of a plasma ultrafiltrate from the glomerular capillaries into Bowman's space

To appreciate the process of ultrafiltration, one must understand the anatomy of the renal corpuscle. The glomerulus consists of a network of capillaries supplied by the afferent arteriole and drained by the efferent arteriole (Figures 35-3 to 35-5). During embryological development, the glomerular capillaries press into the closed end of the proximal tubule, forming the Bowman's capsule of a renal corpuscle. The capillaries are covered by epithelial cells, called **podocytes,** which form the visceral layer of Bowman's capsule (Figures 35-3 to 35-5). The visceral cells face outward at the vascular pole (i.e., where the afferent and efferent arterioles enter and exit Bowman's capsule) to form the parietal layer of Bowman's capsule. The space between the visceral layer and the parietal layer is **Bowman's space,** which at the urinary pole (i.e., where the proximal tubule joins Bowman's capsule) of the glomerulus becomes the lumen of the proximal tubule.

The endothelial cells of glomerular capillaries are covered by a **basement membrane,** which is surrounded by

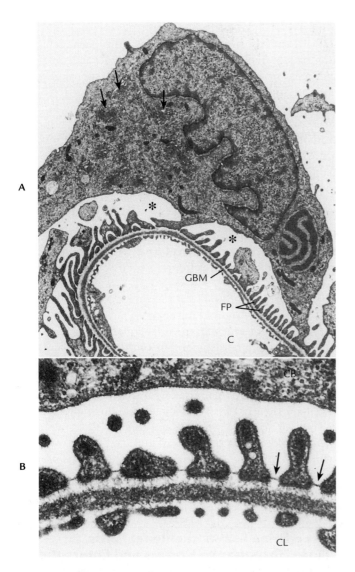

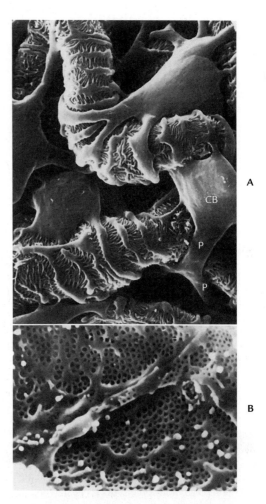

Figure 35-4 A, Electron micrograph of a podocyte surrounding a glomerular capillary. The cell body of the podocyte contains a large nucleus with three indentations. Cell processes of the podocyte form the interdigitating foot processes *(FP)*. The arrows in the cytoplasm of the podocyte indicate the well-developed Golgi apparatus, and the asterisks indicate Bowman's space. *C,* Capillary lumen; *GBM,* glomerular basement membrane. **B,** Electron micrograph of the filtration barrier of a glomerular capillary. The filtration barrier is composed of three layers: the endothelium, basement membrane, and foot processes of the podocytes. Note the diaphragm bridging the floor of the filtration slits *(arrows)*. *CL,* Capillary lumen; *CB,* cell body of a podocyte. *(From Kriz W, Kaissling B. In Seldin DW, Giebisch G, eds: The kidney: physiology and pathophysiology, ed 2, New York, 1992, Raven.)*

Figure 35-5 A, Scanning electron micrograph showing the outer surface of glomerular capillaries. This is the view that would be seen from Bowman's space. Processes *(P)* of podocytes run from the cell body *(CB)* toward the capillaries, where they ultimately split into foot processes. Interdigitation of the foot processes create the filtration slits. **B,** Scanning electron micrograph of the inner surface (blood side) of a glomerular capillary. This view would be seen from the lumen of the capillary. The fenestrations of the endothelial cells are seen as small 700-Å holes. *(From Kriz W, Kaissling B. In Seldin DW, Giebisch G eds: The kidney: physiology and pathophysiology, ed 2, New York, 1992, Raven.)*

podocytes (Figures 35-3 to 35-5). The capillary endothelium, basement membrane, and foot processes of podocytes form the so-called filtration barrier (Figures 35-3 to 35-5). The endothelium is fenestrated (i.e., contains 700-Å holes where $1\text{Å} = 10^{-10}$ m) and is freely permeable to water, small solutes (such as Na^+, urea, and glucose), and even small proteins but is not permeable to cells. Because endothelial cells express negatively charged glycoproteins on their surface, they can retard the filtration of large anionic proteins. The basement membrane, which is a porous matrix of negatively charged proteins, is an important filtration barrier to plasma proteins. The podocytes, which are endocytic, have long fingerlike processes that completely encircle the outer surface of the capillaries (Figure 35-5). The processes of the podocytes interdigitate to cover the basement membrane and are separated by gaps called **filtration slits.** Each filtration slit is bridged by a thin diaphragm, which contains pores with dimensions of 40 × 140 Å. Therefore the filtration slits retard the filtration of some proteins and macromolecules that pass through the endothelium and basement membrane. Because the endothelium, basement membrane, and filtration slits contain negatively charged glycoproteins, some molecules are held back on the basis of size and charge. For molecules with an effective molecular radius between 20 and 42 Å, cationic molecules are filtered more readily than anionic molecules.

The **nephrotic syndrome** is produced by a variety of disorders and is characterized by an increase in the permeability of the glomerular capillaries to proteins. The augmented permeability results in an increase in urinary protein excretion **(proteinuria).** Thus the appearance of proteins in the urine can indicate kidney disease. Individuals with this syndrome may also develop edema and hypoalbuminemia as a result of the proteinuria.

Another important component of the renal corpuscle is the **mesangium,** which consists of **mesangial cells** and the **mesangial matrix** (Figure 35-3). Mesangial cells surround the glomerular capillaries, provide structural support for the glomerular capillaries, secrete the extracellular matrix, exhibit phagocytic activity, and secrete prostaglandins and cytokines. Because they also contract and are adjacent to glomerular capillaries, mesangial cells may influence the GFR by regulating blood flow through the glomerular capillaries or by altering the capillary surface area. Mesangial cells located outside the glomerulus (between the afferent and efferent arterioles) are called **extraglomerular mesangial cells.**

Mesangial cells are involved in the development of immune complex–mediated glomerular disease. Because the glomerular basement membrane does not completely surround all glomerular capillaries, some immune complexes can enter the mesangial area without crossing the glomerular basement membrane. Accumulation of immune complexes induces the infiltration of inflammatory cells into the mesangium and promotes the production of cytokines and autocoids by cells in the mesangium. These cytokines and autocoids enhance the inflammatory response, which can lead to cell scarring and eventually obliteration of the glomerulus.

The juxtaglomerular apparatus is one component of an important feedback mechanism

The structures that make up the juxtaglomerular apparatus (JGA) include (Figure 35-3):
1. The macula densa of the thick ascending limb
2. The extraglomerular mesangial cells
3. The renin-producing granular cells of the afferent arteriole

The cells of the macula densa represent a morphologically distinct region of the thick ascending limb. This re-

gion passes through the angle formed by the afferent and efferent arterioles of the same nephron. The cells of the macula densa contact the extraglomerular mesangial cells and the granular cells of the afferent and efferent arterioles. Granular cells of the afferent arterioles are modified smooth muscle cells that manufacture, store, and release renin. **Renin** is involved in the formation of angiotensin II and ultimately in the secretion of aldosterone (see Chapters 37 and 38). The JGA is one component of the tubuloglomerular feedback mechanism that is involved in the autoregulation of RBF and of GFR.

Renal nerves help regulate renal blood flow, glomerular filtration rate, and salt and water resorption by the nephron

The nerve supply to the kidneys consists of sympathetic nerve fibers that originate in the celiac plexus. There is no parasympathetic innervation. Adrenergic fibers that innervate the kidneys release norepinephrine and dopamine. The adrenergic fibers lie adjacent to the smooth muscle cells of the major branches of the renal artery (interlobar, arcuate, and interlobular arteries) and the afferent and efferent arterioles. Moreover, the renin-producing granular cells of the afferent arterioles are innervated by sympathetic nerves. Renin secretion is stimulated by increased sympathetic activity. Nerve fibers also innervate the proximal tubule, loop of Henle, distal tubule, and collecting duct; activation of these nerves enhances Na^+ resorption by these nephron segments.

Once Urine Leaves the Renal Pelvis, It Flows Through the Ureters and Enters the Urinary Bladder, Where Urine Is Stored

The ureters are muscular tubes about 30 cm long. They enter the bladder at its posterior aspect near the base, above the bladder neck. The **bladder** is composed of two parts: the fundus, or body, which stores urine, and the neck, which is shaped like a funnel and connects with the urethra. The bladder neck, which is 2 to 3 cm long, is also called the posterior urethra. In females, the posterior urethra is the end of the urinary tract and the point of exit of urine from the body. In males, urine flows through the posterior urethra into the anterior urethra, which extends through the penis. Urine leaves the urethra through the external meatus.

The renal calyces, pelvis, ureters, and urinary bladder are lined with a transitional epithelium composed of several layers of cells. This epithelium is surrounded by a mixture of spiral and longitudinal smooth muscle fibers. The bladder is also lined with a transitional epithelium surrounded by a mixture of smooth muscle fibers called the **detrusor muscle.** Muscle fibers in the bladder neck form the **internal sphincter,** which is not a true sphincter but a thickening of the bladder wall formed by converging muscle fibers. The internal sphincter is not under conscious control. Its inherent tone prevents emptying of the bladder until appropriate stimuli initiate urination. The urethra passes through the urogenital diaphragm, which contains a layer of skeletal muscle called the **external sphincter.** This muscle is under voluntary control and can be used to prevent or interrupt urination, especially in males. In females the external sphincter is poorly developed; thus it is less important in voluntary bladder control. The smooth muscle cells in the lower urinary tract are electrically coupled, exhibit spontaneous action potentials, contract when stretched, and are under autonomic control.

The walls of the ureters, bladder, and urethra are highly folded and thereby very distensible. In the bladder and urethra, these folds are called **rugae.** As the bladder fills with urine, the rugae flatten, and the volume of the bladder increases with very little change in intravesical pressure. The volume of the bladder can increase from a minimal volume of 10 ml after urination to 400 ml with a pressure change of only 5 cm H_2O; this illustrates the highly compliant nature of the bladder.

Innervation of the bladder and urethra controls urination

The smooth muscle of the bladder neck receives sympathetic innervation from the hypogastric nerves. (α-Adrenergic receptors, located mainly in the bladder neck and the urethra, cause contraction. Stimulation of these receptors facilitates the storage of urine by inducing closure of the urethra. Sacral parasympathetic fibers (muscarinic) innervate the body of the bladder and cause a sustained bladder contraction. Sensory fibers of the pelvic nerves (visceral afferent pathway) also innervate the fundus. These sensory fibers carry input from receptors that detect bladder fullness, pain, and temperature sensation. The sacral pudendal nerves innervate the skeletal muscle fibers of the external sphincter, and excitatory impulses cause contraction.

Urine passes from the kidneys to the bladder as a result of inherent pacemaker activity

As urine collects in the renal calyces, stretch promotes their pacemaker activity. This pacemaker activity initiates a peristaltic contraction that begins in the calyces and spreads to the pelvis and along the length of the ureter, thereby forcing urine from the renal pelvis toward the bladder. Transmission of the peristaltic wave is caused by action potentials that are generated by the pacemaker and that pass along the smooth muscle syncytium. The ureters are innervated with sensory nerve fibers (pelvic nerves).

Nephrolithiasis (i.e., kidney stones) is a common medical problem. A total of 5% to 10% of Americans develop kidney stones. Most stones (80% to 90%) are composed of calcium salts. The remaining stones are composed of uric acid, magnesium–ammonium acetate, and cysteine. Stones are formed by crystallization in a supersaturated urinary milieu. When the ureter is blocked by a kidney stone, reflex constriction of the ureter around the stone elicits severe flank pain.

Micturition is the process of emptying the urinary bladder

Two processes are involved in micturition: (1) progressive filling of the bladder until the pressure rises to a critical value and (2) a neuronal reflex called the **micturition reflex,** which empties the bladder. The micturition reflex is a spinal cord reflex. However, it can be inhibited or facilitated by centers in the brainstem and cerebral cortex.

Filling of the bladder stretches the bladder wall and triggers a reflex initiated by stretch receptors, which causes the bladder wall to contract. Sensory signals from the bladder fundus enter the spinal cord via pelvic nerves and return directly to the bladder through parasympathetic fibers in the same nerves. Stimulation of parasympathetic fibers causes intense contraction of the detrusor muscle. The smooth muscle in the bladder is a syncytium; therefore stimulation of the detrusor muscle also causes the muscle cells in the neck of the bladder to contract. Because the muscle fibers of the bladder outlet are oriented longitudinally and radially, contraction opens the bladder neck and allows urine to flow through the posterior urethra. Voluntary relaxation of the external sphincter, achieved by cortical inhibition of the pudendal nerve, permits the flow of urine through the external meatus. Voluntary relaxation of the external sphincter is required, and it may be the event that initiates micturition. Interruption of the hypogastric sympathetic nerves and the pudendal nerves to the lower urinary tract does not alter the micturition reflex. In contrast, destruction of the parasympathetic nerves results in complete bladder dysfunction.

The Glomerular Filtration Rate Is Equal to the Sum of the Filtration Rates of All the Functioning Nephrons

The GFR is an index of kidney function. A fall generally means that kidney disease is progressing, whereas a recovery generally suggests recuperation. Thus knowledge of the patient's GFR is essential in evaluating the severity and course of kidney disease.

Creatinine is a by-product of skeletal muscle creatine metabolism, and it can be used to measure the GFR. Creatinine is freely filtered across the glomerulus into Bowman's space, and to a first approximation, it is not resorbed, secreted, or metabolized by the cells of the nephron. Accordingly, the amount of creatinine excreted in the urine per minute equals the amount of creatinine filtered at the glomerulus each minute (Figure 35-6):

$$\text{Amount Filtered} = \text{Amount Excreted} \qquad \textbf{35-1}$$
$$\text{GFR} \times P_{Cr} = U_{Cr} \times \dot{V}$$

where:

P_{Cr} = Plasma concentration of creatinine
U_{Cr} = Urine concentration of creatinine
$\dot{V}$ = Urine flow

If Equation 35-1 is solved for the GFR:

$$\text{GFR} = \frac{U_{Cr} \times \dot{V}}{P_{Cr}} \qquad \textbf{35-2}$$

Thus the clearance of creatinine provides a means for determining the GFR. Clearance has the dimensions of volume/time, and it represents a volume of plasma from which all the substance has been removed and excreted into the urine per unit time.

Creatinine is not the only substance that can be used to measure the GFR. Any substance that meets the fol-

lowing criteria can serve as an appropriate marker for the measurement of GFR. The substance must:

1. Be freely filtered across the glomerulus into Bowman's space
2. Not be resorbed or secreted by the nephron
3. Not be metabolized or produced by the kidney
4. Not alter the GFR

> **Creatinine** is used to estimate the GFR in clinical practice. It is synthesized at a relatively constant rate, and the amount produced is proportional to the muscle mass. However, creatinine is not a perfect substance for measuring GFR because it is secreted to a small extent by the organic cation secretory system in the proximal tubule (see Chapter 36). The error introduced by this secretory component is approximately 10%. Thus the amount of creatinine excreted in the urine exceeds the amount expected from filtration alone by 10%. However, the method used to quantitate the plasma creatinine concentration (P_{Cr}) overestimates the true value by 10%. Consequently, the two errors cancel, and in most clinical situations, creatinine clearance provides a reasonably accurate measure of the GFR.

Not all the creatinine (or other substances used to measure the GFR) that enters the kidney in the renal arterial plasma is filtered at the glomerulus. Likewise, not all of the plasma coming into the kidney is filtered. Although nearly all of the plasma that enters the kidney in the renal artery passes through the glomerulus, approximately 10% does not. The portion of filtered plasma is termed the **filtration fraction** and is determined as:

$$\text{Filtration fraction} = \frac{\text{GFR}}{\text{RPF}} \qquad \textbf{35-3}$$

where *RPF* is **renal plasma flow.** Under normal conditions the filtration fraction averages 0.15 to 0.20. This means that only 15% to 20% of the plasma that enters the glomerulus is actually filtered. The remaining 80% to 85% continues on through the glomerular capillaries and into the efferent arterioles and peritubular capillaries. It is finally returned to the systemic circulation in the renal vein.

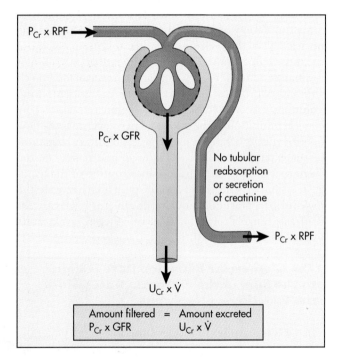

Figure 35-6 Renal handling of creatinine. Creatinine is freely filtered across the glomerulus and is to a first approximation, not resorbed, secreted, or metabolized by the nephron. Note that all the creatinine coming to the kidney in the renal artery does not get filtered at the glomerulus (Normally, 15% to 20% of plasma creatinine is filtered.) The portion that is not filtered is returned to the systemic circulation in the renal vein. *P_{Cr},* Plasma creatinine concentration; *RPF,* renal plasma flow; *U_{Cr},* urinary concentration of creatinine; *$\dot{V}$,* urine flow rate.

> A fall in the GFR may be the first and only clinical sign of kidney disease. Thus measuring the GFR is important when kidney disease is suspected. A 50% loss of functioning nephrons reduces the GFR only by about 25%. The decline in GFR is not 50% because the remaining nephrons compensate. Because measurements of GFR are cumbersome, kidney function is usually assessed in the clinical setting by measuring the P_{Cr} which is inversely re-

lated to the GFR (Figure 35-7). However, as Figure 35-7 shows, the GFR must decline substantially before an increase in the P_{Cr} can be detected in a clinical setting. For example, a fall in GFR from 120 to 100 ml/min is accompanied by an increase in the P_{Cr} from 1.0 to 1.2 mg/dl. This does not appear to be a significant change in the P_{Cr}, but the GFR has actually fallen by almost 20%.

The first step in the formation of urine is ultrafiltration of the plasma by the glomerulus

In normal adults, the GFR ranges from 90 to 140 ml/min for males and from 80 to 125 ml/min for females. Thus in 24 hours, as much as 180 L of plasma is filtered by the glomeruli. The plasma ultrafiltrate is devoid of cellular elements and is essentially protein free. The concentrations of salts and of organic molecules, such as glucose and amino acids, are similar in the plasma and ultrafiltrate. Ultrafiltration is driven by Starling forces across the glomerular capillaries, and changes in these forces alter the GFR (see Chapter 22). The GFR and renal plasma flow are normally held within very narrow ranges by a phenomenon called **autoregulation** (see Chapter 23). This section reviews the composition of the glomerular filtrate, the dynamics of its formation, and the relationship between renal plasma flow and GFR. In addition, the factors that contribute to the autoregulation of GFR and RBF are discussed.

The glomerular filtration barrier determines the composition of the plasma ultrafiltrate

The glomerular filtration barrier restricts the filtration of molecules on the basis of size and electrical charge (Figure 35-8). In general, neutral molecules with a radius smaller than 20 Å are filtered freely, molecules larger than 42 Å are not filtered, and molecules between 20 and 42 Å are filtered to various degrees. For example, serum albumin, an anionic protein that has an effective molecular radius of 35.5 Å, is filtered poorly. Because the filtered albumin is resorbed avidly by the proximal tubule, almost no albumin appears in the urine.

Figure 35-8 shows how electrical charge affects the filtration of macromolecules (e.g., dextrans) by the glomerulus. Dextrans are a family of exogenous polysaccharides manufactured in various molecular weights. They can be electrically neutral or have either negative charges (polyanionic) or positive charges (polycationic). As the size (i.e., effective molecular radius) of a dextran increases, the rate at which it is filtered decreases. For any given molecular radius, cationic molecules are more readily filtered than anionic molecules. The reduced filtration rate for anionic molecules is explained by the presence of negatively charged glycoproteins on the surface of all components of the glomerular filtration barrier. These charged glycoproteins repel similarly charged molecules. Because most plasma proteins are negatively charged, the negative charge on the filtration barrier restricts the filtration of proteins that have a molecular radius of 20 to 42 Å or more.

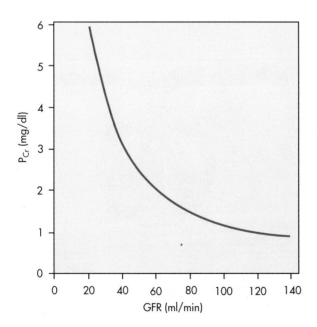

Figure 35-7 Relationship between GFR and P_{Cr}. The amount of creatinine filtered is essentially equal to the amount excreted; thus GFR $\times$ P_{Cr} = $U_{Cr} \times \dot{V}$. Because the production of creatinine is constant, excretion must be constant to maintain creatinine balance. Therefore if the GFR falls from 120 to 60 ml/min, the P_{Cr} must increase from 1 to 2 mg/dl to keep the filtration of creatinine and thus its excretion equal to the production rate.

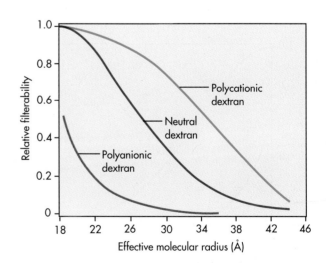

Figure 35-8 Influence of size and electrical charge of dextran on its filterability. A value of one indicates that it is filtered freely, whereas a value of zero indicates that it is not filtered. The filterability of dextrans between approximately 20 and 42 Å depends on charge. Dextrans larger than 42 Å are not filtered regardless of charge, and polycationic dextrans and neutral dextrans smaller than 20 Å are freely filtered.

The importance of the negative charges on the filtration barrier in restricting the filtration of plasma proteins is shown in Figure 35-9. The removal of negative charges from the filtration barrier causes proteins to be filtered solely on the basis of their effective molecular radius. Hence at any molecular radius between approximately 20 and 42 Å, the filtration of polyanionic proteins will exceed the filtration that prevails in the normal state (in which the filtration barrier has anionic charges). In a number of glomerular diseases the negative charge on the filtration barrier is reduced because of immunological damage and inflammation. As a result, the filtration of proteins is increased, and proteins appear in the urine (**protein-uria**).

The forces responsible for the glomerular filtration of plasma are the same as those in all capillary beds

Ultrafiltration occurs because the Starling forces (i.e., hydrostatic and oncotic pressures) drive fluid from the lumen of glomerular capillaries, across the filtration barrier, and into Bowman's space (Figure 35-10). The hydrostatic pressure in the glomerular capillary (P_{GC}) is oriented to promote the movement of fluid from the glomerular capillary into Bowman's space. Because the reflection coefficient (σ) for proteins across the glomerular capillary is essentially one, the glomerular ultrafiltrate is essentially protein free, and the oncotic pressure in Bowman's space (π_{BS}) is near zero. Therefore, P_{GC} is the only force that favors filtration. Filtration is opposed by the hydrostatic pressure in Bowman's space (P_{BS}) and the oncotic pressure in the glomerular capillary (π_{GC}).

As shown in Figure 35-10, a net ultrafiltration pressure (P_{UF}) of 17 mm Hg exists at the afferent end of the glomerulus, whereas at the efferent end, it is 8 mm Hg (where $P_{UF} = P_{GC} - P_{BS} - \pi_{GC}$). Two additional points concerning Starling forces and this pressure change are important. First, P_{GC} decreases slightly along the length of the capillary because of the resistance to flow along the length of the capillary. Second, π_{GC} increases along the length of the glomerular capillary. Because water is filtered and protein is retained in the glomerular capillary, the protein concentration in the capillary rises, and π_{GC} increases.

THE GFR IS PROPORTIONAL TO THE SUM OF THE STARLING FORCES THAT EXIST ACROSS THE CAPILLARIES $[(P_{GC} - P_{BS}) - \sigma(\pi_{GC} - \pi_{BS})]$ MULTIPLIED BY THE ULTRAFILTRATION COEFFICIENT (K_F). That is:

$$GFR = K_f[(P_{GC} - P_{BS}) - \sigma(\pi_{GC} - \pi_{BS})] \quad \textbf{35-4}$$

K_f is the product of the intrinsic permeability of the glomerular capillary and the glomerular surface area available for filtration. The rate of glomerular filtration is considerably greater in glomerular capillaries than in systemic capillaries, mainly because K_f is approximately 100 times greater in glomerular capillaries. Furthermore, the P_{GC} is approximately twice as great as the hydrostatic pressure in systemic capillaries.

The GFR can be altered by changing K_f or by changing any of the Starling forces. In normal individuals, the GFR is regulated by alterations in the P_{GC} that are mediated mainly by changes in afferent or efferent arteriolar resistance. P_{GC} is affected in three ways:

1. Changes in afferent arteriolar resistance: A decrease in resistance increases the P_{GC} and

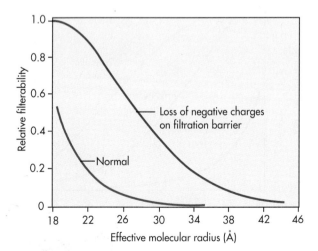

Figure 35-9 Reduction of the negative charges on the glomerular wall results in the filtration of proteins on the basis of size only. In this situation the relative filterability of proteins depends only on the molecular radius. Accordingly, the excretion of polyanionic proteins (20 to 42 Å) in the urine increases because more proteins of this size are filtered.

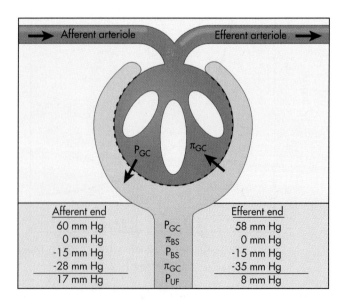

Figure 35-10 Idealized glomerular capillary and the Starling forces across it. The reflection coefficient *(σ)* for protein across the glomerular capillary is one. P_{BS}, Hydrostatic pressure in Bowman's space; P_{GC}, hydrostatic pressure in the glomerular capillary; P_{UF}, net ultrafiltration pressure; π_{GC}, oncotic pressure in the glomerular capillary; π_{BS}, oncotic pressure in Bowman's space.

GFR, whereas an increase in resistance decreases them.

2. Changes in efferent arteriolar resistance: A decrease in resistance reduces the P_{GC} and GFR, whereas an increase in resistance elevates them.

3. Changes in renal arteriolar pressure: An increase in blood pressure transiently increases the P_{GC} (which enhances the GFR), whereas a decrease in blood pressure transiently decreases the P_{GC} (which reduces the GFR).

A reduction in the GFR in disease states is most often due to decreases in K_f because of the loss of filtration surface area. The GFR also changes in pathophysiological conditions because of changes in P_{GC}, π_{GC}, and P_{BS}.

1. Changes in K_f: An increased K_f enhances the GFR, whereas a decreased K_f reduces the GFR. Some kidney diseases reduce the K_f by decreasing the number of filtering glomeruli (i.e., diminished surface area). Some drugs and hormones that dilate the glomerular arterioles also increase the K_f. Similarly, drugs and hormones that constrict the glomerular arterioles also decrease the K_f.

2. Changes in P_{GC}: In acute renal failure, the GFR declines because the P_{GC} falls. As previously discussed, a reduction in the P_{GC} is caused by a decline in renal arterial pressure, an increase in afferent arteriolar resistance, or a decrease in efferent arteriolar resistance.

3. Changes in π_{GC}: An inverse relationship exists between the π_{GC} and the GFR. Alterations in the π_{GC} result from changes in protein synthesis outside the kidneys. In addition, protein loss in the urine caused by some renal diseases can lead to a decrease in the plasma protein concentration and thus in the π_{GC}.

4. Changes in P_{BS}: An increased P_{BS} reduces the GFR, whereas a decreased P_{BS} enhances the GFR. Acute obstruction of the urinary tract (e.g., a kidney stone occluding the ureter) increases the P_{BS}.

Blood Flow Through the Kidneys Serves Several Important Functions

Blood flow through the kidneys:

1. Indirectly determines the GFR
2. Modifies the rate of solute and water resorption by the proximal tubule
3. Participates in the concentration and dilution of urine
4. Delivers oxygen, nutrients, and hormones to the cells of the nephron and returns carbon dioxide and resorbed fluid and solutes to the general circulation
5. Delivers substrates for excretion in the urine

Blood flow through any organ may be represented by the following equation:

$$Q = \Delta P/R \qquad \text{35-5}$$

where:

Q = Blood flow

ΔP = Mean arterial pressure minus venous pressure for that organ

R = Resistance to flow through that organ (see Chapter 20)

Accordingly, RBF is equal to the pressure difference between the renal artery and the renal vein divided by the renal vascular resistance:

$$RBF = \frac{\text{Aortic pressure} - \text{Renal venous pressure}}{\text{Renal vascular resistance}} \qquad \text{35-6}$$

Because the afferent arteriole, efferent arteriole, and interlobular artery are the major resistance vessels in the kidneys, they determine renal vascular resistance. Like most other organs, the kidneys regulate their blood flow by adjusting the vascular resistance in response to changes in arterial pressure (see Chapter 23). As shown in Figure 35-11, these adjustments are so precise that blood flow remains relatively constant as arterial blood pressure changes between 90 and 180 mm Hg. The GFR is also regulated over the same range of arterial pressures. The phenomenon whereby RBF and GFR are maintained relatively constant, namely autoregulation, is achieved by changes in vascular resistance, mainly through the afferent arterioles of the kidneys. Because both the GFR and RBF are regulated over the same range of pressures and because RBF is an important de-

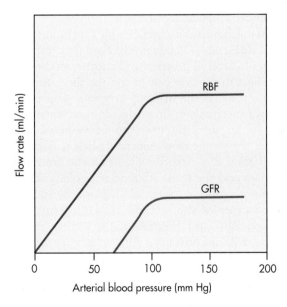

Figure 35-11 Relationship between arterial blood pressure and RBF and between arterial blood pressure and GFR. Autoregulation maintains the GFR and RBF relatively constant as blood pressure changes from 90 to 180 mm Hg.

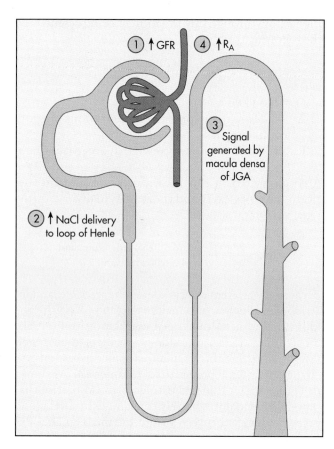

Figure 35-12 Tubuloglomerular feedback. An increase in the GFR *(1)* increases NaCl delivery to the loop of Henle *(2)*, which is sensed by the macula densa and converted into a signal *(3)* that increases the resistance of the afferent arteriole (R_A) *(4)*, which decreases the GFR. *(Modified from Cogan MG: Fluid and electrolytes: physiology and pathophysiology, Norwalk, Conn, 1991, Appleton & Lange.)*

terminant of GFR, it is not surprising that the same mechanisms regulate both flows.

Two mechanisms are responsible for the autoregulation of RBF and GFR: one mechanism that responds to changes in arterial pressure and another that responds to changes in the flow rate of tubular fluid. Both regulate the tone of the afferent arteriole. The pressure-sensitive mechanism, or myogenic mechanism, is related to an intrinsic property of vascular smooth muscle: the tendency to contract when it is stretched (see Chapter 23). Accordingly, when the arterial pressure rises and the renal afferent arteriole is stretched, the smooth muscle contracts. Because the increase in the resistance of the arteriole offsets the increase in pressure, RBF and therefore GFR remain constant. (That is, RBF is constant if $\Delta P/R$ is kept constant [see Equation 35-5].)

The second mechanism responsible for the autoregulation of GFR and RBF is the flow-dependent mechanism known as **tubuloglomerular feedback** (Figure 35-12). This mechanism involves a feedback loop in which the flow of tubular fluid (or some other factor, such as the rate of sodium chloride [NaCl] resorption) is sensed by the macula densa of the JGA. This stimulus is

converted into a signal that affects afferent arteriolar resistance and thus the GFR. When the GFR increases and causes the flow of tubular fluid at the macula densa to rise, the JGA sends a signal that causes renal vasoconstriction, which returns the RBF and GFR to normal levels. In contrast, when the GFR and tubular flow past the macula densa decrease, the JGA sends a signal that causes the RBF and GFR to increase to normal levels. The signal affects the RBF and GFR mainly by changing the resistance of the afferent arteriole. The variable that is sensed at the macula densa and the effector substance that alters the resistance of the afferent arteriole have not been identified. It has been suggested that flow-dependent changes in NaCl resorption are sensed by the macula densa. The effector mechanism may be (1) adenosine, which constricts the afferent arteriole (in contrast to its vasodilator effect on most other vasculature beds); (2) ATP, which selectively vasoconstricts the afferent arteriole; or (3) a metabolite of arachidonic acid. Nitric oxide (NO), a vasodilator produced by the macula densa, may also play a role in tubuloglomerular feedback, but it is not essential for autoregulation. The macula densa may release both a vasoconstrictor and a vasodilator (e.g., NO), which oppose each other's action at the level of the afferent arteriole.

Animals engage in many activities that can change arterial blood pressure. Thus having mechanisms that maintain RBF and GFR relatively constant despite changes in arterial pressure are highly desirable because such changes influence water and salt excretion (see Chapter 36). If the GFR and RBF were to rise or fall suddenly in proportion to changes in blood pressure, urinary excretion of fluid and solute would also change suddenly. Such changes in water and solute excretion without comparable changes in intake would alter the fluid and electrolyte balance. Accordingly, autoregulation of the GFR and RBF provides an effective means for uncoupling renal function from arterial pressure, and it ensures that fluid and solute excretion remain constant.

Three salient points concerning autoregulation are:

1. Autoregulation is absent when arterial pressure is less than 90 mm Hg.
2. Autoregulation is not perfect; the RBF and GFR do change slightly as the arterial blood pressure varies.
3. Despite autoregulation, the RBF and GFR can be changed by certain hormones and by changes in sympathetic nerve activity (Table 35-1).

Individuals with **renal artery stenosis** (narrowing of the artery lumen) caused by atherosclerosis, for example, can have an elevated systemic arterial blood pressure mediated by stimulation of the renin-angiotensin system (see Chapter 37). Pressure in the renal artery proximal to the stenosis is increased, but pressure distal to the stenosis is normal or reduced. Autoregulation is important in main-

Table 35-1   Major Hormones that Influence GFR and RBF

	Stimulus	Effect on GFR	Effect on RBF
Vasoconstrictors			
Sympathetic nerves	↓ECV	↓	↓
AII*	↓ECV, renin	↓	↓
Endothelin	Stretch, AII, BK, Epi	↓	↓
Vasodilators			
Prostaglandins (PGI$_2$, PGE$_2$)	↓ECV, shear force, AII	No change	↑
NO	Shear force, ACh, His, BK, ATP	↑	↑
Bradykinin	PG, ↓ACE	↑	↑

ECV, Extracellular fluid volume; *AII*, angiotensin II; *BK*, bradykinin; *Epi*, epinephrine; *ACh*, acetylcholine; *His*, histamine; *ACE*, angiotensin-converting enzyme.
*High concentrations of angiotensin II affect both afferent and efferent arterioles and decrease the GFR and RBF.

taining RBF, P$_{GC}$, and GFR in the presence of this stenosis. The administration of drugs to lower the systemic blood pressure also lowers the pressure distal to the stenosis; accordingly the RBF, P$_{GC}$, and GFR fall.

Hormones and Sympathetic Nerves Regulate the Glomerular Filtration Rate and Renal Blood Flow

Several factors and hormones affect the GFR and RBF (Table 35-1). The myogenic mechanism and tubuloglomerular feedback play a key role in maintaining GFR and RBF constant. Sympathetic nerves, angiotensin II, prostaglandins, NO, endothelin, bradykinin, and perhaps adenosine exert major control over RBF and GFR. Figure 35-13 shows how changes in afferent and afferent arteriolar resistance modulate the GFR and RBF.

Sympathetic nerves
The afferent and efferent arterioles are innervated by sympathetic neurons: however, sympathetic tone is minimal when the volume of extracellular fluid is normal (see Chapter 36). Norepinephrine is released by sympathetic nerves, and circulating epinephrine is secreted by the adrenal medulla. These substances cause vasoconstriction by binding to α$_1$-adrenoceptors, which are located mainly on the afferent arterioles. Activation of α$_1$-adrenoceptors decreases the GFR and RBF. Dehydration or strong emotional stimuli, such as fear and pain, activate sympathetic nerves and reduce the GFR and RBF.

Angiotensin II
Angiotensin II is produced systemically and within the kidneys. It constricts the afferent and efferent arterioles and decreases the RBF and GFR (see Chapter 37). Figure 35-14 shows how norepinephrine, epinephrine, and angiotensin II act together to decrease the RBF and GFR, as would occur, for example, with hemorrhage.

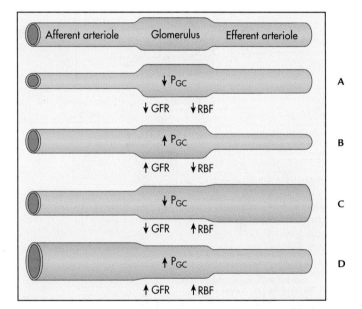

Figure 35-13 Relationship between selective changes in the resistance of either the afferent arteriole or the efferent arteriole on RBF and GFR. Constriction of either the afferent or efferent arteriole increases resistance, and according to Equation 35-5 (Q = ΔP/R), an increase in resistance (R) decreases flow (Q) (i.e., RBF). Dilation of either the afferent or afferent arteriole increases flow (i.e., RBF). Constriction of the afferent arteriole **(A)** decreases the P$_{GC}$ because less of the arterial pressure is transmitted to the glomerulus, thereby reducing the GFR. In contrast, constriction of the efferent arteriole **(B)** elevates the P$_{GC}$ and thus increases the GFR. Dilation of the efferent arteriole **(C)** decreases the P$_{GC}$ and thus decreases the GFR. Dilation of the afferent arteriole **(D)** increases the P$_{GC}$ because more of the arterial pressure is transmitted to the glomerulus, thereby increasing the GFR. *(Modified from Rose BD, Rennke HG: Renal pathophysiology: the essentials, Baltimore, 1994, Williams & Wilkins.)*

Hemorrhage decreases arterial blood pressure and therefore activates the sympathetic nerves to the kidneys via the baroreceptor reflex (Figure 35-14). Norepinephrine causes intense vasoconstriction of the afferent and efferent arterioles and thereby decreases the GFR and RBF. The rise in sympathetic activity also increases the release of epinephrine and angiotensin II, which cause further vasoconstriction and a fall in RBF. The rise in the vascular re-

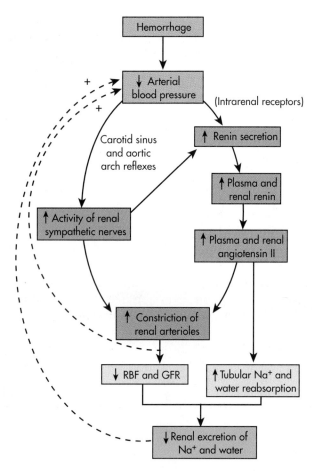

Figure 35-14 Pathway by which hemorrhage activates renal sympathetic nerve activity and stimulates the production of angiotensin II. *(Modified from Vander AJ: Renal physiology, ed 2, New York, 1980, McGraw-Hill.)*

sistance of the kidneys and other vascular beds increases the total peripheral resistance. The resulting tendency for blood pressure to increase (blood pressure = cardiac output × total peripheral resistance) offsets the tendency of blood pressure to decrease in response to hemorrhage. Hence this system works to preserve the arterial pressure at the expense of maintaining a normal GFR and RBF.

Prostaglandins

Prostaglandins may not regulate the RBF or GFR in healthy, resting people. However, during pathophysiological conditions such as hemorrhage, prostaglandins (PGI_2, PGE_2) are produced locally within the kidneys, and they increase RBF without changing the GFR. Prostaglandins increase RBF by dampening the vasoconstrictor effects of sympathetic nerves and angiotensin II. This effect prevents severe and potentially harmful vasoconstriction and renal ischemia. Prostaglandin synthesis is stimulated by dehydration and stress (e.g., surgery, anesthesia), angiotensin II, and sympathetic nerves.

Nitric oxide

NO, an endothelium-derived relaxing factor, is an important vasodilator under basal conditions, and it counteracts the vasoconstriction produced by angiotensin II or catecholamines. When blood flow increases, a greater shear force acts on the endothelial cells in the arterioles and increases the production of NO. Also, a number of vasoactive hormones, including acetylcholine, histamine, bradykinin, and ATP, cause the release of NO from endothelial cells. Increased production causes dilation of the afferent and efferent arterioles in the kidneys. In addition, NO decreases the total peripheral resistance, and inhibition of NO production increases the total peripheral resistance.

The production of abnormal NO is observed in individuals with **diabetes mellitus** and **hypertension.** Excess renal NO production in diabetes may be responsible for glomerular hyperfiltration and damage of the glomerulus, problems characteristic of this disease. Elevated NO levels increase the glomerular capillary pressure secondary to a fall in the afferent arteriolar resistance. The ensuing hyperfiltration may cause glomerular damage. The normal response to an increase in dietary salt intake includes the stimulation of renal NO production, which maintains the blood pressure. In some individuals, NO production may not increase appropriately in response to an increase in salt intake, so blood pressure rises.

Endothelin

Endothelin is a potent vasoconstrictor secreted by endothelial cells of the renal vessels, mesangial cells, and distal tubular cells in response to angiotensin II, bradykinin, epinephrine, and endothelial shear stress. Endothelin causes profound vasoconstriction of the afferent and efferent arterioles and decreases the GFR and RBF. Although this potent vasoconstrictor may not influence the GFR and RBF in resting subjects, endothelin production is elevated in a number of glomerular disease states (e.g., renal disease associated with diabetes mellitus).

Bradykinin

Kallikrein is a proteolytic enzyme produced in the kidneys. Kallikrein cleaves circulating kininogen to bradykinin, which is a vasodilator that acts by stimulating the release of NO and prostaglandins. Bradykinin increases the GFR and RBF.

Adenosine

Adenosine is produced within the kidneys and causes vasoconstriction of the afferent arteriole, thereby reducing the GFR and RBF. As previously mentioned, adenosine may play a role in tubuloglomerular feedback.

Atrial natriuretic peptide

Secretion of atrial natriuretic peptide (ANP) by the heart increases when the volume of extracellular fluid is expanded. This increase dilates the afferent arteriole

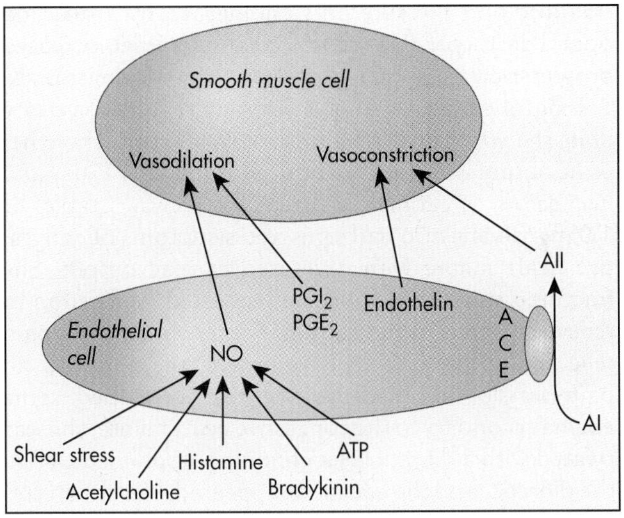

Figure 35-15 Examples of the interactions of endothelial cells with smooth muscle or mesangial cells. *ACE,* Angiotensin converting enzyme; *AI,* angiotensin I; *AII,* angiotensin II. *(Modified from Navar LG et al: Physiol Rev 76:425, 1996.)*

and constricts the efferent arteriole. Therefore the net effect of ANP produces a modest increase in the GFR with little change in RBF.

ATP
Cells release ATP into the renal interstitial fluid. ATP has dual effects on the GFR and RBF. Under some conditions, ATP constricts the afferent arteriole, reduces RBF and GFR, and may play a role in tubuloglomerular feedback. In contrast, ATP may stimulate NO production and increase the GFR and RBF.

Glucocorticoids
Administration of therapeutic doses of glucocorticoids increase the GFR and RBF.

Histamine
The local release of histamine modulates RBF during the resting state and during inflammation and injury. Histamine decreases the resistance of the afferent and efferent arterioles and thereby increases RBF without elevating the GFR.

Dopamine
The proximal tubule produces the vasodilator substance dopamine. Dopamine has several actions within the kidney, such as increasing RBF and inhibiting renin secretion.

As illustrated in Figure 35-15, endothelial cells play an important role in regulating the resistance of the afferent and efferent arterioles by producing a number of paracrine hormones, including NO, prostacyclins (PGI$_2$), endothelin, and angiotensin II. These hormones regulate contraction or relaxation of smooth muscle cells in afferent and efferent arterioles or mesangial cells. Shear stress, acetylcholine, histamine, bradykinin,

and ATP stimulate the production of NO, which increases the GFR and RBF. **Angiotensin-converting enzyme (ACE),** located primarily on the surface of endothelial cells lining the afferent arteriole and glomerular capillaries, converts angiotensin I to angiotensin II, which decreases the GFR and RBF. Angiotensin II may also be produced in juxtaglomerular cells and proximal tubular cells. PGI$_2$ and PGE$_2$ secretion by endothelial cells, stimulated by sympathetic nerve activity or angiotensin II, increases the GFR and RBF. Finally, the release of endothelin from endothelial cells decreases the GFR and RBF.

ACE degrades and thereby inactivates bradykinin, and it converts angiotensin I, an inactive hormone, to angiotensin II. Thus ACE increases angiotensin II levels and decreases bradykinin levels. Drugs called **ACE inhibitors,** which reduce systemic blood pressure in patients with hypertension, decrease angiotensin II levels and elevate bradykinin levels. These effects lower systemic vascular resistance, reduce blood pressure, and decrease renal vascular resistance and thereby increase the GFR and RBF (see Chapter 37).

■ SUMMARY

- The functional unit of the kidney is the nephron. Each nephron consists of a renal corpuscle, proximal tubule, loop of Henle, distal tubule, and collecting duct.
- The renal corpuscle is composed of glomerular capillaries and Bowman's capsule.
- The JGA consists of the macula densa, extraglomerular mesangial cells, and renin-producing granular cells in the afferent arteriole.
- The JGA is one component of an important feedback mechanism that regulates the GFR and RBF.
- The micturition reflex is an automatic spinal cord reflex that can be inhibited or facilitated by centers in the brainstem and cortex.
- The GFR is calculated by measuring creatinine clearance.
- Starling forces across the glomerular capillaries provide the driving force for the ultrafiltration of plasma from the glomerular capillaries into Bowman's space.
- The glomerular ultrafiltrate is devoid of cellular elements and contains very little protein but is otherwise identical to plasma.
- RBF (1.25 L/min) is about 25% of the cardiac output. RBF determines the GFR; modifies solute and water resorption by the proximal tubule; participates in concentration and dilution of the urine; delivers oxygen, nutrients, and hormones to the cells of the nephron; returns carbon dioxide and resorbed fluid and solutes to the general circulation; and delivers substrates for excretion in the urine.

- Autoregulation allows the GFR and RBF to remain constant despite changes in arterial blood pressure between 90 and 180 mm Hg.
- Sympathetic nerves, angiotensin II, prostaglandins, NO, endothelin, bradykinin, and perhaps adenosine exert substantial control over the GFR and RBF.

BIBLIOGRAPHY

Arendshorst WJ, Navar LG: Renal circulation and glomerular hemodynamics. In Schrier RW, Gottschalk CW, eds: *Diseases of the kidney*, ed 5, Boston, 1993, Little, Brown.

Carlson JA, Harrington JT: Laboratory evaluation of renal function. In Schrier RW, Gottschalk CW, eds: *Diseases of the kidney*, ed 5, Boston, 1993, Little, Brown.

Dworkin LD, Brenner BM: Biophysical basis of glomerular filtration. In Seldin DW, Giebisch G, eds: *The kidney: physiology and pathophysiology*, ed 2, New York, 1992, Raven.

Dworkin LD, Brenner BM: The renal circulation. In Brenner BM, ed: *Brenner and Rector's the kidney*, ed 5, Philadelphia, 1996, WB Saunders.

Kriz W, Kaissling B: Structural organization of the mammalian kidney. In Seldin DW, Giebisch G, eds: *The kidney: physiology and pathophysiology*, ed 2, New York, 1992, Raven.

Maddox DA, Brenner BM: Glomerular ultrafiltration. In Brenner BM, ed: *Brenner and Rector's the kidney*, ed 5, Philadelphia, 1996, WB Saunders.

Navar LG, Inscho EW, Majid SA, Imig JD, Harrison-Bernard LM, Mitchell KD: Paracrine regulation of the renal microcirculation, *Physiol Rev* 76(2):425, 1996.

Raji L, Bayliss C: Glomerular actions of nitric oxide, *Kidney Int* 48:20, 1995.

Rose BD: *Clinical physiology of acid-base and electrolyte disorders*, ed 4, New York, 1994, McGraw-Hill.

Steers, WD: Physiology and pharmacology of the bladder and urethra. In Walsh PC et al, eds: *Campbell's urology*, ed 7, Philadelphia, 1998, WB Saunders.

Tanagho EA: Anatomy of the genitourinary tract. In Tanagho EA, McAnich JW, eds: *Smith's general urology*, ed 14, Norwalk, Conn, 1995, Appleton & Lange.

Tisher CC, Madsen KM: Anatomy of the kidney. In Brenner BM, ed: *Brenner and Rector's the kidney*, ed 5, Philadelphia, 1996, WB Saunders.

Tucker MS, Stafford SJ: Disorders of micturition. In Schrier RW, Gottschalk CW, eds: *Diseases of the kidney*, ed 5, Boston, 1993, Little, Brown.

Ulfendahl HR, Wolgast M: Renal circulation and lymphatics. In Seldin DW, Giebisch G, eds: *The kidney: physiology and pathophysiology*, ed 2, New York, 1992, Raven.

Umans JG, Levi R: Nitric oxide in the regulation of blood flow and arterial pressure, *Annu Rev Physiol* 57:771, 1995.

CASE STUDIES

Case 35-1

A 75-year-old woman (body weight = 60 kg) was admitted to the intensive care unit after falling at home 2 days earlier. For the first 4 days in the hospital, her urine output was approximately 400 ml/day. On physical examination, she had orthostatic changes in blood pressure (fall in blood pressure on standing), tachycardia, and poor skin turgor. Her serum creatinine level increased progressively from 1.0 mg/dl on the day of admission to 5.9 mg/dl on day 4. After 2 weeks in the intensive care unit, she was transferred to a medical floor, where her urine output was noted to be approximately 1 L/day and her serum creatinine concentration was stable at 1.0 mg/dl. She also had signs and symptoms of congestive heart failure with decreased cardiac output. She fractured several ribs, and she requested medication to relieve the pain. A nonsteroidal antiinflammatory pain reliever was prescribed. By morning, the patient's rib pain was better. Because she had developed some edema secondary to the congestive heart failure, she was treated with a diuretic. Her condition responded well to the diuretic, and the edema disappeared. Her serum creatinine level was stabilized at 1.0 mg/dl. A 24-hour urine collection was performed to determine her GFR:

Urine (creatinine)	64.8 mg/dl
Urine volume	1 L
Serum (creatinine)	1.0 mg/dl

1. **Why did the serum creatinine level increase during the first 4 days of this patient's hospitalization?**
   A. The RBF decreased.
   B. Her urine output was low.
   C. Her creatinine metabolism decreased.
   D. Her GFR decreased.
   E. Her blood volume decreased.

2. **The nonsteroidal antiinflammatory pain reliever inhibits prostaglandin synthesis. What is an adverse effect of this pain reliever on renal function?**
   A. It increases RBF.
   B. It decreases the GFR.
   C. It increases urine output.
   D. It increase urinary protein excretion.
   E. It increase creatinine excretion.

Case 35-2

The urine of a 13-year-old boy turned dark brown several weeks after a bout of "strep throat." The diagnosis was glomerulonephritis (i.e., inflammation of the glomerular capillaries). The urine was dark brown because red blood cells are in the urine.

1. **Which of the following will also be found in high concentration in this boy's urine? (Hint: Think of the glomerular filtration barrier.)**
   A. Na^+
   B. K^+
   C. Serum albumin
   D. Creatinine
   E. Urea

CHAPTER 36

Solute and Water Transport Along the Nephron: Tubular Function

OBJECTIVES

- Describe how the components of the nephron determine the composition and volume of urine.
- Explain how Na^+, Cl^-, other anions, and organic solutes are resorbed in the nephron.
- Explain how the composition and volume of urine are adjusted.
- Describe how various by-products of metabolism, exogenous organic anions, and bases (e.g., drugs) are secreted into the tubular fluid.
- Describe how hormones, sympathetic nerves, dopamine, and Starling forces regulate sodium chloride resorption by the kidneys.
- Explain how ADH regulates water resorption.

The formation of urine involves three basic processes: (1) **ultrafiltration** of plasma by the glomerulus, (2) **resorption** of water and solutes from the ultrafiltrate, and (3) **secretion** of selected solutes into the tubular fluid. Although an average of 180 L of essentially protein-free fluid is filtered by the human glomeruli each day, less than 1% of the filtered water and sodium chloride (NaCl) and variable amounts of other solutes are excreted in the urine (Table 36-1). Via the processes of resorption and secretion, the renal tubules modulate the volume and composition of urine (Table 36-2). Consequently, the tubules precisely control the volume, osmolality, composition, and pH of the intracellular and extracellular fluid compartments. This chapter discusses NaCl and water resorption and some of the factors and hormones that regulate resorption. Details on acid-base transport and on K^+, Ca^{++}, and inorganic phosphate (Pi) transport and their regulation are provided in Chapters 38 and 39.

Quantitatively, the Resorption of Sodium Chloride and Water Represents the Major Function of Nephrons

Approximately 25,000 mEq/day of Na^+ and 179 L/day of water are resorbed by the renal tubules (Table 36-1). In addition, renal transport of many other important solutes is linked either directly or indirectly to Na^+ resorption.

THE PROXIMAL TUBULE RESORBS APPROXIMATELY **67%** OF FILTERED WATER, Na^+, Cl^-, K^+, AND OTHER SOLUTES. In addition, the proximal tubule resorbs virtually all the glucose and amino acids filtered by the glomerulus. The key element in proximal tubule resorption is Na^+,K^+-ATPase in the basolateral membrane. The resorption of every substance, including water, is linked in some manner to the operation of Na^+,K^+-ATPase.

Na^+ is resorbed by different mechanisms in the first and the second halves of the proximal tubule

In the first half of the proximal tubule, Na^+ is resorbed primarily with bicarbonate (HCO_3^-) and a number of organic molecules (e.g., glucose, amino acids, Pi, lactate). In contrast, in the second half, Na^+ is resorbed mainly with Cl^-. This disparity is mediated by differences in the Na^+ transport systems in the first and second halves of the proximal tubule and by differences in the composition of tubular fluid at these sites.

IN THE FIRST HALF OF THE PROXIMAL TUBULE, Na^+ UPTAKE INTO THE CELL IS COUPLED WITH EITHER H^+ OR ORGANIC SOLUTES (Figure 36-1). Na^+ entry into the cell across the apical membrane is mediated by specific transport proteins. For example, Na^+ entry is coupled with H^+ extrusion from the cell by the Na^+-H^+ antiporter (Figure 36-1, *A*). H^+ secretion results in sodium bicarbonate ($NaHCO_3$) resorption (see also Chapter 39). Na^+ also enters proximal cells via several symporter mechanisms, including Na^+-glucose, Na^+-amino acid, Na^+-Pi, and Na^+-lactate (Figure 36-1, *B*).

Table 36-1   Filtration, Excretion, and Resorption of Water, Electrolytes, and Solutes by the Kidneys

Substance	Measure	Filtered*	Excreted	Resorbed	% Filtered Load Resorbed
Water	L/day	180	1.5	178.5	99.2
Na^+	mEq/day	25,200	150	25,050	99.4
K^+	mEq/day	720	100	620	86.1
Ca^{++}	mEq/day	540	10	530	98.2
Bicarbonate (HCO_3^-)	mEq/day	4,320	2	4,318	99.9+
Cl^-	mEq/day	18,000	150	17,850	99.2
Glucose	mmol/day	800	0	800	100.0
Urea	g/day	56	28	28	50.0

*The filtered amount of any substance is calculated by multiplying the concentration of that substance in the ultrafiltrate by the glomerular filtration rate (GFR); for example, the filtered load of Na^+ is calculated as $[Na^+]_{ultrafiltrate}$ (140 mEq/L) × GFR (180 L/day) = 25,200 mEq/day.

Table 36-2   Composition of Urine

Substance	Concentration
Na^+	50-130 mEq/L
K^+	20-70 mEq/L
Ammonium	30-50 mEq/L
Ca^{++}	5-12 mEq/L
Mg^{++}	2-18 mEq/L
Cl^-	50-130 mEq/L
Inorganic phosphate	20-40 mEq/L
Urea	200-400 mM
Creatinine	6-20 mM
pH	5.0-7.0
Osmolality	500-800 mOsm/kg H_2O
Glucose	0
Amino acids	0
Protein	0
Blood	0
Ketones	0
Leukocytes	0
Bilirubin	0

Modified from Valtin HV: *Renal physiology*, ed 2, Boston, 1983, Little, Brown.
These values represent average ranges. Water excretion ranges between 0.5 and 1.5 L/day.

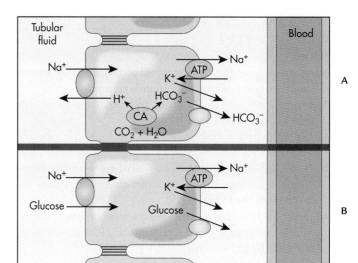

Figure 36-1 Na^+ transport processes in the first half of the proximal tubule. These transport mechanisms are present in all cells in the first half of the proximal tubule but are separated into different cells to simplify the discussion. **A,** Operation of the Na^+-H^+ antiporter in the apical membrane and that of the Na^+,K^+-ATPase and sodium bicarbonate transporter in the basolateral membrane mediate $NaHCO_3$ resorption. Carbon dioxide and water combine inside the cells to form H^+ and HCO_3^- in a reaction facilitated by the enzyme carbonic anhydrase *(CA)*. **B,** Operation of the Na^+-glucose transporter in the apical membrane, in conjunction with the Na^+,K^+-ATPase and glucose transporter in the basolateral membrane, mediates Na^+-glucose resorption. Na^+ resorption is also coupled with other solutes, including amino acids, Pi, and lactate. Resorption of these solutes is mediated by the Na^+–amino acid, Na^+-Pi, and Na^+-lactate antiporters located in the apical membrane and the Na^+,K^+-ATPase, amino acid, Pi, and lactate transporters in the basolateral membrane.

The glucose and other organic solutes that enter the cell with Na^+ leave the cell across the basolateral membrane via passive transport mechanisms. Any Na^+ that enters the cell across the apical membrane leaves the cell and enters the blood via Na^+,K^+-ATPase. In brief, the resorption of Na^+ in the first half of the proximal tubule is coupled to that of HCO_3^- and a number of organic molecules. The resorption of many organic molecules is so avid that they are almost completely removed from the tubular fluid in the first half of the proximal tubule. The resorption of $NaHCO_3$ and Na^+-organic solutes across the proximal tubule establishes a transtubular osmotic gradient that provides the driving force for the passive resorption of water

by osmosis. Because more water than Cl^- is resorbed in the first half of the proximal tubule, the Cl^- concentration in tubular fluid rises along the length of the proximal tubule.

IN THE SECOND HALF OF THE PROXIMAL TUBULE, Na^+ IS MAINLY RESORBED WITH Cl^- ACROSS BOTH THE TRANSCELLULAR AND PARACELLULAR PATHWAYS (Figure 36-2). Na^+ is resorbed with Cl^- rather than organic solutes or HCO_3^- as the accompanying anion because the Na^+-transport mechanisms in the

Table 36-3   NaCl Transport Along the Nephron

Segment	Filtered Load Resorbed (%)	Mechanism of Na$^+$ Entry Across Apical Membrane	Major Regulatory Hormones
Proximal tubule	67	Na$^+$-H$^+$ exchange, Na$^+$ cotransport with amino acids and organic solutes, Na$^+$/H$^+$-Cl$^-$/anion exchange, paracellular	Angiotensin II Norepinephrine Epinephrine Dopamine
Loop of Henle	25	1Na$^+$-1K$^+$-2Cl$^-$ symport	Aldosterone
Distal tubule	~4	NaCl symport	Aldosterone
Late distal tubule and collecting duct	~3	Na$^+$ channels	Aldosterone Atrial natriuretic peptide Urodilatin

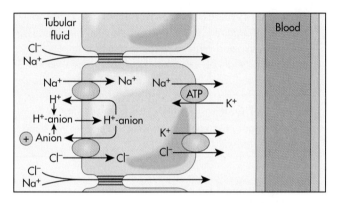

Figure 36-2 Na$^+$-transport processes in the second half of the proximal tubule. Na$^+$ and Cl$^-$ enter the cell across the apical membrane via the operation of parallel Na$^+$-H$^+$ and Cl$^-$-anion antiporters. More than one Cl$^-$-anion antiporter may be involved in this process, but only one is depicted. The secreted H$^+$ and anion combine in the tubular fluid to form an H$^+$-anion complex that can recycle across the plasma membrane. Accumulation of the H$^+$-anion complex in tubular fluid establishes an H$^+$-anion concentration gradient that favors H$^+$-anion recycling across the apical plasma membrane into the cell. Inside the cell, H$^+$ and the anion dissociate and recycle back across the apical plasma membrane. The net result is NaCl uptake across the apical membrane. The anion may be hydroxide ions (OH$^-$), formate (HCO$_2^-$), oxalate$^-$, HCO$_3^-$, or sulfate. The lumen positive transepithelial voltage, indicated by the plus sign inside the green circle in the tubular lumen, is generated by the diffusion of Cl$^-$ (lumen to blood) across the tight junction. The high Cl$^-$ concentration of tubular fluid provides the driving force for Cl$^-$ diffusion.

second half of the proximal tubule differ from those in the first half. Furthermore, the tubular fluid that enters the second half contains very little glucose and amino acids, but the high concentration of Cl$^-$ (140 mEq/L) exceeds that in the first half (105 mEq/L). The high Cl$^-$ concentration is due to the preferential resorption of Na$^+$ with HCO$_3^-$ and organic solutes in the first half of the proximal tubule.

The mechanism of transcellular Na$^+$ resorption in the second half of the proximal tubule is shown in Figure 36-2. Na$^+$ enters the cell across the luminal membrane via the parallel operation of Na$^+$-H$^+$ antiporter and one or more

Cl$^-$-anion antiporters. Because the secreted H$^+$ and anion combine in the tubular fluid and reenter the cell, the operation of the Na$^+$-H$^+$ and Cl$^-$-anion antiporters is equivalent to NaCl uptake from tubular fluid into the cell. Na$^+$ leaves the cell via Na$^+$,K$^+$-ATPase, and Cl$^-$ leaves the cell and enters the blood via a potassium chloride (KCl) symporter in the basolateral membrane.

NaCl is also resorbed across the second half of the proximal tubule via a **paracellular route.** Paracellular NaCl resorption occurs because the rise in the Cl$^-$ concentration in the tubule fluid in the first half of the proximal tubule creates a Cl$^-$ concentration gradient (140 mEq/L in the tubule lumen and 105 mEq/L in the interstitium). This concentration gradient favors the diffusion of Cl$^-$ from the tubular lumen across the tight junctions into the lateral intercellular space. Movement of the negatively charged Cl$^-$ causes the tubular fluid to become positively charged relative to the blood. This positive transepithelial voltage causes the diffusion of positively charged Na$^+$ out of the tubular fluid across the tight junction into the blood. Thus in the second half of the proximal tubule, some Na$^+$ and Cl$^-$ is resorbed across the tight junctions via passive diffusion. The resorption of NaCl establishes a transtubular osmotic gradient that provides the driving force for the passive resorption of water by osmosis.

In brief, the resorption of Na$^+$ and Cl$^-$ in the proximal tubule occurs across paracellular and transcellular pathways. Approximately 67% of the NaCl filtered each day is resorbed in the proximal tubule. Of this, two thirds moves across the transcellular pathway, whereas the remaining third moves across the paracellular pathway (Tables 36-3 and 36-4).

The proximal tubule resorbs 67% of the filtered water

The driving force for water resorption is a transtubular osmotic gradient established by solute resorption (e.g., NaCl, Na$^+$-glucose). The resorption of Na$^+$ along with organic

Table 36-4 Water Transport Along The Nephron

Segment	Filtered Load Reabsorbed (%)	Mechanism of Water Resorption	Hormones That Regulate Water Permeability
Proximal tubule	67	Passive	None
Loop of Henle	15	Descending thin limb only; passive	None
Distal tubule	0	No water resorption	None
Late distal tubule and collecting duct	~8-17	Passive	ADH, ANP*

*Atrial natriuretic peptide (ANP) inhibits ADH-stimulated water permeability.

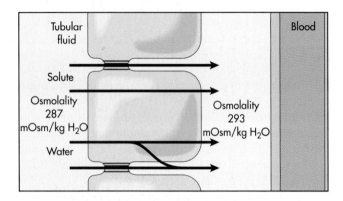

Figure 36-3 Routes of water and solute resorption across the proximal tubule. The transport of solutes, including Na^+, Cl^-, and organic solutes, into the lateral intercellular space increases the osmolality of this compartment, which establishes the driving force for osmotic water resorption across the proximal tubule. This occurs because some Na^+,K^+-ATPase and some transporters of organic solute, HCO_3^-, and Cl^- are located on the lateral cell membranes and deposit these solutes between cells. Furthermore, some NaCl also enters the lateral intercellular space via diffusion across the tight junction (i.e., paracellular pathway). An important consequence of osmotic water flow across the transcellular and paracellular pathways in the proximal tubule is that some solutes, especially K^+ and Ca^{++}, are entrained in the resorbed fluid and are thereby resorbed by the process of solvent drag.

solutes, HCO_3^-, and Cl^- from the tubular fluid into the lateral intercellular spaces reduces the osmolality of the tubular fluid and increases the osmolality of the lateral intercellular space (Figure 36-3). Because the proximal tubule is highly permeable to water, water flows via **osmosis** across both the tight junctions and the proximal tubular cells. The accumulation of fluid and solutes within the lateral intercellular space increases the hydrostatic pressure in this compartment. This increased hydrostatic pressure forces fluid and solutes into the capillaries. Thus water resorption follows solute resorption in the proximal tubule. The resorbed fluid is slightly hyperosmotic to plasma. An important consequence of osmotic water flow across the proximal tubule is that some solutes, especially K^+ and Ca^{++}, are entrained in the resorbed fluid and are thereby resorbed by the process of solvent drag (Figure 36-3). THE RESORPTION OF VIRTUALLY ALL ORGANIC SOLUTES, CL^- AND OTHER IONS, AND WATER IS COUPLED TO NA^+ RESORPTION. THEREFORE CHANGES IN NA^+ RESORPTION INFLUENCE THE RE-

SORPTION OF WATER AND OTHER SOLUTES BY THE PROXIMAL TUBULE.

> **Fanconi's syndrome,** a renal disease that is either hereditary or acquired, is often associated with osteomalacia, acidosis, and hypokalemia. It results from an impaired ability of the proximal tubule to resorb amino acids, glucose, and low-molecular-weight proteins. Because other segments of the nephron cannot resorb these solutes and protein, Fanconi's syndrome results in increased urinary excretion of amino acids, glucose, Pi, and low-molecular-weight proteins.

Proteins filtered by the glomerulus are resorbed in the proximal tubule

As mentioned previously, peptide hormones, small proteins, and small amounts of large proteins such as albumin are filtered by the glomerulus. The glomerulus filters only a small percentage of protein. (The concentration of proteins in the ultrafiltrate is only 40 mg/L.) However, the amount of protein filtered per day is significant because the glomerular filtration rate (GFR) is so high:

$$\text{Filtered protein} = GFR \times [\text{Protein}] \text{ in the ultrafiltrate}$$
$$\text{Filtered protein} = 180 \text{ L/day} \times 40 \text{ mg/L} = 7.2 \text{ g/day}$$

Protein resorption in the proximal tubule begins when the proteins are partially degraded by enzymes on the surface of the proximal tubule cells. These partially degraded proteins are taken into cells via endocytosis. Once they are inside the cell, enzymes digest the proteins and peptides into their constituent amino acids, which then leave the cell across the basolateral membrane and are returned to the blood. Normally, this mechanism resorbs virtually all of the proteins filtered, and hence the urine is essentially protein free. However, because the mechanism is easily saturated, an increase in filtered protein causes **proteinuria** (appearance of protein in the urine). Disruption of the glomerular filtration barrier to proteins increases the filtration of proteins and results in proteinuria. Proteinuria is frequently seen with kidney disease.

During routine urinalysis, the presence of traces of protein in the urine is normal. Protein in the urine can be derived from two sources: (1) filtration and incomplete resorption by the proximal tubule and (2) synthesis by the thick ascending limb of the loop of Henle. Cells in the thick ascending limb produce **Tamm-Horsfall glycoprotein** and secrete it into the tubular fluid. Because the mechanism for protein resorption is "upstream" of the thick ascending limb (i.e., proximal tubule), the secreted Tamm-Horsfall glycoprotein appears in the urine.

Cells of the proximal tubule also secrete organic cations and organic anions

Many of the secreted organic anions and cations (Boxes 36-1 and 36-2) are end-products of metabolism that circulate in the plasma. The proximal tubule also secretes numerous exogenous organic compounds, including p-aminohippuric acid (PAH), penicillin, and pollutants. Many of these organic compounds can be bound to plasma proteins and are not readily filtered. Therefore only a small portion of these potentially toxic substances are eliminated from the body via excretion resulting from filtration alone. Such substances are also secreted from the peritubular capillary into the tubular fluid. These secretory mechanisms are very powerful and remove virtually all organic anions and cations from the plasma that enters the kidneys. Hence these substances are removed from the plasma by both filtration and secretion.

Because all organic anions compete for the same secretory pathway, elevated plasma levels of one anion inhibit the secretion of the others. For example, penicillin secretion by the proximal tubule can be reduced by infusing PAH. Because the kidneys are responsible for eliminating penicillin, the infusion of PAH into individuals who receive penicillin reduces penicillin excretion and thereby extends the biological half life of the drug. In World War II, when penicillin was in short supply, hippurates were given with the penicillin to extend the drug's therapeutic effect.

The histamine H_2-antagonist cimetidine is used to treat gastric ulcers. Cimetidine is secreted by the organic cation pathway in the proximal tubule. It reduces the urinary excretion of procainamide (also an organic cation) by competing with this antiarrhythmic drug for the secretory pathway. The coadministration of organic cations can increase the plasma concentration of both drugs to levels much higher than those seen when the drugs are given alone. This increase can lead to drug toxicity.

Henle's loop resorbs approximately 25% of filtered sodium chloride and K^+

Ca^{++} and HCO_3^- are also resorbed in the loop of Henle (see Chapters 37 and 38 for more details). This resorption occurs almost exclusively in the thick ascending limb. In comparison, the ascending thin limb has a much lower resorptive capacity, and the descending thin limb does not resorb significant amounts of solutes. The loop of Henle resorbs approximately 15% of the filtered water. Water resorption occurs exclusively in the descending thin limb. The ascending limb is impermeable to water.

The key element in solute resorption by the thick ascending limb is the Na^+,K^+-ATPase in the basolateral membrane (Figure 36-4). As with resorption in the proximal tubule, the resorption of every solute by the thick ascending limb is linked somehow to Na^+,K^+-ATPase. This pump maintains a low concentration of cell Na^+, which provides a favorable chemical gradient for the movement of Na^+ from the tubular fluid into the cell. The movement of Na^+ across the apical membrane into the cell is mediated by the $1Na^+$-$1K^+$-$2Cl^-$ symporter, which couples the movement of $1Na^+$ with $1K^+$ and $2Cl^-$. Using the potential energy released by the downhill movement of Na^+ and Cl^-, this symport drives the uphill movement of K^+ into the cell. An Na^+-H^+ antiporter in the apical cell membrane also mediates Na^+ resorption as well as H^+ secretion (HCO_3^- resorption) in the thick ascending limb (see also Chapter 39). Na^+ leaves the cell across the basolateral membrane via Na^+,K^+-ATPase, whereas K^+, Cl^-, and HCO_3^- leave the cell across the basolateral membrane via separate pathways.

The voltage across the thick ascending limb is important for the resorption of several cations. The tubular fluid is positively charged relative to blood because of the unique location of transport proteins in the apical and basolateral membranes. Two points are important: (1) Increased salt transport by the thick ascending limb increases the magnitude of the positive charge in the lumen, and (2) this voltage is an important driving force for the resorption of several cations, including Na^+, K^+, and Ca^{++}, across the paracellular pathway (Figure 36-4). Thus salt resorption across the thick ascending limb occurs via the transcellular and paracellular pathways. A total of 50% of solute transport is transcellular, and 50% is paracellular. Because the thick ascending limb is very impermeable to water, the resorption of NaCl and other solutes reduces the osmolality of tubular fluid to less than 150 mOsm/kg H_2O.

Inhibition of the $1Na^+-1K^+-2Cl^-$ symporter in the thick ascending limb by "loop diuretics" such as **furosemide** inhibits NaCl resorption by the thick ascending limb and thereby increases urinary NaCl excretion. Furosemide also inhibits K^+ and Ca^{++} resorption by reducing the positive lumen voltage that drives the paracellular resorption of these ions. Thus furosemide increases urinary K^+ and Ca^{++} excretion. Furosemide also increases water excretion by reducing the osmolality of the interstitial fluid in the medulla. Water resorption by the descending thin limb of the loop of Henle is passive and driven by the osmotic gradient between the tubular fluid in the descending thin limb and the interstitial fluid in the medulla. (The osmolality is ~290 mOsm/kg H_2O at the beginning of the descending thin limb and ~1200 mOsm/kg H_2O in the medulla.) Thus a reduction of the osmolality of the interstitial fluid reduces water resorption and thereby increases water excretion.

The distal tubule and collecting duct resorb approximately 7% of the filtered NaCl, secrete variable amounts of K^+ and H^+, and resorb a variable amount of water (~8% to 17%)

Water resorption depends on the plasma concentration of ADH. The initial segment of the distal tubule (early distal tubule) resorbs Na^+, Cl^-, and Ca^{++} and is impermeable to water (Figure 36-5). NaCl entry into the cell across the apical membrane is mediated by an Na^+-Cl^- symporter (Figure 36-5). Na^+ leaves the cell via the action of Na^+,K^+-ATPase, and Cl^- leaves the cell via diffusion through channels. NaCl resorption is reduced by **thiazide diuretics,** which inhibit the Na^+-Cl^- symporter. THUS DILUTION OF THE TUBULAR FLUID BEGINS IN THE THICK ASCENDING LIMB AND CONTINUES IN THE EARLY SEGMENT OF THE DISTAL TUBULE.

The last segment of the distal tubule (late distal tubule) and the collecting duct are composed of two cell types: **principal cells** and **intercalated cells.** As illustrated in Figure 36-6, principal cells resorb Na^+ and water and secrete K^+. Intercalated cells secrete either H^+ or HCO_3^-

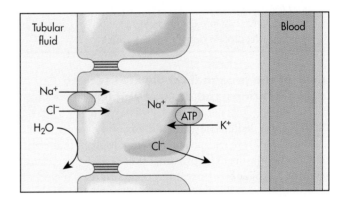

Figure 36-5 Transport mechanism for Na^+ and Cl^- resorption in the early segment of the distal tubule. This segment is impermeable to water.

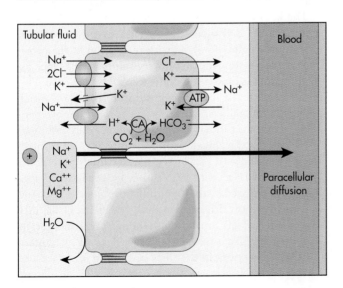

Figure 36-4 Transport mechanisms for NaCl resorption in the thick ascending limb of the loop of Henle. The positive charge in the lumen plays a major role in driving the passive paracellular resorption of cations. *CA,* Carbonic anhydrase.

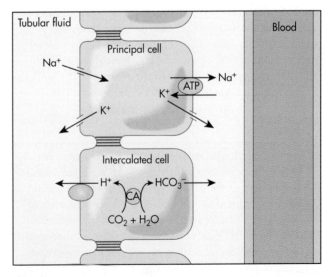

Figure 36-6 Transport pathways in principal cells and intercalated cells of the distal tubule and collecting duct. *CA,* Carbonic anhydrase.

and are thus important in regulating acid-base balance (see Chapter 39). Intercalated cells also resorb K^+. Both Na^+ resorption and K^+ secretion by principal cells depend on the activity of Na^+,K^+-ATPase in the basolateral membrane (Figure 36-6). By maintaining a low concentration of cell Na^+, this pump provides a favorable chemical gradient for the movement of Na^+ from the tubular fluid into the cell. Because Na^+ enters the cell across the apical membrane via diffusion through Na^+-selective channels in the apical membrane, the negative charge inside the cell facilitates Na^+ entry. Na^+ leaves the cell across the basolateral membrane and enters the blood via the action of Na^+,K^+-ATPase. This Na^+ resorption generates a lumen negative charge across the late distal tubule and collecting duct. Cells in the collecting duct resorb significant amounts of Cl^-, most likely across the paracellular pathway. The resorption of Cl^- is driven by the voltage difference across the late distal tubule and collecting duct.

Liddle's syndrome is a rare genetic disorder characterized by an increase in the extracellular fluid volume that causes an increase in blood pressure (i.e., hypertension). Liddle's syndrome is caused by mutations in either the β or γ subunit of the epithelial Na^+ channel. These mutations increase the number of Na^+ channels in the cell membrane and the amount of Na^+ absorbed by each channel. The rate of renal Na^+ absorption is inappropriately high, which leads to an increase in the extracellular fluid volume.

Pseudohypoaldosteronism type I is an uncommon, inherited disorder characterized by an increase in Na^+ excretion, a reduction in the extracellular fluid volume, and hypotension. It is due to mutations in the γ subunit of the epithelial Na^+ channel. These mutations inactivate the channel and thereby diminish renal Na^+ absorption, which reduces the extracellular fluid volume and thereby blood pressure.

K^+ is secreted from the blood into the tubular fluid by principal cells in two steps (Figure 36-6). First, K^+

uptake across the basolateral membrane is mediated via the action of Na^+,K^+-ATPase. Second, K^+ leaves the cell via passive diffusion. Because the K^+ concentration inside the cells is high (~ 150 mEq/L) and the K^+ concentration in tubular fluid is low (~ 10 mEq/L), K^+ diffuses down its concentration gradient across the apical cell membrane into the tubular fluid. Although the negative potential inside the cells tends to retain K^+ within the cell, the electrochemical gradient across the apical membrane favors K^+ secretion from the cell into the tubular fluid (see Chapter 38). The mechanism of K^+ resorption by intercalated cells appears to be mediated by H^+,K^+-ATPase located in the apical cell membrane.

Amiloride is a diuretic that inhibits Na^+ resorption by the distal tubule and collecting duct by directly inhibiting Na^+ channels in the luminal cell membrane. Amiloride also indirectly inhibits Cl^- resorption. The inhibition of Na^+ resorption reduces the negative charge in the lumen, and this diminishes the driving force for paracellular Cl^- resorption and inhibits K^+ secretion. Consequently, amiloride is frequently referred to as a **"K^+-sparing diuretic."** It is most often used in patients who excrete too much K^+ in their urine.

Several Hormones and Factors Regulate Sodium Chloride Resorption

Table 36-5 summarizes the major stimulus for secretion, the nephron site of action, and the effect on transport for each hormone. QUANTITATIVELY, ANGIOTENSIN II AND ALDOSTERONE, AS WELL AS URODILATIN, EPINEPHRINE, AND NOREPINEPHRINE RELEASED BY SYMPATHETIC NERVES, ARE THE MOST IMPORTANT HORMONES THAT REGULATE NaCl RESORPTION AND THEREBY URINARY NaCl EXCRETION. However, other hormones (including dopamine and glucocorticoids), Starling forces, and the phenomenon of glomerulotubular balance influence NaCl resorption. ADH IS THE ONLY MAJOR HORMONE THAT DIRECTLY REGULATES THE AMOUNT OF WATER EXCRETED BY THE KIDNEYS.

Table 36-5	Hormones that Regulate NaCl and Water Resorption		
Hormone*	**Major Stimulus**	**Nephron Site of Action**	**Effect on Transport**
Angiotensin II	↑Renin	PT	↑NaCl and H_2O resorption
Aldosterone	↑Angiotensin II, ↑$[K^+]_p$	TAL, DT/CD	↑NaCl and H_2O resorption†
ANP	↑BP, ↑ECF	CD	↓H_2O and NaCl resorption
Urodilatin	↑BP, ↑ECF	CD	↓H_2O and NaCl resorption
Sympathetic nerves	↓ECF	PT, TAL, DT/CD	↑NaCl and H_2O resorption†
Dopamine	↑ECF	PT	↓H_2O and NaCl resorption
ADH	↑P_{osm}, ↓ECF	DT/CD	↑H_2O resorption†

↑, Increase; *PT*, proximal tubule; $[K^+]_p$, plasma K^+ concentration; *TAL*, thick ascending limb; *DT*, distal tubule; *CD*, collecting duct; *ANP*, atrial natriuretic peptide; *BP*, blood pressure; *ECF*, extracellular fluid; ↓, decrease; P_{osm}, plasma osmolality.
*All of these hormones act within minutes, except aldosterone, which exerts its action on NaCl reabsorption with a delay of 1 hour.
†The effect on H_2O reabsorption does not include the thick ascending limb.

Angiotensin II has a potent stimulatory effect on sodium chloride and water resorption in the proximal tubule

Angiotensin II is one of the most potent hormones that stimulates NaCl and water resorption in the proximal tubule. A decrease in the extracellular fluid volume activates the renin-angiotensin-aldosterone system (see Chapter 37), thereby increasing the plasma concentration of angiotensin II.

Aldosterone is synthesized by the glomerulosa cells of the adrenal cortex, and it stimulates NaCl resorption. It acts on the thick ascending limb of the loop of Henle, distal tubule, and collecting duct. Aldosterone also stimulates K^+ secretion by the distal tubule and collecting duct (see Chapter 38). The two most important stimuli for aldosterone secretion are an increased concentration of angiotensin II and an increased plasma K^+ concentration. Through its stimulation of NaCl resorption in the collecting duct, aldosterone also increases water resorption by this nephron segment.

Some individuals with expanded extracellular fluid volume and elevated blood pressure are treated with drugs that inhibit **angiotensin-converting enzyme (ACE inhibitors [e.g., captopril])** and thereby lower fluid volume and blood pressure. The inhibition of ACE blocks the degradation of angiotensin I to angiotensin II and thereby lowers plasma angiotensin II levels (see Chapter 37). The decline in plasma angiotensin II concentration has three effects. First, NaCl and water resorption by the proximal tubule falls. Second, aldosterone secretion decreases, thus reducing NaCl resorption in the distal tubule and collecting duct. Third, because angiotensin is a potent vasoconstrictor, a reduction in its concentration permits the systemic arterioles to dilate and thereby lower arterial blood pressure. ACE also degrades the vasodilator hormone bradykinin; ACE inhibitors therefore increase the concentration of bradykinin. Thus ACE inhibitors decrease the extracellular fluid volume and the arterial blood pressure by promoting renal NaCl and water excretion and by depressing total peripheral resistance.

Atrial natriuretic peptide and urodilatin are encoded by the same gene and have very similar amino acid sequences

Atrial natriuretic peptide (ANP) is a 28 amino acid hormone secreted by the cardiac atria (see also Chapters 5, 19, 37, and 46). Its secretion is stimulated by a rise in blood pressure and an increase in the extracellular fluid volume. ANP reduces the blood pressure by decreasing the total peripheral resistance and by enhancing urinary NaCl and water excretion. This hormone also inhibits NaCl resorption by the medullary portion of the collecting duct, inhibits

ADH-stimulated water resorption across the collecting duct, and reduces the secretion of ADH from the posterior pituitary.

Urodilatin is a 32 amino acid hormone that differs from ANP by the addition of four amino acids to the amino terminus. Urodilatin is secreted by the distal tubule and collecting duct and is not present in the systemic circulation; thus urodilatin influences only the function of the kidneys. Urodilatin secretion is stimulated by a rise in the blood pressure and an increase in the extracellular fluid volume. It inhibits NaCl and water resorption across the medullary portion of the collecting duct. Urodilatin is a more potent natriuretic and diuretic hormone than ANP because the ANP that enters the kidneys in the blood is degraded by a neutral endopeptidase that has no effect on urodilatin.

Catecholamines stimulate sodium chloride resorption

Catecholamines released from the sympathetic nerves (norepinephrine) and the adrenal medulla (epinephrine) stimulate NaCl and water resorption by the proximal tubule, thick ascending limb of the loop of Henle, distal tubule, and collecting duct. Activation of the sympathetic nerves (e.g., after hemorrhage or a decrease in the extracellular fluid volume) stimulates NaCl and water resorption by these four structures.

Dopamine, a catecholamine, is released from dopaminergic nerves in the kidneys and may also be synthesized by cells of the proximal tubule. The action of dopamine is opposite to that of norepinephrine and epinephrine. Dopamine secretion is stimulated by an increase in extracellular fluid volume, and its secretion directly inhibits NaCl and water resorption in the proximal tubule.

ADH regulates water balance

ADH is the most important hormone that regulates water balance. This hormone is secreted by the posterior pituitary gland in response to an increase in plasma osmolality or a decrease in the extracellular fluid volume. ADH increases the permeability of the collecting duct to water. It also increases water resorption by the collecting duct because of the osmotic gradient that exists across the wall of the collecting duct (see Chapters 37 and 44). ADH has little effect on urinary NaCl excretion.

Starling forces regulate sodium chloride and water resorption across the proximal tubule

As previously described, Na^+, Cl^-, HCO_3^-, amino acids, glucose, and water are transported into the intercellular space of the proximal tubule. Starling forces between this space and the peritubular capillaries facilitate the movement of the reabsorbate into the capillaries. Starling forces across the wall of the peritubular capillaries are the hydrostatic pressures in the peritubular capillary (P_c) and lateral intercellular space (P_{ic}) and the oncotic pressures in the peritubular capillary (π_c) and lateral intercellular space (π_{ic}). Thus the resorption of water, resulting from Na^+ transport from tubular fluid into the lateral intercellular space, is modified by the Starling forces. Thus:

$$Q = K_f[(P_{ic} - P_c) + \sigma(\pi_c - \pi_{ic})]$$

where Q is flow (positive numbers indicate flow from the intercellular space into blood). Starling forces that favor movement from the interstitium into the peritubular capillaries are the π_c and P_{ic} (Figure 36-7). The opposing Starling forces are the π_{ic} and P_c. Normally, the sum of the Starling forces favors the movement of solute and water from the interstitium into the capillary (see also Chapter 22). However, some of the solutes and fluid that enter the lateral intercellular space leak back into the proximal tubular fluid. Starling forces do not affect transport by the loop of Henle, distal tubule, and collecting duct because these segments are less permeable to water than the proximal tubule.

A number of factors can alter the Starling forces across the peritubular capillaries surrounding the proximal tubule. For example, dilation of the efferent arteriole increases the P_c, whereas constriction of the efferent arteriole decreases it. An increase in the P_c inhibits solute and water resorption by increasing the back-leak of NaCl and water across the tight junction, whereas a decrease stimulates resorption by decreasing back-leak across the tight junction.

The π_c is partially determined by the rate of formation of the glomerular ultrafiltrate. For example, if one

assumes a constant plasma flow in the afferent arteriole, the plasma proteins become less concentrated in the plasma that enters the efferent arteriole and peritubular capillary as less ultrafiltrate is formed (i.e., as GFR decreases). Hence the π_c decreases. The π_c is directly related to the **filtration fraction** (FF = GFR/renal plasma flow [RPF]). A fall in the FF resulting from a decrease in GFR at constant RPF decreases the π_c. This in turn increases the backflow of NaCl and water from the lateral intercellular space into the tubular fluid and thereby decreases net solute and water resorption across the proximal tubule. An increase in the FF has the opposite effect.

The importance of Starling forces in regulating solute and water resorption by the proximal tubule is underscored by the phenomenon of **glomerulotubular (G-T) balance.** Spontaneous changes in GFR markedly alter the filtered load of Na^+ (filtered load = GFR × Na^+ concentration). Without rapid adjustments in Na^+ resorption to counter the changes, urine Na^+ excretion would fluctuate widely and disturb the Na^+ balance of the body. However, spontaneous changes in GFR do not alter the Na^+ balance because of the phenomenon of G-T balance. When body Na^+ balance is normal, G-T balance refers to the fact that Na^+ and water resorption increase in proportion to the increase in GFR and filtered load of Na^+. Thus a constant fraction of the filtered Na^+ and water is resorbed from the proximal tubule despite variations in GFR. THE NET RESULT OF G-T BALANCE IS TO REDUCE THE IMPACT OF GFR CHANGES ON THE AMOUNT OF Na^+ AND WATER EXCRETED IN THE URINE.

Two mechanisms are responsible for G-T balance. One is related to the oncotic and hydrostatic pressure differences between the peritubular capillaries and the lateral intercellular space (i.e., Starling forces). For example, an increase in the GFR (at constant RPF) raises the protein concentration in the glomerular capillary plasma above normal. This protein-rich plasma leaves the glomerular capillaries, flows through the efferent arteriole, and enters the peritubular capillaries. The increased π_c augments the movement of solute and fluid from the lateral intercellular space into the peritubular capillaries. This action increases net solute and water resorption by the proximal tubule.

The second mechanism responsible for G-T balance is initiated by an increase in the filtered load of glucose and amino acids. As discussed earlier, the resorption of Na^+ in the first half of the proximal tubule is coupled to that of glucose and amino acids. The rate of Na^+ resorption therefore partially depends on the filtered load of glucose and amino acids. As the GFR and filtered load of glucose and amino acids increase, Na^+ and water resorption also rise.

In addition to G-T balance, another mechanism minimizes changes in the filtered load of Na^+. As discussed in Chapter 35, an increase in the GFR (and thus in the amount of Na^+ filtered by the glomerulus) acti-

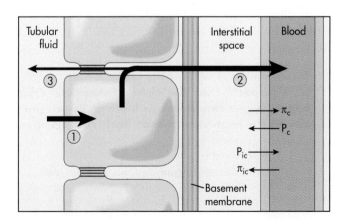

Figure 36-7 Routes of solute and water transport across the proximal tubule and the Starling forces that modify resorption. Solute and water are resorbed across the apical membrane *(1)*. This solute and water then cross the lateral cell membrane. Some of the solute and water reenters the tubule fluid *(3)*, and the remainder enters the interstitial space and then flows into the capillary *(2)*. The width of the arrows is directly proportional to the amount of solute and water moving via the three pathways. Starling forces across the capillary wall determine the amount of fluid flowing through pathway *2* versus pathway *3*. Transport mechanisms in the apical cell membranes determine the amount of solute and water entering the cell *(1)*. Thin arrows across the capillary wall indicate the direction of water movement in response to each force.

vates the tubuloglomerular-feedback mechanism. This action returns the GFR and filtration of Na^+ to normal values. Thus spontaneous changes in the GFR (e.g., caused by changes in posture and blood pressure) increase the amount of Na^+ filtered for only a few minutes. The mechanisms that underlie G-T balance maintain urinary Na^+ excretion constant and thereby maintain Na^+ homeostasis until the GFR returns to normal.

SUMMARY

- The four major segments of the nephron—proximal tubule, loop of Henle, distal tubule, and collecting duct—determine the composition and volume of the urine via the selective resorption of solutes and water and the selective secretion of solutes.
- Tubular resorption allows the kidneys to retain the substances that are essential and to regulate their levels in the plasma by altering their resorption.
- The resorption of Na^+, Cl^-, other anions, organic solutes, and water constitutes the major function of the nephron. The proximal tubule cells resorb 67% of the glomerular ultrafiltrate, and cells of the loop of Henle resorb about 25% of the NaCl that was filtered and about 15% of the water that was filtered.
- The distal segments of the nephron have a more limited resorptive capacity. However, the final adjustments in the composition and volume of the urine and most of the regulation by hormones and other factors occur in distal segments.
- The secretion of substances into tubular fluid is a means of excreting various by-products of metabolism and of eliminating exogenous organic anions and bases (e.g., drugs) and pollutants from the body.
- Various hormones (including angiotensin II, aldosterone, ADH, ANP, and urodilatin), sympathetic nerves, catecholamines, and Starling forces regulate NaCl resorption by the kidneys. ADH is the major hormone that regulates water resorption.

BIBLIOGRAPHY

Aronson PS: 1994 Homer W. Smith Award: from flies to physiology—accidental findings along the trail of renal NaCl transport, *J Am Soc Nephrol* 12:2001, 1995.

Benos DJ et al: Diversity and regulation of amiloride-sensitive Na^+ channels, *Kidney Int* 49:1632, 1996.

Berry CA, Ives HE, Rector FC Jr: Renal transport of glucose, amino acids, sodium, chloride and water. In Brenner BM, ed: *The kidney*, ed 5, Philadelphia, 1996, WB Saunders.

Canessa CM et al: Amiloride-sensitive epithelial Na^+ channel is made of three homologous subunits, *Nature* 367:463, 1994.

Forssmann W-G: Urodilatin: a renal natriuretic peptide, *Nephron* 69:211, 1995.

Hansson JH et al: Hypertension caused by a truncated epithelial sodium channel γ subunit: genetic heterogeneity of Liddle syndrome, *Nature Genet* 11:76, 1995.

Kershaw D, Wiggins RC: Proteinuria. In Shayman JA, ed: *Lippincott's pathophysiology series: renal pathophysiology*, Philadelphia, 1995, JB Lippincott.

Koeppen BK, Stanton BA: Sodium chloride transport: distal nephron. In Seldin DW, Giebisch G, eds: *The kidney: physiology and pathophysiology*, New York, 1992, Raven.

Murer H, Biber J: Renal sodium-phosphate cotransport, *Curr Opin Nephrol Hypertens* 3(5):504, 1994.

Prichard JB, Miller DS: Proximal tubular transport of organic anions and cations. In Seldin DW, Giebisch G, eds: *The kidney: physiology and pathophysiology*, ed 2, New York, 1992, Raven.

Pritchard JB, Miller DS: Mechanisms mediating renal secretion of organic anions and cations, *Physiol Rev* 73(4):765, 1993.

Silbernagel S: Tubular transport of amino acids and small peptides. In Windhager EE, ed: *Handbook of physiology*, section 8: *Renal physiology*, vol 2, New York, 1992, American Physiological Society/Oxford University Press.

Strautnieks SS et al: A novel splice-site mutation in the γ subunit of the epithelial sodium channel gene in three pseudohypoaldosteronism type 1 families, *Nature Genet* 13:248, 1996.

Warnock DG, Bubien JK: Liddle syndrome: clinical and cellular abnormalities, *Hosp Pract* 29(7):95, 1994.

CASE STUDIES

Case 36-1

A 45-year-old woman with breast cancer is enrolled in a clinical research trial to evaluate the effectiveness of a new chemotherapeutic drug. She has no other medical problems. After the second dose of the drug, she reports feeling light-headed when standing. Her blood pressure falls from 145/80 to 110/70 mm Hg when she goes from a supine to a standing position (orthostatic hypotension). In addition, a routine urinalysis shows that her urine contains large quantities of glucose, HCO_3^-, amino acids, phosphate, and organic anions.

1. **Based on the results of the urinalysis, the physician suspects that the chemotherapeutic drug has damaged this woman's kidneys. Which portion of the nephron is mostly likely damaged?**
   - **A.** The glomerulus
   - **B.** The proximal tubule
   - **C.** The thick ascending limb of the loop of Henle
   - **D.** The distal tubule
   - **E.** The collecting duct

2. **The physician attributes the patient's orthostatic hypotension to a decrease in the volume of the extracellular fluid secondary to increased renal Na^+ loss. In response to the decrease in extracellular fluid volume, there will be an increase in which of the following factors that regulate NaCl and water resorption by the nephron?**
   - **A.** Aldosterone
   - **B.** ANP
   - **C.** Urodilatin

D. Dopamine

E. P_c

Case 36-2

A new diuretic agent is developed, and its effect on healthy volunteers is evaluated. After a single dose of this new diuretic, the urine flow rate increased threefold, the fractional excretion of Na^+ increased from 1% to 20%, the excretion of K^+ and Ca^{++} increased, but neither glucose nor amino acids were found in the urine.

1. **Based on the results of the urinalysis, which portion of the nephron is the site of action of this new diuretic agent?**
   A. The glomerulus
   B. The proximal tubule
   C. The thick ascending limb of the loop of Henle
   D. The distal tubule
   E. The collecting duct

2. **Which of the following membrane transport proteins is inhibited by the new diuretic agent?**
   A. Na^+-glucose symporter
   B. Na^+-H^+ antiporter
   C. $1Na^+$-$1K^+$-$2Cl^-$ symporter
   D. Na^+-Cl^- symporter
   E. Na^+ channel

CHAPTER 37

Control of Body Fluid Volume and Osmolality

- Describe the volume and composition of the various body fluid compartments.
- Distinguish among the factors that regulate thirst and cause the secretion of antidiuretic hormone (i.e., body fluid osmolality, extracellular fluid volume, blood pressure).
- Describe the handling of water by the various portions of the nephron, especially the role of antidiuretic hormone in regulating the excretion of water by the kidneys.
- Describe the relationship among extracellular fluid volume, Na^+ balance, and renal Na^+ excretion.
- Describe the handling of Na^+ by the various portions of the nephron and the factors that regulate its excretion.

The kidneys play a critical role in maintaining the volume and composition of the body fluids constant despite daily fluctuations in the intake of water and solutes. The volume of water within the body determines the osmolality of the body fluids. Body fluid osmolality is maintained within a narrow range by regulating water intake (thirst) and by varying the amount of water excreted by the kidneys. The volume of the body fluids also depends on solute balance. The volume of the extracellular fluid determines plasma volume and thus how adequately tissues are perfused. Sodium chloride (NaCl) is the major solute of the extracellular fluid and thus determines the volume of this important body fluid compartment. By regulating the excretion of NaCl, the kidneys maintain extracellular fluid volume within a narrow range. In this chapter the regulation of renal water excretion (urine concentration and dilution) and renal NaCl excretion are discussed. A brief overview of the volumes and composition of the various body fluid compartments is also presented.

Body Fluid Compartments

Water within the body is divided into several compartments that have different compositions

Water accounts for approximately 60% of body weight. The water content of different individuals varies with the amount of adipose tissue; the greater the amount of adipose tissue, the smaller the fraction of body weight attributable to water.

As illustrated in Figure 37-1, the **total body water** is distributed between two major compartments that are separated by the cell membrane. The **intracellular fluid (ICF)** compartment is the larger compartment; it contains approximately two thirds of the total body water. The remaining one third is contained in the **extracellular fluid (ECF)** compartment. The ECF compartment is subdivided into **interstitial fluid** and **plasma;** these compartments are separated by the capillary wall. The interstitial fluid, which represents the fluid surrounding the cells in the various tissues of the body, comprises three fourths of the ECF volume. Included in this compartment is water contained within the bone and dense connective tissue. The plasma volume represents the remaining one fourth of the ECF.

The concentrations of the major cations and anions in the ECF and ICF are summarized in Table 37-1. The ionic composition of the two major compartments of the ECF (interstitial fluid and plasma) is similar because they are separated only by the capillary wall, which is freely permeable to small ions. THE MAJOR DIFFERENCE BETWEEN THE COMPOSITION OF INTERSTITIAL FLUID AND PLASMA IS THAT THE PLASMA CONTAINS SIGNIFICANTLY MORE PROTEIN. Although the presence of protein in the plasma can affect the distribution of cations and anions across the capillary wall by the Gibbs-Donnan effect (see Chapter 2), this effect is normally quite small, and the ionic composition of the interstitial fluid and plasma can be considered identical.

Because of its abundance, Na^+ (and its attendant anions Cl^- and bicarbonate [HCO_3^-]) is the major determinant of the osmolality of the ECF. Accordingly, a rough estimate of ECF osmolality can be obtained by simply doubling the Na^+ concentration. The normal plasma os-

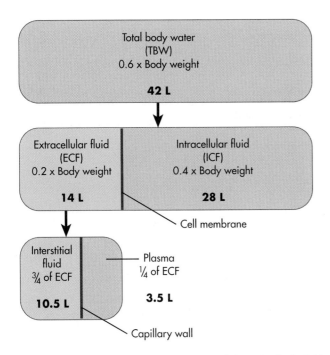

Figure 37-1 Relationship among the volumes of the major body fluid compartments. The values shown are calculated for a 70-kg individual.

Table 37-1	Distribution of Some Cations and Anions in ECF and ICF		
		ECF	ICF*
Na$^+$ (mEq/L)		145	12
K$^+$ (mEq/L)		4	150
Ca^{++} (mEq/L)		5	0.001
Cl$^-$ (mEq/L)		105	5
Bicarbonate (HCO$_3^-$) (mEq/L)		25	12
Inorganic phosphate (Pi)† (mEq/L)		2	100†
pH		7.4	7.1

*The ICF concentrations are estimates from skeletal muscle and include amounts bound to intracellular proteins and free within the cytosol.
†Intracellular phosphate is primarily in the form of organic molecules (e.g., ATP).

effective osmolality that is most important in determining the impact of changes in body fluid osmolality on ICF and ECF volumes.

molality ranges from approximately 280 to 295 mOsm/kg H$_2$O. Because water is in osmotic equilibrium across the capillary wall and across the plasma membrane of cells, measuring the plasma osmolality also provides an estimate of the osmolality of the ECF and ICF.

In clinical situations a more accurate estimate of the plasma osmolality is obtained by also considering the contribution of glucose and urea to the plasma osmolality. Accordingly, plasma osmolality can be estimated as:

Plasma osmolality =

$$2(Plasma\ [Na^+]) + \frac{[Glucose]}{18} + \frac{[Urea]}{2.8}$$

The glucose and urea concentrations are expressed in milligrams per deciliter. (Dividing by 18 for glucose and 2.8 for urea, which is measured as the nitrogen in the urea molecule, allows conversion from the units of milligrams per deciliter to millimoles per liter and thus to milliosmole per kilograms of H$_2$O.) This estimation of plasma osmolality is especially useful when dealing with patients who have elevated plasma glucose concentrations secondary to **diabetes mellitus** and in patients with **chronic renal failure,** whose plasma urea concentration is elevated. However, urea and glucose cross many cell membranes and thus are not **effective osmoles** when considering the effect of changes in plasma osmolality on shifts of fluid between the ICF and ECF. Therefore multiplying the plasma Na$^+$ concentration by two provides the best estimate of the effective osmolality of plasma. It is the

In contrast to the ECF, the Na$^+$ concentration of ICF is extremely low. K$^+$ is the predominant cation of the ICF. This asymmetrical distribution of Na$^+$ and K$^+$ across the plasma membrane is maintained by the activity of the ubiquitous Na$^+$,K$^+$-ATPase (see Chapter 1). The anion composition of the ICF also differs markedly from that of the ECF, with the Cl$^-$ and HCO$_3^-$ concentrations of the ICF being lower in comparison. The major ICF anions are phosphates, organic anions, and protein.

Fluid can shift between body fluid compartments

WATER MOVES FREELY BETWEEN THE VARIOUS BODY FLUID COMPARTMENTS. TWO FORCES DETERMINE THIS MOVEMENT: HYDROSTATIC PRESSURE AND OSMOTIC PRESSURE. Hydrostatic pressure, generated by the pumping of the heart (and the effect of gravity on the column of blood in the vessels), and the osmotic pressure of the plasma proteins (oncotic pressure) are important determinants of fluid movement across the capillary wall (see also Chapter 22), whereas osmotic pressure differences between the ICF and ECF are responsible for fluid movement across cell membranes. Because the plasma membranes of cells are highly permeable to water, a change in the osmolality of either the ICF or ECF moves water rapidly between these compartments. Thus EXCEPT FOR TRANSIENT CHANGES, THE ICF AND ECF COMPARTMENTS ARE IN OSMOTIC EQUILIBRIUM.

In contrast to the movement of water, the movement of ions across cell membranes is more variable and depends on the presence of specific membrane transporters (see Chapter 1). Consequently, as a first approximation, fluid exchange between the ICF and ECF under pathophysiological conditions can be analyzed by assuming that appreciable shifts of ions between the compartments do not occur. Thus fluid shifts between the ICF and the ECF primarily by the movement of water and not ions.

Shifts of fluid between the ICF and ECF can have important consequences when intravenous solutions are administered to patients. Intravenous solutions are available in many formulations. The type of fluid administered is dictated by the patient's need. For example, if the patient's vascular volume is low, a solution containing substances that are poorly permeable across the capillary wall is infused (e.g., 5% albumin solution). The oncotic pressure generated by the albumin molecules retains fluid in the vascular compartment, thus expanding its volume. Expansion of the ECF is accomplished most with isotonic saline solutions (e.g., 0.9% NaCl). The administration of isotonic saline does not induce an osmotic pressure gradient across the plasma membrane of cells. Therefore the entire volume of infused solution remains in the ECF. Patients whose body fluids are hyperosmotic may need hypotonic solutions. These solutions may be hypotonic NaCl (e.g., 0.45% NaCl or 5% dextrose in water [D5W]). The administration of D5W solution is equivalent to infusion of distilled water because the dextrose is ultimately metabolized to carbon dioxide and water. Administration of these fluids increases the volumes of both the ICF and ECF. Finally, patients whose body fluids are hypotonic may need hypertonic solutions. These solutions, which typically contain NaCl (e.g., 3% and 5% NaCl), expand the volume of the ECF but decrease the volume of the ICF by shifting water out of the cells. Other constituents, such as electrolytes (e.g., K^+), or drugs can be added to intravenous solutions to tailor the therapy to the patient's fluid, electrolyte, and metabolic needs.

Control of Body Fluid Osmolality: Urine Concentration and Dilution

The kidneys are responsible for regulating water balance and under most conditions are the major route for the elimination of water from the body (Table 37-2). Another route of water loss from the body includes evaporation from the cells of the skin and the respiratory passages. Collectively, water loss by these routes is termed **insensible water loss** because the individual is unaware of its occurrence. Additional water can be lost through sweat. Water loss via this mechanism can increase dramatically in a hot environment, with exercise, or in the presence of fever (Table 37-3). Finally, water can be lost from the gastrointestinal tract. Fecal water loss is normally small but increases with diarrhea. Gastrointestinal water losses can also occur with vomiting.

Table 37-2	Normal Routes of Water Gain and Loss in Adults at Room Temperature (23° C)	
Route		**ml/day**
Water Intake		
Fluid*		1200
In food		1000
Metabolically produced from food		300
TOTAL		2500
Water Output		
Insensible		700
Sweat		100
Feces		200
Urine		1500
TOTAL		2500

*Fluid intake varies widely for both social and cultural reasons.

Table 37-3	Effect of Environmental Temperature and Exercise on Water Loss and Intake in Adults		
	Normal Temperature	**Hot Weather***	**Prolonged Heavy Exercise***
Water Loss			
Insensible loss			
Skin	350	350	350
Lungs	350	250	650
Sweat	100	1400	5000
Feces	200	200	200
Urine†	1500	1200	500
TOTAL LOSS	2500	3400	6700
Intake	2500	3400	6700

*In hot weather and during prolonged heavy exercise, water balance is maintained only if the individual increases water intake to match the increased loss of water in sweat.

†Decreased water excretion by the kidneys alone is insufficient to maintain water balance.

Renal excretion of water is regulated to maintain water balance

Water loss via sweating, defecation, and evaporation from the lungs and skin is not regulated. In contrast, RENAL EXCRETION OF WATER IS TIGHTLY REGULATED TO MAINTAIN WATER BALANCE. The maintenance of water balance requires that water intake precisely match water loss from the body. If intake exceeds losses, water balance is positive, and the osmolality of the body fluids decreases. Conversely, when intake is less than losses, water balance is negative, and the osmolality of the body fluids increases.

When water intake is low or when water losses increase, the kidneys conserve water by producing a small volume of

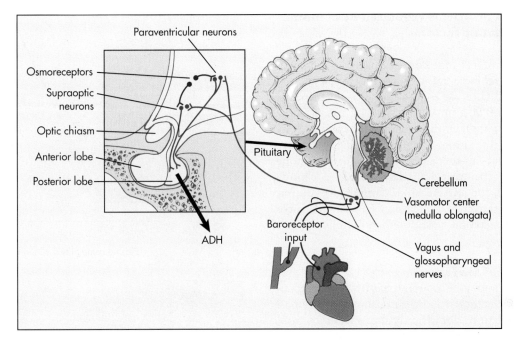

Figure 37-2 Anatomical structures of the hypothalamus and pituitary gland (midsagittal section) depicting the pathways for ADH secretion. Also shown are the pathways involved in regulating ADH secretion. Afferent fibers from the baroreceptors are carried in the vagus and glossopharyngeal nerves. The closed box illustrates an expanded view of the hypothalamus and pituitary gland.

urine that is hyperosmotic with respect to plasma (concentrated urine). When water intake is high, a large volume of hypoosmotic urine is produced (dilute urine). In a normal individual, the urine osmolality can vary from approximately 50 to 1200 mOsm/kg H_2O, and the corresponding urine volume can vary from near 18 to 0.5 L/day.

Disorders of water balance alter the plasma Na⁺ concentration

Disorders of water balance alter the body fluid osmolality, which is usually monitored by measuring plasma osmolality. BECAUSE THE MAJOR DETERMINANT OF PLASMA OSMOLALITY IS Na^+ (WITH ITS ANIONS Cl^- AND HCO_3^-), DISORDERS OF WATER BALANCE ALTER THE PLASMA Na^+ CONCENTRATION. When an abnormal plasma Na^+ concentration is evaluated in an individual, it is tempting to suspect a problem in Na^+ balance. However, the problem most often relates to water balance, not Na^+ balance. CHANGES IN Na^+ BALANCE RESULT IN ALTERATIONS IN THE VOLUME OF ECF, NOT ITS OSMOLALITY (see later section).

Hypoosmolality (a reduction in plasma osmolality) shifts water into cells, and this process results in cell swelling. Symptoms associated with hypoosmolality are related mainly to the swelling of brain cells. For example, a rapid fall in plasma osmolality can alter neurological function and thereby cause nausea, malaise, headache, confusion, lethargy, seizures, and coma. When plasma osmolality is increased (i.e., **hyperosmolality**), water is lost from cells. The symptoms of

increased plasma osmolality are also mainly neurological, and they include lethargy, weakness, seizures, coma, and even death.

The kidneys control water excretion independently of their ability to control the excretion of a number of other physiologically important substances (e.g., Na^+, K^+, H^+, urea). Indeed, this ability is necessary for survival because it allows water balance to be achieved without upsetting the other homeostatic functions of the kidneys.

Antidiuretic hormone regulates renal water excretion

Antidiuretic hormone (ADH), or **vasopressin,** acts on the kidneys to regulate the volume and osmolality of the urine. When plasma ADH levels are low, a large volume of urine is excreted **(water diuresis),** and the urine is dilute. When plasma ADH levels are elevated, a small volume of urine is excreted **(antidiuresis),** and the urine is concentrated.

ADH is a small peptide that is 9 amino acids in length. It is synthesized in neuroendocrine cells located within the **supraoptic** and **paraventricular nuclei** of the hypothalamus (see also Chapter 44). The synthesized hormone is packaged in granules, which are transported down the axon of the cell and stored in the nerve terminals located in the **neurohypophysis (posterior pituitary).** The anatomy of the hypothalamus and pituitary gland is shown in Figure 37-2.

The secretion of ADH is regulated by osmotic and hemodynamic factors

The secretion of ADH by the posterior pituitary can be influenced by several factors. THE TWO PHYSIOLOGICAL REGULATORS OF ADH SECRETION ARE THE OSMOLALITY OF THE BODY FLUIDS (OSMOTIC) AND VOLUME AND PRESSURE OF THE VASCULAR SYSTEM (HEMODYNAMIC). Of these stimuli, a change in body fluid osmolality is the primary regulator of ADH secretion. Other factors that can alter the secretion of this hormone include nausea (stimulates), atrial natriuretic peptide (ANP) (inhibits), and angiotensin II (stimulates). A number of drugs also affect ADH secretion. For example, nicotine stimulates secretion, whereas ethanol inhibits it (see also Chapter 44).

Osmotic control of ADH secretion

A CHANGE IN THE BODY FLUID OSMOLALITY IS THE PRIMARY REGULATOR OF ADH SECRETION. Changes in osmolality as small as 1% are sufficient to significantly alter ADH secretion. Cells located in the hypothalamus but distinct from those that synthesize ADH sense changes in body fluid osmolality. These cells, termed **osmoreceptors,** appear to sense changes in body fluid osmolality by either shrinking or swelling. The osmoreceptors respond only to solutes that are effective osmoles (e.g., NaCl). Urea, which is an ineffective osmole, has little effect on ADH secretion.

When the effective osmolality of the body fluids increases, the osmoreceptors send signals to the ADH-synthesizing cells located in the supraoptic and paraventricular nuclei of the hypothalamus, stimulating ADH secretion. Conversely, when the effective osmolality of the body fluids is reduced, secretion is inhibited. Because ADH is rapidly degraded in the plasma, circulating levels can be reduced to zero within minutes after secretion is inhibited. As a result, the ADH system can respond rapidly to fluctuations in body fluid osmolality.

Figure 37-3, *A,* illustrates the effect of changes in body fluid osmolality (measured as plasma osmolality) on circulating ADH levels. The **set point** of the system is the plasma osmolality value at which ADH secretion begins to increase. Below this set point, virtually no ADH is released. Above the set point, the slope of the relationship is steep, reflecting the sensitivity of this system. The set point varies among individuals and is genetically determined. In healthy adults, it varies from 280 to 295 mOsm/kg H₂O.

Hemodynamic control of ADH secretion

A DECREASE IN THE BLOOD VOLUME OR ARTERIAL PRESSURE ALSO STIMULATES ADH SECRETION. The receptors activated by this response are located in both the low-pressure side (left atrium and pulmonary vessels) and the high-pressure (aortic arch and carotid sinus) side of the circulatory system (see also Chapter 23). Because the low-pressure receptors are located in the high-compliance

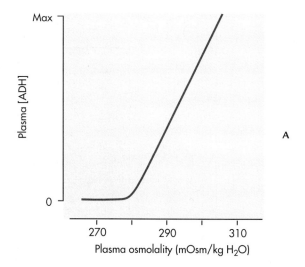

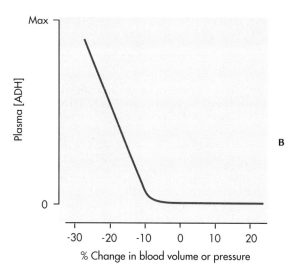

Figure 37-3 Osmotic and hemodynamic control of ADH secretion. **A,** Effect of changes in plasma osmolality (constant blood volume and pressure) on plasma ADH levels. **B,** Effect of changes in blood volume or pressure (constant plasma osmolality) on plasma ADH levels.

side of the circulatory system, they respond to overall vascular volume. The high-pressure receptors respond to arterial pressure. Both groups of receptors are sensitive to stretch of the wall of the structure in which they are located (e.g., cardiac atrial wall, wall of aortic arch) and are termed **baroreceptors** (see also Chapters 19 and 23). Signals from these receptors are carried in afferent fibers of the **vagus** and **glossopharyngeal** nerves to the centers in the brainstem that regulate heart rate and blood pressure. Signals are then relayed from the brainstem to the ADH secretory cells of the supraoptic and paraventricular hypothalamic nuclei. The sensitivity of the baroreceptor system is less than that of the osmoreceptors; a 5% to 10% decrease in blood volume or arterial pressure is required before ADH secretion is stimulated. This is illustrated in Figure 37-3, *B.*

Alterations in blood volume or arterial pressure also affect the response to changes in body fluid osmolality.

With a decrease in blood volume or arterial pressure, the set point is shifted to lower osmolality values, and the slope of the relationship is steeper. With an increase in blood volume or arterial pressure, the opposite occurs; the set point is shifted to higher osmolality values, and the slope is decreased.

Inadequate secretion of ADH results in the excretion of large volumes of dilute urine **(polyuria).** To compensate for this loss of water, the individual must ingest large volumes of water **(polydipsia)** to maintain body fluid osmolality constant. If the individual is deprived of water, the body fluids become hyperosmotic. This condition is called **central diabetes insipidus, neurogenic diabetes insipidus,** or **pituitary diabetes insipidus.** Central diabetes insipidus can be inherited, although this is rare. It occurs more commonly after head trauma, with brain neoplasms, or with brain infections. Individuals with central diabetes insipidus have a urine-concentrating defect that can be corrected by the administration of exogenous ADH. The **syndrome of inappropriate ADH secretion (SIADH)** is a common clinical problem that is characterized by plasma ADH levels that are elevated above what would be expected on the basis of body fluid osmolality and blood volume or arterial pressure (hence the term *inappropriate*). Individuals with SIADH retain water (i.e., reduce renal water excretion). If water intake is not reduced in parallel, their body fluids become progressively hypoosmotic. Characteristically, the urine of these individuals is more concentrated than expected, based on the low body fluid osmolality. SIADH can be caused by infections and neoplasms of the brain, drugs (e.g., antitumor drugs), pulmonary diseases, and carcinoma of the lung.

ADH increases the permeability of the collecting duct to water

THE PRIMARY ACTION OF ADH ON THE KIDNEYS IS TO INCREASE THE PERMEABILITY OF THE COLLECTING DUCT TO WATER. In addition, it increases the permeability of the medullary portion of the collecting duct to urea.

The actions of ADH on water permeability of the collecting duct have been extensively studied. ADH binds to a receptor on the basolateral membrane of the principal cell. This receptor is coupled to adenylyl cyclase (see Chapter 5). In response to ADH-receptor binding, intracellular vesicles containing **water channels (aquaporins)** are inserted into the apical membrane of the cell via exocytosis. With the removal of ADH, the water channels are retrieved from the apical membrane via endocytosis, and the membrane is once again impermeable to water. This shuttling of water channels into and out of the apical membrane provides a mechanism for rapidly controlling membrane water permeability. Because the basolateral membrane is freely permeable to water, any water that enters the cell through apical membrane water channels exits across the basolateral membrane. This transcellular flow of water results in the net absorption of water from the tubule lumen into the peritubular blood.

The collecting ducts of some individuals do not respond normally to ADH. This lack of response can result from defects in the ADH receptor, failure to insert water channels into the apical membrane, or defective water channels. Regardless of the mechanism, these individuals cannot maximally concentrate their urine. Consequently, they suffer from polyuria and polydipsia. This entity is termed **nephrogenic diabetes insipidus** to distinguish it from central diabetes insipidus. Although nephrogenic diabetes insipidus can be inherited, most cases are secondary to other factors such as metabolic disorders (e.g., hypercalcemia) or certain drugs. For example, approximately 35% of individuals who take lithium for bipolar disorder develop nephrogenic diabetes insipidus.

ADH also increases the permeability of the terminal portion of the inner medullary collecting duct to urea. Urea enters the cell across the apical membrane via a specific urea transporter. Acting through adenylyl cyclase, ADH causes the insertion of urea transporters into the apical membrane of the cell. Increased osmolality of the interstitial fluid of the renal medulla also leads to the insertion of urea transporters into the apical membrane. This effect is separate and additive to that of ADH.

Factors that influence ADH secretion also influence the perception of thirst

WHEN BODY FLUID OSMOLALITY IS INCREASED OR THE BLOOD VOLUME OR PRESSURE IS REDUCED, THE INDIVIDUAL PERCEIVES THIRST. Of these stimuli, hyperosmolality is the more potent. An increase of only 2% to 3% in the plasma osmolality produces a strong desire to drink, whereas decreases of 10% to 15% in blood volume or arterial pressure are required to produce the same response.

The neural centers that regulate water intake (thirst center) are located in the anterolateral region of the hypothalamus and are distinct from the osmoreceptors involved in ADH secretion. However, like the osmoreceptors involved in ADH secretion, the cells of the thirst center also respond only to effective osmoles (e.g., NaCl). Even less is known about the pathways involved in the thirst response to decreased blood volume or arterial pressure, but it is believed that the pathways are the same as those involved in the regulation of ADH secretion. Angiotensin II, acting on cells of the thirst center, also evokes the sensation of thirst. Because angiotensin II levels are increased when blood volume and pressure are reduced (see Chapter 36), this effect of angiotensin II contributes to the homeostatic response to restore and maintain the body fluids at their normal volume.

The sensation of thirst is satisfied by drinking even before sufficient water is absorbed from the gastrointestinal tract to correct the plasma osmolality. Oropharyngeal and upper gastrointestinal receptors appear to be involved in this response. However, relief of the thirst sensation via these receptors is short lived. Thirst is only completely satisfied when the plasma osmolality, or blood volume and arterial pressure, is corrected.

The ADH and thirst systems work in concert to maintain water balance. An increase in the plasma osmolality invokes drinking and via ADH action on the kidneys, the conservation of water. Conversely, when the plasma osmolality is decreased, thirst is suppressed, and in the absence of ADH, renal water excretion is enhanced.

The dilution and concentration of urine requires the separation of solute and water excretion

Under normal circumstances the excretion of water is regulated separately from the excretion of solutes (e.g., NaCl). For this to occur the kidneys must be able to excrete urine that is either hypoosmotic or hyperosmotic with respect to the body fluids. This ability to excrete urine of varying osmolality in turn requires that solute be separated from water at some point along the nephron. As discussed in Chapter 36, the reabsorption of solute in the proximal tubule results in the resorption of a proportional amount of water. Hence solute and water are not separated in this portion of the nephron. Moreover, this proportionality between proximal tubule water and solute resorption occurs regardless of whether the kidneys excrete dilute or concentrated urine. Thus the proximal tubule resorbs a large portion of the filtered load of solute and water, but it does not produce dilute or concentrated tubular fluid.

Solute and water are separated in the loop of Henle

The loop of Henle, in particular the thick ascending limb, is the major site where solute and water are separated. Thus the excretion of both dilute and concentrated urine requires normal function of the loop of Henle.

Figure 37-4 summarizes the essential features of the mechanisms whereby the kidneys excrete either a dilute or a concentrated urine. Table 37-4 also summarizes the transport and passive permeability properties of the nephron segments involved in these processes.

First, how the kidneys excrete dilute urine (water diuresis) when ADH levels are low or zero is considered. The following numbers refer to those encircled in Figure 37-4, *A*.

1. Fluid entering the descending thin limb of the loop of Henle from the proximal tubule is isosmotic with respect to plasma. This reflects the es-

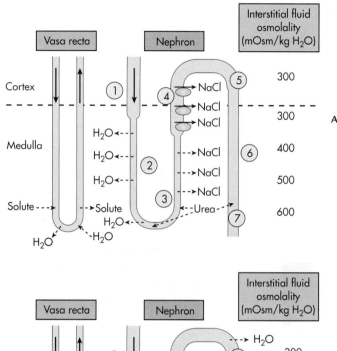

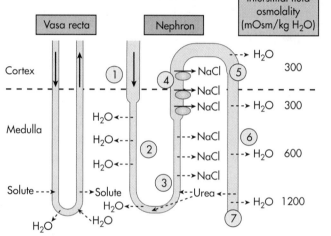

Figure 37-4 A, Mechanism for the excretion of dilute urine (water diuresis). ADH is absent, and the collecting duct is essentially impermeable to water. Note that the osmolality of the medullary interstitium is reduced during water diuresis. **B,** Mechanism for the excretion of a concentrated urine (antidiuresis). Plasma ADH levels are maximal, and the collecting duct is highly permeable to water. Under this condition the medullary interstitial gradient is maximal. See text for details.

sentially isoosmotic nature of solute and water resorption in the proximal tubule (see Chapter 36).

2. The descending thin limb is highly permeable to water and much less so to solutes such as NaCl and urea. (NOTE: Urea is an ineffective osmole in many tissues, but it is an effective osmole in many portions of the nephron.) Consequently, as the fluid descends deeper into the hyperosmotic medulla, water is resorbed owing to the osmotic gradient set up across the descending thin limb by both NaCl and urea. Via this process, fluid at the bend of the loop has an osmolality equal to that of the surrounding interstitial fluid. However, although the osmolality of the tubular and interstitial fluids is similar at the bend of the

Table 37-4   Transport and Permeability Properties of Nephron Segments Involved in Urine Concentration and Dilution

Tubule Segment	Active Transport	Passive Permeability*			Effect of ADH
		NaCl	Urea	H$_2$O	
Loop of Henle					
Descending thin limb	0	+	+	+++	
Ascending thin limb	0	+++	+	0	
Thick ascending limb	+++	+	0	0	
Distal tubule	+	+	0	0	
Collecting duct					
Cortex	+	+	0	0	↑H$_2$O permeability
Medulla	+	+	++	+	↑H$_2$O and urea permeability

*Permeability is proportional to the number of plus signs indicated: +, low permeability; +++, high permeability; 0, impermeable.

loop, their compositions differ. The tubular fluid NaCl concentration is greater than that of the surrounding interstitial fluid. However, the urea concentration of the tubular fluid is less than that of the interstitial fluid (see later section).

3. The ascending thin limb is impermeable to water but permeable to NaCl and urea. Consequently, as tubular fluid moves up the ascending limb, NaCl is passively resorbed (because the luminal NaCl concentration is higher than the interstitial NaCl concentration), whereas urea passively diffuses into the tubular fluid (because the luminal urea concentration is lower than the interstitial urea concentration). The net effect is that the volume of the tubular fluid remains unchanged along the length of the thin ascending limb, but the NaCl concentration decreases and the urea concentration increases. Overall, the movement of NaCl out of the lumen of the thin ascending limb exceeds the movement of urea into the lumen, and the tubular fluid becomes diluted.

4. The thick ascending limb of the loop of Henle is impermeable to water and urea. This portion of the nephron actively resorbs NaCl from the tubular fluid and thereby dilutes it. Dilution occurs to such a degree that this segment is often referred to as the **diluting segment** of the kidney. Fluid leaving the thick ascending limb is hypoosmotic with respect to plasma (approximately 150 mOsm/kg H$_2$O).

5. The distal tubule and cortical portion of the collecting duct actively resorb NaCl and are impermeable to urea. In the absence of ADH, these segments are not permeable to water. Thus when ADH is absent or present at low levels (i.e., decreased plasma osmolality), the distal tubule and cortical collecting duct are impermeable to water. Accordingly, the osmolality of tubule fluid in

these segments is reduced further because NaCl is resorbed without water. Under this condition, fluid leaving the cortical portion of the collecting duct is hypoosmotic with respect to plasma (approximately 100 mOsm/kg H$_2$O).

6. The medullary collecting duct actively resorbs NaCl. Even in the absence of ADH, this segment is slightly permeable to water and urea. Consequently, some urea enters the collecting duct from the medullary interstitium, and a small volume of water is resorbed.

7. The urine has an osmolality as low as approximately 50 mOsm/kg H$_2$O and contains low concentrations of NaCl and urea. The volume of urine excreted can be as much as 18 L/day, or approximately 10% of the glomerular filtration rate.

Second, how the kidneys excrete concentrated urine **(antidiuresis)** when plasma osmolality and plasma ADH levels are high is considered. The following numbers refer to those encircled in Figure 37-4, *B*.

1-4. These steps are similar to those for production of a dilute urine. An important point in understanding how a concentrated urine is produced is that whereas resorption of NaCl by the ascending thin and thick limbs of the loop of Henle dilutes the tubular fluid, the resorbed NaCl accumulates in the medullary interstitium and raises its osmolality. The accumulation of NaCl in the medullary interstitium is crucial for the production of urine hyperosmotic to plasma because it provides the osmotic driving force for water resorption by the collecting duct. The overall process by which the loop of Henle, in particular the thick ascending limb, generates the hyperosmotic medullary interstitial gradient is termed **countercurrent multiplication.** This term derives from both the form and function of the loop of Henle. The loop of Henle consists of two parallel limbs with tubular fluid flowing in opposite directions (countercurrent flow). Fluid flows into the medulla in the descending limb and out of the medulla in the ascending limb. The ascending limb is impermeable to water and resorbs solute from the tubular fluid. Thus fluid within the ascending limb becomes diluted. This separation of solute and water by the ascending limb is termed the **single effect** of the countercurrent multiplication process. The solute removed from the ascending limb tubular fluid accumulates in the surrounding interstitial fluid and raises its osmolality. Because the descending limb is highly permeable to water, the increased osmolality of the medullary interstitium causes water to be absorbed and thereby concentrates the tubular fluid. The countercurrent flow within the descending and ascending limbs of the loop of Henle magnifies, or "multiplies," the osmotic gradient between the tubule fluid in the descending and ascending limbs of the loop of Henle.

5. Because of NaCl resorption by the thick ascending limb of the loop of Henle, the fluid reaching the collecting duct is hypoosmotic with respect to the surrounding interstitial fluid. Thus an osmotic gradient is established across the collecting duct. In the presence of ADH, which increases the water permeability of the collecting duct, water diffuses out of the tubule lumen, and the tubule fluid osmolality increases. This diffusion of water out of the lumen of the collecting duct begins the process of urine concentration. The maximum osmolality that the fluid in the cortical collecting duct can attain is approximately 300 mOsm/kg H_2O, which is the osmolality of the surrounding interstitial fluid and plasma. Although the fluid at this point has the same osmolality as that which entered the descending thin limb, its composition has been altered dramatically. Because of NaCl resorption by the preceding nephron segments, NaCl accounts for a much smaller portion of the total tubular fluid osmolality. Instead, the tubule fluid osmolality reflects the presence of urea (filtered urea plus urea added in the descending thin and ascending thin limbs of the loop of Henle) and other solutes (e.g., K^+, creatinine).

6. The osmolality of the interstitial fluid in the medulla progressively increases from the junction between the renal cortex and medulla, where it is approximately 300 mOsm/kg H_2O, to the papilla, where it approximates 1200 mOsm/kg H_2O. Thus an osmotic gradient exists between tubule fluid and the interstitial fluid along the entire medullary collecting duct. In the presence of ADH, which renders the medullary collecting duct permeable to water, the osmolality of tubule fluid increases as water is resorbed. Because the initial portion of the collecting duct is impermeable to urea, it remains in the tubular fluid, and its concentration increases. In the presence of ADH, the urea permeability of the last portion of the medullary collecting duct is increased. Because the urea concentration of the tubular fluid has been increased by water resorption in the cortex and outer medulla, its concentration in the tubular fluid is greater than its concentration in the interstitial fluid, and some urea diffuses out of the tubule lumen into the medullary interstitium. The maximal osmolality that the fluid in the medullary collecting duct can attain is equal to that of the surrounding interstitial fluid. The major components of the tubular fluid within the medullary collecting ducts are substances that have either escaped resorption or have been secreted into the tubular fluid. Of these, urea is the most abundant.

7. The urine produced when ADH levels are elevated has an osmolality of 1200 mOsm/kg H_2O and contains high concentrations of urea and other nonresorbed solutes. Because urea in the tubular fluid equilibrates with urea in the medullary interstitial fluid, its concentration in the urine is similar to that of the interstitium. The urine volume under this condition can be as low as 0.5 L/day.

As just described, water resorption by the proximal tubule and the loop of Henle is essentially the same regardless of whether the urine is dilute or concentrated. As a result, a relatively constant volume of water (approximately 10% of the filtered load) is delivered to the collecting duct each day. Depending on the plasma ADH concentration, a variable portion of this water is then resorbed along the collecting duct, with water excretion ranging from 0.3% to 10% of the filtered load. During antidiuresis, most of the water is resorbed in the cortical and outer medullary portions of the collecting duct. A much smaller volume is resorbed from the inner medullary collecting duct. This distribution of water resorption along the length of the collecting duct (the cortex more than the outer medulla more than inner medulla) allows for the maintenance of a hyperosmotic interstitial environment in the inner medulla by minimizing the amount of water entering the interstitium of the inner medulla. This in turn allows the urine to be maximally concentrated.

Medullary interstitial fluid osmolality determines the maximal osmolality of urine

As noted, the interstitial fluid of the renal medulla is critically important in concentrating the urine. The osmotic pressure of the interstitial fluid provides the driving force for resorbing water from both the descending thin limb of the loop of Henle and the collecting duct. The principal solutes of the medullary interstitial fluid are NaCl and urea, but the concentration of these solutes is not uniform throughout the medulla (i.e., a gradient exists from cortex to papilla). Other solutes also accumulate in the medullary interstitium (e.g., NH_4^+ [ammonium], K^+), but the most abundant solutes are NaCl and urea. For simplicity, this discussion assumes that NaCl and urea are the only solutes. At the junction of the medulla with the cortex, the interstitial fluid has an osmolality of approximately 300 mOsm/kg H_2O, with virtually all osmoles attributable to NaCl. The concentrations of both NaCl and urea increase progressively with increasing depth into the medulla. When a maximally concentrated urine is excreted, the medullary interstitial fluid osmolality is approximately 1200 mOsm/kg H_2O at the papilla (Figure 37-4 *B*). Of this value, approximately 600 mOsm/kg H_2O is attributed to NaCl and 600 mOsm/kg H_2O to urea. As described later, NaCl is an effective osmole in the inner medulla and thus is responsible for driving water resorption from the medullary collecting duct.

The medullary gradient for NaCl results from the accumulation of NaCl resorbed by the nephron segments in the medulla during countercurrent multiplication. The most important segment in this regard is the ascending limb (the thick limb more than the thin limb) of the loop of Henle. Urea accumulation within the medullary interstitium is more complex and occurs most effectively when a hyperosmotic urine is excreted (i.e., antidiuresis). When a dilute urine is produced, especially over extended periods, the osmolality of the medullary interstitium declines (compare Figure 37-4). This reduced osmolality is almost entirely caused by a decrease in the concentration of urea. This decrease reflects washout by the vasa recta (see later section) and diffusion of urea from the interstitium into the tubular fluid within the medullary portion of the collecting duct. (Recall that the medullary collecting duct is significantly permeable to urea even in the presence of ADH [Table 37-4].)

Urea is not synthesized in the kidney but is generated by the liver as a product of protein metabolism. It enters the tubular fluid via glomerular filtration. As indicated in Table 37-4, the permeability of most nephron segments involved in urinary concentration and dilution to urea is relatively low. The important exception is the medullary collecting duct, which has a relatively high urea permeability that is further increased by ADH. As fluid moves along the nephron and as water is resorbed in the collecting duct, the urea concentration in the tubular fluid increases. When this urea-rich tubular fluid reaches the medullary collecting duct, where the permeability to urea not only is high but is increased by ADH, urea diffuses down its concentration gradient into the medullary interstitial fluid, where it accumulates. When ADH levels are elevated, the urea within the lumen of the collecting duct and the interstitium equilibrates. The resultant urea concentration of the urine is equal to that of the medullary

interstitium at the papilla, or approximately 600 mOsm/kg H_2O.

Some of the urea within the interstitium enters the descending and ascending thin limbs of the loop of Henle. This urea is then trapped in the nephron until it again reaches the medullary collecting duct, where it can reenter the medullary interstitium. Thus UREA RECYCLES FROM THE INTERSTITIUM TO THE NEPHRON AND BACK INTO THE INTERSTITIUM. THIS PROCESS OF RECYCLING FACILITATES THE ACCUMULATION OF UREA IN THE MEDULLARY INTERSTITIUM.

As described, the hyperosmotic medullary interstitium is essential for concentrating the tubular fluid within the collecting duct. Because a hyperosmotic medullary interstitium is essential for urine concentration, any condition that reduces this gradient impairs the ability of the kidneys to maximally concentrate the urine. Urea within the medullary interstitium contributes to the total osmolality of the urine. However, with regard to water resorption across the medullary collecting duct, urea is an ineffective osmole. THE MEDULLARY INTERSTITIAL NaCl CONCENTRATION IS RESPONSIBLE FOR RESORBING WATER FROM THE MEDULLARY COLLECTING DUCT AND THEREBY CONCENTRATING THE NONUREA SOLUTES (E.G., NH_4^+-SALTS, K^+-SALTS, CREATININE) IN THE URINE.

The vasa recta function as countercurrent exchangers

The **vasa recta,** the capillary networks that supply blood to the medulla, are highly permeable to solute and water. As with the loop of Henle, the vasa recta form a parallel set of hairpin loops within the medulla (see Chapter 35). Not only do the vasa recta bring nutrients and oxygen to the medullary nephron segments, but more important, they remove excess water and solute, which are continuously added to the medullary interstitium by these nephron segments. The ability of the vasa recta to maintain the medullary interstitial gradient is flow dependent. A substantial increase in vasa recta blood flow dissipates the medullary gradient (i.e., washout of the medullary interstitial gradient). Alternatively, reduced blood flow reduces oxygen delivery to the nephron segments within the medulla and impairs tubular transport. As a result, the medullary interstitial osmotic gradient cannot be maintained.

Renal water handling is assessed by measuring solute-free water excretion

Assessment of renal water handling includes measurements of urine osmolality and the volume of urine excreted. The range of urine osmolality is from 50 to 1200 mOsm/kg H_2O. The corresponding range in urine volume is 18 L to as little as 0.5 L/day. These ranges are not fixed, but they vary from individual to individual.

As already discussed, total urine osmolality does not accurately reflect the impact of renal water handling on the maintenance of whole-body water balance because urea (which can account for half of the total urine osmolality) is not an effective osmole. As a result, it is often more appropriate to consider the ability of the kidneys to excrete or resorb **solute-free water.** Solute-free water is an abstract term referring to water that does not contain any solute. When a dilute urine is produced, the kidneys excrete solute-free water. When a concentrated urine is produced, solute-free water is resorbed by the kidneys.

The ability of the kidneys to either excrete or resorb solute-free water depends on ADH. When no ADH is present or levels are low, solute-free water is excreted. When ADH levels are high, solute-free water is resorbed. Other factors are also important in determining the ability of the kidneys to excrete or resorb solute-free water:

1. ADH must be absent. This prevents water resorption by the collecting duct.
2. The tubular structures that separate solute from water (i.e., dilute the luminal fluid) must function normally. In the absence of ADH, the following nephron segments can dilute the luminal fluid:
   a. Thin ascending limb of the loop of Henle
   b. Thick ascending limb of the loop of Henle
   c. Distal tubule
   d. Collecting duct

   Because of its high transport rate, the thick ascending limb is quantitatively the most important of these segments that separate solute and water.
3. Adequate delivery of tubular fluid to these nephron sites is required for maximal separation of solute and water. Factors that reduce delivery (e.g., decreased glomerular filtration rate or enhanced proximal tubule resorption) impair the ability of the kidneys to maximally excrete solute-free water

Similar requirements also apply to the resorption of solute-free water by the kidneys. For the kidneys to resorb solute-free water maximally, the following conditions must exist:

1. Adequate delivery of tubular fluid to the nephron segments that separate solute and water. Most important in this regard is the thick ascending limb of the loop of Henle. Delivery of tubular fluid to the loop of Henle in turn depends on the glomerular filtration rate and proximal tubule resorption.
2. Normal resorption of NaCl by the nephron segments. Again the most important segment is the thick ascending limb of the loop of Henle.
3. A hyperosmotic medullary interstitium. The effective interstitial osmolality is maintained by NaCl resorption by the loop of Henle (see 1 and 2).
4. Maximum levels of ADH and responsiveness of the collecting duct to ADH.

Control of Extracellular Fluid Volume and Regulation of Renal NaCl Excretion

The major solutes of the ECF are the salts of Na^+. Of these, NaCl is the most abundant. Because NaCl is also the major determinant of ECF osmolality, alterations in Na^+ balance are commonly assumed to disturb ECF osmolality. However, under normal circumstances, this is not the case because the ADH and thirst systems maintain body fluid osmolality within a very narrow range. For example, the addition of NaCl to the ECF (without water) increases the Na^+ concentration and osmolality of this compartment. (ICF osmolality also increases because of osmotic equilibration with the ECF.) This increase in osmolality in turn stimulates thirst and the release of ADH from the posterior pituitary. The increased ingestion of water in response to thirst, together with the ADH-induced decrease in water excretion by the kidneys, quickly restores ECF osmolality to normal. However, the volume of the ECF increases in proportion to the amount of water ingested, which in turn depends on the amount of NaCl added to the ECF. Thus in the new steady state, the addition of NaCl to the ECF is equivalent to adding an isoosmotic solution, and the volume of this compartment increases. Conversely, a decrease in the NaCl content of the ECF lowers the volume of this compartment.

The kidneys adjust NaCl excretion to match daily intake

The kidneys are the major route for excretion of NaCl from the body. As such, the kidneys are important in regulating the volume of the ECF. Under normal conditions, the kidneys keep the volume of the ECF constant by adjusting the excretion of NaCl to match the amount ingested in the diet. If ingestion exceeds excretion, ECF volume increases above normal, whereas the opposite occurs if excretion exceeds ingestion.

The typical diet contains approximately 140 mEq/day of Na^+ (8 g of NaCl), and thus daily Na^+ excretion is also about 140 mEq/day. However, the kidneys can vary the excretion of Na^+ over a wide range. Excretion rates as low as 10 mEq/day can be attained when individuals are placed on a low-salt diet. Conversely, the kidneys can increase their excretion rate to more than 1000 mEq/day when challenged by the ingestion of a high-salt diet. These changes in Na^+ excretion occur with only modest changes in the steady-state Na^+ content of the body.

The response of the kidneys to abrupt changes in NaCl intake typically takes several hours to several days, depending on the magnitude of the change. During this transition period, the intake and excretion of Na^+ are not matched as they are in the steady state. Thus the individual experiences either a **positive Na^+ balance** (intake higher than excretion) or **negative Na^+ balance** (intake less than excretion). However, by the end of the transition period, a new steady state is established, and intake once again equals excretion. Provided that the ADH and thirst systems are intact and normal, alterations in Na^+ balance change the volume, but not the Na^+ concentration, of the ECF. Changes in ECF volume can be monitored by measuring body weight because 1 L of ECF equals 1 kg of body weight.

Renal NaCl excretion is regulated to maintain a constant ECF volume

As described earlier, the ECF is subdivided into two compartments: blood plasma and interstitial fluid. Plasma volume is a determinant of vascular volume, blood pressure, and thus cardiac output. Therefore these important cardiovascular parameters also depend on ECF volume. The maintenance of Na^+ balance, and thus ECF volume, involves a complex system of sensors and effector signals that act primarily on the kidneys to regulate the excretion of NaCl. As can be appreciated from the dependency of vascular volume, blood pressure, and cardiac output on ECF volume, this complex system is designed to ensure adequate tissue perfusion. Because the primary sensors of this system are located in the large vessels of the vascular system, changes in vascular volume, blood pressure, and cardiac output are the principal factors regulating renal NaCl excretion. In a normal individual, changes in ECF volume result in parallel changes in vascular volume, blood pressure, and cardiac output. Thus a decrease in ECF volume, a situation termed **volume contraction,** results in reduced vascular volume, blood pressure, and cardiac output. Conversely, an increase in ECF volume, a situation termed **volume expansion,** results in increased vascular volume, blood pressure, and cardiac output. When ECF volume is decreased, renal NaCl excretion is reduced. Conversely, an increase in ECF volume results in enhanced renal NaCl excretion, termed **natriuresis.**

In some pathological conditions (e.g., congestive heart failure, hepatic cirrhosis), the renal excretion of NaCl does not reflect the ECF volume. In both of these situations the volume of the ECF is increased. However, instead of increased NaCl excretion, as would be expected, there is a reduction in the renal excretion of NaCl. This paradoxical response can be understood by recognizing that the sensors, because of their location in the vascular system, appear to detect a reduced ECF volume in these situations.

Patients with congestive heart failure frequently have an increase in the volume of the ECF, which is manifested as accumulation of fluid in the lungs (**pulmonary edema**) and peripheral tissues (**generalized edema**). This excess fluid is the result of NaCl and water retention by the kidneys. The kidneys' response (i.e., retention of NaCl and water) is paradoxical because the ECF volume is increased. However, this fluid is not in the vascular system but is in the interstitial fluid compartment. In addition,

blood pressure and cardiac output may be reduced because of poor cardiac performance. Therefore the sensors located in the vascular system respond as they do in ECF volume contraction and cause NaCl and water retention by the kidneys.

Large volumes of fluid accumulate in the peritoneal cavity (**ascites**) of patients with advanced hepatic cirrhosis. This fluid is a component of the ECF and results from NaCl and water retention by the kidneys. Again the response of the kidneys in this situation seems paradoxical if only ECF volume is considered. With advanced hepatic cirrhosis, blood pools in the splanchnic circulation. (The damaged liver impedes the drainage of blood from the splanchnic circulation via the portal vein.) Thus volume and pressure are reduced in the portions of the vascular system where the sensors are found, but venous pressure in the portal system increases, which enhances fluid transudation into the peritoneal cavity. Hence the kidneys respond as they would during ECF volume contraction, which results in NaCl and water retention and the accumulation of ascites fluid.

The remaining portions of this section examine the relationship between ECF volume and renal NaCl excretion in normal adults. Changes in ECF volume result in parallel changes of vascular volume, blood pressure, and cardiac output. The maintenance of a normal volume (**euvolemia**) is reviewed, followed by consideration of the renal response to ECF volume expansion and contraction.

The primary ECF volume sensors are located in the vascular system

The ECF volume is monitored by multiple sensors (Box 37-1). A number of the sensors are located in the vascular system, and they monitor its fullness and blood pressure. These receptors are typically called **volume receptors,** or because they respond to stretch, they are also referred to as **baroreceptors.** The sensors within the liver and central nervous system are less well understood and do not seem

---

Box 37-1 Volume Sensors

Vascular sensors
   Low pressure
      Cardiac atria
      Pulmonary vasculature
   High pressure
      Carotid sinus
      Aortic arch
      Juxtaglomerular apparatus of kidneys
Hepatic sensors
Central nervous system sensors

to be as important as the vascular sensors in monitoring the ECF volume. The hepatic and central nervous system sensors are not considered further.

Low-pressure baroreceptors respond mainly to vascular volume

Baroreceptors are located within the walls of the cardiac atria and pulmonary vessels, and they respond to distention of these structures (see also Chapters 19 and 23). Because the low-pressure side of the circulatory system has a high compliance, the atrial and pulmonary vascular sensors respond mainly to the "fullness" of the vascular system. These baroreceptors send signals to the brainstem via afferent fibers in the vagus nerve. The activity of these sensors modulates both sympathetic nerve outflow and ADH secretion. For example, a decrease in filling of the pulmonary vessels and cardiac atria increases sympathetic nerve activity and stimulates ADH secretion. Conversely, distention of these structures decreases sympathetic nerve activity. In general, 5% to 10% changes in blood volume and pressure are necessary to evoke a response.

The cardiac atria possess an additional mechanism related to the control of renal NaCl excretion. The myocytes of the atria synthesize and store a peptide hormone. This hormone, termed **atrial natriuretic peptide (ANP),** is released when the atria are distended, which via mechanisms outlined later in this chapter reduces blood pressure and increases the excretion of NaCl and water by the kidneys (see also Chapters 19 and 44).

High-pressure baroreceptors respond primarily to arterial blood pressure

Baroreceptors are also present in the arterial side of the circulatory system, located in the wall of the aortic arch, carotid sinus (see also Chapter 23), and afferent arterioles of the kidneys. The aortic arch and carotid baroreceptors send input to the brainstem via afferent fibers in the vagus and glossopharyngeal nerves. The response to this input alters sympathetic outflow and ADH secretion. Thus a decrease in blood pressure increases sympathetic nerve activity and ADH secretion. An increase in pressure tends to reduce sympathetic nerve activity. The sensitivity of the high-pressure baroreceptors is similar to that in the low-pressure side of the vascular system; 5% to 10% changes in pressure are needed to evoke a response.

The **juxtaglomerular apparatus** of the kidneys (see Chapter 35), particularly the afferent arterioles, responds directly to changes in pressure. If perfusion pressure in the afferent arterioles is reduced, renin is released from the myocytes. Renin secretion is suppressed when perfusion pressure is increased. As described later in this chapter, renin determines blood levels of angiotensin II and aldosterone, both of which play an important role in regulating renal NaCl excretion.

Constriction of a renal artery by an atherosclerotic plaque, for example, reduces perfusion pressure to that kidney. This reduced perfusion pressure is sensed by the afferent arterioles and results in the secretion of renin. The elevated renin levels increase the production of angiotensin II, which in turn increases systemic blood pressure via its vasoconstrictor effect on arterioles throughout the vascular system. The increased systemic blood pressure is sensed by the afferent arterioles of the contralateral kidney (i.e., the kidney without stenosis of its renal artery), and renin secretion from that kidney is suppressed. In addition, the high levels angiotensin II act to inhibit renin secretion by the contralateral kidney (negative feedback). The treatment of patients with constricted renal arteries includes surgical repair of the stenotic artery and administration of an inhibitor of angiotensin-converting enzyme (ACE). The ACE inhibitor blocks the conversion of angiotensin I to angiotensin II. As a result, angiotensin II levels decrease, as does the blood pressure. Because angiotensin II inhibits renin secretion, renin levels increase after the administration of the ACE inhibitor. Also, ACE breaks down bradykinin, a potent vasodilator. After the administration of the ACE inhibitor, bradykinin levels increase, which further contributes to the reduction in blood pressure. (See later section for a complete description of the renin-angiotensin-aldosterone system.)

ECF volume sensors send hormonal and neural signals to the kidneys

The volume sensors elicit signals that act on the kidneys to modulate the excretion of NaCl. Both neural and hormonal signals have been identified. These are summarized in Box 37-2, as are their effects on renal NaCl and water excretion.

Renal sympathetic nerves

As described in Chapter 35, sympathetic nerve fibers innervate the afferent and efferent arterioles of the glomerulus, as well as the nephron cells. With a negative Na^+ balance (i.e., ECF volume depletion), the low- and high-pressure vascular baroreceptors stimulate renal sympathetic nerve activity. This has the following effects:

1. The afferent and efferent arterioles are constricted. This vasoconstriction (the effect appears to be greater on the afferent arteriole) decreases the hydrostatic pressure within the glomerular capillary lumen, which results in a decreased glomerular filtration rate. With this decrease, the filtered load of Na^+ to the nephrons is reduced.

2. Renin secretion is stimulated in the cells of the afferent and efferent arterioles. As described later, renin ultimately increases the circulating levels of angiotensin II and aldosterone.

> **Box 37-2**   Signals Involved in the Control of Renal NaCl and Water Excretion
>
> ### Renal Sympathetic Nerves (↑Activity: ↓NaCl Excretion)
> ↓Glomerular filtration rate
> ↑Renin secretion
> ↑Proximal tubule, thick ascending limb of the loop of Henle, distal tubule, and collecting duct NaCl resorption
>
> ### Renin-Angiotensin-Aldosterone (↑Secretion: ↓NaCl Excretion)
> ↑Angiotensin II levels stimulate proximal tubule NaCl resorption
> ↑Aldosterone levels stimulate the thick ascending limb of the loop of Henle, distal tubule, and collecting duct NaCl resorption
> ↑ADH secretion
>
> ### Atrial Natriuretic Peptide (↑Secretion: ↑NaCl Excretion)
> ↑Glomerular filtration rate
> ↓Renin secretion
> ↓Aldosterone secretion
> ↓NaCl and water resorption by the collecting duct*
> ↓ADH secretion
>
> ### ADH (↑Secretion: ↓H_2O Excretion)
> ↑H_2O absorption by the collecting duct

*Urodilatin may contribute to this effect.

3. NaCl resorption along the nephron is directly stimulated. Quantitatively, the most important segment influenced by sympathetic nerve activity is the proximal tubule.

As a result of these actions, INCREASED RENAL SYMPATHETIC NERVE ACTIVITY DECREASES NaCl EXCRETION, an adaptive response that works to restore euvolemia. With a positive Na^+ balance (i.e., ECF volume expansion), renal sympathetic nerve activity is reduced. This generally reverses the effects just described.

Renin-angiotensin-aldosterone system

Smooth muscle cells in the afferent arterioles are the site of synthesis, storage, and release of **renin.** Three factors are important in stimulating renin secretion:

1. **Perfusion pressure.** The afferent arteriole behaves as a high-pressure baroreceptor. When perfusion pressure to the kidneys is reduced, renin secretion is stimulated. Conversely, an increase in perfusion pressure inhibits renin release.
2. **Sympathetic nerve activity.** Activation of the sympathetic nerve fibers that innervate the afferent arterioles increases renin secretion. Renin secretion is decreased as renal sympathetic nerve activity is decreased.
3. **Delivery of NaCl to the macula densa.** Delivery of NaCl to the macula densa regulates the glomerular filtration rate by a process termed **tubuloglomerular feedback** (see Chapter 36). Via this feedback mechanism, increased NaCl delivery to the macula densa decreases the glomerular filtration rate. Conversely, decreased NaCl delivery increases the glomerular filtration rate. In addition, the macula densa plays a role in renin secretion. When NaCl delivery to the macula densa is decreased, renin secretion is enhanced. Conversely, an increase in NaCl delivery inhibits renin secretion. It is likely that macula densa–mediated renin secretion maintains systemic arterial pressure under conditions of a reduced vascular volume. For example, when vascular volume is reduced, perfusion of body tissues (including the kidneys) decreases. This in turn decreases the glomerular filtration rate and the filtered load of NaCl. The reduced delivery of NaCl to the macula densa then stimulates renin secretion, which acts through angiotensin II (a potent vasoconstrictor) to increase the blood pressure and thereby maintain tissue perfusion. However, this macula densa–mediated secretion of renin may not be involved in the alterations in glomerular hemodynamics that underlie the phenomenon of tubuloglomerular feedback (see Chapter 36).

Figure 37-5 summarizes the essential components of the renin-angiotensin-aldosterone system. Renin alone does not have a physiological function; it functions solely as a proteolytic enzyme. Its substrate is a circulating protein, **angiotensinogen,** which is produced by the liver. Angiotensinogen is cleaved by renin to yield a 10 amino acid peptide, **angiotensin I.** Angiotensin I also has no known physiological function, and it is further cleaved to an 8 amino acid peptide, **angiotensin II,** by a converting enzyme **(ACE)** found on the surface of vascular endothelial cells. (Pulmonary and renal endothelial cells are important sites for the conversion of angiotensin I to angiotensin II.) Angiotensin II has several important physiological functions, including:

1. Stimulation of aldosterone secretion by the adrenal cortex
2. Arteriolar vasoconstriction, which increases blood pressure
3. Stimulation of ADH secretion and thirst
4. Enhancement of NaCl resorption by the proximal tubule

Angiotensin II is an important secretagogue for **aldosterone;** an increase in the plasma K^+ concentration is the other important stimulus for aldosterone secretion (see Chapters 38 and 46). Aldosterone is a steroid hormone produced by the glomerulosa cells of the adrenal

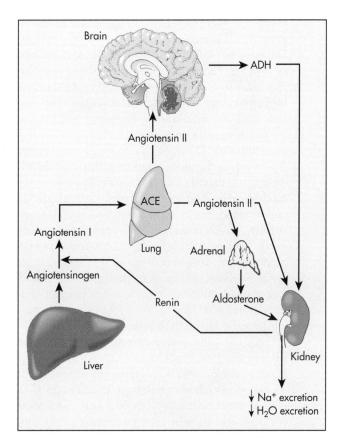

Figure 37-5 Essential components of the renin-angiotensin-aldosterone system. Activation of this system results in decreased excretion of Na$^+$ and water by the kidneys. Angiotensin I is converted to angiotensin II by ACE, which is present on all vascular endothelial cells. The endothelial cells within the lungs play a significant role in this conversion process. See text for details. *ACE,* Angiotensin converting enzyme.

cortex. Aldosterone acts in a number of ways on the kidneys (see also Chapters 38 and 39). With regard to the regulation of the ECF volume, aldosterone reduces NaCl excretion by stimulating its resorption by the thick ascending limb of the loop of Henle, distal tubule, and collecting duct. The effect of aldosterone on renal NaCl excretion depends mainly on its ability to stimulate Na$^+$ resorption in the distal tubule and collecting duct.

Aldosterone stimulates Na$^+$ resorption by the principal cells of the late portion of the distal tubule and collecting duct by increasing Na$^+$ entry into the cell across the apical membrane as well as increasing the exit of Na$^+$ from the cell across the basolateral membrane. The increase in apical membrane Na$^+$ entry occurs via Na$^+$-selective channels, and the increased extrusion of Na$^+$ from the cell across the basolateral membrane occurs by Na$^+$,K$^+$-ATPase. Thus aldosterone increases the resorption of Na$^+$ from the tubular fluid. Reduced levels of aldosterone decrease the amount of Na$^+$ resorbed by the principal cells.

Aldosterone also enhances Na$^+$ resorption by cells of the thick ascending limb of the loop of Henle. This action may reflect an increased entry of Na$^+$ into the cell

across the apical membrane (probably by the apical membrane 1Na$^+$-1K$^+$-2Cl$^-$ symporter) and an increased extrusion from the cell by the basolateral membrane Na$^+$,K$^+$-ATPase.

> Diseases of the adrenal cortex can alter aldosterone levels and thereby impair the ability of the kidneys to maintain Na$^+$ balance and euvolemia. With decreased secretion of aldosterone **(hypoaldosteronism),** the resorption of Na$^+$, mainly by the collecting duct, is reduced, and NaCl is lost in the urine. Because urinary NaCl loss can exceed the amount of NaCl ingested in the diet, a negative Na$^+$ balance ensues, and the ECF volume decreases. In response to the ECF volume contraction, sympathetic tone is increased, and levels of renin, angiotensin II, and ADH are elevated. With increased aldosterone secretion **(hyperaldosteronism),** the effects are the opposite; Na$^+$ resorption, especially by the collecting duct, is enhanced, and excretion of NaCl is reduced. Consequently, ECF volume is increased, sympathetic tone is decreased, and the levels of renin, angiotensin II, and ADH are decreased. As described later, ANP levels are also elevated in this setting.

As summarized in Box 37-2, ACTIVATION OF THE RENIN-ANGIOTENSIN-ALDOSTERONE SYSTEM, AS OCCURS WITH ECF VOLUME DEPLETION, DECREASES THE EXCRETION OF NACL BY THE KIDNEYS. This system is suppressed with ECF volume expansion, and renal NaCl excretion is therefore enhanced.

Atrial natriuretic peptide

Atrial myocytes produce and store the peptide hormone **ANP,** which relaxes vascular smooth muscle and promotes NaCl and water excretion by the kidney. ANP is released with atrial stretch, as would occur with a positive Na$^+$ balance and ECF volume expansion. The circulating form of ANP is 28 amino acids in length. In general, ANP actions, as they relate to renal NaCl and water excretion, antagonize those of the renin-angiotensin-aldosterone system. The actions of ANP include:

1. Vasodilation of the afferent and vasoconstriction of the efferent arterioles of the glomerulus. This increases the glomerular filtration rate and the filtered load of Na$^+$.
2. Inhibition of renin secretion by the afferent arterioles.
3. Inhibition of aldosterone secretion by the glomerulosa cells of the adrenal cortex. ANP reduces aldosterone secretion via two mechanisms: (a) It acts on the juxtaglomerular cells to inhibit renin secretion and thereby reduces angiotensin II–induced aldosterone secretion, and (b) it acts on the glomerulosa cells of the adrenal cortex to inhibit aldosterone secretion.

4. Inhibition of NaCl resorption by the collecting duct, which is also caused in part by reduced levels of aldosterone. However, ANP also acts on the collecting duct cells. Through its second messenger, cyclic GMP, ANP inhibits Na^+ channels in the apical membrane of the cell and thereby decreases Na^+ resorption. This effect occurs predominantly in the medullary portion of the collecting duct.

5. Inhibition of ADH secretion by the posterior pituitary and ADH action on the collecting duct. This decreases water resorption by the collecting duct and thus increases excretion of water in the urine.

THESE EFFECTS INCREASE THE EXCRETION OF NaCl AND WATER BY THE KIDNEYS. Hypothetically, a reduction in the circulating levels of ANP would be expected to decrease NaCl and water excretion, but convincing evidence for this effect has not been reported.

Antidiuretic hormone

As already discussed, a decreased ECF volume stimulates ADH secretion by the posterior pituitary. The elevated levels of ADH decrease water excretion by the kidneys, which serves to reestablish euvolemia.

During euvolemia, renal NaCl excretion equals dietary NaCl intake

The maintenance of Na^+ balance and therefore euvolemia requires the precise balance between the amount of NaCl ingested and that excreted from the body. IN A EUVOLEMIC INDIVIDUAL, DAILY URINE NaCl EXCRETION EQUALS DAILY NaCl INTAKE.

The amount of NaCl excreted by the kidneys can vary widely. Under conditions of salt restriction (i.e., low-NaCl diet), virtually no Na^+ appears in the urine. Conversely, in individuals who ingest large quantities of NaCl, renal Na^+ excretion can exceed 1000 mEq/day. The renal response to variations in dietary NaCl intake may take several days. During the transition period, excretion does not match intake, and the individual is in either positive (intake exceeds excretion) or negative (intake is lower than excretion) Na^+ balance. When Na^+ balance is altered during these transition periods, the ECF volume changes in parallel. (Water excretion, regulated via the ADH system, is also adjusted to keep plasma osmolality constant, resulting in an isoosmotic change in ECF volume.) Thus with a positive Na^+ balance, the ECF volume expands (detected as an increase in body weight), whereas with a negative Na^+ balance, the ECF volume contracts (detected as a decrease in body weight). Ultimately, renal excretion reaches a new steady state, and euvolemia is reestablished as NaCl excretion once again is matched to intake. The time course for the adjustment of renal NaCl excretion to intake varies and depends on the magnitude of the change in NaCl intake. Adaptation to large changes in NaCl intake requires a longer time than adaptation to small changes in intake.

The general features of Na^+ handling along the nephron must be understood to comprehend how renal Na^+ excretion is regulated. (See Chapter 36 for the cellular mechanisms of Na^+ transport along the nephron.) Most (67%) of the filtered load of Na^+ is resorbed by the proximal tubule. An additional 25% is resorbed by the thick ascending limb of the loop of Henle and the remainder by the distal tubule and collecting duct.

In a normal adult, the filtered load of Na^+ is approximately 25,000 mEq/day. With a typical diet, less than 1% of this filtered load is excreted in the urine (approximately 140 mEq/day). Because of the large filtered load of Na^+, small changes in Na^+ resorption by the nephron can profoundly affect the Na^+ balance and thus the volume of the ECF. For example, an increase in Na^+ excretion from 1% to 3% of the filtered load represents an additional loss of approximately 500 mEq/day of Na^+. Because the ECF Na^+ concentration is 140 mEq/L, such an Na^+ loss would decrease the ECF volume by more than 3 L. (Water excretion would parallel the loss of Na^+ to maintain body fluid osmolality constant: 500 mEq/day ÷ 140 mEq/L = 3.6 L/day of fluid loss.)

During euvolemia, the resorption of Na^+ by the collecting duct is regulated to reflect dietary NaCl intake

IN EUVOLEMIC SUBJECTS, THE COLLECTING DUCT IS THE MAIN NEPHRON SEGMENT WHERE Na^+ RESORPTION IS ADJUSTED TO MAINTAIN EXCRETION AT A LEVEL APPROPRIATE FOR DIETARY INTAKE. However, other portions of the nephron are also involved in this process. Because the resorptive capacity of the collecting duct is limited, these other portions of the nephron must resorb the bulk of the filtered load of Na^+. Thus during euvolemia, Na^+ handling by the nephron can be explained by two general processes:

1. Na^+ resorption by the proximal tubule, loop of Henle, and distal tubule is regulated so that a relatively constant portion of the filtered load of Na^+ is delivered to the collecting duct. The combined action of these nephron segments resorbs approximately 96% of the filtered load of Na^+, and thus 4% of the filtered load is delivered to the beginning of the collecting duct.

2. Resorption of this remaining portion of the filtered load of Na^+ by the collecting duct is regulated so that the amount of Na^+ excreted in the urine matches the amount ingested in the diet. Thus the collecting duct makes final adjustments in Na^+ excretion to maintain the euvolemic state.

Mechanisms for maintaining constant Na^+ delivery to the collecting duct

A number of mechanisms maintain delivery of a constant fraction of the filtered load of Na^+ to the beginning of the collecting duct. These processes are autoregulation of the glomerular filtration rate (and thus the filtered load of Na^+), glomerulotubular balance, and load dependency of Na^+ resorption by the loop of Henle and the distal tubule.

Autoregulation of the glomerular filtration rate (see Chapter 35) allows maintenance of a relatively constant filtration rate over a wide range of perfusion pressures. Because the filtration rate is constant, the filtered load of Na^+ to the nephrons is also kept constant.

Despite the autoregulatory control of the glomerular filtration rate, small variations occur. If these changes were not compensated for by an appropriate adjustment in Na^+ resorption by the nephron, Na^+ excretion would change markedly. Fortunately, Na^+ resorption in the euvolemic state, especially by the proximal tubule, changes in parallel with changes in glomerular filtration rate. This phenomenon is termed **glomerulotubular (G-T) balance** (see Chapter 36). Thus if the glomerular filtration rate increases, the amount of Na^+ resorbed by the proximal tubule also increases. The opposite occurs if the glomerular filtration rate decreases.

The final mechanism that helps maintain the constant delivery of Na^+ to the beginning of the collecting duct involves the ability of the loop of Henle and the distal tubule to increase their resorptive rates in response to increased delivery of Na^+. Of these two segments, the loop of Henle, particularly the thick ascending limb, has the greater capacity to increase resorption in response to increased Na^+ delivery.

Regulation of Na^+ resorption by the collecting duct

When delivery of Na^+ is constant, small adjustments in collecting duct resorption are sufficient to balance excretion with intake. A 2% change in the fractional excretion of Na^+ produces more than a 3-L change in the volume of the ECF. Aldosterone is the primary regulator of Na^+ resorption by the collecting duct and thus of Na^+ excretion under this condition. When aldosterone levels are elevated, Na^+ resorption by the principal cells of the collecting duct is increased (excretion decreased). When aldosterone levels are decreased, Na^+ resorption is decreased (excretion increased).

In addition to aldosterone, a number of other factors, including ANP, urodilatin, and sympathetic nerves, alter Na^+ resorption by the collecting duct. However, the relative effects of these other factors on the regulation of Na^+ resorption by the collecting duct during euvolemia are unclear.

As long as variations in the dietary intake of NaCl are minor, the mechanisms previously described can regulate renal Na^+ excretion appropriately and thereby maintain euvolemia. However, these mechanisms cannot effectively handle significant changes in NaCl intake. When NaCl intake changes significantly, ECF volume expansion or ECF volume depletion occurs. In such cases, additional factors are invoked to act on the kidneys to adjust Na^+ resorption and thereby reestablish the euvolemic state.

Renal NaCl excretion is increased in response to an increase in ECF volume

During ECF volume expansion, the volume sensors send signals to the kidneys. These signals result in increased excretion of NaCl and water. The signals acting on the kidneys include:

1. Decreased activity of the renal sympathetic nerves
2. Release of ANP from atrial myocytes
3. Inhibition of ADH secretion from the posterior pituitary and decreased ADH action on the collecting duct
4. Decreased renin secretion and thus decreased production of angiotensin II
5. Decreased aldosterone secretion, which is caused by reduced angiotensin II levels, and elevated ANP levels

The integrated response of the nephron to these signals is illustrated in Figure 37-6. Three general responses to ECF volume expansion occur (the numbers correlate with those encircled in Figure 37-6):

1. **The glomerular filtration rate increases.** The glomerular filtration rate increases mainly as a result of the decrease in sympathetic nerve activity. Sympathetic fibers innervate the afferent and efferent arterioles of the glomerulus and control their diameter. Decreased sympathetic nerve activity leads to arteriolar dilation. Because the effect appears to be greater on the afferent arterioles, the hydrostatic pressure within the glomerular capillary is increased, thereby increasing the glomerular filtration rate. ANP increases the glomerular filtration rate by dilating the afferent and constricting the efferent arterioles. Thus the increased ANP levels that occur during ECF volume expansion may contribute to this response. With the increase in the glomerular filtration rate, the filtered load of Na^+ increases.

2. **The resorption of Na^+ decreases in the proximal tubule.** Several mechanisms may act to reduce Na^+ resorption by the proximal tubule, but the precise role of each of these mechanisms remains controversial. Because activation of the sympathetic nerve fibers that innervate this nephron segment stimulates Na^+ resorption, the decreased sympathetic nerve activity that results from ECF volume expansion may act to decrease Na^+ resorption. In addition, angiotensin II directly stimulates Na^+ resorption by the proximal tubule. Because angiotensin II levels are also reduced under this condition, proximal tubule Na^+ resorption may decrease as a result. The increased hydrostatic pressure within the glomerular capillaries also tends to increase the hydrostatic pressure within the peritubular capil-

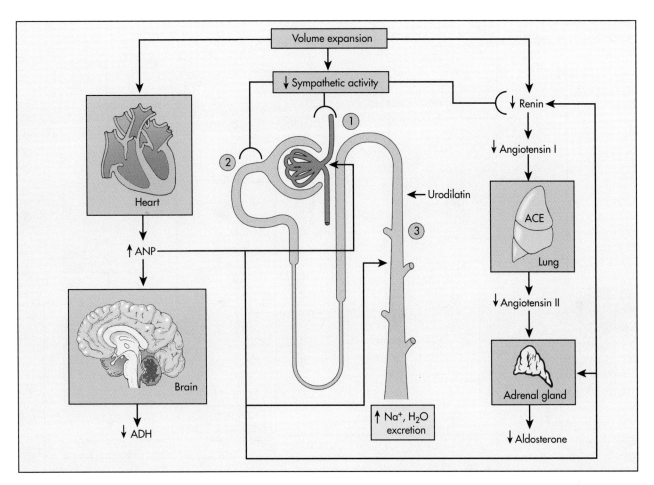

Figure 37-6 Integrated response to the expansion of ECF volume. Numbers refer to the description of the response in the text. *ACE,* Angiotensin converting enzyme.

laries. This alteration in the capillary Starling forces reduces the absorption of solute (e.g., NaCl) and water from the lateral intercellular space and thus reduces tubular resorption. (See Chapter 36 for a complete description of this mechanism.)

3. **Na$^+$ resorption decreases in the collecting duct.** Both the increase in the filtered load and the decrease in NaCl resorption by the proximal tubule result in the delivery of large amounts of NaCl to the loop of Henle and distal tubule. Because activation of the sympathetic nerves and aldosterone stimulates NaCl resorption by the loop of Henle and the distal tubule, the reduced nerve activity and low aldosterone levels that occur with ECF volume expansion could reduce NaCl resorption by these nephron segments. However because resorption by the thick ascending limb and distal tubule is load dependent, these effects are offset, and the fraction of the filtered load of Na$^+$ resorbed is actually increased. Nevertheless, the amount of Na$^+$ delivered to the beginning of the collecting duct exceeds that observed in the euvolemic state. The amount of Na$^+$ delivered to the beginning of the collecting duct varies in proportion to the degree of ECF volume expansion. This increased load of Na$^+$ overwhelms the resorptive capacity of the collecting duct, and this capacity is even further impaired by the actions of ANP (and perhaps urodilatin) and by the decrease in the circulating levels of aldosterone.

The final component in the response to ECF volume expansion is the excretion of water. As Na$^+$ excretion increases, plasma osmolality begins to fall. This decreases the secretion of ADH. ADH secretion is also decreased in response to the elevated levels of ANP. In addition, ANP (and perhaps urodilatin) inhibits the action of ADH on the collecting duct. Together, these effects decrease water resorption by the collecting duct and thereby increase water excretion by the kidneys. Thus the excretion of Na$^+$ and water occurs in concert; euvolemia is restored, and body fluid osmolality remains constant. As already noted, the time course of this response (hours to days) depends on the magnitude of the ECF volume expansion. Thus if the degree of ECF volume expansion is small, the mechanisms just described generally restore euvolemia within 24 hours. However, with

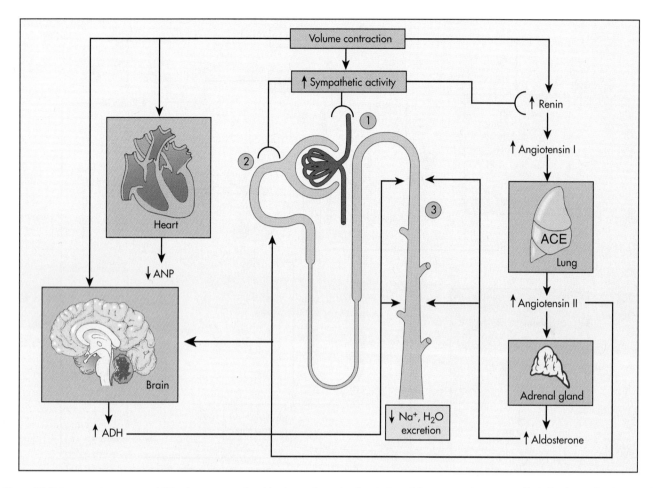

Figure 37-7 Integrated response to ECF volume contraction. Numbers refer to the description of the response in text. Urodilatin levels are also decreased (not depicted). *ACE,* Angiotensin converting enzyme.

large degrees of ECF volume expansion, the response can take several days.

In brief, the renal response to ECF volume expansion involves the integrated action of all parts of the nephron; (1) the filtered load of Na^+ is increased, (2) proximal tubule resorption is reduced (the glomerular filtration rate is increased, whereas proximal resorption is decreased; thus G-T balance does not occur under this condition), and (3) the delivery of Na^+ to the beginning of the collecting duct is increased. This increased delivery, along with the inhibition of collecting duct resorption, results in the excretion of a larger fraction of the filtered load of Na^+ and thus restores euvolemia.

Renal NaCl excretion is decreased in response to a decrease in ECF volume

During ECF volume contraction, the volume sensors send signals to the kidneys, which reduce NaCl and water excretion. The signals that act on the kidneys include:

1. Increased renal sympathetic nerve activity
2. Increased secretion of renin, which results in elevated angiotensin II levels and thus increased secretion of aldosterone by the adrenal cortex

3. Inhibition of ANP secretion by the atrial myocytes
4. Stimulation of ADH secretion by the posterior pituitary

The integrated response of the nephron to these signals is illustrated in Figure 37-7. The general response is as follows (the numbers correlate with those encircled in Figure 37-7):

1. **The glomerular filtration rate decreases.** Afferent and efferent arteriolar constriction occurs as a result of increased renal sympathetic nerve activity. The effect appears to be greater on the afferent than on the efferent arteriole. This disparity causes the hydrostatic pressure in the glomerular capillary to fall and thereby decreases the glomerular filtration rate. This decrease in the glomerular filtration rate reduces the filtered load of Na^+.

2. **Na^+ resorption by the proximal tubule is increased.** Several mechanisms augment Na^+ resorption in this segment. For example, increased sympathetic nerve activity and angiotensin II levels directly stimulate Na^+ resorption by the proximal tubule. The decreased hydrostatic pressure within the glomerular capillaries also leads

to a decrease in the hydrostatic pressure within the peritubular capillaries. This alteration in the capillary Starling forces facilitates the movement of fluid from the lateral intercellular space into the capillary and thereby stimulates the resorption of solute (e.g., NaCl) and water by the proximal tubule. (See Chapter 36 for a complete description of this mechanism.)

3. **Na$^+$ resorption by the collecting duct is enhanced.** The reduced filtered load and enhanced proximal tubule resorption decrease the delivery of Na$^+$ to the loop of Henle and the distal tubule. Increased sympathetic nerve activity and aldosterone stimulate Na$^+$ resorption by the thick ascending limb and distal tubule. Because sympathetic nerve activity is increased and aldosterone levels are elevated during ECF volume contraction, increased Na$^+$ resorption by these segments is expected. However because Na$^+$ transport by the thick ascending limb and distal tubule is load dependent, the stimulatory effects of increased sympathetic nerve activity and aldosterone are offset. Therefore the fraction of the filtered load of Na$^+$ resorbed by these segments is actually less than that which occurs in the euvolemic state. Nevertheless, the result is that less Na$^+$ is delivered to the beginning of the collecting duct, and the small amount of Na$^+$ delivered to the collecting duct is almost completely resorbed because transport in this segment is enhanced. This stimulation of Na$^+$ resorption by the collecting duct is mainly induced by increased aldosterone levels. In addition, ANP (and perhaps urodilatin), which inhibits collecting duct resorption, is not present.

Finally, water resorption by the collecting duct is enhanced by ADH, the levels of which are elevated through activation of the low- and high-pressure vascular baroreceptors as well as by the elevated levels of angiotensin II. As a result, water excretion is reduced; with the Na$^+$ retained by the kidneys, euvolemia is reestablished, and body fluid osmolality remains constant. The time course of this reexpansion (hours to days) and the degree to which euvolemia is attained depend on the magnitude of the ECF volume contraction as well as the dietary intake of Na$^+$. Thus the kidneys can reduce Na$^+$ excretion, and euvolemia is restored as NaCl is ingested. (That is, increasing the NaCl intake reestablishes euvolemia more quickly.)

In brief, the nephron's response to ECF volume contraction involves the integrated action of all its segments: (1) The filtered load of Na$^+$ is decreased, (2) proximal tubule resorption is enhanced (the glomerular filtration rate is decreased, whereas proximal resorption is increased; thus G-T balance does not occur under this condition), (3) and the delivery of Na$^+$ to the beginning of the collecting duct is reduced. This decreased delivery, together with enhanced Na$^+$ resorp-

tion by the collecting duct, virtually eliminates Na$^+$ from the urine.

SUMMARY

- The osmolality and volume of the body fluids are maintained within a narrow range despite wide variations in the intake of water and solute (mainly NaCl). The kidneys are central to this regulatory process by virtue of their ability to vary the excretion of water and solutes.

- The regulation of body fluid osmolality requires that water intake match water loss from the body. When body fluid osmolality increases, ADH secretion and thirst are stimulated, and renal water excretion decreases. When body fluid osmolality decreases, ADH secretion and thirst are suppressed, and renal water excretion increases.

- Central to the process of concentrating and diluting the urine is the loop of Henle. The resorption of NaCl by the loop of Henle allows the separation of solute and water, a process essential for the elaboration of dilute urine. By this same mechanism, the interstitial fluid in the renal medulla is rendered hyperosmotic. This hyperosmotic medullary interstitial fluid in turn provides the osmotic driving force for the resorption of water from the lumen of the collecting duct when ADH is present and thus allows the kidney to concentrate the urine.

- Disorders of water balance alter body fluid osmolality. Changes in body fluid osmolality are manifested by a change in the plasma Na$^+$ concentration. A positive water balance (intake exceeds excretion) decreases the body fluid osmolality and causes hyponatremia. A negative water balance (intake is lower than excretion) increases the body fluid osmolality and causes hypernatremia.

- Maximal excretion of solute-free water by the kidneys requires normal nephron function (especially the thick ascending limb of the loop of Henle), the adequate delivery of tubular fluid to the nephrons, and the absence of ADH. Maximal resorption of solute-free water by the kidneys requires normal nephron function (especially the thick ascending limb of the loop of Henle), adequate delivery of tubular fluid to the nephrons, a hyperosmotic medullary interstitium, the presence of ADH, and responsiveness of the collecting duct to ADH.

- The volume of the ECF is determined by Na$^+$ balance. When Na$^+$ intake exceeds excretion, a positive Na$^+$ balance exists, and ECF volume expansion occurs. Conversely, when Na$^+$ excretion exceeds Na$^+$ intake, a negative Na$^+$ balance exists, and ECF volume depletion occurs. The kidneys are the primary route for Na$^+$ excretion from the body.

- During euvolemia, Na$^+$ excretion by the kidneys is matched to the amount of Na$^+$ ingested in the diet.

■ With ECF volume expansion, low- and high-pressure volume sensors initiate a response that ultimately leads to the increased excretion of NaCl and water by the kidneys and the reestablishment of euvolemia. The components of this response include a decrease in sympathetic outflow to the kidneys, suppression of the renin-angiotensin-aldosterone system, and release of ANP from the cardiac atria. At the level of the kidneys, the glomerular filtration rate is enhanced, and therefore the filtered load of Na^+ increases. In addition, Na^+ resorption by the proximal tubule and collecting duct is reduced. Together, these changes in renal Na^+ handling enhance Na^+ excretion. With ECF volume contraction, this sequence of events is reversed.

BIBLIOGRAPHY

Bichet DG: Vasopressin receptors in health and disease, *Kidney Int* 49:1706, 1996.

Gunning ME et al: Vasoactive peptides and the kidney. In Brenner BM, ed: *The kidney,* ed 5, Philadelphia, 1996, WB Saunders.

Harris HW Jr, Zeidel ML: Cell biology of vasopressin. In Brenner BM, ed: *The kidney,* ed 5, Philadelphia, 1996, WB Saunders.

Knepper MA: Molecular physiology of urinary concentrating mechanism: regulation of aquaporin water channels by vasopressin, *Am J Physiol Renal Physiol* 272:F3, 1997.

Knepper MA, Gottschalk CW: Regulation of water balance: urine concentration and dilution. In Schrier RW, Gottschalk CW, eds: *Diseases of the kidney,* ed 6, Boston, 1997, Little, Brown.

Knepper MA, Rector FC Jr: Urine concentration and dilution. In Brenner BM, ed: *The kidney,* ed 5, Philadelphia, 1996, WB Saunders.

Knepper MA et al: Renal aquaporins, *Kidney Int* 49:1712, 1996.

Levin ER et al: Mechanisms of disease: natriuretic peptides, *New Engl J Med* 339:321, 1998.

Matsusaka T, Ichikawa I: Biological functions of angiotensin and its receptors, *Annu Rev Physiol* 59:395, 1997.

Miller JA et al: Control of extracellular fluid volume and the pathophysiology of edema. In Brenner BM, ed: *The kidney,* ed 5, Philadelphia, 1996, WB Saunders.

Robertson GL, Berl T: Pathophysiology of water metabolism. In Brenner BM, ed: *The kidney,* ed 5, Philadelphia, 1996, WB Saunders.

Sands JM et al: Urea transporters in kidney and erythrocytes, *Am J Physiol Renal Physiol* 273:F321, 1997.

Teitelbaum I et al: Diabetes insipidus and the syndrome of inappropriate antidiuretic hormone secretion. In Brenner BM, ed: *The kidney,* ed 5, Philadelphia, 1996, WB Saunders.

Wagner C, Kurtz A: Regulation of renal renin release, *Curr Opin Nephrol Hyperten* 7:437, 1998.

▷ **CASE STUDIES**

Case 37-1

A previously healthy 45-year-old man is admitted to the hospital with pneumonia. His blood pressure is 140/75 mm Hg, and his plasma Na^+ concentration is 142 mEq/L; both are within the normal range. His condition is treated with intravenous antibiotics and fluids. On the third hospital day, his blood pressure is unchanged, but his plasma Na^+ concentration is 130 mEq/L. His urine osmolality is 450 mOsm/kg H_2O. He has no edema, and his blood pressure does not change when he goes from a reclining to a standing position.

1. **What is the most likely cause for the development of hyponatremia in this man?**
   A. Decreased ingestion of NaCl
   B. Increased renal excretion of NaCl
   C. Positive water balance
   D. Shift of water from the ICF to the ECF
   E. Shift of Na^+ from the ECF to the ICF

2. **What would be the most appropriate way to return the plasma Na^+ concentration to its normal value?**
   A. Administer ADH.
   B. Restrict water intake.
   C. Increase water intake.
   D. Restrict NaCl intake.
   E. Increase NaCl intake.

Case 37-2

A 56-year-old woman has a history of congestive heart failure. Because of poor cardiac output, she is easily fatigued and has developed generalized edema (i.e., increased interstitial fluid volume) with swelling of her ankles and legs. Her plasma Na^+ concentration has decreased from a normal value of 145 to 130 mEq/L. As part of her therapy, she receives a drug that inhibits ACE.

1. **What would be the most appropriate change in this woman's intake of NaCl and water?**

	Water Intake	NaCl Intake
A.	Increase	Increase
B.	Increase	Restrict
C.	Restrict	Increase
D.	Restrict	Restrict
E.	No change	No change

2. **Administration of an ACE inhibitor would be expected to have which of the following effects on circulating levels of renin, aldosterone, and bradykinin?**

	Renin	Aldosterone	Bradykinin
A.	Decreased	Decreased	Decreased
B.	Decreased	Decreased	Increased
C.	Increased	Increased	Decreased
D.	Increased	Decreased	Increased
E.	Increased	Increased	Increased

CHAPTER 38

Potassium, Calcium, and Phosphate Homeostasis

OBJECTIVES

- Explain how K^+ is crucial for many cellular functions.
- Describe how K^+ homeostasis is maintained by hormones and the kidneys.
- Describe the regulation of K^+ excretion by the kidneys.
- Describe how pathophysiological factors alter K^+ homeostasis.
- Explain how Ca^{++} and inorganic phosphate subserve many important cellular functions.
- Describe how the kidneys regulate Ca^{++} and inorganic phosphate homeostasis.
- Describe how hormones regulate plasma levels of Ca^{++} and inorganic phosphate.
- Describe how the kidneys regulate the excretion of Ca^{++} and inorganic phosphate.

The kidneys play an essential role in regulating the amount of several important inorganic ions in the body including K^+, Ca^{++}, and phosphate (Pi). So that appropriate balance, or homeostasis, can be maintained, the excretion of these electrolytes must be equal to their daily intake. If the intake of an electrolyte exceeds its excretion, the amount of this electrolyte in the body increases, and the individual is in positive balance for that electrolyte. Conversely, if excretion of an electrolyte exceeds its intake, its amount in the body decreases, and the individual is in negative balance for that electrolyte. For K^+, Ca^{++}, and Pi the kidneys are the sole or primary route of excretion from the body. Accordingly, this chapter focuses on how the kidneys maintain K^+, Ca^{++}, and Pi homeostasis.

K^+, One of the Most Abundant Cations in the Body, Is Critical for Many Cell Functions

Despite wide fluctuations in dietary K^+ intake, its concentration ($[K^+]$) in cells and extracellular fluid (ECF) remains remarkably constant. Two sets of regulatory mechanisms safeguard K^+ homeostasis. First, several mechanisms regulate the $[K^+]$ in the ECF. Second, other mechanisms maintain the amount of K^+ in the body constant by adjusting renal K^+ excretion to match dietary K^+ intake. It is the kidneys that regulate K^+ excretion.

Total body K^+ is 50 mEq/kg of body weight, or 3500 mEq for a 70-kg individual. A total of 98% of the K^+ in the body is located within cells, where its average $[K^+]$ is 150 mEq/L. A high intracellular $[K^+]$ is required for many cell functions, including cell growth and division and volume regulation. Only 2% of total body K^+ is located in the ECF, where its normal concentration is approximately 4 mEq/L. A $[K^+]$ in the ECF that exceeds 5.0 mEq/L constitutes **hyperkalemia.** Conversely, a $[K^+]$ in the ECF of less than 3.5 mEq/L constitutes **hypokalemia.**

The large concentration difference of K^+ across cell membranes (approximately 146 mEq/L) is maintained by the operation of Na^+,K^+-ATPase. This K^+ gradient is important in maintaining the potential difference across cell membranes (see Chapters 2 and 17). Thus K^+ is critical for the excitability of nerve and muscle cells as well as for the contractility of cardiac, skeletal, and smooth muscle cells.

Cardiac arrhythmias are produced by both hypokalemia and hyperkalemia. The first sign of hyperkalemia is the appearance of tall, thin T waves. Further increases in the plasma $[K^+]$ prolong the PR interval, depress the ST segment, and lengthen the QRS interval. Finally, as the plasma $[K^+]$ approaches 10 mEq/L, the P wave disappears, the QRS interval broadens, the electrocardiogram (ECG) appears as a sine wave, and the ventricles fibrillate (i.e., manifest rapid, uncoordinated contractions of muscle fibers). Hypokalemia prolongs the QT interval, inverts the T wave, and lowers the ST segment. The ECG is a fast and easy way to determine whether changes in the plasma $[K^+]$ influence the heart and other excitable cells. In contrast, measurements of the plasma $[K^+]$ by the clinical laboratory require a blood sample, and values are often not immediately available.

After a meal, the K^+ absorbed by the gastrointestinal tract enters the ECF within minutes (Figure 38-1). If the K^+ ingested during a normal meal ($\approx$33 mEq) were to remain in the ECF compartment, the plasma $[K^+]$ would increase by a potentially lethal 2.4 mEq/L (33 mEq added to 14 L of ECF):

$$\frac{33 \text{ mEq}}{14 \text{ L}} = \Delta 2.4 \text{ mEq/L}$$

This rise in the plasma $[K^+]$ is prevented by the rapid uptake of K^+ into cells. Because the excretion of K^+ by the kidneys after a meal is relatively slow (hours), the uptake of K^+ by cells is essential to prevent life-threatening hyperkalemia. Maintaining total body K^+ constant requires that all the K^+ absorbed by the gastrointestinal tract must eventually be excreted by the kidneys. This process requires about 6 hours.

Several Hormones Promote the Uptake of K^+ into Cells After a Rise in Plasma K^+ Concentration

As illustrated in Figure 38-1, several hormones, including epinephrine, insulin, and aldosterone, increase K^+ uptake into skeletal muscle, liver, bone, and red blood cells by stimulating Na^+,K^+-ATPase. Acute stimulation of K^+ uptake (i.e., within minutes) is mediated by an increased turnover rate of existing Na^+,K^+-ATPase, whereas the chronic increase in K^+ uptake (i.e., within hours to days) is mediated by an increase in the quantity of Na^+,K^+-ATPase. A rise in the plasma $[K^+]$ that follows K^+ absorption by the gastrointestinal tract stimulates insulin secretion from the pancreas, aldosterone release from the adrenal cortex, and epinephrine secretion from the adrenal medulla. In contrast, a decrease in the plasma $[K^+]$ inhibits the release of these hormones. Whereas insulin and epinephrine act within a few minutes, aldosterone requires about an hour to stimulate K^+ uptake into cells.

Epinephrine
Catecholamines affect the distribution of K^+ across cell membranes by activating α- and β_2-adrenergic receptors. The stimulation of α-receptors releases K^+ from cells, especially in the liver, whereas the stimulation of β_2-receptors promotes K^+ uptake by cells.

For example, the activation of α-receptors after exercise is important in preventing hypokalemia. The rise in plasma $[K^+]$ after a K^+-rich meal is greater if the patient has been pretreated with propranolol, a β-adrenergic receptor antagonist. Furthermore, the release of epinephrine during stress (e.g., myocardial ischemia) can rapidly lower the plasma $[K^+]$.

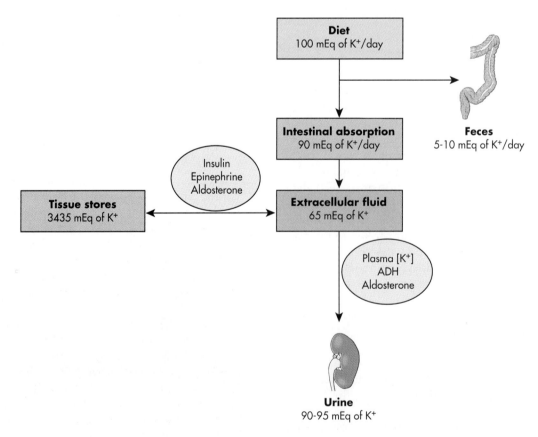

Figure 38-1 Overview of K^+ homeostasis. See text for details.

Insulin

Insulin also stimulates K^+ uptake into cells (see also Chapter 42). The importance of insulin is illustrated by two observations. First, the rise in plasma $[K^+]$ after a K^+-rich meal is greater in patients with diabetes mellitus (i.e., insulin deficiency) than in normal people. Second, insulin (and glucose to prevent insulin-induced hypoglycemia) can be infused to correct hyperkalemia. Insulin is the most important hormone that shifts K^+ into cells after the ingestion of K^+ in a meal.

Aldosterone

Aldosterone, like catecholamines and insulin, also promotes K^+ uptake into cells. A rise in aldosterone levels (e.g., primary aldosteronism) causes hypokalemia, whereas a fall in aldosterone levels (e.g., Addison's disease) causes hyperkalemia. As discussed later, aldosterone also stimulates urinary K^+ excretion. Thus aldosterone alters the plasma $[K^+]$ by acting on K^+ uptake into cells and by altering urinary K^+ excretion.

Some Hormones and Factors Disturb Normal K^+ Uptake by Cells

Acid-base balance

In general, metabolic acidosis increases the plasma $[K^+]$, whereas metabolic alkalosis decreases it. In contrast, respiratory acid-base disorders have little or no effect on the plasma $[K^+]$. Metabolic acidosis produced by the addition of inorganic acids (e.g., HCl, H_2SO_4) increases the plasma $[K^+]$ much more than an equivalent acidosis produced by the accumulation of organic acids (e.g., lactic acid, acetic acid, keto acids). The reduced pH (i.e., increased H^+ concentration $[H^+]$) promotes the movement of H^+ into cells and the reciprocal movement of K^+ out of cells. Metabolic alkalosis has the opposite effect; the plasma $[K^+]$ decreases as K^+ moves into cells and H^+ exits. The mechanism responsible for this shift is not fully understood. The movement of H^+ may occur as the cells buffer changes in the $[H^+]$ of the ECF. As H^+ moves across the cell membranes, K^+ moves in the opposite direction, and thus cations are neither gained nor lost across cell membranes. Although organic acids produce a metabolic acidosis, they do not cause significant hyperkalemia.

Two explanations have been suggested for the reduced ability of organic acids to cause hyperkalemia. First, the organic anion may enter the cell with H^+ and thereby eliminate the need for K^+/H^+ exchange across the membrane. Second, organic anions may stimulate insulin secretion, which moves K^+ into cells. This movement may counteract the direct effect of the acidosis, which moves K^+ out of cells.

Plasma osmolality

The osmolality of the plasma also influences the distribution of K^+ across cell membranes. An increase in the osmolality of the ECF enhances K^+ release by cells and thus increases extracellular $[K^+]$. The plasma K^+ level may increase by 0.4 to 0.8 mEq/L for an elevation of 10 mOsm/kg H_2O in plasma osmolality. Hypoosmolality has the opposite action. The alterations in plasma $[K^+]$ associated with changes in osmolality are related to changes in cell volume. For example, as plasma osmolality increases, water leaves cells because of the osmotic gradient across the plasma membrane. Water leaves cells until the intracellular osmolality equals that of the ECF. This loss of water shrinks cells and causes the cell $[K^+]$ to rise. The rise in intracellular $[K^+]$ provides a driving force for the exit of K^+ from cells. This sequence increases plasma $[K^+]$. A fall in plasma osmolality has the opposite effect.

Cell lysis

Cell lysis causes hyperkalemia, which results from the addition of intracellular K^+ to the ECF. Severe trauma (e.g., burns) and some diseases such as **tumor lysis syndrome** and **rhabdomyolysis** (i.e., destruction of skeletal muscle) destroy cells and release K^+ and other cell solutes into the ECF. In addition, gastric ulcers may cause the seepage of red blood cells into the gastrointestinal tract. The blood cells are digested, and the K^+ released from the cells is absorbed and can cause hyperkalemia.

Exercise

During exercise, more K^+ is released from skeletal muscle cells than during rest. The ensuing hyperkalemia depends on the degree of exercise. In people walking slowly the plasma $[K^+]$ increases by 0.3 mEq/L. The plasma $[K^+]$ may increase by at least 2.0 mEq/L with vigorous exercise.

Exercise-induced changes in the plasma $[K^+]$ usually do not produce symptoms and are reversed after several minutes of rest. However, exercise can lead to life-threatening hyperkalemia in individuals (1) who have endocrine disorders that affect the release of insulin, epinephrine, or aldosterone; (2) whose ability to excrete K^+ is impaired (e.g., renal failure); or (3) who take certain medications, such as β-adrenergic blockers. For example, during exercise, the plasma $[K^+]$ may increase by at least 2 to 4 mEq/L in individuals who take β-adrenergic receptor antagonists for hypertension.

BECAUSE ACID-BASE BALANCE, PLASMA OSMOLALITY, CELL LYSIS, AND EXERCISE DO NOT MAINTAIN THE PLASMA $[K^+]$ AT A NORMAL VALUE, THEY DO NOT CONTRIBUTE TO K^+ HOMEOSTASIS. The extent to which these pathophysiological states alter the plasma $[K^+]$ depends on the integrity of the homeostatic mechanisms that regulate plasma $[K^+]$ (e.g., the secretion of epinephrine, insulin, and aldosterone).

The Kidneys Play a Major Role in Maintaining K⁺ Balance

As illustrated in Figure 38-1, the kidneys excrete 90% to 95% of the K⁺ ingested in the diet. Excretion equals intake even when intake increases by as much as tenfold. This balance of urinary excretion and dietary intake underscores the importance of the kidneys in maintaining K⁺ homeostasis. Although small amounts of K⁺ are lost each day in the stool and sweat (approximately 5% to 10% of the K⁺ ingested in the diet), this amount is essentially constant, is not regulated, and therefore is relatively less important than the K⁺ excreted by the kidneys. K⁺ secretion from the blood into the tubular fluid by the cells of the distal tubule and collecting duct system is the key factor in determining urinary K⁺ excretion (Figure 38-2).

Because K⁺ is not bound to plasma proteins, it is freely filtered by the glomerulus. When normal individuals have an average diet, urinary K⁺ excretion is about 15% of the amount filtered. Accordingly, K⁺ must be resorbed along the nephron. When dietary K⁺ intake increases, however, K⁺ excretion can exceed the amount filtered. Thus K⁺ can also be secreted.

The proximal tubule resorbs about 67% of the filtered K⁺ under most conditions. Approximately 20% of the filtered K⁺ is resorbed by the loop of Henle, and as with the proximal tubule, the amount resorbed is a constant fraction of the amount filtered. In contrast to these segments, which can only resorb K⁺, the distal tubule and collecting duct are able to resorb or secrete K⁺. The rate of K⁺ resorption or secretion by the distal tubule and collecting duct depends on a variety of hormones and factors. When K⁺ intake is normal (100 mEq/day), K⁺ is secreted. A rise in dietary K⁺ intake increases K⁺ secretion. K⁺ secretion can increase the amount of K⁺ that appears in the urine so that it approaches 80% of the amount filtered (Figure 38-2). In contrast, a low-K⁺ diet activates K⁺ resorption along the distal tubule and collecting duct so that urinary excretion falls to about 1% of the K⁺ filtered by the glomerulus (Figure 38-2). The kidneys cannot reduce K⁺ excretion to the same low levels as they can for Na⁺ (0.2%). Therefore hypokalemia can develop in individuals placed on a K⁺-deficient diet. Because the magnitude and direction of K⁺ transport by the distal tubule and collecting duct are variable, the overall rate of urinary K⁺ excretion is determined by these tubular segments.

> In individuals with advanced renal disease, the kidneys are unable to eliminate K⁺ from the body. The plasma [K⁺] therefore rises. The resulting hyperkalemia reduces the resting membrane potential (i.e., the voltage becomes less negative), which decreases the excitability of neurons, cardiac cells, and muscle cells by inactivating fast Na⁺ channels in the membrane. Severe, rapid increases in the plasma [K⁺] can lead to cardiac arrest and death. In con-

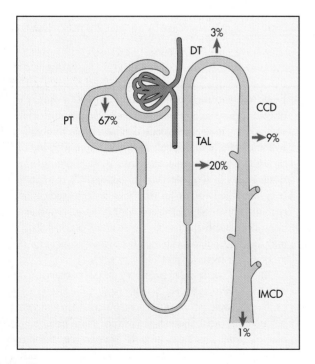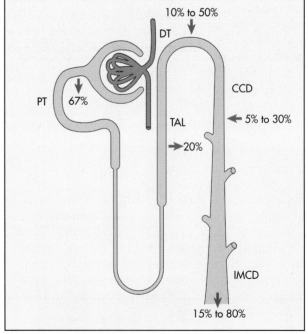

Figure 38-2 K⁺ transport along the nephron. K⁺ excretion depends on the rate and direction of K⁺ transport by the distal tubule and collecting duct. Percentages refer to the amount of filtered K⁺ resorbed or secreted by each nephron segment. *Left,* Dietary K⁺ depletion. An amount of K⁺ equal to 1% of the filtered load of K⁺ is excreted. *Right,* Normal and increased dietary K⁺ intake. An amount of K⁺ equal to 15% to 80% of the filtered load is excreted. *CCD,* Cortical collecting duct; *DT,* distal tubule; *IMCD,* inner medullary collecting duct; *PT,* proximal tubule; *TAL,* thick ascending limb.

trast, in patients taking diuretic drugs for hypertension, urinary K^+ excretion often exceeds dietary K^+ intake. Accordingly, the K^+ balance is negative, and hypokalemia develops. This decline in the extracellular $[K^+]$ hyperpolarizes the resting cell membrane (i.e., the voltage becomes more negative) and reduces the excitability of neurons, cardiac cells, and muscle cells. Severe hypokalemia can lead to paralysis, cardiac arrhythmias, and death. Hypokalemia can also impair the ability of the kidneys to concentrate the urine and can stimulate the renal production of NH_4^+. Therefore the maintenance of a high intracellular $[K^+]$, a low extracellular $[K^+]$, and a high K^+ concentration gradient across cell membranes is essential for a number of cellular functions.

The cellular mechanism of K^+ secretion by principal cells in the distal tubule and collecting duct is a two-step process

The two processes of cellular K^+ secretion are: (1) K^+ uptake from blood across the basolateral membrane by Na^+,K^+-ATPase and (2) diffusion of K^+ from the cell into the tubular fluid. Na^+,K^+-ATPase creates a high intracellular $[K^+]$, which provides the chemical driving force for K^+ exit across the apical membrane through K^+ channels. Although K^+ channels are also present in the basolateral membrane, K^+ preferentially leaves the cell across the apical membrane and enters the tubular fluid. K^+ transport follows this route for two reasons. First, the electrochemical gradient of K^+ across the apical membrane favors its downhill movement into the tubular fluid. Second, the permeability of the apical membrane to K^+ is greater than that of the basolateral membrane. Therefore K^+ preferentially diffuses across the apical membrane into the tubular fluid. The three major factors that control the rate of K^+ secretion by the distal tubule and the collecting duct are:

1. The activity of Na^+,K^+-ATPase
2. The driving force (electrochemical gradient) for K^+ movement across the apical membrane
3. The permeability of the apical membrane to K^+

Every change in K^+ secretion results from an alteration in one or more of these factors.

In contrast, the cellular pathways and mechanisms of K^+ resorption in the distal tubule and collecting duct are not as well understood. Intercalated cells may resorb K^+ via an H^+,K^+-ATPase transport mechanism located in the apical membrane. This transporter mediates K^+ uptake in exchange for H^+. However, the pathway of K^+ exit from intercalated cells into the blood is unknown. The resorption of K^+ is activated by a low K^+-diet.

THE REGULATION OF K^+ EXCRETION IS ACHIEVED MAINLY BY ALTERATIONS IN K^+ SECRETION BY PRINCIPAL CELLS OF THE DISTAL TUBULE AND COLLECTING DUCT. Plasma $[K^+]$ and aldosterone are the major physiological regulators of K^+ secretion. Antidiuretic hormone (ADH) also stimulates K^+ secretion; however, it is less important than the plasma

$[K^+]$ and aldosterone. Other factors, including the flow rate of tubular fluid and acid-base balance, influence K^+ secretion by the distal tubule and collecting duct. However, they are not homeostatic mechanisms because they disturb K^+ balance.

Hormones and the plasma K^+ concentration regulate urinary K^+ excretion

Plasma K^+ concentration

Plasma $[K^+]$ is an important determinant of K^+ secretion by the distal tubule and collecting duct. Hyperkalemia (e.g., resulting from a high-K^+ diet or from rhabdomyolysis) stimulates secretion within minutes. Several mechanisms are involved. First, hyperkalemia stimulates Na^+,K^+-ATPase and thereby increases K^+ uptake across the basolateral membrane. This uptake raises the intracellular $[K^+]$ and increases the electrochemical driving force for K^+ exit across the apical membrane. Second, hyperkalemia also increases the permeability of the apical membrane to K^+. Third, hyperkalemia stimulates aldosterone secretion by the adrenal cortex, which, as discussed later, acts synergistically with the plasma $[K^+]$ to stimulate K^+ secretion. Fourth, hyperkalemia also increases the flow rate of tubular fluid, which, as discussed later, stimulates K^+ secretion by the distal tubule and collecting duct.

Hypokalemia (e.g., caused by a low-K^+ diet or diarrhea) decreases K^+ secretion via actions opposite to those described for hyperkalemia. Hence hypokalemia inhibits Na^+,K^+-ATPase, decreases the electrochemical driving force for K^+ efflux across the apical membrane, reduces the permeability of the apical membrane to K^+, and reduces plasma aldosterone levels.

Chronic hypokalemia (plasma $[K^+] < 3.5$ mEq/L) occurs most often in patients who receive diuretics for hypertension. Hypokalemia also occurs in patients who vomit, have nasogastric suction, have diarrhea, abuse laxatives, or have hyperaldosteronism. Hypokalemia occurs because the excretion of K^+ by the kidneys exceeds the dietary intake of K^+. Vomiting, nasogastric suction, diuretics, and diarrhea all can decrease the ECF, which in turn stimulates aldosterone secretion. Because aldosterone stimulates K^+ excretion by the kidneys, its action contributes to the development of hypokalemia.

Chronic hyperkalemia (plasma $[K^+] > 5.0$ mEq/L) occurs most frequently in individuals with reduced urine flows, low plasma aldosterone levels, and renal disease in which the glomerular filtration rate falls to below 20% of normal. In these individuals, hyperkalemia occurs because the excretion of K^+ by the kidneys is less than the dietary intake of K^+. Less common causes for hyperkalemia occur in people with deficiencies of insulin, epinephrine, and aldosterone secretion or people with metabolic acidosis caused by inorganic acids.

Aldosterone

A chronic (i.e., ≥24 hours) elevation in the plasma aldosterone concentration enhances K^+ secretion across the distal tubule and collecting duct by increasing the amount of Na^+,K^+-ATPase in principal cells. This increase elevates the cell $[K^+]$. Aldosterone also increases the driving force for K^+ exit across the apical membrane and increases the permeability of the apical membrane to K^+. Aldosterone secretion is increased by hyperkalemia and by angiotensin II (after activation of the renin-angiotensin system). Aldosterone secretion is decreased by hypokalemia and atrial natriuretic peptide.

Although an acute (i.e., within hours) increase in aldosterone levels enhances the activity of Na^+,K^+-ATPase, K^+, excretion does not increase. The reason for this lack of increase relates to the effect of aldosterone on Na^+ resorption and tubular flow. Aldosterone stimulates Na^+ resorption and thereby water resorption and thus decreases tubular flow. The decrease in flow in turn decreases K^+ secretion (as discussed in more detail later). However, chronic stimulation of Na^+ resorption expands the ECF and thereby returns tubular flow to normal. These actions allow the direct stimulatory effect of aldosterone on the distal tubule and collecting duct to increase K^+ excretion.

Glucocorticoids

Glucocorticoids also stimulate K^+ excretion. However, this effect is indirect and is mediated by an increase in the glomerular filtration rate, which increases tubular flow.

Antidiuretic hormone

ADH increases the electrochemical driving force for K^+ exit across the apical membrane of principal cells by stimulating Na^+ uptake across the apical membrane of principal cells. The increased Na^+ uptake reduces the electrical potential difference across the apical membrane (i.e., the interior of the cell becomes less negatively charged). Despite this effect, ADH does not change K^+ secretion by these nephron segments. The reason for this relates to the effect of ADH on tubular fluid flow. ADH decreases tubular fluid flow by stimulating water resorption. The decrease in tubular flow in turn decreases K^+ secretion (explained later). The inhibitory effect of a decreased flow of tubular fluid offsets the stimulatory effect of ADH on the electrochemical driving force for K^+ exit across the apical membrane. If ADH did not increase the electrochemical gradient, favoring K^+ secretion, urinary K^+ excretion would fall as ADH levels increase, and urinary flow rates decrease. Hence K^+ balance would change in response to alterations in water balance. Thus the effects of ADH on the electrochemical driving force for K^+ exit across the apical membrane and tubule flow enable urinary K^+ excretion to be maintained constant despite wide fluctuations in water excretion.

K^+ excretion is perturbed by changes in the flow of tubular fluid and disorders of acid-base balance

Flow of tubular fluid

A rise in the flow of tubular fluid (e.g., with diuretic treatment, ECF volume expansion) stimulates K^+ secretion within minutes, whereas a fall (e.g., ECF volume contraction caused by hemorrhage, severe vomiting, or diarrhea) reduces K^+ secretion by the distal tubule and collecting duct. Increments in tubular fluid flow are more effective in stimulating K^+ secretion as dietary K^+ intake is increased. Alterations in tubular fluid flow influence K^+ secretion by changing the driving force for K^+ exit across the apical membrane. As K^+ is secreted into the tubular fluid, the $[K^+]$ of the fluid increases. This increase reduces the electrochemical driving force for K^+ exit across the apical membrane and thereby reduces the rate of K^+ secretion. An increase in tubular fluid flow minimizes the rise in tubular fluid $[K^+]$ as the secreted K^+ is washed downstream.

A second mechanism responsible for the flow-dependent stimulation of K^+ secretion is related to Na^+ resorption. A rise in flow increases the amount of Na^+ that enters the distal tubule and collecting duct, and this in turn enhances Na^+ resorption. The increase in Na^+ resorption stimulates K^+ uptake across the basolateral membrane by increasing the activity of Na^+,K^+-ATPase, and this action promotes K^+ secretion. Because diuretic drugs increase the flow of tubular fluid through the distal tubule and collecting duct, they also enhance urinary K^+ excretion. In contrast, a decline in tubular fluid flow inhibits K^+ secretion. This response occurs because a decline in the tubular fluid flow facilitates the rise in tubular fluid $[K^+]$ and thereby reduces secretion.

Acid-base balance

Another factor that modulates K^+ secretion is the $[H^+]$ of the ECF. Acute alterations (within minutes to hours) in the pH of the plasma influence K^+ secretion by the distal tubule and collecting duct. Alkalosis (i.e., a plasma pH above normal) increases K^+ secretion, whereas acidosis (i.e., a plasma pH below normal) decreases it. An acute acidosis reduces K^+ secretion via two mechanisms: (1) It inhibits Na^+,K^+-ATPase and thereby reduces the cell $[K^+]$ and the electrochemical driving force for K^+ exit across the apical membrane, and (2) it reduces the permeability of the apical membrane to K^+. Alkalosis has the opposite effects.

The effect of metabolic acidosis on K^+ excretion is time dependent. When metabolic acidosis lasts for several days, urinary K^+ excretion is stimulated. This occurs because chronic metabolic acidosis decreases the resorption of water and sodium chloride (NaCl) by the proximal tubule by inhibiting Na^+,K^+-ATPase. Hence the flow of tubular fluid is augmented through the distal tubule and collecting duct. The inhibition of proxi-

Table 38-1	Effects of Hormones and Other Factors on K$^+$ Secretion by the Distal Tubule and Collecting Duct		
Condition	**Direct or Indirect**	**Flow**	**Urinary Excretion**
Hyperkalemia	↑	↑	↑
Aldosterone			
Acute	↑	↓	NC
Chronic	↑	NC	↑
Glucocorticoids	NC	↑	↑
ADH	↑	↓	NC
Acidosis			
Acute	↓	NC	↓
Chronic	↓	↑↑	↑
Alkalosis	↑	↑	↑↑

Modified from Field MJ, Berliner RW, Giebisch GH. In Narins R, ed: *Textbook of nephrology: clinical disorders of fluid and electrolyte metabolism,* ed 5, New York, 1994, McGraw-Hill.
NC, No change.

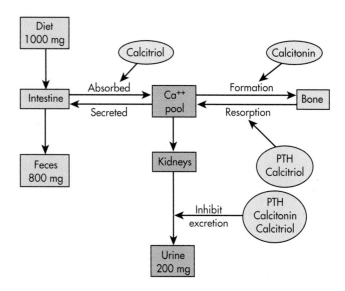

Figure 38-3 Overview of Ca^{++} homeostasis. See text for details. *PTH,* Parathyroid hormone.

mal tubular water and NaCl resorption also decreases the ECF and thereby stimulates aldosterone secretion. In addition, chronic acidosis, caused by inorganic acids, increases the plasma [K$^+$], which stimulates aldosterone secretion. The rise in tubular fluid flow, plasma [K$^+$], and aldosterone levels offsets the effects of acidosis on the cell [K$^+$] and apical membrane permeability, and K$^+$ secretion rises. Thus metabolic acidosis may either inhibit or stimulate K$^+$ excretion, depending on the duration of the disturbance.

As discussed earlier, the rate of urinary K$^+$ excretion is frequently determined by simultaneous changes in hormone levels, acid-base balance, or flow (Table 38-1). The powerful effect of flow often enhances or opposes the response of the distal tubule and collecting duct to hormones and changes in acid-base balance. This interaction can be beneficial in the case of hyperkalemia, in which the change in flow enhances K$^+$ excretion and thereby restores K$^+$ homeostasis. However, this interaction can also be detrimental, as in the case of alkalosis, in which changes in flow and acid-base status alter K$^+$ homeostasis.

Ca^{++} and Inorganic Phosphate Are Multivalent Ions that Have Many Complex and Vital Functions

In a normal adult, the renal excretion of Ca^{++} and Pi is balanced by gastrointestinal absorption. If the plasma concentrations decline substantially, gastrointestinal absorption, bone resorption, and renal tubular resorption increase and return plasma concentrations of Ca^{++} and Pi to normal levels. During growth and during pregnancy, intestinal absorption exceeds urinary excretion, and these ions accumulate in newly formed fe-

tal tissue and bone. In contrast, bone disease (e.g., **osteoporosis**) or a decline in lean body mass increases urinary loss of multivalent ions without a change in intestinal absorption. In these conditions, Ca^{++} and Pi are lost from the body. In conjunction with the gastrointestinal tract and bones, the kidneys play a major role in maintaining plasma Ca^{++} and Pi levels.

Ca^{++} plays a major role in many cellular processes

Cellular processes in which Ca^{++} plays a part include bone formation, cell division and growth, blood coagulation, hormone-response coupling, and electrical stimulus-response coupling (e.g., muscle contraction, neurotransmitter release). A total of 99% of Ca^{++} is stored in bone, approximately 1% is found in the intracellular fluid (ICF), and 0.1% is located in the ECF. The total Ca^{++} concentration ([Ca^{++}]) in plasma is 10 mg/dl (2.5 mM or 5 mEq/L), and its concentration is normally maintained within very narrow limits. A low ionized plasma [Ca^{++}] **(hypocalcemia)** increases the excitability of nerve and muscle cells and can lead to hypocalcemic **tetany,** which is characterized by skeletal muscle spasms. An elevated ionized plasma [Ca^{++}] **(hypercalcemia)** may decrease neuromuscular excitability or produce cardiac arrhythmias, lethargy, disorientation, and even death.

Ca^{++} HOMEOSTASIS DEPENDS ON TWO FACTORS: (1) THE TOTAL AMOUNT OF Ca^{++} IN THE BODY AND (2) THE DISTRIBUTION OF Ca^{++} BETWEEN BONE AND THE ECF. The total body Ca^{++} level is determined by the relative amounts of Ca^{++} absorbed by the gastrointestinal tract and excreted by the kidneys (Figure 38-3). Ca^{++} is absorbed by the gastrointestinal tract through an active, carrier-mediated transport mechanism that is stimulated by **calcitriol,** a metabolite of vitamin D_3 (see also Chapters 34 and 43). Net Ca^{++} absorption is normally 200 mg/day, but it can increase to 600 mg/day when calcitriol levels rise. In adults, Ca^{++} excretion by the kidneys equals the amount absorbed by the gastrointestinal tract (200 mg/day), and it changes in parallel with the resorption of Ca^{++} by the gastrointestinal tract. Thus in adults, Ca^{++} balance is maintained because the amount of Ca^{++} ingested in an average diet (1000 mg/day) equals the amount lost in the feces (800 mg/day, the amount that escapes absorption by the gastrointestinal tract) plus the amount excreted in the urine (200 mg/day).

The second factor that controls Ca^{++} homeostasis is the distribution of Ca^{++} between bone and the ECF. Three hormones (parathyroid hormone [PTH], calcitriol, and calcitonin) are the most important hormones that regulate the distribution of Ca^{++} between bone and the ECF and thereby regulate the plasma $[Ca^{++}]$. In humans, however, calcitonin may not participate much in Ca^{++} homeostasis. PTH is secreted by the parathyroid glands, and its secretion is stimulated by a decline in the plasma $[Ca^{++}]$ (i.e., hypocalcemia). PTH increases the plasma $[Ca^{++}]$ by (1) stimulating bone resorption, (2) increasing Ca^{++} resorption by the kidneys, and (3) stimulating the production of calcitriol, which in turn increases Ca^{++} absorption by the gastrointestinal tract and stimulates bone resorption. The production of calcitriol is stimulated by hypocalcemia and hypophosphatemia. The effect of hypocalcemia is secondary to the increased levels of PTH resulting from the decrease in plasma $[Ca^{++}]$. Calcitriol increases the plasma $[Ca^{++}]$ via actions similar to those of PTH. Calcitonin is secreted by parafollicular C-cells, and its secretion is stimulated by hypercalcemia. Calcitonin decreases the plasma $[Ca^{++}]$ mainly by stimulating bone formation (i.e., deposition of Ca^{++} in bone). Figure 38-4 illus-

trates the relationship between the plasma $[Ca^{++}]$ and plasma levels of PTH and calcitonin.

> Conditions that lower PTH levels (i.e., vitamin D_3 deficiency, hypoparathyroidism after parathyroidectomy for an adenoma) reduce the plasma $[Ca^{++}]$, which can cause hypocalcemic tetany (intermittent muscular contractions). In severe cases, **hypocalcemic tetany** can cause death by asphyxiation. Hypercalcemia can also cause lethal cardiac arrhythmias and decreased neuromuscular excitability. Clinically, the most common causes of hypercalcemia are primary hyperparathyroidism and malignancy-associated hypercalcemia. Primary hyperparathyroidism results from the overproduction of PTH caused by a tumor of the parathyroid glands. In contrast, malignancy-associated hypercalcemia, which occurs in 10% to 20% of all patients with cancer, is caused by the secretion of **parathyroid hormone–related peptide (PTHRP),** a PTH-like hormone secreted by carcinomas in various organs. Increased levels of PTH and PTHRP cause hypercalcemia and hypercalcinuria.

Approximately 50% of the Ca^{++} in plasma is ionized, 45% is bound to plasma proteins (mainly albumin), and 5% is complexed to several anions, including HCO_3^-, citrate, Pi, and $SO_4^=$. The pH of plasma influences this distribution. Acidosis increases the percentage of ionized Ca^{++} at the expense of Ca^{++} bound to proteins, whereas alkalosis decreases the percentage of ionized Ca^{++}, again by altering the Ca^{++} bound to proteins. Individuals with alkalosis are susceptible to tetany, whereas individuals with acidosis are less susceptible to tetany, even when total plasma Ca^{++} levels are reduced. The increase in the $[H^+]$ in patients with metabolic acidosis causes more H^+ to bind to plasma proteins, HCO_3^-, citrate, Pi, and $SO_4^=$, thereby displacing Ca^{++}. This displacement increases the plasma concentration of ionized Ca^{++}. In alkalosis the $[H^+]$ of plasma decreases. Some H^+ ions dissociate from plasma proteins, HCO_3^-, citrate, Pi, and $SO_4^=$ in exchange for Ca^{++}, thereby decreasing the plasma concentration of ionized Ca^{++}. The Ca^{++} available for glomerular filtration consists of the ionized fraction and the amount complexed with anions. Thus about 55% of the Ca^{++} in the plasma is available for glomerular filtration.

Ca^{++} is resorbed along the nephron

Normally, 99% of the filtered Ca^{++} (i.e., ionized and complexed) is resorbed by the nephron. The proximal tubule resorbs 70% of the filtered Ca^{++}. Another 20% is resorbed in the loop of Henle (mainly the thick ascending limb), about 9% is resorbed by the distal tubule, and <1% is resorbed by the collecting duct. About 1% (200 mg/day) is excreted in the urine. This fraction is equal to the net

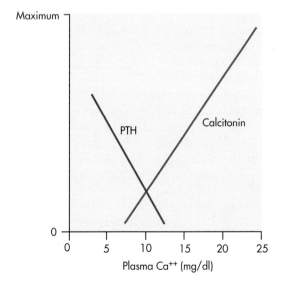

Figure 38-4 Effect of the plasma $[Ca^{++}]$ on plasma levels of PTH and calcitonin. *(Modified from Azria M: The calcitonins: physiology and pharmacology, Basel, Switzerland, 1989, Karger.)*

amount absorbed daily by the gastrointestinal tract. Figure 38-5 summarizes the handling of Ca^{++} by the different portions of the nephron.

Ca^{++} resorption by the proximal tubule occurs via two pathways: transcellular and paracellular. Ca^{++} resorption across the cellular pathway accounts for 20% of proximal resorption. Ca^{++} resorption through the cell is an active process that occurs in two steps. First, Ca^{++} diffuses down its electrochemical gradient across the apical membrane through Ca^{++} channels and into the cell. Second, Ca^{++} is extruded across the basolateral membrane against its electrochemical gradient. The extrusion of Ca^{++} is thought to occur by a Ca^{++}-ATPase and a $3Na^+$-Ca^{++} antiporter. A total of 80% of Ca^{++} is resorbed between cells across the tight junctions (i.e., paracellular pathway). This passive, paracellular resorption of Ca^{++} occurs via solvent drag along the entire length of the proximal tubule and is also driven by the positive luminal voltage in the second half of the proximal tubule. Thus approximately 80% of Ca^{++} resorption is paracellular, and approximately 20% is transcellular in the proximal tubule.

Ca^{++} resorption by the loop of Henle is restricted to the thick ascending limb. Ca^{++} is resorbed by cellular and paracellular routes via mechanisms similar to those described for the proximal tubule but with one difference. Ca^{++} is not resorbed by solvent drag in this segment. (The thick ascending limb is impermeable to water.) In the thick ascending limb, Ca^{++} and Na^+ resorption parallel each other. These processes are parallel because of the significant component of Ca^{++} resorption that oc-

curs via passive paracellular mechanisms secondary to Na^+ resorption and via the generation of the lumen-positive transepithelial voltage. Therefore Na^+ resorption also changes in parallel with Ca^{++} resorption by the proximal tubule and the thick ascending limb of the loop of Henle.

In the distal tubule, where the voltage in the tubule lumen is electrically negative with respect to the blood, Ca^{++} resorption is entirely active because Ca^{++} is resorbed against its electrochemical gradient. Ca^{++} resorption by the distal tubule is exclusively transcellular, and the mechanism is similar to that in the proximal tubule and thick ascending limb: uptake across the apical membrane by Ca^{++}-permeable ion channels and extrusion across the basolateral membrane by Ca^{++}-ATPase and the $3Na^+$-Ca^{++} antiporter. Na^+ and Ca^{++} excretion usually change in parallel. However, these processes are not always parallel because the resorption of Ca^{++} and Na^+ by the distal tubule is independent and is differentially regulated. For example, **thiazide diuretics** inhibit Na^+ resorption by the distal tubule and stimulate Ca^{++} resorption by this segment. Accordingly, the net effects of thiazide diuretics are to increase urinary Na^+ excretion and to reduce urinary Ca^{++} excretion.

Urinary Ca^{++} excretion is regulated by parathyroid hormone, calcitonin, and calcitriol

PTH exerts the most powerful control on renal Ca^{++} excretion, and it is responsible for maintaining Ca^{++} homeostasis. Overall, this hormone stimulates Ca^{++} resorption by the kidneys (i.e., reduces Ca^{++} excretion). Although PTH inhibits the resorption of NaCl and fluid, and therefore Ca^{++} by the proximal tubule, PTH stimulates Ca^{++} resorption by the thick ascending limb of the loop of Henle and the distal tubule. As a result, urinary Ca^{++} excretion declines. Calcitonin and calcitriol also stimulate Ca^{++} resorption by the kidneys. Calcitonin stimulates Ca^{++} resorption by the thick ascending limb and distal tubule, but it is less effective than PTH. Calcitriol either directly or indirectly enhances Ca^{++} resorption by the distal tubule. It is also less effective than PTH.

Several factors disturb Ca^{++} excretion. An increase in plasma Pi concentrations ([Pi]) (e.g., caused by an increased dietary intake of Pi) elevates PTH levels and thereby decreases Ca^{++} excretion. A decline in the plasma [Pi] (e.g., caused by dietary Pi depletion) has the opposite effect. Changes in the ECF volume alter Ca^{++} excretion mainly by affecting NaCl and fluid resorption in the proximal tubule. Volume contraction increases NaCl and water resorption by the proximal tubule and thereby enhances Ca^{++} resorption. Accordingly, urinary Ca^{++} excretion declines. Volume expansion has the opposite effect. Acidosis increases Ca^{++} excretion, whereas alkalosis decreases excretion. The regulation of Ca^{++} resorption by pH occurs in the distal tubule via an unknown mechanism.

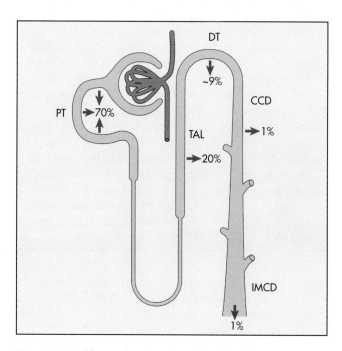

Figure 38-5 Ca^{++} transport along the nephron. Percentages refer to the amount of the filtered Ca^{++} resorbed by each segment. Approximately 1% of the filtered Ca^{++} is excreted. *CCD,* Cortical collecting duct; *DT,* distal tubule; *IMCD,* inner medullary collecting duct; *PT,* proximal tubule; *TAL,* thick ascending limb.

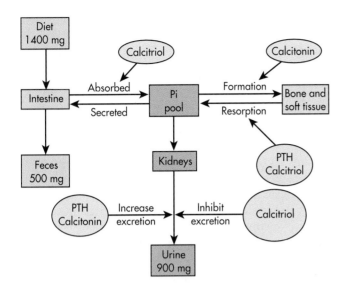

Figure 38-6 Overview of Pi homeostasis. See text for details.

Inorganic phosphate is an important component of many organic molecules

Pi is an important component of many organic molecules, including DNA, RNA, ATP, and intermediates of metabolic pathways. It is also a major constituent of bone. Its concentration in plasma is an important determinant of bone formation and resorption. In addition, urinary Pi is an important buffer (titratable acid) for the maintenance of acid-base balance (see Chapter 39). A total of 86% of Pi is located in bone, approximately 14% is located in the ICF, and 0.03% is located in the ECF. The normal plasma [Pi] is 4 mg/dl. Approximately 10% of the Pi in the plasma is protein-bound and is therefore unavailable for ultrafiltration by the glomerulus. Accordingly, the [Pi] in the ultrafiltrate is 10% less than that in plasma.

A general scheme of Pi homeostasis is shown in Figure 38-6. The maintenance of Pi homeostasis depends on two factors: (1) the amount of Pi in the body and (2) the distribution of Pi between the ICF and ECF compartments. Total body Pi levels are determined by the relative amount of Pi absorbed by the gastrointestinal tract versus the amount excreted by the kidneys. Pi absorption by the gastrointestinal tract occurs via active and passive mechanisms; Pi absorption increases as dietary Pi rises, and it is stimulated by calcitriol. Despite variations in Pi intake between 800 and 1500 mg/day, the kidneys keep the total body Pi balance constant by excreting an amount of Pi in the urine equal to the amount absorbed by the gastrointestinal tract. Thus the kidneys play a vital role in maintaining Pi homeostasis.

The second factor that maintains Pi homeostasis is the distribution of Pi among bone and the ICF and ECF compartments. PTH, calcitriol, and calcitonin regulate the distribution of Pi between bone and the ECF. As with Ca^{++} homeostasis, calcitonin is the least important of the hormones involved in Pi homeostasis in humans. The release

of Pi from intracellular stores is stimulated by the same hormones (i.e., PTH, calcitriol) that release Ca^{++} from this pool. Thus the release of Pi is always accompanied by a release of Ca^{++}. In contrast, calcitonin increases bone formation and thereby decreases the plasma [Pi].

The kidneys also make an important contribution to the regulation of the plasma [Pi]. A small rise in the plasma [Pi] increases the amount of Pi filtered by the glomerulus. Because the kidneys normally resorb Pi at a maximum rate, any increase in the amount filtered leads to a rise in urinary Pi excretion. In fact, an increase in the amount of Pi filtered enhances urinary Pi excretion to a value above that caused by Pi absorption by the gastrointestinal tract. This process results in a net loss of Pi from the body and decreases plasma [Pi]. In this way the kidneys regulate the plasma [Pi]. The maximum resorptive rate for Pi varies and is regulated by dietary Pi intake. A high-Pi diet decreases the maximum resorptive rate of Pi by the kidneys, and a low-Pi diet increases it. This effect is independent of changes in PTH levels.

In patients with **chronic renal failure,** the kidneys cannot excrete Pi. Because of continued Pi absorption by the gastrointestinal tract, Pi accumulates in the body, and the plasma [Pi] rises. The excess Pi complexes with Ca^{++} and reduces the plasma [Ca^{++}]. Pi accumulation also decreases the production of calcitriol. This response reduces Ca^{++} absorption by the intestine, an effect that further reduces the plasma [Ca^{++}]. This reduction increases PTH secretion and Ca^{++} release from bone. These actions result in **osteitis fibrosa cystica** (i.e., increased bone resorption with replacement by fibrous tissue, which renders bone more susceptible to fracture). Chronic hyperparathyroidism (i.e., elevated PTH levels) during chronic renal failure can lead to metastatic calcifications in which Ca^{++} and Pi precipitate in arteries, soft tissues, and viscera (see also Chapter 43). The deposition of Ca^{++} and Pi in heart and lung tissue may cause myocardial failure and pulmonary insufficiency, respectively. The prevention and treatment of hyperparathyroidism and Pi retention include a low-Pi diet or the administration of a "phosphate binder" (i.e., an agent that forms insoluble Pi salts and thereby renders Pi unavailable for absorption by the gastrointestinal tract). Supplemental Ca^{++} and calcitriol are also prescribed.

Figure 38-7 summarizes Pi transport by the various portions of the nephron. The proximal tubule resorbs 80% of the Pi filtered by the glomerulus, and the distal tubule resorbs 10%. In contrast, the loop of Henle and the collecting duct resorb negligible amounts of Pi. Therefore 10% of the filtered load of Pi is excreted.

Pi resorption by the proximal tubule occurs mainly, if not exclusively, via a transcellular route. Pi uptake

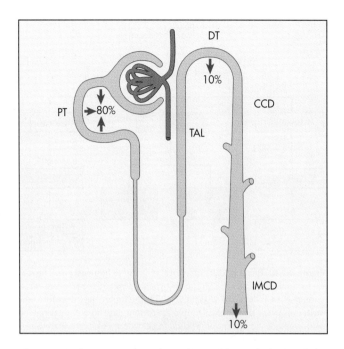

Figure 38-7 Pi transport along the nephron. Pi is resorbed primarily by the proximal tubule. Percentages refer to the amount of the filtered Pi resorbed by each nephron segment. Approximately 10% of the filtered Pi is excreted. *CCD,* Cortical collecting duct; *DT,* distal tubule; *IMCD,* inner medullary collecting duct; *PT,* proximal tubule; *TAL,* thick ascending limb.

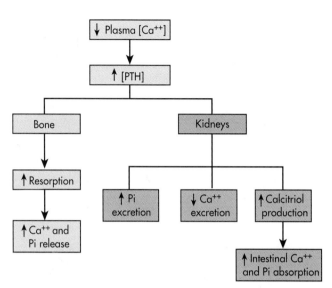

Figure 38-8 Effect of PTH on Ca^{++} and Pi homeostasis. The major stimulus of PTH secretion is hypocalcemia. *(Modified from Rose BD, Rennke HG, eds: Renal pathophysiology: the essentials, Baltimore, 1994, Williams & Wilkins.)*

across the apical membrane occurs via a $2Na^+$-Pi symport mechanism. Pi exits across the basolateral membrane, most likely by a Pi-anion antiporter. The cellular mechanism of Pi resorption by the distal tubule has not been characterized.

Parathyroid hormone is the most important hormone that controls Pi excretion

PTH inhibits Pi resorption by the proximal tubule and thereby increases Pi excretion. Dietary Pi intake also regulates Pi excretion by mechanisms unrelated to changes in PTH levels. Pi loading increases excretion, whereas Pi depletion decreases it. Changes in dietary Pi intake modulate Pi transport by altering the transport rate of each $2Na^+$-Pi symporter and by increasing the number of transporters.

ECF volume also affects Pi excretion. Volume expansion increases excretion, and volume contraction decreases it. The effect of ECF volume on Pi excretion is indirect and may involve changes in the levels of hormones other than PTH. Acid-base balance also influences Pi excretion; acidosis increases Pi excretion, and alkalosis decreases it. Glucocorticoids increase the excretion of Pi. Glucocorticoids increase the delivery of Pi to the distal tubule and collecting duct by inhibiting Pi resorption by the proximal tubule. This inhibition enables the distal tubule and collecting duct to secrete more H^+ and to generate more HCO_3^- because Pi is an important urinary

buffer (see Chapter 39). Finally, growth hormone decreases Pi excretion.

> In the absence of glucocorticoids (e.g., in **Addison's disease**), Pi excretion is depressed, as is the ability of the kidneys to excrete titratable acid and to generate new HCO_3^-. Growth hormone increases the resorption of Pi by the proximal tubule. As a result, growing children have a higher plasma [Pi] than adults, and this elevated [Pi] is important for the formation of bone.

Integrative review of parathyroid hormone, calcitriol, and calcitonin on Ca^{++} and Pi homeostasis

Hypocalcemia is the major stimulus of PTH secretion. As summarized in Figure 38-8, PTH has numerous effects on Ca^{++} and Pi homeostasis. PTH stimulates bone resorption (i.e., release of Ca^{++} and Pi from bone), increases urinary Pi excretion, decreases urinary Ca^{++} excretion, and stimulates the production of calcitriol, which stimulates Ca^{++} and Pi absorption by the intestine. Because changes in Pi handling in bone, the intestines, and the kidneys tend to balance out, PTH increases the plasma [Ca^{++}] while having little effect on the plasma [Pi]. Overall, a rise in the plasma PTH levels increases the plasma [Ca^{++}] and decreases the plasma [Pi]. A decline in plasma PTH levels has the opposite effect.

Calcitriol also plays an important role in Ca^{++} and Pi

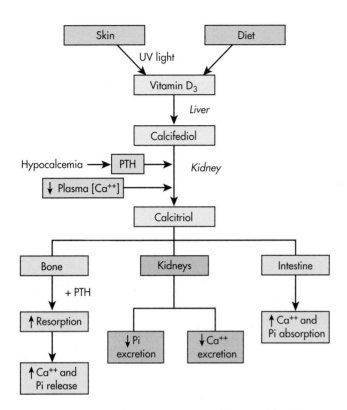

Figure 38-9 Activation of vitamin D_3 and its effect on Ca^{++} and Pi metabolism. Hypocalcemia, via PTH, and hypophosphatemia are the major stimuli of the metabolism of calcifediol to calcitriol in the kidneys. The net effect of calcitriol is to increase the plasma $[Ca^{++}]$ and $[Pi]$. *(Modified from Rose BD, Rennke HG, eds: Renal pathophysiology: the essentials, Baltimore, 1994, Williams & Wilkins.)*

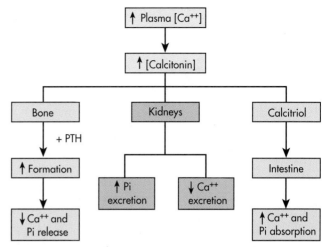

Figure 38-10 Effect of calcitonin on Ca^{++} and Pi homeostasis. The major stimulus of calcitonin secretion is hypercalcemia. The net effect of calcitonin is to reduce the plasma $[Ca^{++}]$. Quantitatively, therefore, the most important effects of calcitonin are to stimulate bone formation and to decrease bone resorption. Although calcitonin reduces urinary Ca^{++} excretion and intestinal Ca^{++} absorption, these effects are relatively minor and have little effect on the plasma $[Ca^{++}]$. The effects of calcitonin on the kidneys and calcitriol production are relatively minor compared with its effect on bone. *(Modified from Rose BD, Rennke HG, eds: Renal pathophysiology: the essentials, Baltimore, 1994, Williams & Wilkins.)*

> Estrogen replacement therapy, which should be accompanied by progesterone, is useful for women at high risk for developing osteoporosis.

homeostasis (Figure 38-9). Calcitriol stimulates Ca^{++} and Pi absorption by the intestine and Ca^{++} and Pi release from bone and decreases Ca^{++} and Pi excretion by the kidneys. The net effect of calcitriol is to increase the plasma $[Ca^{++}]$ and $[Pi]$. Thus the major stimuli of calcitriol production are hypocalcemia via PTH and hypophosphatemia (i.e., a low plasma $[Pi]$).

Calcitonin is also an important hormone in Ca^{++} homeostasis because it blocks bone resorption and stimulates Ca^{++} deposition in bone (Figure 38-10). Calcitonin's modest direct effect on decreasing urinary Ca^{++} excretion is a relatively minor action of the hormone. The major stimulus of calcitonin secretion is an increase in the plasma $[Ca^{++}]$. Because changes in Pi handling in bone, the intestines, and the kidneys tend to balance out, calcitonin decreases the plasma $[Ca^{++}]$ while having little effect on the plasma $[Pi]$.

> **Estrogens** defend against PTH-mediated resorption of bone. In estrogen-deficient conditions, most prominently after menopause, the unabated effect of PTH on bone contributes significantly to the development of osteoporosis.

SUMMARY

- K^+ homeostasis is maintained by the kidneys, which adjust K^+ excretion to match dietary K^+ intake, and by the hormones insulin, epinephrine, and aldosterone.
- Other events, such as cell lysis, exercise, and changes in acid-base balance and plasma osmolality, disturb the plasma $[K^+]$.
- K^+ excretion by the kidneys is determined by the rate of K^+ secretion by the distal tubule and collecting duct. K^+ secretion by these tubular segments is regulated by the plasma $[K^+]$, aldosterone, and ADH. In contrast, changes in tubular fluid flow and acid-base disturbance perturb K^+ excretion by the kidneys.
- The kidneys, in conjunction with the gastrointestinal tract and bone, play a vital role in regulating the plasma $[Ca^{++}]$ and $[Pi]$.
- Plasma Ca^{++} is regulated by PTH, calcitriol, and calcitonin. Ca^{++} excretion by the kidneys is determined by (1) the net rate of intestinal Ca^{++} absorption, (2) the balance between bone formation and resorption, and (3) the net rate of Ca^{++} resorption by the

distal tubule and thick ascending limb of the loop of Henle.

- Ca^{++} resorption by the thick ascending limb is regulated by PTH, calcitriol, and calcitonin, all of which stimulate Ca^{++} resorption.
- The plasma [Pi] is regulated by the maximal resorptive capacity of Pi by the kidneys. A fall in the [Pi] stimulates the production of calcitriol, which releases Pi from bone into the ECF, increases Pi absorption by the intestine, and decreases urinary Pi excretion.

BIBLIOGRAPHY

Berndt TJ, Knox FG: Renal regulation of phosphate excretion. In Seldin DW, Giebisch G, eds: *The kidney: physiology and pathophysiology,* ed 2, New York, 1992, Raven.

Friedman PA, Gesek FA: Cellular calcium transport in renal epithelia: measurement, mechanisms, and regulation, *Physiol Rev* 75(3):429, 1995.

Giebisch G, Malnic G, Berliner RW: Control of renal potassium excretion. In Brenner BM, ed: *The kidney,* ed 5, Philadelphia, 1996, WB Saunders.

Hebert SC: An ATP-regulated, inwardly rectifying potassium channel from rat kidney (ROMK), *Kidney Int* 48(4):1010, 1995.

Knochel JP, Agarwal R: Hypophosphatemia and hyperphosphatemia. In Brenner BM, ed: *The kidney,* ed 5, Philadelphia, 1996, WB Saunders.

Murer H, Biber J: Renal sodium-phosphate cotransport, *Curr Opin Nephrol Hypertens* 3(5):504, 1994.

Rose BD, Rennke HG: Disorders of potassium balance. In Rose BD, Rennke HG, eds: *Renal pathophysiology: the essentials,* Baltimore, 1994, Williams & Wilkins.

Seldin DW, Giebisch G, eds: *The regulation of potassium balance,* New York, 1989, Raven.

Stanton BA, Giebisch G: Renal potassium transport. In Windhager EE, ed: *Handbook of physiology,* section 8, *Renal physiology,* vol 2, New York, 1992, American Physiological Society/ Oxford University Press.

Suki WN, Rouse D: Renal transport of calcium, magnesium and phosphate. In Brenner BM, ed: *The kidney,* ed 5, Philadelphia, 1996, WB Saunders.

Sutton RAL, Dirks JH: Disturbances of calcium and magnesium metabolism. In Brenner BM, ed: *The kidney,* ed 5, Philadelphia, 1996, WB Saunders.

Wright FS, Giebisch G: Regulation of potassium excretion. In Seldin DW, Giebisch G, eds: *The kidney: physiology and pathophysiology,* ed 2, New York, 1992, Raven.

▷ CASE STUDIES

Case 38-1

An 18-year-old man with insulin-dependent diabetes mellitus was seen in the emergency department. He did not take his insulin during the previous 24 hours because he did not feel well and was not eating. He was weak, nauseated, and thirsty, and he urinated frequently. On physical examination, he had deep and rapid respira-

tions (Kussmaul's respiration). The following laboratory data were obtained:

Plasma [Na^+]	135 mEq/L
Serum [Cl^-]	99 mEq/L
Plasma [K^+]	8.0 mEq/L
Plasma [HCO_3^-]	7 mEq/L
Blood pH	6.99
Partial pressure of arterial carbon dioxide	30 mm Hg
Plasma [glucose]	1200 mg/dl
Urine	Contains glucose and ketones

The diagnosis of diabetic ketoacidosis was made, and the patient was admitted to the hospital. After insulin was administered, the plasma [K^+] decreased.

1. What caused hyperkalemia in this patient?
 A. Frequent urination
 B. Ketoacidosis
 C. Increased plasma glucose levels
 D. Glucose and ketones in the urine
 E. Metabolic alkalosis

2. Why did the plasma [K^+] decrease after the administration of insulin?
 A. Promotion of K^+ uptake into cells
 B. Correction of the ketoacidosis, which allows K^+ to enter cells in exchange for H^+
 C. Decrease in polyuria, which stimulates the amount of K^+ excreted in the urine
 D. Stimulation of glucose uptake by cells, which increases plasma osmolality and thereby causes K^+ to enter cells
 E. Insulin inhibition of Na^+,K^+-ATPase and thereby K^+ uptake into cells

Case 38-2

A 55-year-old woman came to the emergency department with severe flank pain caused by a renal stone lodged in her right ureter. Tests revealed that the renal stone formed because of demineralization of bone and elevated serum levels of PTH. A benign, PTH-secreting adenoma of the parathyroid gland was identified.

1. What values of serum [Ca^{++}] and [Pi] would be predicted for this patient?
 A. Increased serum [Ca^{++}], decreased serum [Pi]
 B. Increased serum [Ca^{++}], increased serum [Pi]
 C. Unchanged serum [Ca^{++}], unchanged serum [Pi]
 D. Decreased serum [Ca^{++}], decreased serum [Pi]
 E. Decreased serum [Ca^{++}], increased serum [Pi]

2. **The high levels of serum PTH concentration in this woman would be expected to increase Ca^{++} resorption in which segment of the nephron?**
   - **A.** The glomerulus
   - **B.** The proximal tubule
   - **C.** The thick ascending limb of the loop of Henle
   - **D.** The distal tubule
   - **E.** The collecting duct

3. **The high levels of serum PTH in this woman would be expected to decrease Pi resorption in which segment of the nephron?**
   - **A.** The glomerulus
   - **B.** The proximal tubule
   - **C.** The thick ascending limb of the loop of Henle
   - **D.** The distal tubule
   - **E.** The collecting duct

CHAPTER 39

Role of the Kidneys in Acid-Base Balance

OBJECTIVES

- Indicate the impact of diet and cellular metabolism on acid-base balance.
- Distinguish among the roles of the kidneys, lungs, and liver in acid-base balance.
- Describe the mechanisms for H^+ transport in the various segments of the nephron and ways that these mechanisms are regulated.
- Distinguish between the resorption of the filtered load of bicarbonate and the generation of new bicarbonate.
- Describe the importance of urine buffers, especially ammonia production and excretion, in the process of new bicarbonate formation.
- Indicate the defense mechanisms the body uses to minimize the impact of acid and alkali on the pH of body fluids.
- Distinguish between metabolic and respiratory acid-base disorders.
- Distinguish between simple and mixed acid-base disorders.

Virtually all cellular, tissue, and organ processes are sensitive to pH. Indeed, life cannot exist outside of a range of body fluid pH from 6.8 to 7.8 (160 to 16 nEq/L of H^+). Each day, acid and alkali are ingested in the diet. Also, cellular metabolism produces a number of substances that have an impact on the pH of body fluids. Without appropriate mechanisms to deal with this daily acid and alkali load and thereby maintain acid-base balance, many processes necessary for life could not occur. This chapter reviews the maintenance of whole-body acid-base balance. Although the emphasis is on the role of the kidneys in this process, the roles of the lungs and liver are also considered. In addition, the impact of diet and cellular metabolism on acid-base balance is presented. Finally, disorders of acid-base balance are considered, primarily to illustrate the physiological processes involved. Throughout this chapter, **acid** is defined as any substance that adds H^+ to the body fluids, whereas **alkali** is defined as a substance that removes H^+ from the body fluids.

Overview of Acid-Base Balance

The diet of humans contains many constituents that are either acid or alkali. In addition, cellular metabolism produces acid and alkali. Finally, alkali is normally lost each day in the feces. As described later, the net effect of these processes is the addition of acid to the body fluids. For acid-base balance to be maintained, acid must be excreted from the body at a rate equivalent to its addition. If acid addition exceeds excretion, **acidosis** results. Conversely, if acid excretion exceeds addition, **alkalosis** results.

Diet determines metabolically produced acid and alkali

The major constituents of the diet are carbohydrates and fats. When tissue perfusion is adequate, O_2 is available to tissues, insulin is present at normal levels, and carbohydrates and fats are metabolized to CO_2 and H_2O. On a daily basis, 15 to 20 moles of CO_2 are generated through this process. Normally, this large quantity of CO_2 is effectively eliminated from the body by the lungs, so this metabolically derived CO_2 has no impact on acid-base balance. CO_2 is usually termed **volatile acid,** reflecting the fact that it has the potential to generate H^+ after hydration with H_2O (see Equation 39-4). Acid not derived directly from the hydration of CO_2 is termed **nonvolatile acid** (e.g., lactic acid).

The cellular metabolism of other dietary constituents also has an impact on acid-base balance. For example, cysteine and methionine, sulfur-containing amino acids, yield sulfuric acid when metabolized, whereas hydrochloric acid results from the metabolism of lysine, arginine, and histidine. A portion of this nonvolatile acid load is offset by the production of bicarbonate (HCO_3^-) through the metabolism of the amino acids, aspartate and glutamate. On average the metabolism of dietary amino acids yields net nonvolatile acid production. Finally, the metabolism of certain organic anions (e.g., citrate) results in the production of HCO_3^-, which offsets nonvolatile acid production to some degree. In balance, in individuals ingesting a meat-containing diet, acid production exceeds HCO_3^- production. In addition to the metabolically derived acids and alkalis, the foods ingested contain acid and alkali. For example, the presence of phosphate ($H_2PO_4^-$) in ingested food increases the dietary acid load. Finally, during digestion, some HCO_3^- is normally lost in the feces (see Chapter 34). This loss is equivalent to the addition of nonvolatile acid to the body. Together, dietary intake, cellular metabolism, and fecal HCO_3^- loss result in the addition of approximately 1 mEq/kg body weight of nonvolatile acid to the body each day (50 to100 mEq/day for most adults).

> When insulin levels are normal, carbohydrates and fats are completely metabolized to CO_2 + H_2O. However, if insulin levels are abnormally low (e.g., **diabetes mellitus**), the metabolism of carbohydrates leads to the production of several organic ketoacids (e.g., β-hydroxybutyric acid).
>
> In the absence of adequate levels of O_2 **(hypoxia)**, anaerobic metabolism by cells can also lead to the production of organic acids (e.g., lactic acid) rather than CO_2 + H_2O. This frequently occurs in normal individuals during vigorous exercise. Poor tissue perfusion, such as that which occurs with reduced cardiac output, can also lead to anaerobic metabolism by cells and thus to acidosis. In these conditions, the organic acids accumulate, and the pH of the body fluids decreases (acidosis). Treatment (e.g., administration of insulin in the case of diabetes) or improved delivery of adequate levels of O_2 to the tissues (e.g., in the case of poor tissue perfusion) results in the metabolism of these organic acids to CO_2 + H_2O and thereby helps correct the acid-base disorder.

Nonvolatile acids are rapidly buffered

Nonvolatile acids do not circulate throughout the body but are immediately buffered. As discussed later, HCO_3^- in the extracellular fluid (ECF) is an important buffer species. Thus the buffering of nonvolatile acids results in the following:

$$H_2SO_4 + 2NaHCO_3 \leftrightarrow Na_2SO_4 + 2CO_2 + 2H_2O \qquad \textbf{39-1}$$

$$HCl + NaHCO_3 \leftrightarrow NaCl + CO_2 + H_2O \qquad \textbf{39-2}$$

This buffering process yields the Na^+ salts of the strong acid anions and removes HCO_3^- from the ECF. The kidneys must excrete these Na^+ salts and replenish the HCO_3^- lost by neutralization of the nonvolatile acids.

Renal Acid Excretion

TO MAINTAIN ACID-BASE BALANCE, THE KIDNEYS MUST EXCRETE AN AMOUNT OF ACID EQUAL TO THE NONVOLATILE ACID PRODUCTION. In addition, they must prevent the loss of HCO_3^- in the urine. This task is quantitatively more important be-

cause the filtered load of HCO_3^- is approximately 4320 mEq/day (24 mEq/L × 180 L/day = 4320 mEq/day), compared with only 50 to 100 mEq/day needed to balance nonvolatile acid production.

The resorption of filtered bicarbonate and the excretion of acid occur via H^+ secretion

BOTH THE RESORPTION OF FILTERED HCO_3^- AND THE EXCRETION OF ACID ARE ACCOMPLISHED VIA H^+ SECRETION BY THE NEPHRONS. Thus in a single day the nephrons must secrete approximately 4390 mEq of H^+ into the tubular fluid. Most of the secreted H^+ is resorbed with the filtered load of HCO_3^-. Only 50 to 100 mEq of H^+, an amount equivalent to nonvolatile acid production, is excreted in the urine. As a result of this acid excretion, the urine is normally acidic.

Theoretically, the kidneys could excrete the nonvolatile acids and replenish the HCO_3^- lost during extracellular buffering by reversing the reactions shown in Equations 39-1 and 39-2. However, the equilibrium constants of these nonvolatile acids are so low that this process would require a urine pH of 1.0, and the minimum urine pH attainable by the kidneys is only 4.0 to 4.5. Consequently, the kidneys cannot excrete the free acids. Instead, they must excrete the salts of these acids and excrete H^+ with urinary buffers such as phosphate ($HPO_4^=/H_2PO_4^-$). Other constituents of the urine can also serve as buffers (e.g., creatinine), although their role is less important than phosphate. Collectively, the various urinary buffers are termed **titratable acids.** This term is derived from the method by which these buffers are quantitated in the laboratory. Typically, alkali (OH^-) is added to a urine sample to titrate its pH to that of plasma (i.e., 7.4). The amount of alkali added is equal to the H^+ titrated by these urine buffers and is termed titratable acid.

The excretion of H^+ as a titratable acid is insufficient to balance the daily nonvolatile acid load. An additional and important mechanism by which the kidneys contribute to the maintenance of acid-base balance is through the synthesis and excretion of **ammonium (NH_4^+).** The mechanisms involved in this process are discussed in more detail later in this chapter. With regard to the renal regulation of acid-base balance, each NH_4^+ excreted in the urine results in the return of an HCO_3^- to the systemic circulation, which replenishes the HCO_3^- lost during neutralization of the nonvolatile acid. Thus the production and excretion of NH_4^+ are equivalent to the excretion of acid by the kidneys.

Net acid excretion equals nonvolatile acid production

In brief, THE KIDNEYS CONTRIBUTE TO ACID-BASE HOMEOSTASIS BY RESORBING THE FILTERED LOAD OF HCO_3^- AND EXCRETING AN AMOUNT OF ACID EQUIVALENT TO THE AMOUNT OF NONVOLATILE ACID PRODUCED EACH DAY. This overall process is termed

net acid excretion (NAE), and it can be quantitated as follows:

$$NAE = [(U_{NH_4^+} \times \dot{V}) + (U_{TA} \times \dot{V})] - (U_{HCO_3^-} \times \dot{V}) \quad \textbf{39-3}$$

where $(U_{NH_4^+} \times \dot{V})$ and $(U_{TA} \times \dot{V})$ are the rates of excretion (mEq/day) of NH_4^+ and titratable acid (TA) and $(U_{HCO_3} \times \dot{V})$ is the amount of HCO_3^- lost in the urine (equivalent to adding H^+ to the body). Again, maintenance of acid-base balance means that the NAE must equal nonvolatile acid production. Under most conditions, very little HCO_3^- is excreted in the urine. Thus NAE essentially reflects titratable acid and NH_4^+ excretion. Quantitatively, titratable acid accounts for approximately one third and NH_4^+ two thirds of NAE.

The filtered load of bicarbonate must be resorbed

As indicated by Equation 39-3, the NAE is maximized when little or no HCO_3^- is excreted in the urine. Indeed, under most circumstances, very little HCO_3^- appears in the urine. Because HCO_3^- is freely filtered at the glomerulus, approximately 4320 mEq/day is delivered to the nephrons and is then resorbed. The majority of this HCO_3^- is resorbed in the proximal tubule (80% of the filtered load), an additional 15% is resorbed by the thick ascending limb of the loop of Henle, and the remainder (5%) is resorbed by the distal tubule and collecting duct.

The proximal tubule resorbs most of the filtered load of bicarbonate

Figure 39-1 summarizes the primary transport processes responsible for HCO_3^- resorption in the proximal tubule. H^+ secretion across the apical membrane of the cell occurs by both an Na^+-H^+ antiporter and an H^+-ATPase. The Na^+-H^+ antiporter is the predominant pathway for H^+ secretion and uses the lumen-to-cell Na^+ gradient to drive this process (i.e., secondary active secretion of H^+). Within the cell, H^+ and HCO_3^- are produced in a reaction catalyzed by **carbonic anhy-**

drase. The H^+ is secreted into the tubular fluid, whereas the HCO_3^- exits the cell across the basolateral membrane and returns to the peritubular blood. Although the electrochemical gradient for HCO_3^- favors its passive movement out of the cell across the basolateral membrane, simple diffusion does not occur to a significant degree. Instead, HCO_3^- movement out of the cell across the basolateral membrane is coupled to other ions. The majority of HCO_3^- exits via a symporter that couples the efflux of $1Na^+$ with $3HCO_3^-$. In addition, some of the HCO_3^- exits in exchange for Cl^- (via a Cl^--HCO_3^- antiporter). As noted in Figure 39-1, carbonic anhydrase is also present in the brush border of the proximal tubule cells. This enzyme catalyzes the dehydration of H_2CO_3 in the luminal fluid, and thereby facilitates the resorption of HCO_3^-.

The cellular mechanism for HCO_3^- resorption by the thick ascending limb of the loop of Henle is virtually identical to that in the proximal tubule. The only difference is that carbonic anhydrase is not present in the brush border of the cells of the thick ascending limb.

The distal tubule and collecting duct resorb the small amount of HCO_3^- that escapes resorption by the proximal tubule and loop of Henle. Figure 39-2 shows the cellular mechanism of HCO_3^- resorption by the collecting duct, where H^+ secretion occurs via the intercalated cell (see Chapter 35). Within the cell, H^+ and HCO_3^- are produced by the hydration of CO_2; this reaction is catalyzed by carbonic anhydrase. H^+ is secreted into the tubular fluid via two mechanisms. The first involves an apical membrane H^+-ATPase. The second couples the secretion of H^+ with the resorption of K^+ via an H^+-

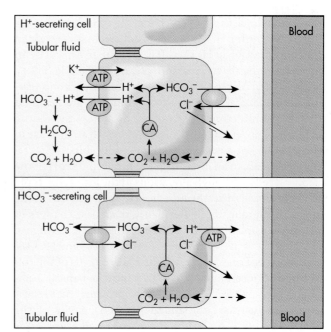

Figure 39-2 Cellular mechanisms for the resorption and secretion of HCO_3^- by the intercalated cells of the collecting duct. See text for details. *CA*, Carbonic anhydrase.

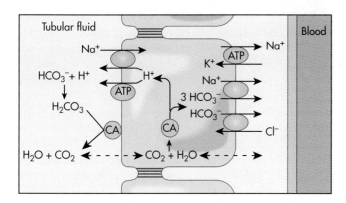

Figure 39-1 Cellular mechanism for the resorption of filtered HCO_3^- by the cells of the proximal tubule. See text for details. *CA*, Carbonic anhydrase.

K^+-ATPase similar to that found in the stomach (see Chapter 34). The HCO_3^- exits the cell across the basolateral membrane in exchange for Cl^- (via a Cl^--HCO_3^- antiporter) and enters the peritubular capillary blood.

A second population of intercalated cells within the collecting duct secrete HCO_3^- rather than H^+ into the tubular fluid. In these intercalated cells, in contrast to the intercalated cells previously described, the H^+-ATPase is located in the basolateral membrane, and a Cl^--HCO_3^- antiporter is located in the apical membrane (Figure 39-2). Their activity can be increased during metabolic alkalosis, when the kidneys must excrete excess HCO_3^-. However, under normal conditions H^+ secretion predominates in the collecting duct.

The apical membrane of the cells of the collecting duct is not very permeable to H^+, and the pH of the tubular fluid can become quite acidic. Indeed, the most acidic tubular fluid along the nephron (pH = 4.0 to 4.5) is produced there. In comparison, the permeability of the proximal tubule to H^+ and HCO_3^- is much higher, and the tubular fluid pH falls to only 6.5 in this segment. As explained later, the ability of the collecting duct to lower the pH of the tubular fluid is critically important for the excretion of urinary buffers and NH_4^+.

Systemic acid-base balance regulates nephron H^+ secretion

A number of factors regulate the secretion of H^+ by the cells of the nephron (Table 39-1). FROM A PHYSIOLOGICAL PERSPECTIVE THE PRIMARY FACTOR THAT REGULATES H^+ SECRETION BY THE NEPHRON IS CHANGE IN THE SYSTEMIC ACID-BASE BALANCE. At the cellular level, this reflects changes in the cell-to-tubular fluid gradient for H^+. Whether produced by a decrease in the concentration of HCO_3^- ($[HCO_3^-]$) in plasma or by an increase in the partial pressure of carbon dioxide (Pco_2), acidosis decreases the pH of the cells of the nephron, creating a more favorable cell-to-tubular fluid H^+ gradient and thereby stimulating H^+ secretion along the entire nephron. Conversely, alkalosis secondary to an increase in the $[HCO_3^-]$ or a decrease in the Pco_2 inhibits H^+ secretion secondary to an increase in the intracellular pH of the nephron cells. Although alterations in the intracellular pH of nephron cells directly influence H^+ secretion across the apical membrane, there is evidence that these changes in pH, perhaps mediated by other intracellular messengers, also alter the activity and expression of key H^+ and HCO_3^- transporters. For example, the intercalated cells of the collecting duct insert more H^+-ATPase into their apical membranes in response to acidosis. In the proximal tubule, acidosis also increases the abundance and activity of the apical membrane Na^+-H^+ antiporter as well as the Na^+-$3HCO_3^-$ symporter in the basolateral membrane. It is likely that the effects of inhibited H^+ secretion caused by systemic alkalosis are also mediated in part by the

Table 39-1	Factors Influencing H^+ Secretion by the Nephron	
Factor	**Principal Site of Action**
Increased H^+ Secretion	
Primary	
Decrease in plasma HCO_3^- concentration ($\downarrow$pH)	Entire nephron
Increase in partial pressure of arterial carbon dioxide	Entire nephron
Secondary (not directed at maintaining acid-base balance)	
Increase in filtered load of HCO_3^-	Proximal tubule
Decrease in ECF volume	Proximal tubule
Increase in angiotensin II	Proximal tubule
Increase in aldosterone	Collecting duct
Hypokalemia	Proximal tubule
Decreased H^+ Secretion	
Primary	
Increase in plasma HCO_3^- concentration ($\uparrow$pH)	Entire nephron
Decrease in partial pressure of arterial carbon dioxide	Entire nephron
Secondary (not directed at maintaining acid-base balance)	
Decrease in filtered load of HCO_3^-	Proximal tubule
Increase in ECF volume	Proximal tubule
Decrease in aldosterone	Collecting duct
Hyperkalemia	Proximal tubule

reduced activity and expression of these H^+ and HCO_3^- transporters.

Other factors can alter nephron H^+ secretion

Table 39-1 also lists other factors that influence the secretion of H^+ by the cells of the nephron. However, these factors are not directly related to the maintenance of acid-base balance. Because H^+ secretion in the proximal tubule and thick ascending limb of the loop of Henle is linked to the resorption of Na^+ (via the Na^+-H^+ antiporter), factors that alter Na^+ resorption secondarily effect H^+ secretion. For example, the process of glomerulotubular balance ensures that the resorption rate of the proximal tubule is matched to the glomerular filtration rate (see Chapter 36). Thus when the glomerular filtration rate is increased, the filtered load to the proximal tubule is increased, and more fluid (including HCO_3^-) is resorbed. Conversely, a decrease in the filtered load results in the decreased resorption of fluid and thus HCO_3^-.

Alterations in Na^+ balance, through changes in the ECF

volume, also have an impact on H^+ secretion. With volume depletion (negative Na^+ balance), H^+ secretion is enhanced. This occurs via several mechanisms. First, the renin-angiotensin-aldosterone system is activated by volume depletion, and Na^+ resorption by the nephron is enhanced (see Chapter 37). Angiotensin II acts on the proximal tubule and thick ascending limb of the loop of Henle to stimulate the apical membrane Na^+-H^+ antiporter and thereby stimulate H^+ secretion. Aldosterone's primary action on the collecting duct is to stimulate Na^+ resorption. However, it also stimulates the intercalated cells to secrete H^+. Second, the peritubular Starling forces across the proximal tubule are altered during volume depletion to enhance overall proximal tubule resorption (see Chapter 36). With volume expansion (positive Na^+ balance), H^+ secretion is reduced because of low levels of angiotensin II and aldosterone, as well as because of alterations in the peritubular Starling forces (reduced resorption by the proximal tubule).

Parathyroid hormone (PTH) also inhibits HCO_3^- resorption by the proximal tubule. PTH is mainly involved in the maintenance of Ca^{++} and phosphate balance (see Chapters 38 and 43). However, PTH inhibits the Na^+-H^+ antiporter in the apical membrane of proximal tubule cells. Finally, K^+ balance influences the secretion of H^+ by the proximal tubule, with hypokalemia stimulating and hyperkalemia inhibiting secretion. It is thought that K^+-induced changes in intracellular pH are responsible for this effect, with hypokalemia acidifying and hyperkalemia alkalinizing the cells.

Ammonium production and excretion forms new bicarbonate

As discussed previously, resorption of the filtered load of HCO_3^- is important for maximizing the NAE. However, HCO_3^- resorption alone does not replenish the HCO_3^- lost during the buffering of the nonvolatile acids produced during metabolism. To maintain acid-base balance, the kidneys must replace this lost HCO_3^- with new HCO_3^-. A portion of the new HCO_3^- is produced while urinary buffers (primarily phosphate) are being excreted. This process is illustrated in Figure 39-3. In the collecting duct, when the tubular fluid contains little or no HCO_3^- because HCO_3^- is resorbed in "upstream" tubular segments, H^+ secreted into the tubular fluid combines with a urinary buffer. Thus H^+ secretion results in the excretion of H^+ with a buffer, and the HCO_3^- produced in the cell from the hydration of CO_2 is added back to the blood. The amount of phosphate excreted each day and therefore available to serve as a urinary buffer is not sufficient to allow adequate generation of new HCO_3^-. Moreover, the amount of phosphate excreted is regulated in response to the need to maintain phosphate balance (see Chapters 38 and 44), and not in response to the need to maintain acid-base balance. In contrast, NH_4^+ is produced by the kidneys, and its synthesis and subsequent excretion can be regulated in response

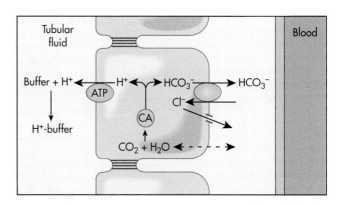

Figure 39-3 Excretion of H^+ with non-HCO_3^- urine buffers. The primary urine buffer is phosphate (HPO_4^-). Another buffer is creatinine. Collectively, the urine buffers are termed **titratable acids.** For simplicity, only H^+-ATPase is shown. H^+ secretion by H^+,K^+-ATPase also titrates urine buffers. *CA,* Carbonic anhydrase.

to the acid-base requirements of the body. Because of this, NH_4^+ excretion is critically involved in the formation of new HCO_3^-.

NH_4^+ is produced in the kidneys via the metabolism of glutamine. Essentially, the kidneys metabolize glutamine, excrete NH_4^+, and return HCO_3^- to the body. However, the formation of new HCO_3^- via this process depends on the kidneys' ability to excrete NH_4^+ in the urine. If NH_4^+ is not excreted in the urine but enters the systemic circulation instead, it is converted into urea by the liver. This conversion process generates H^+, which is then buffered by HCO_3^-. Thus the production of urea from NH_4^+ consumes HCO_3^- and negates the formation of HCO_3^- through the synthesis and excretion of NH_4^+ by the kidneys.

The process by which the kidneys excrete NH_4^+ is complex. Figure 39-4 illustrates the essential features of this process. NH_4^+ is produced from glutamine in the cells of the proximal tubule. Each glutamine molecule produces two molecules of NH_4^+ and a divalent anion. The metabolism of this anion ultimately provides two molecules of HCO_3^-. The HCO_3^- exits the cell across the basolateral membrane and enters the peritubular blood as new HCO_3^-. NH_4^+ exits the cell across the apical membrane and enters the tubular fluid. The primary mechanism for the secretion of NH_4^+ into the tubular fluid involves the Na^+-H^+ antiporter, with NH_4^+ substituting for H^+. In addition, NH_3 can diffuse out of the cell into the tubular fluid, where it is protonated to NH_4^+.

A significant portion of the NH_4^+ secreted by the proximal tubule is resorbed by the loop of Henle. The thick ascending limb is the primary site of this NH_4^+ resorption, with NH_4^+ substituting for K^+ on the $1Na^+$-$1K^+$-$2Cl^-$ symporter. In addition, the lumen positive transepithelial voltage in this segment drives the paracellular resorption of NH_4^+.

The NH_4^+ resorbed by the thick ascending limb of the loop of Henle accumulates in the medullary interstitium, where it exists in chemical equilibrium with NH_3 (pK_a =

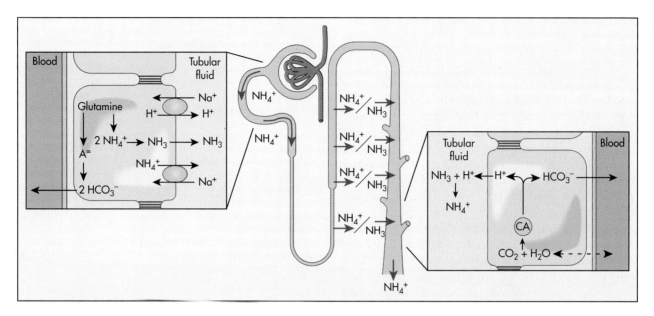

Figure 39-4 Production, transport, and excretion of NH_4^+ by the nephron. For every NH_4^+ excreted in the urine an HCO_3^- is returned to the systemic circulation. See text for details.

9.0). NH_4^+ then reenters the tubular fluid of the collecting duct. The mechanism by which this occurs involves the processes of **nonionic diffusion** and **diffusion trapping.** The collecting duct does not have a specific transport mechanism for the secretion of NH_4^+, nor do the cells have a significant passive permeability to it. However, the cells of the collecting duct are permeable to NH_3, which can diffuse from the medullary interstitium into the lumen of the collecting duct. As previously described, H^+ secretion by the intercalated cells of the collecting duct acidifies the luminal fluid. (A luminal fluid pH as low as 4.0 to 4.5 can be achieved.) Consequently, NH_3 diffusing from the medullary interstitium into the collecting duct lumen (nonionic diffusion) is protonated to NH_4^+ by the acidic tubular fluid. Because the collecting duct is less permeable to NH_4^+ than to NH_3, NH_4^+ is trapped in the tubule lumen (diffusion trapping) and eliminated from the body in the urine.

H^+ secretion by the collecting duct is critical for the excretion of NH_4^+. If collecting duct H^+ secretion is inhibited, the NH_4^+ resorbed by the thick ascending limb will not be excreted in the urine. Instead, it will be returned to the systemic circulation, where as described previously, it will be converted to urea by the liver and consume HCO_3^- in the process. Thus new HCO_3^- is produced during the metabolism of glutamine by cells of the proximal tubule. However, the overall process is not complete until the NH_4^+ is excreted (i.e., the production of urea from NH_4^+ by the liver is prevented). Thus NH_4^+ EXCRETION CAN BE USED AS A "MARKER" OF GLUTAMINE METABOLISM IN THE PROXIMAL TUBULE. BECAUSE OF THE STOICHIOMETRY OF THIS REACTION, ONE NEW HCO_3^- IS RETURNED TO THE SYSTEMIC CIRCULATION FOR EACH NH_4^+ EXCRETED IN THE URINE.

An important feature of the renal NH_4^+ system is that it can be regulated by systemic acid-base balance. Alterations in the pH of ECF, presumably caused by affecting the pH of intracellular fluid, change glutamine metabolism (NH_4^+ production) in the cells of the proximal tubule. During systemic acidosis, the enzymes in the proximal tubule cell responsible for the metabolism of glutamine are stimulated. This involves the synthesis of new enzyme and requires several days for complete adaptation. With increased levels of this enzyme, NH_4^+ production is increased, allowing enhanced production of new HCO_3^-. Conversely, glutamine metabolism is reduced with alkalosis.

The K^+ concentration ($[K^+]$) of plasma also alters NH_4^+ production. When hyperkalemia exists, NH_4^+ production is inhibited, whereas hypokalemia stimulates NH_4^+ production. The mechanism by which plasma K^+ alters NH_4^+ production is not fully understood. Alterations in the plasma $[K^+]$ may change the intracellular pH by exchanging H^+ for K^+ (see Chapter 38), and the change in intracellular pH may then control glutamine metabolism. Via this mechanism, the exchange of extracellular K^+ for intracellular H^+ during hyperkalemia would raise intracellular pH and thereby inhibit glutamine metabolism. The opposite would occur during hypokalemia.

> **Renal tubule acidosis (RTA)** refers to conditions in which NAE by the kidneys is impaired. Under these conditions the kidneys are unable to excrete a sufficient amount of net acid to balance nonvolatile acid production, and acidosis results. RTA can be caused by a defect in H^+ secretion in the proximal tubule (**proximal RTA**)

or distal tubule (**distal RTA**) or by inadequate production of NH_4^+.

Proximal RTA can be caused by a variety of hereditary and acquired conditions (e.g., **cystinosis, Fanconi's** syndrome, administration of carbonic anhydrase inhibitors). H^+ secretion by the cells of the proximal tubule is impaired, resulting in decreased resorption of the filtered load of HCO_3^-. Consequently, HCO_3^- is lost in the urine, the plasma $[HCO_3^-]$ decreases, and acidosis ensues.

Distal RTA also occurs in a number of hereditary and acquired conditions (e.g., **medullary sponge kidney,** certain drugs such as **amphotericin B,** and conditions secondary to urinary obstruction). Depending on the cause, the secretion of H^+ by the intercalated cells of the collecting duct may be impaired, or the permeability of the collecting duct to H^+ may be increased. In either case, the ability to acidify the tubular fluid is impaired. Consequently, titratable acid excretion is reduced, and nonionic diffusion and diffusion trapping of NH_4^+ are impaired. This in turn decreases NAE, with the subsequent development of acidosis.

Failure to produce and excrete sufficient quantities of NH_4^+ can also reduce the amount of NAE by the kidneys. In this situation, H^+ secretion by the proximal tubule is normal (as is H^+ secretion by the distal tubule and collecting duct), and the urine pH is maximally acidic. However, because of the lack of sufficient quantities of NH_4^+, NAE is less than net acid production, and metabolic acidosis develops. This form of RTA is usually seen in individuals who have a reduced number of nephrons (i.e., mild to moderate renal failure). If the acidosis that results from any of these forms of RTA is severe, individuals must ingest alkali (e.g., $NaHCO_3$) to maintain acid-base balance. In this way, the HCO_3^- lost each day in the buffering of nonvolatile acid is replenished by new HCO_3^- ingested in the diet.

Acid-Base Disorders

The diagnosis of and approach to patients with acid-base disorders frequently involves the measurement and interpretation of arterial blood gases. This analysis, which includes measurements of the partial pressure of oxygen (Po_2), Pco_2, and pH, focuses on the components of the HCO_3^- buffer system and the following reaction:

$$CO_2 + H_2O \xrightarrow{\text{CA}} H_2CO_3 \leftrightarrow H^+ + HCO_3^- \qquad \textbf{39-4}$$

The first reaction (hydration/dehydration of CO_2) is the rate-limiting step. This reaction, which is normally slow, is greatly accelerated in the presence of the enzyme **carbonic anhydrase (CA).** The second reaction, the ionization of H_2CO_3 to H^+ and HCO_3^-, is virtually instantaneous. From the measurements of Pco_2 and pH,

the $[HCO_3^-]$ can be calculated using the Henderson-Hasselbalch equation:

$$pH = 6.1 + \log \frac{[HCO_3^-]}{0.03\, Pco_2} \qquad \textbf{39-5}$$

The pH of the ECF is maintained within a very narrow range (7.35 to 7.45). Inspection of Equation 39-5 shows that the pH of the ECF varies when either the $[HCO_3^-]$ or Pco_2 is altered. Disturbances of acid-base balance that result from a change in the $[HCO_3^-]$ of ECF are termed **metabolic acid-base disorders,** whereas those resulting from a change in the Pco_2 are termed **respiratory acid-base disorders.** These disorders are considered in more detail later in this chapter. The kidneys are primarily responsible for regulating the $[HCO_3^-]$, whereas the lungs regulate the Pco_2.

For simplicity of presentation in this chapter, the value of 7.40 for body fluid pH is used as normal, even though the normal reference range is from 7.35 to 7.45. Similarly, the normal range for Pco_2 is 35 to 45 mm Hg. However, a Pco_2 of 40 mm Hg is used as the normal reference value. Finally, a value of 24 mEq/L is considered a normal ECF $[HCO_3^-]$, even though the normal range is 22 to 28 mEq/L.

Defense mechanisms minimize changes in the pH of body fluid

When an acid-base disturbance develops, the body uses a series of mechanisms to defend against the change in the pH of the ECF. THESE DEFENSE MECHANISMS DO NOT CORRECT THE ACID-BASE DISTURBANCE BUT MERELY MINIMIZE THE CHANGE IN pH IMPOSED BY THE DISTURBANCE. RESTORATION OF THE BLOOD pH TO ITS NORMAL VALUE REQUIRES CORRECTION OF THE UNDERLYING PROCESS OR PROCESSES THAT PRODUCED THE ACID-BASE DISORDER. The body has three general mechanisms to defend against changes in body fluid pH produced by acid-base disturbances: (1) extracellular and intracellular buffering, (2) adjustments in blood Pco_2 via alterations in the ventilatory rate of the lungs, and (3) adjustments in the renal NAE.

Extracellular and intracellular buffers act quickly to minimize changes in body fluid pH

THE FIRST LINE OF DEFENSE AGAINST ACID-BASE DISORDERS IS EXTRACELLULAR AND INTRACELLULAR BUFFERING. The response of the extracellular buffers is virtually instantaneous, whereas that to intracellular buffering is slower and can take several minutes.

Metabolic disorders that result from the addition of nonvolatile acid or alkali to the body fluids are buffered in both the extracellular and intracellular fluids. The HCO_3^- buffer system is the principal ECF buffer. When nonvolatile acid is added to the body fluids (or base is lost from the body), HCO_3^- is consumed during the process of neutralizing the acid load, and the $[HCO_3^-]$

of the ECF is reduced. Conversely, when nonvolatile base is added to the body fluids (or acid is lost from the body), H^+ is consumed, causing more HCO_3^- to be produced from the dissociation of H_2CO_3. Consequently, the $[HCO_3^-]$ increases.

Although the HCO_3^- buffer system is the principal ECF buffer, phosphate and plasma proteins provide additional extracellular buffering. The combined action of the buffering processes for HCO_3^-, phosphate, and plasma protein accounts for approximately 50% of the buffering of a nonvolatile acid load and 70% of a nonvolatile alkali load. The remainder of the buffering under these two conditions occurs intracellularly. Intracellular buffering involves the movement of H^+ into cells (during buffering of nonvolatile acid) or the movement of H^+ out of cells (during buffering of nonvolatile alkali). H^+ is titrated inside the cell by HCO_3^-, phosphate, and the histidine groups on proteins.

Bone represents an additional source of extracellular buffering. With acidosis, buffering by bone results in its demineralization because Ca^{++} released from bone as Ca^{++}-containing salts binds H^+ in exchange for Ca^{++}.

When respiratory acid-base disorders occur, the pH of body fluid changes as a result of alterations in the P_{CO_2} (see Equation 39-5). Virtually all buffering in respiratory acid-base disorders occurs intracellularly. When the P_{CO_2} rises (respiratory acidosis), CO_2 moves into the cell, where it combines with H_2O to form H_2CO_3. H_2CO_3 rapidly dissociates, and the H^+ concentration ($[H^+]$) increases. Some of the H^+ is then buffered by cellular protein. This process is reversed when the P_{CO_2} is reduced (respiratory alkalosis).

The ventilatory rate of the lungs changes in response to acid-base disorders

THE LUNGS ARE THE SECOND LINE OF DEFENSE AGAINST ACID-BASE DISORDERS. As indicated by the Henderson-Hasselbalch equation (see Equation 39-5), changes in the P_{CO_2} alter the blood pH: A rise decreases the pH, and a reduction increases the pH.

The ventilatory rate determines the P_{CO_2}. Increased ventilation decreases P_{CO_2}, whereas decreased ventilation increases it. The blood P_{CO_2} and pH are important regulators of the ventilatory rate (see Chapter 31). When metabolic acidosis occurs, a rise in the $[H^+]$ (decrease in pH) increases the ventilatory rate. Conversely, during metabolic alkalosis, a decreased $[H^+]$ (increase in pH) leads to a reduced ventilatory rate. With maximal hyperventilation, the P_{CO_2} can be reduced to approximately 10 mm Hg. Because hypoxia, a potent stimulator of ventilation, also develops with hypoventilation, the degree to which the P_{CO_2} can be increased is limited. In an otherwise normal individual, hypoventilation cannot raise the P_{CO_2} above 60 mm Hg. The respiratory response to metabolic acid-base disturbances may be initiated within minutes but may require several hours to complete.

Renal net acid excretion changes in response to acid-base disorders

THE THIRD AND FINAL LINE OF DEFENSE AGAINST ACID-BASE DISORDERS IS THE KIDNEYS. In response to an alteration in the plasma pH and P_{CO_2}, the kidneys make appropriate adjustments in the excretion of HCO_3^- and net acid. The renal response may require several days to reach completion because it takes hours to days to increase the synthesis and activity of the proximal tubule enzymes involved in NH_4^+ production. In the case of acidosis (increased $[H^+]$ or P_{CO_2}), the secretion of H^+ by the nephron is stimulated, and the entire filtered load of HCO_3^- is resorbed. The production and excretion of NH_4^+ are also stimulated, and thus the NAE by the kidneys is increased (see Equation 39-3). The new HCO_3^- generated during the process of NAE is returned to the body, and the plasma $[HCO_3^-]$ increases.

When alkalosis exists (decreased $[H^+]$ or P_{CO_2}), the secretion of H^+ by the nephron is inhibited. As a result, NAE and HCO_3^- resorption are reduced. HCO_3^- appears in the urine. Also, some HCO_3^- is secreted into the urine by the collecting duct. With enhanced excretion of HCO_3^-, the plasma $[HCO_3^-]$ decreases.

The loss of gastric contents from the body (i.e., vomiting, nasogastric suction) produces metabolic alkalosis secondary to the loss of HCl. If the loss of gastric fluid is significant, volume contraction occurs. Under this condition, the kidneys cannot excrete sufficient quantities of HCO_3^- to compensate for the metabolic alkalosis. HCO_3^- is not excreted because the volume contraction enhances Na^+ resorption by the proximal tubule and increases aldosterone levels (see Chapter 37). These responses in turn limit HCO_3^- excretion because Na^+ resorption in the proximal tubule is coupled to H^+ secretion via the Na^+-H^+ antiporter. As a result, HCO_3^- is resorbed because of the need to reduce Na^+ excretion. In addition, the elevated aldosterone levels stimulate H^+ secretion by the collecting duct. Thus in individuals who lose gastric contents, metabolic alkalosis and paradoxically acidic urine characteristically occur. Correction of the alkalosis occurs only when euvolemia is reestablished. With restoration of euvolemia, HCO_3^- resorption by the proximal tubule decreases, as does H^+ secretion by the collecting duct. As a result, HCO_3^- excretion increases, and the plasma $[HCO_3^-]$ returns to normal

---

Table 39-2 summarizes the primary alterations and the subsequent defense mechanisms of the various simple acid-base disorders. The defense mechanisms are commonly referred to as **compensatory responses.** In all acid-base disorders the compensatory

Table 39-2   Mechanisms of Defense Against Acid-Base Disorders

Disorder	Plasma pH	Primary Alteration	Defense Mechanisms
Metabolic acidosis	↓	↓Plasma [HCO_3^-]	ICF and ECF buffers Hyperventilation (↓P_{CO_2}) ↑Renal NAE
Metabolic alkalosis	↑	↑Plasma [HCO_3^-]	ICF and ECF buffers Hypoventilation (↑P_{CO_2}) ↓Renal NAE
Respiratory acidosis	↓	↑P_{CO_2}	ICF buffers ↑Renal NAE
Respiratory alkalosis	↑	↓P_{CO_2}	ICF buffers ↓Renal NAE

ICF, Intracellular fluid.

response does not correct the underlying disorder but simply reduces the magnitude of the change in pH. Correction of the acid-base disorder requires treatment of its cause.

Metabolic acidosis is characterized by a low plasma bicarbonate concentration and a low pH

Metabolic acidosis can develop via the addition of non-volatile acid to the body (e.g., diabetic ketoacidosis), the loss of nonvolatile base (e.g., that caused by diarrhea), or the failure of the kidneys to excrete sufficient net acid to replenish the HCO_3^- used to neutralize nonvolatile acids (e.g., renal tubular acidosis, renal failure). As previously described, the buffering of H^+ occurs in both the ECF and the intracellular fluid (ICF). When the pH falls, the respiratory centers are stimulated, and the ventilatory rate is increased (respiratory compensation). This reduces the P_{CO_2}, which further minimizes the fall in plasma pH. Finally, renal excretion of net acid is increased. This occurs via the elimination of all HCO_3^- from the urine (enhanced resorption of filtered HCO_3^-) and via increased NH_4^+ excretion (enhanced production of new HCO_3^-). If the process that initiated the acid-base disturbance is corrected, the enhanced excretion of acid by the kidneys will ultimately return the pH and [HCO_3^-] to normal. After correction of the pH, the ventilatory rate also returns to normal.

When nonvolatile acid is added to the body fluids, as in **diabetic ketoacidosis,** the [H^+] increases (pH decreases), and the [HCO_3^-] decreases. In addition, the concentration of the anion associated with the nonvolatile acid increases. This change in the anion concentration provides a convenient way of analyzing the cause of a metabolic acidosis by calculating what is termed the **anion gap.** The anion gap represents the difference between the concentration of the major plasma cation (Na^+) and the major plasma anions (Cl^- and HCO_3^-):

$$\text{Anion gap} = [Na^+] - ([Cl^-] + [HCO_3^-]) \qquad \textbf{39-6}$$

Under normal conditions the anion gap ranges from 8 to 16 mEq/L. It is important to recognize that an anion gap does not actually exist. All cations are balanced by anions. The gap simply reflects the parameters that are measured. In reality:

$$[Na^+] + [\text{Unmeasured cations}] = [Cl^-] + \qquad \textbf{39-7}$$
$$[HCO_3^-] + [\text{Unmeasured anions}]$$

If the anion of the nonvolatile acid is Cl^-, the anion gap will be normal. (That is, the decrease in the [HCO_3^-] is matched by an increase in the [Cl^-].) The metabolic acidosis associated with diarrhea or renal tubular acidosis has a normal anion gap. In contrast, if the anion of the nonvolatile acid is not Cl^- (e.g., lactate, β-hydroxybutyrate), the anion gap will increase. (That is, the decrease in the [HCO_3^-] is not matched by an increase in the [Cl^-] but rather by an increase in the concentration of the unmeasured anion.) The anion gap is increased in metabolic acidosis associated with renal failure, diabetes mellitus (ketoacidosis), lactic acidosis, and the ingestion of large quantities of aspirin. Thus CALCULATION OF THE ANION GAP IS A USEFUL WAY OF IDENTIFYING THE ETIOLOGY OF METABOLIC ACIDOSIS.

Metabolic alkalosis is characterized by an elevated plasma bicarbonate concentration and an elevated pH

Metabolic alkalosis can occur via the addition of nonvolatile base to the body (e.g., ingestion of antacids), as a result of volume contraction (e.g., hemorrhage), or more commonly, from the loss of nonvolatile acid (e.g., loss of gastric HCl because of vomiting). Buffering occurs predomi nantly in the ECF and to a lesser degree in the ICF. The increase in the pH inhibits the respiratory centers, the ventilatory rate is reduced, and thus the P_{CO_2} is elevated (respiratory compensation). The renal compensatory response to metabolic alkalosis is to increase the excretion of HCO_3^- by reducing its resorption along the nephron. Normally, this occurs quite rapidly and effectively. However, as already noted, when alkalosis occurs with volume depletion (e.g., vomiting in which fluid loss occurs with H^+ loss), HCO_3^- is not excreted. Renal excretion of HCO_3^- is enhanced, and alkalosis is corrected only with restoration of euvolemia. Enhanced renal excretion of HCO_3^- eventually returns the pH and $[HCO_3^-]$ to normal, provided that the underlying cause of the initial acid-base disturbance is corrected. When the pH is corrected, the ventilatory rate also returns to normal.

Respiratory acidosis is characterized by an elevated partial pressure of carbon dioxide and a reduced pH

Respiratory acidosis results from decreased gas exchange across the alveoli, as a result of either inadequate ventilation (e.g., drug-induced depression of the respiratory centers) or impaired gas diffusion (e.g., pulmonary edema, such as that which occurs in cardiovascular or lung disease). In contrast to the metabolic disorders, buffering during respiratory acidosis occurs almost entirely in the ICF. The increase in the P_{CO_2} and the decrease in pH stimulate both HCO_3^- resorption by the nephron and NH_4^+ excretion (renal compensation). Together, these responses increase NAE and generate new HCO_3^-. The renal compensatory response takes several days to occur. Consequently, respiratory acid-base disorders are commonly divided into acute and chronic phases. In the acute phase, the time for the renal compensatory response is not sufficient, and the body relies on intracellular buffering to minimize the change in pH. Correction of the underlying disorder returns the P_{CO_2} to normal, and the renal excretion of acid decreases to its initial level.

Respiratory alkalosis is characterized by a reduced partial pressure of carbon dioxide and an elevated pH

Respiratory alkalosis results from increased gas exchange in the lungs, usually caused by increased ventilation from stimulation of the respiratory centers (e.g., via drugs or disorders of the central nervous system). Hyperventilation can also occur as a result of anxiety, pain, or fear. As noted, buffering is primarily in the ICF. As with respiratory acidosis, respiratory alkalosis has both acute and chronic phases reflecting the time required for renal compensation to occur. With renal compensation, the elevated pH and reduced P_{CO_2} inhibit HCO_3^- resorption by the nephron and reduce NH_4^+ production and excretion. As a result of these

two effects, NAE is reduced. Correction of the underlying disorder returns the P_{CO_2} to normal, and renal excretion of acid then increases to its initial level.

Analysis of Acid-Base Disorders

The analysis of an acid-base disorder is directed at identifying the underlying cause so that appropriate therapy can be initiated. The patient's medical history and associated physical findings often provide valuable clues about the nature and origin of an acid-base disorder. In addition, the analysis of an arterial blood sample is frequently required. Such an analysis is straightforward if approached systematically. For example, consider the following data:

pH	7.35
$[HCO_3^-]$	16 mEq/L
P_{CO_2}	30 mm Hg

The acid-base disorder represented by these values, or any other set of values, can be determined using the following three-step approach (Figure 39-5):

1. Examination of the pH: When the pH is considered first, the underlying disorder can be classified as either an acidosis or an alkalosis. The defense mechanisms of the body cannot correct an acid-base disorder by themselves. Thus even if the defense mechanisms are completely operative, the pH still indicates the origin of the initial disorder. In the example provided, the pH of 7.35 indicates acidosis.

2. Determination of metabolic versus respiratory disorder: Simple acid-base disorders are either metabolic or respiratory. To determine which disorder is present, the clinician must next examine the $[HCO_3^-]$ and P_{CO_2}. As previously discussed, acidosis could be the result of a decrease in the $[HCO_3^-]$ (metabolic) or an increase in the P_{CO_2} (respiratory). Alternatively, alkalosis could be the result of an increase in the $[HCO_3^-]$ (metabolic) or a decrease in the P_{CO_2} (respiratory). For the example provided, the $[HCO_3^-]$ is reduced from normal (normal = 24 mEq/L), as is the P_{CO_2} (normal = 40 mm Hg). The disorder must therefore be metabolic acidosis; it cannot be a respiratory acidosis because the P_{CO_2} is reduced.

3. Analysis of compensatory response: Metabolic disorders result in compensatory changes in ventilation and thus in the P_{CO_2}, whereas respiratory disorders result in compensatory changes in renal acid excretion and thus the $[HCO_3^-]$. In an appropriately compensated metabolic acidosis, the P_{CO_2} is decreased, whereas it is elevated in compensated metabolic alkalosis. With respira-

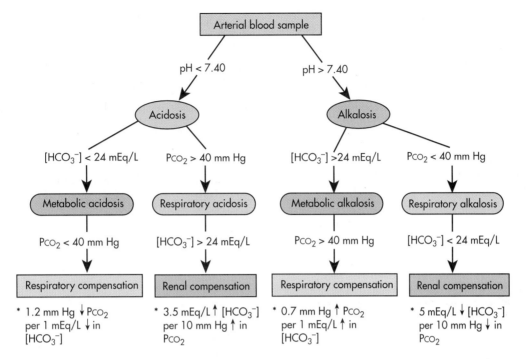

Figure 39-5 Approach for the analysis of simple acid-base disorders.

tory acidosis, complete compensation results in an elevation of the $[HCO_3^-]$. Conversely, the $[HCO_3^-]$ is reduced in response to respiratory alkalosis. In this example, the P_{CO_2} is reduced from normal, and the magnitude of this reduction is as expected (Figure 39-5). Therefore the acid-base disorder is a simple metabolic acidosis with appropriate respiratory compensation.

Multiple acid-base disorders can exist in a patient

If the appropriate compensatory response is not present, a **mixed acid-base disorder** should be suspected. Such a disorder reflects the presence of two or more underlying causes for the acid-base disturbance. A mixed disorder should be suspected when analysis of the arterial blood gas indicates that appropriate compensation has not occurred. For example, consider the following data:

pH	6.96
$[HCO_3^-]$	12 mEq/L
P_{CO_2}	55 mm Hg

When the three-step approach is followed, it is evident that the disturbance is an acidosis that has both a metabolic component ($[HCO_3^-] < 24$ mEq/L) and a respiratory component ($P_{CO_2} > 40$ mm Hg). Thus this disorder is mixed. These disorders can occur, for example, in an individual who has a history of a chronic pulmonary disease such as emphysema (i.e., chronic respiratory acidosis) and who develops an acute gastrointestinal illness with diarrhea. Because diarrhea fluid contains HCO_3^-, its loss from the body results in the development of metabolic acidosis.

A MIXED ACID-BASE DISORDER IS ALSO INDICATED WHEN A PATIENT HAS ABNORMAL P_{CO_2} AND $[HCO_3^-]$ VALUES, BUT THE pH IS NORMAL. Such a condition can develop in a patient who has ingested a large quantity of aspirin. The salicylic acid (active ingredient in aspirin) produces metabolic acidosis, and at the same time, it stimulates the respiratory centers, causing hyperventilation and respiratory alkalosis. Thus the patient has a reduced plasma $[HCO_3^-]$ and a reduced P_{CO_2}.

SUMMARY

- The pH of the body fluids is maintained within a narrow range by the coordinated function of the lungs, liver, and kidneys. These organs maintain acid-base balance by balancing the excretion of acid and alkali with the amounts ingested in the diet and produced by metabolism.
- The kidneys maintain acid-base balance through the excretion of an amount of acid equal to the amount of nonvolatile acid produced by metabolism and ingested in the diet. The kidneys also prevent the loss of HCO_3^- in the urine by resorbing virtually all the HCO_3^- filtered at the glomeruli. Both the resorption of filtered HCO_3^- and the excretion of acid are accomplished by the secretion of H^+ by the nephrons.

- Renal NAE is quantitated as:

$$NAE = [(U_{NH_4^+} \times \dot{V}) + (U_{TA} \times \dot{V})] - (U_{HCO_3^-} \times \dot{V})$$

- Phosphate is the primary urinary buffer (titratable acid). The production (from glutamine metabolism) and excretion of NH_4^+ are critical to the generation of new HCO_3^- by the kidneys and is regulated in response to acid-base disturbances.
- The body uses three lines of defense to minimize the impact of acid-base disorders on body fluid pH: (1) ECF and ICF buffering, (2) respiratory compensation, and (3) renal compensation.
- Metabolic acid-base disorders result from primary alterations in the $[HCO_3^-]$, which in turn results from the addition of acid to or loss of alkali from the body. In response to metabolic acidosis, pulmonary ventilation is increased, which decreases the P_{CO_2}. An increase in the $[HCO_3^-]$ causes alkalosis. This decreases pulmonary ventilation, which elevates the P_{CO_2}. The pulmonary response to metabolic acid-base disorders occurs in a matter of minutes.
- Respiratory acid-base disorders result from primary alterations in the P_{CO_2}. Elevation of the P_{CO_2} produces acidosis, and the kidneys respond with an increase in the excretion of net acid. Conversely, the reduction of P_{CO_2} produces alkalosis, and renal acid excretion is reduced. The kidneys respond to respiratory acid-base disorders over several hours to days.

BIBLIOGRAPHY

Alpern RJ, Preisig PA: Renal acid-base transport. In Schrier RW, Gottschalk CW, eds: *Diseases of the kidney,* ed 6, Boston, 1997, Little, Brown.

Alpern RJ, Rector FC Jr: Renal acidification mechanisms. In Brenner BM, ed: *The kidney,* ed 5, Philadelphia, 1996, WB Saunders.

Bianchini L, Pouyssegur J: Na$^+$/H$^+$ exchangers: structure, function, and regulation. In Schlondorf D, Bonventre JV, eds: *Molecular nephrology,* New York, 1995, Marcel Dekker.

DuBose TD Jr et al: Acid-base disorders. In Brenner BM, ed: *The kidney,* ed 5, Philadelphia, 1996, WB Saunders.

Gamble JL Jr: Moving more closely to acid-base relationships in the body as a whole, *Perspect Biol Med* 39:593, 1996.

Gluck SL et al: Renal plasma membrane vacuolar H$^+$ ATPases: properties and function in acid-base homeostasis, In Schlondorf D, Bonventre JV, eds: *Molecular nephrology,* New York, 1995, Marcel Dekker.

Gluck SL et al: Distal urinary acidification from Homer Smith to the present, *Kidney Int* 49:1660, 1996.

Gluck SL et al: Physiology and biochemistry of the kidney vacuolar H$^+$-ATPase, *Annu Rev Physiol* 58:427, 1996.

Moe OW: Sodium-hydrogen exchange in renal epithelia: mechanisms of acute regulation, *Curr Opin Nephrol Hyperten* 6:440, 1997.

Wakabayashi S et al: Molecular physiology of vertebrate Na$^+$/H$^+$ exchangers, *Physiol Rev* 77:51, 1997.

Wingo CS, Smolka AJ: Function and structure of H-K-ATPase in the kidney, *Am J Physiol Renal Fluid Electrolyte Physiol* 269:F1, 1995.

▷ CASE STUDIES

Case 39-1

A 22-year-old man with insulin-dependent diabetes mellitus is seen in the emergency department. He reports that he "has had the flu for the past couple days." Because he has not felt well and was not eating, he has not taken any insulin during the previous 24 hours. He also reports taking two aspirin tablets before coming to the emergency department because of a headache. On examination, he is found to have rapid and deep respirations. The following laboratory data are obtained:

pH	7.32	(normal: 7.40)
P$_{O_2}$	100 mm Hg	(normal: 100 mm Hg)
P$_{CO_2}$	30 mm Hg	(normal: 40 mm Hg)
[HCO$_3^-$]	15 mEq/L	(normal: 24 mEq/L)

1. What type of acid-base disorder does this man have?
  A. Metabolic acidosis
  B. Metabolic alkalosis
  C. Respiratory acidosis
  D. Respiratory alkalosis
  E. Mixed disorder (metabolic acidosis and respiratory alkalosis)

2. Why are this man's respirations rapid and deep?
  A. They will increase his P$_{CO_2}$.
  B. They have occurred in response to his hypoxemia.
  C. They are a normal respiratory response to his acid-base disturbance.
  D. There is poor pulmonary gas exchange caused by an infection in his lungs.
  E. Aspirin has stimulated his respiratory center.

3. What is the most important component of the compensatory response of this man's kidneys to his acid-base disorder?
  A. Increased filtered load of HCO$_3^-$
  B. Decreased secretion of H$^+$ by the proximal tubule
  C. Increased production and excretion of NH$_4^+$
  D. Decreased H$^+$ secretion by the collecting duct
  E. Increased secretion of HCO$_3^-$ by the collecting duct

Case 39-2

A 50-year-old woman with a history of a duodenal ulcer comes to the emergency room because she has had intermittent vomiting for several days. She is admitted to the hospital, and a nasogastric tube is introduced to continuously remove the stomach contents. After 24 hours, the woman has signs of volume depletion. The following laboratory values are obtained:

pH	7.50	(normal: 7.40)
P_{O_2}	100 mm Hg	(normal: 100 mm Hg)
P_{CO_2}	47 mm Hg	(normal: 40 mm Hg)
$[HCO_3^-]$	35 mEq/L	(normal: 24 mEq/L)
Urine pH	6.0	

1. What type of acid-base disorder does this woman have?
   A. Metabolic acidosis
   B. Metabolic alkalosis
   C. Respiratory acidosis
   D. Respiratory alkalosis
   E. Mixed disorder (metabolic alkalosis and respiratory acidosis)

2. Why is this woman's urine acidic?
   A. Collecting duct H^+ secretion is stimulated by aldosterone.
   B. H^+ secretion by the proximal tubule is impaired (i.e., proximal renal tubular acidosis).
   C. The filtered load of HCO_3^- is increased.
   D. NH_4^+ production and excretion are increased.
   E. Titratable acid excretion is increased.

VIII

ENDOCRINE SYSTEM

Saul M. Genuth

General Principles of Endocrine Physiology

OBJECTIVES

- Describe the overall workings of the endocrine system.
- Differentiate various modes of hormone synthesis.
- Explain the multiple mechanisms of hormone actions.
- Indicate how hormone production is measured.
- Explain the factors that determine whole-body responsiveness to hormones.

The endocrine system relates to all of the preceding chapters because it regulates the functioning of every cell, tissue, and organ in the body. Although the endocrine system has numerous components with individual diverse characteristics, this chapter sets forth a set of basic themes that underlie the processes of hormone secretion and action.

The Endocrine System Is a Key Component in Environmental Adaptation

The endocrine system is a key component in the adaptation of the human organism to alterations in the internal and external environment. THE ENDOCRINE SYSTEM ACTS TO MAINTAIN A STABLE INTERNAL MILIEU IN THE FACE OF CHANGES IN INFLOW OR OUTFLOW OF SUBSTRATES, MINERALS, WATER, ENVIRONMENTAL SUBSTANCES, HEAT, AND SO ON. Specific endocrine cells, usually grouped in glands, sense the disturbance and respond by secreting chemical substances called **hormones** into the bloodstream. These special molecules are carried via the circulation to various tissues, where they signal and act on their target cells. As a result the target cells respond in a manner that usually opposes the direction of change that evoked hormone secretion and thereby restores the organism toward its original state. In addition to this fundamental role in maintaining **homeostasis,** the endocrine system helps initiate, mediate, and regulate the processes of growth, development, maturation, reproduction, and senescence.

A hormone was originally defined as a substance that was elaborated by one type of cell and that carried a signal through the bloodstream to distant target cells. However, this sophisticated method of signaling prob-

ably evolved from a more primitive one (Figure 40-1). Hormone molecules secreted by endocrine cells can also reach and act on target cells within the same locale simply by diffusing through the interstitial fluid separating them; this process is called **paracrine function.** Hormone molecules can even act back on their cells of origin to modulate their own secretion or other intracellular processes; this is called **autocrine function.**

Classic endocrine cells reside in the pituitary, thyroid, adrenal, and parathyroid glands; in the gonads; and in the pancreatic islets. However, hormone-like signaling molecules are also elaborated by other nonclassic endocrine cells such as neurons, renal cells, cardiac atrial and ventricular cells, endothelial cells, immune system cells, adipose cells, mesenchymal cells, and platelets.

The endocrine system may act independently of or may be integrated with the nervous system

The endocrine and nervous systems are the major components in the organism's adaptability to change (Figure 40-2). These two signaling systems have several characteristics in common:

1. Both neurons and endocrine cells are capable of secreting.
2. Both endocrine cells and neurons generate electrical potentials and can be depolarized.
3. Some molecules serve as both a neurotransmitter and a hormone.
4. The mechanism of action of both hormones and neurotransmitters requires interaction with specific receptors in target cells.

Although the endocrine system responds more often to chemical stimuli and the nervous system more often to physical or mechanical stimuli, considerable overlap exists. For example, changes in the quantity of light and changes in plasma substrate concentrations may evoke responses by both systems. Interaction between the two systems takes several forms:

1. Some stimuli that cause hormone release are first sensed by the nervous system, which in turn signals an appropriate endocrine cell to respond.

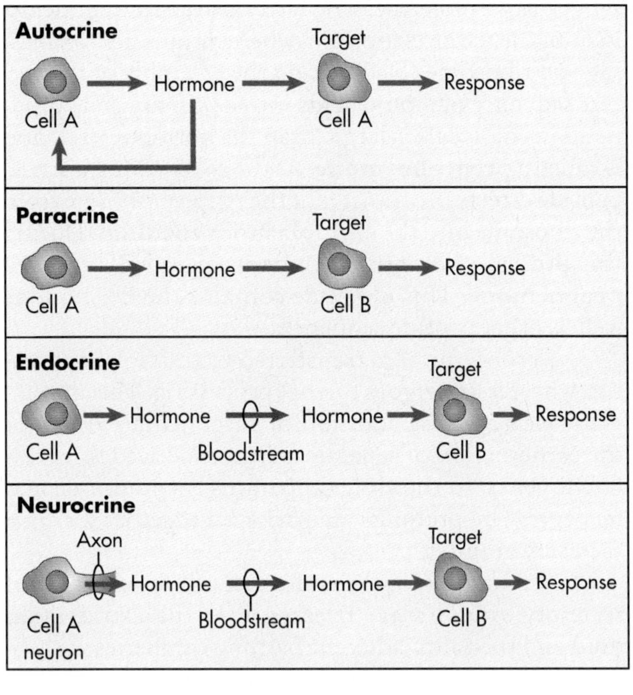

Autocrine

Cell A → Hormone → Target Cell A → Response

Paracrine

Cell A → Hormone → Target Cell B → Response

Endocrine

Cell A → Hormone → Bloodstream → Hormone → Target Cell B → Response

Neurocrine

Cell A neuron, Axon → Hormone → Bloodstream → Hormone → Target Cell B → Response

Figure 40-1 Mechanisms for cell-to-cell signaling via hormone molecules. In autocrine function the hormone signal acts back on the cell of origin or adjacent identical cells. In paracrine function the hormone signal is carried to an adjacent target cell over short distances via the interstitial fluid. In endocrine function the signal is carried to a distant target cell via the bloodstream. In neurocrine function the hormone signal originates in a neuron and after axonal transport to the bloodstream, is carried to a distant target cell.

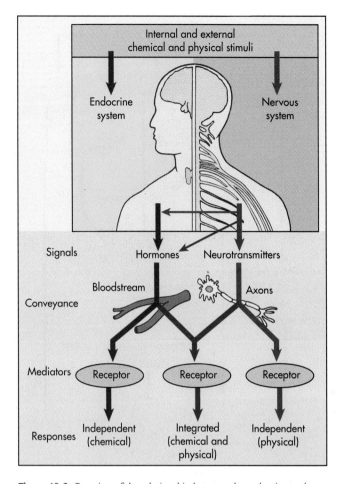

Figure 40-2 Overview of the relationship between the endocrine and nervous systems. Similar stimuli may elicit activity of both systems. Hormones secreted by endocrine cells and conveyed via the bloodstream are analogous to neurotransmitters released by neurons after being conveyed by their axons. Neurotransmitters may also stimulate hormone release and themselves act as hormones. Responses are mediated by receptors in each system and may consist of either chemical or physical changes.

2. Some neurons extend their axons in bundles or tracts that terminate adjacent to capillaries. Stimulation releases their neurotransmitters into the bloodstream. This hybrid form of signal transmission is called **neurocrine function** (Figure 40-1), and the signaling molecules are called **neurohormones.** For example, **antidiuretic hormone (ADH)** is synthesized in the cell body of a hypothalamic neuron but is released from the end of the neuron's axon into blood bathing the posterior pituitary gland. ADH then acts on distant cells in the kidney and causes the retention of free water. The stimulus for axonal release of ADH is water deprivation, sensed in the hypothalamus as an increase in plasma osmolality, a decrease in volume, or both reactions.

3. Some stimuli evoke integrated endocrine and nervous system responses that augment each other in restoring homeostasis.

The principle of chemical homeostasis and the fundamental relationship of the endocrine system to the nervous system are well illustrated by the response of the organism to a lowered plasma concentration of glucose **(hypoglycemia),** such as that which can occur with very strenuous and prolonged exercise (Figure 40-3). Because a supply of glucose is absolutely required to sustain brain function, hypoglycemia cannot be tolerated for long. Endocrine cells in the pancreas respond to hypoglycemia by secreting a hormone called **glucagon** that stimulates the release of stored glucose from the liver. Other endocrine cells in the pancreas respond in the opposite way to hypoglycemia by diminishing the secretion of the hormone **insulin,** thereby reducing use of glucose by tissues other than the brain.

Certain neurons in the hypothalamus sense hypoglycemia and augment the release of stored glucose directly by transmitting sympathetic neural impulses to liver cells and indirectly by transmitting sympathetic nervous system impulses to the adrenal medulla. This neuroendocrine gland secretes the hormone **epinephrine,** which acts on the liver to release stored glucose and on other tissues to reduce glucose use. Finally, other neurons in the hypothalamus also sense hypoglycemia and via combined neurocrine and endocrine pathways,

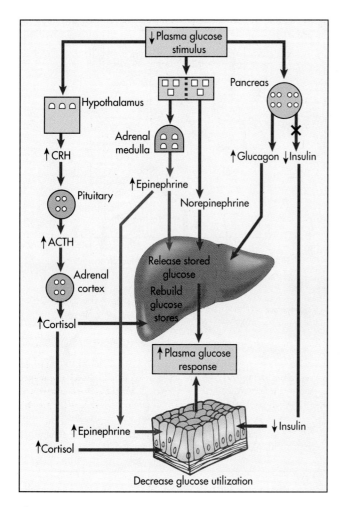

Figure 40-3 Integrated endocrine and neural response to hypoglycemia. The anterior pituitary gland, adrenal cortex, adrenal medulla, and pancreatic islets participate in the main endocrine components of the response. The hypothalamus and the sympathetic nervous system participate in the neural components of the response. See text for details on how each component acts to restore the plasma glucose concentration to normal. *ACTH,* Adrenocorticotropic hormone; *CRH,* corticotropin-releasing hormone.

stimulate the adrenal cortex to secrete the hormone **cortisol.** This hormone augments the synthesis of glucose in the liver to maintain the supply in case initial stores become depleted. Cortisol also inhibits the insulin-stimulated use of glucose by tissues other than the brain. Together these endocrine and neural responses to hypoglycemia promptly raise plasma glucose levels back to normal.

Hormones Are Synthesized, Stored, and Secreted in a Variety of Ways

Peptide and **protein hormones** are synthesized by a general process that characterizes the synthesis of all secreted proteins (Figure 40-4). The gene or DNA molecule that directs hormone synthesis transcribes a mes-

senger RNA molecule. The latter traverses the nuclear membrane to the cytoplasm, where it translates its message on ribosomes by directing the assembly of the correct sequence of amino acids into a primary gene product. This molecule is larger than the hormone itself and is called a **preprohormone.** At the N-terminus, a signal peptide directs the transfer of the preprohormone from the ribosome into the **endoplasmic reticulum.** During this process, the signal peptide is degraded, leaving a **prohormone.** This molecule contains the hormone as well as other peptide sequences.

The prohormone is transferred to the Golgi apparatus, where it undergoes further processing. This may include cleavage, the addition of carbohydrate units, or the combination of separate subunits derived from different genes. In the Golgi apparatus the hormone and its peptide by-products are packaged together within a secretory granule.

On stimulation of the endocrine cell the contents of secretory granules are released into the extracellular fluid and then into adjacent bathing capillaries via exocytosis (Figure 40-5). By the contraction of microfilaments and guidance by microtubules, the secretory granules move to the plasma membrane of the cell and fuse with it. A **GTP-binding protein** helps attach the granules to specific sites. The mechanisms of granule release require an increase in the intracytoplasmic Ca^{++} concentration; the Ca^{++} is derived from both extracellular fluid and intracellular stores within the endoplasmic reticulum and other organelles. Exocytosis is also often preceded by increases in **cyclic AMP** concentration.

Catecholamine hormones (epinephrine, norepinephrine, dopamine) are synthesized from the amino acid tyrosine through a series of enzymatic reactions. However, they are stored in secretory granules and secreted in a manner similar to that of peptide hormones.

Thyroid hormones (thyroxine, triiodothyronine) are synthesized from tyrosine and iodide in a series of reactions that occur with the amino acid already incorporated via peptide linkage into a large protein molecule. The hormones are then sequestered within the protein molecule in a storage space (follicle) shared by a group of surrounding endocrine cells. The secretion of thyroid hormone requires retrieval from the follicle and enzymatic release from its protein storage form.

Steroid hormones (cortisol, aldosterone, androgens, estrogens, progestins, vitamin D) are synthesized from cholesterol by a series of enzymatic reactions. However, they are not stored to any appreciable extent within the gland of origin. Thus increases in the secretion of a steroid hormone are accomplished by the activation of the entire biosynthetic sequence from cholesterol. In effect, the storage form of all steroid hormones is the intracellular depot of cholesterol.

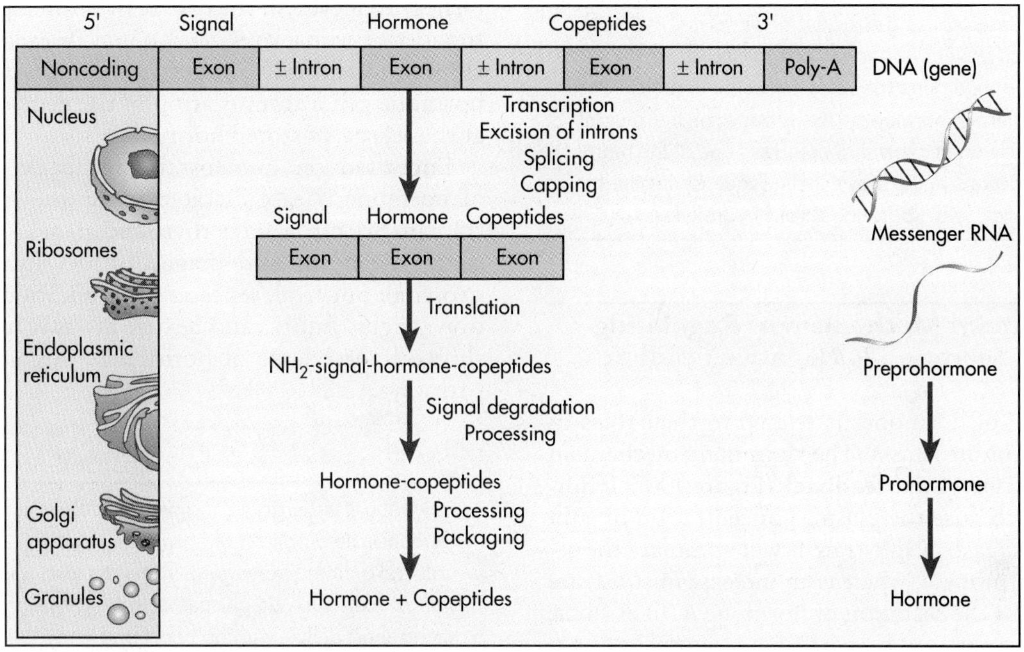

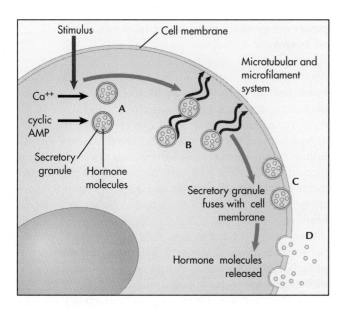

5'	Signal	Hormone	Copeptides	3'	
Noncoding	Exon	± Intron	Exon	± Intron	Exon	± Intron	Poly-A	DNA (gene)

Transcription
Excision of introns
Splicing
Capping

Signal	Hormone	Copeptides
Exon	Exon	Exon

Messenger RNA

Translation

NH₂-signal-hormone-copeptides

Signal degradation
Processing

Hormone-copeptides

Processing
Packaging

Hormone + Copeptides

Preprohormone

Prohormone

Hormone

Nucleus
Ribosomes
Endoplasmic reticulum
Golgi apparatus
Granules

Figure 40-4 Peptide hormone synthesis. In the nucleus the primary gene transcript undergoes excision of introns (noncoding regions), splicing of the exons (coding regions), and capping. The resultant mature messenger RNA enters the cytoplasm, where it directs the synthesis of a precursor peptide sequence (preprohormone) on ribosomes. In this process the N-terminus signal is removed, and the resultant prohormone is transferred into the endoplasmic reticulum. The prohormone undergoes further processing and is then packaged into secretory granules in the Golgi apparatus. After final cleavage of the prohormone within the granules, the hormone and copeptides are secreted by exocytosis.

Stimulus
Cell membrane
Microtubular and microfilament system
Ca⁺⁺
cyclic AMP
A
B
C
Secretory granule
Hormone molecules
Secretory granule fuses with cell membrane
D
Hormone molecules released

Figure 40-5 Secretion of peptide hormones via exocytosis. **A,** Secretion is initiated by the application of a stimulus that raises the cytosolic Ca^{++} level and also usually raises the intracellular level of cyclic AMP. **B,** The secretory granules are lined up and translocated to the plasma membrane via activation of a microtubular and microfilament system. **C,** The membrane of the secretory granule fuses with that of the cell. **D,** The common membrane is lysed, releasing the hormone into the interstitial space.

Genetic diseases causing deficient or abnormal synthesis of peptide or protein hormones are rare and usually involve the hormone gene itself (e.g., insulin). In the case of thyroid or steroid hormones, the product of the mutant gene is usually an enzyme that catalyzes one of the many separate reactions in the biosynthetic sequence for the affected hormone (e.g., adrenal steroid hydroxylases).

The Dominant Mechanism of Regulating Hormone Secretion Is Negative Feedback

The secretion of hormones is related to their roles in maintaining homeostasis. The dominant mechanism of regulation is **negative feedback** (Figure 40-6). If hormone A acts to raise the plasma concentration of substrate B, a decrease in substrate B will stimulate the secretion of hormone A, whereas an increase in substrate B will suppress the secretion of hormone A. In essence, PHYSIOLOGICAL CONDITIONS THAT REQUIRE THE ACTION OF A HORMONE ALSO STIMULATE ITS RELEASE; CONDITIONS OR PRODUCTS RESULTING FROM PRIOR HORMONE ACTION SUPPRESS FURTHER HORMONE RELEASE. This homeostatic partnership may exist between a hormone and one or more substrates, minerals, other hormones, or even physical factors such as fluid volume.

Occasionally, positive feedback is observed. In such circumstances a product of initial hormone action stimulates further hormone secretion. When the product eventually reaches appropriate concentrations, it may then exert negative feedback on hormone secretion. This mechanism of regulation occurs when a biological process begins at a very low level, yet must reach

rather high levels in the course of normal physiological function. Feedback regulation may be exerted at all levels of endocrine cell function (i.e., at transcription of the hormone gene, at translation of the gene message, and at the release of stored hormone).

Engrafted on homeostatic feedback are patterns of hormone release dictated by diurnal (daily) or ultradian (within a day) rhythms, stages of sleep, seasonal variation, and stages of development (fetal, neonatal, pubertal, senescent). In addition, pain, emotion, fright, injury, and sexual arousal may evoke or shut off the release of hormones via complex neural pathways.

Individuals undergoing major medical or surgical stress demonstrate a pattern of hormonal release (e.g., cortisol, catecholamines, glucagon) that stimulates the mobilization of fuels such as glucose or free fatty acids and augments their delivery to the heart and musculature. In contrast, growth and reproductive processes are suppressed. Hormones also modulate immune responses to stress.

Hormone Turnover

The binding of hormones by plasma proteins greatly influences hormonal rates of turnover

After secretion into the blood, catecholamine, peptide, and most protein hormones circulate unbound to other plasma constituents. In contrast, thyroid and steroid hormones circulate largely bound to specific globulins as well as to albumin. The extent of this protein binding greatly influences the rates at which hormones exit from plasma into interstitial fluid and gain access to target cells. A hormone's plasma half-life (the time required for a 50% decrease in concentration) is increased by strong protein binding.

Larger protein hormones with carbohydrate components have longer half-lives than smaller protein and peptide hormones. After exiting from plasma, hormone molecules may return from other compartments via lymphatic channels, sometimes after dissociation from target cells.

The sum of a hormone's removal processes is expressed as its metabolic clearance rate

Irreversible removal of a hormone from the body results from target cell uptake, metabolic degradation, and urinary or biliary excretion. The sum of all removal processes is expressed in the concept of **metabolic clearance rate (MCR),** or the volume of plasma cleared of hormone per unit of time. In a steady state this equals the mass of

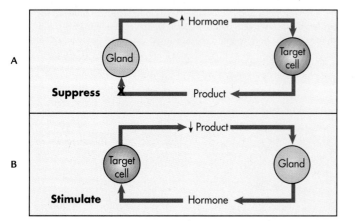

Figure 40-6 Negative feedback principle. **A,** If an increase in hormone secretion stimulates a greater output of product from the target cell, the product feeds back on the gland to suppress further hormone secretion. In this way, hormone excess is limited or prevented. **B,** If a decrease in the output of product from the target cell stimulates hormone secretion, the hormone in turn stimulates the output of product by the target cell. In this way, product deficiency is limited or corrected.

hormone removed per unit of time divided by its plasma concentration:

$$MCR = \frac{mg/min \text{ (removed)}}{mg/ml \text{ (plasma)}} = \frac{ml \text{ plasma (cleared)}}{min} \quad \textbf{40-1}$$

MCR is an expression of the overall efficiency with which a hormone is removed from plasma irrespective of the mechanism. Its derivation is conceptually analogous to that of **renal clearance,** which is explained in Chapter 35. In the latter case, milligram per minute (mg/min) removed, the measured numerator in Equation 40-1, is the urinary excretion of the substance.

The kidney and liver are the major sites of the metabolic degradation of hormones. Renal clearance of a hormone (e.g., thyroid hormone) is extremely low if it is bound to specific plasma globulins. Although peptide and smaller protein hormones are filtered to some degree by the renal glomeruli, they usually undergo tubular reabsorption and subsequent degradation within the kidney so that only a minute amount appears in the urine.

Metabolic degradation of hormones occurs via enzymatic processes that include proteolysis, oxidation, reduction, hydroxylation, decarboxylation, and methylation. Hormones or their metabolites may also be conjugated to water-soluble molecules, such as glucuronides and sulfates, and then excreted in the bile or urine.

The amount of hormone secreted can be estimated from plasma and urine measurements

With the use of isotopic techniques, the total amount of hormone secreted into the bloodstream per unit time can be measured. For clinical purposes, the measurement of hormone in plasma or urine must usually suffice. However, these measurements are valid indices of hormone production if certain conditions exist. In a steady state, the amount of hormone entering the plasma is equal to the amount of hormone exiting the plasma.

$$\text{Secretion rate} = \text{Disposal rate} = \text{Metabolic clearance} \times \quad \textbf{40-2}$$
$$\text{Plasma concentration}$$

If the MCR can be taken as a constant (i.e., MCR is assumed to be normal), then the secretion rate is proportional to the plasma level. This is the theoretical basis for using only the plasma hormone measurement as an index of secretory rate. However, the secretion of many hormones is characterized by diurnal variation and episodic spurts. In such instances, multiple plasma samples may be necessary for a valid estimate.

Similarly, hormone secretion can sometimes be assessed by measuring its urinary excretion in accurately timed collections. This serves to average plasma fluctuations over the collection interval. Urinary excretion is a valid index of secretion rate when kidney function and kidney handling of the hormone are normal.

Hormone Responses Require Recognition by the Target Cell, Generation of Second Messengers, and Various Intracellular Effector Mechanisms

Three major sequential steps are involved in eliciting responses to hormones (Figure 40-7):

1. The hormone must be recognized by the target cell.
2. An intracellular signal must then be generated.
3. One or more intracellular processes (e.g., enzyme reactions, ion movements, cytoskeletal rearrangements, gene transcription) must be increased or decreased.

The binding of hormones to specific receptors causes hormone recognition

Recognition takes place via binding of the hormone to a specific receptor that may be located within the plasma membrane, cytoplasm, nucleus, or possibly other organelles of the target cell. The receptor has a specific binding site with a high affinity for the hormone. The two molecules associate in reversible fashion to form a hormone-receptor complex. The receptor confers specificity to the interaction of a hormone with its target cells. Only cells that have the receptor can respond to the hormone; only hormones for which the cell possesses receptors can affect the cell.

Certain individuals susceptible to **autoimmune diseases** develop antibodies to some of their own hormone receptors. When such antibodies react with the receptor molecules, they may simply block access of the hormone to the receptor and cause biological deficiency (e.g., **hypothyroidism** caused by chronic **autoimmune thyroiditis**). Alternatively, the antibody-receptor combination mimics the hormone-receptor interaction and causes hyperfunction of the gland (e.g., **hyperthyroidism** caused by **Graves' disease**). These conditions are described in Chapter 45.

The reaction between hormone and receptor is the initial determinant of the rate of hormone action

The reaction between a hormone and its receptor can be expressed in classic chemical terms:

$$[H] + [R] \leftrightarrow [HR] \quad \textbf{40-3}$$

$$K = \frac{[HR]}{[H][R]} \quad \textbf{40-4}$$

$$[HR] = K[H][R] \quad \textbf{40-5}$$

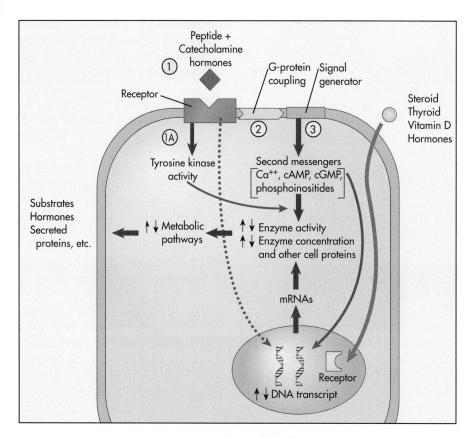

Figure 40-7 Hormone actions on target cells. Hormones interact with either the plasma membrane or intracellular receptors. Hormones may generate second messengers within the receptor (e.g., tyrosine kinase activity), cytoplasm (e.g., cyclic AMP *[cAMP]*), or nucleus (i.e., gene expression). Metabolic pathways can be regulated by altering the activities or the concentrations of enzymes. Cell growth and architecture may also be modulated. *cGMP,* Cyclic GMP.

where:

[H] = Free hormone concentration

[R] = Free or unoccupied receptor concentration

[HR] = Hormone-receptor complex or bound hormone concentration

K = Affinity (association) constant

The amount of receptor occupied by hormone ([HR]) is the critical component that governs the magnitude of hormone action at this first step. As can be seen from Equation 40-5, [HR] is increased when the receptor has a high affinity (K) for the hormone, when the cell is exposed to high hormone concentrations [H], or when the receptor number [R] is high.

In some cases, [HR] is the rate-limiting step in the whole sequence of hormone action; therefore the maximal biological response to these hormones is directly proportional to the number of receptors. In cases in which [HR] is not rate limiting, the biological response can sometimes be maximal when only a small proportion of the available receptors is occupied by hormone.

Receptor molecules undergo continuous, regulated turnover

Receptor molecules are continually synthesized, translocated to sites of association with hormone molecules, and degraded. These processes can be influenced by their respective hormone partners. Most hormones decrease or "down-regulate" the number of their own receptors; this helps prevent excess hormone action on the cell. Other hormones recruit their own receptors and thereby amplify hormone action on the cell.

Receptors are large protein molecules that may also contain carbohydrate units. The receptors incorporated into plasma membranes have extracellular portions that bind their hormones; transmembrane and intracellular portions interact with signal-generating mechanisms that initiate intracellular actions (see Chapter 5).

Signal generation is the next step in hormone action

When hormone-receptor association occurs within the plasma membrane of the cell, the resultant complex is often coupled to other plasma membrane components (see Chapter 5). These generate within the cell a variety of signal molecules, or "second messengers," which then regulate metabolic and other processes (see Figures 5-1 and 40-7). In this situation the essential information for triggering the cell's response resides in the receptor molecule; this information is transmitted to the cytoplasm when the hormone occupies and changes the conformation of the extracellular domain of the membrane receptor. The hormone is essentially an extra-

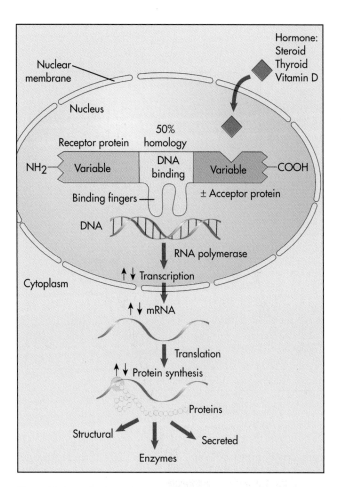

Figure 40-8 Mechanism of action of vitamin D, steroid, and thyroid hormones. The hormone combines with a nuclear protein receptor. The carboxy-terminal portion of the receptor varies for each hormone. The midportion of the receptor molecule has considerable similarity among hormones and contains DNA-binding fingers. Binding of the hormone-receptor complex to hormone regulatory elements in DNA molecules either stimulates or suppresses the transcription of target genes. The result is increased or decreased synthesis of cell proteins.

cellular signal that is greatly amplified by the second messengers.

In contrast, when hormone-receptor association occurs within the cytoplasm or nucleus, the hormone-receptor complex ultimately interacts with specific DNA molecules and alters gene expression (Figures 40-7 and 40-8). There, the second messengers are transcribed RNA molecules that direct the synthesis of protein molecules. In this situation, essential information for triggering the cell's response resides in the hormone molecule itself as well as in the receptor. The hormone is an intracellular signal.

Plasma membrane–generated second messengers

A variety of mechanisms are used to transduce initial hormone-receptor signals arising within the plasma membrane. These signals lead to the generation of a variety of second messengers within the cytoplasm. They include cy-

clic AMP; cyclic GMP; Ca^{++}; inositol 1,4,5-trisphosphate; diacylglycerol; tyrosine kinases; protein tyrosine phosphatases; and nitric oxide. All of these mechanisms are presented in detail in Chapter 5 and should be reviewed before proceeding.

None of the membrane-generated second messengers is unique to any particular hormone, and a single hormone may operate through multiple messengers. In addition, a messenger such as cyclic AMP can also modulate gene expression by binding to a specific protein transcription factor. The combination then binds a regulatory element on target DNA molecules. Thus peptide and protein hormones can also increase or decrease the synthesis of target enzymes and other proteins.

Nuclear second messengers modulate gene expression

Hormones that directly enter the cell (steroids, vitamin D, thyroid hormones) combine with receptor proteins in the cytoplasm and nucleus (Figure 40-8). These receptor proteins are organized into distinct functional domains. A specific C-terminus domain of the receptor molecule binds the hormone. Another domain in the middle portion of the receptor binds to DNA. This second domain exhibits considerable homology among the various receptors and is coded for by a superfamily of genes related to oncogenes (growth-regulating genes). After binding, this hormone-receptor complex undergoes an activation process, during which the hormone ligand displaces an inactivating or blocking protein from the receptor. After transformation, the complex can then enter the nucleus, or if already there, can associate with regulatory elements on target DNA molecules.

The DNA site with which the hormone-receptor complex interacts is termed the **hormone regulatory element;** it is usually "upstream" from the basal promotor site at the 5′ end of the gene. After the hormone-receptor complex has been bound, transcription of the primary gene message by RNA polymerase is either induced or repressed. Thus by raising or lowering the levels of specific RNA molecules and thereby the rate of translation of the gene message, the hormone increases or decreases the concentration of specific cell proteins. When the latter are enzymes, the rates of specific metabolic reactions are likewise increased or decreased by the hormone.

The onset of hormone actions mediated by nuclear second messengers is generally slower than that mediated by cytoplasmic second messengers. There is also a more graded response to increasing the hormone concentration, rather than amplification, because each hormone-receptor unit engages a single DNA molecule. The magnitude of action may be influenced by the concentrations of RNA polymerase, enzymes of protein synthesis or processing, transfer RNA, or amino acids and by the number and activity of ribosomes.

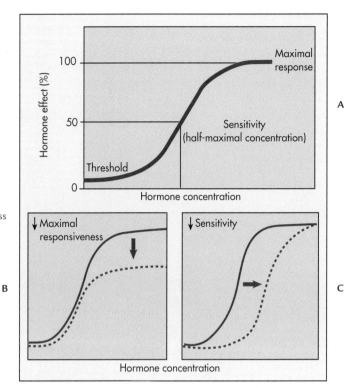

Figure 40-9 General shape of a hormone dose-response curve (**A**). Alterations in this curve can take the form of a change in maximal responsiveness (**B**) or a change in sensitivity (**C**).

Although rare, diseases caused by mutant genes for receptors or G proteins have provided much insight into the mechanisms of hormone action. For example, the reduced activity of a mutant α subunit of a stimulatory G protein leads to diminished cyclic AMP levels, resulting in **deficient action of parathyroid hormone** and then **hypocalcemia** (see Chapter 43). Another mutant G protein, which is constitutively overactive, is associated with continuous **hypersecretion of growth hormone,** or **acromegaly** (see Chapter 44). Mutant nuclear receptors for thyroid hormone lead to **hypothyroidism** caused by the inability of thyroid target cells to respond normally to the hormone (see Chapter 45). Mutant plasma membrane receptors for insulin cause **diabetes mellitus** (see Chapter 42).

The outcome of hormone action depends on many factors

The final quantitative outcome of the interaction of a hormone with its target cells depends on several factors. These include hormone concentration; receptor number; duration of exposure to hormone; intervals between consecutive exposures; intracellular conditions such as concentrations of rate-limiting enzymes, cofactors, or substrates; and the concurrent effects of antagonistic or synergistic hormones.

The dose-response curve for the action of a hormone is often sigmoidal (Figure 40-9). An intrinsic basal level of cell activity may be observed independent of the hormone. A certain minimal threshold concentration of hormone is required to elicit a measurable response. The effect produced by saturating doses of hormone is defined as the **maximal responsiveness** of the target cells. The concentration of hormone required to elicit a half-maximal response is an index of the **sensitivity** of the target cells to that hormone.

Alterations in the dose-response curve in vivo can take two general forms (Figure 40-9):

1. A decrease in maximal responsiveness may be caused (a) by a decrease in the number of functional target cells, in the total number of receptors per cell, or in the concentration of an enzyme activated by the hormone or (b) by an increase in the concentration of a noncompetitive inhibitor.
2. A decrease in hormone sensitivity may be caused (a) by a decrease in hormone-receptor affinity or number, (b) by an increase in the rate of hormone degradation, or (c) by an increase in the concentration of antagonistic and competitive hormones.

Obesity is a good example of a condition in which sensitivity to a hormone, insulin, is considerably diminished. In **type 2 diabetes** (non–insulin dependent diabetes), both sensitivity and maximal responsiveness to insulin are reduced, factors that play a major role in causing high plasma glucose levels.

SUMMARY

- The function of the endocrine system is to regulate metabolism, fluid status, growth, and sexual development. The endocrine and nervous systems work together to maintain homeostasis.

- Hormones are signaling molecules conveyed by the bloodstream (endocrine), by neural axons and the bloodstream (neurocrine), or by local diffusion (paracrine, autocrine). Hormones may be proteins, peptides, catecholamines, steroids, or iodinated tyrosine derivatives.

- Protein or peptide hormone synthesis begins with the generation of a primary gene product called a prohormone. The latter undergoes processing via proteolytic cleavage and glycosylation to yield the hormone.

- Thyroid hormone and catecholamines are synthesized from tyrosine and steroid hormones from cholesterol, both via multiple enzyme reactions.

- Peptide and protein hormones and catecholamines are stored in granules and secreted by exocytosis. Thyroid hormone is stored within protein molecules in large quantities; steroid hormones are not stored at all. Both are released by diffusion.

- Protein, peptide, and catecholamine hormones act on target cells via specific protein receptors located in the plasma membranes. Stimulatory or inhibitory G proteins link the hormone-receptor complex to membrane mechanisms that generate cyclic AMP; cyclic GMP; Ca^{++}; diacylglycerol; inositol 1,4,5-trisphosphate; tyrosine kinases; and protein tyrosine phosphatases that act as second messengers.

- Thyroid and steroid hormones act via protein receptors located in the nucleus. The hormone-receptor complex interacts with hormone-regulatory units in DNA molecules to alter the expression of target genes.

- Plasma levels and urinary excretion rates of a hormone are used clinically as indirect indices of the hormonal secretion rate; these indices are valid as long as metabolic and renal clearance of the hormone is normal. The binding of some hormones to plasma proteins also influences their availability to target cells.

- The sensitivity of an organism to hormone action can be influenced by changes in receptor number or affinity, the hormone degradation rate, or competitive antagonists.

- The maximal effect produced by saturating concentrations of hormone can be influenced by the number of target cells, number of receptors, concentration of target enzymes, or noncompetitive antagonists.

BIBLIOGRAPHY

Birnbaumer L et al: Molecular basis of regulation of ionic channel by G proteins, *Rec Prog Horm Res* 45:121, 1989.

Carson-Jurica MA et al: Steroid receptor family: structure and function, *Endocr Rev* 11:201, 1990.

Combarnous Y: Molecular basis of the specificity of binding of glycoprotein hormones to their receptors, *Endocr Rev* 13:670, 1992.

Freedman LP: Anatomy of the steroid receptor zinc finger region, *Endocr Rev* 13:129, 1992.

Glass CK: Differential recognition of target genes by nuclear receptor monomers, dimers, and heterodimers, *Endocr Rev* 15:391, 1994.

Habener JF: Genetic control of hormone formation. In Wilson JD, Foster DF, eds: *Textbook of endocrinology,* ed 9, Philadelphia, 1998, WB Saunders.

Kahn CR, Smith RJ, Chin WW: Mechanism of action of hormones that act at the cell surface. In Wilson JD, Foster DF, eds: *Textbook of endocrinology,* ed 9, Philadelphia, 1998, WB Saunders.

Lacy PE: Beta cell secretion: from the standpoint of a pathobiologist, *Diabetes* 19:895, 1970.

Schuchard M et al: Steroid hormone regulation of nuclear proto-oncogenes, *Endocr Rev* 14:659, 1993.

Spaulding SW: The ways in which hormones change cyclic adenosine 3'-5'-monophosphate–dependent protein kinase subunits, and how such changes affect cell behavior, *Endocr Rev* 14:632, 1993.

Spiegel AM, Shenker A, Weinstein LS: Receptor-effector coupling by G proteins: implications for normal and abnormal signal transduction, *Endocr Rev* 13:536, 1992.

CASE STUDY

Case 40-1

A patient comes to a physician with symptoms suggesting deficiency of protein hormone X. However, the measurement of hormone X in the plasma demonstrates an elevated level. When hormone X is administered to the patient, a normal maximal biological response is elicited but only with a higher-than-normal dose.

1. **Which of the following is *not* a likely explanation for this patient's symptoms?**
   - **A.** A mutant receptor for hormone X
   - **B.** A 50% deficiency of receptors for hormone X
   - **C.** Excessive secretion of a competitive antagonist to hormone X
   - **D.** A 95% deficiency of an enzyme that generates the key second messenger involved in the action of hormone X
   - **E.** The secretion of a mutant hormone X

2. **For which of the following possible causes of the patient's hormone resistance syndrome would the administration of an inhibitor of hormone X secretion be helpful?**
   - **A.** A mutant receptor for hormone X
   - **B.** A 50% deficiency of receptors for hormone X
   - **C.** Excessive secretion of a competitive antagonist to hormone X
   - **D.** A 95% deficiency of an enzyme that generates the key second messenger involved in the action of hormone X
   - **E.** The secretion of a mutant hormone X

CHAPTER 41

Whole Body Metabolism

OBJECTIVES

- Indicate the sources of energy and the forms in which energy is expended in humans.
- Explain the basic metabolic pathways of energy production and expenditure.
- Explain the principles of carbohydrate, protein, and fat metabolism and their interrelationships.
- Describe the patterns of metabolic responses and adaptations to fasting and exercise.
- Explain the concepts of how energy storage and body weight are regulated.

Metabolism may be broadly defined as the sum of all the chemical and physical processes involved (1) in producing and expending energy from exogenous and endogenous sources, (2) in synthesizing and degrading structural and functional tissue components, and (3) in disposing of resultant waste products. These processes are of fundamental importance to all cells, tissues, organs and systems discussed throughout this book. REGULATING THE RATE AND DIRECTION OF THE VARIOUS COMPONENTS OF METABOLISM IS ONE OF THE MAJOR FUNCTIONS OF THE ENDOCRINE SYSTEM. Therefore a firm grasp of the basic elements of metabolism is essential for understanding the important influence of hormones on body functions.

Energy Metabolism

Energy input equals energy output

The laws of thermodynamics require that total energy balance be constantly maintained in living organisms. However, energy may be obtained in various forms, stored in other forms, and expended in many different ways. Therefore numerous interconversions of chemical, mechanical, and thermal energy are possible. However, the basic rule is that IN THE STEADY STATE, WHEN BODY WEIGHT AND BODY COMPOSITION ARE STABLE, ENERGY INPUT MUST ALWAYS EQUAL ENERGY OUTPUT. Figure 41-1 illustrates this overall flow of energy through the human organism.

Energy is derived from the oxidation of carbon and hydrogen in dietary molecules

Energy input consists of foodstuffs, which are classified into three major chemical categories: carbohydrate, fat, and protein. The complete combustion of each chemical type to CO_2 and water yields characteristic amounts of energy, expressed as joules or kilocalories per gram (1 kcal = 4184 J). The combustion of each type also requires characteristic amounts of O_2 per gram, depending on the proportions of carbon, hydrogen, and O_2 in the substance. However, for each class of foodstuff, the energy yield per liter of O_2 used is quite similar because the ratio of carbon to hydrogen atoms is quite similar in each class. WITHIN THE BODY THE CARBON SKELETONS OF CARBOHYDRATE AND PROTEIN CAN BE CONVERTED TO FAT, AND THEIR POTENTIAL ENERGY CAN BE STORED MORE EFFICIENTLY IN THAT MANNER. THE CARBON SKELETONS OF PROTEIN CAN ALSO BE CONVERTED TO CARBOHYDRATE WHEN THAT ENERGY SOURCE IS SPECIFICALLY NEEDED. HOWEVER, IN THE HUMAN, CARBON ATOMS FROM FAT ARE NOT CONVERTED TO CARBOHYDRATE TO ANY SIGNIFICANT EXTENT.

There are several distinct components of energy output

Energy output can be divided into several distinct, measurable components:

First, in individuals at rest, energy is expended in a myriad of synthetic and degradative chemical reactions; in the generation and maintenance of chemical and electrical gradients of ions and other molecules across cell and organelle membranes; in the creation and conduction of signals, particularly in the nervous system; in the mechanical work of respiration and circulation of the blood; and in obligate heat loss to the environment. This absolute minimal energy expenditure is called the **basal** or **resting metabolic rate (BMR or RMR)**. In the adult human, the BMR amounts to an average daily expenditure of 20 to 25 kcal (84 to 105 kJ)/kg of body weight (1.0 to 1.2 kcal/min), and this uses approximately 200 to 250 ml O_2 per minute.

The BMR is linearly related to lean body mass and body surface area. The central nervous system and muscle mass together account for 60% to 70% of the BMR. The BMR declines in the elderly, partly because lean body mass declines with age. The BMR increases when environmental temperature rises. During sleep, it falls 10% to 15%. Part of the

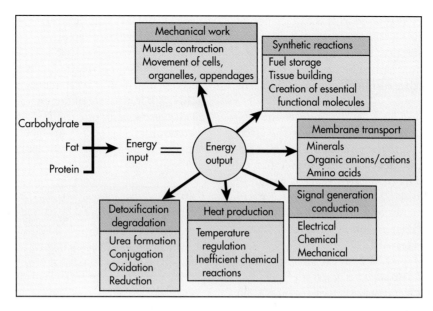

Figure 41-1 Energy balance. In a steady state, input as caloric equivalents of food equals output as caloric equivalents of various forms of mechanical and chemical work and heat.

interindividual variation in the BMR is genetically determined. Women have slightly lower BMRs than men.

Second, the ingestion of food causes a small obligate increase in energy expenditure referred to as **diet-induced thermogenesis.** This is explained by the disposition of the ingested calories, such as the storage of glucose in the large-molecule glycogen or by enhanced protein synthesis from amino acids.

Third, **nonshivering thermogenesis** refers to energy expended specifically to produce heat and maintain the core temperature of the body. Some of this is **obligatory** and contributed to by essentially all tissues. It is **facultative** when evoked by acute exposure to a cold environment. Impulses from the sympathetic nervous system are important mediators of this response to a fall in temperature (see Chapter 10). Facultative thermogenesis may also be used to adjust for prolonged excesses or deficits of energy intake.

Fourth, energy is also expended by sedentary individuals in unconscious and seemingly purposeless activity, such as fidgeting. Fifth, the additional energy expended in occupational labor and purposeful exercise varies greatly among individuals and from day to day. This component generates the greatest variation in daily caloric intake and underscores the importance of energy stores for buffering temporary discrepancies between energy output and intake.

Of a total average daily expenditure of 2300 kcal (9700 kJ) in a typical sedentary adult, basal metabolism accounts for 60% to 70%, dietary thermogenesis for 5% to 15%, and spontaneous physical activity for 20% to 30%. As many as 3000 additional kilocalories may be used in daily physical work. During short periods of high-intensity exercise, energy expenditure can increase more than tenfold.

Energy Generation

Chemical pathways

Adenosine triphosphate is the major molecular intermediary of usable chemical energy
The basic chemical currency of energy in all living cells consists of the two high-energy phosphate bonds contained in **ATP.** To a much lesser extent, guanosine triphosphate, cytosine triphosphate, uridine triphosphate, and inosine triphosphate also serve as energy sources after energy from ATP is transferred to them.

The two terminal P-O bonds of ATP each contain about 12 kcal of potential energy per mole under physiological conditions of temperature and pH. These bonds are in constant flux. They are generated by substrate oxidation and are consumed as the energy is (1) transferred into other high-energy bonds such as creatine phosphate in muscle, (2) expended in creating lower-energy phosphorylated metabolic intermediates such as glucose-6-phosphate, or (3) converted to mechanical work such as the propulsion of spermatozoa. Because the production and transfer of energy is only 65% efficient, about 18 kcal worth of substrate is required to generate each terminal P-O bond of ATP. If 2300 kcal is turned over in a typical day, about 128 moles, or 63 kg, of ATP (a mass approximating body weight) is generated and expended.

The combustion of carbohydrates, chiefly as glucose, includes two major phases
At the end of a cytoplasmic anaerobic phase known as **glycolysis** (Embden-Meyerhof pathway), each glucose molecule has been degraded to two molecules of pyru-

vate (Figure 41-2) but has yielded only 8% of its potential energy content. Glycolysis can serve as a sole source of energy only briefly because (1) the supply of glucose is limited and (2) the pyruvate must be siphoned off via reduction to lactate, which is ultimately noxious if the lactate accumulates.

During the mitochondrial aerobic phase, the two pyruvate molecules are degraded to CO_2 via the **citric acid cycle** (Krebs cycle), and the remaining energy is liberated. In this pathway, **acetyl coenzyme A (acetyl CoA),** initially formed by oxidative decarboxylation of pyruvate, is condensed with oxaloacetate to form citrate. Through a cyclic series of reactions the carbons of acetyl CoA appear as CO_2, oxaloacetate is regenerated, and much more ATP is formed.

Fatty acids are oxidized, two carbons at a time
The combustion of fat as fatty acids first requires their transfer from the cytoplasm to the mitochondria, where as fatty acyl CoAs, they are oxidized via the biochemical sequence known as **β-oxidation.** This process yields two carbons at a time as acetyl CoA until the entire fatty acid molecule is broken down. The resulting acetyl CoA is disposed of via the citric acid cycle. A variable portion of fatty acid oxidation in the liver stops at the last four carbons and yields **acetoacetic** and **β-hydroxybutyric acids.** When the rate of fatty acid delivery to the liver exceeds the capacity of the citric acid cycle, more of these water-soluble ketoacids are generated and released by the liver to be oxidized in other tissues.

> The condition known as **ketosis** occurs when fasting is prolonged beyond the usual overnight period or when carbohydrate intake is low and ketoacids accumulate. It develops to an extreme degree in **diabetes mellitus** when the hormone insulin is very deficient.

The combustion of protein first requires its hydrolysis to yield the component amino acids. Each of these amino acids undergoes degradation by individual path-

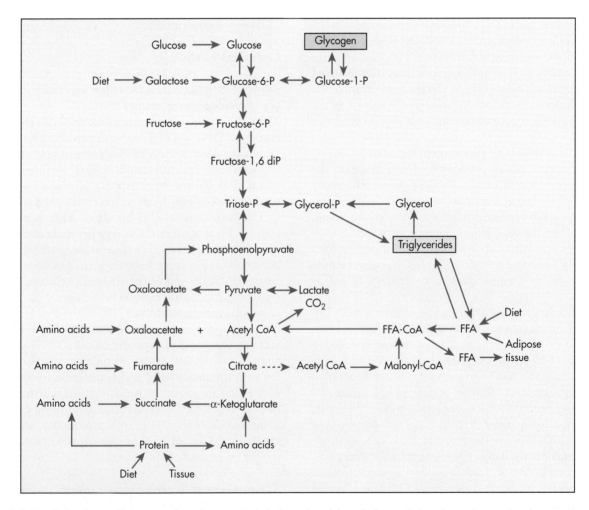

Figure 41-2 Chemical pathways of energy transfer and storage. Carbohydrates funnel through glucose-6-phosphate to be stored as glycogen. Alternatively, they can undergo glycolysis to pyruvate and are used for the synthesis of fatty acids. The latter, regardless of source, are esterified with glycerol-phosphate and stored as triglycerides. Amino acids from endogenous or exogenous proteins are converted to glucose via oxaloacetate or pyruvate. *CoA,* Coenzyme A; *diP,* diphosphate; *FFA,* free fatty acid; *P,* phosphate.

ways, which ultimately lead to intermediate compounds of the citric acid cycle and then to acetyl CoA and CO_2.

The oxidation of all substrates yields large numbers of hydrogen atoms. These atoms are oxidized to water in the mitochondrion in link with phosphorylation of ADP to ATP. In this process, three high-energy P-O bonds are formed for each atom of O_2 used. This usually yields an overall efficiency of 60% to 65% for the recovery of usable chemical energy.

Respiratory quotient

Substrates yield various amounts of CO_2 for each unit of O_2 consumed

In oxidation, the proportion of CO_2 produced and exhaled ($\dot{V}CO_2$) to O_2 used and inhaled ($\dot{V}O_2$) is characteristic of each major substrate. The ratio of $\dot{V}CO_2$ to $\dot{V}O_2$ is known as the **respiratory quotient (RQ).** As indicated by the following equations, the RQ equals 1.0 for the oxidation of carbohydrate (e.g., glucose), whereas it equals 0.70 for the oxidation of fat (e.g., palmitic acid). For carbohydrates:

$$C_6H_{12}O_6 + 6O_2 \rightarrow 6CO_2 + 6H_2O \qquad \textbf{41-1}$$

Glucose:

$$RQ = 6CO_2/6O_2 = 1.0$$

For fats:

$$C_{15}H_{31}COOH + 23O_2 \rightarrow 16CO_2 + 16H_2O \qquad \textbf{41-2}$$

Palmitic acid:

$$RQ = 16CO_2/23O_2 = 0.70$$

The RQ for protein reflects that of the individual RQs of the amino acids and averages 0.80. Ordinarily, however, protein is only a minor energy source.

Normal humans can vary their fuel mix and RQ from 0.7 to 1.0 without difficulty. Patients with very poor pulmonary function who cannot excrete CO_2 efficiently benefit from a low RQ. They are therefore given a higher proportion of fat calories as an energy source so that the least amount of CO_2 is produced for the quantity of O_2 used.

Energy Storage and Transfers

Energy can be transformed from one chemical type to another and transferred from site to site

The intake of energy in the form of food is periodic. Its time course does not match either the constant rate of energy expenditure in the basal state or the variable rate during intermittent muscle work. Therefore the organism must have mechanisms for storing ingested energy for future needs. The greatest part of these energy reserves (75%) is in the form of fat, stored as triglycerides, in adipose tissue. In humans of normal weight, fat constitutes 10% to 30% of body weight, but it can reach 80% in very obese individuals. Fat is a particularly efficient storage fuel because it has a high caloric density (i.e., 9 kcal/g) and it engenders little additional weight as intracellular water.

Triglycerides are formed by the esterification of free fatty acids with α-glycerol phosphate. Free fatty acids arise largely from the digestion of dietary fat, but they can also be synthesized from acetyl CoA derived from the oxidation of glucose (Figure 41-2). Thus dietary carbohydrate can be converted to fat in the liver and transferred to adipose tissue for storage in that more efficient form.

Protein (4 kcal/g) constitutes almost 25% of the potential energy reserves, and the component amino acids can contribute to the glucose supply. However, because proteins have vital structural and functional roles, their use as a major source of energy is not desirable.

Carbohydrate (4 kcal/g) in the form of the glucose polymer **glycogen** forms less than 1% of total energy reserves. However, this portion is critical for the support of metabolism of the central nervous system and for short bursts of intense muscle work. Approximately one fourth of the glycogen stores (75 to 100 g) is in the liver, and about three fourths (300 to 400 g) is in the muscle mass. Liver glycogen can be made available to other tissues via the process of **glycogenolysis** and glucose release. Muscle glycogen can be used only by muscle because this tissue lacks the enzyme glucose-6-phosphatase, which is required for the dephosphorylation of glucose before its entrance into the bloodstream (Figure 41-2).

Glycogen can be formed from all three major dietary sugars: glucose, galactose, and fructose. In addition, in the liver (and to a much lesser extent in the kidney), glucose itself can also be synthesized de novo from the three carbon precursors pyruvate, lactate, and glycerol and from parts of the carbon skeleton of the 20 amino acids in protein, except leucine. This process, known as **gluconeogenesis,** converts two pyruvate molecules to glucose.

Gluconeogenesis is not a simple reversal of all the reactions of glycolysis

The chemical free energy change is too large to permit an efficient backward flow of the glycolytic reactions at three steps (Figure 41-2): (1) pyruvate to phosphoenolpyruvate, (2) fructose-1,6-diphosphate to fructose-6-phosphate, and (3) glucose-6-phosphate to glucose. The first step requires energy input in the form of ATP and GTP. Simple phosphatase reactions reverse the last two steps.

Net glucose synthesis cannot occur from acetyl CoA formed from the β-oxidation of fat, even though carbon atoms from acetyl CoA can become part of glucose molecules via oxaloacetate and the citric acid cycle. Thus fat can contribute to carbohydrate stores only via conversion

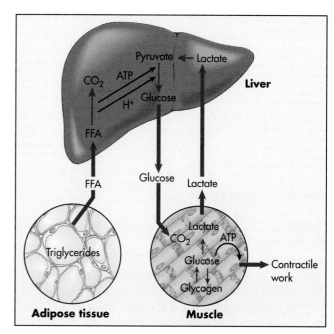

Figure 41-3 Interorgan energy transfers. Energy contained in free fatty acid *(FFA)* can be transferred to energy contained in glucose in the liver. Lactate released from muscle glycogen by glycolysis can carry energy back to the liver, where the lactate is built back into new glucose molecules (and glycogen).

of the 3-carbon glycerol moiety of triglycerides (via glycerol phosphate) to glucose.

The processes of energy storage and transfer themselves expend energy

The assimilation of dietary sources of energy partly accounts for the stimulation of O_2 use after a meal (i.e., diet-induced thermogenesis). Storing dietary fatty acids as triglycerides in adipose tissue costs only 3% of the original calories, and storing glucose as glycogen costs only 7% of the original calories. In contrast, the conversion of carbohydrate to fat uses 23% of the original calories, and a similar amount is expended in storing dietary amino acids as protein or in converting them to glycogen.

The metabolism of glucose and fatty acids is interrelated

Because glucose and fatty acids are alternative and in effect competing energy substrates, some relationship between their use and their synthesis and storage within cells could be expected. For example, when dietary glucose is plentiful, glycolysis is augmented, more acetyl CoA is generated from pyruvate, and more citrate is formed (Figure 41-2). Citrate then activates the first step in the synthesis of fatty acids (acetyl CoA → malonyl CoA). In addition, glycolysis produces more glycerol phosphate from triose phosphates (Figure 41-2). The combination of increased fatty acid synthesis and glycerol phosphate availability results in the accentuated synthesis of triglycerides and the reduced oxidation of fat. Thus INCREASED CARBOHYDRATE USE SHIFTS FAT METABOLISM FROM OXIDATION TO STORAGE. Conversely, under circumstances in which the fatty acid supply is augmented, β-oxidation increases. Several of its products (e.g., acyl CoA) then retard glycolysis and enhance gluconeogenesis and glycogen synthesis. Thus THE INCREASED USE OF FAT AS

FUEL SHIFTS CARBOHYDRATE METABOLISM FROM OXIDATION TO STORAGE. Many of these intrinsic chemical checks and balances are reinforced by hormonal signals.

The transfer of energy between organs also occurs (Figure 41-3). The stored energy contained within adipose tissue triglycerides is transported as free fatty acids to the liver. There, part of the energy (not the carbon atoms) is effectively transferred to glucose molecules. This is because as fatty acids are oxidized and yield ATP, gluconeogenesis is stimulated concurrently and uses the ATP that was generated. The newly synthesized glucose molecules can then be transported to muscle tissue, where their energy is released during glycolysis and applied to muscle contraction. Furthermore, if the lactate produced exceeds the ability of the muscle to oxidize it rapidly enough in the citric acid cycle, the lactate can be returned to the liver, where it may again be built back up into glucose molecules. From this viewpoint THE LIVER IS A FLEXIBLE AND VERSATILE ORGAN THAT CAN TRANSMUTE AND TRANSFER ENERGY FROM FUEL DEPOTS TO WORKING TISSUES. Hormones help regulate this process.

> When liver disease causes severe hepatic insufficiency (e.g., **alcoholic hepatitis, cirrhosis**), energy metabolism can be markedly distorted. An inability to store glucose as glycogen leads to hypoglycemia during fasting. Inability to take up lactate produced by peripheral anaerobic glycolysis can cause high plasma levels of lactic acid and serious metabolic acidosis.

Carbohydrate Metabolism

In addition to providing energy, sugar components of glycoproteins, glycopeptides, and glycolipids have structural and functional roles. Examples include basement membrane collagen, mucopolysaccharides, nerve cell myelin, hormones, and hormone receptors.

Glucose is the central molecule in carbohydrate metabolism

Postabsorptive plasma glucose concentration averages 80 mg/dl (4.5 mM), with a range of 60 to 110 mg/dl.

> When the plasma glucose level falls below 60 mg/dl, as may occur with an overdose of insulin taken by a patient with diabetes, the uptake of the sugar and use of O_2 by the brain decrease in parallel. Central nervous system function becomes progressively impaired, leading to convulsions, coma, and even death.

The major products of glycolysis, lactate and pyruvate, circulate at average plasma concentrations of 0.7 and 0.07 mM, respectively. However, when tissues are deprived of O_2, the equilibrium between the two shifts further toward lactate, the reduced molecule. Plasma concentration ratios rise from 10:1 to as high as 30:1. Ischemia may produce very high concentrations of lactate that cause metabolic acidosis (see Chapters 30 and 39).

In the basal state, glucose turnover is about 225 g/day in adults. Approximately 55% of glucose use results in terminal oxidation to CO_2, of which the brain accounts for the greatest part. Another 20% stops at lactate, which then returns to the liver for resynthesis into glucose (Cori cycle) (Figure 41-3). Reuptake by the liver and other splanchnic tissues accounts for the remaining 20% of glucose use. Most of the glucose used ($\approx$70%) in the basal state is independent of insulin, a hormone with otherwise important regulatory effects on glucose metabolism.

The circulating pool of glucose (11 g), which is only slightly larger than the liver output in 1 hour (9 g), can maintain brain oxidation for only 3 hours. This is why the continuous hepatic production of glucose is critical in the fasting state. About 80% of this production results from glycogenolysis and 20% from gluconeogenesis. Lactate is the source of more than half the glucose supplied by gluconeogenesis. The remainder is largely accounted for by amino acids. The supply of lactate comes from glycolysis largely in muscle, red blood cells, and white blood cells. The amino acid precursors come from proteolysis of muscle.

The fate of ingested glucose is largely storage as glycogen

When an individual ingests glucose after overnight fasting, approximately 70% of the load is assimilated by peripheral tissues, mainly muscle, and about 30% by splanchnic tissues, mainly liver. Only 25% is oxidized during the 3 to 5 hours required for complete glucose absorption from the gastrointestinal tract. The remainder is stored as glycogen in muscle and liver. Glucose initially stored as muscle glycogen can later be transferred to the liver by undergoing glycolysis to lactate, which is released into the circulation; the lactate is then taken up by the liver, rebuilt into glucose, and stored as glycogen (Figure 41-3). During absorption of exogenous glucose, hepatic output of the sugar is largely unnecessary and is greatly reduced from basal levels.

Protein Metabolism

Intake of proteins, especially those containing amino acids that cannot be synthesized in the body, is vital to health

The average adult body contains 10 kg of protein, of which about 6 kg is metabolically active. Amino acids are released daily by proteolysis from muscle, the main endogenous repository. A portion of each amino acid quantity is reused for protein synthesis, and the rest is degraded. A daily dietary protein intake of 0.8 g/kg is ordinarily sufficient for an adult human to remain in balance. When accretion of lean body mass is taking place (e.g., in growing children, pregnant women, and persons recovering from prior illness-induced weight loss), daily protein requirements increase to 1.5 to 2.0 g/kg.

All proteins are composed of the same 20 amino acids. Half of these are called **essential amino acids** because their carbon skeletons, the corresponding α-ketoacids, cannot be synthesized by humans. Once present, however, these ketoacids can be converted to the essential amino acids by transamination. The other half, the **nonessential amino acids,** can be synthesized endogenously because the appropriate carbon skeletons can be built from glucose metabolites in the citric acid cycle. The essential amino acids must be supplied in the diet in amounts that range from 0.5 to 1.5 g/day. A deficiency of even one essential amino acid disrupts normal protein synthesis.

Milk and egg proteins are particularly rich in essential amino acids, but properly combined vegetable sources can also provide all of them. About 40% of the protein intake of infants and children should consist of essential amino acids to support growth. In adults, this requirement falls to 20%. Many amino acids, including the essential ones, are also precursors for important molecules such as purines, pyrimidines, polyamines, phospholipids, creatine, carnitine, methyl donors, thyroid and catecholamine hormones, and neurotransmitters. Some of these neurotransmitters are amino acids.

> A deficiency of protein intake is a worldwide problem. When people are chronically deprived of both protein and calories, marked loss of muscle mass and adipose tissue results. When calories are sufficient but protein is de-

ficient over relatively short periods, a syndrome known as **kwashiorkor** occurs. This is characterized by low plasma albumin levels, edema caused by low plasma oncotic pressure, fragile hair, depressed immune function, deficiency of lymphocytes, reduced wound healing, increased infections, and fatty infiltration of the liver.

Amino acids can be converted to glucose, can be completely oxidized, or can give rise to ketoacids

After the removal of the amino group, all 20 amino acids are completely oxidized to CO_2 and water. Each amino acid traverses a specific degradative pathway. (Refer to standard biochemistry textbooks for details.) However, all these pathways converge into three general metabolic processes: gluconeogenesis, ketogenesis, and ureagenesis. Except for leucine, all the amino acids can contribute carbon atoms for the synthesis of glucose. Five ketogenic amino acids give rise to acetoacetate. In the degradation of all amino acids, ammonia is released. Ammonia, incorporated mainly into glutamine and alanine molecules, is then transported to the liver. In the liver, ammonia is "detoxified" through incorporation into urea, a metabolically inert molecule. The urea that results from protein degradation is excreted by the kidney (see Chapter 37).

Protein balance is reflected by nitrogen balance

In the healthy adult under steady-state conditions, the total daily level of nitrogen excreted in the urine as urea plus ammonia, along with minor losses of nitrogen in the feces (0.4 g/day) and skin (0.3 g/day), is equal to that released during the metabolism of exogenous and endogenous protein. Such an individual is said to be in **nitrogen balance.** When no protein is ingested, the sum of urea plus ammonia nitrogen in the urine reflects almost quantitatively the rate of endogenous protein degradation. When protein breakdown is greatly accelerated by tissue trauma or disease (e.g., after major gastrointestinal surgery or with sepsis), the urea plus ammonia nitrogen in the urine may exceed the protein nitrogen intake. In these cases the individual is said to be in **negative nitrogen balance.** In a growing child or a previously malnourished individual undergoing protein repletion and a gain in lean body mass, urea plus ammonia nitrogen excretion in the urine is less than the intake of protein nitrogen. This individual is said to be in **positive nitrogen balance.**

Fat Metabolism

Body fat has multiple components and functions

Fat represents almost half the total daily substrate for oxidation ($\approx$100 g, or 900 kcal). The usual daily intake of fat in the United States is approximately 100 g, or about 40% of total calories. The major component of both dietary and storage fat is triglycerides. These consist largely of long-chain saturated and monounsaturated fatty acids (chiefly palmitic, stearic, and oleic acids) esterified to glycerol. ABOUT 3% TO 5% OF FATTY ACIDS ARE POLYUNSATURATED AND CANNOT BE SYNTHESIZED IN THE BODY. These are termed **essential fatty acids** (linoleic, linolenic, and arachidonic) because they are required as precursors for certain membrane phospholipid and glycolipid substances as well as for important intracellular mediators known as **prostaglandins.** Another component of fat is the steroid molecule **cholesterol,** which serves a variety of functions in membranes and is the precursor for bile acids and steroid hormones. Cholesterol is both ingested and synthesized by most cells.

The typical fat intake previously cited is now deemed excessive for good health, particularly because it promotes **atherosclerosis.** In this common condition, plaques laden with lipid form in the walls of the arteries and are often the sites of thrombosis, which obstructs the flow of blood and causes necrosis of vital tissue such as heart muscle or cerebral cortex. Current nutritional recommendations are for the intake of fat not to exceed 30% and saturated fat (usually animal fat) not to exceed 10% of total calories. The intake of monounsaturated fat should modestly exceed that of polyunsaturated fat. Cholesterol intake should be less than 600 mg/day and reduced to below 300 mg/day if the plasma cholesterol level is elevated.

The transport of water-insoluble lipids in plasma requires that they be incorporated into complex lipoprotein particles. The protein portion of each particle is derived from several **apoproteins** synthesized in the liver and intestine. These apoproteins serve catalytic functions and interact with specific cell receptors. Figure 41-4 summarizes the metabolic pathways and interactions of the lipoprotein particles.

Plasma lipid components are associated with specific proteins and have various functions and rates of turnover

Chylomicrons, formed from dietary fat (see Chapter 34), are the lowest-density lipoproteins. After their absorption from the gastrointestinal tract, they disappear from plasma rapidly. Their major component is triglycerides, which are partly hydrolyzed by the key enzyme, **lipoprotein lipase,** on capillary endothelial surfaces. This enzyme is activated by apoprotein C-II and transferred to the chylomicron by **high-density lipoprotein (HDL)** particles (see later section). The resulting free fatty acids are taken up by adipose cells for resynthesis into triglycerides and storage and by other cells for oxidation. The residual lipoprotein particles, which are higher in cholesterol content and are known as **chylomicron remnants,** are taken

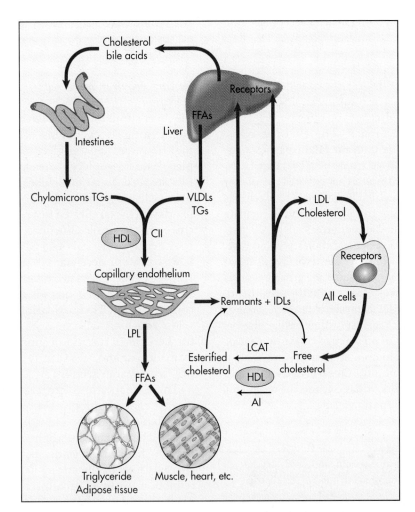

Figure 41-4 Lipoprotein metabolism and major aspects of lipid turnover in humans. Exogenous triglycerides *(TGs)* in the form of chylomicrons absorbed from the intestine and endogenous triglycerides (very low-density lipoproteins *[VLDLs]*) produced in the liver both give rise to free fatty acids *(FFAs)* for storage in adipose tissue and oxidation in muscle. High-density lipoprotein *(HDL)* particles facilitate the liberation of free fatty acids from triglycerides, and the enzyme lipoprotein lipase *(LPL)* directly catalyzes this process. The resultant particles, called remnants from chylomicrons and intermediate-density lipoproteins *(IDLs)* from very-low-density lipoproteins, undergo further change in the circulation, which also is facilitated by high-density lipoprotein. The ratio of esterified cholesterol to free cholesterol is increased in the remnant and IDL particles by the enzyme lecithin-cholesterol acyltransferase *(LCAT)*. The remnant particles are then taken up by the liver for further metabolism. The intermediate-density lipoprotein particles are partly taken up by the liver and partly converted to cholesterol-rich, low-density lipoprotein *(LDL)* particles. The latter are then taken up by virtually all cells after interaction with specific low-density lipoprotein receptors. Cholesterol, either synthesized in the liver or extracted from remnant and IDL particles, is also excreted into the intestine, partly as bile acids. *AI,* Apoprotein A-I; *CII,* Apoprotein C-II.

up by the liver for further degradation. This uptake is directed by apoproteins E and B-48, which react with specific hepatic receptors.

In contrast, **very-low-density lipoprotein (VLDL)** particles are formed in the postabsorptive state by endogenous synthesis in the liver and to a lesser extent in the intestine. They are denser, contain somewhat more cholesterol than chylomicrons, and have a longer plasma half-life. The initial metabolism of VLDL is the same as that of chylomicrons. The product of lipoprotein lipase action consists of particles called **intermediate-density lipoprotein (IDL).** About half the IDLs return to the liver and are taken up, like chylomicron remnants. The other half of the IDLs are further enriched with cholesterol to form **low-density lipoprotein (LDL)** particles. Circulating LDL is responsible for transferring cholesterol into other cells. The uptake of LDL, IDL, and remnant particles takes place

through initial interaction between apoproteins E and B-100 and specific cell receptors; this process is then followed by endocytosis.

The uptake of LDL cholesterol by cells has important regulatory actions on intracellular cholesterol metabolism. Cholesterol uptake from plasma down-regulates the LDL receptor and thereby reduces further entrance of the sterol. The uptake of cholesterol also suppresses its own intracellular synthesis.

High-density lipoprotein particles play key roles in fat metabolism

HDL particles are synthesized in the liver and intestine and have a long half-life. Different types facilitate the major steps in fat metabolism just described. HDL particles exchange key apoproteins with the other lipoprotein particles. The smaller, denser HDL_3 particles accept free cholesterol molecules from chylomicrons; from VLDL, IDL, and remnant particles; and from peripheral cells (Figure 41-4). The cholesterol is esterified via the enzyme lecithin-cholesterol acyltransferase (LCAT); the esterification is activated by apoprotein A-I. The resulting cholesterol esters are then exchanged for triglycerides on other particles via a cholesterol-ester transfer protein. The HDL_3 is transformed to the larger, more buoyant HDL_2 particle. The triglycerides are later removed from the HDL_2 particle by the action of hepatic lipase, and this restores the denser HDL_3. The net effect of such HDL cycling is to accelerate the clearance of triglycerides from plasma and to regulate the ratios of free to esterified cholesterol.

The plasma concentration of total cholesterol (average, 185 mg/dl) and especially of LDL cholesterol (average, 120 mg/dl) is a very important risk factor for atherosclerosis and death from cardiovascular events. On the other hand, a higher plasma level of HDL cholesterol (average, 50 mg/dl) exerts a protective effect against cardiovascular disease. Free fatty acids circulate in an average concentration of 400 µmol/L bound to albumin molecules and with a plasma half-life of only 2 minutes. One half of the turnover of free fatty acids represents oxidation, and the other half represents reesterification to triglycerides.

Genetic abnormalities in apoprotein and lipid receptor particles account for a substantial number of **dyslipidemias.** The premature development of coronary artery disease is often the consequence. For example, mutant apoprotein E molecules cause familial forms of **hyperlipidemia,** which is characterized by elevations of both triglyceride and cholesterol levels caused by the accumulation of IDL and remnant particles. An excessive apoprotein B-100 content of VLDL and LDL particles characterizes **familial combined hyperlipidemia,** in which cholesterol and often triglyceride levels are high. In **familial hypercholesterolemia,** mutant LDL receptors prevent the normal cellular uptake of cholesterol; this diminished uptake results in extremely high plasma cholesterol concentrations (>700 mg/dl) in homozygotes, visible and palpable deposits of cholesterol in skin and tendons, and even coronary thrombosis in children.

Metabolic Adaptations

Fasting

In the fasting state the individual totally depends on endogenous substrates for energy. The mobilization of glucose provides essential fuel for the central nervous system; the release of free fatty acids provides for the oxidative needs of the other tissues. An increase in protein degradation to amino acids is also a fundamental feature of this response.

THE FASTING INDIVIDUAL IS SAID TO BE IN A STATE OF CATABOLISM BECAUSE CARBOHYDRATE, FAT, AND PROTEIN STORES ARE ALL DECREASING.

Fasting requires increased glucose production and fat oxidation

The liver supplies glucose to the circulation initially by augmenting glycogenolysis. After 12 to 15 hours of fasting, however, hepatic glycogen stores are almost depleted, and a rapid enhancement of gluconeogenesis fills the void. To supply glucose precursors, 75 to 100 g of muscle protein is broken down daily during the first few days. This is reflected in a rising excretion of urea nitrogen in the urine. Gluconeogenesis is also supported by the daily provision of 15 to 20 g of glycerol, which is released by the accelerated lipolysis of triglycerides in adipose tissue. Glucose oxidation in muscle and liver is spared as increasing quantities of free fatty acids become available. Their oxidation in the liver yields ketoacids, which can also be oxidized by muscle cells, and further spares the use of glucose. The net shift away from glucose and toward fatty acid oxidation lowers the RQ (see previous section).

These adaptations are also reflected in changing plasma concentrations of substrates. Levels of glucose and alanine, a major gluconeogenic amino acid, decrease, whereas the levels of free fatty acids, glycerol, and branch-chain amino acids, such as leucine, increase. Increased levels of the strong ketoacids produce a slight reduction in the plasma bicarbonate levels and blood pH (i.e., mild metabolic acidosis [see Figure 39-5]).

When fasting is prolonged beyond a few days, other important adaptations occur. Total energy expenditure, which is reflected in the BMR, decreases 10% to 20% and thereby limits the drain on energy stores. The central nervous system no longer depends entirely on glucose as an energy source, and much of its needs are eventually met by the ketoacids. Gluconeogenesis therefore diminishes, and protein breakdown declines to 25 g/day. In long-term fasting, body weight diminishes by an average of 300 g/day; two thirds of the lost weight is accounted for by fat and one third by lean tissue, 25% of which is protein.

Circumstances such as accidental isolation in areas totally lacking in food sources evoke these adaptations to prolonged fasting. As long as sufficient water is available to prevent dehydration, the adipose stores of a normal human ($\approx$10 kg) can sustain the reduced basal energy needs and greatly limited physical activity ($\approx$1400 kcal/day) for up to 60 days. Likewise, the mobilizable protein stores ($\approx$6 kg) can supply the diminished requirements for glucose oxidation. However, the loss of protein leads to progressive muscle weakness, apathy, organ dysfunction, and ultimately death.

Exercise

Exercise stimulates the production of glucose and the oxidation of fuels

The metabolic response to exercise resembles the response to fasting in that the mobilization and generation of fuels for oxidation are dominant factors. The types and amounts of substrate vary with the intensity and duration of the exercise (Figure 41-5). For very intense, short-term exercise (e.g., a 10- to 15-second sprint), stored creatine phosphate and ATP provide the energy at a rate of approximately 50 kcal/min. When these stores are depleted, additional intensive exercise for up to 2 minutes can be sustained via the breakdown of muscle glycogen to glucose-6-phosphate, and glycolysis yields the necessary energy (at a rate of 30 kcal/min). This anaerobic phase is limited by the accumulation of lactic acid in the exercising muscles and circulation.

> Several muscle diseases resulting from defects in energy generation are caused by a deficiency of an enzyme in the pathway from glycogen to pyruvate/lactate. An example is **McArdle's disease,** or **muscle phosphorylase deficiency.** Such patients experience pain and weakness after exercise. The glycogen mobilization is evidenced by a failure of lactate levels to increase in the antecubital vein after brief forearm muscle exercise during which the arterial inflow is excluded by a cuff.

After several minutes of exhaustive anaerobic exercise, an O_2 debt of 10 to 12 L can be built up. This must be repaid before the exercise can be repeated: (1) The accumulated lactic acid must be oxidized or rebuilt into glucose, (2) muscle ATP and creatine phosphate contents must be restored, and (3) the O_2 normally present in the lungs, body fluids, myoglobin, and hemoglobin must be replenished.

For less intense but longer periods of exercise, the aerobic oxidation of substrates is required to produce the necessary energy (at ≈12 kcal/min). Substrates from the blood circulation are added to muscle glycogen. Glucose uptake from plasma increases manyfold in some muscle groups. Hepatic glucose production increases, initially largely because of glycogenolysis, to meet this need, but gluconeogenesis becomes increasingly important as liver glycogen stores become depleted. However, endurance can be improved by high-carbohydrate feedings for several days before prolonged exercise (e.g., a marathon run) because this increases stores of both liver and muscle glycogen. To support gluconeogenesis, amino acids are increasingly released by muscle proteolysis. Eventually, fatty acids, liberated from adipose tissue triglycerides, form the predominant substrate, which supplies two thirds of the energy needs during sustained exercise. Except for the increases in circulating pyruvate and lactate that result from enhanced glycolysis, the pattern of change in plasma substrates is similar to that of fasting, only occurring more quickly.

> Genetic defects in the oxidation of fatty acids lead to reduced exercise capacity and muscle pain or even progressive muscle weakness. Cardiac muscle dysfunction may occur. Deficiencies of **carnitine** or the enzyme **carnitine palmityl transferase** impair the transfer of fatty acids from the cytoplasm into the mitochondria. Deficiencies of β-oxidation enzymes cause even more severe con-

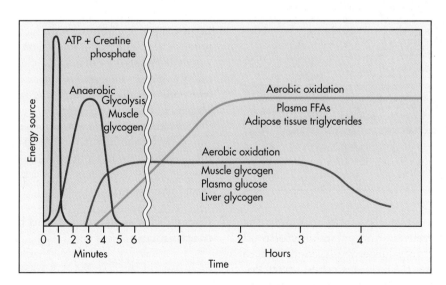

Figure 41-5 Energy sources during exercise. Note the sequential use of stored high-energy phosphate bonds as creatine phosphate and glycogen for short-term intensive exercise. Circulating glucose and free fatty acids (FFAs) become increasingly important with time, and the latter dominate in sustained exercise.

sequences in infants who cannot tolerate even short fasts because an overdependence on glucose for fuel leads to hypoglycemia.

Regulation of Energy Stores

The amounts and percentages of body weight accounted for by energy stored as fat in adipose tissue vary greatly among individuals. Studies of human monozygotic twins and animal models of obesity have provided indisputable evidence for a genetic influence on fat mass. Certain mutant genes inexorably cause obesity in animal models. Analogues of the normal animal regulatory genes have been found in the normal human genome. Mutations of these genes, a rare occurrence in humans, are associated with and probably cause obesity.

Environmental and cultural influences, specifically the quality and quantity of the food available, also modulate fat mass. Another factor that may contribute to the propensity for obesity is that humans have more energy-storage adipose cells per unit body mass than most other species.

Energy stores are held close to particular levels in human adults

Some data suggest the existence of a particular set point for energy stores in each individual. Once adult weight is reached, it tends to be rather constant until middle age, at which point most humans incur at least a modest weight gain that leads to a higher proportion of body fat. Abdominal fat particularly increases with age and more so in men. Normal and obese individuals subjected to overfeeding or underfeeding experiments return to their starting weight and degree of fatness when again allowed free access to food. This compensatory control of appetite (caloric and nutrient intake) resides in the hypothalamus, which contains a hunger center and a satiety center.

Humans who suffer damage to the hypothalamus from neoplasms or infiltrative disorders, such as **sarcoidosis,** sometimes gain large amounts of weight, which they maintain. Conversely, in the hypothalamic dysfunction of **anorexia nervosa,** weight is maintained at low, even life-threatening levels.

Many signals to the hypothalamus, including the sight, smell, taste, sweetness, and palatability of food and a reduction in plasma glucose levels, contribute to the stimulation of appetite. Eating is inhibited by glucose in the duodenum or portal vein. A variety of neuropeptides in the brain, some also with gastrointestinal location and function, and a variety of neurotransmitters carry appetite regulatory signals to and within the central nervous system. Some are nutrient specific, such as serotonin (glucose) and enterostatin (fat). Some are under hormonal regulation. For example, insulin strongly inhibits the synthesis of neuropeptide Y, a potent hypothalamic stimulator of food intake; insulin deficiency is associated with an excessive appetite (polyphagia). Cortisol inhibits the synthesis of corticotropin-releasing hormone, an appetite suppressor; a corticol excess stimulates appetite and weight gain.

Energy expenditure is adjusted to a long continuation of a change in energy intake

Homeostatic setting of energy stores and body weight also occurs via the regulation of energy expenditure. Thus experimental weight gain and loss evokes an increase and a decrease, respectively, of energy expenditure. In animals, **brown adipose tissue (BAT)** seems specifically designed for such purposes. The large mitochondria in BAT are stimulated by an **uncoupling protein (UCP),** also called **thermogenin,** that disassociates ATP production from O_2 use and thereby generates heat without producing useful chemical or mechanical work. UCP production is regulated by sympathetic nervous system signals (i.e., norepinephrine interacting with β_3-adrenergic receptors). BAT is clearly present and probably functional in human newborns who must adapt to a sudden lowering of environmental temperature from that in utero to that outside the mother by increasing heat production. However, this type of adipose tissue is difficult to detect and even harder to quantitate in adult humans. New homologous UCPs have been found in white adipose tissue and in the muscles of humans, and they may mediate obligatory and facultative thermogenesis.

If a hypothalamic set point for energy stores exists in each individual, how does the hypothalamus sense and quantitate peripheral fat mass? One answer is now clear. **Leptin,** a peptide hormone produced and secreted by adipose tissue, plays such a role. In one mouse model, leptin was deficient because of a mutant leptin gene, and the animal was obese. This animal overate, had a low BMR and low body temperature, and was inactive physically. Replacement therapy with leptin corrected all of these abnormalities and caused weight loss. In another mouse model, the obese animal had elevated levels of leptin, but the leptin receptor in the hypothalamus was defective because of a mutant gene. Treatment with leptin had no effect, as would be expected.

Energy stores are regulated by hormonal mechanisms

A schema for the regulation of energy stores is depicted in Figure 41-6. When adipose tissue mass expands beyond a designated set point (because of an increased number of cells with normal triglyceride content, a normal number of

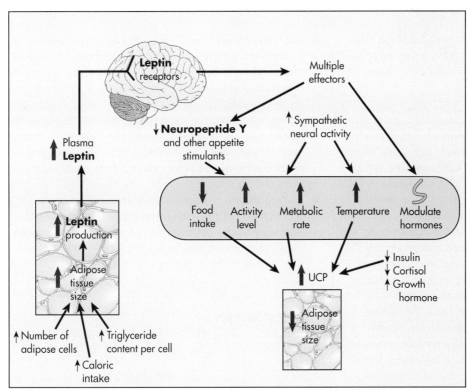

Figure 41-6 One schema for the regulation of energy stores. Leptin production, secretion, and plasma levels are proportional to adipose mass and "report" the size of the adipose mass to the hypothalamus and other brain areas. If excessive caloric intake leads to an undue increase in adipose mass, the plasma level of leptin increases. Greater occupancy of the leptin receptor initiates a series of effector mechanisms that adjust the adipose mass downward when it increases beyond a physiologically optimal set point. These effector mechanisms decrease food intake and increase the basal energy expenditure and obligatory thermogenesis via an increase in the levels of UCP and modulate the secretion of hormones to decrease the lipogenic activity and increase the lipolytic activity of adipose tissue.

cells with increased triglyceride content, or both), leptin synthesis and secretion increase. The resulting elevated plasma leptin concentration leads to a greater occupancy of leptin plasma membrane receptors in the hypothalamus and other areas of the brain. Leptin stimulation sets into motion multiple response mechanisms that decrease adipose tissue mass. These endocrine, neural, and neurocrine mechanisms include (1) decreasing food intake by increasing the production of appetite suppressors and decreasing the production of appetite stimulators, (2) increasing energy expenditure by increasing the BMR and body temperature via increasing UCP levels and physical activity, and (3) changing the hormonal set point to reduce lipogenesis and increase lipolysis in adipose tissue cells.

Plasma leptin levels do not increase acutely after food intake; thus leptin probably does not act as an immediate regulator of energy turnover. Fasting for several days decreases leptin levels, whereas continuous hyperinsulinemia stimulated by glucose or food increases leptin levels. These responses may be the result of subtle changes in adipose mass as well as insulin's direct stimulatory effect on leptin production.

> The pathological accumulation of energy stores as fat (i.e., obesity) is a major health problem in many countries. A body weight 20% above desirable or a **body mass index (BMI)** of 25 to 27 (see equation in next column) increases the risk of diabetes, hypertension, and cardiovascular disease; a body weight 40% to 50% above the desirable level or a BMI above 30 increases the risk of death.

> The accumulation of fat in abdominal and particularly visceral depots confers especially high risk.
>
> $$BMI = Weight\ (kg) \div Height\ (m^2)$$

The exact cause or causes of human obesity are not known. Some obese individuals overeat and recognize an inability to control it, but most believe that their caloric intakes are less than they are actually ingesting.

Many obese individuals also behave as if they have an elevated set point for energy stores. These individuals appear to tenaciously "defend" this set point by decreasing energy expenditure when caloric intake is reduced and significant amounts of weight are lost. Nonobese infants or adults with lower BMRs are at greater risk for future weight gain. However, once obesity is present and static, the BMR, the diet-induced thermogenesis (both adjusted for body weight), and the energy cost of exercise are generally equal to the respective values in individuals of normal weight.

In obese animals and humans, the profile of certain hormones involved in the regulation of fat metabolism (increased insulin and cortisol levels, decreased growth hormone levels) generally favors the deposition rather than the mobilization of fat. Endorphin levels are elevated, which may reflect abnormal central appetite stimulation. In addition, the adipose tissue of obese humans contains elevated levels of lipoprotein lipase, the key enzyme that transfers circulating triglycerides into cells. None of these abnormalities has been proved to be the primary cause of the common form of human obesity.

The initial studies of leptin in obese humans suggest that absolute leptin deficiency is an extremely rare cause of obesity. In obese humans, the plasma leptin levels and leptin messenger RNA levels in adipose cells are usually increased and correlate with fat mass. Hence the peripheral signal indicating that energy stores are too large is usually being generated, but it is not being received or acted on normally in the hypothalamus. However, only very rarely has a mutant leptin receptor been found as a cause for obesity. Thus human obesity is likely to result from defects in the generation of a leptin second messenger or effector mechanism within the leptin target cells or in the effector pathways further "downstream" (Figure 41-6). Whether partial resistance to leptin action can be overcome by sufficient exogenous leptin therapy is under study. The present treatment for fighting obesity—dieting, disciplined exercise, behavior modification, and drugs that may act favorably at some point in the complex system that sets energy stores—is palliative but not curative.

SUMMARY

- Energy input as carbohydrate, fat, and protein calories must equal energy expenditure. The latter is composed of basal, diet-induced, and nonshivering thermogenesis and sedentary activity components plus exercise.
- Fatty acids are the major fuel in most tissues except for the central nervous system and red blood cells, where glucose is the major and obligatory oxidative substrate.
- The metabolism of glucose to pyruvate (anaerobic glycolysis), β-oxidation of fatty acids, and the disposal of acetyl CoA by the citric acid cycle lead to the mitochondrial generation of ATP via oxidative phosphorylation.
- Energy is stored mainly as adipose tissue triglycerides, with lesser amounts as protein. Carbohydrate stores as glycogen are very small.
- During long-term fasting, gluconeogenesis from amino acids and glycerol is required to sustain central nervous system metabolism and its critical functions. The pathway of gluconeogenesis is partly a reversal of glycolysis, but it requires special steps from pyruvate to fructose-6-phosphate. Increased use of fatty acids during fasting greatly increases the production of the ketoacids, β-hydroxybutyrate, and acetoacetate.
- Endogenous protein turnover obligates a daily ingestion of proteins, in particular those containing essential amino acids, such as leucine.
- Fat metabolism involves a variety of circulating lipoprotein particles, apoproteins, and their receptors. These transfer triglycerides and cholesterol, either originating in the diet or from hepatic synthesis, to and from various tissues.
- Energy needs during exercise are met in sequence by stored muscle creatine phosphate plus ATP, stored muscle glycogen, anaerobic glycolysis, and finally, aerobic oxidation of glucose and fatty acids taken up from the plasma.
- The regulation of energy stores at individual set points is complex. Leptin, a secreted adipose tissue product, interacts with hypothalamic receptors to down-regulate appetite and to up-regulate energy expenditure and thereby prevents excessive accumulation of fat.

BIBLIOGRAPHY

Bouchard C, Despres JP, Mauriege P: Genetic and nongenetic determinants of regional fat distribution, *Endocr Rev* 14:72, 1993.

Cahill GF: Starvation in man, *N Engl J Med* 282:668, 1970.

Considine RV et al: Serum immunoreactive-leptin concentrations in normal-weight and obese humans, *N Engl J Med* 334:292, 1996.

Ferrannini E et al: The disposal of an oral glucose load in healthy subjects: a quantitative study, *Diabetes* 34:580, 1985.

Harris RBS: Role of set-point theory in regulation of body weight, *FASEB J* 4:3310, 1990.

Kimball SR et al: Protein metabolism. In Rifkin H, Porte D, eds: *Diabetes mellitus*, ed 4, New York, 1990, Elsevier.

Leibel RL, Rosenbaum M, Hirsch J: Changes in energy expenditure resulting from altered body weight, *N Engl J Med* 332:621, 1995.

Leibowitz SF: Brain neurotransmitters and hormones in relation to eating behavior and its disorders. In Bjorntorp P, Brodoff BN, eds: *Obesity*, Philadelphia, 1992, JB Lippincott.

McGarry JD, Foster DW: Ketogenesis. In Porte D Jr, Sherwin RS, eds: *Ellenberg & Rifkin's diabetes mellitus*, ed 5, Stamford, Conn, 1997, Appleton & Lange.

Ravussin E et al: Determinants of 24-hour energy expenditure in man: methods and results using a respiratory chamber, *J Clin Invest* 78:1568, 1986.

Roberts SB et al: Dietary energy requirements of young adult men, determined by using the doubly labeled water method, *Am J Clin Nutr* 54:499, 1991.

Rohner-Jeanrenaud F, Jeanrenaud B: Obesity, leptin, and the brain, *N Engl J Med* 334:324, 1996.

Seifter S, England S: Carbohydrate metabolism. In Rifkin H, Porte D, eds: *Diabetes mellitus*, ed 4, New York, 1990, Elsevier.

Shulman GI, Barrett EJ, Sherwin RS: Integrated fuel metabolism. In Porte D Jr, Sherwin RS, eds: *Ellenberg & Rifkin's diabetes mellitus*, ed 5, Stamford, Conn, 1997, Appleton & Lange.

Sims EAH, Danforth E Jr: Expenditure and storage of energy in man, *J Clin Invest* 79:1019, 1987.

Tall AR: Plasma high density lipoproteins. *J Clin Invest* 86:379, 1990.

Wolfe BM et al: Effect of elevated free fatty acids on glucose oxidation in normal humans, *Metabolism* 37:323, 1988.

Woods SC et al: Food intake and energy balance. In Porte D Jr, Sherwin RS, eds: *Ellenberg & Rifkin's diabetes mellitus*, ed 5, Stamford, Conn, 1997, Appleton & Lange.

CASE STUDIES

Case 41-1

A 25-year-old man weighing 70 kg and in fit condition embarks on a solo mountain climb in winter. He is injured in an avalanche and fractures both legs. This immobilized person survives for 15 days without calories by drinking melted snow. He is then rescued. On examination, his body temperature is 34° C.

1. At the time of rescue, which of the following findings would be expected?

   A. Decreased plasma alanine level
   B. Increased urine nitrogen level
   C. Decreased plasma free fatty acids
   D. Decreased plasma ketoacid levels
   E. Increased plasma glucose level

2. Approximately how many grams of adipose tissue fat might he likely have lost?

   A. 2550 g
   B. 1550 g
   C. 1450 g
   D. 3500 g
   E. 5750 g

Case Study 41-2

A 28-year-old woman sees a physician for obesity, which has been present since early infancy. Of her 10 siblings, 2 have a similar history of obesity. Neither parent is obese, but one grandparent on each side of the family was obese. The patient's height is 5'2", and her weight is 242 pounds. Her body mass index is $120/1.55^2 = 46$. The family history suggests a genetic form of obesity with an autosomal recessive pattern of inheritance.

1. Which of the following is a candidate gene for causing this syndrome?

   A. An inactivating mutant gene for neuropeptide Y synthesis
   B. An inactivating mutant gene for a β-adrenergic receptor in adipose tissue
   C. A hyperactivating mutant gene for the leptin receptor
   D. A hyperactivating mutant gene for UCP
   E. An inactivating mutant gene for lipoprotein lipase

2. With great effort, the patient loses 50 pounds in 6 months on a low-calorie diet and regular exercise. However, she gradually slips back into ad lib eating and her former sedentary ways; and over 3 years, her weight restabilizes at 250 pounds. Which of the following is correct?

   A. She has an abnormal appetite setting.
   B. She has an abnormal low set point for leptin secretion.
   C. She has an abnormal low set point for energy expenditure.
   D. She has an abnormal low set point for UCP production.
   E. She has an abnormal set point for energy stores.

CHAPTER 42

Hormones of the Pancreatic Islets

OBJECTIVES

- Describe the synthesis and secretion of the two major pancreatic islet hormones: insulin and glucagon.
- Explain the powerful effects of insulin and glucagon on glucose, fatty acid, and amino acid metabolism and the feedback effects of these substrates on insulin and glucagon secretion.
- Identify the mechanisms of action of insulin and glucagon on their target cells.
- Explain the interrelationships between insulin and glucagon, particularly their mutually antagonistic effects on substrate flow in the liver.
- Describe the respective roles of insulin and glucagon in metabolic adaptations to fasting and exercise.

The major pancreatic islet hormones, **insulin** and **glucagon,** are rapid and powerful regulators of metabolism. Their secretion is determined primarily by plasma substrate levels. TOGETHER, GLUCAGON AND INSULIN COORDINATE THE DISPOSITION OF NUTRIENT INPUT FROM MEALS AS WELL AS THE FLOW OF ENDOGENOUS SUBSTRATES DURING FASTING VIA ACTIONS ON THE LIVER, ADIPOSE TISSUE, AND MUSCLE MASS. In turn, these hormones form regulatory feedback loops with critical substrates. Insulin and glucagon directly or indirectly influence the metabolism and hence the function of all the organ systems described earlier in this book.

Functional Anatomy

The cells of origin of insulin and glucagon are interspersed in small islets scattered throughout the pancreas. This proximity permits each hormone to influence the other's secretion. The islets are composed of 60% β-cells, the source of insulin, and 25% α-cells, the source of glucagon. The remaining islet cells secrete various neuropeptides with gastrointestinal functions.

The strategic location of the islets reflects their functional role

Insulin and glucagon are secreted in response to nutrient inflow and to gastrointestinal secretagogues, as are the enzymes of the acinar pancreas (see Chapter 33). The islet hormones may have paracrine effects on nearby acinar cells as well as on each other through tight junctions and gap junctions between the endocrine cells. The location of the islets (Figure 42-1) leads to the secretion of insulin and glucagon into the pancreatic veins and then into the portal vein, where they join the influx of nutrients from meals in the splanchnic circulation. This arrangement permits the liver, the central organ in nutrient traffic, to be exposed to higher concentrations of these pancreatic islet hormones than peripheral tissues. It also permits the liver to modulate the availability of insulin and glucagon to peripheral tissues by extracting variable amounts of these hormones during first passage through that organ.

INSULIN AND GLUCAGON ARE OFTEN SECRETED RECIPROCALLY AND ACT RECIPROCALLY. WHEN ONE IS NEEDED, THE OTHER USUALLY IS NOT. The consequences of isolated insulin deficiency—the common disease **type 1 diabetes mellitus**—are so devastating that insulin has dominated physiological thinking. In contrast, isolated glucagon deficiency is virtually unknown in medicine; moreover, it can be compensated for by other mechanisms.

Insulin is synthesized from a prohormone and secreted by exocytosis

Insulin is a peptide hormone with a molecular weight of 6000. It is composed of two straight chains linked by disulfide bridges. The B chain contains the core of biological activity, whereas the A chain contains most of the species-specific sites. Human insulin and molecular variants produced by recombinant DNA techniques have virtually replaced animal insulins for the treatment of diabetes.

The synthesis of insulin by the β-cell follows the same general pattern as that for peptide hormones described in Chapter 40. The gene directs the synthesis of a preprohormone, from which the signal peptide is cleaved to yield the

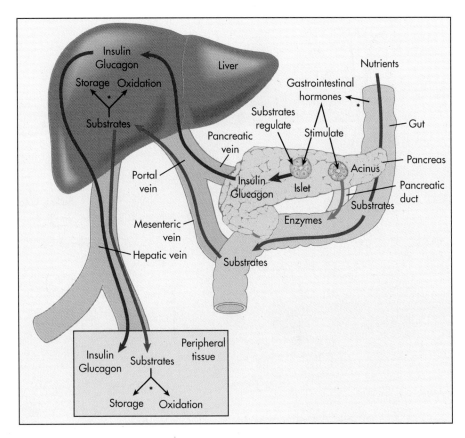

Figure 42-1 View of the pivotal location of the pancreatic islets. Secretion of the islet hormones, insulin and glucagon, is coordinated with the secretion of exocrine pancreatic enzymes. Both are stimulated by the entry of nutrients into the gastrointestinal tract and by gastrointestinal hormones. Pancreatic enzymes reach the intestinal lumen via the pancreatic duct. Islet hormones are secreted into the portal vein and thereby reach the liver with the substrates resulting from nutrient digestion. Within the liver, these hormones direct the storage or oxidation of the ingested substrates. Islet hormones that pass through the liver with substrates similarly affect the metabolism of these substrates by peripheral tissues. Asterisks indicate the action sites.

single-chain **proinsulin.** Establishment of the disulfide links is followed by the excision of a connecting peptide known as **C peptide.** The Golgi apparatus packages insulin and C peptide together in the secretory granules. These granules also contain zinc, which acts to join six insulin molecules into hexamers.

Insulin is secreted via exocytosis (see Figure 40-5) of its granules, which are arrayed in parallel with microtubules in the β-cell cytoplasm. The microtubules are associated with a web of microfilaments that contain myosin and actin near the plasma membrane. On application of a stimulus, contraction of microfilaments draws the granules to the plasma membrane, where they fuse with it, rupture, and release equimolar amounts of insulin and C peptide.

The metabolism of glucose in the β-cell stimulates insulin secretion

The single most important stimulator of insulin release is glucose (Figure 42-2). The mechanism involves the following sequence:

1. A specific glucose transporter (GLUT2) facilitates rapid diffusion into the β-cell and maintains an intracellular glucose concentration equal to that of interstitial fluid.

2. The enzyme glucokinase, which has a K_m of 5 mM for glucose (the average fasting concentration), acts as a glucose sensor that controls the rates of glucose use.

3. The products of glucose metabolism, including ATP, nicotine-adenine dinucleotide phosphate (NADH), and the reduced form of NADH (NADPH), increase, and an ATP-sensitive K^+ channel closes.

4. This triggers the opening of voltage-regulated Ca^{++} channels. The intracellular Ca^{++} increases and triggers exocytosis (see Figure 40-5).

5. G proteins linked to adenylyl cyclase and to phospholipase C mediate the stimulatory and inhibitory actions of other modulators of insulin release via alterations in the levels of cyclic AMP, phosphatidylinositol products, and diacylglycerols (Figure 42-2). In addition to causing insulin release, glucose stimulates the synthesis of hormone by increasing the transcription rate of the insulin gene and the translation rate of its mature messenger RNA.

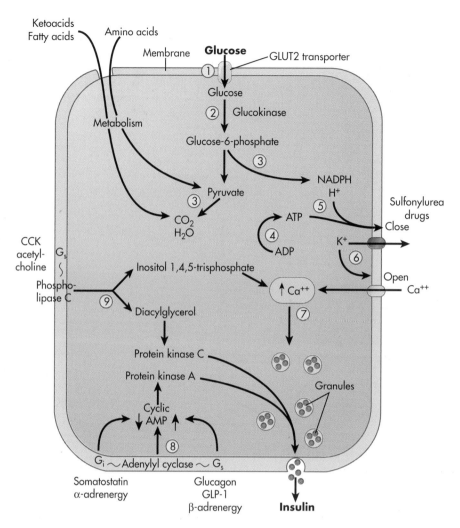

Figure 42-2 Regulation of insulin secretion by the β-cell. Glucose transport *(1)* and glucokinase-catalyzed phosphorylation *(2)* raise glucose-6-phosphate levels. The metabolism of glucose-6-phosphate *(3)* subsequently leads to increased levels of ATP *(4)* and reduced nicotine-adenine dinucleotide phosphate *(NADPH), (5)* that inhibit or close a potassium channel *(6)* and open a calcium channel *(6)*. Increased calcium levels then trigger exocytosis of insulin granules *(7)*. Other modulators of secretion act via the adenylyl cyclase–cyclic AMP–protein kinase pathway *(8)* and the phospholipase-phosphoinositide pathway *(9)*. *CCK,* Cholecystokinin; *GLP-1,* glucagon-like peptide-1.

Type 1 diabetes mellitus results from the complete destruction of β-cells and the ultimate loss of all insulin. However, in rare instances, much milder diabetes mellitus is caused by genetic abnormalities in insulin synthesis and secretion; such abnormalities include mutant glucokinase, insulin promoter factor-1, and insulin genes.

Regulation of insulin secretion

In the broadest sense, insulin secretion is governed by a feedback relationship with the exogenous nutrient supply
When the supply of nutrients is abundant (Figure 42-3), insulin is secreted in response to their inflow; the hormone then stimulates the use of these same incoming nutrients as it inhibits the mobilization of endogenous substrates. When the nutrient supply is low or absent, insulin secretion is dampened, and the mobilization of endogenous fuels is enhanced.

The central regulating molecule is glucose. At plasma glucose levels lower than 50 mg/dl, little or no insulin is secreted, whereas the response is maximal at plasma levels higher than 250 mg/dl. Brief exposure of the β-cell to glucose induces a rapid but transient release of insulin. With continuous glucose exposure, this initial response fades, only to be replaced later by a more prolonged second phase.

Glucose entry from the gastrointestinal tract follows digestion of the carbohydrate components of a meal. Under these circumstances, more insulin is released than can be accounted for by the extent to which plasma glucose levels rise. This phenomenon results from the release of insulinogenic gastrointestinal peptide hormones such as gastric inhibitory peptide, gastrin, secretin, cholecystokinin, and most notably a glucagon-like peptide (GLP-1) from intestinal cells. In addition, digestion of the protein in a meal yields amino acids, some of which synergize with glucose in stimulating the β-cells.

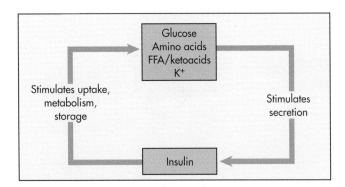

Figure 42-3 Feedback relationship between insulin and nutrients. The nutrients that stimulate insulin secretion are the same as those whose disposal is facilitated by insulin. *FFA*, Free fatty acids.

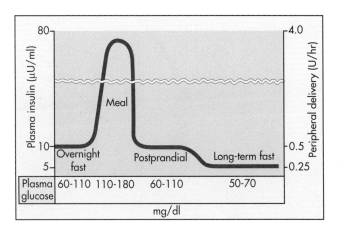

Figure 42-4 Pattern of plasma insulin levels and the corresponding insulin-delivery rates to the peripheral circulation in various physiological states (10 μU/ml = 7 × 10⁻¹¹ M). The usual prevailing plasma glucose levels are also indicated. Fasting insulin levels regulate the mobilization of endogenous substrates at appropriate rates. Levels after meals stimulate the storage of substrates.

Lipids and their products contribute little directly to the β-cell response to a meal. When the digestion and absorption of nutrients are completed, plasma glucose and amino acid levels return to baseline, and insulin secretion subsides to a rate that is maintained steadily during periods between meals and overnight fasting. An intrinsic cyclic oscillation every 14 minutes characterizes basal secretion.

If fasting is extended for days, insulin secretion declines below the basal rate and then resets at a lower level. In this state, secretion is maintained by lower, but still stimulatory, plasma glucose levels, with contributions from greatly elevated levels of ketoacids and free fatty acids. Insulin secretion is also modulated by cholinergic and β-adrenergic stimulatory and α-adrenergic inhibitory influences. All these factors cause physiological fluctuations in peripheral plasma insulin levels and in the average equivalent rates of insulin delivery into the peripheral circulation. These changes are summarized in Figure 42-4.

> **Type 2 diabetes mellitus** is the most common form of the disease. One important factor in this type of diabetes is an early subtle disturbance in the pattern of insulin secretion. This is characterized by altered cyclicity, diminished pulse frequency, and delayed response to rising glucose levels. Eventually, glucose is no longer recognized as a stimulus. The primary cause of such β-cell dysfunction remains unknown.

β-Cell function is quantitated by measurements of C peptide

Peripheral plasma insulin levels are about 7 × 10⁻¹¹ M. Insulin concentration in the portal vein ranges from two to ten times higher than in the peripheral circulation. The liver extracts about half the insulin reaching it, but this varies with the nutritional state. Thus actual β-cell secre-

tory rates are better estimated by measuring plasma (or even urine) levels of C peptide because this cosecreted molecule is not removed by the liver. Such estimates yield values of 1.0 to 2.5 mg/day (25 to 40 units/day) for insulin secretion. C peptide and the small quantity of proinsulin secreted by β-cells as yet have no known physiological actions.

Insulin has a short plasma half-life (6 to 8 minutes), mainly because of specific degradation in the kidney and liver. However, insulin is also degraded in conjunction with its actions on its target cells after receptor binding and internalization of the hormone. Very little intact insulin is excreted in the urine.

Actions of insulin

Insulin is a strongly anabolic hormone

THE OVERALL THRUST OF INSULIN ACTION IS TO FACILITATE THE STORAGE OF SUBSTRATES AND INHIBIT THEIR RELEASE (Figure 42-5). As a result, secreted or administered insulin decreases the plasma concentrations of glucose, of free fatty acids and ketoacids, and predominantly of the essential branch-chain amino acids (i.e., leucine, isoleucine, valine). The major sites of insulin action are the liver, muscle, and adipose tissue. In each target tissue, carbohydrate, lipid, and protein metabolism are regulated coordinately.

Under maximal insulin stimulation, the usual rate of glucose use by peripheral tissues increases fivefold to sixfold. Simultaneously, the output of glucose by the liver drops to considerably below half. Most of the extra glucose uptake occurs in muscle, with a small fraction occurring in adipose tissue. Approximately 75% of this glucose is converted to glycogen, and about 25% undergoes glycolysis and terminal oxidation to carbon dioxide. The absolute rate of glucose oxidation, however, is increased threefold by insulin.

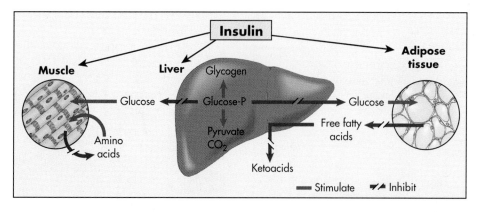

Figure 42-5 Effect of insulin on the overall flow of fuels. Tissue uptake of glucose and amino acids is stimulated by insulin; tissue release of glucose, amino acids, and free fatty acids is inhibited by insulin, as is ketogenesis. The net result is a decrease in plasma levels of these substrates.

The hypersecretion of insulin by a β-cell tumor causes **hypoglycemia.** The latter produces central nervous system dysfunction, which ranges from mild difficulty in concentrating to severe behavioral disturbances, psychosis, convulsions, and coma. Symptoms are typically worse in the fasting state and are countered by overeating carbohydrates, with resulting weight gain. The diagnosis is established by demonstrating inappropriately high levels of plasma insulin and C peptide when the plasma glucose concentration is low.

The basal rate of free fatty acid inflow to plasma from adipose tissue is also markedly decreased by insulin. (At the same time, the inflow of glycerol, the other product of triglyceride hydrolysis, is decreased sharply.) As a result, insulin reduces the basal rate of lipid oxidation more than 90%. Because insulin also stimulates triglyceride synthesis and storage, it facilitates weight gain.

The action of insulin on protein turnover can be assessed by determining the hormone's effect on the flux of the essential amino acid leucine. Maximum doses decrease leucine's rate of inflow into plasma to almost half. Because the only source of leucine in the basal state is endogenous protein, insulin must inhibit proteolysis. In addition, insulin decreases leucine's rate of oxidation. The result of these insulin effects is a net gain in body protein.

Insulin stimulates glucose uptake by cells and storage as glycogen

IN MUSCLE AND ADIPOSE TISSUE, INSULIN STIMULATES THE TRANSPORT OF GLUCOSE FROM THE PLASMA INTO THE CYTOPLASM, WHERE IT IS RAPIDLY PHOSPHORYLATED. IN MUSCLE AND LIVER, INSULIN LARGELY STIMULATES GLYCOGEN FORMATION FROM GLUCOSE-6-PHOSPHATE. To a much lesser extent, insulin stimulates the glycolysis and oxidation of glucose. In adipose tissue, insulin's most important carbohydrate effect is to stimulate the production of α-glycerol phosphate from the triose phosphate intermediates of glycolysis. The α-glycerol phosphate is used to esterify free

fatty acids and thus store them as triglycerides (see Figure 41-3).

Insulin stimulates the conversion of glucose to glycogen and inhibits the reverse reaction, the breakdown of glycogen to glucose, by increasing the activities or concentrations of glycogen synthase and decreasing those of phosphorylase, respectively (see Figure 41-3). The equilibrium between glucose and glucose-6-phosphate is shifted toward the latter because the concentration of the phosphorylating enzyme glucokinase is increased by insulin. (In only the liver, the level of the dephosphorylating enzyme glucose-6-phosphatase is decreased by insulin.) Insulin also shifts the balance between glycolysis and gluconeogenesis toward the former and away from the latter. Glycolysis is accelerated because insulin increases the key enzymes phosphofructokinase, pyruvate kinase, and pyruvate dehydrogenase; gluconeogenesis is retarded because insulin decreases the enzymes phosphoenolpyruvate carboxykinase, pyruvate carboxylase, and fructose 1,6-diphosphatase (see Figure 41-3).

In the liver, glucose availability reinforces the effects of insulin that lead toward glycogen storage or glycolysis and away from glucose release. Conversely, if plasma glucose levels decline below normal, these effects become attenuated by intrahepatic autoregulatory phenomena as well as by the secretion of hormones whose actions are antagonistic to insulin (e.g., glucagon, epinephrine, cortisol, growth hormone).

Insulin stimulates fat storage

IN ADIPOSE TISSUE, INSULIN FACILITATES TRANSFER OF CIRCULATING FAT INTO THE ADIPOSE CELL BY INDUCING THE ENZYME LIPOPROTEIN LIPASE (see Figure 41-5). More free fatty acid is thereby liberated from circulating triglyceride and is rapidly taken up into the adipose cell, where it is reesterified. Thus dietary fat not needed for immediate energy generation is stored. OF EQUAL OR GREATER IMPORTANCE, INSULIN PROFOUNDLY INHIBITS THE REVERSE REACTION (I.E., LIPOLYSIS OF STORED TRIGLYCERIDE) BY INHIBITING THE NECESSARY ENZYME, HORMONE-SENSITIVE ADIPOSE TISSUE LIPASE. In this manner, the release and delivery of free fatty acids to other tissues are greatly suppressed.

In the liver, insulin favors shunting of incoming free fatty acids away from β-oxidation by inhibiting their transfer into mitochondria and directing them toward esterification by increasing the production of β-glycerol phosphate. Because β-oxidation is diminished, less β-hydroxybutyrate and acetoacetate are produced. Thus INSULIN IS POWERFULLY ANTIKETOGENIC.

> Virtually complete loss of insulin and its actions causes the striking manifestations of type 1 diabetes mellitus. Over a period of weeks, **hyperglycemia** develops to a point exceeding the renal threshold of glucose (see Chapter 36). Large amounts of glucose are lost in the urine; the high urinary glucose concentration creates a continuous osmotic diuresis, **polyuria,** thirst, and dehydration. This drain of carbohydrate calories along with catabolic losses of adipose triglyceride stores and lean body mass causes weight loss despite increased food intake (**polyphagia**). Uninhibited lipolysis leads to high plasma levels of free fatty acids, the stimulation of ketogenesis, and very high plasma levels of β-hydroxybutyrate and acetoacetate. The plasma level of bicarbonate and the pH fall, and a profound metabolic acidosis ensues (see Chapters 30 and 39). Coma and death follow unless treatment with insulin, intravenous fluids, and electrolytes is provided.

Insulin also stimulates de novo synthesis of free fatty acids from glucose. Cytoplasmic acetyl coenzyme A (acetyl CoA) derived from pyruvate is shunted toward fatty acid formation because insulin increases the key enzymes: acetyl CoA carboxylase and fatty acid synthase. In addition, insulin stimulates the synthesis of cholesterol from acetyl CoA by activating the key enzyme, hydroxymethylglutaryl-CoA reductase. The net effect of insulin is therefore to increase the fat content of the liver and in some circumstances to increase the release of very-low-density lipoprotein from that organ.

Insulin stimulates protein storage

In muscle, insulin stimulates the sodium-dependent transport of certain amino acids from the plasma, across the cell membrane, and into the cytoplasm, all independently of the transport of glucose. When amino acids are abundant, the overall synthesis of proteins is also increased via the stimulation of transcription and translation. Specific examples are the stimulation of the synthesis of albumin in the liver and of amylase (by insulin) in the exocrine pancreas. These anabolic effects are reinforced by important anticatabolic effects (i.e., by inhibiting the enzymes of proteolysis and the inhibition of amino acid release from the cell). Moreover, in cartilage and osseous tissue, insulin and structurally related insulin growth factors (see Chapter 44) enhance the

general synthesis of proteins as well as of DNA, RNA, and other macromolecules. Thus INSULIN IS AN IMPORTANT CONTRIBUTOR TO GROWTH, TISSUE REGENERATION, AND BONE REMODELING.

Insulin regulates plasma cation and anion concentrations

Both glycogen and protein synthesis require the concurrent cellular uptake of potassium, phosphate, and magnesium. The translocation of all three of these electrolytes from the extracellular to the intracellular space is stimulated by insulin. Insulin also stimulates their reabsorption by the renal tubules. Preventing the urinary loss of potassium and phosphate also contributes to anabolism, whereas conserving sodium may be related to the need for the additional formation of extracellular fluid to accompany the expansion of lean body mass.

> When insulin is administered to patients in **diabetic ketoacidosis,** increased transport into cells can cause profound drops in plasma phosphate, potassium, and magnesium levels. Potassium always, phosphate occasionally, and magnesium rarely must be given intravenously to prevent the serious or even fatal consequences of hypokalemia, hypophosphatemia, or hypomagnesemia.

Insulin has other actions that are relevant to total body energy turnover and stores

Diet-induced thermogenesis, particularly after carbohydrate ingestion, is enhanced by insulin, probably through the stimulation of glycogen formation. Insulin also increases the energy expenditure by stimulating Na^+,K^+-ATPase. Although most parts of the brain are unresponsive to insulin, this hormone probably acts on the hypothalamus. Insulin decreases the synthesis of neuropeptide Y (see Chapter 41). By this action—and by increasing leptin levels—insulin is an appetite suppressant. Since leptin inhibits insulin secretion, leptin and insulin form a negative-feedback loop that regulates energy stores in adipose tissue. If insulin lowers plasma glucose levels to below those needed for normal brain metabolism (i.e., <55 mg/dl), hunger is stimulated by other mechanisms.

Insulin acts through a plasma membrane tyrosine kinase receptor

The initial step in all actions of insulin is binding of the hormone to its plasma membrane receptor (Figure 42-6). This receptor is a glycoprotein composed of two symmetrical units connected by disulfide bonds. Each of these main units is made up of an α subunit that extends externally and binds the hormone and a β subunit that traverses the cell membrane and terminates in an intracytoplasmic tail. Receptor molecules cycle between a cytoplasmic pool and the plasma membrane, and their number is down-regulated by insulin.

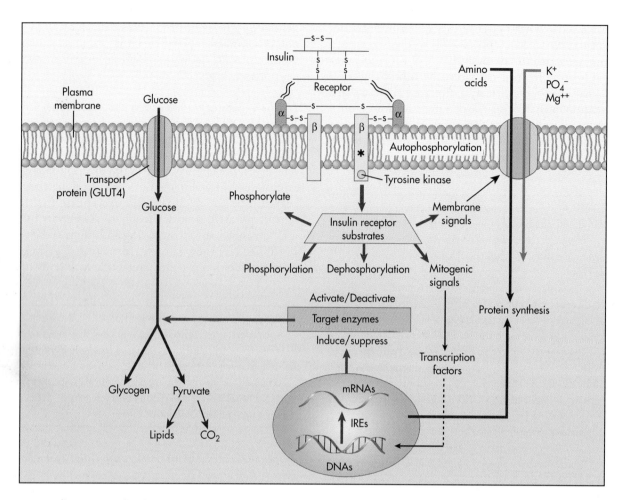

Figure 42-6   Insulin action on cells. The binding of insulin to its receptor causes autophosphorylation of the receptor, which then itself acts as a tyrosine kinase that phosphorylates tyrosines in insulin receptor substrates. As a result, these substrates phosphorylate serine and threonine residues in other proteins and enzymes. Numerous target enzymes are ultimately activated or inactivated, and the result is to shift the metabolism of glucose toward glycogen and pyruvate. The glucose transporter, GLUT4, is recruited to the plasma membrane, where it facilitates glucose entry into the cell. The transport of amino acids, potassium, magnesium, and phosphate into the cell is also facilitated by other mechanisms. The synthesis of various enzymes is induced or suppressed and cell growth is regulated by signal molecules that modulate gene expression. Numerous intermediary molecules are involved. *IREs,* Insulin regulatory elements; *mRNA,* messenger RNA.

After insulin binds to its receptor, the following steps occur:

1. The β subunit of the receptor undergoes autophosphorylation with ATP at specific tyrosine sites.
2. The phosphorylated receptor itself becomes a tyrosine kinase, which then phosphorylates tyrosines in several large proteins called **insulin receptor substrates (IRSs).**
3. The activation of IRSs initiates a cascade of serine and threonine phosphorylations in multiple intermediary molecules such as phosphatidylinositol-3-kinase, growth receptor–binding protein-2, and mitogen-activated protein kinase. Metabolic and mitogenic pathways are thereby altered in parallel though not necessarily synchronously.
4. The target enzymes previously described are rapidly activated or deactivated, by both phosphorylation and dephosphorylation. The same enzymes

may be induced or repressed more slowly by modulating gene transcription.

5. Plasma membrane carrier mechanisms are activated.
6. DNA transcription factors related to cell growth are modified.
7. In some target cells (e.g., adipose tissue) cyclic AMP levels are lowered by insulin's stimulation of **phosphodiesterase;** this contributes to some of the hormone's actions (e.g., the inhibition of lipolysis).

Insulin stimulates a specific glucose carrier system within the plasma membrane of target cells

A particular glucose transporter (GLUT4) facilitates the diffusion (not the active transport) of extracellular glucose into the cytosol of muscle and adipose cells, down an already existing, large concentration gradient. Insulin rapidly increases transfer of GLUT4 from its cytoplasmic depots to the plasma membrane and later increases GLUT4 synthesis. The crucial importance of this action is that at basal physiological insulin concentrations, the transport of glucose into muscle and adipose tissue cells is often the rate-limiting step in glucose metabolism. In comparison, the phosphorylation of glucose is so rapid that intracellular concentrations of free glucose are usually negligible. At the high insulin concentrations that prevail after a meal, the rate-limiting step in glucose metabolism shifts to an intracellular point that also governs insulin actions.

In rare instances, deletions as well as missense and nonsense mutations in the insulin receptor gene cause receptor malfunction and marked resistance to the action of insulin. In affected infants, this can lead to diabetes mellitus, profound disorders of growth, and death. Impaired insulin action (as well as inadequate insulin secretion) is also a major factor, producing hyperglycemia in the very common type 2 diabetes mellitus. Because most of these patients are obese and seldom exhibit increased ketogenesis, insulin resistance may be greater in muscle than in adipose tissue.

Insulin secretion is correlated with the appropriate actions of insulin

The major actions of insulin form a hierarchy that is related to successive increases in plasma insulin concentration. The low insulin concentrations that prevail in humans who have fasted overnight are able to partially restrain and thereby regulate the endogenous release rates of free fatty acids and amino acids. Somewhat higher insulin concentrations elicited by incoming dietary nutrients are required to completely shut off unneeded glucose production by the liver. The peak insulin concentrations elicited by a meal greatly stimulate glucose and amino acid uptake by peripheral tissues, especially muscle, and fatty acid uptake by adipose tissue. These actions of insulin ensure that those substrates may be stored for future use.

Glucagon

Glucagon is synthesized and secreted in response to a lowering of plasma glucose levels

GLUCAGON IS AN IMPORTANT REGULATOR OF INTRAHEPATIC GLUCOSE AND FREE FATTY ACID METABOLISM. This hormone is a straight-chain peptide with a molecular weight of 3500. The N-terminus residues 1 to 6 are essential for biological activity. The glucagon gene directs the synthesis of a preproglucagon in the α-cells of the pancreatic islets. Preproglucagon is processed to a prohormone that subsequently yields glucagon and other peptides of still unknown function. In certain cells of the intestinal tract, the alternative

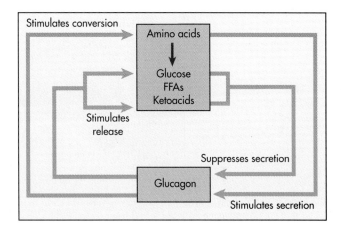

Figure 42-7 Feedback relationship between glucagon and nutrients. Glucagon stimulates the production and release of glucose, free fatty acids *(FFAs)*, and ketoacids, which in turn suppress glucagon secretion. Amino acids stimulate glucagon secretion, and glucagon in turn stimulates amino acids' conversion to glucose.

processing of preproglucagon yields glucagon-like peptides with different functions. IN CONTRAST TO INSULIN, GLUCAGON SYNTHESIS IS INHIBITED BY HIGH GLUCOSE LEVELS AND IS STIMULATED BY LOW GLUCOSE LEVELS.

The secretion of glucagon is related in feedback fashion to the principal function of the hormone, namely the stimulation of glucose output by the liver and the maintenance of plasma glucose levels (Figure 42-7). Thus hypoglycemia promptly evokes a twofold to fourfold increase in plasma glucagon concentrations from basal levels of about 100 pg/ml (3×10^{-11} M), whereas hyperglycemia suppresses glucagon secretion by more than 50%. These effects of glucose are independently reinforced by insulin, possibly through paracrine action within the islet. Thus insulin (stimulated by glucose) directly inhibits glucagon secretion; conversely, when insulin is absent, the stimulatory effect of low glucose levels on glucagon secretion is exaggerated.

The other major energy substrate, free fatty acids, also suppresses glucagon release, whereas a sharp decline in plasma levels of free fatty acids is stimulatory. A protein meal and amino acids, which are the substrates for glucose production, stimulate glucagon secretion, but this response is dampened by concurrent glucose or insulin action. As a result, the usual mixed meal produces only small and variable increases in plasma glucagon levels, in contrast to the large and consistent increases in plasma insulin levels (Figure 42-4).

Prolonged fasting and sustained exercise, circumstances that require glucose mobilization, increase glucagon secretion. Under stressful conditions such as major infection or surgery, glucagon secretion is often greatly augmented. This probably occurs through sympathetic nervous system stimulation of the α-cells via α-adrenergic receptors.

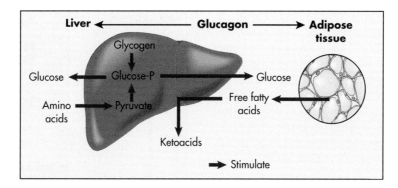

Figure 42-8 Effect of glucagon on the overall flow of fuels. The tissue release of glucose, free fatty acids, and ketoacids raises the plasma levels of these fuels, whereas the uptake of amino acids by the liver lowers them. *Pi,* Phosphate.

Glucagon is extracted by the liver on the first pass, and it has a short half-life in peripheral plasma. The hormone is degraded in the kidney and liver.

In almost all respects, the actions of glucagon are opposite to those of insulin

Glucagon promotes the mobilization rather than the storage of fuels, especially glucose (Figure 42-8). Both glucagon and insulin act at numerous similar control points for glucose metabolism in the liver. Indeed, glucagon can be viewed as the primary hormone that regulates hepatic glucose production and ketogenesis, whereas insulin's main hepatic role is that of a glucagon antagonist. GLUCAGON EXERTS AN IMMEDIATE AND PROFOUND GLYCOGENOLYTIC EFFECT THROUGH THE ACTIVATION OF HEPATIC GLYCOGEN PHOSPHORYLASE. Simultaneously, the resynthesis of phosphorylated glucose molecules back to glycogen is prevented by the inhibition of glycogen synthase. Glucagon also stimulates gluconeogenesis via several mechanisms. The hepatic extraction of amino acid precursors is increased. The activities of key gluconeogenic enzymes—pyruvate carboxylase, phosphoenolpyruvate carboxykinase, and fructose 1,6-diphosphatase—are increased, whereas activities of the key glycolytic enzymes—phosphofructokinase and pyruvate kinase—are decreased (see Figure 41-3).

Fructose 2,6-bisphosphate is a mediator of glucagon action

The enzyme pair, phosphofructokinase/fructose 1,6-diphosphatase, determines the flow between fructose 6-phosphate and fructose 1,6-diphosphate (see Figure 41-2). Thus this enzyme pair determines the relative rates of gluconeogenesis and glycolysis. The activities of these two enzymes in turn are reciprocally regulated by the hepatic level of another metabolite, **fructose 2,6-bisphosphate.** GLUCAGON DECREASES THE CONCENTRATION OF FRUCTOSE 2,6-BISPHOSPHATE, an action that favors the flow

from fructose 1,6-diphosphate to fructose 6-phosphate, AND THEREBY STIMULATES GLUCONEOGENESIS. Insulin has the opposite effect, probably by inhibiting the action of glucagon.

The importance of glucagon is shown by the sharp decline in hepatic glucose output that occurs when glucagon secretion is inhibited. Conversely, increasing glucagon concentrations rapidly raise the plasma glucose level. This occurs even in the presence of modestly elevated insulin levels. However, after an initial increase, hepatic glucose production wanes during continuous glucagon administration, probably because rising intracellular glucose levels within the liver feed back to autoregulate glucose synthesis. In addition, insulin release is stimulated by both glucose and glucagon. If glucagon is given in a more physiological fluctuating pattern, however, each increment in the hormone increases hepatic glucose output.

> In type 1 diabetes, the loss of α-cell responsiveness to a drop in the plasma glucose level (i.e., functional glucagon deficiency) often develops. Patients with such a condition become increasingly vulnerable to the risk of severe hypoglycemia if too large a dose of insulin is administered or if a meal is missed. If hypoglycemia severe enough to impair consciousness occurs, glucagon can be injected to raise plasma glucose levels and restore function of the central nervous system.

Glucagon is a ketogenic hormone

Another key intrahepatic action of glucagon is to direct incoming free fatty acids toward β-oxidation and away from triglyceride synthesis. The mechanism involves the intermediate malonyl CoA, which is an inhibitor of the transfer of free fatty acid into the mitochondria. Glucagon suppresses the synthesis of malonyl CoA by inhibiting the enzyme acetyl-CoA carboxylase. The lower levels of malonyl

CoA then allow a greater influx of free fatty acids into the mitochondria for conversion to ketoacids.

> In diabetic ketoacidosis (see previous section), high plasma glucagon levels provide important contributions to the overproduction of the ketoacids. The suppression of glucagon secretion by insulin administration helps restore normal ketoacid levels and pH.

Glucagon actions on adipose tissue or muscle are rather insignificant unless insulin is virtually absent. Peripheral glucose use is largely unaffected by glucagon. However, glucagon can activate hormone-sensitive adipose tissue lipase and thereby increase lipolysis, the delivery of free fatty acids to the liver, and ketogenesis. Another action of glucagon, opposite to that of insulin, is to inhibit renal tubular sodium reabsorption and thus to cause natriuresis.

Glucagon acts through a plasma membrane G protein that stimulates the production of adenylyl cyclase and cyclic AMP

The molecular mechanism of glucagon action begins with hormone binding to a plasma membrane receptor in the liver. The glucagon receptor complex causes a rapid increase in intracellular cyclic AMP (see Figure 5-3). This is followed by a specific enzymatic cascade. Protein kinase A activity increases and converts inactive phosphorylase kinase to active phosphorylase kinase. The latter then converts inactive phosphorylase to active phosphorylase, and glycogenolysis results. Other enzymes in glucose metabolism, whose functional state depends on the addition or removal of covalently bound phosphate, are likewise regulated by glucagon.

Insulin/Glucagon Ratio

Substrate fluxes are very sensitive to the relative availability of insulin and glucagon

The usual molar ratio of insulin to glucagon in plasma is about 2.0. Under circumstances that require the mobilization and increased use of endogenous substrates, the insulin/glucagon ratio drops to 0.5 or less. This occurs in fasting, in prolonged exercise (see Chapter 41), and in the neonatal period when the infant is abruptly cut off from maternal fuel supplies but is not yet able to efficiently assimilate exogenous fuel. The ratio usually drops because of both decreased insulin secretion and increased glucagon secretion. Conversely, when substrate storage is advantageous, such as after a pure carbohydrate load or a mixed meal, this ratio rises to 10 or more, mainly because of increased insulin secretion.

SUMMARY

- The pancreatic islets contain insulin-secreting β-cells and glucagon-secreting α-cells. The microarchitecture and circulation permit paracrine and neurocrine functioning as well as direct cell-to-cell communication.
- Insulin is a major glucoregulatory, antilipolytic, antiketogenic, and anabolic hormone. It consists of two straight-chain peptides held together by disulfide bonds.
- Insulin secretion is stimulated by glucose, protein, gastrointestinal peptides, and cholinergic and β-adrenergic stimuli. Its release is inhibited by α-adrenergic stimuli and by circumstances that require fuel mobilization, such as fasting and exercise.
- Insulin promotes fuel storage. It inhibits adipose tissue lipolysis, ketogenesis, hepatic glycogenolysis, gluconeogenesis, glucose release, and muscle proteolysis. It stimulates muscle glucose uptake and storage as glycogen, and it stimulates protein synthesis.
- Insulin acts through a plasma membrane receptor with tyrosine kinase activity. This leads to modulation of the activities of the enzymes involved in glucose and fatty acid metabolism. Insulin also affects gene expression of numerous enzymes and proteins.
- Insulin decreases plasma levels of glucose, free fatty acids, ketoacids, and branch-chain amino acids. Insulin deficiency leads to hyperglycemia, loss of lean body and adipose tissue mass, growth retardation, and ultimately to metabolic ketoacidosis.
- Glucagon is a single-chain peptide released in response to hypoglycemia and to amino acids. Glucagon secretion increases during prolonged fasting and exercise.
- Glucagon promotes the mobilization of glucose by stimulating hepatic glycogenolysis and gluconeogenesis. It also increases fatty acid oxidation and ketogenesis. Cyclic AMP is the second messenger for glucagon, and the modification of enzyme activities by phosphorylation is the main mechanism of action. Glucagon increases the plasma levels of glucose, free fatty acids, and ketoacids, but it decreases amino acid levels.
- The insulin/glucagon ratio controls the relative rates of glycolysis and gluconeogenesis by altering hepatic fructose 2,6-bisphosphate levels. The two hormones have antagonistic effects at numerous steps in hepatic glucose and fatty acid metabolism.

BIBLIOGRAPHY

Cheatham B, Kahr CR: Insulin action and the insulin signaling network, *Endocr Rev* 16:117, 1995.
Cook DL, Taborsky GJ: β-Cell function and insulin secretion. In Rifkin H, Porte D, eds: *Diabetes mellitus,* ed 5, New York, 1997, Elsevier Scientific.

Fehmann H-C, Göke R, Göke B: Cell and molecular biology of the incretin hormones glucagon-like peptide-I and glucose-dependent insulin releasing polypeptide, *Endocr Rev* 16:390, 1995.

Flakoll P, Carlson MG, Cherrington A: Physiologic action of insulin. In LeRoith D, Taylor SI, Olefsky JM, eds: *Diabetes mellitus,* Philadelphia, 1996, Lippincott-Raven.

Kahn SE: Regulation of β-cell function in vivo, *Diabetes Metab Rev* 4:372, 1996.

Kimball SR, Vary TC, Jefferson LS: Regulation of protein synthesis by insulin, *Annu Rev Physiol* 56:321, 1994.

Matschinsky FM, Sweet IR: Annotated questions and answers about glucose metabolism and insulin secretion of β-cells, *Diabetes Metab Rev* 4:130, 1996.

O'Brien RM, Granner DK: Insulin action: gene regulation. In LeRoith D, Taylor SI, Olefsky JM, eds: *Diabetes mellitus,* Philadelphia, 1996, Lippincott-Raven.

Philippe J: Structure and pancreatic expression of the insulin and glucagon genes, *Endocr Rev* 12:252, 1991.

Polonsky KS, O'Meara NM: Secretion and metabolism of insulin, proinsulin and C peptide. In DeGroot LJ, ed: *Endocrinology,* ed 3, Philadelphia, 1995, WB Saunders.

Polonsky KS, Given BD, Van Cauter E: Twenty-four-hour profiles and pulsatile patterns of insulin secretion in normal and obese subjects, *J Clin Invest* 81:442, 1988.

Saad MF et al: Physiological insulinemia acutely modulates plasma leptin, *Diabetes* 47:544, 1998.

Schwartz MW et al: Insulin in the brain: a hormonal regulator of energy balance, *Endocr Rev* 13:387, 1992.

Steiner DF et al: Chemistry and biosynthesis of the islet hormones: insulin, islet amyloid polypeptide (amylin), glucagon, somatostatin and pancreatic polypeptide. In DeGroot LJ, ed: *Endocrinology,* ed 3, Philadelphia, 1995, WB Saunders.

Unger RH, Orci L: Glucagon. In Rifkin H, Porte D, eds: *Diabetes mellitus,* ed 5, New York, 1997, Elsevier Scientific.

Weir GC, Bonner-Weir S: Islets of Langerhans: the puzzle of intraislet interactions and their relevance to diabetes, *J Clin Invest* 85:983, 1990.

▷ CASE STUDIES

Case 42-1

A 25-year-old woman with type 1 diabetes comes to the emergency department complaining of thirst, frequent urination, and weakness. She feels "lightheaded" when she stands. Because of nausea and vomiting after a meal in a restaurant the previous day, she stopped eating and taking her insulin. On examination, she is dehydrated and hypotensive. Her breathing is rapid and deep.

1. Which of the following is likely to be lower than normal?
    A. Urinary urea levels
    B. Plasma levels of glucagon
    C. Plasma levels of free fatty acids
    D. Blood partial pressure of carbon dioxide
    E. Plasma acetoacetate levels

2. Which of the following will increase after insulin administration?
    A. Plasma triglyceride levels
    B. Plasma potassium levels
    C. Lipoprotein lipase activity
    D. Adipose tissue lipase activity
    E. Plasma phosphate levels

Case 42-2

A 40-year-old woman wins the Boston Marathon in record time.

1. Which of the following describes her hormone balance as she crosses the finish line?
    A. Insulin high, glucagon high
    B. Insulin high, glucagon low
    C. Insulin low, glucagon low
    D. Insulin low, glucagon high
    E. Insulin equal to glucagon

2. Which of the following molecules is decreased in concentration or activity in her liver?
    A. Fructose 6-phosphate
    B. Phosphoenolpyruvate carboxykinase
    C. Fructose 2,6-disphosphate
    D. Glucose 6-phosphatase
    E. Phosphorylase

CHAPTER 43

Endocrine Regulation of the Metabolism of Calcium and Phosphate

OBJECTIVES

- Explain the functions of calcium and phosphate in human biology.
- Describe the dynamic role of bone in calcium and phosphate metabolism.
- Describe the sources of vitamin D and its actions on calcium metabolism.
- Define the pattern and regulation of parathyroid hormone synthesis and secretion.
- Explain parathyroid hormone's actions on the kidneys, bones, and gastrointestinal tract.
- Evaluate the potential roles for parathyroid-related protein and calcitonin in calcium metabolism.

Calcium and phosphate homeostasis is essential for health and life. The physiological functioning of all other systems described elsewhere in this textbook depends on calcium and phosphate availability. A complex system acts to maintain normal body contents and extracellular fluid levels of these minerals in the face of environmental (e.g., diet) and internal (e.g., pregnancy) changes. The key elements in the regulatory system are **vitamin D** and **parathyroid hormone (PTH),** with subsidiary participation by **calcitonin (CT)** and other hormones. THE INTESTINAL TRACT, KIDNEYS, SKELETON, SKIN, AND LIVER ARE ALL INVOLVED IN THE HOMEOSTATIC REGULATION OF CALCIUM AND PHOSPHATE METABOLISM.

Calcium and Phosphate Turnover

Calcium

Intracellular free calcium concentration is maintained by the extracellular calcium concentration and intracellular bound calcium stores

The calcium ion (Ca^{++}) is of fundamental importance to all biological systems. Calcium, usually complexed to calmodulin (see Chapter 40), participates in numerous important enzymatic reactions. This ion is a vital component in the mechanisms of hormone secretion and hormone action. CALCIUM IS INTIMATELY INVOLVED IN NEUROTRANSMISSION, MUSCLE CONTRACTION, MITOSIS AND CELL DIVISION, FERTILIZATION, AND BLOOD CLOTTING. IT IS THE MAJOR CATION IN THE CRYSTALLINE STRUCTURE OF BONE AND TEETH. For these reasons, it is vital that cells be bathed with fluid in which the calcium concentration is kept within narrow limits.

Calcium metabolism may be viewed as having two parts: an intracellular microcomponent and an extracellular macrocomponent. Each is regulated differently and somewhat independently. The crucial intracellular calcium functions are carried out at an average basal cytosolic free calcium concentration of 10^{-7} M (range 5×10^{-8} to 3×10^{-7} M). In contrast, the free calcium concentration in extracellular fluid is approximately 10^{-3} M, or 10,000-fold higher. This large extracellular/intracellular gradient is maintained by a low permeability of the plasma cell membrane to Ca^{++} and by the regulated activities of a Ca^{++}-ATPase pump and a Ca^{++}/Na^{+} exchange system (see Chapters 1, 12, 17, and 18). Within the cell a much larger store of Ca^{++} is bound to various proteins and membranes, to the endoplasmic reticulum, and within the mitochondria. If it were in solution, this Ca^{++} content would be equivalent to an intracellular concentration of 10^{-2} M.

The cytosolic free Ca^{++} concentration can be altered as needed, both by regulating influx from outside the cell and by mobilizing intracellular stores. When Ca^{++} is required to function as a second messenger, the free Ca^{++} concentration can rise from 10^{-7} M to as high as 10^{-5} M. In absolute terms, however, this represents the movement of only small amounts of extra Ca^{++} into the cytoplasmic fluid. Such changes are transient (seconds to minutes). The excess cytosolic Ca^{++} is either rapidly extruded from the cell or returned to the intracellular reservoirs. The influx and efflux are so finely balanced that Ca^{++} can serve as an internal cell signal with a large dynamic range of gain and sensitivity.

Extracellular calcium levels are made up of free, complexed, and protein-bound fractions

The concentration of calcium in the extracellular fluid and plasma normally fluctuates little. This helps maintain intracellular calcium at a proper level. When concentrations of calcium in plasma and extracellular fluid are either above or below the normal range, intracellular function can be widely and severely affected. Abnormalities in neurotransmission and in the growth and renewal of the skeleton are prominent examples.

The normal range of total calcium concentration in plasma is 8.6 to 10.6 mg/dl, or 2.15 to 2.65×10^{-3} M. Because Ca^{++} is a divalent ion, this is equivalent to 4.3 to 5.3 mEq/L. Individual day-to-day variation is less than 10%. Approximately 50% of total plasma calcium is in the ionized form, Ca^{++}, which is biologically active; 40% is bound to proteins, mainly albumin; and 10% is complexed in nonionic but ultrafiltrable forms, such as calcium bicarbonate. The total plasma calcium concentration rises or falls with plasma albumin levels, but this has no biological consequence as long as the Ca^{++} concentration remains in the normal range. The equilibrium between ionized and protein-bound calcium depends on the blood pH. Alkalosis increases the protein-bound and decreases the Ca^{++} concentration, whereas acidosis has the opposite effect.

> When the calcium concentration drops below normal, neuromuscular irritability develops. This is manifested by numbness and paresthesias ("pins and needles" sensation) and by tetanic contractions of muscles in the hands and feet (**carpopedal spasm**) and most dangerously, in the larynx. The latter can cause **airway obstruction. Epileptic seizures** may also occur. When the calcium concentration is excessive, depressed neurotransmission can cause impaired mentation or consciousness, muscle weakness, and decreased gastrointestinal motility. Individuals who hyperventilate to the point of severe respiratory alkalosis can lower the Ca^{++} level enough (without changing the total concentration) to produce the sensory symptoms described.

Calcium balance reflects dietary intake, gastrointestinal absorption, and renal excretion

The normal turnover of calcium in the body is complex (see Figure 38-6). Daily dietary calcium intake may range from 200 to 2000 mg. The percentage of dietary calcium absorbed from the gut is inversely related to the calcium intake in a curvilinear manner. Thus in the face of dietary calcium deprivation, one important mechanism for maintaining a normal plasma calcium concentration and body calcium stores is an adaptive increase in the percentage of ingested calcium that is absorbed. At a daily intake of 1000 mg, about 35% is absorbed. In a steady state, the same amount of calcium, 350 mg, is ex-

creted. Approximately 150 mg is secreted into intestinal juices and excreted in stools, along with the unabsorbed fraction from the diet. The remaining 200 mg is excreted in the urine. Although the kidney filters about 10,000 mg of non-protein-bound Ca^{++} per day, approximately 98% is reabsorbed by the renal tubules. Therefore any alteration in renal tubular Ca^{++} transport provides a very sensitive means for maintaining calcium balance.

> These control mechanisms are clinically important when calcium conservation is needed, such as in aged people, whose calcium intakes typically fall, causing an increase in the danger of **osteoporosis.** These mechanisms protect the mother from hypocalcemia and bone loss during pregnancy, when calcium stores are drained by the fetus. In contrast, these mechanisms act to protect against lethal **hypercalcemia** (e.g., that can occur when metastatic cancer causes the rapid destruction of bone).

Bone formation and resorption help maintain normal plasma levels of calcium

The extracellular pool of calcium is only 1000 mg. The largest store of calcium, about 1.2 kg, is in the skeleton. Of this, 4000 mg is available for rapid buffering of plasma calcium without dissolution of bone. Nonetheless, bone is a dynamic tissue that undergoes daily structural turnover. In this process, approximately 500 mg of calcium is extracted from the extracellular pool as new bone is formed, and a like amount is returned to this pool as old bone is broken down.

Phosphate

The phosphate ion is of critical importance to all biological systems and is the major intracellular anion

The phosphate ion ($PO_4^{\equiv}$) is a component of many intermediates in glucose metabolism. It is part of the structure of all high-energy transfer compounds such as ATP, cofactors such as nicotinic acid dinucleotide, and lipids such as phosphatidylcholine. Phosphate functions as a covalent modifier of the activity of numerous enzymes. PHOSPHATE IS ALSO AN INTEGRAL PART OF THE CRYSTALLINE STRUCTURE OF BONE. The normal concentration of phosphate in the plasma is 2.4 to 4.5 mg/dl, or 0.81 to 1.45×10^{-3} M. Because the valence of phosphate changes with the pH, it is less useful to express normal concentrations in milliequivalents per liter.

Phosphate balance reflects dietary intake, gastrointestinal absorption, and renal excretion

The daily turnover of phosphate is as complex as that of calcium (see Figure 38-9). In contrast to calcium, the percentage of phosphate absorbed from the diet is relatively constant, and thus the net absorption of phosphate from the gut is more linearly related to intake. Therefore urinary excretion provides the major mechanism for regulating phosphate balance (see Chapter 38). The daily filtered load is approximately 7000 mg, but renal tubular reabsorption can vary from 70% to 100% to compensate for fluctuations in dietary intake. Large stores of phosphate (about 100,000 mg) in the soft tissue, as in muscle, are a source for rapid regulation of the plasma concentration. Approximately 200 to 250 mg of phosphate enters and leaves the extracellular fluid daily in the course of bone turnover. Severe depletion of phosphate can result in serious cardiac and skeletal muscle dysfunction, hemolysis, and abnormal bone growth.

Bone Turnover

Bone formation and resorption are normally coupled to each other in a steady state

Bone is a major and dynamic reservoir for calcium and phosphate (see Figures 38-6 and 38-9). Therefore it is essential that the clinician understand the aspects of bone structure and function pertinent to the regulation of calcium and phosphate metabolism. Bone is broadly divided into two types: cortical and trabecular. **Cortical,** or **compact bone,** represents 80% of the total mass and is typified by the thick shafts of the appendicular skeleton (arms and legs). **Trabecular,** or **spongy bone,** constitutes 20%; it makes up most of the axial skeleton (vertebrae, skull, ribs, pelvis) and bridges the centers of the long bones. Trabecular bone has a fivefold greater surface area than cortical bone, making it more important in the regulation of calcium metabolism even though it has a lesser mass.

Bone formation occurs on the outer surface of cortical bone, whereas bone resorption occurs on its inner surface. Both formation and resorption also take place in specialized nutrient canals within cortical bone and on the surfaces of trabecular bone. Throughout life, the processes of bone formation and resorption are tightly regulated. During growth phases, formation exceeds resorption, and the skeletal mass increases. Linear growth occurs between the heads and the shafts of long bones in specialized areas known as **epiphyseal growth plates.** These close off at the end of puberty, when the adult height is reached. Bone width increases by adding bone to the outer surfaces.

Bone mass varies with stages of life

Total bone mass reaches a peak between ages 20 and 30 years. Thereafter, equal rates of formation and resorption prevail until age 40 to 50 years, at which time resorption begins to exceed formation and the total bone mass slowly decreases. The continual process of bone turnover in the adult, known as **remodeling,** involves 10% of the total bone mass per year.

Bone contains several types of cells with different functions

Three major cell types exist in bone: **osteoblasts, osteocytes,** and **osteoclasts** (Figure 43-1). The first two arise from primitive mesenchymal cells, called **osteoprogenitor cells,** within the investing connective tissue. Various bone proteins, known as **skeletal growth factors,** attract osteoprogenitor cells, direct their differentiation into osteoblasts, and stimulate their further growth. Osteoclasts arise from the same precursors as circulating monocytes and tissue macrophages. Together the three major cell types form the **osteon,** or bone modeling unit.

> Women have a smaller bone mass than men, and during the perimenopausal period, they lose bone rapidly as ovarian function declines. This is caused by estrogen deficiency, but lifelong calcium intakes that are only marginally adequate also contribute. The resultant **osteoporosis** leads to fractures of the spine and wrist. Later in life, senescent osteoporosis leads to hip fractures in both genders.

Bone formation

Bone formation is carried out by active osteoblasts, which synthesize and secrete type 1 collagen. The collagen fibrils line up in regular arrays, creating an organic matrix known as **osteoid,** within which calcium phosphate is deposited in amorphous masses. The slow addition of hydroxide and bicarbonate ions to the mineral phase produces mature

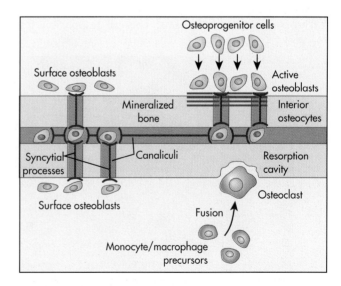

Figure 43-1 Relationship between bone cells and bone remodeling. Note that the canaliculi provide channels through which calcium and phosphate can be transferred from the interior to the exterior of bone. These minerals may be used for new bone formation or may be transported into the circulation. *(Redrawn from Avioli LV et al. In Bondy PK, Rosenberg LE: Metabolic control and disease, Philadelphia, 1980, WB Saunders.)*

hydroxyapatite crystals, which have a molar calcium-phosphate ratio of 1.7. As this completely mineralized bone accumulates and surrounds the osteoblast, that cell loses its synthetic activity and becomes an interior osteocyte (Figure 43-1). Osteoblastic activity therefore is observed only on the surfaces of bone, along which resting cells wait to be activated.

THE MINERALIZATION PROCESS CRITICALLY REQUIRES NORMAL PLASMA CONCENTRATIONS OF CALCIUM AND PHOSPHATE. The enzyme **alkaline phosphatase** and other proteins from the osteoblast also participate. **Osteocalcin** is a major bone protein with a strong affinity for calcium and for uncrystallized hydroxyapatite. Alkaline phosphatase and osteocalcin circulate in plasma, and their concentrations correlate well with quantitative histological assessments of osteoblastic activity.

Osteolysis

Within each **osteon,** or bone unit, minute fluid-containing channels called **canaliculi** traverse the mineralized bone; through these channels the interior osteocytes remain connected with surface cells via syncytial cell processes (Figure 43-1). This arrangement provides an enormous surface area for the transfer within minutes of calcium from the interior to the exterior of the osteons and from there to the extracellular fluid. This transfer process, carried out by the osteocytes, is known as **osteocytic osteolysis.** It does not significantly decrease mature bone mass but simply removes calcium from the surface crystal layer.

Bone resorption

THE PROCESS OF BONE RESORPTION DOES NOT MERELY EXTRACT CALCIUM; IT DESTROYS THE ENTIRE ORGANIC MATRIX AS WELL, THEREBY DIMINISHING BONE MASS. The cell responsible for

bone resorption is the osteoclast, which is a giant multinucleated cell formed by the fusion of several precursors (Figure 43-1). The osteoclast contains large numbers of mitochondria and lysosomes. It attaches to the surface of the osteon and creates at this point a ruffled border by infolding its plasma membrane. Within this enclosed zone the process of dissolution is carried out by collagenase and other enzymes as well as protons secreted by the osteoclast. During this process, the osteoclast literally tunnels its way into the mineralized bone. Calcium, phosphate, magnesium, **pyridinolines** and **pyridiniums** (fluorescent products of collagen cross-linkages), *N*-**telopeptides** of collagen, and the constituent amino acids (including hydroxyproline and hydroxylysine, which are unique to collagen) are all released into the extracellular fluid. Urine levels of the organic products reflect the bone resorption rate.

In the bone remodeling process, resorption precedes and initiates formation

As already emphasized, the resorption and formation of bone are closely coordinated locally. In a complex sequence, resting osteoblasts are stimulated to recruit and activate osteoclasts, probably via paracrine signaling. The resultant resorption cavity created by the osteoclast then becomes the site of subsequent osteoblastic activity, which fills in the recently formed cavity with new bone. Thus bone resorption precedes and subsequently triggers replacement bone formation.

The recruitment of osteoblasts and osteoclasts from precursors and the activity of each cell type are regulated by various local factors, including lymphokines, tissue growth and transforming factors, prostaglandins, and an array of hormones. GENERALLY, WHETHER THE PRIMARY EFFECT OF A HORMONE IS ON THE FORMATION OR THE RESORPTION OF BONE, THE PHENOMENON OF COUPLING SECOND-

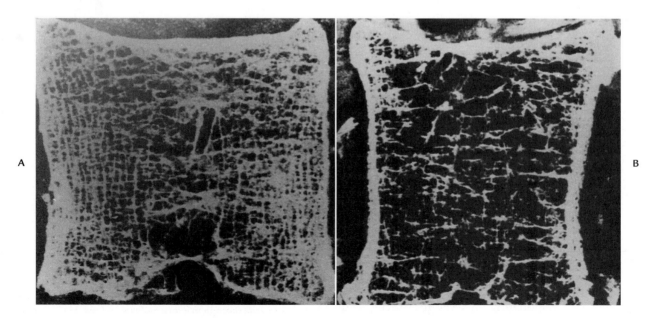

Figure 43-2 A, Radiograph of a normal vertebra from a 40-year-old woman. **B,** Radiograph of a vertebra from a 92-year-old woman. Note the marked loss of trabecular bone with relatively less loss of cortical bone. *(From Atkinson P: Calcif Tissue Res 1:24, 1967.)*

ARILY ALTERS THE OTHER PROCESS IN THE SAME DIRECTION. Therefore the net effect of a hormone excess or deficiency partly depends on the degree to which the coupling phenomenon defends the total bone mass. As a result of the aging process, the balance shifts toward resorption, and bone mass declines (Figure 43-2).

Vitamin D

Vitamin D, through its active metabolites, is a major regulator of calcium and phosphate metabolism. VITAMIN D ACTS TO SUSTAIN NORMAL PLASMA CONCENTRATIONS OF CALCIUM AND PHOSPHATE BY INCREASING THEIR INFLOW FROM THE INTESTINAL TRACT, AND IT ALSO IS REQUIRED FOR NORMAL BONE FORMATION. It is a hormone in the sense that it is synthesized in the body, although not by an endocrine gland; after further processing, it is transported through the circulation to act on target cells. It is also a vitamin in the sense that when it cannot be synthesized in sufficient quantities, it must be ingested for health to be maintained.

Vitamin D is synthesized in the skin and ingested largely from animal sources

The sterol structure of the synthesized form of vitamin D (D_3) is shown in Figure 43-3. The ingested form (D_2), which is prepared by irradiating plant or milk ergosterol, differs only slightly. Vitamins D_3 and D_2 are essentially prohormones that undergo metabolic conversion to molecules with identical qualitative and quantitative actions. Henceforth, the term **vitamin D** will refer to both.

The minimum daily requirement of vitamin D is approximately 2.5 µg (100 units). Endogenously, it is synthesized in the skin from the precursor, **7-dehydrocholesterol,** by ultraviolet (UV) irradiation of specific frequencies. Exogenously, the fat-soluble vitamin D is available in fish, liver, and milk, and it is absorbed from the gut, like fats. Vitamin D is stored in the body in amounts normally sufficient for several months.

Vitamin D is activated by successive hydroxylations

Once vitamin D enters the circulation from the skin or gut, it is concentrated in the liver. There, it is hydroxylated to 25-hydroxyvitamin D (25-OH-D). This molecule is transported to the kidney, where it undergoes alternative fates (Figure 43-4). Hydroxylation in the 1 position produces the metabolite 1,25-dihydroxyvitamin D (1,25-$(OH)_2$-D), which unquestionably expresses most if not all of the biological activity of vitamin D. Alternatively, 25-OH-D may be hydroxylated in the 24 position. 24,25-Dihydroxyvitamin D (24,25-$(OH)_2$-D) is only one twentieth as potent as 1,25-$(OH)_2$-D, and it mainly serves to dispose of excess vitamin D.

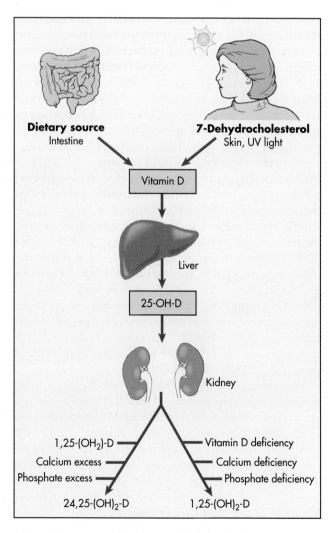

Figure 43-4 Vitamin D metabolism. Whether synthesized in the skin or absorbed from the diet, vitamin D undergoes hydroxylation of position 25 in the liver. In the kidney, it is further hydroxylated in position 1 when more biological activity is required or in position 24 when less biological activity is required.

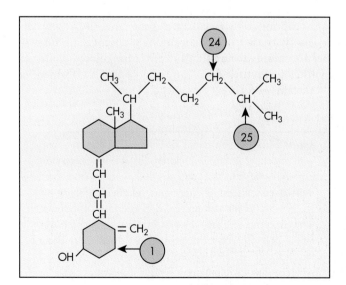

Figure 43-3 Structure of vitamin D. Positions 1, 24, and 25 are important sites of hydroxylation that affect biological activity.

Vitamin D deficiency can occur in several ways. If individuals who live in sunny climates (e.g., India) and are dependent on vitamin D synthesis move to cloudy countries (e.g., England), they may become deficient in vitamin D if they do not alter their dietary habits or ingest supplementary vitamin D. In urban centers overcast with smog, black infants who are breast-fed are also at risk because less effective UV radiation reaches sites of vitamin D synthesis. When a subject's exposure to sunlight is inadequate, deficiency also results from gastrointestinal diseases that cause malabsorption of fats, such as pancreatic insufficiency. Liver disease leads to diminished rates of 25-hydroxylation and hence to deficient vitamin D action. A common cause of deficient vitamin D action is kidney failure, in which the production of the most active metabolite, 1,25-(OH)$_2$-D, is almost totally lost.

The activation of vitamin D occurs in response to calcium or phosphate deficiency

Feedback control of vitamin D activation occurs through regulation of the renal tubule mitochondrial 1-hydroxylase and 24-hydroxylase enzyme activities (Figure 43-4). 25-OH-D is preferentially directed toward the active metabolite, 1,25-(OH)$_2$-D, whenever calcium, phosphate, or vitamin D itself is lacking. Calcium deprivation leads to a compensatory secretion of **PTH.** This hormone then stimulates 1-hydroxylation. A lowering of plasma phosphate and renal phosphate content also augments 1-hydroxylase activity. In addition, because 1,25-(OH)$_2$-D is a feedback inhibitor of its own synthesis, in vitamin D deficiency there is lack of inhibition and compensatory enhancement of 1-hydroxylase activity. In contrast, 24-hydroxylase activity is stimulated by normal to elevated calcium or phosphate concentrations and by 1,25-(OH)$_2$-D. The net result of this regulation is that the supply of active 1,25-(OH)$_2$-D is increased (and that of inactive 24,25-(OH)$_2$-D is decreased) whenever homeostasis requires increasing calcium and phosphate intake from dietary sources or skeletal stores. If an excess of 1,25-(OH)$_2$-D develops, it too can be 24-hydroxylated to 1,24,25-trihydroxyvitamin D (1,24,25-(OH)$_3$-D) and thereby virtually inactivated.

Vitamin D, 25-OH-D, and 1,25-(OH)$_2$-D circulate bound to a protein carrier. 1,25-(OH)$_2$-D has by far the lowest concentration (0.03 μg/L) and the shortest half-life of the three (6 hours). However, regulation is powerful enough to maintain the appropriate concentration of 1,25-(OH)$_2$-D even when the concentrations of its precursors are quite reduced.

Vitamin D acts on target tissues by modulating gene expression

The active form of vitamin D (1,25-(OH)$_2$-D) acts through the general mechanism outlined for steroid hormones (see Chapter 40). After binding to a cytosolic receptor, the hormone receptor complex enters the nucleus, where it stimulates or represses the transcription of messenger RNA for several products. One is **calbindin,** a calcium-binding protein found in cells of the intestinal mucosa, bone, kidney, and parathyroid glands. Calbindin has significant homology with calmodulin and a high affinity for calcium. Calbindin is not essential for vitamin D stimulation of calcium transport because this process precedes the appearance of the protein in intestinal cells. However, calbindin probably protects the cells from the effect of high cytoplasmic concentrations of calcium during enhanced transport.

Vitamin D increases calcium absorption from the gut and calcium availability for bone mineralization

The major action of 1,25-(OH)$_2$-D is to stimulate the absorption of calcium from the intestinal lumen against a concentration gradient (see Chapter 34). 1,25-(OH)$_2$-D localizes in the nuclei of intestinal villus and crypt cells, where it acts on the brush border. It probably stimulates the production of a plasma membrane calcium transporter protein. 1,25-(OH)$_2$-D is responsible for the adaptation whereby the intestinal absorption of calcium increases in response to decreases in dietary intake, as previously described. 1,25-(OH)$_2$-D also augments the active absorption of phosphate across the intestinal cell membrane. In addition, 1,25-(OH)$_2$-D stimulates bone resorption by interacting with its receptor in **osteoblasts,** thereby driving the resorptive action of the osteoclast by an osteoblast-derived factor. This effect of 1,25-(OH)$_2$-D is physiologically important in sensitizing the bone to the resorptive effects of PTH.

The normal mineralization of newly formed osteoid along a regular advancing front is critically dependent on vitamin D. The major mechanism for this action is augmentation of the supply of calcium and phosphate. However, in osteoblasts, 1,25-(OH)$_2$-D represses transcription of the collagen gene and decreases collagen synthesis. In the hormone's absence, unmineralized osteoid accumulates from unregulated collagen synthesis (Figure 43-5), and the bone so formed is weakened.

The skeletal manifestations of vitamin D deficiency vary with the stage of life. In children, the growth centers are preferentially affected, and the failure of normal bone mineralization leads to abnormal epiphyses (Figure 43-5), bowing of the extremities, and collapse of the chest wall—a disease called **rickets.** In adults, bone pain, vertebral collapse, and fractures along stress lines occur. Plasma calcium and phosphate levels are decreased, whereas the alkaline phosphatase concentration is increased. Therapy with vitamin D or the appropriate metabolite is curative.

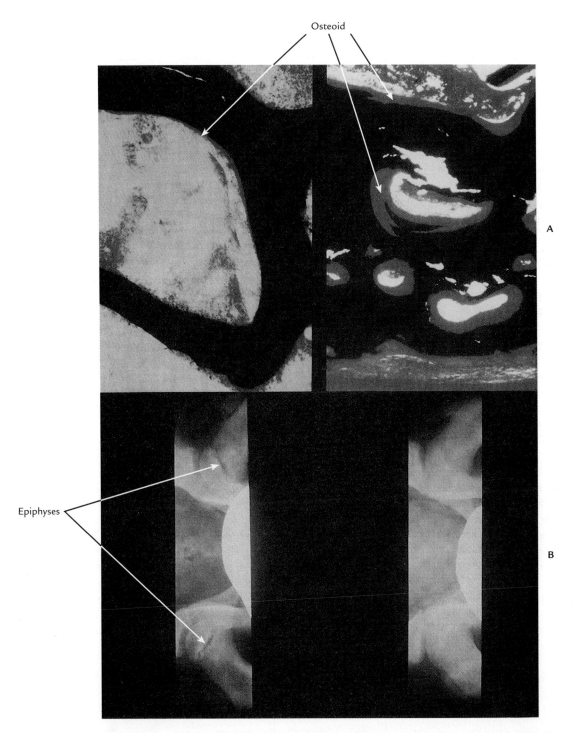

Figure 43-5 A, Histological section. *Left,* Normal trabecular bone showing a very low ratio of unmineralized osteoid to mineralized bone. *Right,* Trabecular bone from an individual with vitamin D deficiency, showing a much higher proportion of osteoid to mineralized bone (i.e., excess osteoid). **B,** X-ray film of a child's hip. *Left,* Hip with deficient vitamin D action, showing a widened, irregular epiphysis. *Right,* Same hip after effective treatment with vitamin D mineralized the area normally.

Skeletal muscle is another target tissue for vitamin D. It increases calcium transport and uptake by the sarcoplasmic reticulum as well as the cellular uptake of phosphate. A deficiency of vitamin D leads to muscle weakness, electrophysiological evidence of abnormal contraction and relaxation, and altered cytoarchitecture.

The skin cells (keratinocytes) that synthesize vitamin D also 1-hydroxylate 25-(OH)-D. This locally produced 1,25-(OH)$_2$-D has paracrine effects that regulate the orderly formation of the outer cornified layer of the epidermis.

A role for vitamin D in immunomodulation has also emerged. Monocytes and macrophages can also synthesize 1,25-(OH)$_2$-D from 25-OH-D. The hormone can decrease the production of numerous lymphokines and the proliferation of lymphocytes. It is likely that these phenomena are part of the autocrine or paracrine regulation of immunoactivity engendered by tissue injury or invasion.

> In diseases characterized by the formation of granulomas (i.e., **sarcoidosis** or **tuberculosis**) the component macrophages may synthesize excessive amounts of 1,25-(OH)$_2$-D. This can result in hypercalcemia and hypercalciuria.

Parathyroid Gland Function

The four parathyroid glands are major regulators of plasma calcium and phosphate concentrations and flux. These four glands develop from branchial pouches at 5 to 14 weeks of fetal life. They descend to lie just posterior to the thyroid gland in the neck. The total weight of adult parathyroid tissue is about 130 mg.

The predominant cell of the parathyroid gland is known as the **chief cell.** These cells are present throughout life and are the source of PTH. A second and related cell type, the **oxyphil cell,** first appears at puberty and increases in number with age. Each active chief cell has a granular endoplasmic reticulum and a large, convoluted Golgi apparatus with vacuoles and vesicles. During hormone secretion, numerous granules undergo exocytosis.

THE PARAMOUNT EFFECT OF PTH IS TO SUSTAIN OR INCREASE THE PLASMA CALCIUM LEVEL. THIS IS ACCOMPLISHED BY DIRECTLY STIMULATING THE ENTRY OF CALCIUM INTO PLASMA FROM BONE AND TUBULAR URINE AND INDIRECTLY FROM THE INTESTINAL TRACT (VIA 1,25-(OH)$_2$-D). AN IMPORTANT SECOND EFFECT IS TO DECREASE OR PREVENT AN UNDUE RISE IN THE PLASMA PHOSPHATE LEVEL BY INCREASING THE EXCRETION OF PHOSPHATE INTO THE URINE.

Parathyroid hormone is synthesized from a prohormone and secreted in response to hypocalcemia

PTH is a single-chain protein (molecular weight, 9600) that contains 84 amino acids. The biological activity of the hormone resides in the N-terminus portion of the molecule within amino acids 1 to 34.

The gene for PTH directs the synthesis of **prepro-PTH.** A total of 25 amino acids are enzymatically cleaved from the N-terminal end, leaving **pro-PTH.** Pro-PTH is then transported to the Golgi apparatus, where another six amino acids are cleaved. The resulting PTH is packaged for storage in secretory granules. The degradation of PTH also occurs within the gland; therefore not all synthesized molecules reach the circulation.

THE DOMINANT REGULATOR OF PARATHYROID GLAND ACTIVITY IS THE PLASMA CALCIUM LEVEL. PTH AND CALCIUM FORM A NEGATIVE-FEEDBACK PAIR, AND THE SECRETION OF PTH IS INVERSELY RELATED TO THE PLASMA CALCIUM CONCENTRATION (Figure 43-6). Maximum secretory rates are achieved when the plasma Ca^{++} concentration falls below 3.5 mg/dl. PTH secretion increases within minutes if plasma Ca^{++} is selectively decreased by chelation, even though the plasma total calcium concentration remains unchanged. Conversely, as the Ca^{++} concentration increases to 5.5 mg/dl, PTH secretion is progressively diminished. However, secretion reaches a persistent basal rate that is not suppressible by further elevation of the ambient calcium concentration.

A plasma membrane calcium receptor regulates parathyroid hormone secretion

The regulation of PTH represents an exception to the general rule that hormone secretion by exocytosis is stimulated by calcium. A unique **calcium receptor** within the plasma membrane of the parathyroid cell responds rapidly to alterations in extracellular calcium levels. A FALL IN THE EXTRACELLULAR Ca^{++} LEVEL ACTIVATES THE RECEPTOR, WHICH VIA G PROTEINS STIMULATES ADENYLYL CYCLASE AND INHIBITS PHOSPHOLIPASE C (SEE CHAPTER 5). THE RESULTANT INCREASE IN CYCLIC AMP AND DECREASE IN CYTOPLASMIC Ca^{++} LEAD TO EXOCYTOSIS OF PTH-CONTAINING GRANULES (Figure 43-7). When the extracellular calcium level is high, the reverse sequence occurs, and PTH secretion is inhibited (Figure 43-7). The parathyroid cells respond similarly to small variations in plasma magnesium levels.

Calcium also modulates PTH turnover within the gland. Prolonged exposure to a high ambient calcium concentration lowers the rate of PTH synthesis and stimulates the intraglandular degradation of PTH. Calcium also regulates the size of the parathyroid cells. THE NET EFFECT OF CALCIUM EXCESS IS A DECREASE IN BOTH THE GLANDULAR STORES AND THE RELEASE RATES OF PTH. CONVERSELY, CALCIUM DEFICIENCY

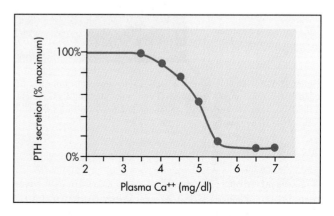

Figure 43-6 Inverse relationship between PTH secretion and plasma Ca^{++} concentration in humans. Note the maintenance of some PTH secretion even at high calcium levels. *(Redrawn from Brent GA et al: J Clin Endocrinol Metab 67:944, 1988.)*

INCREASES PTH STORES, SECRETORY RATES, AND ULTIMATELY, GLAND SIZE.

Phosphate exerts no direct effect on PTH secretion in vitro. However, via the complexing of calcium and a decreasing Ca^{++} concentration, a rise in the plasma phosphate concentration indirectly causes a transient increase in PTH secretion. 1,25-$(OH)_2$-D directly feeds back on the parathyroid gland to inhibit transcription of the PTH gene, reduce PTH secretion, and decrease the proliferation of parathyroid cells. Severe magnesium depletion also inhibits PTH synthesis and release.

PTH secretion is pulsatile; it increases at night and with aging. The plasma PTH concentration is about 30 pg/ml (3×10^{-12} M). Whereas the hormone has a short half-life, its C-terminus metabolites circulate with half-lives of many hours.

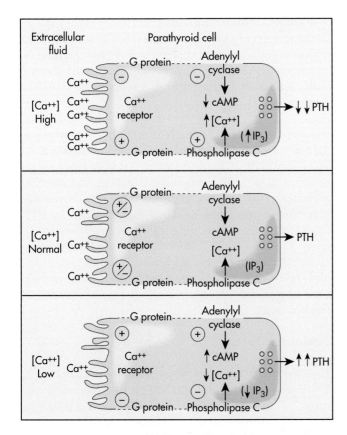

Figure 43-7 Mechanism of regulation of PTH secretion by changes in Ca^{++} concentrations ($[Ca^{++}]$) in the extracellular fluid. An increase in the calcium concentration is sensed by a plasma membrane Ca^{++} receptor in the parathyroid cell *(top)*. The activated receptor is linked to an inhibitory G protein, which inhibits adenylyl cyclase. As a result, intracellular levels of cyclic AMP *(cAMP)* fall. The activated receptor is also linked to a stimulatory G protein that stimulates phospholipase C. As a result, levels of inositol 1,4,5-trisphosphate *(IP₃)* increase and transduce a rise in the intracellular calcium concentration. Exocytosis of PTH secretory granules and PTH release are *decreased*. The opposite sequence occurs when there is a decrease in the calcium concentration in the extracellular fluid *(bottom)*; in that case, exocytosis of PTH secretory granules and PTH release are increased. +, Disinhibited or stimulated; −, inhibited or unstimulated; +/−, balanced between stimulated and inhibited.

Intracellular effects

OVERALL, PTH INCREASES PLASMA CALCIUM LEVELS AND DECREASES PLASMA PHOSPHATE LEVELS BY ACTING ON THREE MAJOR TARGET ORGANS: THE KIDNEYS, THE BONES, AND INDIRECTLY, THE GASTROINTESTINAL TRACT. Actions on all three targets ultimately increase the calcium influx into the plasma and raise its concentration (Figure 43-8). In contrast, PTH acts on the kidney to increase the exit of phosphate from plasma; this action overwhelms the effect on bone and gut, which increases phosphate entry into the plasma; therefore the plasma phosphate concentration falls (Figure 43-8).

Parathyroid hormone acts through cyclic AMP as a second messenger

PTH action is initiated by binding to a G protein–linked plasma membrane receptor. IN ALL TARGET CELLS, THE ACTIVATION OF ADENYLYL CYCLASE AND AN INCREASE IN CYCLIC AMP LEVELS FOLLOW. The second messenger then triggers a protein kinase cascade (see Chapter 5), which ultimately leads to the phosphorylation of proteins necessary for the expression of PTH action.

PTH also stimulates the uptake of calcium into the cytoplasm of its target cells. This may be mediated by increases in phosphoinositide second messengers (see Chapter 5). The initial uptake of calcium is reflected in a slight transient hypocalcemia, which immediately follows PTH administration and precedes the classic hypercalcemia. The presence of 1,25-$(OH)_2$-D is required for maximal responsiveness to PTH. A sufficient intra-

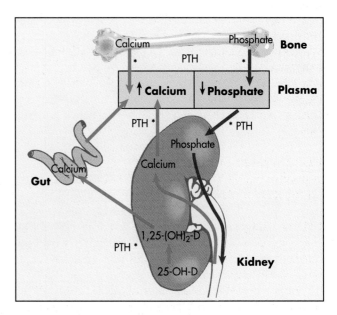

Figure 43-8 Overview of PTH actions. PTH acts directly on bone and kidney to increase calcium influx into plasma. By stimulating 1,25-$(OH)_2$-D synthesis, it also indirectly increases calcium absorption from the gut. Thus the plasma calcium level increases. In contrast, PTH inhibits the renal tubular reabsorption of phosphate, thereby increasing urinary phosphate excretion. This effect quantitatively offsets the entry of phosphate from bone and gut. Therefore the plasma phosphate level decreases.

cellular concentration of magnesium is also necessary for PTH to act maximally.

Renal effects

Parathyroid hormone stimulates calcium reabsorption and inhibits phosphate reabsorption by the renal tubules

PTH increases the reabsorption of calcium in the proximal tubule and ascending loop of Henle. Magnesium reabsorption is also increased. In contrast, PTH decreases the reabsorption of phosphate in the proximal and distal tubules (see Chapter 38). These effects are mediated by PTH's stimulation of the production of cyclic AMP at the capillary surface of the renal tubular cell. The cyclic AMP is transported to the luminal surface, where it activates protein kinases that are located in the membranes of the brush border and are involved in calcium and phosphate reabsorption. During this process, cyclic AMP is released into the tubular lumen. THEREFORE THE EARLIEST OBSERVABLE RENAL EFFECT OF PTH IN VIVO IS A DRAMATIC INCREASE IN THE URINARY EXCRETION OF CYCLIC AMP. The previously described calcium receptor also modulates calcium reabsorption by renal tubular cells.

The relationship between urinary calcium excretion and plasma calcium concentration is altered by PTH (Figure 43-9). At any given plasma calcium concentration, PTH diminishes the amount of calcium lost in the urine and thus counters hypocalcemia. Conversely, the suppression of PTH secretion by an excess calcium

load increases calcium excretion and helps prevent hypercalcemia.

The net effect of prolonged alterations in PTH secretion on urinary calcium excretion is eventually dominated by the influence of PTH on bone and gut. A continuous excess of PTH eventually elevates the plasma calcium level and with it, the load of calcium filtered by the glomerulus. Therefore the absolute amount of calcium excreted in the urine eventually increases despite the stimulation of tubular reabsorption by PTH.

In contrast, the relationship between urinary phosphate excretion and the plasma phosphate level is shifted in the opposite direction by PTH (Figure 43-9). This phosphaturic effect of PTH allows disposal of the extra phosphate released when the hormone stimulates bone resorption (see next section). Otherwise, PTH would simultaneously elevate plasma calcium and phosphate levels and thereby create the danger of precipitating calcium-phosphate complexes in tissue.

PTH also inhibits the reabsorption of sodium and bicarbonate in the proximal tubule (see Chapter 36). This action may prevent metabolic alkalosis, which could result from the release of bicarbonate during the dissolution of hydroxyapatite crystals in bone, as discussed later.

Parathyroid hormone directly stimulates the synthesis of 1,25-dihydroxyvitamin D_2 from 25-hydroxyvitamin D

PTH stimulates the synthesis of 1,25-$(OH)_2$-D by increasing cyclic AMP levels and producing a cascade that activates a key cofactor, **renoredoxin**. The decrease in plasma and renal phosphate content caused by PTH further augments this direct action on 1-hydroxylase activity. The increase in 1,25-$(OH)_2$-D stimulates calcium absorption from the gut and raises plasma calcium levels (Figure 43-8). This important indirect effect of PTH on the intestinal tract again serves the major function of the hormone.

Skeletal effects

Parathyroid hormone mobilizes calcium from bone

The major action of PTH on bone is to accelerate the removal of calcium. The initial effect of PTH is to stimulate osteocytic osteolysis, which causes a transfer of calcium from the bone canalicular fluid into the osteocyte and then out the opposite side of the cell into interstitial fluid. The replenishment of calcium in the canalicular fluid probably then occurs from the surface of partially mineralized bone.

A SECOND, MORE SLOWLY DEVELOPING EFFECT OF PTH IS TO STIMULATE THE OSTEOCLASTS TO RESORB COMPLETELY MINERALIZED BONE. In this process, both calcium and phosphate are released for transfer ultimately into the extracellular fluid; in addition, the organic bone matrix is hydrolyzed by PTH activation of collagenase and lysosomal enzymes. PTH initially increases the active resorptive ruffled border of the osteoclasts. This is followed by

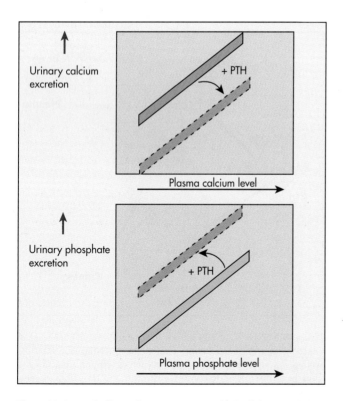

Figure 43-9 Renal effects of PTH. At any given level of plasma calcium, PTH decreases urinary calcium excretion. At any given level of plasma phosphate, PTH increases urinary phosphate excretion.

PTH stimulation of osteoclast size, number of nuclei, fusion, and proliferation from precursors. PTH also induces increases in the enzymes, acid phosphatase and carbonic anhydrase, and the accumulation of an acidic environment. The resultant lowering of bone pH contributes to the resorptive process. Because of collagen degradation, PTH increases the release of hydroxyproline and other bone collagen products into plasma and urine (see section on bone resorption).

Parathyroid hormone's effects on osteoclasts are partly mediated by osteoblasts

The dramatic effects of PTH on osteoclasts in vitro are not evident in the absence of osteoblasts. Therefore an initial action of PTH on osteoblasts may be required to stimulate local factors that secondarily recruit and activate the osteoclasts (e.g., interleukins, macrophage colony–stimulating factor). PTH receptors are present on osteoblasts as well as on osteoclasts. When exposed to the hormone, osteoblasts immediately change shape. Later, PTH inhibits the synthesis of collagen by the osteoblasts, probably at the level of transcription. The stimulation of osteoclastic bone resorption and the inhibition of osteoblastic bone formation are achieved by the elevated concentrations of hormone that result from stimulation of the parathyroid glands through hypocalcemia. Thus these actions of PTH are part of its general mission to rapidly restore the plasma calcium level to normal.

Paradoxically, PTH in lower amounts also has anabolic actions on bone. In part, increases in bone formation may reflect coupling to enhanced resorption. However, by stimulating the production of local growth factors, PTH increases the number and activity of osteoblasts. The intermittent administration of PTH to humans in small doses increases trabecular bone mass but still decreases cortical bone.

> Prolonged excess secretion of PTH occurs in **primary hyperparathyroidism,** usually because of a benign neoplasm in one parathyroid gland. The plasma calcium concentration is high (with attendant symptoms, as previously described), and the phosphate concentration is usually low. The increased renal excretion of calcium can cause kidney stones. Modest loss of cortical bone may result. In hyperparathyroidism secondary to kidney failure, both 1,25-(OH)$_2$-D and calcium concentrations decrease, and the parathyroid glands enlarge. Massive bone resorption by osteoclasts can result, with attendant pain, fractures, and deformities. Cure of hyperparathyroidism requires removal of the excess parathyroid tissue.

PTH-related protein

PTH-related peptide or protein (PTH$_{rp}$) was originally discovered as a product of human cancers that were of squamous cell origin and that were associated with hypercalcemia. However, normal skin keratinocytes, lactating mammary epithelium, placenta, and fetal parathyroid glands also synthesize PTH$_{rp}$.

The gene for PTH$_{rp}$ and the gene for PTH evolved from a common ancestor. Because of the striking homology in their N-terminus amino acids, PTH$_{rp}$ exhibits most of the actions of PTH on bone and kidney by binding to the PTH receptor. PTH$_{rp}$, however, does not stimulate renal 1-hydroxylase. Hence patients with hypercalcemia caused by PTH$_{rp}$ do not have elevated plasma 1,25-(OH)$_2$-D levels.

There is likely a normal physiological role for PTH$_{rp}$ during intrauterine life and early infancy. PTH$_{rp}$ in the placenta and in the fetus may maintain the 30% to 40% increased Ca^{++} concentration gradient that exists between fetal and maternal plasma. It may regulate calcium concentration in breast milk and calcium homeostasis early in neonatal life. PTH$_{rp}$ in skin contributes to regular cellular differentiation.

Calcitonin

Calcitonin is secreted in response to an increased plasma calcium level

CT decreases plasma calcium levels, largely by antagonizing the actions of PTH on bone. CT is secreted by a small population of neuroendocrine cells, known as **C cells,** or **parafollicular cells,** in the thyroid gland. CT is a straight-chain peptide of 32 amino acids, synthesized from a preprohormone. The hormone is packaged in granules along with N-terminus and C-terminus copeptides of unknown function. Although its role in normal human physiology is uncertain, C-cell neoplasms and other tumors of neural crest origin often secrete great amounts of CT.

The major stimulus of CT secretion is a rise in the plasma calcium concentration of as little as 1 mg/dl. The stimulating effect of calcium on CT secretion involves the calcium receptor previously described and an increase in cyclic AMP. The ingestion of food also increases CT secretion, a response mediated by gastrin and other gastrointestinal hormones. CT circulates in humans at concentrations of 10 to 100 pg/ml (10^{-11} M).

The major effect of calcitonin is to decrease plasma calcium levels

The binding of CT to its plasma membrane receptors stimulates adenylyl cyclase production and elevates cyclic AMP levels. This second messenger initiates at least a portion of CT action in all target cells. THE HYPOCALCEMIC ACTION OF CT IS CAUSED BY THE INHIBITION OF OSTEOCYTIC OSTEOLYSIS AND OSTEOCLASTIC BONE RESORPTION, PARTICULARLY WHEN THEY ARE STIMULATED BY PTH. Continued exposure to CT eventually decreases the number of osteoclasts and alters their morphological features. Since bone formation is also stimulated, denser bone with fewer resorption cavities eventually results.

The importance of CT in humans is controversial. CT deficiency does not lead to overt hypercalcemia, and CT hypersecretion rarely produces hypocalcemia. It may be that abnormal CT secretion is easily compensated for by adjustments in PTH and vitamin D levels. A role for CT in fetal bone development and in protection against the declining bone mass of aging has been proposed.

CT is used therapeutically to block bone resorption in situations in which the resorption rate is high (e.g., **Paget's disease**). The hormone is also used to treat **osteoporosis.**

Integrated Regulation of Calcium and Phosphate

An integrated system maintains normal concentrations of calcium and phosphate. Calcium deprivation (Figure 43-10) stimulates PTH secretion. PTH increases urinary phosphate excretion and thereby decreases the plasma and renal cortical phosphate content. Excess PTH secretion, together with the decreased phosphate concentration, stimulates the production of 1,25-(OH)$_2$-D. The latter raises the plasma calcium concentration back toward normal by increasing the absorption of calcium from the gut. PTH also increases bone resorption and calcium reabsorption from the renal tubular urine. TOGETHER THEN, PTH AND 1,25-(OH)$_2$-D RESPOND TO CALCIUM DEPRIVATION BY INCREASING THE FLUX OF CALCIUM INTO THE PLASMA. SIMULTANEOUSLY, THE EXTRA PHOSPHATE THAT ENTERS WITH THE CALCIUM IS ELIMINATED IN THE URINE VIA PTH ACTION.

Phosphate deprivation (Figure 43-11) directly stimulates 1,25-(OH)$_2$-D production, which increases the flux of phosphate into plasma by stimulating bone resorption and phosphate absorption from the gut. The extra calcium that enters simultaneously raises the plasma calcium level. This suppresses PTH secretion, and the absence of PTH causes urinary phosphate excretion to diminish and thus aids in the restoration of plasma phosphate levels back to normal. At the same time the suppression of PTH diminishes renal tubular calcium reabsorption and increases urinary calcium excretion. THUS THE EXTRA CALCIUM THAT WAS MOBILIZED IS ELIMINATED MORE EASILY.

THIS COMBINED ARRANGEMENT OF DUAL HORMONE REGULATION AND DUAL HORMONE ACTION BY PTH AND VITAMIN D PERMITS A SELECTIVE DEFENSE OF EITHER THE PLASMA CALCIUM LEVEL OR THE PLASMA PHOSPHATE LEVEL WITHOUT CREATING A CIRCULATORY EXCESS OF THE OTHER. The same principles apply in reverse when excess loads of calcium or phosphate are imposed on the body.

The renal responses to PTH provide the most rapid (within minutes) defense against sudden changes in calcium or phosphate levels. The gastrointestinal responses to 1,25-(OH)$_2$-D occur over days. Bone responses to regulation by PTH and 1,25-(OH)$_2$-D are rapid when produced by osteocytic osteolysis and relatively slow when caused by osteoclastic resorption. However, the capacity for calcium and phosphate uptake and release by the skeleton is enormous.

The compensatory responses of the kidney and the gut defend the total body and bone stores of calcium and phosphate against erosion. In contrast, the skeletal mechanisms that defend the plasma calcium and phosphate levels have the important disadvantage that they eventually sacrifice the chemical and structural integrity of the bone mass.

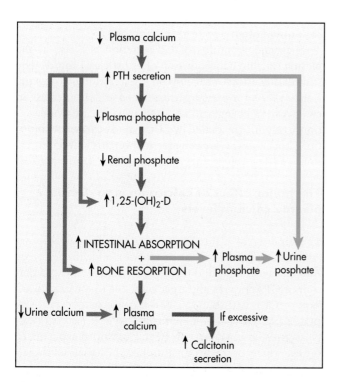

Figure 43-10 Compensatory response to a decrease in the plasma calcium concentration. See text for explanation.

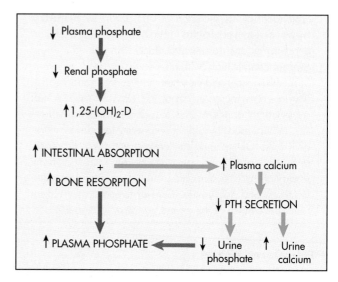

Figure 43-11 The compensatory response to a decrease in the plasma phosphate concentration. See text for explanation.

SUMMARY

- Calcium is critically involved in numerous functions, including neurotransmission, hormone secretion and action, enzyme activities, muscle contraction, and blood clotting. It is also the chief mineral that contributes to the structural integrity of the skeleton.

- Extracellular calcium concentration is closely controlled, in part to help regulate the wide transient swings in intracellular concentration, which is 10,000-fold lower.

- Phosphate participates in the major enzymatic pathways of energy generation, substrate flux, and protein and other macromolecule synthesis. Phosphate is also the anion partner of calcium in bone structure.

- The calcium balance depends on dietary intake, gastrointestinal absorption, renal excretion, and internal transfers between extracellular calcium and the skeletal reservoir.

- The phosphate balance reflects dietary intake, gastrointestinal absorption, renal excretion, and internal shifts among extracellular fluid, large soft tissue contents, and the skeletal reservoir.

- Bone is a complex organ with several cell types that are specifically devoted to a continuous process of remodeling. Mineralized bone is resorbed by osteoclasts (which release calcium and phosphate), followed by osteoblasts reforming new bone (which reassimilates calcium and phosphate). This coupled process is augmented during growth periods and slows with aging.

- Vitamin D is a steroid molecule that is both synthesized in the skin by UV light and absorbed from the diet. It undergoes successive hydroxylations in the liver and kidney to $1,25\text{-}(OH)_2\text{-D}$, the active metabolite.

- $1,25\text{-}(OH)_2\text{-D}$ acts via its intestinal epithelial nuclear receptor to increase the absorption of ingested calcium (and phosphate). The hormone is therefore critical for supplying calcium for bone formation and maintaining the normal plasma levels required for other calcium-dependent processes. Overall, $1,25\text{-}(OH)_2\text{-D}$ increases both plasma calcium and plasma phosphate levels.

- PTH is a straight-chain peptide synthesized as a preprohormone in four parathyroid glands. PTH and calcium form a classic negative-feedback pair. PTH is released in response to the decreased plasma calcium level perceived by a plasma membrane calcium receptor; PTH synthesis and secretion are suppressed by calcium (and $1,25\text{-}(OH)_2\text{-D}$).

- PTH acts via a plasma membrane receptor and cyclic AMP to increase osteoclastic bone resorption, to increase the renal tubular reabsorption of calcium and decrease that of phosphate, and to increase $1,25\text{-}(OH)_2\text{-D}$ synthesis in the kidney. Overall, PTH increases levels of plasma calcium and decreases levels of plasma phosphate.

- Calcium deficiency evokes a synergistic sequence that increases levels of PTH and $1,25\text{-}(OH)_2\text{-D}$. Their combined actions restore plasma calcium levels to normal.

- Phosphate deprivation evokes a synergistic sequence that increases $1,25\text{-}(OH)_2\text{-D}$ secretion but decreases PTH secretion. The result is the restoration of plasma phosphate levels to normal.

- CT is a peptide hormone synthesized in C-cells within the thyroid gland. It is secreted in response to hypercalcemia and acts as a PTH antagonist that inhibits bone resorption and lowers the plasma level of calcium.

BIBLIOGRAPHY

Bell NH: Vitamin D metabolism, aging, and bone loss, *J Clin Endocrinol Metab* 80:1051, 1995 (editorial).

Bouillon R, Okamura WH, Norman AW: Structure-function relationships in the vitamin D endocrine system, *Endocr Rev* 16:200, 1995.

Brent GA et al: Relationship between the concentration and rate of change of calcium and serum intact parathyroid hormone levels in normal humans, *J Clin Endocrinol Metab* 67:944, 1988.

Bringhurst FR: Calcium and phosphate distribution, turnover, and metabolic actions. In DeGroot LJ, ed: *Endocrinology,* ed 3, Philadelphia, 1995, WB Saunders.

Chattopadhyay N, Mithal A, Brown EM: The calcium-sensing receptor: a window into the physiology and pathophysiology of mineral ion metabolism, *Endocr Rev* 17:289, 1996.

Coleman DT, Fitzpatrick LA, Bilezikian J: Biochemical mechanisms of parathyroid hormone action. In Bilezikian J, ed: *The parathyroids: basic and clinical concepts,* New York, 1994, Raven.

Holick MF: Skin: site of the synthesis of vitamin D and a target tissue for the active form, 1,25-dihydroxyvitamin D_3, *Ann NY Acad Sci* 548:14, 1988.

Martin TJ, Moseley JM: Parathyroid hormone–related protein. In DeGroot LJ, ed: *Endocrinology,* ed 3, Philadelphia, 1995, WB Saunders.

Potts JT Jr et al: Parathyroid hormone: physiology, chemistry, biosynthesis, secretion, metabolism, and mode of action. In DeGroot LJ, ed: *Endocrinology,* ed 3, Philadelphia, 1995, WB Saunders.

Roodman GD: Advances in bone biology: the osteoclast, *Endocr Rev* 17:308, 1996.

Ross TK, Darwish HM, Deluca HF: Molecular biology of vitamin D action, *Vitam Horm* 49:281, 1994.

Schmid C: IGFs: function and clinical importance to the regulation of osteoblast function by hormones and cytokines with special reference to insulin-like growth factors and their binding proteins, *J Intern Med* 234:535, 1993.

Stern PH: Vitamin D and bone, *Kidney Int* 29:S17, 1990.

CASE STUDIES

Case 43-1

A 50-year-old overstressed businessman treats frequent "heartburn" with large daily doses of antacids containing aluminum hydroxide. The latter binds phosphate in the gastrointestinal tract and causes the patient to have severe phosphate deficiency.

1. Which of the following would increase?
   A. Plasma PTH levels
   B. Urine phosphate levels
   C. Plasma 24,25-$(OH)_2$-D levels
   D. Plasma 1,25-$(OH)_2$-D levels
   E. Bone formation

2. Which of the following would decrease?
   A. Gastrointestinal absorption of calcium
   B. Plasma PTH levels
   C. Urine hydroxyproline levels
   D. Urine calcium levels
   E. Plasma calcitonin levels

Case 43-2

A well-nourished, otherwise healthy 35-year-old woman who had three kidney stones in 18 months has an elevated plasma calcium level of 13 mg/dl and is found to have hyperparathyroidism. X-ray films show bone resorption.

1. Which of the following would be decreased?
   A. Urine cyclic AMP levels
   B. Urine phosphate levels
   C. Number of osteoclasts
   D. Bone formation
   E. Plasma phosphate levels

2. After removal of a large parathyroid tumor, which of the following would increase rapidly?
   A. Plasma phosphate levels
   B. Nerve excitability
   C. Urine calcium levels
   D. Heart rate
   E. Plasma Ca^{++} levels

CHAPTER 44

Hypothalamus and Pituitary Gland

- Describe the anatomical and functional relationships between the hypothalamus and the posterior and anterior pituitary gland.
- Explain the regulation of antidiuretic hormone and oxytocin (posterior pituitary hormones) secretion.
- Identify the actions of antidiuretic hormone and oxytocin on their target tissues.
- Explain the regulation of growth hormone and prolactin (anterior pituitary hormones) secretions.
- Identify the actions of growth hormone and prolactin on their target tissues.

The pituitary gland, once called *the master gland,* retains a preeminent position in endocrinology, even though it is now known to be under neural regulation by products from the hypothalamus and under feedback control by circulating products of its target glands. The pituitary gland and hypothalamus, with their associated neural and vascular connections, form a complex functional unit that epitomizes the subtle interrelationship between the endocrine and nervous systems. THIS UNIT REGULATES WATER METABOLISM, MILK SECRETION, BODY GROWTH, REPRODUCTION, LACTATION, AND THE GROWTH AND SECRETORY ACTIVITIES OF THE THYROID, ADRENAL, AND REPRODUCTIVE GLANDS, THEREBY AFFECTING THE PHYSIOLOGICAL FUNCTIONING OF VIRTUALLY ALL OTHER ORGAN SYSTEMS IN THE BODY.

The neurons of the hypothalamus synthesize and secrete neurohormones (Figure 44-1). Two of these neurohormones are transferred down the cell axons and are stored in secretory vesicles at the ends of the axons within the posterior pituitary gland, also known as the **neurohypophysis.** From there, they are released into the bloodstream and reach the general circulation to act on distant target cells (**neurocrine** function). Other hypothalamic neurohormones are transported down the cell axons to end in a neurovascular region known as the **median eminence,** which is situated just below the hypothalamus (Figure 44-1). From terminal secretory storage vesicles in the median eminence, these neurohormones are released into the bloodstream, and via local circulation, they reach the nearby anterior pituitary gland, also known as the **adenohypophysis.** There, they stimulate or inhibit endocrine target cells (again, neurocrine function). The endocrine cells in the adenohypophysis synthesize, store, and secrete a variety of peptide and protein hormones that are released into the bloodstream and reach the general circulation to act on distant peripheral target cells (**endocrine** function). In addition, the hormones of these closely intertwined endocrine cells may act on neighboring target cells within the adenohypophysis (**paracrine** function).

The Anatomy and Embryological Development of the Hypothalamus and Pituitary Gland Subserve Their Close Functional Relationship

The pituitary gland sits beneath the hypothalamus in a socket of bone (**sella turcica**) within the skull. The gland represents a fusion of two tissues. The posterior portion, or neurohypophysis, develops as a downward outpouching of neuroectoderm from brain tissue in the floor of the third ventricle. This differentiates into the neurons of the hypothalamus. The lower part of the downward-growing neural stalk forms the bulk of the posterior pituitary. The upper part of the neural stalk expands to form the median eminence. Both the posterior pituitary and the median eminence consist largely of the terminals of various hypothalamic neurons. Both tissues are highly vascularized, and their capillaries contain fenestrations (intercellular windows) that allow the influx and efflux of protein molecules.

The posterior pituitary is supplied by the **inferior hypophyseal artery,** whose capillary plexus invests the terminal swellings of axons from the supraoptic and paraventricular areas of the hypothalamus. These terminals are the immediate source of the peptide neurohormones, **antidiuretic hormone (ADH)** and **oxytocin (OCT);** ADH is also known as **arginine vasopressin (AVP).** These neurohormones are released into the capillary plexus, which carries them into the systemic circulation via draining veins (Figure 44-1).

The anterior pituitary develops from an upward outpouching of ectoderm from the floor of the oral cavity. After pinching off, the pouch becomes separated from

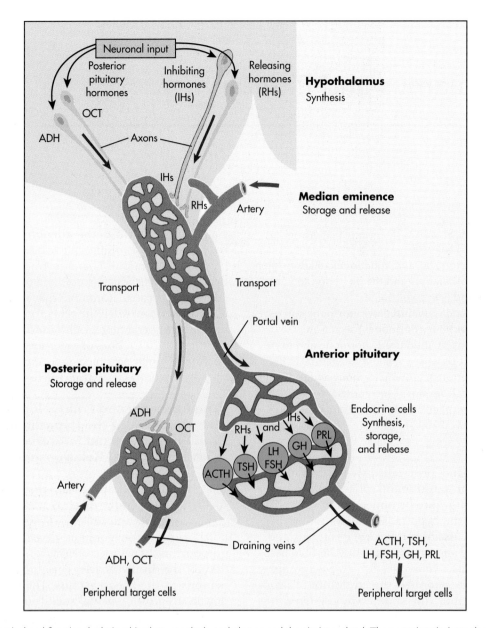

Figure 44-1 Anatomical and functional relationships between the hypothalamus and the pituitary gland. The posterior pituitary gland is an extension of neural tissue that stores neurohormones and has its own arterial blood supply. In contrast, the anterior pituitary gland is endocrine tissue with a blood supply derived largely from veins that first drain neural tissue in the median eminence. Because of this arrangement the endocrine cells are exposed to high concentrations of neurohormones that originate in the hypothalamus and are stored in the median eminence. The hormones secreted by the posterior and anterior pituitary gland reach and act on peripheral target cells. *ACTH,* Adrenocorticotropic hormone; *ADH,* antidiuretic hormone; *FSH,* follicle-stimulating hormone; *GH,* growth hormone; *LH,* luteinizing hormone; *OCT,* oxytocin; *PRL,* prolactin; *TSH,* thyroid-stimulating hormone.

the mouth by the sphenoid bone of the skull. At the junction of the anterior and posterior lobes of the pituitary gland is an intermediate zone, minuscule in humans but well developed in animals, from which another peptide hormone, **melanocyte-stimulating hormone (MSH),** is produced.

The median eminence is supplied mainly by the superior hypophyseal artery (and to a lesser extent, the inferior hypophyseal artery). Its capillary plexus invests terminal swellings of axons from a variety of hypothalamic neurons. These neurons are the source of hypothalamic **releasing** and **inhibiting hormones** that

regulate anterior pituitary function. The capillary plexus of the median eminence forms a set of **portal veins** that descend into the anterior pituitary (Figure 44-1). These veins then give rise to a second fenestrated capillary plexus, which has a dual role. Hypothalamic releasing and inhibiting hormones, which are carried down from the median eminence, exit the second plexus and regulate secretion by the endocrine cells in the anterior pituitary. The protein hormone products of these cells then enter the same capillary plexus and are delivered via the circulation to distant target cells.

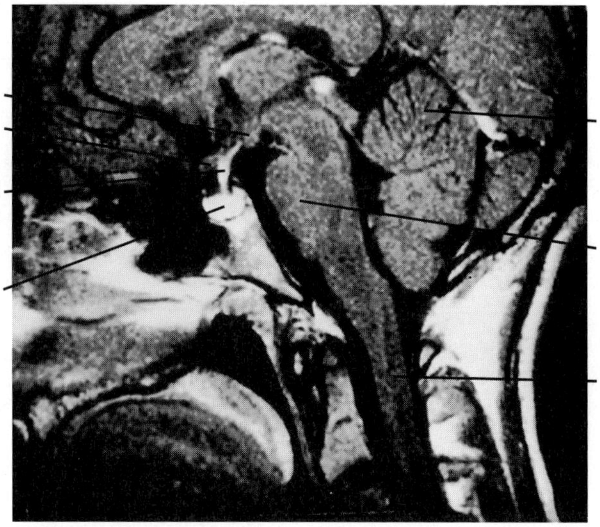

Figure 44-2 Magnetic resonance image of the brain, showing the proximity of the hypothalamus and pituitary gland and their connection by a neurohypophyseal stalk. Also, note the proximity of the optic chiasm (crossing of optic nerves) to the pituitary gland.

The anterior pituitary derives 90% of its blood supply in this manner and has little direct arterial input. Furthermore, its endocrine cells lie outside the blood-brain barrier. The reversal of flow upward in the portal veins may permit high concentrations of anterior pituitary hormones to reach the median eminence and even the hypothalamus, where they could feed back on neurons without impedance from the blood-brain barrier.

> Just above the pituitary gland and sella turcica lies the crossing of the optic nerves as they course from the retina to the cerebral cortex. Any upward tumorous growth of the pituitary out of the sella turcica can compress the optic nerves and cause a characteristic loss of visual fields and acuity. This anatomy can be well visualized by magnetic resonance imaging (Figure 44-2).

Hypothalamic Function Regulates Pituitary Gland Secretions to Coordinate with the Essential Needs of the Organism

A comprehensive discussion of the hypothalamus is provided in Chapter 10. From an endocrine standpoint, however, the hypothalamus may be viewed as a central relay station for collecting and integrating signals from diverse sources and funneling them to the pituitary gland (Figure 44-3). The hypothalamus receives input from the thalamus, the reticular activating substance, the limbic system (amygdala, olfactory bulb, hippocampus, and habenula), the eyes, and remotely the neocortex. Through this input, PITUITARY FUNCTION CAN BE INFLUENCED BY SLEEP OR WAKEFULNESS, PAIN, EMOTION, FRIGHT, SMELL, LIGHT, AND POSSIBLY EVEN THOUGHT.

It can be coordinated with other behavior such as mating responses. INTERHYPOTHALAMIC AXONAL CONNECTIONS ALLOW THE OUTPUT OF PITUITARY HORMONES TO RESPOND TO CHANGES IN AUTONOMIC NERVOUS SYSTEM ACTIVITY AND TO THE NEEDS OF TEMPERATURE REGULATION, WATER BALANCE, AND ENERGY REQUIREMENTS.

The proximity of these various areas of the hypothalamus to one another has functional logic. For example, hormones of the thyroid gland increase energy expenditure, metabolic rate, and thermogenesis. The neurons that ultimately control thyroid gland output are located close to neurons that regulate temperature and energy intake via appetite control.

Separation of the hypothalamus into individual nuclei or distinct anatomical centers of endocrine function is relatively imprecise, with two exceptions. The supraoptic nucleus is a collection of large neurons that secrete mainly ADH, and the paraventricular nucleus is a similar collection of neurons that secrete mainly OCT. These two neuronal pools overlap only slightly. In contrast, the small neurons that secrete the hypothalamic releasing and inhibiting hormones are more loosely aggregated in various areas, and they overlap more. As a general but not absolute rule, only one cell type secretes each neurohormone. In some hypothalamic neurons, monoamine neurotransmitters are also produced.

Each hypothalamic anterior pituitary releasing or inhibiting hormone can be assigned a primary target for which it has been named, such as **thyrotropin-releasing hormone** (a hormone that releases **thyrotropin,** an anterior pituitary hormone, which then stimulates the thyroid gland) or **somatostatin** (*soma,* "body growth"; *statin,* "halting of function"). However, some of these neuropeptides act on more than one anterior pituitary cell.

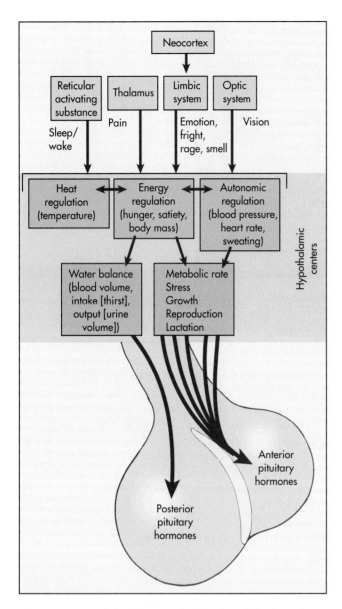

Figure 44-3 Interrelationships among various hypothalamic regulatory centers, their inputs from various parts of the brain, and their outputs to the pituitary gland. Note that sleep, pain, stressors, energy needs, temperature, and signals from the autonomic nervous system, as well as other factors, influence pituitary function.

In addition to the hypothalamic neurons whose axons end in the posterior pituitary and median eminence, other neurons have axons that project to different parts of the brain. In these instances the same hypothalamic peptides serve as neurotransmitters. (These neuropeptides have also been found in the spinal cord, sympathetic ganglia, sensory neurons, pancreatic islets, and neuroendocrine cells of the gastrointestinal tract.)

Hypothalamic neurohormones are synthesized from preprohormones (see Chapter 40) and are typically secreted in pulses generated by an intrinsic neural oscillator (Figure 44-4). This pulsatile pattern of signaling is necessary for optimal effects on target cells.

In women who are infertile because of hypothalamic dysfunction, ovulatory menstrual cycles can be restored only if the appropriate hypothalamic releasing hormone is administered in pulses of the correct size and frequency throughout the day. If the releasing hormone is administered continuously, the necessary anterior pituitary response is ultimately lost because of the down-regulation of the releasing hormone receptor. The same phenomenon is observed with regard to spermatogenesis in men.

Releasing and inhibiting hormones react with plasma membrane receptors in anterior pituitary cells; Ca^{++}, phosphatidylinositol products, and cyclic AMP are generated as second messengers. The releasing hormones all stimulate the exocytosis of granules containing tropic hormones. In addition, they stimulate the transcription of tropic hormone genes and enhance hormone activity via posttranslational modification. Inhibiting hormones have the opposite effects. Hypothalamic neurohormones can also regulate the numbers of their own receptors.

Various neurotransmitters subserve hypothalamic function

Afferent impulses to hypothalamic neurons are transmitted via norepinephrine, serotonin, acetylcholine, the amino acid neurotransmitters (glutamate, aspartate, glycine, and γ-aminobutyric acid) and numerous neuropeptides. From some hypothalamic neurons, dopamine and β-endorphin transmit signals to neighboring neurons via intrahypothalamic tracts and to the median eminence via efferent tracts. These signals directly or indirectly modulate the discharge of releasing and inhibiting hormones. In addition, neurotransmitters from the hypothalamus (e.g., dopamine) may themselves reach the portal vein blood and directly influence the output of anterior pituitary hormones.

The hypothalamus and pituitary gland respond to feedback control

The pituitary hypothalamic axis is under feedback control from its peripheral targets (Figure 44-5). Tropic hormones from the adenohypophysis regulate the concentrations of (1) hormones secreted by the thyroid, adrenal, and reproductive glands; (2) peripherally generated peptide products; and (3) substrates such as glucose or free fatty acids. These in turn feed back to regulate the output of both the hypothalamus and the anterior pituitary. This is known as **long-loop feedback,** and it is usually negative, although it can transiently be positive. Negative feedback can also be exerted by the anterior pituitary hormones on the synthesis or discharge of the related hypothalamic releasing or inhibiting hormones. This is known as **short-loop feedback.** Because these hormones do not ordinarily cross the blood-brain barrier, short-loop feedback may occur either

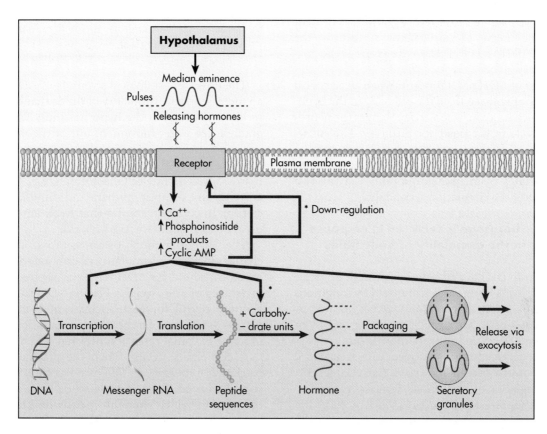

Figure 44-4 Action of hypothalamic releasing or inhibiting hormones on anterior pituitary cells. Characteristically the neurohormones are released in pulses, bind to plasma membrane receptors, and act through Ca^{++} and other second messengers. They regulate gene expression, posttranslational processes, and secretion of anterior pituitary tropic hormones.

via fenestrated cells of the capillaries that bathe hypothalamic neurons or via retrograde flow through pituitary portal veins. Finally, a hypothalamic releasing hormone may even inhibit its own synthesis and discharge or synthesis of a paired hypothalamic inhibiting hormone. This is called **ultrashort-loop feedback.**

The Posterior Pituitary Gland Regulates Water Metabolism and Breast Milk Secretion

ADH and OCT, two small homologous peptides with molecular weights of approximately 1000, are secreted by the posterior pituitary gland. THE PRIMARY ROLE OF ADH IS TO CONSERVE WATER AND REGULATE THE TONICITY OF BODY FLUIDS (SEE CHAPTER 37). A SECONDARY ROLE IS TO HELP MAINTAIN VASCULAR VOLUME. THE PRIMARY ROLE OF OCT IS TO EJECT MILK FROM THE LACTATING MAMMARY GLAND; AN ADDITIONAL ROLE IS TO STIMULATE CONTRACTION OF THE UTERUS. Although their main functions are very different, both hormones are synthesized, stored, and secreted in similar fashion.

The similar genes that direct synthesis of the prepro-hormones for ADH and OCT likely have a common ancestor gene. In addition to the two neuropeptides, the gene products include distinctive small proteins known as **neurophysins.** Neurophysin-1 for OCT and neurophysin-2 for ADH are very similar. After processing, ADH and OCT are packaged with their respec-

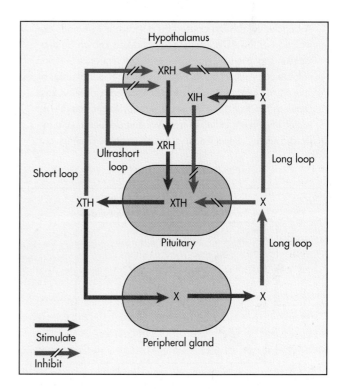

Figure 44-5 Negative-feedback loops regulating hormone secretion in a typical hypothalamus–pituitary–peripheral gland axis. Note that feedback from the periphery can regulate both hypothalamic and pituitary function. Ultrashort-loop feedback may be intrahypothalamic. *X,* Peripheral gland hormone; *XIH,* hypothalamic inhibiting hormone; *XRH,* hypothalamic releasing hormone; *XTH,* pituitary tropic hormone.

tive neurophysins in neurosecretory granules. The neurophysins may serve as carrier proteins during the transport of ADH and OCT down the axons to the posterior pituitary gland.

The release of ADH or OCT occurs when an electrical discharge is transmitted from the cell body in the hypothalamus down its axon, where it depolarizes the neurosecretory vesicle in the posterior pituitary. The subsequent influx of calcium into the vesicles releases the hormones via exocytosis. During this process, each hormone dissociates from its neurophysin, and the two molecules enter the circulation separately.

Antidiuretic hormone is secreted in response to changes in the osmolality of body fluids

The secretion of ADH illustrates the homeostatic principle that the release of a hormone is stimulated by conditions that require its action (Figure 44-6). WATER DEPRIVATION RAISES THE PLASMA OSMOLALITY, WHICH EVOKES THE RELEASE OF ADH. IN TURN, ADH CAUSES THE RETENTION OF FREE WATER BY THE KIDNEY AND AN INCREASE IN URINE OSMOLALITY, RESULTING IN A PLASMA OSMOLALITY DECLINE TO NORMAL (see Chapter 37). Conversely, ingestion of a water load decreases plasma osmolality. This suppresses ADH release, which increases water excretion and raises the plasma osmolality to normal. Thus water and ADH form a negative-feedback loop, which operates to defend total body water and osmolality.

A deficiency of ADH caused by disease or traumatic destruction of the ADH neurons, a condition known as **diabetes insipidus,** has dramatic consequences. Urine volume can reach 500 to 1000 ml/hr, with osmolalities as low as 50 mOsm/kg. This forces frequent urination and requires the individual to drink equally large volumes of water to prevent collapse from volume depletion and hyperosmolality. Impairment of thirst or consciousness can

therefore lead to death from dehydration. Treatment with ADH provides rapid relief.

The direct physiological stimulus of ADH release is an increase in the osmolality of fluids that bathe osmoreceptor neurons in the hypothalamus. This creates a gradient for water movement out of the neurons, and the consequent rise in intracellular osmolality triggers the release of ADH. Any administered solute that does not readily penetrate cell membranes (e.g., sodium) creates the same osmotic gradient and stimulates ADH secretion. In contrast, solutes that freely enter cells (e.g., urea) do not stimulate ADH release.

The hypothalamic osmoreceptors respond to changes in plasma osmolality of only 1% to 2%. The osmolar threshold for ADH release is approximately 280 mOsm/kg of body weight. Plasma ADH then increases about 1 pg/ml for each increase of 3 mOsm/kg in plasma osmolality. The generation of sufficient ADH to produce maximal retention of water and maximal urinary osmolality occurs when the plasma osmolality reaches 294 mOsm/kg. The osmolar threshold for the stimulation of thirst is close to or somewhat higher than that for ADH. Therefore in defending normal body water content and tonicity, ADH secretion may precede the activation of thirst.

Antidiuretic hormone is secreted in response to changes in body fluid volume

ADH release is also stimulated by hypovolemia and hypotension (Figure 44-6). This is a much less sensitive response because a decrease of 5% to 10% in blood volume, cardiac output, or blood pressure is required. Hemorrhage, quiet standing, and positive-pressure breathing, all of which reduce cardiac output and central blood volume, increase ADH secretion. Conversely, an increase in the central blood volume, which is caused by the administration of blood or isotonic saline solution, suppresses ADH release. Hypovolemia is perceived by several pressure (rather than volume) sensors (see Chapters 19 and 23). These include carotid and aortic baroreceptors and stretch receptors in the walls of the left atrium and pulmonary veins. Normally, these pressure receptors tonically inhibit ADH release. A reduction in circulating blood volume decreases pressure on the baroreceptors and reduces the flow of inhibitory impulses to the hypothalamus. This increases ADH secretion. Hypovolemia also directly stimulates the generation of **renin** and **angiotensin** within the brain. Angiotensin augments the release of ADH and stimulates thirst. In contrast, **atrial natriuretic peptide,** which is generated in response to volume or pressure overload, inhibits ADH release. Plasma ADH concentrations rise much more in response to hypovolemia than in response to hyperosmolality. This correlates with the lesser sensitivity of the vascular system than of the kidney to ADH action.

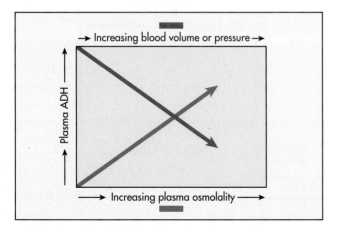

Figure 44-6 Positive correlation between the plasma ADH and increasing plasma osmolality. Negative correlation between plasma ADH and increasing blood volume or pressure.

The two major stimuli of ADH secretion interact (see Figure 37-3, C). Increases or decreases in volume or pressure reinforce the osmolar responses by raising or lowering, respectively, the threshold for the osmotic release of ADH. Thus HYPOVOLEMIA OR HYPERTENSION SENSITIZES THE SYSTEM TO HYPEROSMOLARITY. When hypovolemia is severe, baroregulation can override osmotic regulation. Consequently, ADH secretion can be stimulated even though plasma osmolality may be below the threshold of 280 mOsm/kg. The result can even be an expanded extracellular fluid volume (edema) with a low serum sodium level and osmolality.

Pain, emotional stress, nausea and vomiting, heat, and a variety of drugs also stimulate ADH release. Ethanol, on the other hand, is a frequently encountered inhibitor that causes diuresis. Cortisol and thyroid hormone restrain ADH release; when they are deficient, ADH may be secreted even though the plasma osmolality is low.

In patients with severe congestive heart failure, increased secretion of ADH may be stimulated by a low effective circulating pressure and volume. The ADH causes water retention, which simultaneously causes or worsens edema and leads to dilutional hyponatremia. A clinical syndrome of secretion of excess ADH in amounts inappropriate to the plasma osmolality occurs in a variety of other settings. These include psychiatric or cerebral disease and pulmonary disease or tumor; it also occurs after major surgery and use of psychotropic drugs. The plasma osmolality is chronically low and sometimes reaches a point at which the patient becomes obtunded or has seizures. The restriction of water intake or the inhibition of ADH action is required to correct this situation, known as the **syndrome of inappropriate ADH (SIADH).**

ADH circulates at basal concentrations of about 1 pg/ml (10^{-12} M). The plasma half-life is very short. During water deprivation, ADH secretion increases threefold to fivefold, and synthesis of the hormone is augmented. Plasma levels of cosecreted neurophysin-2 also rise and fall in parallel with plasma levels of ADH.

Antidiuretic hormone acts on renal tubules to conserve water

The major action of ADH is on the renal tubular mechanism for concentrating the urine (i.e., for reabsorbing osmotically unencumbered water from the glomerular filtrate [see Chapter 37]). ADH stimulates the two phases in the countercurrent concentrating mechanism. First, the hormone increases the transport of sodium out of the thick ascending portion of the loop of Henle and into the medullary interstitium and thus helps create the osmotic gradient for water. Second and more important, ADH increases the permeability of the collecting duct membranes to water and thus facilitates the diffusion of water back into the medulla. The maximal effect of ADH increases the osmolality of urine to a value four times higher than that of plasma, or about 1200 mOsm/kg. Urine osmolality also correlates directly with plasma ADH concentration. Without the hormone, urine osmolality falls to less than 100 mOsm/kg, and free water clearance reaches 10 to 15 ml/min (see Chapter 37).

The intracellular mechanism of ADH action in the kidney requires binding to a plasma membrane receptor on the capillary (basal) side of the renal tubular cell. This is followed by the generation of cyclic AMP as second messenger and the subsequent phosphorylation of proteins mediated by a protein kinase on the luminal (apical) side of the cell. In the collecting ducts, this leads to the insertion of specific proteins called **aquaporins** into the cell membrane. The aquaporins form water-conducting channels that increase water permeability. The flow of water is governed by the high osmolality of the medullary interstitium (see Figure 37-4). ADH stimulates the insertion of aquaporin-2 into the plasma membrane.

Several factors can blunt the action of ADH on tubular cells. These include an inactivating, mutant, stimulating G protein; solute diuresis; chronic water loading (which reduces medullary hyperosmolality); potassium deficiency; calcium excess; cortisol excess; and lithium administration. When any of these circumstances exist, the ineffectiveness of ADH leads to **nephrogenic diabetes insipidus.**

In addition to its major role in water metabolism, ADH may have other functions. It contributes in a minor way to increasing vascular tone in response to hemorrhage. When administered systemically in large doses, it elevates the blood pressure and constricts the coronary and splanchnic beds. This action requires binding to a different receptor in vascular cells and is mediated by the phosphatidylinositol–protein kinase C second-messenger system. ADH also functions as a hypothalamic releasing factor via axons that project to the median eminence and stimulate the secretion of pituitary adrenocorticotropin, which in turn stimulates the secretion of adrenal cortisol.

Oxytocin is secreted in response to various reproductive needs

OCT is required for normal nursing. Known biologically as the *milk letdown factor*, it is secreted within seconds in response to suckling. Sensory receptors in the nipple generate afferent impulses that reach the hypothalamic paraventricular and supraoptic nuclei via various relays. A final cholinergic synapse causes the discharge of OCT and neurophysin-1 from the posterior pituitary in a manner similar to that of ADH. Continued suckling further stimulates the synthesis and transport of OCT to the posterior pituitary. In humans, there is little crossover secretion of

ADH with suckling or of secretion of OCT with increased plasma osmolality. OCT secretion can also be stimulated by vaginal distention during sexual intercourse. The inhibition of OCT release by emotional distress can interfere with nursing.

Oxytocin acts on the breast and uterus

OCT causes the myoepithelial cells of the alveoli in the breast to contract. This forces the milk from the alveoli into the ducts and nipple, from where it is extracted by the infant. OCT acts via plasma membrane receptors and the generation of phosphoinositide products and calcium in target cells. The binding of OCT to the receptor is increased by estrogen. Although basal plasma levels of OCT are similar in men and women, no role for the circulating hormone in men is known.

OCT also stimulates contraction of the uterus. Low doses cause rhythmic contractions, whereas higher doses cause sustained tetanic contraction. OCT and its receptor are also present in the human ovary and testis, where the locally produced hormone may play a role in reproduction.

> There is controversial evidence regarding the function of maternal OCT in normal labor in humans, but the sustained contractions produced by OCT may be important in reducing blood loss from the uterus after the delivery of the conceptus. OCT in large doses is often used therapeutically to induce labor or to stop excessive postpartum bleeding.

The Anterior Pituitary Gland Secretes Numerous Hormones with Various Functions

The **anterior pituitary gland,** or **adenohypophysis,** makes up most of the 500 mg of pituitary tissue. It contains at least five types of endocrine cells, each being the source of a different hormone with a distinct function after which it is named. These cell types, their relative proportions in the pituitary, and their major secretory products are shown in Figure 44-7. Although the five types of functional cells aggregate in regions, they do not form unique enclaves but are also interspersed among one another. They vary somewhat in size and in the characteristics of their secretory granules, but they can be identified with certainty only by immunohistochemical staining of the hormones within. Cells that contain no known hormone are called **null cells.** They show evidence of protein hormone synthesis and contain a few secretory granules.

Each anterior pituitary cell is regulated by one or more hypothalamic neurohormones that reach it through the portal veins, as described previously. Three of the cell types produce hormones that regulate the

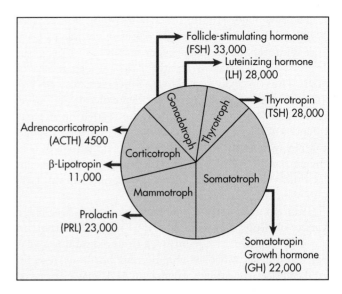

Figure 44-7 The relative proportions of cell types in the anterior pituitary gland, their major hormonal products, and the molecular weights of the latter. Note the preponderance of cells secreting growth hormone and prolactin.

function of the thyroid gland **(thyroid-stimulating hormone [TSH]),** the adrenal glands **(adrenocorticotropic hormone [ACTH]),** and the gonads **(luteinizing hormone [LH]** and **follicle-stimulating hormone [FSH]).** For purposes of better integration, the synthesis, secretion, and actions of these tropic hormones are presented in conjunction with their peripheral target glands (see Chapters 45, 46, and 48). The differentiation of several types of anterior pituitary endocrine cells is stimulated by **Pit-1,** a transcription factor whose synthesis is increased by hypothalamic releasing hormones via cyclic AMP as second messenger.

Growth hormone (somatotropin)

The major physiological effect of **growth hormone (GH)** is stimulation of postnatal somatic growth and development. Once childhood growth and puberty have been completed, GH continues to modulate the metabolism, body composition, and functional capabilities of adults.

The synthesis and secretion of GH are stimulated and inhibited by hypothalamic factors and peripheral metabolic signals

Somatotrophs are the most numerous cells of the pituitary and are concentrated in its lateral wings (Figure 44-8). Their product, GH, is a single, large polypeptide chain with 191 amino acids and two disulfide bridges. Helical tertiary structures within the molecule are important in the binding of GH to its receptor. The human genome contains multiple genes that code for a family of closely related GH molecules. Only one of these is expressed as normal pituitary GH. Messenger RNA directs the synthesis of a prehormone. After the removal of a signal peptide, the complete hormone is stored in gran-

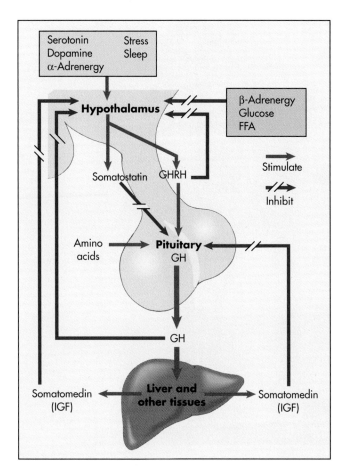

Figure 44-8 Regulation of GH secretion. Note that two hypothalamic peptides, one stimulatory and one inhibitory, regulate GH release. Negative feedback by insulin growth factor *(IGF)*, the peripheral product, is exerted at the hypothalamic and the pituitary levels. There is also complex regulation by substrates and neural influences. *FFA,* Free fatty acid; *GHRH,* GH–releasing hormone.

ules. GH synthesis is increased by the specific hypothalamic releasing hormone, **growth hormone–releasing hormone (GHRH)** and by thyroid hormone and cortisol.

GH secretion via exocytosis is stimulated by GHRH, which is a hypothalamic peptide with 44 amino acids. GHRH interacts with its plasma membrane receptor, after which calcium, phosphatidylinositol products, and cyclic AMP are generated as second messengers.

Somatostatin, a hypothalamic peptide in either a 14 or a 28 amino acid form, is a powerful inhibitor of GH release. Somatostatin blocks GHRH stimulation non-competitively. The inhibitor acts through its own plasma membrane receptor, in part by decreasing both the entry of calcium into the cells and the levels of cyclic AMP. GH is secreted in pulses caused by the intermittent release of GHRH into portal pituitary vein blood. Somatostatin also diminishes the frequency and amplitude of GHRH pulses.

The secretion of GH is influenced by many factors (Figure 44-8). However, THE FINAL COMMON PATHWAY FOR MOST STIMULATORS OF GH IS AN INCREASE IN THE LEVELS OF

GHRH, A DECREASE IN THE LEVELS OF SOMATOSTATIN, OR BOTH CHANGES. CONVERSELY, THE SUPPRESSORS OF GH DECREASE THE LEVELS OF GHRH, INCREASE THE LEVELS OF SOMATOSTATIN, OR CAUSE BOTH EFFECTS. Some agents can alter GH secretion via direct effects on the somatotroph.

The release of GH is regulated metabolically by the energy substrates glucose and free fatty acids and by amino acids. A sharp drop in the levels of either glucose or free fatty acid stimulates a large increase in the plasma levels of GH, whereas an elevation of the levels of either considerably reduces plasma GH levels. Protein ingestion or intravenous amino acid infusion stimulates GH release. Arginine is an especially effective amino acid. BOTH SHORT-TERM FASTING AND PROLONGED PROTEIN-CALORIE DEPRIVATION INCREASE GH SECRETION. IN CONTRAST, OBESITY REDUCES GH RESPONSES TO ALL STIMULI, INCLUDING GHRH.

Central nervous system regulation of GH secretion takes several forms. A nocturnal surge in GH occurs 1 to 2 hours after the onset of deep sleep. Conversely, light sleep, which is associated with rapid eye movements (REM sleep), inhibits GH release. Various stresses, including trauma, surgery, anesthesia, fever, and even simple venipuncture, elevate plasma GH. Exercise is also a potent stimulant. These conditions influence hypothalamic GHRH and somatostatin neurons through a variety of monoamine neurotransmitters (Figure 44-8).

CHILDREN SECRETE MORE GH THAN ADULTS, ESPECIALLY DURING PUBERTY, WHEN ESTRADIOL AND TESTOSTERONE LEVELS RISE SHARPLY. IN AGED INDIVIDUALS, GH SECRETION DECLINES. Females are usually more responsive to GH stimuli than males.

> Children who cannot secrete GH or respond to its actions grow at a reduced rate and are delayed in skeletal and sexual maturation. They are short in stature and modestly obese (Figure 44-9). In some short children, deficiency is easily established because of the failure of plasma GH to rise acutely with any stimulus. In others, a fairly specific loss of nocturnal peaks or a diminution of total daily integrated secretion is used as evidence for a more subtle GH deficiency that justifies replacement therapy. GH secretion is reduced by a deficiency of thyroid hormone or by an excess of cortisol. In both conditions, the growth and maturation of children are also impaired.

Resting basal plasma levels of GH are 1 to 5 ng/ml (10^{-10} M). The hormone circulates bound to a binding protein that is identical to the extracellular domain of plasma membrane GH receptors. Daily GH secretion is approximately 600 mg in prepubertal children, 1800 mg in individuals in late puberty, and 300 to 500 mg in adults.

Feedback regulation of GH secretion occurs at all levels (Figure 44-8). Long-loop negative feedback is exerted

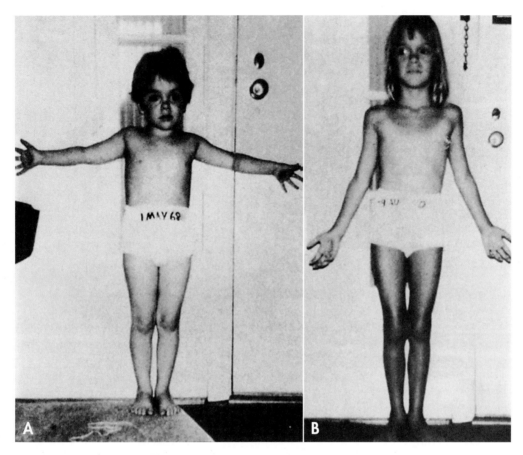

Figure 44-9 Effect of 15 months of GH replacement on a 6-year-old child with GH deficiency. Note that GH increases linear growth and decreases adiposity. *(From Foster D, Wilson J, eds:* Williams textbook of endocrinology, *Philadelphia, 1985, WB Saunders.)*

by **somatomedin,** which is a peripheral product of GH action. Somatomedin inhibits the release of GHRH, inhibits GHRH's action on the pituitary somatotroph, and stimulates somatostatin release. Short-loop negative feedback is exerted by GH itself via the stimulation of somatostatin release. Ultrashort-loop negative feedback is exerted by GHRH, possibly via synapses with somatostatin neurons.

Growth hormone acts through peripherally generated peptide mediators

GH interacts with several distinct plasma membrane receptors in target cells throughout the body. One GH molecule binds two neighboring receptor molecules. The intracellular tails of the receptors then "dock" and activate intracytoplasmic tyrosine kinases. The kinases phosphorylate transcription factor proteins, which mediate GH's effects on gene expression. However, much of the growth-promoting effect of GH requires the peripheral generation of an entirely different family of peptides known as **somatomedins.** These peptides, which have a molecular weight of 7000, resemble proinsulin in structure (see Chapter 42). They were originally discovered in plasma and are also termed **insulin growth factors (IGFs).**

Two principal IGFs, their receptors, and the respective genes are well characterized. IGF-1 has 50% and IGF-2 has 70% amino acid homology with the A and B chains of insulin (see Chapter 42). IGFs are produced by many tissues in response to GH. However, circulating IGFs originate mainly in the liver, and the lag between the administration of GH and the subsequent increase in plasma IGF-1 and IGF-2 is about 12 hours. Both types of IGF circulate bound to a number of large binding proteins that regulate their availability to tissues. GH stimulates the production of some of these binding proteins in the liver. The IGF binding proteins account for the relatively stable concentration and much longer half-lives of IGFs than that of GH itself. The IGF binding proteins are also found and expressed in many tissues where they may modulate IGF actions. BOTH IGFs, BUT ESPECIALLY IGF-1, ARE GREATLY REDUCED IN THE PLASMA OF GH-DEFICIENT SUBJECTS.

Although IGFs may function as circulating hormones in classic endocrine fashion, they also function as locally produced hormones in paracrine and even autocrine fashion. GH probably induces the differentiation of precursor cells in target tissues (e.g., prechondrocytes in cartilage) into mature cells (chondrocytes), which then express the IFG-1 gene under further GH stimulation. IGF-1 then acts through its own plasma membrane receptor, which has structural similarity to the insulin receptor (see Chapter 42). The IGF-2 receptor is dissimilar to the IGF-1 and insulin receptors.

Insulin growth factors mediate the processes of growth

IGFs mediate the typical GH responses of cartilage, bone, muscle, adipose tissue, fibroblasts, and tumor cells in vitro. INDIVIDUALS WHO LACK THE ABILITY TO PRODUCE IGFS EXPERIENCE RETARDED GROWTH DESPITE HIGH GH LEVELS. Although fetal GH is not required for intrauterine growth, IGFs generated in the placenta or other fetal tissues may participate in regulating prenatal growth. A GH variant produced in the placenta likely stimulates the production of these growth factors. The IGF-2 gene and its receptor gene are expressed very early in fetal development.

During adolescence, plasma IGF-1 levels rise because of increases in GH secretion, with which they correlate. The progression of pubertal growth correlates with the increase in the levels of plasma IGF-1. Very tall people have a hyperresponsiveness to GHRH, which suggests that the GH secretory capacity is one determinant of final height.

In states of fasting and protein-calorie malnutrition, IGF levels in plasma are diminished; this finding correlates with the negative nitrogen balance in these conditions. Because GH levels are elevated in these catabolic states, factors other than GH must also regulate IGF production. In turn, the high GH levels most likely result from negative feedback caused by low IGF levels (Figure 44-8). IGF production is also diminished by cortisol and estrogens, hormones that antagonize GH action.

Insulin growth factors stimulate the processes of anabolism

GH, via IGFs, is a hormone with overall anabolic action (see Chapter 41). When it is administered to GH-deficient children or adults, it decreases plasma amino acid levels and urea production because the amino acids are shunted toward protein synthesis and away from oxidative degradation (see Chapter 41). The total body nitrogen balance, along with the related balances of the intracellular minerals potassium and phosphate, becomes positive. Lean body mass increases, whereas fat mass decreases. Bone formation is enhanced. The resting metabolic rate, exercise capacity, and sense of well-being all increase. These changes suggest that GH is essential to optimal health, even in adults. The decrease in GH with aging may play a role in the changes of senescence.

The multiplicity of GH targets and effects is indicated in Figure 44-10. The most striking and specific effect is the acceleration of linear growth (Figure 44-9)

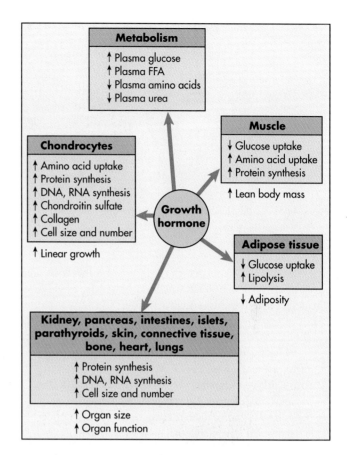

Figure 44-10 Overview of GH actions. *FFA*, Free fatty acid.

that results from GH action on the epiphysial cartilage growth centers of long bones (see Chapter 43). All aspects of the metabolism of chondrocytes, the cartilage-forming cells, are stimulated. This includes the synthesis of collagen and the proteoglycan chondroitin, which together, form the resilient extracellular matrix of cartilage. In addition, GH stimulates the synthesis and proliferation of proteins, RNA, and DNA in these cells. In support of the augmented protein synthesis, GH also stimulates the cellular uptake of amino acids.

Many tissues share in the anabolic response to GH. The width of bones increases, and in children, bone length increases. The visceral organs (i.e., liver, kidney, pancreas, intestines), endocrine glands (i.e., adrenals, parathyroids, pancreatic islets), skeletal muscle, heart, skin, and connective tissue all enlarge. This is also reflected in enhanced function of these organs.

Growth hormone opposes insulin actions

GH affects carbohydrate and lipid metabolism. It stimulates the expression of the insulin gene. HOWEVER, GH ALSO INDUCES RESISTANCE TO THE ACTION OF INSULIN. Glucose uptake by muscle and adipose cells is inhibited, and the plasma glucose concentration rises. Hyperinsulinemia results in compensation. In addition, GH enhances lipolysis and antagonizes insulin-stimulated li-

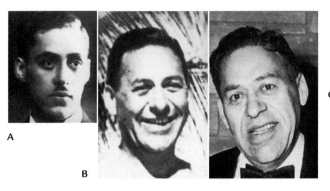

C

Figure 44-11 Coarsening of the face in a patient who developed GH hypersecretion (acromegaly). **A,** Age 24. **B,** Age 50. **C,** Age 58.

pogenesis. These actions increase plasma levels of free fatty acids and ketoacids and decrease adipose tissue. Thus GH is a diabetogenic hormone.

> Sustained hypersecretion of GH from a slow-growing somatotroph tumor produces a unique syndrome called **acromegaly**, which reflects all these actions. In adults, the accumulation of excess soft tissue and the widening of bones lead to coarser features (Figure 44-11) and spadelike digits. Thick skin, enlarged muscles such as that in the tongue, and decreased subcutaneous fat are seen. Glomerular filtration and cardiac output are increased. Glucose intolerance or frank diabetes occurs in some individuals. Life expectancy is reduced via accelerated atherosclerosis. The diagnosis is confirmed by elevated plasma GH and IGF levels. If surgery is not curative, somatostatin analogues are effective treatment.

Growth hormone and insulin actions are also correlated

The secretion and actions of GH and insulin are metabolically coordinated:

1. When protein and energy intake is ample, amino acids can be used for protein synthesis and growth. Thus protein ingestion stimulates the secretion of both GH and insulin, and together, the hormones augment the production of IGFs. The IGFs in turn stimulate accretion of lean body mass. At the same time, the insulin-antagonistic effect of GH helps prevent hypoglycemia, which might otherwise result from the increased insulin secretion in the absence of ingested carbohydrate.

2. When carbohydrate is ingested alone, insulin secretion is increased, but GH secretion is suppressed. In the absence of amino acids, the accelerated generation of IGFs is not advantageous. Insulin antagonism also is not necessary; on the contrary, unopposed expression of insulin action permits the efficient storage of excess carbohydrate calories.

3. With fasting, insulin secretion falls, GH secretion rises, but IGF levels still decline. This combination seems appropriate in a situation in which protein catabolism is essential and protein synthesis must decline (see Chapter 41). However, the increase in GH is beneficial because it contributes to enhanced lipolysis and decreases peripheral tissue glucose use. This helps mobilize free fatty acids for oxidative purposes and helps provide glucose for central nervous system needs.

Prolactin

Prolactin (PRL) is a protein hormone principally concerned with stimulating breast development and milk production in women. In addition, it may play a role in reproductive function in both genders. The PRL-producing cells, called **mammotrophs,** are the second most prevalent in the pituitary gland (Figure 44-7). They increase in number during pregnancy and lactation.

Pregnancy regulates the synthesis and secretion of prolactin

PRL is a single-chain protein with 198 amino acids and 3 disulfide bridges. It is structurally similar to GH, and the two genes are thought to have arisen from a common ancestor. The synthesis of PRL proceeds from a prehormone in the manner described for GH. Some molecules are also *N*-glycosylated and are then secreted constitutively. A small number of pituitary cells called **mammosomatotrophs** secrete both PRL and GH. The transcription of the PRL gene is regulated by the same factors that regulate the secretion of the hormone.

THE MOST IMPORTANT INFLUENCE ON PRL SECRETION IS THE COMBINATION OF PREGNANCY, ELEVATED ESTROGEN LEVELS, AND NURSING (Figure 44-12). In preparation for lactation, PRL secretion increases steadily during pregnancy to a twentyfold plasma elevation. This is probably mediated by the high estrogen levels of pregnancy, which stimulates hyperplasia of the mammotrophs and transcription of the PRL gene. Although estrogen does not directly stimulate the release of PRL, it does enhance its release in response to other stimuli. If a new mother does not nurse her child, the plasma PRL level declines to the range that prevails in nonpregnant women by 6 weeks after delivery. Suckling, however, maintains elevated PRL levels for 8 to 12 weeks. PRL secretion rises at night and in conjunction with major stresses. The functional significance of such increases in PRL in these situations is unclear.

The hypothalamic regulation of prolactin secretions is both positive and negative

UNIQUE AMONG THE ANTERIOR PITUITARY HORMONES, THE SECRETION OF PRL IS PREDOMINANTLY UNDER INHIBITION BY HYPOTHALAMIC FACTORS (Figure 44-12). Disruption of pituitary

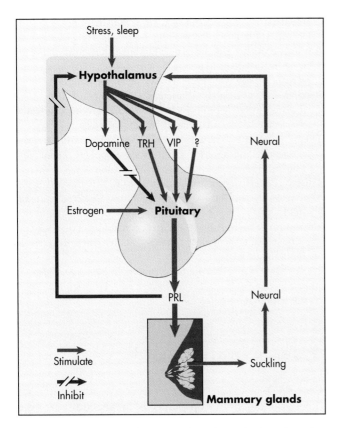

Figure 44-12 Regulation of PRL secretion. The predominant hypothalamic influence is normally inhibitory via dopamine. Pregnancy, high estrogen levels, and nursing (sucking) are the major physiological stimulators. *VIP,* Vasoactive intestinal peptide.

connections to the hypothalamus leads to a great increase in PRL secretion, whereas the secretion rate of all other anterior pituitary hormones decreases. **Dopamine** released from the median eminence into the portal veins is the major hypothalamic inhibitory factor that suppresses the release and synthesis of PRL. An additional PRL-inhibiting factor may be a copeptide synthesized with the hypothalamic peptide: LH-releasing hormone. Short-loop negative feedback also operates because PRL inhibits its own secretion by stimulating the synthesis and release of hypothalamic dopamine (Figure 44-12).

The hypothalamus is also the source of PRL-releasing factors. Thyrotropin-releasing hormone (TRH) strongly stimulates the synthesis and release of PRL by acting through its receptors in mammotrophs. However, TRH probably does not primarily mediate the PRL response to nursing. Numerous other hypothalamic peptides, such as vasoactive intestinal peptide (VIP), have PRL-releasing activity, but their roles are unknown.

Actions of prolactin

PRL PARTICIPATES IN STIMULATING THE ORIGINAL DIFFERENTIATION OF BREAST TISSUE AND ITS FURTHER EXPANSION DURING PREGNANCY. IT IS THE PRINCIPAL HORMONE RESPONSIBLE FOR LACTOGENESIS (MILK PRODUCTION). Together with estrogen, progesterone, cortisol, and GH, PRL stimulates the proliferation and branching of the breast ducts. During pregnancy, PRL, estrogen, and progesterone cause the development of glandular tissue (alveoli), within which milk production will occur. After parturition, milk synthesis and secretion require PRL along with cortisol and insulin.

PRL acts by combining with a plasma membrane receptor similar to that of GH and subsequently activating intracytoplasmic tyrosine kinases. The result is a rapid transcription of RNAs for the milk proteins (casein, lactalbumin, and β-lactoglobulin) and enzymes such as galactosyl transferase—all of which are necessary for the synthesis of lactose, the major sugar in milk. These actions are antagonized by estrogen and progesterone.

A second area of PRL action may be on the reproductive axis. An excess of PRL blocks the synthesis and release of gonadotropin-releasing hormone and thus inhibits gonadotropin secretion. PRL also has immunomodulatory actions.

> Although the exact role of PRL in normal human reproduction is uncertain, an excess of PRL from a pituitary tumor has major consequences. Because the secretion of pituitary gonadotropins is suppressed, ovulation and menstruation are prevented in women, and spermatogenesis is blocked in men. Nonpregnant women secrete milk, and men may have breast enlargement. Surgical removal of the tumor and treatment with dopamine agonists reverse these effects.

SUMMARY

- The hypothalamic-pituitary unit regulates water metabolism, growth, lactation, and the functions of the thyroid gland, adrenal glands, and gonads.
- Peptide hormones synthesized in some hypothalamic neurons pass down their axons to be stored in and released into the circulation from the posterior pituitary gland. Other hypothalamic peptides travel down axons to the median eminence, from which they are released into a portal venous circulation that carries them to the anterior pituitary gland. There, they stimulate or inhibit the release of target hormones.
- Hypothalamic releasing and inhibiting peptides are secreted in pulses and induce effects via Ca^{++}, cyclic AMP, and phosphatidylinositol products as messengers. They stimulate or inhibit transcription, modulate translation, and stimulate or inhibit the secretion of target anterior pituitary hormones.

- The anterior pituitary gland contains five functional cell types: thyrotrophs, adrenocorticotrophs, gonadotrophs, somatotrophs, and mammotrophs.
- ADH is a small peptide that is synthesized in the hypothalamus and is secreted from the posterior pituitary in response to an increase in plasma osmolality or to a decrease in plasma volume or blood pressure.
- ADH acts on renal tubule cells using cyclic AMP as a second messenger to increase the reabsorption of free water and thus the final urine osmolality.
- OCT is structurally similar to ADH, but it acts specifically on the mammary gland to cause the release of milk. It is secreted in response to suckling.
- GH is a protein hormone with anabolic effects. It stimulates cartilage development, bone growth, and the accretion of lean body mass, largely via a peptide mediator (IGF, or somatomedin) produced in the liver and many other target cells.
- GH secretion is stimulated by GHRH and inhibited by somatostatin. Glucose, free fatty acids, and the peripheral mediator IGF inhibit GH secretion.
- GH excess produces the disease acromegaly. GH deficiency in childhood leads to short stature and delayed maturation.
- PRL is structurally similar to GH, but it specifically stimulates the growth of mammary glands and the production of milk. Normally, PRL is tonically inhibited by dopamine from the hypothalamus.

BIBLIOGRAPHY

Amato G et al: Body composition, bone metabolism, and heart structure and function in growth hormone (GH) deficient adults before and after GH replacement therapy at low doses, *J Clin Endocrinol Metab* 77:1671, 1993.

Brixen K et al: A short course of recombinant human growth hormone treatment stimulates osteoblasts and activates bone remodeling in normal human volunteers, *J Bone Miner Res* 5:609, 1990.

Corpas E, Harman SM, Blackman MR: Human growth hormone and human aging, *Endocr Rev* 14:20, 1993.

Daughaday WH, Rotwein P: Insulin-like growth factors I and II: peptide, messenger ribonucleic acid and gene structures, serum, and tissue concentrations, *Endocrinol Rev* 10:68, 1989.

Horseman ND, Yu-Lee L-Y: Transcriptional regulation by the helix bundle peptide hormones: growth hormone, prolactin, and hematopoietic cytokines, *Endocr Rev* 15:627, 1994.

Kelly PA et al: The prolactin/growth hormone receptor family, *Endocr Rev* 12:235, 1991.

Kerrigan JR, Rogol AD: The impact of gonadal steroid hormone action on growth hormone secretion during childhood and adolescence, *Endocr Rev* 13:281, 1992.

Knepper MA: Molecular physiology of urinary concentrating mechanism: regulation of aquaporin water channels by vasopressin, *Am J Physiol* 272:F3, 1997.

Lamberts SW, Macleod RM: Regulation of prolactin secretion at the level of the lactotroph, *Physiol Rev* 70:279, 1990.

Müller EE: Role of neurotransmitters and neuromodulators in the control of anterior pituitary hormone secretion. In DeGroot LJ, ed, *Endocrinology,* ed 3, Philadelphia, 1995, WB Saunders.

Reeves WB, Bichet DB, Anderoli TE: The posterior pituitary and water metabolism. In Foster D, Wilson J, eds: *Williams textbook of endocrinology,* ed 9, Philadelphia, 1998, WB Saunders.

Riskind PN, Martin JB: Functional anatomy of the hypothalamic-anterior pituitary complex. In Degroot LJ, ed: *Endocrinology,* ed 3, Philadelphia, 1995, WB Saunders.

Theill LE, Karin M: Transcriptional control of growth hormone expression and anterior pituitary development, *Endocr Rev* 14:670, 1993.

Thissen JP, Ketelslegers JM, Underwood LE: Nutritional regulation of the insulin-like growth factors, *Endocr Rev* 15:80, 1994.

Thompson CJ, Selby P, Baylis PH: Reproducibility of osmotic and nonosmotic tests of vasopressin secretion in men, *Am J Physiol* 260:R533, 1991.

Thorner MO et al: The anterior pituitary. In Foster D, Wilson J, eds: *Williams textbook of endocrinology,* ed 9, Philadelphia, 1998, WB Saunders.

▶ CASE STUDIES

Case 44-1

A 49-year-old man complains of headache, sore feet from wearing the same shoes too many years ("Could my feet be growing?"), and a change in his facial appearance. His dentist has had to remake dental plates frequently. The patient's features appear coarse, and his hands are large and spade-like. Investigation for acromegaly reveals a very elevated plasma GH level and a very large pituitary tumor on magnetic resonance imaging.

1. **Which of the following genetic abnormalities could have produced this condition?**
   - **A.** A mutant hyperactivating IGF gene
   - **B.** A mutant hyperactivating IGF receptor gene
   - **C.** A mutant inactivating IGF-1 gene
   - **D.** A mutant hyperactivating GHRH receptor gene
   - **E.** A mutant inactivating IGF-1 receptor gene

2. **Assuming the pituitary lesion is a monoclonal autonomous secreting GH-producing tumor, which of the following would you expect to find?**
   - **A.** Increased GHRH release and increased IGF release
   - **B.** Decreased GHRH release and decreased IGF release
   - **C.** Decreased GHRH release and increased IGF release
   - **D.** Increased GHRH release and decreased IGF release
   - **E.** No change in GHRH or IGF release

3. **Which of the following metabolic changes from normal would be expected in the patient if he was**

maintained on a constant isocaloric and fixed-protein diet?

A. Decreased levels of IGF-1 binding protein

B. Decreased levels of urea in urine

C. Decreased plasma glucose levels after an oral glucose load

D. Decreased plasma insulin levels after an oral glucose load

E. Decreased plasma GH levels after an oral glucose load

Case 44-2

A 17-year-old girl sustains a severe head injury in a motorcycle accident and is virtually comatose for 3 days, requiring intravenous fluids (5% glucose in water) for maintenance. Beginning on the second day, she is noted to have a sharp increase in urine volume to 8 L/day. A quick check shows no glucose in her urine.

1. Which of the following would be expected?

A. Decreased serum osmolality

B. Decreased serum sodium levels

C. Decreased blood urea nitrogen levels

D. Increased plasma atrial natriuretic hormone levels

E. Decreased urine osmolality

2. The patient is treated with an intravenous infusion of ADH. This would result in which of the following?

A. Decreased cyclic AMP levels in urine

B. Increased blood pressure

C. Increased serum osmolality

D. Decreased serum potassium levels

E. Decreased plasma cortisol levels

CHAPTER 45

Thyroid Gland

OBJECTIVES

- Explain the synthesis of thyroid hormones and the unique role of iodide therein.
- Explicate the regulation of thyroid hormone secretion by the hypothalamic–anterior pituitary axis and the reciprocal negative feedback of thyroid hormone on this axis.
- Describe how binding to serum proteins and the metabolism of thyroid hormone are important determinants of the hormone's effect on tissue.
- Describe the overriding effects of thyroid hormone on general metabolic processes.
- Delineate the profound effects of thyroid hormone on human physical and mental development.

The thyroid gland was the first endocrine gland to be recognized as such. Its absence or enlargement was correlated with altered biological findings at distant body sites, providing the clue that it produces a substance reaching tissue targets via the bloodstream. Extracts of the thyroid gland were subsequently shown to correct the striking disease state that resulted from its absence. The thyroid gland produces two hormones, **thyroxine (T_4)** and **triiodothyronine (T_3),** at a rather steady pace. THESE HORMONES INCREASE THE RATE OF BASAL O_2 USE AND METABOLISM AND THE CONSEQUENT RATE OF HEAT PRODUCTION SO THAT THEY ARE ADJUSTED TO ALTERATIONS IN ENERGY NEED, CALORIC SUPPLY, AND ENVIRONMENTAL TEMPERATURE. Thyroid hormones concordantly modulate the delivery of substrates and O_2 by the cardiovascular and respiratory systems to sustain the metabolic rate in target tissues. The actions of thyroid hormone are critical for the normal growth and maturation of the fetus and the child. Virtually all other previously described organ systems in the body are affected by thyroid hormone.

Functional Anatomy

The thyroid gland develops from the endoderm of the pharyngeal gut. The gland descends to the anterior neck, where it lies adjacent to both sides of the trachea and can often be palpated (Figure 45-1, *A*). It can also be visualized using several imaging techniques (e.g., ultrasonography). By 12 weeks of human gestation, the gland synthesizes and secretes thyroid hormones under the stimulus of the fetal hypothalamus and pituitary gland. THIS ENTIRE AXIS IS REQUIRED FOR SUBSEQUENT NORMAL INTRAUTERINE DEVELOPMENT OF THE CENTRAL NERVOUS SYSTEM AND SKELETON because neither maternal thyroid hormone nor its pituitary-stimulating hormone can cross the placenta in sufficient quantities after the first trimester.

The thyroid gland in adults weighs approximately 20 g. The histological structure is shown schematically in Figure 45-1, *B*. The cuboidal endocrine cells are surrounded by a basement membrane, and they form single-layered circular **follicles.** The lumina of the follicles contain thyroid hormones stored in the form of a **colloid** material. When stimulated, the endocrine cells enlarge and assume a columnar shape with the nuclei at their base. Because it is undergoing resorption, the colloid material in the lumen appears scalloped. Also scattered within the thyroid gland are the parafollicular cells, or C-cells, which secrete calcitonin (see Chapter 43).

The synthesis and secretion of thyroid hormones is a stepwise process requiring iodine

Thyroid hormones are unique in that they incorporate an inorganic element, iodine, into an organic structure made up of two molecules of the amino acid tyrosine. The secretory products of the thyroid gland are known as **iodothyronines.** THE MAJOR PRODUCT IS **3,5,3′,5′-TETRAIODOTHYRONINE,** KNOWN AS **THYROXINE** AND REFERRED TO AS **T_4.** This molecule functions largely as a circulating prohormone. Secreted in much less quantity is **3,5,3′-triiodothyronine,** known simply as **triiodothyronine** and referred to as **T_3.** This molecule, which provides almost all thyroid hormone activity in target cells, is produced mostly in various tissues from the circulating supply of the prohormone T_4. A trivial secretory product with no identified hormonal action is **3,3′,5′-triiodothyronine.** This is known as **reverse T_3 (rT_3)** because it differs from T_3 only in the location of one of the three iodine atoms. This inactive molecule is an alternative product of the prohormone T_4 and is produced when less thyroid hormone action is needed. The structures of T_4, T_3, and rT_3 are shown in Figure 45-2.

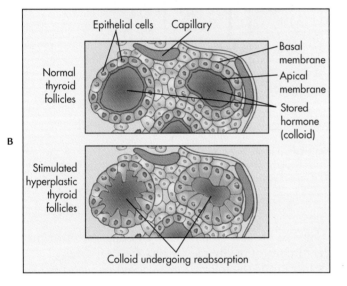

Figure 45-1 A, The anterior location of the thyroid gland permits visualization and palpation when it is enlarged and forms a goiter. **B,** Basic thyroid unit. A normal follicle consists of a central core of colloid material surrounded by a single layer of cuboidal cells. When stimulated by thyrotropin, the cells elongate, and the central core becomes scalloped because of resorption of the colloid.

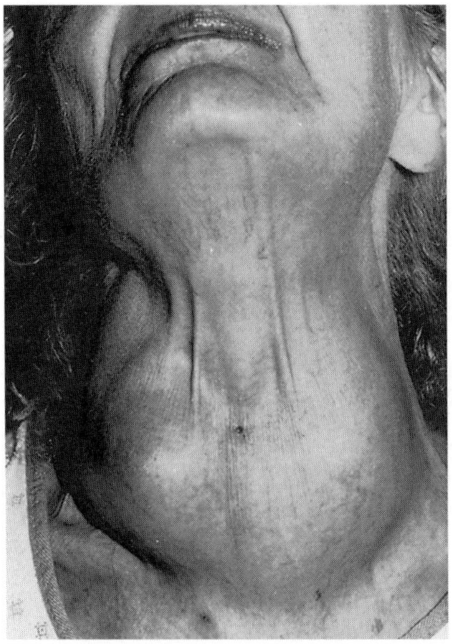

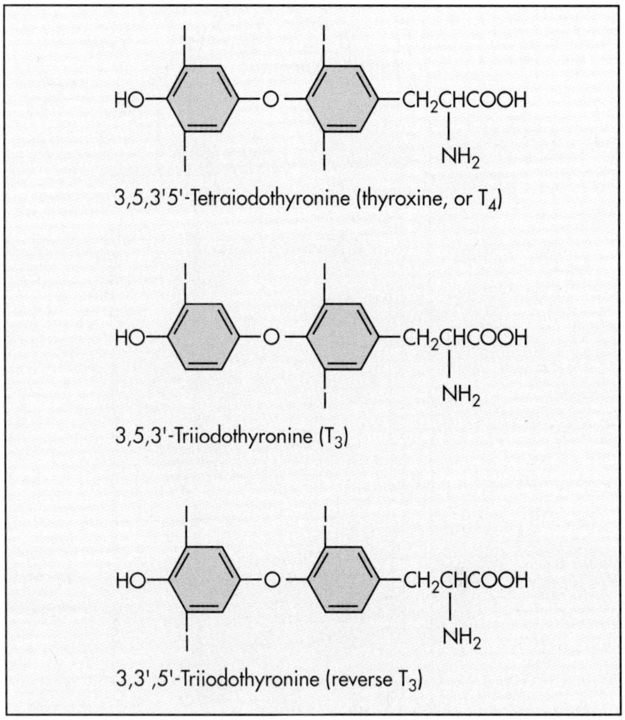

Figure 45-2 Structures of T_4, T_3, and rT_3. Note that T_3 and rT_3 differ only in the position from which an iodine atom was removed from T_4.

thyroglobulin, and their release into the circulation requires proteolytic cleavage of the peptide bonds.

Step 1: Iodide metabolism is an intrinsic component of thyroid hormone synthesis

Iodide is an essential dietary element because of its thyroid role. The minimum daily iodide requirement for hormone synthesis is about 75 μg. In the United States the average daily intake is 300 to 400 μg, and almost the same amount is excreted in the urine. About 80 μg, or 20% of the extrathyroidal iodide pool, is taken up daily by the gland. With iodide deficiency the extrathyroidal pool size shrinks; however, the gland can increase the daily percentage uptake to 80% to 90% and thereby still acquire sufficient iodide for hormone synthesis. A decrease in urinary excretion helps conserve iodide, as does the preferential synthesis of T_3 over T_4. Under steady-state conditions, about 80 μg of iodide is released from the gland daily, 90% in the form of T_4. The content of iodide within the thyroid gland is 100 times greater than the amount needed daily for hormone production. Because all this iodide is stored in the form of iodinated thyroglobulin, the human is protected for approximately 2 months from the effects of iodide deficiency.

IODIDE IS ACTIVELY TRANSPORTED INTO THE THYROID GLAND AGAINST CHEMICAL AND ELECTRICAL GRADIENTS BY AN Na^+-I^- COTRANSPORT SYSTEM LOCATED IN THE BASAL MEMBRANE OF THE CELLS (see Chapter 36). This process, known as the **iodide trap,** maintains a high ratio of free iodide concen-

Three major steps are involved in the synthesis of thyroid hormones: (1) the uptake and concentration of iodide within the gland, (2) the oxidation and incorporation of the iodide into the phenol ring of tyrosine, and (3) the coupling of two iodinated tyrosine molecules to form either T_4 or T_3 (Figure 45-3).

Before iodination and coupling, the tyrosine molecules must first be incorporated by standard peptide linkage into a protein known as **thyroglobulin.** Thyroglobulin is the substance actually iodinated on specific constituent tyrosines that are brought into proximity for coupling by the three-dimensional structure of the protein. The thyroid hormones formed remain in peptide linkage within

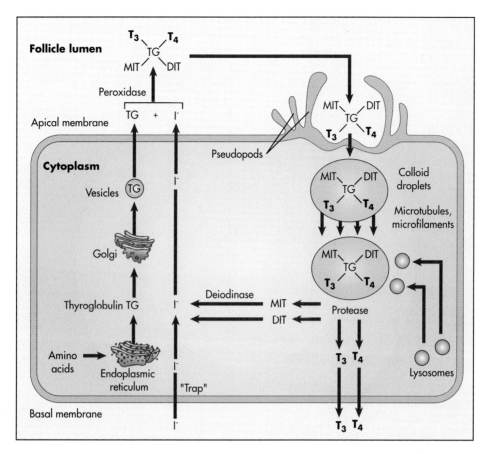

Figure 45-3 Thyroid hormone synthesis and release. T_4 and T_3 synthesis occurs within the protein molecule thyroglobulin *(TG)* at the border of the cytoplasm and the follicle lumen. The retrieval of stored hormone requires endocytosis of the colloid followed by intracytoplasmic proteolysis by lysosomes. Iodide in the precursor molecules monoiodotyrosine *(MIT)* and diiodotyrosine *(DIT)* is recovered by the action of the enzyme deiodinase.

tration in the gland to the iodide concentration in the plasma. The trapping mechanism for iodide requires energy generation via oxidative phosphorylation and is linked to Na^+,K^+-ATPase. Various anions, such as thiocyanate (CNS^-), perchlorate (ClO_4^-), and pertechnetate (TcO_4^-), act as competitive inhibitors of iodide transport.

Small increases in dietary iodide intake lead to increases in the rate of thyroid hormone synthesis. However, as the daily dosage of iodide exceeds 2000 μg, the intraglandular concentration of free iodide or some iodinated product reaches a level that inhibits the iodide trap and the biosynthetic mechanism; thus the hormone production declines back to normal. A severe lack of dietary iodide (endemic in certain parts of the world) ultimately leads to thyroid hormone deficiency despite maximal operation of the iodide trap.

Step 2: Tyrosine is iodinated within a storage protein called thyroglobulin

Thyroglobulin is a large glycoprotein that is synthesized as two separate peptide units. These combine and are then glycosylated in transit to the Golgi apparatus. The completed protein, incorporated in small vesicles,

moves to the apical membrane and then into the adjacent lumen of the follicle (Figure 45-3).

Just inside the follicle lumen, iodide is incorporated into particular tyrosine molecules at specific sites within thyroglobulin. An enzyme complex known as **thyroid peroxidase** is bound to and traverses the apical membrane. This hemoprotein enzyme simultaneously catalyzes the oxidation of iodide and its substitution for a hydrogen in the benzene ring of tyrosine. The immediate oxidant of iodide is hydrogen peroxide (H_2O_2). This is probably generated via the reduction of O_2 by reduced nicotinamide adenosine dinucleotide phosphate (NADPH) and flavoproteins. Both monoiodotyrosine (MIT) and diiodotyrosine (DIT) result from iodination.

Step 3: Two iodinated tyrosine molecules are combined to form an iodothyronine molecule

The coupling of two iodinated tyrosines is also carried out within thyroglobulin by the same enzyme, peroxidase. One DIT molecule is juxtaposed either with another DIT molecule to form T_4 or with an MIT molecule to form T_3. The tertiary structure of thyroglobulin facilitates these juxtapositions. The usual ratio of T_4 to T_3 in the gland is 10:1. When iodide availability is restricted or when the thyroid gland is hyperstimulated, the formation of T_3 is favored; in this way, relatively more active hormone is provided.

Step 4: Secretion of thyroid hormone requires its retrieval from storage in the follicle

Once thyroglobulin has been iodinated, it is stored within the follicle as **colloid.** The release of peptide-bonded T_4 and T_3 into the bloodstream first requires the retrieval of the thyroglobulin, which is transferred from the lumen of the follicle into the endocrine cell via **micropinocytosis** or **endocytosis** (Figure 45-3). In this process, the cell membrane forms pseudopods that engulf a pocket of colloid that is pinched off by the cell membrane and becomes a colloid droplet within the cytoplasm. The droplet moves in a basal direction, probably as a result of microtubule and microfilament function. At the same time, lysosomes move from the base toward the apex of the cell and fuse with the colloid droplets. Lysosomal proteases then release free T_4 and T_3, which leave the cell through the basal membrane and enter the adjacent capillary blood (Figure 45-3).

The uncoupled MIT and DIT molecules, which are also released from thyroglobulin, are rapidly deiodinated within the cell by the enzyme **deiodinase** (Figure 45-3). Because these compounds are metabolically inactive and if secreted, would be lost in the urine, their deiodination conserves iodide for recycling into hormone synthesis. Normally, only minor amounts of intact thyroglobulin itself leave the cell.

> Any step in the sequence from iodide trapping to thyroglobulin proteolysis may be defective in congenital biosynthetic disorders, and these defects result in thyroid hormone deficiency. A group of drugs known as **thiouracils** block the enzyme peroxidase and are very useful in treating states of thyroid hyperfunction. A large excess of iodide itself, its competitive anion perchlorate, or lithium (widely used in the treatment of manic-depressive disorders) also inhibits T_4 synthesis. Iodide is sometimes used to treat **hyperthyroidism** for short periods until more definitive therapy takes hold.

Thyroid Gland Activity Is Regulated by the Hypothalamus and Anterior Pituitary Gland

The thyroid gland is the effector component of a classic hypothalamic–anterior pituitary–peripheral gland axis (Figure 45-4) (see Chapter 44). The major stimulator of thyroid hormone secretion is **thyrotropin,** or **thyroid-stimulating hormone (TSH),** which is secreted by the anterior pituitary gland. The direct stimulator of TSH secretion is **thyrotropin-releasing hormone (TRH)** from the hypothalamus. Via negative feedback, the thy-

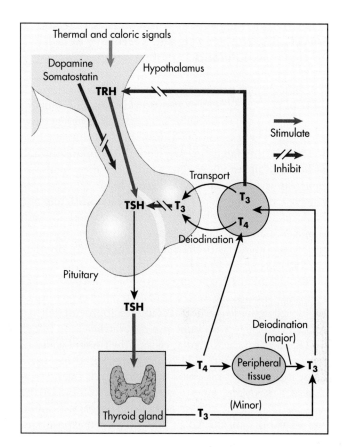

Figure 45-4 Hypothalamic-pituitary-thyroid axis. Thyrotropin-releasing hormone *(TRH)* stimulates the release of thyrotropin *(TSH)* from the pituitary gland. Thyrotropin stimulates T_4 secretion and to a minor degree T_3 secretion by the thyroid gland. T_3 arising from T_4 in peripheral tissues or within the pituitary gland itself blocks the effect of thyrotropin-releasing hormone and suppresses the release of thyrotropin via negative feedback. Dopamine and somatostatin also tonically inhibit thyrotropin release.

roid hormones T_4 and T_3 inhibit the synthesis and release of TSH from the pituitary gland as well as TRH synthesis and release from the hypothalamus.

Thyrotropin-releasing hormone stimulates the synthesis and release of thyroid-stimulating hormone

TRH is a tripeptide, pyroglutamine-histidine-proline-amide. The TRH gene codes for a large precursor molecule that contains the small tetrapeptide glutamine-histidine-proline-glycine. After translation, the glutamic acid undergoes cyclization, and the terminal glycine is replaced with an amino group. TRH is stored in the median eminence (see Chapter 44) and reaches its target cells via the pituitary portal vein. TRH binding to its plasma membrane receptor triggers increases in calcium and phosphatidylinositol product second messengers, which elicit TSH release via exocytosis. Prolonged stimulation with TRH also increases TSH synthesis and via glycosylation, its bioactivity. TRH eventually down-regulates its own receptors and thereby diminishes its effectiveness.

Thyrotropin stimulates numerous processes involved in the growth and secretory activity of the thyroid gland

TSH is a glycoprotein hormone whose molecular weight is 28,000. It is composed of two peptide subunits, each of which is coded for by separate genes on two different chromosomes. The α subunit is "nonspecific" because it is also part of two unrelated pituitary hormones (luteinizing and follicle-stimulating hormones) and chorionic gonadotropin from the placenta, all with reproductive function. In contrast, the β subunit of TSH is completely different and contains the specific biologically active sites of the hormone. Nonetheless, via noncovalent forces, the β-subunit must be combined with the α subunit for TSH to stimulate thyroid cells.

TSH circulates in concentrations of about 10^{-11} M. For technical reasons, these are usually reported in units of biological activity; the normal range is approximately 0.4 to 5.5 μU/ml. The α subunit also circulates.

TSH acts on the follicular cells of the thyroid gland to produce many effects, which are summarized in Figure 45-5. THE PROCESSES OF IODIDE TRAPPING AND OF EACH STEP IN T_4 AND T_3 SYNTHESIS, AS WELL AS THE ENDOCYTOSIS OF COLLOID AND THE PROTEOLYTIC RELEASE OF T_4 AND T_3 FROM THE GLAND, ARE ALL RAPIDLY STIMULATED BY TSH. Sustained exposure to TSH leads to hyperplasia and hypertrophy of the follicular cells (Figure 45-1, *B*), which is manifested by increases in endoplasmic reticulum, ribosomes, the size and complexity of the Golgi apparatus, and DNA synthesis. In the absence of TSH the gland atrophies, although it still maintains a low basal level of thyroid hormone secretion. The

trophic effects of TSH on the thyroid gland may be mediated by the local generation of growth factors such as insulin growth factors (IGF-1, IGF-2) (see Chapter 44). TSH binding to its plasma membrane receptor activates adenylyl cyclase via a stimulatory G protein (see Chapter 5). Cyclic AMP then mediates the stimulation of iodide uptake by the cell. The phosphatidylinositol system may participate with cyclic AMP in rapidly stimulating the peroxidase-catalyzed subsequent steps in thyroid hormone synthesis. Concurrently, TSH increases glucose oxidation, which may provide the NADPH needed for the peroxidase reaction. After several hours, TSH increases nucleic acid, protein, and phospholipid synthesis, actions that underlie the growth-promoting effects of TSH.

> The trophic effects of TSH are commonly expressed pathophysiologically. A genetic biosynthetic defect, an acquired impairment of thyroid hormone synthesis caused by inflammation or drugs, and iodide deficiency all increase TSH secretion via negative feedback. Chronic stimulation of the thyroid gland by TSH hypersecretion may then produce a spectacular enlargement of the gland, known as a **goiter** (Figure 45-1, *A*).

Thyroid hormone output is under sensitive feedback control

Negative feedback keeps plasma levels of T_4 and T_3 relatively constant. INCREASES AND DECREASES IN THYROID HORMONE LEVELS OF ONLY 10% TO 30% ARE ENOUGH TO CHANGE TSH LEVELS (AND THEIR RESPONSE TO TRH) IN THE OPPOSITE DIRECTION. NEGATIVE FEEDBACK IS EXERTED PREDOMINANTLY AT THE PITUITARY LEVEL (Figure 45-4).

> Individuals with long-standing deficiencies of thyroid hormone from thyroid gland disease have high plasma TSH levels as well as enlarged pituitary glands that contain increased numbers of thyrotroph cells and an elevated TSH content. Conversely, a pathological excess of thyroid hormone causes very low plasma TSH levels and atrophy of the thyrotroph cells.

The effector molecule of negative feedback is T_3, which can enter the thyrotroph cell from the plasma. However, the T_3 generated within the pituitary gland from the deiodination of T_4 taken up from the plasma is more important (Figure 45-4). T_3 suppresses TSH release, represses expression of the TSH gene, and downregulates TRH receptors.

TSH secretion is also tonically inhibited by dopamine and somatostatin from the hypothalamus. Cortisol and growth hormone reduce TSH secretion as well, the latter probably by stimulating somatostatin release (see Chapter 44).

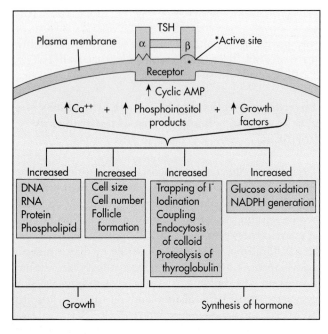

Figure 45-5 TSH actions on the thyroid cell. Cyclic AMP along with Ca^{++} and phosphoinositol products act as second messengers generated by TSH binding to its receptor. All steps in thyroid hormone production, as well as many aspects of thyroid cell metabolism and growth, are stimulated by TSH. α, α Subunit; β, β subunit.

The operation of the hypothalamic-pituitary-thyroid axis results in a slightly pulsatile plasma TSH level and steady plasma T_4 and T_3 levels. This befits hormones, whose actions on metabolism wax and wane slowly. Physiological conditions that alter TSH levels (and therefore T_4 and T_3 levels) are consonant with the action of thyroid hormones on energy use and thermogenesis. During total fasting, TSH responsiveness to TRH stimulation and possibly TRH release itself are diminished; T_3 levels also fall. This coincides with an advantageous decrease in the resting metabolic rate (see Chapter 41). In contrast, the ingestion of excess calories, especially carbohydrates, tends to increase T_3 availability. In animals, exposure to cold increases the secretion of TSH and thyroid hormone. In humans, this response is observed shortly after birth, when the change in temperature from the maternal to external environment is accompanied by a sharp rise in plasma TSH and T_4 levels. The latter remains above adult levels for some weeks.

The Metabolism of Thyroid Hormone Contributes to Its Actions

T_4 serves largely as a prohormone for T_3, but T_4 also provides some intrinsic intracellular action of its own. The average daily secretion of T_4 is 90 µg. The circulating storage function of plasma T_4 is reflected in its large pool size and long half-life (6 days). In contrast, the major portion of T_3 (35 µg per day) and virtually all rT_3 come from the deiodination of circulating T_4. T_3 has a much smaller pool size and a shorter half-life (1 day). Average plasma concentrations are:

T_4	8 µg/dl
T_3	0.12 µg/dl
rT_3	0.04 µg/dl

> The replacement of thyroid hormone in deficient individuals is almost always carried out with the prohormone T_4 and not with the more active metabolite, T_3. This is done to mimic the physiological situation. The biochemical targets are a normal level of T_4 and a reduction to normal (via negative feedback) of elevated TSH levels.

Protein binding of thyroid hormones determines their availability to tissues

T_4 and T_3 circulate almost entirely bound to proteins. The major binding protein is **thyroxine-binding globulin (TBG),** a glycoprotein that is synthesized in the liver. Each TBG molecule binds one molecule of T_4. About 70% of T_4 and T_3 is bound to TBG. The remainder is bound to **transthyretin** (thyroxine-binding prealbumin) and albumin. Transthyretin, which has a lower affinity for T_4 than TBG, more readily transfers the hormone to target cells by

dissociation. By creating a circulating reservoir of T_4, TBG and transthyretin buffer against acute changes in thyroid gland function. Even the sudden addition to the plasma of an entire day's thyroid gland output would cause only a 10% increase in the circulating T_4 concentration. After removal of the gland, it would take nearly 1 week for the plasma T_4 concentration to fall 50%.

Only 0.03% of total T_4 and 0.3% of total T_3 are in the free state. However, these are the critical biologically active fractions. Free T_4 and T_3 not only exert the thyroid hormone effects on target tissues but are also responsible for pituitary feedback. A chemical equilibrium between T_4 and TBG governs the distribution of the hormone between the free T_4 and bound $T_4 \cdot$ TBG fractions:

$$T_4 + TBG \leftrightarrow T_4 \cdot TBG \qquad \textbf{45-1}$$

$$Keq = \frac{[T_4 \cdot TBG]}{[T_4][TBG]} \qquad \textbf{45-2}$$

$$\frac{Free\ T_4}{Bound\ T_4} = \frac{[T_4]}{[T_4 \cdot TBG]} = \frac{1}{Keq[TBG]} \qquad \textbf{45-3}$$

where K_{eq} is the equilibrium constant.

A temporary decrease in free T_4 caused by a decrease in thyroid gland secretion can be rapidly reversed via a dissociation of bound T_4 (see Equation 45-1). Likewise, a temporary increase in free T_4 can be rapidly compensated for by the association of the excess T_4 with TBG, which has additional unoccupied binding sites. Sustained decreases or increases in the daily T_4 supply caused by thyroid disease, however, eventually lead to sustained alterations in both the bound and free fractions.

A primary change in the TBG concentration itself disturbs the ratio of free to bound T_4 (see Equation 45-3). In this situation the normal thyroid gland must increase or decrease its rate of hormone secretion until the new equilibrium state restores the absolute free T_4 level to normal.

> Acute hepatic disease, pregnancy, or estrogen therapy raises serum TBG levels. In severe chronic hepatic disease (such as **cirrhosis**) or kidney disease (such as the **nephrotic syndrome**), serum TBG levels fall, because of either reduced synthesis or loss of TBG in the urine. Any resultant changes in free T_4 levels are transient because negative feedback alters TSH secretion and thyroid gland secretion so that free T_4 levels can be restored to normal.

The metabolic fate of thyroid hormones determines their action

The liver, kidney, and skeletal muscle are the major sites of degradation of thyroid hormones. The rate of disposal of T_4 is proportional to the free T_4 concentration in plasma.

Because T_4 is only 25% as hormonally active as T_3, the initial step of converting it either to the active metabolite

T_3 (by outer-ring deiodination [Figure 45-2]) or to the inactive metabolite rT_3 (by inner-ring deiodination) is an important means of adjusting thyroid hormone action on tissues. Normally, the split between T_3 and rT_3 is equal. When it is physiologically desirable to have more thyroid hormone action, as in exposure to cold, more T_3 and less rT_3 are generated. The opposite, less T_3 and more rT_3, commonly occurs in critically ill persons and portends a poor outcome. The activity of the enzyme **5′ monodeiodinase**, which catalyzes the conversion of T_4 to T_3, is an important regulator of this distribution. The rare trace element, selenium, is necessary for the activity of this enzyme.

The Intracellular Actions of Thyroid Hormone Are Mediated by Nuclear Receptors and Changes in Gene Expression

T_4 and T_3 enter target cells via carrier-mediated, energy-dependent transport, after which most of the T_4 undergoes deiodination to T_3 (Figure 45-6). Both T_4 and T_3 are transferred to the nucleus, where T_3 binds to a nuclear receptor with much greater affinity than T_4. Two distinct forms of the T_3 receptor are expressed in a tissue-specific manner. The T_3 receptor complex interacts with DNA to stimulate or inhibit the transcription of numerous messenger RNAs. The latter then direct the increased or decreased synthesis of many specific proteins in different tissues. Examples include enzymes, growth hormone, myosin chains, TSH, and T_3 receptors.

> The critical importance of the T_3 receptor is clinically illustrated by individuals whose hypothyroidism is caused by resistance to thyroid hormone. These patients have either mutant receptors that are unable to transduce the hormone signal efficiently or a single allele for a mutant receptor that blocks T_3 binding to the normal receptor.

The quantitative responses of tissues to T_3 correlate well with their nuclear receptor content and with the degree of receptor occupancy (see Chapter 40). Normally, about half the available receptor sites are occupied by T_3. Because T_3 acts largely through gene transcription, a 12- to 48-hour delay occurs before its effects become evident in vivo. Several weeks of hormone replacement are required before all the consequences of a deficiency state are corrected.

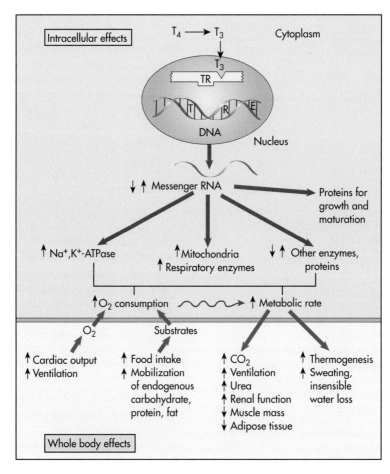

Figure 45-6 Thyroid hormone effects. *Top,* Intracellular actions resulting from T_3 binding to its nuclear receptor *(TR),* which is linked to thyroid regulatory elements *(TRE)* in target DNA molecules. *Bottom,* All the various whole body effects of thyroid hormone that sustain increased O_2 consumption and permit disposal of the excess CO_2, heat, and metabolic products.

THE MOST OBVIOUS EFFECT OF THYROID HORMONE IS TO STIMU-LATE O_2 CONSUMPTION AND SUBSTRATE USE (Figure 45-6). A number of mechanisms are probably involved. T_3 increases mitochondria's number, size, and membrane areas and increases the concentrations of certain key respiratory enzymes. T_3 also stimulates the activity of the Na^+,K^+-ATPase pump, which is responsible for membrane cation transport (see Chapter 1). Because large amounts of ATP are thereby consumed and much ADP is correspondingly generated by Na^+,K^+-ATPase, the extra ADP could be one "messenger" by which thyroid hormone stimulates mitochondrial O_2 use. Another possibility is that thyroid hormone simultaneously stimulates the synthesis and oxidation of fatty acids and glucose, processes that create futile, wasteful cycles requiring energy input and heat generation. In brain tissue, O_2 consumption is not stimulated by T_3, but the hormone increases the synthesis of specific structural and functional proteins.

The whole body actions of thyroid hormone subserve an increase in O_2 use

In humans, O_2 use at rest is approximately 225 to 250 ml/min (see Chapter 41). It falls to about 150 ml/min in the absence of thyroid hormone and can increase to 400 ml/min with thyroid hormone excess. Of necessity, thermogenesis and body temperature increase or decrease concomitantly with O_2 use. Temperature changes, however, are moderated by thyroid hormone–induced increases or decreases in heat loss through appropriate changes in cutaneous blood flow, sweating, and ventilation.

Thyroid hormone could not stimulate O_2 use for long without augmenting O_2 supply to the tissues (Figure 45-6). Thus thyroid hormone increases the resting rate of ventilation sufficiently to maintain a normal arterial O_2 pressure despite increased O_2 use and a normal CO_2 pressure in the face of increased CO_2 production. In addition, the O_2-carrying capacity of the blood is enhanced by a small increase in red cell mass.

ANOTHER IMPORTANT ACTION OF THYROID HORMONE IS TO IN-CREASE CARDIAC OUTPUT, WHICH ENSURES SUFFICIENT O_2 DELIV-ERY TO THE TISSUES. The resting heart rate and stroke volume are both increased, and the speed and force of myocardial contractions are enhanced (see Chapter 19). These effects are partly indirect, via adrenergic stimulation. However, thyroid hormone directly increases myocardial Ca^{++} uptake, adenylyl cyclase activity, and the active form of myosin-stimulated ATPase. The systolic blood pressure rises and diastolic blood pressure falls, reflecting the combined effects of the increased stroke volume with a substantial reduction in peripheral vascular resistance. The latter results from blood vessel dilation produced by the increased tissue metabolism (see Chapter 23).

The stimulation of O_2 use also requires the provision of substrates for oxidation. Thyroid hormone potentiates the stimulatory effects of other hormones on glucose absorption from the gastrointestinal tract, on gluconeogenesis, on lipolysis, on ketogenesis, and on proteolysis of the labile protein pool. THE OVERALL METABOLIC EFFECT OF THYROID HOR-MONE HAS THEREFORE APTLY BEEN DESCRIBED AS ACCELERATING THE METABOLIC RESPONSE TO STARVATION.

Thyroid hormone also stimulates the biosynthesis of cholesterol and its oxidation, conversion to bile acids, and biliary secretion. The net effect is to decrease the body pool and plasma level of cholesterol. The rate of metabolic disposal of steroid hormones, B vitamins, and administered drugs is increased. Therefore to maintain effective plasma levels of these substances in the presence of increased thyroid hormone, their endogenous production or their exogenous administration must be increased.

Thyroid hormone interacts with the sympathetic nervous system

A MAJOR INTERMEDIARY IN SOME THYROID HORMONE ACTIONS IS THE SYMPATHETIC NERVOUS SYSTEM. The activity of the sympathetic nervous system is diminished by thyroid hormone, as evidenced by decreased plasma levels and urinary excretion of the specific neurotransmitter, norepinephrine. However, the sensitivity of tissues to the thermogenic, lipolytic, glycogenolytic, and gluconeogenic effects of epinephrine and norepinephrine is enhanced. Thyroid hormone may modestly reinforce the cardiovascular responses to catecholamine hormones by increasing the number of β-adrenergic receptors, coupling them to adenylyl cyclase, and increasing cyclic AMP levels. In this manner, T_3 amplifies the induction of uncoupling protein (see Chapter 41) by norepinephrine in adipose tissue.

Hyperthyroidism presents a striking clinical picture because of the described effects. The increase in metabolic rate leads to weight loss, which is characteristically accompanied by an **increased** intake of food. The excessive generation of heat causes discomfort in warm environments, fever if the condition is severe, excessive sweating, thirst, and increased ventilation. Muscle weakness, atrophy, and even osteoporosis can result from increased protein degradation. The increase in β-adrenergic responsivity is manifested by tremor, nervousness, insomnia, and an anxious stare. The heart rate is rapid, atrial fibrillation may occur, and a high-cardiac-output form of heart failure may develop in extreme cases. The use of β-adrenergic antagonists ameliorates the sympathetic nervous system manifestations.

Thyroid hormone modulates skeletal growth and central nervous system development

IN HUMANS, THYROID HORMONE STIMULATES THE LINEAR GROWTH, DEVELOPMENT, AND MATURATION OF BONE. A direct effect of T_3 on the activity of chondrocytes in the growth plate of bone may result from increases in IGF production and activity (see Chapter 44). T_3 also accelerates growth by stimulating the secretion of growth hormone. Although thyroid hormone is not required for linear bone growth until after birth, it is already essential for maturation of the growth centers in fetal bones. The regular progression of tooth development and eruption depends on thyroid hormone, as does the normal renewal cycle of the epidermis and hair follicles. Because thyroid hormone stimulates degradative processes in structural and integumentary tissues, elevated levels cause the resorption of bone, which is manifested by increased urinary levels of hydroxyproline, an increased number of pyridinium cross-links (see Chapter 43), and accelerated shedding of the skin and hair. The synthesis of the mucopolysaccharides that form the intercellular ground substance is inhibited by thyroid hormone.

Normal skeletal muscle function also requires thyroid hormone. This may be related to the regulation of energy production and storage in this tissue. The muscle content of creatine phosphate is reduced by an excess of thyroid hormone.

THYROID HORMONE HAS CRITICAL EFFECTS ON THE DEVELOPMENT OF THE CENTRAL NERVOUS SYSTEM. If thyroid hormone is deficient in utero, growth of the cerebral and cerebellar cortex, the proliferation of axons and branching of dendrites, and myelinization are all impaired. Irreversible brain damage results when the deficiency of thyroid hormone is not recognized and treated immediately after birth. These ana-

tomical defects are paralleled by biochemical abnormalities. Without thyroid hormone, RNA and protein content, protein synthesis, the levels of enzymes necessary for DNA synthesis, the protein and lipid content of myelin, neurotransmitter receptors, and neurotransmitter synthesis are decreased in various areas of the brain. In children and adults, thyroid hormone enhances the speed and amplitude of reflexes, wakefulness, alertness, responsiveness to various stimuli, awareness of hunger, memory, and learning capacity. Normal emotional tone also depends on appropriate thyroid hormone levels.

> The clinical effects of hypothyroidism (Figure 45-7) may be severe, especially in a newborn, in whom the condition is known as **cretinism.** The central nervous system manifestations can include mental retardation and delayed developmental milestones such as sitting, standing, and walking. Lethargy, growth retardation, skeletal immaturity, and poor school performance occur. In children and adults the decreased metabolic rate causes intolerance of cold, decreased sweating, dry skin, a low cardiac output, and weight gain. The latter results from both excess adipose tissue and edema fluid that accumulates in association with ground substance mucopolysaccharides (Figure 45-7). All these abnormalities vanish with thyroid hor-

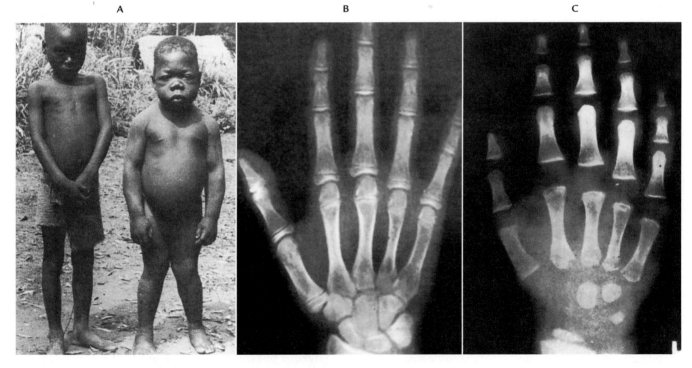

A   B   C

Figure 45-7 Normal 6-year-old child *(left)* and congenitally hypothyroid 17-year-old child *(right)* from the same village in an area of endemic cretinism **(A).** Note especially the short stature, obesity, malformed legs, and dull expression of the mentally retarded hypothyroid child. Other features are a prominent abdomen; a flat, broad nose, a hypoplastic mandible; dry, scaly skin; delayed puberty; and muscle weakness. Hand x-ray films of a 13-year-old normal child **(B)** and a 13-year-old hypothyroid child **(C).** Note that the hypothyroid child has a marked delay in development of the small bones of the hands, in growth centers at either end of the fingers, and in the growth center of the distal end of the radius. *(A from Delange FM. In Braverman LE, Utiger RD, eds:* Werner and Ingbar's the thyroid, *ed 7, Philadelphia, 1996, Lippincott-Raven.* **B** *from Tanner JM et al:* Assessment of skeletal maturity and prediction of adult height [TW2 method], *New York, 1975, Academic.* **C** *from Andersen HJ. In Gardner LI, ed:* Endocrine and genetic diseases of childhood and adolescence, *Philadelphia, 1975, WB Saunders.)*

> mone replacement (except any signs resulting from irreversible central nervous system damage).

Thyroid hormone contributes to the regulation of reproductive function in both genders. The normal process of sperm production; the ovarian cycle of follicular development, maturation, and ovulation; and the maintenance of a healthy pregnant state are all disrupted by significant deviations of thyroid hormone levels from normal. In part, these may be caused by alterations in the metabolism of sex steroid hormones.

Summary

- The basic endocrine unit of the thyroid gland is a follicle that consists of a single circular layer of epithelial cells surrounding a central lumen containing stored thyroid hormones (colloid). These hormones are tetraiodothyronine (thyroxine or T_4) and triiodothyronine (T_3).
- T_4 and T_3 are synthesized from tyrosine and iodine by the enzyme complex, peroxidase. The tyrosine is incorporated in peptide links within the protein thyroglobulin. After iodination, two iodotyrosine molecules are coupled to yield the iodothyronines.
- The secretion of stored T_4 and T_3 requires the retrieval of thyroglobulin from the follicle lumen via endocytosis. To support hormone synthesis, iodide is actively concentrated by the gland.
- Thyrotropin (TSH) acts on the thyroid gland, largely via cyclic AMP, to stimulate all steps in hormone production as well as growth of the epithelial cells. The secretion of TSH from the anterior pituitary is stimulated by thyrotropin-releasing hormone from the hypothalamus and is inhibited by T_4 and T_3.
- More than 99.5% of the T_4 and T_3 circulate bound to various proteins. Only the free fractions of T_4 and T_3 are biologically active.
- T_4 functions largely as a prohormone. Peripheral monodeiodination of the outer ring yields most of the T_3, which is the principal active hormone.
- Thyroid hormone increases the basal metabolic rate. A nuclear T_3-receptor complex interacts with many target DNA molecules to induce or suppress the synthesis of a variety of enzymes and other proteins. The result is to increase O_2 use and thermogenesis by numerous mechanisms.
- Additional important actions of thyroid hormone are to increase the heart rate, cardiac output, and ventilation and to decrease peripheral resistance. These subserve the increased tissue O_2 demand.
- Other effects of thyroid hormone on the central nervous system and skeleton are crucial to normal

growth and development. In the absence of thyroid hormone, brain development is retarded, and cretinism results. Linear growth is restricted, and the bones fail to mature normally.

BIBLIOGRAPHY

Brent GA: Mechanisms of disease: the molecular basis of thyroid hormone action, *N Engl J Med* 331:847, 1994.

Brown D et al: Amphibian metamorphosis: a complex program of gene expression changes controlled by the thyroid hormone, *Recent Prog Horm Res* 50:309, 1995.

Chin WW: Hormonal regulation of thyrotropin and gonadotropin gene expression, *Clin Res* 36:484, 1988.

Dunn AD: Release and secretion of thyroid hormone. In Braverman LE, Utiger RD, eds: *Werner and Ingbar's the thyroid,* ed 7, Philadelphia, 1996, Lippincott-Raven.

Kohn LD et al: The thyrotropin receptor, *Vitam Horm* 50:287, 1995.

Larsen PR, Silva JE, Kaplan MM: Relationships between circulating and intracellular thyroid hormones: physiological and clinical implications, *Endocr Rev* 2:87, 1981.

Lazar MA: Thyroid hormone receptors: multiple forms, multiple possibilities, *Endocr Rev* 14:184, 1993.

Mariotti S et al: The aging thyroid, *Endocr Rev* 16:686, 1995.

Oppenheimer JH, Schwartz HL, Strait KA: The molecular basis of thyroid hormone actions. In Braverman LE, Utiger RD, eds: *Werner and Ingbar's the thyroid,* ed 7, Philadelphia, 1996, Lippincott-Raven.

Polikar R et al: The thyroid and the heart, *Circulation* 87:1435, 1993.

Porterfield SP, Hendrich CE: The role of thyroid hormones in prenatal and neonatal neurological development: current perspectives, *Endocr Rev* 14:94, 1993.

Scanlon MF, Toft AD: Regulation of thyrotropin secretion. In Braverman LE, Utiger RD, eds: *Werner and Ingbar's the thyroid,* ed 7, Philadelphia, 1996, Lippincott-Raven.

Taurog A: Hormone synthesis: thyroid iodine metabolism. In Ingbar SH, Braverman LE, eds: *Werner and Ingbar's the thyroid,* Philadelphia, 1996, JB Lippincott.

Case Studies

Case 45-1

A 45-year-old recently divorced, obese male pharmacist complains of a rapid heart rate, a 20-pound weight loss in 2 months, and heat intolerance. His pulse rate is 110 beats/min at rest. The serum T_4 level is elevated, confirming the clinical impression of hyperthyroidism. On further questioning, the patient finally admits to taking large doses of exogenous T_4 tablets to help him lose weight so that he can more easily remarry.

1. Which of the following would be decreased?
    A. Serum T_3 levels
    B. Serum rT_3 levels
    C. Serum TSH levels
    D. Serum free T_4 levels
    E. Serum free T_3 levels

2. **Which one of the following cardiovascular factors would be increased?**
   - **A.** Cardiac β-adrenergic receptors
   - **B.** Muscle creatine phosphate levels
   - **C.** Plasma norepinephrine levels
   - **D.** Systemic vascular resistance
   - **E.** Diastolic blood pressure

3. **Which of the following might initially be increased in the thyroid gland?**
   - **A.** Iodide trap activity
   - **B.** Content of colloid
   - **C.** Peroxidase activity
   - **D.** Height of thyroid epithelial cells
   - **E.** Thyroglobulin synthesis

Case 45-2

A 16-month-old girl appears to be growing more slowly than normal. Her apathetic appearance alerts the pediatrician to the possibility of hypothyroidism. Her thyroid gland is greatly enlarged. Her serum T_4 level is low, and her serum TSH level is high.

1. **Which of the following could *not* be true?**
   - **A.** Iodide deficiency caused her hypothyroidism.
   - **B.** An inactive mutant peroxidase enzyme caused her hypothyroidism.
   - **C.** She has the skeletal maturation of a 22-month-old child.
   - **D.** She has excess body water.
   - **E.** She has made no attempt to walk.

2. **As a result of T_4 therapy, which of the following would be expected?**
   - **A.** Her heart rate would be reduced.
   - **B.** Her systolic blood pressure would be reduced.
   - **C.** Her height would be unchanged.
   - **D.** Her weight would be unchanged.
   - **E.** Her respiratory rate would be increased.

Adrenal Cortex

- Delineate the general biochemical pathway for the synthesis of all adrenal steroid hormones.
- Explain the complex regulation of adrenocortical function by the hypothalamic-pituitary-adrenal axis.
- Emphasize the extreme importance to life of the multiple effects of cortisol on body tissues.
- Describe the specific mechanisms of regulating aldosterone secretion in contrast to cortisol secretion.
- Explain how aldosterone affects kidney function and blood pressure.

Adrenal Hormones from Separate Anatomical Zones Regulate or Modulate Many Essential Physiological Processes

The adrenal glands are multifunctional endocrine organs that secrete a variety of hormones. Abundant experimental and clinical evidence has demonstrated that the adrenal glands are essential to life. THEIR SECRETIONS SUBSERVE A WIDE VARIETY OF PHYSIOLOGICAL FUNCTIONS, INCLUDING BLOOD GLUCOSE REGULATION; PROTEIN TURNOVER; FAT METABOLISM; SODIUM, POTASSIUM, AND CALCIUM BALANCE; MAINTENANCE OF CARDIOVASCULAR TONE; MODULATION OF TISSUE RESPONSE TO INJURY OR INFECTION; AND MOST IMPORTANT, SURVIVAL AS A RESULT OF STRESS. These actions require modulation of the other organ systems whose functions are described elsewhere in this book.

Each adrenal gland is located just above the ipsilateral kidney (Figure 46-1), and their combined weight is 6 to 10 g. Each gland is a combination of two separate functional entities (Figure 46-2). The outer zone, or **cortex,** comprises 80% to 90% of the weight. It is derived from mesodermal tissue and is the source of corticosteroid hormones. The inner zone, or **medulla,** comprises the other 10% to 20%. It is derived from neuroectodermal cells of the sympathetic ganglia and is the source of catecholamine hormones. Paracrine actions between the inner cortical cells and the neighboring medullary cells are possible. The adrenal glands have one of the highest rates of blood flow per gram of tissue. Arterial blood enters the outer cortex and breaks up into capillaries; venous drainage is into the medulla. This exposes the inner cells of the cortex and the cells of the medulla to high concentrations of steroid hormones from the outer cortex.

The outermost **zona glomerulosa** of the adrenal cortex is only a few cells thick (Figure 46-2). The middle **zona fasciculata** is the widest layer and consists of long cords of columnar cells. The innermost **zona reticularis** contains networks of interconnecting cells. TYPICAL STEROID-SECRETING CELLS ARE RICH IN LIPID DROPLETS AND CONTAIN NUMEROUS LARGE MITOCHONDRIA WITH VESICLES IN THEIR MEMBRANES.

The major hormones of the cortex are (1) the **glucocorticoid, cortisol,** which has critical roles in carbohydrate and protein metabolism and in the adaptation to stress; (2) the **mineralocorticoid, aldosterone,** which is vital to maintaining normal extracellular fluid volume and potassium levels; and (3) **sex steroid precursors,** which contribute to maintaining secondary sexual characteristics.

> The discovery and synthesis of cortisol were medical landmarks. Cortisol was lifesaving for patients whose adrenal glands were destroyed by disease, and it dramatically reversed their debilitation. Cortisol also has potent antiinflammatory and antiimmune effects that are used to treat diseases in which autoimmunity plays an important pathogenetic role and to prevent rejection of organ transplants.

The synthesis of corticosteroid hormones proceeds from cholesterol and is catalyzed by P-450 enzymes in the mitochondria and microsomes

THE PRECURSOR FOR ALL ADRENOCORTICAL HORMONES IS CHOLESTEROL, WHICH IS TAKEN UP FROM THE PLASMA VIA A SPECIFIC PLASMA MEMBRANE RECEPTOR FOR LOW-DENSITY LIPOPROTEINS (see Chapter 41). After transfer into the cell, the cholesterol is largely esterified and stored in vacuoles within the cytoplasm. Under basal conditions, cholesterol just taken up from plasma is immediately used for hormone synthesis. However, when hormone production is stimulated, stored cholesterol is rapidly mobilized and transferred to the mitochondria for the first synthetic step.

Most of the reactions in corticosteroid synthesis are catalyzed by **cytochrome P-450 enzymes** (Figure 46-3).

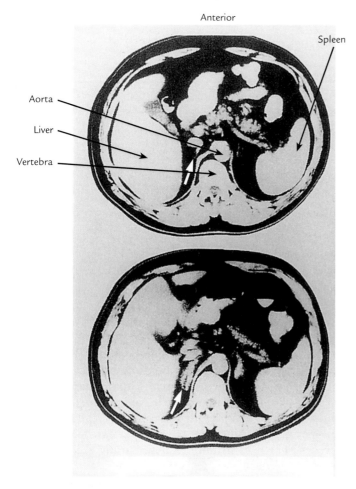

Figure 46-1 Computed axial tomographic (CAT) scans of the abdomen. *Top,* Small size of the left adrenal gland *(white arrow)* relative to other organs. *Bottom,* Marked hyperplasia of the left adrenal gland *(white arrow)* that occurred after 1 week of stimulation by an excess of endogenous adrenocorticotrophic hormone. The right adrenal gland was less well seen on these images, but it also enlarged after excess amounts of this hormone. *(From Mastorakos G et al: J Clin Endocrinol Metab 77:1690, 1993.)*

The genes that direct their synthesis have considerable similarity. A single P-450 enzyme may catalyze more than one reaction depending on its location in the cortex and on substrate availability. These enzymes catalyze hydroxylations of the steroid nucleus (Figure 46-3). The reactions require molecular oxygen, reduced nicotine-adenine dinucleotide phosphate, a flavoprotein enzyme, and an iron-containing protein called **adrenoxin.**

Cortisol synthesis uniquely requires the addition of an 11-hydroxyl group to the steroid molecule

The synthesis of cortisol, the major glucocorticoid in humans (Figure 46-3), occurs largely in the zona fasciculata. The initial and rate-limiting reaction converts cholesterol to **pregnenolone** and is catalyzed by the mitochondrial side-chain-cleaving enzyme complex P-450scc (also known as 20,22-desmolase). The pregnenolone is then converted to **progesterone,** after which hydroxyls are successively

added at the 17 and 21 positions. These reactions take place within the endoplasmic reticulum. The resultant 11-deoxycortisol is transferred to the mitochondria and hydroxylated in the 11 position, the final and critical step in creating a glucocorticoid molecule.

NEITHER THE FINAL PRODUCT, CORTISOL, NOR ITS PRECURSORS ARE STORED IN THE ADRENOCORTICAL CELL. Thus an acute need for increased cortisol secretion requires rapid activation of the initial controlling step: side-chain-cleavage of stored cholesterol.

Aldosterone synthesis uniquely requires oxidation of the 18 position on the steroid molecule

The synthesis of aldosterone, the major mineralocorticoid (Figure 46-3), is performed exclusively in the zona glomerulosa. The reactions from cholesterol to **corticosterone** (a glucocorticoid) occur as in the zona fasciculata. In the subsequent key step, the C_{18} methyl group of corticosterone is oxidized to yield aldosterone (by the same or very similar mitochondrial enzyme that catalyzes 11-hydroxylation). **11-Deoxycorticosterone** and 18-hydroxydeoxycorticosterone also have mineralocorticoid activity and are synthesized in small quantities in the zona fasciculata.

Androgen and estrogen precursors are 17-hydroxylated steroid molecules

The synthesis of sex steroids occurs largely in the zona reticularis. The potent androgen, **testosterone,** and the potent estrogen, **estradiol,** are normally secreted only in trace amounts by the adrenal cortex. However, substantial amounts of adrenal precursor steroids with weak androgenic activity are secreted and converted to testosterone and estradiol by peripheral tissues. These precursors—**androstenedione, dehydroepiandrosterone (DHEA),** and **dehydroepiandrosterone sulfate (DHEA-S)**—are synthesized from 17-hydroxyprogesterone and 17-hydroxypregnenolone, respectively, as shown in Figure 46-3 and in greater detail in Figure 48-1. In women the adrenal precursors supply 50% of the androgenic hormone requirements. In men, they are unimportant because the testes produce testosterone.

Genetic defects in cortisol biosynthesis have important and varied consequences for infants. A defect in either the 21- or 11-hydroxylase enzyme gene (Steps D and E in Figure 46-3) leads to overproduction of androgenic steroids from the accumulated precursors, 17-hydroxyprogesterone and 17-hydroxypregnenolone. This causes masculinization of female fetuses in utero and early secondary sexual changes in male infants and young boys. A severe deficiency of 21-hydroxylase activity may also cause manifestations of cortisol (glucocorti-

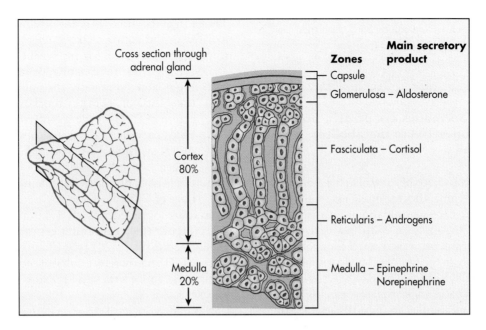

Figure 46-2 Structure and main secretory products of the adrenal gland.

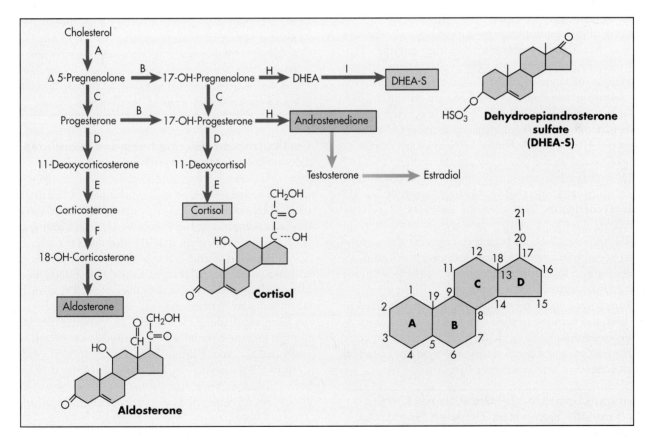

Figure 46-3 Sequence of reactions in the synthesis of adrenocorticosteroid hormones from the common precursor cholesterol. Step A is overall rate limiting. Step E is critical to glucocorticoid activity. Step G is critical to mineralocorticoid activity. Step B is essential to the formation of sex steroid precursors. *DHEA*, Dehydroepiandrosterone; *OH*, hydroxy; *A*, 20,22-desmolase (P-450scc); *B*, 17-hydroxylase (P-450c17); *C*, 3β-ol-dehydrogenase, Δ^{4,5}-isomerase; *D*, 21-hydroxylase (P-450c21); *E*, 11-hydroxylase (P-450c11); *F*, 18-hydroxylase; *G*, 18-OH-dehydrogenase; *H*, 17,20-desmolase (P-450c17); *I*, sulfotransferase.

coid) and aldosterone (mineralocorticoid) deficiency. Deficiency of 11-hydroxylase leads to overproduction of the mineralocorticoid 11-deoxycorticosterone (Figure 46-3), which causes hypertension and hypokalemia.

Corticosteroid hormones are protein-bound in serum and converted to metabolites excreted in urine

Basal plasma concentrations of cortisol in the morning are 5 to 20 µg/dl; by evening, they are often less than 5 µg/dl. The hormone circulates largely bound to a specific corticosteroid-binding globulin called **transcortin.** The concentrations of transcortin and total plasma cortisol are increased during pregnancy and estrogen administration. However, only free cortisol is biologically active, and the physiological effects of changes in transcortin levels are determined by principles similar to those discussed with regard to changes in thyroid binding globulin levels (see Chapter 45). Free cortisol is filtered by the kidney, and the small amount of daily urinary cortisol excretion (10 to 100 µg) is usually a valid index of cortisol secretion (see Chapter 40).

Cortisol is in equilibrium with its biologically inactive 11-keto analogue, **cortisone,** via the enzyme 11β-hydroxydehydrogenase. This ubiquitous enzyme renders exogenous cortisone an effective source of cortisol activity. The reverse conversion of cortisol to cortisone in the kidney is important in preventing cortisol from exerting mineralocorticoid activity via aldosterone receptors to which it binds (see later section). Almost all cortisol and cortisone is metabolized in the liver; they are then conjugated and excreted in the urine as glucuronides. The measurement of these urinary metabolites, known generally as **17-hydroxycorticoids,** also provides an index of cortisol secretion.

Aldosterone circulates bound to a specific aldosterone binding globulin as well as to transcortin and albumin. Aldosterone and its liver-generated metabolites are excreted in the urine as glucuronide conjugates.

Adrenal androgen precursors are also metabolized in the liver and excreted in the urine in a fraction known as **17-ketosteroids.** However, these products are not specific for the adrenal gland because they also arise from gonadal androgens.

Cortisol Secretion by the Adrenal Cortex Is Basically Regulated Through Negative Feedback on the Hypothalamus and Pituitary Gland

The pattern of cortisol secretion is very complex (Figure 46-4). The immediate stimulator of cortisol secretion is **adrenocorticotropin (ACTH)** from the anterior pituitary gland. The most important immediate stimulator of ACTH secretion is the neuropeptide **corticotropin-releasing hormone (CRH),** from the hypothalamus.

Thus a hypothalamic–anterior pituitary–adrenal cortex axis exists and forms a classic negative-feedback loop (Figure 46-4). Cortisol (or any synthetic glucocorticoid analogue [e.g., **dexamethasone, prednisone**]):

1. Feeds back (long loop) within minutes to inhibit the release of ACTH by blocking the stimulatory action of CRH on the corticotroph cells
2. Feeds back more slowly (within hours) to inhibit ACTH synthesis by blocking the transcription of its gene
3. Feeds back on the hypothalamus to block the release of CRH

In short-loop feedback, ACTH inhibits the release of CRH (Figure 46-4). Antidiuretic hormone (ADH) (arginine vasopressin [AVP]) (see Chapter 44) also stimulates ACTH and therefore cortisol secretion in stressful situations, and cortisol feeds back to restrain ADH release.

When given in large doses for long periods, synthetic glucocorticoids profoundly suppress the function of the CRH neurons, the corticotroph cells, and consequently the cells of the zona fasciculata and zona reticularis. The ACTH-dependent adrenal cortex atrophies. After such therapy is withdrawn, full recovery of the inactivated hypothalamic–anterior pituitary–adrenal axis can take up to 1 year. During this time, patients must be protected against deficient responses to stress by receiving supplemental cortisol.

Corticotropin-releasing hormone stimulates adrenocorticotropin synthesis and release

CRH is a 41 amino acid peptide synthesized from a prepro-CRH. CRH enters the pituitary portal veins and travels to the corticotroph cells (see Figure 44-1). After binding to a plasma membrane receptor, CRH stimulates the release of ACTH via calcium and cyclic AMP as second messengers and also stimulates ACTH synthesis. CRH exhibits diverse other actions in the central nervous system. These include stimulating sympathetic nervous system activity, decreasing fever, suppressing food intake, suppressing reproductive function and sexual activity, suppressing growth hormone release, and altering behavior. Peripheral plasma levels of CRH are very low, but they mirror negative feedback because they are slightly increased by cortisol deficiency and decreased by glucocorticoid administration.

Adrenocorticotropin stimulates adrenocortical cell hyperplasia and corticosteroid hormone synthesis and release

ACTH is a 39 amino acid peptide that increases the synthesis and immediate release of cortisol, adrenal androgens, their precursors, and aldosterone. However, only cortisol feeds back negatively as previously described. ACTH is synthesized from a large precursor called **preproopiomela-**

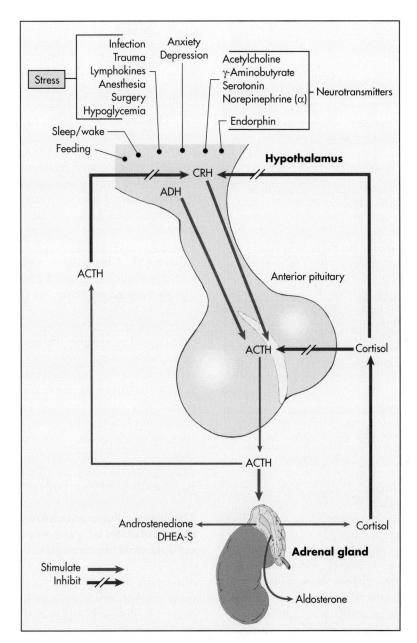

Figure 46-4 Regulation of cortisol secretion by the hypothalamic–anterior pituitary–adrenal cortex axis. A variety of stimuli to the hypothalamus activate the secretion of corticotropin-releasing hormone *(CRH)*, which in turn increases the secretion of adrenocorticotropin *(ACTH)* and thence cortisol. Antidiuretic hormone *(ADH)* has an auxiliary stimulating effect on ACTH secretion. Cortisol exerts negative feedback at both the hypothalamic and the pituitary levels.

nocortin, which gives rise to a number of cosecreted products, including **β-endorphin** and **melanocyte stimulating hormone (MSH);** the latter increases skin pigmentation. After binding to its adrenal plasma membrane receptor, ACTH stimulates the generation of cyclic AMP, which is the major second messenger for its actions (Figure 46-5). The ultimate effects of ACTH are mediated by protein products that result from a cascade of enzyme phosphorylations catalyzed by protein kinases A and C. These products include enzyme activators, transcription factors, and growth factors. ACTH acutely stimulates cholesterol uptake by the cell, cholesterol ester hydrolysis, cholesterol transfer to the mitochondria, the rate-limiting P-450scc desmolase reaction, and the critical 11-

hydroxylation step in cortisol synthesis. ACTH also alters the shape of the adrenocortical cell by affecting its cytoskeleton and by bringing the cholesterol vacuoles into contact with the mitochondria. Continuous stimulation with ACTH causes hyperplasia of the adrenal cortex (Figure 46-1).

Cortisol secretion is pulsatile, diurnal, and stimulated by stresses

Bursts of cortisol secretion are induced by pulses of ACTH, which are caused by the pulsatile release of CRH. Peak plasma ACTH and cortisol levels are achieved about 2 hours before awakening; the nadir of plasma ACTH and

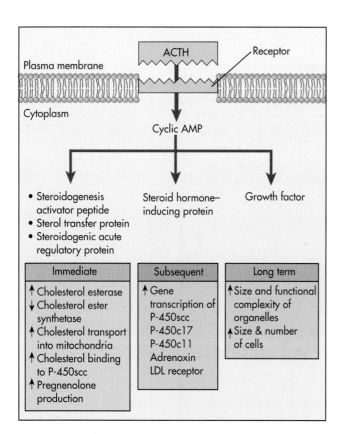

Figure 46-5 ACTH actions on target adrenocortical cells. Through cyclic AMP as second messenger, ACTH activates and induces steroidogenic enzymes and stimulates adrenocortical cell growth. See text for details. *LDL,* Low-density lipoprotein.

cortisol is reached just before a person falls asleep. The morning peak of cortisol constitutes 50% of its total daily secretion. The clock time of this peak can be altered by systematically shifting the sleep-wake cycle. THIS PHENOMENON IS OF OCCUPATIONAL SIGNIFICANCE, SUCH AS IN TRANSOCEANIC AIRLINE FLIGHTS. The circadian rhythm is intrinsic and generated within the hypothalamus, probably by the suprachiasmatic nucleus. Negative feedback affects the setting of this center: Exogenous glucocorticoid suppresses and prior cortisol deficiency accentuates the early morning ACTH peak. Loss of consciousness and constant exposure to either dark or light also blunt the circadian rhythm.

Cortisol is required for survival of the "stressed" organism. Severe pain and prolonged exercise also cause the release of cortisol, whereas the state of analgesia induced by endorphins (endogenous opiates) blocks the cortisol response. Stress can override the diurnal pattern of cortisol secretion as well as the suppressive effects of negative feedback. Several neurotransmitters mediate the stressful inputs that stimulate CRH (plus AVP) release (Figure 46-4).

Extra cortisol is secreted in patients with serious medical illnesses (such as **sepsis**) or major fractures, those undergoing surgery or electroconvulsive therapy, and those experiencing hypoglycemia. In patients in intensive care units, plasma cortisol levels are elevated twofold to fivefold; there is an increased risk of mortality in patients with the highest levels.

Activation of cell-mediated immunity also increases ACTH and cortisol release. Lymphokines, such as various interleukins, stimulate ACTH secretion (see Figure 47-4). Because infection and tissue trauma are accompanied by cell-mediated immune responses and because cortisol is an important modulator of those responses (see following discussion), a significant feedback relationship exists between the immune and endocrine systems.

Cortisol (Glucocorticoids) Actions Permit Many Physiological Processes To Be Maintained at Normal Levels

CORTISOL IS REQUIRED TO SUSTAIN GLUCOSE PRODUCTION FROM PROTEIN AND TO SUPPORT VASCULAR RESPONSIVENESS. IN ADDITION, THIS HORMONE MODULATES CENTRAL NERVOUS SYSTEM FUNCTION, SKELETAL TURNOVER, HEMATOPOIESIS, MUSCLE FUNCTION, RENAL FUNCTION, AND IMMUNE RESPONSES. The term **permissive,** which has been used to describe cortisol's action, implies that the hormone may not directly initiate, so much as allow, critical processes to occur. For example, cortisol does not itself directly stimulate glycogenolysis. However, if cortisol is present, glycogenolysis stimulated by glucagon is enhanced.

The intracellular mechanism of cortisol action is modulation of gene expression via a cytoplasmic/nuclear protein receptor

Almost all effects of cortisol are mediated via transcriptional mechanisms (see Figure 40-8). Cortisol enters target cells via facilitated diffusion and binds to either a type 1 or type 2 receptor in the cytoplasm or nucleus. The cortisol-receptor complex must undergo cytoplasmic activation before it can move into the nucleus and bind to a target DNA molecule. The final response is an increase or a decrease in the gene transcription of specific messenger RNAs. Although other steroid hormones can bind to a cortisol receptor and other steroid receptors may bind to a similar regulatory element on the same DNA molecule, THE COMBINATION OF CORTISOL, ONE OF ITS RECEPTORS, AND A RESPONSIVE DNA MOLECULE IS REQUIRED TO ELICIT SPECIFIC CORTISOL ACTION.

Effects on metabolism

Cortisol causes the conversion of protein to glucose and a negative nitrogen balance
THE MOST IMPORTANT OVERALL EFFECT OF CORTISOL IS TO STIMULATE THE CONVERSION OF PROTEIN TO GLUCOSE AND THE STORAGE OF GLUCOSE AS GLYCOGEN, thus the term **glucocorticoid** (Figure 46-6). The type 2, or glucocorticoid, receptor mediates such actions. All phases of this process—

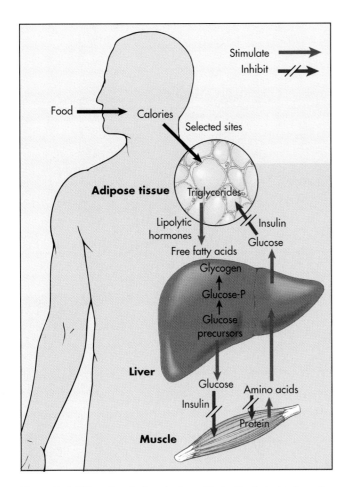

Figure 46-6 Effect of cortisol on the flow of fuels. Cortisol stimulates the mobilization of amino acids and their conversion to glucose. The glucose is preferentially but not exclusively stored as glycogen. Insulin-mediated glucose uptake by the peripheral tissues is inhibited. Cortisol facilitates the storage of fat in selected adipose tissue sites but also facilitates the release of free fatty acids.

mobilization of protein from muscle stores, entrance of the released amino acids into the hepatic gluconeogenetic pathway, conversion of pyruvate to glycogen, and disposition of the ammonia released from metabolism of the precursor amino acids—are augmented. Cortisol increases the activity of the enzymes involved in each of these steps. In some of these instances, the hormone "permits" substrate induction of its enzyme; in others, cortisol directly increases transcription of the target enzyme gene.

If the glucocorticoid effect is excessive and lengthy, the continuous drain on body protein produces serious deleterious effects because muscle, bone, connective tissue, and skin lose mass. This is exacerbated by the inhibitory effects of cortisol on the synthesis of constitutive proteins, such as collagen.

The clinical expression of the negative nitrogen balance that results from prolonged cortisol excess (**Cushing's** syndrome) is striking (Figure 46-7). Skin becomes so thin

from loss of connective tissue that the capillaries show through, and because of fragile walls, they rupture spontaneously, causing bruises. Muscle weakness and atrophy are prominent. Osteoporosis results in atraumatic fractures and bone necrosis.

THE PRESENCE OF CORTISOL IS ESSENTIAL FOR THE MAINTENANCE OF PLASMA GLUCOSE LEVELS AND FOR SURVIVAL DURING PROLONGED FASTING. Without this hormone, death may occur from hypoglycemia once glycogen stores are gone. However, only a small increase in cortisol secretion occurs with fasting; the previous normal levels of the hormone help make possible the early mobilization of amino acids and gluconeogenesis. On the other hand, plasma cortisol levels increase sharply in response to acute hypoglycemia. In this situation, cortisol amplifies the glycogenolytic actions of glucagon and epinephrine, and it synergizes with them in rebuilding liver glycogen stores.

Cortisol opposes the key effects of insulin

Consonant with its role in preventing hypoglycemia, cortisol is a strong antagonist to insulin (Figure 46-6). Cortisol inhibits insulin-stimulated glucose uptake by muscle and adipose tissue and blocks the suppressive effect of insulin on hepatic glucose output. The interaction between cortisol and insulin is complex. Both hormones favor hepatic glycogen storage by increasing glycogen synthase activity (see Figure 41-3). However, they have opposite effects on the expression of genes for the gluconeogenetic enzyme, phosphoenolpyruvate carboxykinase, and the glucose-releasing enzyme, glucose-6-phosphatase. Thus cortisol favors glucose synthesis and output by the liver, whereas insulin inhibits both processes. The net result of cortisol excess is a rise in plasma glucose concentration and a compensatory increase in plasma insulin levels. WHEN THE INSULIN RESPONSE IS INSUFFICIENT, DIABETES MELLITUS CAN DEVELOP, OR IF ALREADY PRESENT, IT CAN BE GREATLY WORSENED.

Cortisol also plays a complex role in fat metabolism (Figure 46-7). The presence of cortisol "permits" maximal stimulation of fat mobilization by growth hormone, epinephrine, and other lipolytic factors during fasting. However, the hormone also greatly increases appetite and stimulates lipogenesis in certain adipose tissue depots. THEREFORE IN CUSHING'S SYNDROME AN EXCESS OF CORTISOL ALSO RESULTS IN THE ACCUMULATION OF FAT, BUT THE OBESITY HAS A PECULIAR DISTRIBUTION, FAVORING THE FACE AND TRUNK BUT SPARING THE EXTREMITIES (Figure 46-7).

Thus cortisol is a catabolic, antianabolic, and diabetogenic hormone. In stress situations, cortisol accentuates the hyperglycemia produced by other hormones and greatly accelerates the loss of body protein. These actions are amplified if insulin secretion is simultaneously deficient.

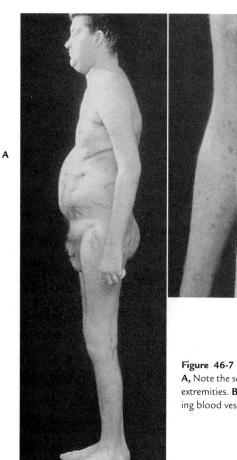

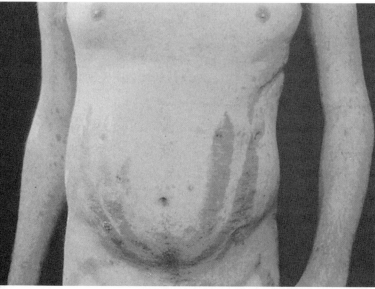

Figure 46-7 Individual suffering from Cushing's syndrome, an excess of cortisol. **A,** Note the selective accumulation of abdominal fat and the loss of musculature in the extremities. **B,** The extreme thinness of the skin reveals blood flowing through underlying blood vessels.

Cortisol affects diverse tissues and organs

Cortisol affects muscle, bone, the vascular system, the kidneys, and the central nervous system (Figure 46-8). It also affects the maturation of various systems and organs in the fetus.

Muscle
Basal levels of cortisol are required for the maintenance of normal contractility and for maximal performance of skeletal and cardiac muscle. In contrast, excess cortisol produces muscle atrophy and weakness through protein wastage.

Bone
The major effect of cortisol is to decrease bone formation. Less prominently, cortisol increases bone resorption. THE NET OUTCOME OF CORTISOL EXCESS CAN BE A PROFOUND REDUCTION IN BONE MASS AND IN CHILDREN, A REDUCTION IN LINEAR GROWTH AS WELL. Several actions contribute to this outcome. Cortisol decreases the synthesis of 1,25-hydroxyvitamin D and blocks its action; therefore calcium absorption from the gastrointestinal tract is defective (see Chapter 43). At the same time, urinary calcium excretion is increased. Thus less calcium is available for the mineralization of bone. Cortisol also inhibits the dif-

ferentiation of mesenchymal precursors into osteoblasts and the synthesis of collagen by these cells.

Vascular system
Cortisol is required for the maintenance of normal blood pressure. This hormone permits an enhanced responsiveness of arterioles to the constrictive action of adrenergic stimulation and also optimizes myocardial performance. Cortisol helps maintain blood volume by decreasing the permeability of the vascular endothelium. IN CUSHING'S SYNDROME, HYPERTENSION FREQUENTLY IS PRESENT.

Kidney
Cortisol increases the rate of glomerular filtration. It is also essential for the rapid excretion of a water load because it inhibits both the secretion of ADH and its action on the collecting duct tubules (see Chapter 44). CLINICALLY, THE ABSENCE OF CORTISOL MAY LEAD TO WATER RETENTION AND RESULTANT HYPONATREMIA.

Central nervous system
The type 1 receptor for cortisol (which is identical to the mineralocorticoid receptor) is present throughout the brain, and it is concentrated in the hippocampus, reticular activating substance, and autonomic nuclei of

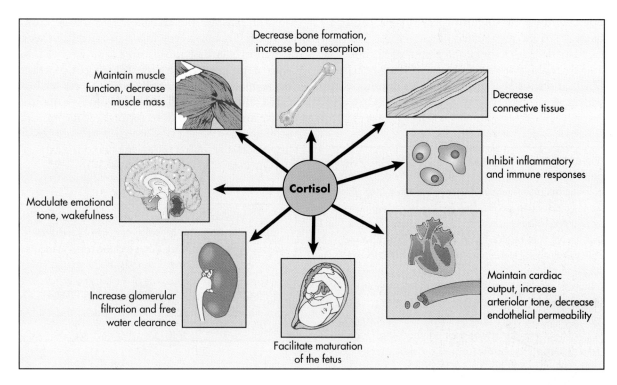

Figure 46-8 Cortisol's effects on various tissues and organs.

the brainstem. Cortisol modulates perceptual and emotional functioning. A deficiency of cortisol accentuates auditory, olfactory, and gustatory acuity. The increase in CRH pulses and cortisol levels just before awakening is important for normal arousal and initiation of daytime activity. CLINICALLY, AN EXCESS OF CORTISOL CAN CAUSE INSOMNIA AND EITHER EUPHORIA OR DEPRESSION.

Fetus

Cortisol facilitates in utero maturation of the lungs, gastrointestinal tract, central nervous system, retina, and skin. The development rate of the pulmonary alveoli, flattening of the lining cells, and thinning of the lung septa are increased. Most important, the synthesis of surfactant, a phospholipid vital for maintaining alveolar surface tension, is increased. These actions permit satisfactory breathing immediately after birth. Cortisol also facilitates the maturation of the enzyme capacity of the intestinal mucosa from a fetal to an adult pattern. This permits the newborn to digest the disaccharides in milk.

Cortisol inhibits inflammatory and immune responses

Cortisol has a profound influence on the complex set of reactions evoked by trauma, chemical irritants, foreign proteins, and infection. The overriding effect is to inhibit many important steps in the response to tissue injury.

Cortisol impedes the ability of tissues either to eliminate immediately noxious substances and invaders or to wall them off from the rest of the body. Thus long-term treatment with pharmacological doses of any glucocorticoid increases a patient's susceptibility to opportunistic infections, allows their dissemination, and masks them. Normal wound healing after injury may also be prevented.

The mechanisms by which cortisol suppresses these responses are shown in the following examples:

1. Cortisol induces a phosphoprotein called **lipocortin** that inhibits the enzyme phospholipase A_2. This enzyme generates arachidonic acid. Because the latter serves as the precursor for the synthesis of prostaglandins and related compounds, the production of these mediators of inflammation is reduced. The production of **nitric oxide** and **platelet activating factor** is also decreased.
2. Cortisol decreases the production of **interleukin-1, interleukin-2, interleukin-6,** and **tumor necrosis factor.** This blocks the entire cascade of cell-mediated immunity as well as the generation of fever.
3. Cortisol stabilizes lysosomes and thereby reduces the release of enzymes capable of degrading foreign substances.
4. Cortisol blocks the recruitment of neutrophils by inhibiting their ability to bind chemotactic peptides. The production of stimulatory **leukotri-**

enes is inhibited, impairing the phagocytic and bacterial capacity of neutrophils.

5. Cortisol decreases the proliferation of fibroblasts and their ability to synthesize and deposit tissue fibrils and thus prevents the encapsulation of invaders.

The therapeutic use of glucocorticoids represents a two-edged sword. Glucocorticoids are dramatically beneficial when inflammatory reactions are so severe that they are functionally disabling or life threatening (e.g., during a severe asthma attack) or when the rejection of transplanted tissues must be prevented. However, their adverse effects—vulnerability to serious infection, diabetes, osteoporosis, and psychiatric disorders—require physicians to PRESCRIBE GLUCOCORTICOIDS CAUTIOUSLY AND ONLY WHEN NO SAFER FORM OF TREATMENT EXISTS.

This injunction does not apply to the use of replacement doses of cortisol in patients who lack adrenocortical function (**Addison's disease**). Cortisol deficiency leads to anorexia, weight loss, fatigue, poor tolerance of stress, fever, hypoglycemia, and in women, loss of sexual hair. The loss of negative feedback causes hypersecretion of ACTH and darkening of the skin through its melanocyte-stimulating activity. Suitable replacement therapy can reverse these findings without adverse effects.

Aldosterone Secretion Is Regulated Primarily in Response to Changes in Sodium Availability and Extracellular Fluid Volume

ALDOSTERONE, THE MAJOR PRODUCT OF THE ZONA GLOMERULOSA, HAS TWO PRINCIPAL FUNCTIONS: (1) SUSTAINING EXTRACELLULAR FLUID VOLUME BY CONSERVING BODY SODIUM AND (2) PREVENTING THE OVERLOAD OF POTASSIUM BY ACCELERATING ITS EXCRETION (see Chapters 37 and 38). Thus aldosterone is secreted largely in response to a reduced circulating fluid volume and an increased plasma potassium (Figure 46-9).

When the sodium concentration is depleted, the fall in extracellular fluid and plasma volume causes a decrease in the arterial blood pressure and renal blood flow. The juxtaglomerular cells in the kidney respond by secreting the enzyme **renin** into the peripheral circulation (see Chapter 37). Renin acts on its substrate, **angiotensinogen,** to form **angiotensin I.** The latter is further cleaved by **angiotensin-converting enzyme** to the potent vasoconstrictors **angiotensin II** and **angiotensin III.** These bind to receptors in the zona glomerulosa and stimulate the key enzymatic steps in the synthesis (Figure 46-3) and release of aldosterone (Figure 46-9). The calcium and the phosphatidylinositol messenger systems are mediators.

Basal plasma aldosterone levels range from 5 to 15 ng/dl. When hypovolemia is produced, either rapidly by hemorrhage or acute diuresis or slowly by chronic sodium deprivation, the aldosterone concentration increases markedly. Conversely, when excess sodium is ingested and the extracellular fluid volume expands, renin release and aldosterone secretion are suppressed. Thus THE JUXTAGLOMERULAR CELLS AND ZONA GLOMERULOSA FORM A PHYSIOLOGICAL FEEDBACK SYSTEM TO DEFEND THE EXTRACELLULAR FLUID VOLUME (see Chapters 36 and 37).

This physiological feedback system plays an important role in disease states in which effective blood flow to the kidney is reduced. These states include cardiac failure, hepatic failure, renal artery stenosis, and hypoalbuminemia with transudation of fluid out of the plasma space. In each of these conditions, the hypersecretion of aldosterone is stimulated, and sodium retention occurs; this causes or augments edema.

The atrial natriuretic peptide hormones, which are released by atrial myocytes in response to increased vascular volume, decrease aldosterone secretion directly by acting on the zona glomerulosa and indirectly by reducing the release of renin (see Chapter 37).

Potassium excess stimulates aldosterone secretion

Aldosterone also participates in a vital feedback relationship with potassium (Figure 46-9). Aldosterone facilitates the clearance of potassium from the extracellular fluid, and concordantly potassium is an important stimulator of aldosterone secretion. In humans, raising the plasma potassium concentration only 0.5 mEq/L immediately increases plasma aldosterone levels. Conversely, potassium depletion lowers aldosterone secretion. Potassium acts by depolarizing the zona glomerulosa cell membrane, thereby allowing an influx of calcium and the activation of aldosterone biosynthesis.

Other factors that influence renin release or angiotensin II formation secondarily affect aldosterone secretion. β-Adrenergic stimulation of the kidney in response to hypovolemia increases the output of renin and aldosterone. Certain prostaglandins produced within the kidney also increase renin release. Conversely, inhibitors of angiotensin-converting enzyme decrease aldosterone secretion.

Therefore β-adrenergic–blocking agents (e.g., **propranolol**) used in the treatment of hypertension or angina, inhibitors of prostaglandin synthesis (e.g., **indomethacin**) used in the treatment of inflammatory conditions, and angiotensin-converting enzyme inhibitors (e.g., **capto-**

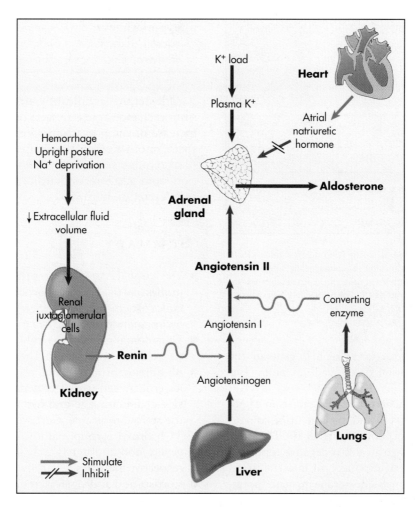

Figure 46-9 Regulation of aldosterone secretion. Activation of the renin-angiotensin system in response to hypovolemia is the predominant stimulus for aldosterone production. The kidney, liver, and lungs are required for the production of angiotensin II, the direct stimulator. An elevation of plasma potassium levels is the other major stimulus of aldosterone secretion. Atrial natriuretic hormones inhibit aldosterone secretion.

pril) used in the treatment of hypertension or congestive heart failure can all depress aldosterone secretion and elevate plasma potassium levels (see later section).

Aldosterone secretion is also stimulated by ACTH. However, this effect wanes after several days because as sodium is retained and extracellular fluid volume rises, renin and angiotensin levels decrease, whereas atrial natriuretic hormone levels increase. These responses return aldosterone secretion back to basal levels. When ACTH is deficient, the aldosterone response to sodium depletion is modestly diminished.

Aldosterone (mineralocorticoids) causes sodium retention and potassium excretion by the kidney

The kidney is the major site of mineralocorticoid activity. In renal tubular cells, aldosterone binds to the mineralocorticoid receptor, which is identical to the type l cortisol receptor. Messenger RNAs and proteins are induced and must mediate the hormone's actions, which require hours

to appear. Aldosterone stimulates the active reabsorption of sodium from the distal tubular urine; the sodium is transported through the tubular cell and back into the capillary blood (Figure 46-10) (see Chapter 36). Thus net urinary sodium excretion is diminished, and the vital extracellular cation is conserved. Because water is passively reabsorbed with the sodium, plasma sodium concentration increases only slightly, and extracellular fluid volume expands isotonically. ALTHOUGH ONLY A SMALL FRACTION OF TOTAL SODIUM REABSORPTION IS REGULATED BY ALDOSTERONE, DEFICIENCY OF THE HORMONE PRODUCES A CRITICAL NEGATIVE SODIUM BALANCE. Hypovolemia and hypotension result unless a large intake of sodium and water is maintained.

Aldosterone acts at various sites in distal renal tubular and collecting duct cells

Aldosterone acts (1) at the apical (luminal) surface to increase the number of membrane channels through which sodium enters the cell along an electrochemical gradient; (2) at the basal (capillary) surface of the cell to activate Na^+,K^+-ATPase, which pumps the sodium back into the interstitial fluid and plasma; and (3) in the mitochondria

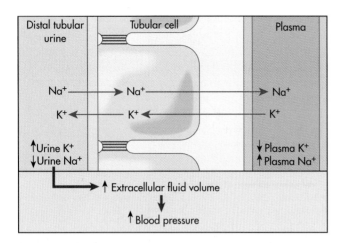

Figure 46-10 Action of aldosterone on the renal tubule. Sodium reabsorption from tubular urine is stimulated. Simultaneously, potassium secretion into the tubular urine is increased via responses to the electronegative gradient created by sodium movement. The net result is the expansion of extracellular fluid and kaliuresis.

to stimulate Krebs cycle reactions that help generate the energy needed for operation of the sodium pump (see Chapter 37).

Aldosterone also stimulates the active secretion of potassium from the tubular cell and into the urine concurrently with sodium reabsorption (Figure 46-10). The latter creates in the tubular lumen an electronegative condition that facilitates the transfer of potassium into the urine. Therefore the extent to which aldosterone increases potassium secretion depends greatly on the delivery of sodium to the distal tubule. Aldosterone cannot significantly increase potassium excretion in a sodium-depleted subject; conversely, a high sodium intake exaggerates the urinary potassium loss caused by aldosterone. Unlike sodium flux, potassium flux does not entrain the movement of water. Therefore POTASSIUM RETENTION CAUSED BY ALDOSTERONE DEFICIENCY OR BY DRUGS THAT BLOCK ALDOSTERONE ACTION CAN RESULT IN A RISE IN PLASMA POTASSIUM TO DANGEROUS LEVELS. Aldosterone also enhances the tubular secretion of H^+ in conjunction with sodium reabsorption.

Continued administration of aldosterone produces only a limited retention of sodium, which then ceases. This escape is caused by expansion of the extracellular fluid and is mediated in part by atrial natriuretic hormones. In contrast, the potassium loss induced by aldosterone continues because sodium delivery to the distal tubule is maintained.

The net clinical effect of **primary hyperaldosteronism** is modest fluid retention without detectable edema. Hypertension, **hypokalemia,** and metabolic alkalosis are the dominant signs. This situation can be ameliorated by the administration of aldosterone antagonists (e.g., **spironolactone**). In contrast, **aldosterone deficiency** leads to natriuresis, dehydration, hypotension,

---

hyperkalemia, hyponatremia, and hyperchloremic acidosis. These findings are also present in **Addison's disease,** which is caused by adrenocortical destruction.

Aldosterone significantly affects sodium and potassium exchange across muscle cells. The net result is an increase in the potassium content of the intracellular space, another effect that helps prevent hyperkalemia. Aldosterone also modestly stimulates sodium reabsorption from gastrointestinal fluids and enhances potassium excretion in the feces.

SUMMARY

- The adrenal cortex secretes three types of steroid hormones: cortisol, a glucocorticoid; aldosterone, a mineralocorticoid; and androgen precursors, largely dehydroepiandrosterone.
- The adrenal glands are richly vascularized and essential to survival because of the cortisol they produce.
- All adrenocorticosteroids are synthesized from cholesterol by sequential enzymatic steps consisting of side-chain cleavage and hydroxylation of key sites in the steroid molecule. Cortisol specifically requires an 11-hydroxyl group; aldosterone, an 18-hydroxyl group; and androgens, a 17-hydroxyl group for their respective activities.
- Cortisol and androgen secretion are stimulated by adrenocorticotropin (ACTH) from the pituitary gland. ACTH secretion is stimulated by CRH from the hypothalamus. Cortisol feeds back negatively to suppress the release of both ACTH and CRH.
- ACTH, via cyclic AMP as second messenger, stimulates the cellular uptake of cholesterol, its movement from storage vacuoles into mitochondria, and all subsequent biosynthetic steps to cortisol.
- Cortisol acts via a nuclear receptor and modulates gene expression of numerous enzymes and proteins. Cortisol increases muscle proteolysis and hepatic conversion of the liberated amino acids into glucose and its storage as glycogen. Cortisol also inhibits insulin-stimulated glucose uptake by muscle.
- Cortisol stimulates caloric intake and favors the deposition of fat in selected sites. By inhibiting collagen synthesis, cortisol reduces bone formation and causes thinning of the skin and capillary walls.
- Cortisol strongly inhibits the entire process of inflammation, including the recruitment and function of neutrophils and the release of prostaglandin and leukotriene mediators. It also inhibits the immune system and prevents the proliferation of thymus-derived lymphocytes and the production of some lymphokines.
- Aldosterone is a major regulator of sodium, potassium, and fluid balance. It acts on the renal tubule via

a nuclear receptor. Sodium reabsorption is increased, and there is concomitant expansion of extracellular fluid. Renal potassium excretion is concurrently increased, and plasma potassium concentration is lowered.

■ Aldosterone secretion is regulated primarily by the renin-angiotensin system.

BIBLIOGRAPHY

Chrousos GP: The hypothalamic-pituitary-adrenal axis and immune-mediated inflammation, *N Engl J Med* 332:1351, 1995.

Chrousos GP, Gold PW: The concepts of stress and stress system disorders, *JAMA* 267:1244, 1992.

Darmaun D, Matthews DE, Bier DM: Physiological hypercortisolemia increases proteolysis, glutamine, and alanine production, *Am J Physiol* 255:E366, 1988.

Gustafsson J et al: Biochemistry, molecular biology and physiology of the glucocorticoid receptor, *Endocr Rev* 8:185, 1987.

Horrocks PM et al: Patterns of ACTH and cortisol pulsatility over twenty-four hours in normal males and females, *Clin Endocrinol (Oxf)* 32:127, 1990.

Keith LD, Kendall JW: Regulation of ACTH secretion. In Imura H: *The pituitary gland*, New York, 1985, Raven.

Mastorakos G, Chrousos GP, Weber JS: Recombinant interleukin-6 activates the hypothalamic-pituitary-adrenal axis in humans, *J Clin Endocrinol Metab* 77:1690, 1993.

Meikle AW: Secretion and metabolism of the corticosteroids and adrenal function and testing. In DeGroot LJ, ed: *Endocrinology*, ed 3, Philadelphia, 1995, WB Saunders.

Miller WL: Molecular biology of steroid hormone synthesis, *Endocr Rev* 9:295, 1988.

Mortensen RM, Williams GH: Aldosterone action: physiology. In DeGroot LJ, ed: *Endocrinology*, ed 3, Philadelphia, 1995, WB Saunders.

Munck A, Náray-Fejes-Tóth A: Glucocorticoid action: physiology. In DeGroot LJ, ed: *Endocrinology*, ed 3, Philadelphia, 1995, WB Saunders.

Numa S, Imura H: ACTH and related peptides: gene structure and biosynthesis. In Imura H: *The pituitary gland*, New York, 1985, Raven.

Orth DN, Kovacs WJ, Debold CR: The adrenal cortex. In Wilson JD, Foster DW, eds: *Williams textbook of endocrinology*, Philadelphia, 1992, WB Saunders.

Stocco DM, Clark BJ: Regulation of the acute production of steroids in steroidogenic cells, *Endocr Rev* 17:221, 1996.

Wick G et al: Immunoendocrine communication via the hypothalamus-pituitary-adrenal axis in autoimmune diseases, *Endocr Rev* 14:539, 1993.

▷ **CASE STUDIES**

Case 46-1

A 56-year-old woman with a 40-year history of heavy tobacco use has recently begun coughing. She has gained 20 pounds in 6 months, mostly in the face and abdomen, and has noticed increasing facial hair. Her blood pressure is 160/108 mm Hg. She has bilateral edema of her legs. A chest x-ray film shows a large mass in her right lung. Her physician suspects a lung cancer that is an ectopic source of ACTH production.

1. **Which of the following would be increased?**
   - **A.** Serum potassium levels
   - **B.** Skin pigmentation
   - **C.** Pituitary ACTH secretion
   - **D.** Hypothalamic CRH secretion
   - **E.** Serum renin levels

2. **The patient undergoes surgery to remove the tumor. On the first day after surgery, she develops a high fever, hypotension, profound anorexia, and hyponatremia. What is the diagnosis?**
   - **A.** She has acute cortisol deficiency resulting from atrophy of the adrenal zona fasciculata.
   - **B.** She has acute ACTH deficiency resulting from atrophy of the adrenocorticotrophs.
   - **C.** She has acute ADH deficiency.
   - **D.** She has acute aldosterone deficiency resulting from atrophy of the adrenal zona glomerulosa.
   - **E.** She has acute DHEA deficiency resulting from atrophy of the adrenal zona reticularis.

Case 46-2

A 65-year-old man with severe atherosclerosis abruptly develops hypertension. His blood pressure is 220/122 mm Hg. On auscultation, a harsh bruit (sound of blood flowing past an obstruction) is heard over the right kidney. His serum potassium concentration is low. The diagnosis of a partial occlusion of the renal artery is confirmed radiographically.

1. **Which of the following would be decreased?**
   - **A.** Serum potassium levels
   - **B.** Serum aldosterone levels
   - **C.** Serum angiotensin levels
   - **D.** Serum renin levels
   - **E.** Serum atrial natriuretic hormone levels

2. **Which of the following does *not* contribute to the patient's hypertension?**
   - **A.** Calcium
   - **B.** Angiotensin-converting enzyme
   - **C.** Protein kinase C
   - **D.** Na^+,K^+-ATPase
   - **E.** Cyclic AMP

CHAPTER 47

Adrenal Medulla

- Explain the relationship between the neural and endocrine functions of catecholamine hormones.
- Describe the biochemistry and intracellular sites of catecholamine hormone synthesis.
- Describe the factors that regulate epinephrine and norepinephrine secretion by the adrenal medulla.
- Examine the wide array of epinephrine and norepinephrine actions.
- Explain the concept of the stress reaction and the complex interplay of adrenocortical and medullary hormones in response to stress.

The Adrenal Medulla Functions Partly as a Sympathetic Nervous System Ganglion and Partly as an Endocrine Gland

The adrenal medulla forms the inner core of the adrenal gland (see Figure 46-2). It is the source of the circulating catecholamine hormone, **epinephrine.** The medulla also secretes **norepinephrine,** primarily a neurotransmitter that can also function as a hormone. The catecholamine hormones are important mediators of rapid fuel mobilization; they increase the release of both glucose and free fatty acids, especially during acute stress. They also stimulate the cardiovascular system and cause contraction or relaxation of smooth muscles in the respiratory, gastrointestinal, and genitourinary tracts.

The adrenal medulla is essentially a specialized sympathetic ganglion (see Figure 10-2). However, the neuronal cells of the medulla do not have axons; instead, they discharge their products directly into the bloodstream, and thus they function in true endocrine fashion. The medulla is often activated with the sympathetic portion of the autonomic nervous system and acts in concert with it in the "fight-or-flight" reaction. Some of the neurotransmitter actions of norepinephrine are duplicated and amplified by the hormone actions of epinephrine, which reaches similar targets via the circulation. However, epinephrine has other effects of its own, some of which modulate those of norepinephrine.

The adrenal medulla is formed in parallel with the peripheral sympathetic nervous system. At about 7 weeks of gestation, neuroectodermal cells invade the adrenal cortex, where they develop into the medulla. The development of this tissue and the induction of hormone synthesis are stimulated by nerve growth factor.

The adult adrenal medulla weighs about 1 g and is composed of **chromaffin cells.** These are organized in cords in intimate relationship with venules that drain the adrenal cortex. THE CHROMAFFIN CELLS ARE INNERVATED BY CHOLINERGIC PREGANGLIONIC FIBERS OF THE SYMPATHETIC NERVOUS SYSTEM. Within these cells are numerous granules similar to those found in postganglionic sympathetic nerve terminals. These contain catecholamines, ATP, proopiomelanocortin products (see Chapter 46), and other neuropeptides. Approximately 85% of the chromaffin granules store epinephrine, and 15% store norepinephrine.

Catecholamine Hormones Are Synthesized in Sequential Steps Alternating Between the Cytoplasm and Storage Granules of the Adrenomedullary Cells

The catecholamines are synthesized by the series of reactions shown in Figure 47-1. The intermediates move back and forth in sequence between the cytoplasm and the storage granules. The first, rate-limiting step is the conversion of tyrosine to dihydroxyphenylalanine (DOPA). It occurs in the cytoplasm and requires molecular O_2, a tetrahydropteridine, and reduced nicotinamide-adenine dinucleotide phosphate. The subsequent decarboxylation of DOPA to dopamine in the cytoplasm uses pyridoxal phosphate as a cofactor. The dopamine must then be taken up into the chromaffin granules, where the next enzyme in the sequence, dopamine β-hydroxylase, catalyzes the formation of norepinephrine from dopamine, molecular O_2, and a hydrogen donor. With a few granules the sequence ends there, and the norepinephrine remains stored.

In most granules, norepinephrine reenters the cytoplasm, where it is *N*-methylated to epinephrine, with *S*-adenosylmethionine as the methyl donor. The epinephrine is then taken back up into the chromaffin granules for storage. Granule uptake of catecholamines and their storage at high concentrations require ATP. A total of 1 mole of the nucleotide complexes with 4 moles of catecholamine hormone and a protein known as **chromogranin.**

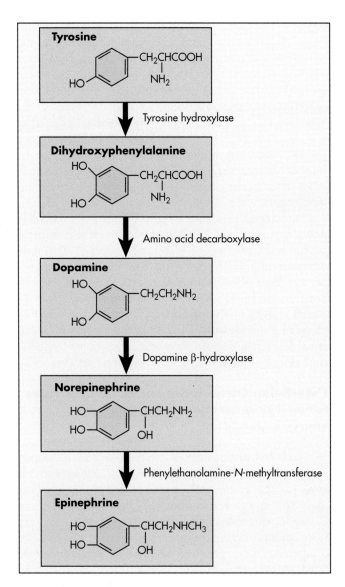

Figure 47-1 Pathway of catecholamine hormone synthesis in the adrenal medulla.

The synthesis and secretion of catecholamine hormones are regulated by sympathetic nerve impulses and cortisol

The synthesis of epinephrine and norepinephrine is regulated by several factors. Acute sympathetic stimulation of the medulla activates the initial rate-limiting step. Chronic stimulation induces an increased concentration of tyrosine hydroxylase, and thereby catecholamine output is maintained in the face of continuous demand. Cyclic AMP mediates both of these effects. Cortisol specifically induces the last enzyme in the sequence, *N*-methyltransferase, and selectively stimulates epinephrine synthesis. The perfusion of the adrenal medulla with cortisol-enriched blood from the cortex facilitates this induction.

The effector pathway for the release of adrenal medullary hormones consists of **cholinergic** preganglionic fibers in the splanchnic nerves. On nerve stimulation, **ace-**tylcholine, which is released from the nerve terminals, depolarizes the chromaffin cell membrane by increasing its permeability to sodium. This in turn induces an influx of Ca^{++}, which causes aggregation of the chromaffin granules. Exocytosis follows with the secretion of epinephrine, norepinephrine, ATP, dopamine β-hydroxylase, neuropeptides, and chromogranin.

In a complex set of reactions, catecholamine hormones are metabolized to products excreted in the urine

All the circulating epinephrine is derived from adrenal medullary secretion. Basal plasma epinephrine levels are 25 to 50 pg/ml. In contrast, almost all the circulating norepinephrine is derived from sympathetic nerve terminals and from the brain; this represents norepinephrine that escaped local reuptake from the synaptic clefts. Basal norepinephrine levels are 100 to 350 pg/ml. Both catecholamines have plasma half-lives of about 2 minutes, which allows rapid turnoff of their dramatic effects. Only 2% to 3% of catecholamines, the majority of which is norepinephrine, are excreted unchanged in the urine.

Epinephrine and norepinephrine are metabolized by *O*-methylation and oxidative deamination, predominantly in the liver and kidney. The major end products, **vanillylmandelic acid** and **metanephrines,** are excreted in the urine. They serve as indices of activity of the sympathetic nervous system or of pathological hypersecretion of the catecholamine hormones by **pheochromocytomas,** or tumors of the adrenal medulla.

Adrenal medullary secretion is stimulated by many factors related to stress

As previously noted, secretion from the adrenal medulla is part of the fight-or-flight reaction (Figure 46-2). Thus THE PERCEPTION OR EVEN ANTICIPATION OF DANGER, FEAR, EXCITEMENT, TRAUMA, PAIN, HYPOVOLEMIA, HYPOTENSION, ANOXIA, HYPOTHERMIA, HYPOGLYCEMIA, AND INTENSE EXERCISE CAUSE THE RAPID RELEASE OF EPINEPHRINE AND NOREPINEPHRINE (see Chapter 26). These stimuli are sensed at various levels in the sympathetic nervous system, and responses are initiated in the hypothalamus and brainstem (see Chapter 10). Epinephrine secretion may follow activation of the sympathetic nervous system by more intense stimuli. However, epinephrine secretion specifically increases in response to mild hypoglycemia, moderate hypoxia, and fasting even though sympathetic nervous system activity may remain constant or may decrease.

Mild hypoglycemia causes a fivefold to tenfold increase in the plasma epinephrine concentration but little change in the norepinephrine concentration. The resulting epinephrine concentration can stimulate a compensatory increase in the plasma glucose level; the norepinephrine level cannot. The reduction in central venous pressure produced by a person assuming the upright position (see

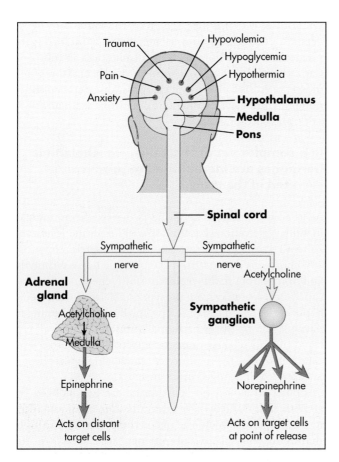

Figure 47-2 Activation of catecholamine effects via the sympathetic nervous system and the adrenal medulla. The adrenal medulla is homologous to a sympathetic ganglion, but the adrenal medulla releases its catecholamines into the bloodstream rather than into a synaptic cleft.

Chapter 24) increases both plasma epinephrine and norepinephrine concentrations twofold. However, only the epinephrine concentration is high enough to increase the heart rate and blood pressure. Thus epinephrine functions as a true hormone in both situations, whereas norepinephrine does not. Norepinephrine, however, contributes as a neurotransmitter to the compensatory response to hypovolemia and to more severe hypoglycemia because the higher concentration necessary for its action is generated locally at the effector site (Figure 47-2). IN STATES OF MAJOR METABOLIC DECOMPENSATION, SUCH AS DIABETIC KETOACIDOSIS, THE CIRCULATING CONCENTRATIONS OF BOTH CATECHOLAMINES RISE HIGH ENOUGH TO EVOKE RESPONSES.

Catecholamine Hormones Work Through Several Plasma Membrane Receptors and Second Messengers

Epinephrine and norepinephrine exert their many effects via several plasma membrane receptors, designated β_1, β_2, β_3, α_1, and α_2. The β_1-, β_2-, and β_3- receptors are structurally similar glycoproteins. Each winds in and out of the plasma membrane so that more than one surface is presented extracellularly for hormone

binding and intracellularly for signal generation (see Figure 5-5). The β_1- and β_2-receptors are coupled to the stimulating G protein of adenylyl cyclase, and hormone binding increases cyclic AMP levels. In contrast, the α_2-receptor is coupled to the inhibiting G protein of adenylyl cyclase, and hormone binding decreases cyclic AMP levels. Catecholamine hormones therefore either trigger (β_1 or β_2) or suppress (α_2) a cascade of protein phosphorylations catalyzed by protein kinase A. The α_1-receptor is structurally different and is coupled to calcium and phosphatidylinositol products as second messengers.

Continuous exposure to catecholamines eventually down-regulates the number of receptors and induces partial refractoriness to hormone action. A distinctly different phenomenon—acute desensitization to successive doses of catecholamine hormones—is caused by hormone-induced activation of protein kinase A or C, which results in the phosphorylation of the receptor molecules themselves. This desensitization process constitutes a form of rapid intracellular negative feedback that almost immediately limits hormone actions.

Catecholamine hormones mobilize substrates for energy generation and increased energy expenditure

THE MAJOR METABOLIC EFFECT OF CATECHOLAMINES IS FUEL MOBILIZATION (Figure 47-3). Glycogenolysis in the liver is stimulated via the cyclic AMP–mediated activation of phosphorylase, and glucose output increases. In the absence of glucagon, this epinephrine action is critical to recovery from insulin-induced hypoglycemia in type 1 diabetes (see Chapter 42). Glycogenolysis in muscle is similarly stimulated. This increases muscle glucose supply and glycolysis. Lactate is released and serves as a substrate for hepatic gluconeogenesis. In addition, gluconeogenesis is stimulated directly by catecholamines, through α_1-receptors in the liver. Plasma glucose levels also rise because catecholamines inhibit insulin secretion as well as insulin-stimulated glucose uptake by muscle tissue. The availability of free fatty acids is increased by activating the enzyme, adipose tissue lipase. The enhanced lipolysis in turn leads to increased free fatty acid oxidation in the liver and ketogenesis.

> Thus the catecholamine hormones are diabetogenic. They contribute materially to the development of hyperglycemia and ketonemia in diabetic ketoacidosis, particularly when an intercurrent stress has provoked this metabolic emergency.

Catecholamines increase the basal metabolic rate by stimulating facultative, or nonshivering, thermogenesis (see Chapter 41). This action is an important part

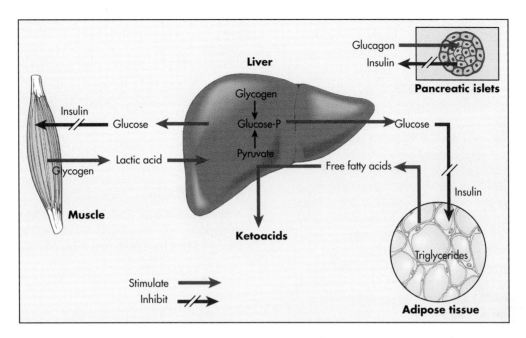

Figure 47-3 Metabolic effects of epinephrine. The hormone stimulates glucose production and inhibits glucose uptake. Lipolysis and ketogenesis are stimulated. The result is an increase in plasma levels of glucose, free fatty acids, and ketoacids.

of the response to cold exposure. In adipose tissue, catecholamines stimulate energy expenditure and increase heat production by inducing transcription of the gene for an uncoupling protein (see Figure 41-7). Catecholamines also increase diet-induced thermogenesis.

Sympathetic nervous system activity decreases during fasting and increases after feeding. In this way, norepinephrine adapts total energy use to energy availability and helps maintain balance between them. In contrast, epinephrine secretion increases slightly during prolonged fasting and also 4 to 5 hours after a meal, when the plasma glucose level is declining. This response serves a different purpose: sustaining glucose production for use by the central nervous system.

> The activity of the sympathetic nervous system tends to be decreased in obese individuals. This characteristic favors storage of energy as fat when dietary calories are plentiful.

Epinephrine and norepinephrine activate the cardiovascular system

The cardiovascular and visceral effects of epinephrine are consonant with its metabolic actions (Table 47-1). For example, during exercise, epinephrine increases cardiac output by increasing the cardiac contractile force and heart rate (see Chapters 19 and 26). At the same time, muscle arterioles dilate, whereas renal, splanchnic, and cutaneous arterioles constrict. Systolic blood pressure increases. The net effect is to shunt blood to exercising muscles and away

Table 47-1	Actions of Catecholamine Hormones
β	**α**
Metabolic	
↑ Glycogenolysis	↑ Gluconeogenesis (α_1)
↑ Glucose use	
↑ Lipolysis and ketosis (β_1)	
↑ Calorigenesis (β_1)	
↑ Insulin secretion (β_2)	↓ Insulin secretion (α_2)
↑ Glucagon secretion (β_2)	
↑ Muscle K$^+$ uptake (β_2)	
Cardiovascular	
↑ Cardiac contractility (β_1)	
↑ Heart rate (β_1)	
↑ Conduction velocity (β_1)	
↑ Arteriolar dilation (β_2) (muscle)	↑ Arteriolar vasoconstriction (α_1) (splanchnic, renal, cutaneous, genital)
↓ Blood pressure	↑ Blood pressure
Visceral	
↑ Muscle relaxation (β_2) Gastrointestinal Urinary Bronchial	↑ Sphincter contraction (α_1) Gastrointestinal Urinary
Other	
—	Sweating (adrenergic) Dilation of pupils Platelet aggregation (α_2)

↑, Increased; ↓, decreased.

from other tissues while essential coronary and cerebral blood flows (see Chapter 26). This guarantees the delivery of O_2 and substrate for energy production to the critical tissues in situations of danger or during whole body exercise.

> In severe or prolonged states of shock, the compensatory hypersecretion of catecholamines can eventually contribute to fatal ischemic kidney and hepatic failure and to lactic acidosis (see Chapter 26). The catecholamine response to exercise may also be disadvantageous in patients who have coronary artery disease and who cannot adequately increase myocardial blood flow. β-Adrenergic antagonists are used to good therapeutic advantage in this situation; by decreasing heart rate, cardiac contractility, and systolic blood pressure, these drugs improve the balance between myocardial work and O_2 supply and prevent **angina pectoris** (chest pain).

Catecholamine hormones have effects that mimic those of the sympathetic nervous system

During exposure to cold, the constriction of cutaneous vessels helps conserve heat and reinforces epinephrine's thermogenic action. Other responses useful to the threatened individual are (1) relaxation of the bronchioles, which improves alveolar gas exchange; (2) dilation of the pupils, which permits better distant vision; and (3) inhibition of temporarily unneeded gastrointestinal and genitourinary motor activity.

> During acute asthma attacks, constriction of the bronchioles increases airway resistance (see Chapter 28) and causes wheezing and hypoxia. Synthetic β-adrenergic agonists of epinephrine, administered through inhalers, relax the bronchioles and provide critical relief to patients in respiratory distress.

The catecholamines also have significant actions on mineral metabolism. They increase sodium reabsorption by the kidney by stimulating renal tubular sodium transport and by stimulating renin release and consequently aldosterone secretion. They also stimulate the influx of potassium into muscle cells via $β_2$-receptors and help prevent hyperkalemia.

> Pathological hypersecretion of epinephrine and norepinephrine from a tumor of the chromaffin cells **(pheochromocytoma)** results in a distinct and dangerous syndrome. Bursts of catecholamine release can cause sudden tachycardia, extreme anxiety with a sense of impending death, cold perspiration, skin pallor resulting from vasoconstriction, blurred vision, headache, and chest pain. The blood pressure may rise greatly and cause stroke or heart failure. In addition to such episodes, chronic catecholamine excess may produce weight loss (as a result of the increased metabolic rate) and hyperglycemia. Prompt surgical removal of the tumor is mandatory.

The Hypothalamic-Pituitary-Adrenocortical Axis, Adrenal Medulla, and Sympathetic Nervous System Together Integrate the Response to Stress

The adrenal medulla and adrenal cortex are both major participants in the adaptation to stress. Their intimate anatomical juxtaposition mirrors a fundamental functional relationship between the sympathetic nervous system and the corticotropin-releasing hormone–adrenocorticotropic hormone–cortisol axis (Figure 47-4). Stress is perceived by many areas of the brain, from the cortex down to the brainstem. Major stresses almost simultaneously activate corticotropin-releasing hormone (CRH) and ADH neurons and adrenergic neurons in the hypothalamus. The activation is mutually reinforcing because norepinephrine input increases CRH release and CRH increases adrenergic discharge (Figure 47-4). The release of CRH (and ADH) elevates plasma cortisol levels; adrenergic stimulation elevates plasma catecholamine levels. Together, these hormones increase glucose production and shift glucose use toward the central nervous system and away from peripheral tissues. Epinephrine also rapidly augments the supply of free fatty acid to the heart and to muscles, and cortisol facilitates this lipolytic response. Both hormones raise the blood pressure and cardiac output and improve the delivery of substrates to tissues critical to the immediate defense of the organism. If the stress involves tissue trauma or invasion by microorganisms, high cortisol levels eventually act to restrain the initial inflammatory and immune responses so that they do not lead to irreparable damage.

Norepinephrine and CRH produce other adaptive responses to stress. A general state of arousal and vigilance, an activation of defensively useful behavior, and appropriate aggressiveness result from norepinephrine stimulation of pertinent brain centers. At the same time, CRH input to other hypothalamic neurons inhibits appetite, sexual activity, and growth hormone and gonadotropin release. This is reinforced by the excess of cortisol, which also suppresses growth and ovulation. Thus the adaptation to stress represents a prime example of the integration between the nervous system and the endocrine system.

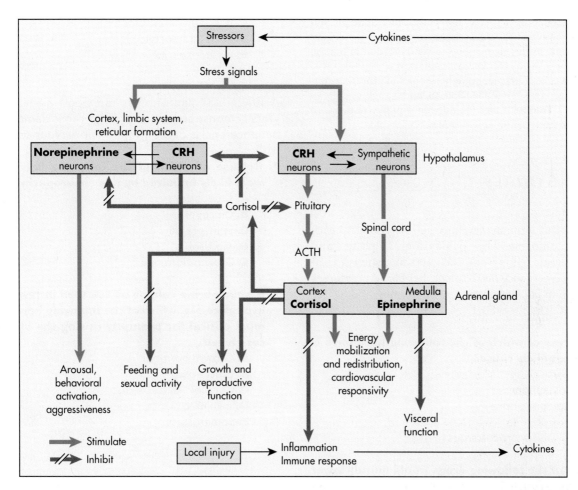

Figure 47-4 Integrated responses to stress mediated by the sympathetic nervous system and the hypothalamic-pituitary-adrenocortical axis. The responses are mutually reinforcing at both the central and peripheral levels. Negative feedback by cortisol also can limit an overresponse that might be harmful to the individual.

SUMMARY

- The adrenal medulla is an enlarged, specialized sympathetic ganglion that synthesizes epinephrine and norepinephrine from tyrosine and stores them in granules.
- Catecholamines are released from the medulla in response to activity in preganglionic cholinergic fibers of the sympathetic nervous system that are stimulated by hypoglycemia, hypovolemia, hypotension, exercise, or stress.
- Circulating epinephrine increases the concentrations of plasma glucose, free fatty acids, and ketoacids by stimulating glycogenolysis and lipolysis and by inhibiting glucose uptake by muscle. The metabolic rate also rises. Cyclic AMP and Ca^{++} are second messengers.
- Cardiovascular actions include increases in heart rate and cardiac contractility and variable effects on different vascular beds.
- Circulating norepinephrine contributes to the above effects, but more often the effects of epinephrine are reinforced by concurrent activation of the sympathetic nervous system, with norepinephrine as the neurotransmitter.

BIBLIOGRAPHY

Clutter WE et al: Epinephrine plasma metabolic clearance rates and physiologic thresholds for metabolic and hemodynamic actions in man, *J Clin Invest* 66:94, 1980.

Cryer PE: Physiology and pathophysiology of the human sympathoadrenal neuroendocrine system, *N Engl J Med* 303:436, 1980.

Landsberg L, Young JB: The role of the sympathetic nervous system and catecholamines in the regulation of energy metabolism, *Am J Clin Nutr* 36:1018, 1983.

Landsberg L, Young JB: Catecholamines and the adrenal medulla. In Wilson JD, Foster DW, eds: *Williams textbook of endocrinology*, ed 9, Philadelphia, 1998, WB Saunders.

Lefkowitz RJ, Caron MG: Adrenergic receptors: molecular mechanisms of clinically relevant recognition, *Clin Res* 33:395, 1985.

Matthews DE, Pesola G, Campbell RG: Effect of epinephrine on amino acid and energy metabolism in humans, *Am J Physiol* 258:E948, 1990.

Santiago JV et al: Epinephrine, norepinephrine, glucagon, and growth hormone release in association with physiological decrements in the plasma glucose concentration in normal and diabetic man, *J Clin Endocrinol Metab* 51:877, 1980.

Silverberg A et al: Norepinephrine: hormone and neurotransmitter in man, *Am J Physiol* 234:E252, 1978.

Wortsman J, Frank S, Cryer PE: Adrenomedullary response to maximal stress in humans, *Am J Med* 77:779, 1984.

▷ CASE STUDIES

Case 47-1

A 25-year-old woman develops sudden, severe headaches accompanied by palpitations, anxiety, and clammy sweat. During one such episode, she is examined in an emergency department; her blood pressure is 260/140 mm Hg, her pulse is 56 beats/min, and her serum K^+ value is 3.4 mEq/L.

1. An excess of which of the following hormones is the most likely cause?
   A. Cortisol
   B. Epinephrine
   C. Norepinephrine
   D. Aldosterone
   E. 11-Deoxycorticosterone

2. Which of the following drugs would quickly lower her dangerously high systolic and diastolic blood pressures?
   A. An α_1-adrenergic blocker
   B. A β_1-adrenergic blocker
   C. A β_2-adrenergic blocker
   D. An α_2-adrenergic blocker
   E. An aldosterone antagonist

Case Study 47-2

A 40-year-old man who has had type 1 diabetes for 30 years demonstrates severe hyperglycemic damage to the peripheral parts of the sympathetic nervous system.

1. Release of which of the following hormones is most likely impaired by this "neuropathy"?
   A. C peptide
   B. Glucagon
   C. Epinephrine
   D. Cortisol
   E. Growth hormone

2. If epinephrine cannot be released in response to hypoglycemia, which of the following hormones is most critical for promptly raising the blood glucose level?
   A. Growth hormone
   B. Glucagon
   C. Cortisol
   D. Insulin
   E. Somatostatin

CHAPTER 48

Overview of Reproductive Function

OBJECTIVES

- Identify the synthetic pathway for androgens and estrogens, the gonadal steroid hormones.
- Identify the common elements of the hypothalamic pituitary gonadal axis in males and females.
- Describe the common hormonal components of puberty and senescence in males and females.
- Explain the differences between genetic sex, gonadal sex, and phenotypic (genital) sex.

The endocrine glands in general are essential to maintaining the life and well-being of the individual. In contrast, the endocrine function of the gonads is also concerned with the perpetuation and well-being of the species. Human reproduction requires highly complex patterns of hypothalamic-pituitary-gonadal function that ensure the development and maintenance of mature gametes, **ova** and **spermatozoa,** from primordial germ cells; their subsequent successful union **(fertilization);** and finally the growth and development of the conceptus within the body of the mother. Gonadal hormones also influence many other functions and structures described elsewhere in this book (e.g., hepatic function, skeletal structure). Although certain fundamental differences exist between male and female gonadal function, important conceptual similarities and operational homologies are also present. The gender differences are better appreciated if the common aspects of gonadal function are first understood.

The Gonads Contain Several Cell Types with Different Reproductive and Hormonal Functions

The gonad, whether ovary or testis, consists of two distinct anatomical and functional parts. One part encloses the developing germ cell line, with specialized membrane and cytoplasmic barriers that prevent its indiscriminate exposure to all constituents of plasma and interstitial fluid. In the ovary the germ cell enclosure is the **follicle;** in the testis, it is the **spermatogenic (seminiferous) tubule.** The other part is composed of surrounding endocrine cells that secrete sex steroid hormones, protein hormones, and other products necessary for germ cell development. The most important sex steroids are **estradiol** and **progesterone** in the female and **testosterone** in the male. Protein hormones produced by the gonads include **inhibin, activin, follistatin, antimüllerian hormone (AMH),** and **oocyte meiosis inhibitor,** as well as various derivatives of proopiomelanocortin (see Chapter 46).

Acting locally in paracrine and autocrine fashion, the gonadal hormones stimulate the development of the respective germ cells into ova and spermatozoa. Acting systemically in endocrine fashion, these hormones (1) stimulate the development and function of the secondary sex organs essential for the support and delivery of the ova and spermatozoa to the site of fertilization, (2) regulate the secretion of hypothalamic-pituitary hormones essential to gonadal function, (3) modify somatic shape and regulate certain physiological functions within each gender, and (4) support the conceptus in the early phase of pregnancy in the female.

There are two principal types of endocrine cells in the gonads. Those immediately encompassing the germ cells are called **granulosa cells** in the ovary and **Sertoli cells** in the testis. Those more distant from the germ cells and separated from them by a basement membrane are called **theca** or **interstitial cells** in the ovary and **Leydig cells** in the testis. The homologous granulosa and Sertoli cells secrete mainly estrogens, whereas the homologous theca and Leydig cells secrete mainly androgens. Only in females, progesterone is secreted in large amounts by transformed granulosa and theca cells known as **luteal cells.** The protein products come mostly from granulosa and Sertoli cells.

Synthesis of Sex Steroid Hormones

The gonads synthesize androgens and estrogens by the same biochemical steps used in the adrenal cortex

THE BIOSYNTHESIS OF GONADAL STEROID HORMONES FOLLOWS A COMMON PATHWAY IN BOTH GENDERS (Figure 48-1). THE ENZYMES, THEIR ORGANELLE LOCALIZATION, AND THEIR COFACTOR REQUIREMENTS ARE THE SAME AS THOSE DESCRIBED FOR THE ADRENAL CORTEX (see Chapter 46). Furthermore, the go-

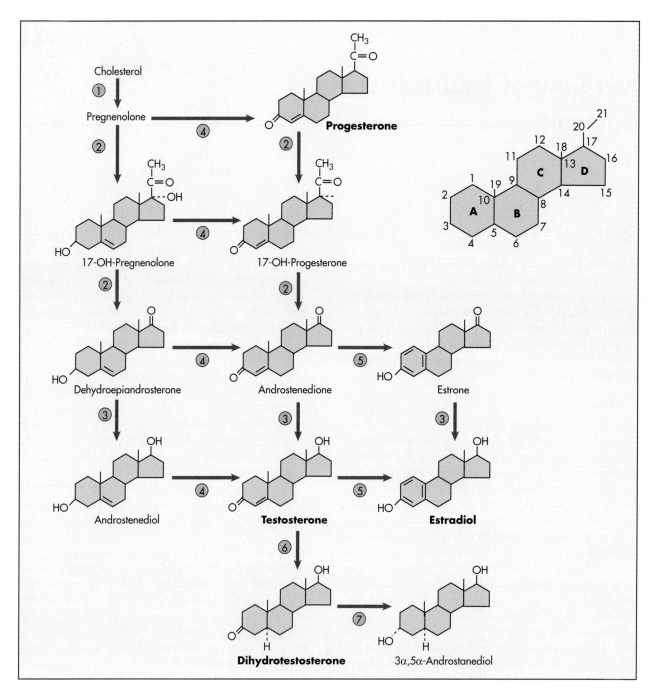

Figure 48-1 Pathways of synthesis of steroid hormones in the gonads. Testosterone is the major product of the testis. Estradiol and progesterone are the major products of the ovary. *OH,* Hydroxy. The enzymes are: *1,* 20,22-desmolase (P-450scc); *2,* 17-hydroxylase/17,20-desmolase; *3,* 17β-hydroxysteroid dehydrogenase; *4,* 3β-ol-dehydrogenase, Δ^{4,5}-isomerase; *5,* aromatase; *6,* 5α-reductase; *7,* 3α-reductase.

nadal enzymes are identical to the adrenal enzymes, and the same genes direct their synthesis. Cholesterol, either synthesized in situ from acetyl coenzyme A or taken up from the low-density lipoproteins in plasma, is the starting compound. P-450scc (20,22-desmolase) catalyzes side-chain cleavage of cholesterol and is the rate-limiting step for the synthesis of progesterone, androgens, and estrogens. Within the testes a small quantity of testosterone undergoes 5α-reduction to **di-** **hydrotestosterone (DHT),** a potent androgen. However, a much larger and more important conversion of testosterone to DHT, catalyzed by the enzyme 5α-reductase, occurs in target tissues. Estradiol and estrone are synthesized from their respective obligate androgen precursors by the P-450 **aromatase** enzyme complex. This sequentially catalyzes the hydroxylation and oxidation of the 19-methyl group, the creation of a 1-2 double bond, the decarboxylation of position 19, and the formation of the characteristic benzene ring of estrogens.

Regulation of Gonadal Steroid Hormone Secretion

A hypothalamic releasing hormone and two pituitary gonadotropins regulate the synthesis and secretion of sex hormones

A hypothalamic–anterior pituitary–gonadal axis, analogous to those involved in thyroid and adrenal function, is the basis for gonadal regulation (Figure 48-2). The components are **gonadotropin-releasing hormone (GnRH)** and two pituitary gonadotropins, designated **luteinizing hormone (LH)** and **follicle-stimulating hormone (FSH).** A single pituitary cell type, the gonadotroph, generally produces both LH and FSH, although occasional gonadotrophs contain only one or the other.

Gonadotropin-releasing hormone

GnRH, also known as **luteinizing hormone–releasing hormone,** stimulates both LH and FSH secretion but LH more so. GnRH, a decapeptide synthesized from a much larger preprohormone, is produced in two clusters of neurons in the arcuate and preoptic nuclei of the hypothalamus. From there, the hormone is transported axonally for storage in the median eminence. Input from other areas of the brain to the hypothalamus (see Chapter 44) permits reproduction to be influenced by light-dark cycles (likely via melatonin), by stress hormones such as corticotropin-releasing hormone, and by olfactory stimuli via airborne molecules known as **pheromones.** Dopaminergic and endorphinergic tracts within the hypothalamus and the median eminence transmit important inhibitory influences on the release of GnRH (Figure 48-2). GnRH is released into the pituitary portal veins in pulses driven by a primary generator. Men have 8 to 10 pulses per day, whereas in women the frequency and periodicity of pulses vary with the menstrual cycle. In prepubertal children, pulsatility is greatly reduced.

Properly programmed GnRH pulses stimulate the secretion of an appropriate balance of FSH and LH

GnRH binds to its plasma membrane receptor and triggers an influx of extracellular calcium into the gonadotroph cells. Complexed to calmodulin, the calcium acts as the major second messenger (see Figure 5-9), and phosphatidylinositol products play a subsidiary role. GnRH stimulates the simultaneous release of LH and FSH from their secretory granules. The ratio of FSH to LH increases when the frequency of GnRH pulses declines. GnRH also stimulates the transcription of genes that direct the synthesis of the two gonadotropins and the subsequent processing of their prohormones via

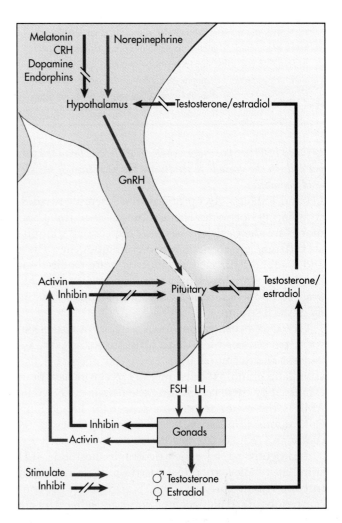

Figure 48-2 Hypothalamic–anterior pituitary–gonadal axis. The hypothalamic peptide gonadotropin-releasing hormone *(GnRH)* stimulates the release of two gonadotropins, luteinizing hormone *(LH)* and follicle-stimulating hormone *(FSH),* from the pituitary gland. The gonadotropins in turn stimulate gonadal secretion of primarily testosterone in males and primarily estradiol in females. These feed back negatively at both the pituitary and hypothalamic levels to inhibit the secretion of luteinizing hormone and follicle-stimulating hormone. In addition, follicle-stimulating hormone stimulates the gonadal release of inhibin, which feeds back negatively to preferentially block the release of follicle-stimulating hormone. In contrast, estradiol (in women) and the gonadal protein activin have positive feedback effects on pituitary secretion. *CRH,* Corticotropin-releasing hormone.

glycosylation. A GnRH infusion typically produces a biphasic LH response.

Prolonged stimulation by GnRH causes the downregulation of its receptor, consequent desensitization of the gonadotroph to GnRH, and resulting profound inhibition of gonadotropin secretion. Long-acting GnRH superagonists are commonly used therapeutically when gonadotropin secretion and androgen or estrogen production by the gonad must be suppressed. Such situations include

carcinoma of the prostate in men and **endometriosis** in women. In participants of in vitro fertilization programs, it may be easier to produce ova at a specified time with an external program of FSH and LH administration (see Chapter 50) if endogenous secretion of these hormones is eliminated.

LH and FSH act via cyclic AMP on different primary target cells in the gonads to stimulate the secretion of sex steroid hormones

LH and FSH are glycoproteins that resemble thyroid-stimulating hormone. The α subunits of all three hormones are identical, whereas their respective β subunits are different and are determined by unique genes. The α and β subunits in each gonadotropin are required for binding to its gonadal receptor, and proper carbohydrate components are necessary for full biological activity of the β subunits.

LH MAINLY STIMULATES THE THECA CELLS OF THE FEMALE AND THE LEYDIG CELLS OF THE MALE TO SYNTHESIZE AND SECRETE ANDROGENS and to a much lesser extent, estrogens. LH also stimulates granulosa cells, once LH receptors have been expressed by these cells during the female cycle. Cyclic AMP is the major second messenger for LH actions. Continuous stimulation by LH down-regulates its receptor and reduces responsivity to the hormone.

Analogous to adrenocorticotropic hormone, LH stimulates cholesterol transfer to the mitochondria and its conversion to pregnenolone. Subsequently the concentrations of steroidogenic enzymes and adrenoxin are increased by stimulating transcription of their genes. Most important, LH INCREASES THE LEVELS OF 17-HYDROXYLASE/17,20-DESMOLASE, WHICH IS THE ESSENTIAL STEP IN ANDROGEN SYNTHESIS (Figure 48-1).

FSH stimulates **granulosa** and **Sertoli cells** to secrete estrogens. Acting via its plasma membrane receptor and cyclic AMP as a second messenger, FSH INCREASES TRANSCRIPTION OF THE GENE FOR **AROMATASE,** THE ENZYME SPECIFIC TO ESTRADIOL SYNTHESIS. Another important effect of FSH is to increase the number of LH receptors in target cells and thereby to amplify their sensitivity to LH. FSH also stimulates the secretion of **inhibin** and other protein products of the granulosa and Sertoli cells (Figure 48-2).

Sex steroid hormones and protein products of the gonads feed back to regulate the release of gonadotropin-releasing hormone and the secretion of pituitary gonadotropins

The regulation of gonadotropin secretion, sex steroid hormone production, and other aspects of gonadal function is complex, and those aspects distinctive to each gender are described in later sections. However, certain common principles exist (Figure 48-2). TESTOSTERONE IN MEN AND ESTRADIOL IN WOMEN INHIBIT THE SECRETION OF LH AND FSH. In this basic negative-feedback loop, the sex steroids act at the pituitary level by blocking the actions of GnRH on gonadotropin release and synthesis. They also act at the hypothalamic level by recruiting endorphin neurons to decrease GnRH levels. Both the frequency and the amplitude of LH and FSH pulses are diminished.

Negative feedback forms the basis for the use of current contraceptive drugs by women. Combinations of relatively small doses of estrogens and synthetic progestational agents, given orally, decrease the secretion of pituitary gonadotropins to levels below those needed to produce a mature ovum monthly. The cessation of oral contraceptives is generally followed by rapid reinstitution of fertility. Analogous administration of androgens for this purpose has not yet been successfully formulated for safe and effective use as a male contraceptive.

In women, an additional specific positive-feedback effect of estradiol on LH secretion is included in the basic framework (see Chapter 50). This effect depends on the dose, time, and duration of exposure to estradiol.

Another negative-feedback loop relates **inhibin** from granulosa and Sertoli cells to FSH secretion. IN-HIBIN REDUCES GnRH RELEASE, FSH β SUBUNIT SYNTHESIS, AND THE STIMULATORY EFFECT OF GnRH ON FSH SECRETION. In contrast, from the same gonadal cells, **activin** exerts a positive-feedback effect to stimulate FSH secretion. Thus the output of LH and FSH from the pituitary gland can be exquisitely and differentially regulated by interactions among hypothalamic and gonadal products. At various times the critical influence may be from either site. In this sense the gonad can be viewed as much more self-regulatory than either the adrenal cortex or the thyroid. This is most apparent in women, as discussed later.

The Secretion Pattern of Sex Steroid Hormones Varies Markedly at Different Stages of Life

The hypothalamic-pituitary-gonadal axis changes markedly throughout human life. Although the female and male patterns differ, certain common aspects bear emphasis (Figure 48-3).

Intrauterine and childhood pattern

In humans, GnRH is present in the hypothalamus by 4 weeks of gestation, and FSH and LH are present in the pituitary gland by 10 to 12 weeks of gestation. A peak of gonadotropin concentrations occurs in fetal plasma at midgestation. The concentrations drop to low levels before birth and then transiently increase (more prolonged in females) again at about 2 months of age. For the rest of

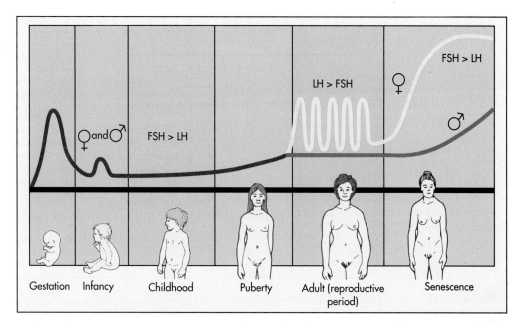

Figure 48-3 Pattern of gonadotropin secretion throughout life. Note the transient peaks during gestation and early infancy and low levels thereafter in childhood. Women subsequently develop monthly cyclic bursts, with LH concentrations exceeding FSH concentrations; men do not develop such a pattern. Both genders show increased gonadotropin production after 50 years of age, with FSH levels exceeding LH levels.

childhood, FSH and LH are secreted at very low levels. These changes are mirrored by similar fluctuations of plasma testosterone in males and of plasma estradiol in females.

Puberty

THE TRANSITION FROM A NONREPRODUCTIVE TO A REPRODUCTIVE STATE REQUIRES THE PUBERTAL MATURATION OF THE ENTIRE HYPOTHALAMIC-PITUITARY-GONADAL AXIS. Before a child reaches 10 years of age, plasma LH and FSH levels are low despite very low concentrations of gonadal hormones. Therefore either the negative-feedback system is inoperative or the hypothalamus and pituitary gland are exquisitely sensitive to testosterone, estradiol, and inhibin. One factor in puberty may thus be the gradual maturing of hypothalamic neurons, and this process leads to an increased synthesis and release of GnRH. Two biological factors that initiate this process may be (1) maturation of the bones to a certain stage and (2) an increase in adipose tissue to a particular level. A preceding increase in adrenal androgen secretion marked by increasing plasma levels of dehydroepiandrosterone sulfate may stimulate the required bone development. An increase in plasma leptin levels may signal GnRH neurons that an adequate amount of adipose tissue is present.

The age at which this reproductive maturational process begins ranges from 9 to 17 years. It may also be genetically preprogrammed because familial patterns are apparent. As puberty approaches, a pulsatile pattern of LH and FSH secretion appears. The ratio of plasma LH to FSH rises as the pulse frequency increases. Furthermore, during early and middle puberty but not usually thereafter, a dis-

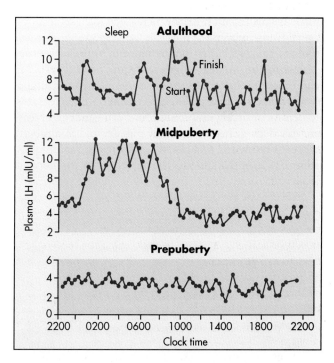

Figure 48-4 Changing pattern of diurnal LH secretion from childhood to adulthood. During puberty, LH secretion becomes much more pulsatile. In addition, a nocturnal peak appears early in puberty and then disappears when puberty is completed. Males and females both undergo these changes. Each day's sampling started and finished at approximately 10 AM. (Redrawn from Boyar RM et al: N Engl J Med 287:582, 1972.)

tinct nocturnal peak in LH secretion is observed (Figure 48-4). This coincides with, but is not proved to be the result of, a decrease in nocturnal melatonin secretion. These changes in GnRH and gonadotropins occur even in the absence of the gonads.

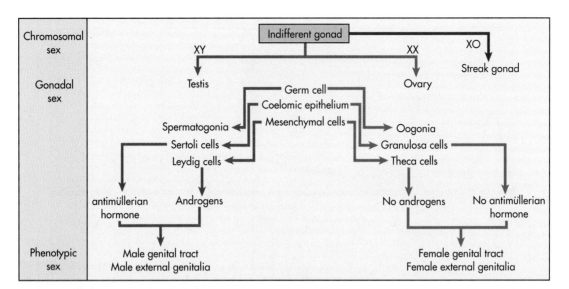

Figure 48-5 Overview of the development of the cells of the ovary and testis from the primitive indifferent gonad. Androgens and AMH from the normal testis induce the male pattern of differentiation of the genital tract and external genitalia. It is the lack of secretion of these products from the normal ovary at the critical times that determines differentiation of the genital tract and the external genitalia into the female pattern.

During early puberty, the responsiveness of the pituitary gland to GnRH changes so that LH exceeds FSH output. This may result from the increased synthesis and storage of LH in response to pulsatile GnRH secretion because the latter allows better maintenance of GnRH receptors. Although the gonadal target cells can respond to LH in childhood, their responsiveness is augmented during puberty. Therefore plasma levels of estradiol in females, testosterone in males, and inhibin in both genders increase sharply during these years. Early puberty and midpuberty can thus be viewed as a cascade of increasing maturation from the hypothalamic to the pituitary to the gonadal level.

> Clinical endocrine testing often fails to distinguish between a late onset of normal puberty and a disorder of the hypothalamus that prevents the increased secretion of LH and FSH. Because failure to show physical signs of puberty by age 13 or 14 (see Chapters 49 and 50) is psychologically distressing to the child, treatment with sufficient testosterone or estradiol to induce such changes and a growth spurt may be warranted. Such hormonal support can be withdrawn after an appropriate period to determine whether normal puberty has finally begun.

Once the adult pattern of gonadotropin secretion is established, the basal plasma concentrations of LH and FSH (approximately 10^{-11} M) are similar in men and women. An important distinguishing feature between the genders is the additional establishment of a dramatic monthly gonadotropin cycle in females only (see Chapter 50); this is when the LH bursts greatly exceed the FSH bursts (Figure 48-3).

Climacteric

In both genders, a loss of gonadal responsiveness to gonadotropin stimulation develops around the fifth decade of life. In males, this is gradual, and some reproductive capacity usually persists even into the ninth decade. In females, reproductive capacity is eventually lost completely, and menopause occurs. In both genders, negative feedback leads to elevated plasma gonadotropin levels. The FSH level rises more than the LH level, and the increase in both gonadotropins is more distinct in females (Figure 48-3).

The Two Genders Are Normally Differentiated by Genetic, Gonadal, and Genital (Phenotypic) Factors

The most fundamental and obvious difference between the genders lies in the anatomy and consequent physiology of their reproductive tracts. During the first 5 weeks of gestation, however, the gonads of males and females are indistinguishable, and their genital tracts are unformed. From this stage of the "indifferent gonad" to that of the completed normal individual of either gender lies the process of sexual differentiation (Figures 48-5 and 48-6). The final maleness or femaleness is best characterized in terms of differences in genetic, gonadal, and genital (phenotypic) sex.

Maleness versus femaleness is determined positively and predominantly by the presence of the Y chromosome

The normal male has a chromosome complement of 44 autosomes and two sex chromosomes, XY. WITHOUT THE Y CHROMOSOME (OR IN RARE INSTANCES, DNA TRANSLOCATED

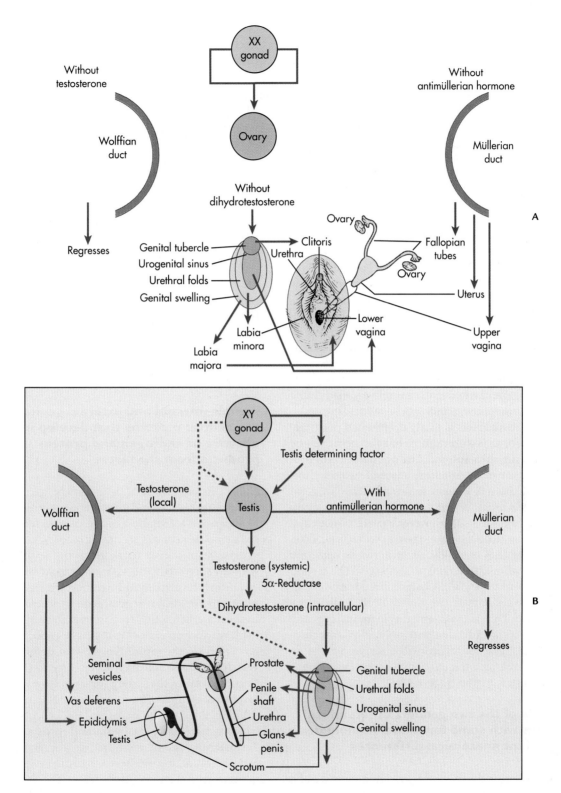

Figure 48-6 A, Development of the female reproductive organs. Note that this development does not require hormonal products from the ovary. Therefore in the absence of gonads, the female pattern results. **B,** Development of the male reproductive organs. Note that the complete male pattern requires the secretion and local action of testosterone on the wolffian duct, the reduction of testosterone to DHT to provide androgen action in the anlage cells of the external genitalia, and the secretion of AMH to suppress development of the müllerian duct.

FROM THE Y TO THE X CHROMOSOME), NEITHER TESTICULAR DE-VELOPMENT NOR MASCULINIZATION OF THE GENITAL TRACTS AND EXTERNAL GENITALIA CAN OCCUR. The organization of the indifferent gonad into the characteristic spermatogenic tubules of the male is directed by a 14-kilobase segment known as the **sex-determining region of the Y-chromosome (SRY gene),** which encodes the **testis determining factor (TDF).** This gene is located on the short arm of the Y chromosome (Figures 48-5 and 48-6, *B*). Either identical to or closely linked to the SRY or TDF gene is one that codes for the **H-Y antigen.** This glycoprotein is present on the surface of all male cells except diploid germ cells, and it is one factor that can cause rejection of male tissues by female recipients. The H-Y antigen causes virilization of the cells of an indifferent gonad or of disaggregated early ovarian cells in vitro. Other loci on the Y chromosome are probably involved in guiding an orderly process of spermatogenesis. Even though it is essential, the Y chromosome by itself is not sufficient for maleness. Located on the X chromosome is the gene for the **androgen receptor,** which sensitizes the genital ducts and the external genitalia to the masculinizing effects of testosterone and DHT. Autosomal genes may also participate in directing the initial organization of the primitive gonad into a functioning reproductive gland.

In contrast, femaleness is partly determined positively by the presence of an X chromosome but also negatively by the absence of a Y chromosome. The normal female chromosome complement is 44 autosomes and two sex chromosomes, XX. Both X chromosomes are active in germ cells and are essential for the genesis of a normal ovary (Figures 48-5 and 48-6, *A*). However, FEMALE DIFFERENTIATION OF THE GENITAL DUCTS AND EXTERNAL GENITALIA REQUIRES THAT ONLY A SINGLE X CHROMOSOME BE ACTIVE IN DIRECTING TRANSCRIPTION WITHIN THEIR CONSTITUENT CELLS. The second X chromosome of a normal XX female is randomly inactivated in all tissues outside the gonad. Both X alleles are equally affected. Thus if an abnormality in **meiosis** or early **mitosis** produces an individual with only a single sex chromosome (an X), that individual will undergo normal female genital development even though her gonad is abnormal and without function (Figure 48-5).

The gonads of the two genders differentiate into organs with some functional homologies but important anatomical differences

The indifferent gonad of 5 weeks' gestation consists of a primordial mesonephric ridge with several components: (1) coelomic epithelium, the precursor of granulosa and Sertoli cells; (2) mesenchymal stromal cells, the precursors of theca and Leydig cells; and (3) germ cells that have migrated there from the yolk sac endoderm (Figure 48-5). This assembly is organized as an outer cortex and an inner medulla.

In a normal male fetus, the spermatogenic tubules begin to form at 6 weeks, followed by differentiation of the

Sertoli cells at 7 weeks and the Leydig cells at 8 to 9 weeks. At this point the testis is structurally recognizable, and testosterone secretion has begun. The germ cells have become enclosed within the medulla, whereas the cortex has regressed. No known hormonal influences are required for this differentiation of the indifferent gonad into a testis.

In a normal female fetus, differentiation of the indifferent gonad into an ovary does not start until 9 weeks' gestation. At this time, ACTIVITY OF BOTH X CHROMOSOMES WITHIN THE GERM CELLS IS ESSENTIAL. The germ cells begin to undergo mitosis, giving rise to daughter cells called **oogonia,** which continue to proliferate. Shortly thereafter, meiosis is initiated in some oogonia, and each is surrounded by differentiating granulosa cells and precursor theca cells to form a **follicle.** The germ cells, now known as **primary oocytes,** remain in the first stage, or **prophase,** of meiosis until they are activated many years later. In contrast to the male arrangement of gonadal zones, the cortex, which contains the follicles, predominates in the developed ovary, whereas the medulla regresses. The primitive ovary begins to synthesize estrogenic hormones concurrent with these developments, and these hormones may contribute to later ovarian differentiation by blocking androgen actions.

Female internal and external genitalia are the neutral patterns that develop in the absence of androgen and protein products from the testes

Up to this point in fetal development, sexual differentiation is largely independent of known hormonal products. However, DIFFERENTIATION OF THE GENITAL DUCTS AND EXTERNAL GENITALIA REQUIRES SPECIFIC HORMONAL SIGNALS FROM THE NORMAL MALE GONAD TO PRODUCE THE MASCULINE FORMAT. WITHOUT SUCH INPUT, THE FEMININE FORMAT WILL RESULT.

During the sexually indifferent stage, from 3 to 7 weeks' gestation, two different genital ducts develop on each side. In the male, at about 9 to 10 weeks, the wolffian, or mesonephric, duct on each side begins to grow. Together, they give rise to the **epididymis, vas deferens, seminal vesicles,** and **ejaculatory duct** by 12 weeks (Figure 48-6, *B*). This constitutes the system for delivering sperm from the testis to the female. The growth and differentiation of each wolffian duct in the male are induced by testosterone, which is secreted by the **ipsilateral testis** and acts locally. Testosterone is not converted to the active metabolite DHT before acting on the wolffian duct cells, as it must be in other genital tissues. In the female the wolffian ducts regress at 10 to 11 weeks because the ipsilateral ovary does not secrete testosterone.

Each müllerian duct arises parallel to the wolffian duct on its side. In the male the müllerian ducts begin to regress at 7 to 8 weeks, about the same time that the Sertoli cells of the testis appear. These cells produce a glycoprotein, AMH, which causes atrophy of the müllerian ducts. AMH belongs to a superfamily of growth-regulating factors that are coded for by genes similar to each other and to the

AMH gene; these include transforming growth factors (TGF-α, TGF-β), epidermal growth factor, and inhibin. AMH also initiates the descent of the testes into the inguinal area. The early critical secretion of AMH in the male may be initiated by a product of the SRY gene. Although the homologous granulosa cells of the ovary produce AMH, they do not do so until after the müllerian ducts have already developed to the point where AMH can no longer cause their regression. Therefore in the female, these ducts grow and differentiate into fallopian tubes at their upper ends and join at their lower ends to form a single uterus, cervix, and upper vagina (Figure 48-6, A). This process does not require any known ovarian hormone.

The external genitalia of both genders begin to differentiate at 9 to 10 weeks. They are derived from the same primitive structures: the genital tubercle, genital swelling, urethral or genital folds, and urogenital sinus (Figure 48-6). FOR THE EXTERNAL GENITALIA TO DIFFERENTIATE INTO THE MASCULINE FORMAT, TESTOSTERONE MUST BE SECRETED INTO THE FETAL CIRCULATION AND MUST SUBSEQUENTLY BE CONVERTED TO DHT WITHIN THESE TISSUES With DHT stimulation the genital tubercle grows into the glans penis, the genital swellings fold and fuse into the scrotum, the urethral folds enlarge and enclose the penile urethra and corpora spongiosa, and the urogenital sinus gives rise to the prostate gland (Figure 48-6, B).

In the normal XX female, in an individual with an XO chromosome karyotype, or in an individual who has no gonads, the external genitalia develop into the clitoris, labia majora, labia minora, and lower vagina without significant positive androgenic influence (Figure 48-6, A). The critical importance of androgen molecules to the development of masculine external genitalia is emphasized by the presence of adequate androgen receptors in female urogenital tract cells. Estrogen molecules in the female may play a role by offsetting the possible virilizing actions of normal adrenal androgens in that gender.

Initially, a placental gonadotropin and later a fetal pituitary gonadotropin stimulate the androgen secretion involved in sexual differentiation

The initial androgen production necessary for male sexual differentiation does not depend on fetal pituitary gonadotropins. An LH-like hormone, **chorionic gonadotropin** from the placenta, stimulates early testosterone production by the Leydig cells of the testis. On the other hand, the continued growth of the male genitalia in the last 6 months of gestation requires fetal pituitary LH to support the necessary testicular androgen production. Similarly, the later molding of the female genitalia in utero may be modulated by ovarian estrogen production, which also depends on fetal pituitary gonadotropins.

Other aspects of phenotypic sexual differentiation are not evident until long after birth. These include differences between the unchanging daily pattern of gonadotropin secretion in the male versus the monthly cyclic pattern in the female, the degree of breast development, and psychological identification with one gender. What factors imprint or regulate these traits in humans are not certain. Evidence from rodents suggests that circulating androgens program the fetal hypothalamus to set the ultimate noncycling pattern of gonadotropin secretion in the postpubertal male. (To do so, testosterone may paradoxically require conversion to estradiol within the target neurons.) Without androgens, the ultimate cyclic pattern of the female results. This would constitute another instance in which the female pattern was the "neutral pattern" but the male pattern required an action derived from the Y chromosome.

Mammary gland development in the rodent embryo also is clearly regulated by androgens. In its absence, a normal female breast develops; in its presence, the elaborated ductal system is suppressed. In the human, however, male/female differences in breast tissue are not apparent until puberty. At that time, increased estrogen in the female induces the growth and differentiation of breast tissue; increased androgens in the male suppresses these processes.

Limited evidence suggests that psychological gender identification is mostly independent of hormonal regulation or even of the phenotype of the genitalia. Instead, it appears to depend more on rearing cues, which of course can be influenced by parental perceptions of phenotypic/genital sex. However, a few XY individuals with ambiguous genitalia resulting from congenital deficiency of DHT, who had been raised as girls, experienced significant growth of the penis at puberty and reversed their psychosocial gender from female to male. Nonetheless, even this reversal could reflect an alteration in the way that such individuals were perceived by others after pubertal changes occurred.

SUMMARY

- Female and male gonadal structure and function have important homologous characteristics. In each gender, germ cells develop within sheltered and hormonally conditioned environments provided by granulosa cells (estrogens) and theca cells (androgens) in the female and by Sertoli cells (estrogens) and Leydig cells (androgens) in the male.

- Gonadal steroids are synthesized from cholesterol via the same enzymatic pathways that adrenal steroids use. The predominant products are estradiol in the female and testosterone in the male. An important protein hormone product is inhibin.

- Testosterone production is stimulated by LH, and estradiol and inhibin production by FSH, from the anterior pituitary gonadotrophs.

- LH and FSH are secreted in response to a pulsatile hypothalamic release of a GnRH.
- Estradiol and testosterone feed back negatively on the hypothalamus and pituitary to decrease LH and FSH release, and inhibin feeds back negatively on FSH release.
- Gonadotropin and sex steroid production have fetal peaks, are low during childhood, and rise to adult levels during puberty. Sex steroid levels decline during senescence, whereas gonadotropin levels increase because of negative feedback.
- Gender differences in reproductive function derive from the process of sexual differentiation. The Y chromosome is a positive determinant of the development of the indifferent gonad into a testis and of spermatogenesis. Two active X chromosomes are required for normal development of the ovary and for oogenesis.
- Regardless of karyotype, masculinization of the internal genital ducts and the external genitalia into a delivery system for sperm requires normal testosterone production and action. Suppression of the development of the female internal ducts requires AMH from the testis.
- In the absence of these testicular hormones, the internal ducts develop into organs for receiving sperm and housing a conceptus, and the external genitalia are feminized.

BIBLIOGRAPHY

Brzezinski A: Mechanisms of disease: melatonin in humans, *N Engl J Med* 336:186, 1997.

Friedman RC, Downey J: Neurobiology and sexual orientation: current relationships, *J Neuropsychiatr Clin Neurosci* 5:131, 1993.

Hawkins JR: The *SRY* gene, *Trends Endocrinol Metab* 4:328, 1993.

Josso N: Anatomy and endocrinology of fetal sex differentiation. In DeGroot LJ, ed: *Endocrinology*, ed 3, Philadelphia, 1995, WB Saunders.

Lee MM, Donahoe PK: Müllerian inhibiting substance: a gonadal hormone with multiple functions, *Endocr Rev* 14:152, 1993.

Lindzey J et al: Molecular mechanisms of androgen action, *Vitam Horm* 49:383, 1994.

Müller U, Lattermann U: H-Y antigens, testis differentiation, and spermatogenesis, *Exp Clin Immunogenet* 5:176, 1988.

Odell WD: Endocrinology of sexual maturation. In DeGroot LJ, ed: *Endocrinology*, ed 3, Philadelphia, 1995, WB Saunders.

Odell WD: Genetic basis of sexual differentiation. In DeGroot LJ, ed: *Endocrinology*, ed 3, Philadelphia, 1995, WB Saunders.

Reichlin S: Neuroendocrinology. In Foster D, Wilson J, eds: *Williams textbook of endocrinology*, ed 9, Philadelphia, 1998, WB Saunders.

Southworth MB et al: The importance of signal pattern in the transmission of endocrine information: pituitary gonadotropin responses to continuous and pulsatile gonadotropin-releasing hormone, *J Clin Endocrinol Metab* 72:1286, 1991.

Veldhuis JD: The hypothalamic pulse generator: the reproductive core, *Clin Obstet Gynecol* 33:538, 1990.

Wu FCW et al: Ontogeny of pulsatile gonadotropin releasing hormone secretion from midchildhood, through puberty, to adulthood in the human male: a study using deconvolution analysis and an ultrasensitive immunofluorometric assay, *J Clin Endocrinol Metab* 81:1798, 1996.

Yen SSC: Neuroendocrinology of reproduction. In Yen SSC, Jaffe RB, eds: *Reproductive endocrinology*, Philadelphia, 1999, WB Saunders.

▷ CASE STUDIES

Case 48-1

A 22-year-old woman has never menstruated. Otherwise, she has been well. She is 5 feet 6 inches tall and weighs 130 pounds. Physical examination reveals well-developed, rather full breasts. There is no pubic or axillary hair. The external genitalia are feminine in pattern. The vagina is shortened and ends in a blind pouch without a recognizable cervix. No uterus or ovaries are felt or seen on an ultrasound examination. A small mass was felt in each inguinal area.

1. The biological effects of which of the following hormones are missing?
   A. Estrogen
   B. Androgen
   C. AMH
   D. FSH
   E. Insulin growth factor-1

2. Measurement of plasma testosterone levels shows the value to be very high for a female. Which of the following is a likely finding?
   A. Her chromosome karyotype is XX.
   B. The inguinal masses are ovaries.
   C. Her plasma LH level is low.
   D. She has an inactivating mutation of the androgen receptor.
   E. She has an inactivating mutation of the estrogen receptor.

Case 48-2

A 15-year-old boy delivered by a midwife in Appalachia develops inflammatory bowel disease for which he is treated with high doses of glucocorticoids for 6 months. To his and his parents' consternation, he notes two episodes of bleeding from an orifice adjacent to his urethra for several days every month. On physical examination, he has a masculine adult voice, early beard growth, and a masculine format of pubic hair. Careful examination of the genitalia reveals incomplete fusion of the urethral folds around the shaft of what was thought to be a penis but is belatedly recognized to be an enlarged clitoris. The scrotum is also incompletely fused and deeply pigmented. A persistent urogenital sinus and a small orifice to an apparent vagina are noted. No testes are felt. The chromosome karyotype is XX.

1. **Which of the following structures might be absent?**
   A. Vas deferens (spermatic cord)
   B. Ovaries
   C. Uterus
   D. Fallopian tubes
   E. Adrenal zona reticularis

2. **What caused the pigmented "scrotum"?**
   A. Dehydroepiandrosterone
   B. Testosterone
   C. 17-Hydroxyprogesterone
   D. Luteinizing hormone
   E. Adrenocorticotropic hormone

CHAPTER 49

Male Reproduction

OBJECTIVES

- Describe the structural arrangement that subserves the reproductive function of the testis.
- Describe the biology of spermatogenesis and its hormonal regulation.
- Explain the pattern of secretion and metabolism of testosterone.
- Identify the various actions of androgenic hormones.

The testis is the site in which male gametes, spermatozoa, are formed and matured in a specialized hormonal environment dominated by testosterone. This potent androgen also influences numerous processes described in other sections of the book, including skeletal development, hepatic protein synthesis, red blood cell production, and renal tubular function.

The Anatomy of the Testis Creates Special Conditions Conducive to the Maturation of Germ Cells Under Endocrine, Paracrine, and Autocrine Regulation

The testes are situated in the scrotum, where they are maintained at 1° to 2° C below the body core temperature, a situation that facilitates sperm production. Each adult testis weighs about 40 g and has a long diameter of 4.5 cm. A total of 80% of the testis is made up of the **spermatogenic** or **seminiferous tubules;** the remaining 20% is composed of connective tissue containing the **Leydig cells.** The spermatogenic tubules, a coiled mass of loops, empty into a ductal system that eventually drains into the **epididymis,** a maturation and storage site for spermatozoa. From there, spermatozoa are carried via the **vas deferens** and **ejaculatory duct** into the penis for emission.

The structure of the spermatogenic tubule is shown in Figure 49-1. Each tubule is bounded by a basement membrane that separates it from the Leydig cells, the **peritubular (myoid) cells,** and the adjacent capillaries. Beneath this membrane are **Sertoli cells** and immature germ cells, the **spermatogonia.** As the spermatogonia divide and develop around the circumference of the tubule, columns of maturing germ cells are formed below them. These columns reach from the basement

membrane to the lumen and culminate in the spermatozoa. Each column lies between the cytoplasms of two adjoining Sertoli cells, which extend from the basement membrane to the lumen (Figure 49-1). SPECIAL PROCESSES OF THE CYTOPLASMS OF ADJACENT SERTOLI CELLS FUSE INTO TIGHT JUNCTIONS THAT CREATE TWO COMPARTMENTS OF INTERCELLULAR SPACE BETWEEN THE BASEMENT MEMBRANE AND THE LUMEN OF THE TUBULE. The spermatogonia lie within the proximal or **basal** compartment, whereas their descendants that arise from subsequent stages in spermatozoan development lie in the distal **adluminal** compartment.

The compartmentalization of intercellular space between germ cells accomplishes two important functions

THE BASEMENT MEMBRANE, THE OVERLAPPING PERITUBULAR CELLS, AND THE SERTOLI CELL CYTOPLASM TOGETHER FORM A BLOOD-TESTIS BARRIER WITH TWO IMPORTANT FUNCTIONS: First, this barrier can exclude harmful circulating substances from the intercellular fluid that bathes the maturing germ cells and from the tubular fluid surrounding the spermatozoa. Conversely, products from the later stages of spermatogenesis are prevented from diffusing back into the bloodstream and producing antibodies. Second, THIS ARRANGEMENT ALSO PROVIDES GERM CELLS WITH HIGH LOCAL CONCENTRATIONS OF TESTOSTERONE FROM THE LEYDIG CELLS as well as protein and other products from the Sertoli cells. Such high concentrations are essential for spermatogenesis.

Biology of Spermatogenesis

Spermatozoa are the products of a complex process of development from spermatogonia

Sperm production continues virtually throughout the normal male's life. At peak, 100 to 200 million sperm can be produced daily. To generate this large number, the spermatogonia must renew themselves continuously through cell division. This differs from the situation in the female, who at birth has a fixed number of germ cells that continually decreases throughout her life.

The descendants of the spermatogonia undergo an extraordinary metamorphosis to spermatozoa as they

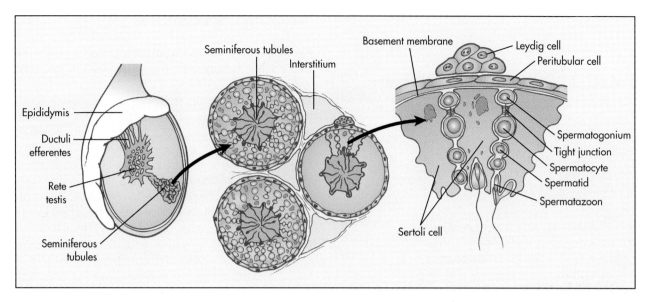

Figure 49-1 Architecture of the testis. The Leydig cells and peritubular cells are separated from the spermatogenic tubules. Within the tubules, the germ cell line is completely invested by the cytoplasm of the surrounding Sertoli cells. In addition, tight junctions between adjacent Sertoli cells separate the ancestral spermatogonia from their descendant spermatocytes, spermatids, and spermatozoa. Thus a blood-testis barrier effectively filters plasma, permitting only selected substances to reach the developing germ cells from the cytoplasm of the Sertoli cells. *(Redrawn from Skinner MK: Endocr Rev 12:45, 1991.)*

move from the basement membrane to the tubule. This process of differentiation depends on support from the abutting functional Sertoli cells. Within the basal compartment (Figure 49-1) a spermatogonium undergoes two mitotic divisions that give rise to three active cells and a single resting cell; the resting cell will be the "ancestor" of a later generation of spermatozoa. The active cells divide further to yield type B spermatogonia, which then generate a number of **primary spermatocytes** (Figure 49-2). These enter the prophase of meiosis, the first reduction division, in which they remain for about 20 days.

The complex process of chromosomal reduplication, synapsis, crossover, division, and separation completes meiosis. Within the adluminal compartment (Figure 49-1) the daughter cells, **secondary spermatocytes,** divide again. The products, called **spermatids** (Figure 49-2), then contain 22 autosomes and either an X or a Y chromosome. The spermatids lie near the lumen of the tubule and are attached to the abutting Sertoli cells by specialized junctions. They also remain connected to spermatocytes through intercellular bridges. The spermatids undergo nuclear condensation, shrinkage of cytoplasm, formation of an **acrosome,** and development of a tail, and then they emerge as flagellated spermatozoa (Figure 49-2). In the end, 64 spermatozoa arise from each spermatogonium. The spermatozoa are then extruded into the tubular lumen, and most of their cytoplasm is imbedded in Sertoli cells, where it is phagocytized and degraded. Movement of the spermatozoa into the epididymis is facilitated by fluid currents generated by the peritubular myoid cells.

The components of spermatozoa are a head with penetrating power, a midportion with energy-generating capacity, and a tail with motile power

The mature spermatozoa are linear structures with several components (Figure 49-2). The head contains the nucleus and an acrosomal cap with concentrated hydrolytic and proteolytic enzymes that facilitate penetration of the ovum. The middle piece, or body, contains mitochondria, which generate the motile energy of the spermatozoa. The chief, or principal, piece contains stored ATP and pairs of contractile microtubules down its entire length. Cross-bridging arms contain **dynein,** an ATPase that transfers the energy of ATP bonds into a sliding movement between the microtubules. This imparts flagellar motion to the spermatozoa. Both Ca^{++} and cyclic AMP promote sperm motility.

Spermatogenesis is an orderly, partially self-regulating process that occurs throughout the length of the tubule

A total of 60 to 70 days are required for the entire sequence of spermatozoal development. However, INDIVIDUAL RESTING SPERMATOGONIA DO NOT BEGIN THE PROCESS OF SPERMATOGENESIS RANDOMLY. Groups of adjacent spermatogonia initiate a cycle of development about every 16 days, which constitutes one "generation." At about the same time that the primary spermatocytes of one cycle enter prophase, a second cycle of spermatogonia is activated. A third cycle begins about the time spermatids from the first cycle appear.

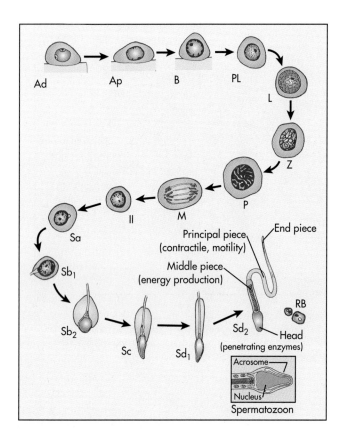

Figure 49-2 Development of spermatozoa from spermatogonia in the human. The final spermatozoan is almost devoid of cytoplasm. *II,* Secondary spermatocyte; *Ad,* dark spermatogonium; *Ap,* pale spermatogonium; *B,* type B spermatogonium; *L,* leptotene spermatocyte; *M,* meiotic division; *P,* pachytene spermatocyte; *PL,* preleptotene primary spermatocyte; *RB,* residual body; *Sa, Sb, Sc, Sd,* spermatids; *Z,* zygotene spermatocyte. (*Redrawn from De Kretser DM et al. In DeGroot LJ, ed:* Endocrinology, *ed 3, vol 3, Philadelphia, 1995, WB Saunders.*)

When these spermatids have completed their transformation into spermatozoa, a fourth cycle of spermatogonia has begun. The individual descendants of any one type B spermatogonium that lie within the adluminal compartment of the tubule may not be totally separated. Continuity of cytoplasm and possibly cell-to-cell intercommunication may exist. Because of this and because of the regular topographical association of particular stages of spermatogenesis in neighboring cycles around the circumference of the tubule, the products of germ cells in one stage of spermatogenesis may modulate events in other stages.

The spermatozoa traverse the epididymis in 2 to 4 weeks. During this time, they lose their remaining cytoplasm and become increasingly motile. The epididymis is lined by specialized epithelial cells whose function includes progressive modulation of the chemical and osmotic environment in which the sperm advance. Proteins produced by these cells bind to sperm membranes and enhance their forward mobility and their ultimate ability to fertilize an ovum. After reaching the vas deferens, sperm may be stored viably for several months.

Delivery of Spermatozoa

Erectility of the penis and ejaculation of sperm are under autonomic nervous system control

The process of ejaculation delivers spermatozoa from the vas deferens out of the penile urethra and for reproductive purposes, into the female genital tract. ERECTION OF THE PENIS, A PROCESS THAT RESULTS FROM FILLING OF ITS VENOUS SINUSES, IS ACCOMPLISHED THROUGH SIMULTANEOUS DILATION OF ARTERIOLES AND CONSTRICTION OF VEINS AND IS UNDER PARASYMPATHETIC CONTROL. NITRIC OXIDE, CYCLIC GMP, AND PROSTAGLANDIN E MEDIATE THE CHANGES IN VESSEL TONE THAT RESULT IN PENILE ENGORGEMENT. EJACULATION IS THEN EFFECTED BY SYMPATHETIC ACTIVATION. Just before ejaculation, successive fluids are added to the contents of the vas deferens. The initial alkaline secretions from the **prostate** gland help neutralize the acid pH of the female genital secretions. The terminal portion of the ejaculate is composed of secretions from the **seminal vesicles.** These contain fructose, an important oxidative substrate for the spermatozoa, and prostaglandins. Seminal fluid also contains calcium, zinc, luteinizing hormone (LH), follicle-stimulating hormone (FSH), prolactin, testosterone, estradiol, inhibin, oxytocin, endorphins, and a variety of enzymes. Their exact source and the role of each in fertilization remain to be determined.

A typical seminal emission contains 200 to 400 million spermatozoa in a volume of 3 to 4 ml. Once they are within the vagina, the spermatozoa rapidly move inward. Their life span in the female genital tract is approximately 2 days. The transport of sperm to the ovum requires mechanical assistance by smooth muscle contractions of the female reproductive organs. The contractions may be stimulated by prostaglandins in the semen.

THE FERTILIZING ABILITY OF SPERMATOZOA NORMALLY REQUIRES EXPOSURE TO FEMALE GENITAL SECRETIONS. In vivo, human sperm cannot fertilize an ovum until they have been in contact with the female reproductive tract for several hours; the process is termed **capacitation.** In vitro, however, fertilization can occur after the ejaculated sperm have been washed free of seminal fluid. This observation suggests that washing has removed inhibitory substances. Although the process of capacitation is incompletely understood, it increases motility and enhances the ability of sperm to penetrate the ovum. Penetration requires the **acrosomal reaction** in which the acrosomal membrane and the outer sperm membrane fuse to create pores through which the enclosed proteolytic enzymes can escape and degrade the protective wall of the ovum.

During Puberty, Males Develop Adult Levels of Androgenic Hormones and Full Reproductive Function

Puberty begins at an average age of 10 to 11 years and ends at about 15 to 17 years. Activation of the testes results in adult size and function of the accessory organs of reproduction, complete secondary sexual character-

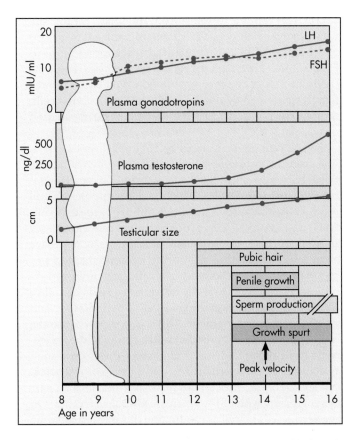

Figure 49-3 Average chronological sequence of hormonal and biological events in normal male puberty. The secretion of FSH and LH initiates testicular enlargement and testosterone secretion, respectively. Testosterone then stimulates somatic growth and skeletal development as well as maturation of the organs of reproduction. *(Data from Marshall WA, Tanner JM: Arch Dis Child 45:13, 1970; and Winter JSD et al: Pediatr Res 6:126, 1972.)*

istics, and adult musculature. Boys undergo a linear growth spurt, and the epiphyseal growth centers (see Chapter 43) close when adult height is attained. A composite picture of the sequence is shown in Figure 49-3.

Enlargement of the testes is the first physical sign of puberty. This principally represents an increase in the volume of the spermatogenic tubules, and it is preceded by small increases of plasma FSH. Leydig cells appear, and testosterone secretion rises secondary to increases of the plasma LH level. The plasma testosterone level climbs rapidly over a 2-year period, during which time pubic and axillary hair appear, the penis enlarges, muscle mass increases, and the peak velocity of linear growth is achieved (Figure 49-3). When the boy is about age 13, sperm production begins. Growth ceases 1 to 2 years after adult testosterone levels are reached. In about one third of boys, a transient stimulation of breast growth occurs, probably reflecting increased production of estradiol. As testosterone levels become dominant, the breast tissue regresses.

Hormonal Regulation of Spermatogenesis

For various reasons, the hormonal regulation of spermatogenesis is more difficult to elucidate and less com-

pletely understood than that of oogenesis. Numerous hormones and hormonal products are involved, and circumstances exist for paracrine and autocrine interactions among Leydig, peritubular, Sertoli, and germ cells.

For normal sperm production, the adult gonadotropin-releasing hormone—luteinizing hormone—follicle stimulating hormone—testosterone axis must function normally

THE PULSATILITY OF GONADOTROPIN-RELEASING HORMONE (GNRH) RELEASE AND OF FSH/LH ACTIONS ON THEIR TARGET CELLS AND THE PRODUCTION OF VERY HIGH INTRATESTICULAR CONCENTRATIONS OF TESTOSTERONE ARE ESSENTIAL COMPONENTS IN SPERMATOGENESIS. In normal adults, experimental production of transient FSH and LH deficiency via total suppression of the pituitary gonadotrophs almost completely halts sperm production. Selective replacement of either FSH or LH then reinitiates sperm production but not to normal levels, which can only be achieved by restoring FSH and LH together. Adult males who lack GnRH neurons can be made fertile by properly programmed multiple pulses of GnRH delivered daily. A suitable period of pubertal exposure to FSH is essential to spermatogenesis; however, after that, sperm production can sometimes be maintained adequately by LH or high levels of testosterone alone in adults with hypopituitarism.

FSH, LH, and testosterone may also coordinate with local estradiol, other sterols, inhibin, and activin, as well as pituitary-secreted prolactin and growth hormone in the regulation of spermatogenesis. For example, growth hormone deficiency delays the onset of reproductive function, probably because of a resulting lack of local production of insulin-like growth factors (somatomedins) (see Chapter 44).

During intrauterine development of the testis, testosterone, which is stimulated by the surge of fetal gonadotropins (see Figures 48-3 and 49-4), may condition the transformation of primordial germ cells into resting spermatogonia. From then until puberty, the spermatogonia normally remain dormant, presumably because gonadotropin secretion and testosterone levels in the testis are low. Activation of the spermatogonia, which may possess FSH receptors, then starts shortly after FSH secretion begins its pubertal increase. Subsequently, plasma concentrations of LH and testosterone also rise. However, TESTOSTERONE REACHES LEVELS MANY TIMES HIGHER IN THE TESTIS THAN IN THE PLASMA because of LH action on the Leydig cells. In men who lack LH, the provision of testosterone in amounts only sufficient to raise plasma levels to the normal range is unable to promote spermatogenesis. This critical action of LH may also be facilitated by prolactin, which increases the number of LH receptors on the Leydig cells. The extent to which local testosterone regulates spermatogenesis or requires intratesticular conversion to dihydrotestosterone (DHT) or even estradiol is uncertain. Whether testosterone or its products directly act on the spermatocytes and spermatids is also uncertain, since

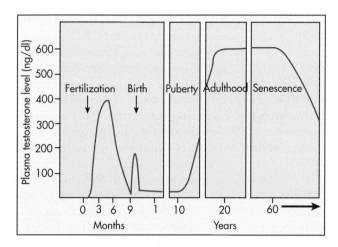

Figure 49-4 Plasma testosterone profile during the life span of a normal male. The intrauterine surge corresponds with completion of masculinization of the external genitalia in the fetus. The adult plateau is achieved rapidly during puberty. The senescent decline is relatively modest, and there is slight if any loss of androgen effects. *(Data from Griffin JE et al. In Bondy PK, Rosenberg LE: Metabolic control and disease, Philadelphia, 1980, WB Saunders; and Winter JSD et al: J Clin Endocrinol Metab 42:679, 1976.)*

these germ cells appear to lack receptors for the steroid hormones. Testosterone does clearly stimulate Sertoli cell function, and this may be the principal means whereby the hormone regulates the maturation of germ cell precursors to spermatozoa.

Follicle-stimulating hormone, probably in conjunction with testosterone, acts critically on the Sertoli cells, whose role is vital and complex

The only known Sertoli function before puberty is secretion of antimüllerian hormone in early fetal life (see Chapter 48). After puberty, each Sertoli cell is in contact with numerous germ cells in various stages of development through ectoplasmic invaginations within their respective plasma membranes. In association with the cycle of spermatogenesis, the Sertoli cells show regular changes (1) in activity, (2) in the shape of the nucleus and cytoplasmic processes, (3) in concentrations of lipid and glycogen, (4) in mitochondrial function, and (5) in enzyme content. These Sertoli cell changes and cell division depend on FSH stimulation. The Sertoli cell cytoplasm also acts as a conduit through which the germ cells move from the basal to the adluminal compartment. Thus the tight junctions between adjacent Sertoli cells must be induced to open regularly to permit maturing primary spermatocytes to pass. The junctions then close again behind the spermatocytes, and thus maintain the blood-testis barrier (Figure 49-1).

FSH stimulates Sertoli cell production of a **stem cell factor** that interacts with a specific receptor on the spermatogonium. This factor stimulates mitosis and inhibits **apoptosis** (programmed cell death) of spermatogonia, thereby increasing their number. Another Sertoli cell prod-

uct, activin (bound to follistatin), modulates mitochondrial changes that occur as spermatogonia enter meiosis and become primary spermatocytes (Figure 49-2). Thus FSH, ACTING AT LEAST IN PART VIA THE SERTOLI CELLS, ENHANCES THE EARLY STAGES OF SPERM PRODUCTION. Epidermal growth factor, elaborated by nearby Leydig and peritubular cells, inhibits the proliferation but increases the differentiation of spermatogonia.

Sertoli cells are stimulated by FSH to synthesize estradiol from testosterone, which is provided by the Leydig cells. FSH also stimulates the synthesis of **androgen-binding protein (ABP),** which is a unique Sertoli cell product that complexes with high affinity to testosterone, DHT, and estradiol. This protein may concentrate the sex steroids in the Sertoli cells and thereby create a storage form for controlled release during appropriate stages of spermatogenesis. Although germ cells lack androgen receptors, testosterone and the other sex steroids bound to ABP may be able to enter the germ cells via endocytosis and influence their development. ABP is also secreted into the tubular fluid, where it prevents reabsorption of the sex steroids from the epididymis and ensures their continuing availability to the spermatozoa during transit. TESTOSTERONE SUPPORTS THE LATER STAGES OF SPERMATOGENESIS, in part by synergizing with FSH to increase androgen receptors in the Sertoli cells as well as production of ABP. Testosterone inhibits the degeneration of spermatocytes and of the early forms of round spermatids. Testosterone also stimulates the adherence of round spermatids to Sertoli cells by increasing **N-cadherin** production and then stimulates the elongation of these round spermatids (Figure 49-2).

FSH induces the production of binding proteins for iron, copper, and vitamin A. The binding proteins allow these and other substances necessary for spermatogenesis to be extracted more readily from plasma and transferred to germ cells. Other products of FSH actions on Sertoli cells provide energy sources, such as lactic acid, to the germ cells and facilitate the expulsion of spermatozoa into the lumen of the tubule.

Local feedback loops operate within and between the Sertoli, Leydig, and peritubular cells. FSH stimulates inhibin B and estradiol production, but inhibin feeds back to block the critical aromatase reaction in estradiol synthesis. Testosterone from the Leydig cells stimulates inhibin secretion by the Sertoli cells, whereas activin and estradiol from the Sertoli cells feed back negatively to block testosterone synthesis in the Leydig cells. Testosterone also stimulates the differentiation and proliferation of peritubular cells. Protein products from Sertoli and peritubular cells modulate each other's function. The timing of these actions must somehow be coordinated to produce an optimal balance of the molecules that foster spermatogenesis.

Approximately 10% of otherwise normal males are completely or relatively infertile because of anatomical abnormalities (e.g., **varicocele**), inadequate spermatogenesis, or rejection of their sperm by elements of the female genital tract or the ova of their partners. The ejaculate may contain (1) no sperm **(azoospermia),** (2) an inadequate number of sperm (<10,000,000/ml) **(oligospermia),** (3) a high percentage of sperm with reduced mobility, or (4) a high percentage of sperm with immature or abnormal morphological characteristics. With azoospermia, the serum FSH level is elevated secondary to loss of negative feedback by inhibin, which is deficient. However, in other situations, basal measurements of plasma gonadotropin and testosterone levels and their responsiveness to GnRH administration are often normal. Yet testicular biopsies can show spermatogenic arrest at various stages from spermatogonia to spermatids, with few normal-appearing spermatozoa. The failure of Sertoli cells to form properly functioning junctional complexes with germ cells is another abnormality that can be seen on testicular biopsy analysis. It is not clear whether hormonal stimulation is at fault (e.g., the timing, frequency, or amplitude of FSH/LH pulses may be abnormal), whether the production of local paracrine and autocrine regulatory factors may be defective, or whether the Y chromosome genes that modulate spermatogenesis are ineffective mutants. Even when the sperm count and morphological characteristics are normal, other potential causes of male infertility could exist; these include absence of a necessary protein (e.g., an acrosomal enzyme, a surface binding protein) in the sperm, inadequate contents of prostatic or seminal vesicle secretions, and the presence in the female of antibodies directed at a normal or mutant sperm surface protein.

Androgens

Secretion and metabolism

Testosterone is in part only a circulating prohormone

Testosterone, the major androgenic hormone, is synthesized as described in Chapter 48. In adults, plasma testosterone levels show small pulses throughout the day that correspond to pulses of LH. Much of androgen action is supplied by the reduction of testosterone to DHT in target tissues. In addition, circulating testosterone and androstenedione are the major sources of systemic estradiol and estrone, respectively, in men. The estrogens are produced by aromatization in such sites as adipose tissue and the liver. In certain instances, estradiol may even be the actual mediator of an apparent testosterone action. Only 1% to 2% of plasma testosterone is in a free form. Testosterone and DHT circulate mostly bound to a sex steroid–binding globulin (SSBG), which is identical in amino acid sequence to ABP of Sertoli cell origin. The remaining testosterone is bound to albumin. Only the free and possibly the loosely bound albumin fractions of the androgens are biologically active.

Thus SSBG-bound fractions serve as circulating androgen reservoirs, similar to those of thyroid hormone and cortisol. SSBG concentration is itself decreased by androgens and increased by estrogens. Thus androgens increase their own biological availability by increasing the percentage of available circulating unbound hormone. Most testosterone is metabolized to products oxidized at the 17 position (see Figure 48-1) and excreted in the urine; these products constitute 30% of the 17-ketosteroid fraction (see Chapter 46).

Plasma testosterone levels vary throughout life. As shown in Figure 49-4, the plasma testosterone level rises to adult values in the fetus at the same time as plasma gonadotropins (see Figure 48-3) and when the external genitalia are undergoing differentiation. By birth, however, the testosterone levels have declined greatly. After a brief postnatal surge, plasma testosterone (and LH) levels fall to low values throughout childhood, and Leydig cells cannot even be identified in the testis. At the age of about 11 years, Leydig cells reappear, and plasma testosterone concentration begins a steep rise to approximately 600 ng/dl at about age 17 (Figure 49-4). This plateau is sustained for some 50 years. During the late decades of life, the plasma testosterone level gradually declines somewhat, this time because the Leydig cells lose their responsiveness to LH stimulation. Because of negative feedback, plasma LH levels rise slowly. Although there may be a decline in libido and sperm production, spermatogenesis still occurs in most octogenarians.

Outside the testis androgens act on reproductive organs, produce secondary sexual characteristics, stimulate somatic growth and maturation, and influence metabolism

Testosterone diffuses into target cells, where in most males it is usually reduced to DHT. A single receptor binds androgens with a greater affinity for DHT than for testosterone. The androgen receptor complex interacts with DNA molecules (see Figure 40-8), probably assisted by nuclear accessory proteins. This results in induction or repression of the synthesis of specific proteins. RNA and DNA polymerase levels are increased. Androgens stimulate the growth and differentiation of the epididymis and male accessory organs of reproduction. These effects are manifested by hypertrophy and hyperplasia of the epithelial cells, stromal components, and blood vessels in target organs such as the prostate.

The major androgen effects, classified according to the probable effector molecule, are shown in Figure 49-5. DHT is specifically required in the fetus for differentiation of the penis, scrotum, penile urethra, and prostate (see Figure 48-6). DHT is required again during puberty for growth of the scrotum and prostate and for the stimulation of prostatic secretions. DHT stimulates the hair follicles to pro-

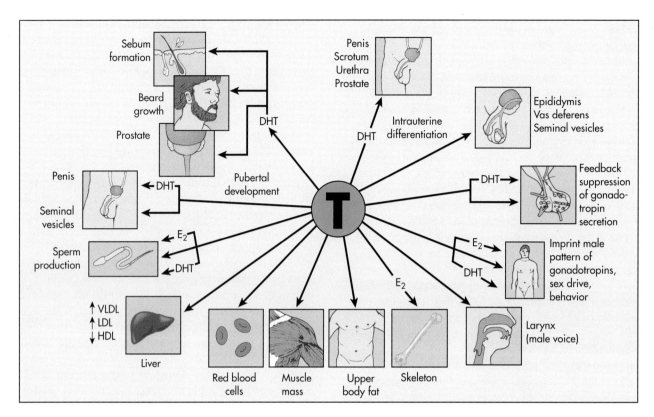

Figure 49-5 Spectrum of androgen effects. The final or most important effector molecule is not known with certainty in all cases. Some effects, such as increases in muscle mass, result from the action of testosterone *(T)* itself. Other effects, such as prostate growth and development, are definitely mediated by DHT. The role of estradiol *(E₂)* produced from testosterone in the testis itself is uncertain, but estradiol does mediate skeletal actions. *HDL,* High-density lipoprotein; *LDL,* low-density lipoprotein; *VLDL,* very-low-density lipoprotein.

duce the typical masculine beard growth, diamond-shaped pubic hair, and recession of the temporal hairline. Growth of the sebaceous glands and their production of sebum also results from DHT action. Testosterone stimulates fetal differentiation of the epididymis, vas deferens, and seminal vesicles (see Figure 48-6). During puberty, testosterone and DHT cause enlargement of the penis and seminal vesicles and stimulate the latter to secrete. Spermatozoa can be produced by adults with 5α-reductase deficiency who secrete testosterone but lack DHT. However, this observation does not preclude the normal participation of DHT in spermatogenesis.

Testosterone first stimulates the growth spurt and bone lengthening during puberty, but it ultimately halts linear growth by closing the epiphyseal growth centers (see Chapter 43). Estradiol also participates in these actions in males. Without closure of the epiphyses, a tall but sexually immature adult results **(eunuchoidal habitus).** Testosterone both potentiates growth hormone secretion and synergizes with growth hormone by stimulating the local production of transforming growth factor in osteoblasts. Testosterone causes enlargement of the muscle mass in boys during puberty by increasing the size of muscle fibers. It enlarges the larynx, thickens the vocal cords, and thereby deepens the voice. In

adult life, the administration of testosterone to either gender causes nitrogen retention, which reflects protein anabolism.

Feedback suppression of gonadotropin secretion is largely an effect of testosterone because the hypothalamus cannot produce DHT. Circulating DHT and estradiol generated from testosterone within the hypothalamus may also participate to some extent in negative feedback. Libidinous drives, the ability to maintain an erection for a sufficient period of time, and aggressive behavior are likely fostered by androgens, but they are also influenced by other factors that may partially sustain them after testosterone has become deficient.

Androgens also increase red blood cell mass by stimulating erythropoietin synthesis (see Chapter 16) and by directly affecting the maturation of erythroid precursors. Androgens regulate the synthesis of many hepatic proteins; in particular, they decrease all hormone-binding globulins. More important, androgen action increases plasma levels of very-low-density lipoproteins but decreases plasma levels of high-density lipoproteins. This is partly responsible for the much higher risk of coronary artery disease in men. On the other hand, androgens create a greater bone mass in men than in women, which results in a protective effect against osteoporosis.

SUMMARY

- The anatomical arrangement of the testis permits spermatogenesis to occur in a protective and conditioned environment within the spermatogenic tubules behind a blood-testis barrier.
- Sertoli cells are stimulated by FSH to provide ABP, growth factors, inhibin, mineral and vitamin binding proteins, and enzymes required for the development, sustenance, and transit of spermatozoa.
- Leydig cells in the interstitium of the testis are stimulated by LH to secrete testosterone, which in high local concentrations is essential for spermatogenesis.
- Testosterone and its active product DHT are required for pubertal masculinization to occur.
- Testosterone also increases muscle mass and linear body growth but ultimately halts any further increase in height by closing the epiphyseal growth centers of bones.

BIBLIOGRAPHY

Andersson K-E, Wagner G: Physiology of penile erection, *Physiol Rev* 75:191, 1995.

De Kretser DM, Risbridger GP, Kerr JB: Basic endocrinology of the testis. In DeGroot LJ, ed: *Endocrinology*, ed 3, Philadelphia, 1995, WB Saunders.

De Kretser DM et al: Spermatogenesis, *Hum Reprod* 13:1, 1998.

Fawcett DW: Ultrastructure and function of the Sertoli cell. In Hamilton DW, Greep RO, eds: *Handbook of physiology* section 7, vol 5, Bethesda, Md, 1975, American Physiological Society.

Johnson MD: Genes related to spermatogenesis: molecular and clinical aspects, *Semin Reprod Endocrinol* 9:72, 1991.

Joseph DR: Structure, function, and regulation of androgen-binding protein/sex hormone–binding globulin, *Vitam Horm* 49:197, 1994.

Kierszenbaum AL: Mammalian spermatogenesis in vivo and in vitro: a partnership of spermatogenic and somatic cell lineages, *Endocr Rev* 15:116, 1994.

Lindzey J et al: Molecular mechanisms of androgen action, *Vitam Horm* 49:383, 1994.

McLachlan RI et al: The endocrine regulation of spermatogenesis: independent roles for testosterone and FSH, *J Endocrinol* 148:1, 1996.

Saez JM: Leydig cells: endocrine, paracrine, and autocrine regulation, *Endocr Rev* 15:574, 1994.

Skinner MK: Cell-cell interactions in the testis, *Endocr Rev* 12:45, 1991.

Spiteri-Grech J, Nieschlag E: The role of growth hormone and insulin-like growth factor I in the regulation of male reproductive function, *Horm Res* 38(suppl 1):22, 1992.

Steinberger E, Steinberger A: Hormonal control of spermatogenesis. In DeGroot LJ et al, eds: *Endocrinology*, vol 3, Philadelphia, 1995, WB Saunders.

Tapanainen JS, Aittomäki K, Huhtaniemi IT: New insights into the role of follicle-stimulating hormone in reproduction, *Ann Med* 29:265, 1997.

Yamamoto M, Turner TT: Epididymis, sperm maturation, and capacitation. In Lipshultz LI, Howards SS, eds: *Infertility in the male*, St Louis, 1991, Mosby.

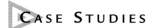

CASE STUDIES

Case 49-1

A 32-year-old XY male has a congenital deficiency of GnRH caused by the intrauterine failure of GnRH neurons to send their axons to the median eminence.

1. Which of the following abnormalities would be expected?

    A. Relatively short arms and legs

    B. Female external genitalia

    C. Prostatic hypertrophy

    D. Small testes

    E. Arrest of spermatogenesis at the spermatid stage

2. Which would be the optimal treatment to make this man fertile?

    A. Testosterone injections

    B. FSH injections

    C. LH injections

    D. A long-acting GnRH agonist injected daily

    E. GnRH injected by a pump programmed to deliver multiple pulses daily

Case 49-2

A 46-year-old man with multiple autoimmune diseases developed an autoantibody to the FSH receptor that blocked FSH activity.

1. Which of the following plasma levels would be higher than normal?

    A. Inhibin

    B. Antimüllerian hormone

    C. LH

    D. FSH

    E. Testosterone

2. Which of the following would be lower than normal?

    A. Plasma testosterone level

    B. Plasma low-density lipoprotein level

    C. Sperm count

    D. Red blood cell count

    E. Bone density

Female Reproduction

OBJECTIVES

- Describe the complex developmental sequence of ovarian follicles.
- Explain the hormonal regulation of oogenesis.
- Delineate the critical actions of estradiol on reproductive and other tissues.
- Identify the many functions of the placenta.
- Describe the changes in maternal metabolism caused by pregnancy.
- Explain the concepts of parturition.

The ovaries are the site where the female gametes, ova, develop and mature in a sheltering and supportive environment. In addition, the ovaries secrete estrogens, hormones that act on numerous peripheral tissues and organs described earlier in this book. Estrogens affect the cardiovascular system, renal function, skeletal structure, and hepatic protein synthesis.

The ovaries, along with the fallopian tubes and uterus, are situated in the pelvis. In adults, each ovary weighs approximately 15 g and consists of three zones. The dominant zone is the **cortex,** which is lined by **germinal epithelium** and contains all the **oocytes,** each enclosed in a **follicle.** Follicles in various stages of development and regression are present throughout the cortex (Figure 50-1). The surrounding stroma is composed of connective tissue elements and **interstitial cells.** The other two zones of the ovary, the **medulla** and the **hilum,** contain scattered steroid-producing cells whose function is unknown. The ovaries and follicle development can be visualized using ultrasonography.

The **granulosa** and **theca cells** of the ovary produce hormones and other substances that act locally to modulate the development of the ovum and its extrusion from the follicle. The hormones are also secreted into the blood and act on the fallopian tubes, uterus, vagina, breasts, hypothalamus, pituitary gland, adipose tissue, liver, kidney, bones, and vasculature. Many of these endocrine effects also subserve the process of reproduction. THE FUNDAMENTAL REPRODUCTIVE UNIT IN THE OVARY IS THE FOLLICLE, WHICH CONSISTS OF ONE OOCYTE SURROUNDED BY A CLUSTER OF GRANULOSA AND THECA CELLS. When fully developed, the follicle (1) maintains, nurtures, and matures the oocyte and releases it at the proper time and (2) provides hormonal support for the fetus until the placenta can assume this function.

Biology of Oogenesis

Germ cells initially differentiate into oocytes suspended in the prophase of meiosis

Oogonia arise from primordial germ cells that migrate to the genital ridge at 5 to 6 weeks of gestation. In the developing ovary, they undergo mitosis until 20 to 24 weeks have elapsed, when the total number of oogonia has reached a maximum of 7 million. Beginning at 8 to 9 weeks and continuing until 6 months after birth, oogonia start into the prophase of meiosis and become primary oocytes. The latter grow from 10 to 25 μm in diameter when meiosis begins and reach 50 to 120 μm at maturity. The process of meiosis is kept suspended in prophase by inhibitory hormones, at least until sexual maturation of the individual and in some primary oocytes, until menopause. Thus primary oocytes have life spans of up to 50 years.

Oocytes undergo attrition

From the start of oogenesis, a process of oocyte attrition occurs simultaneously so that by birth, only 2 million primary oocytes exist and by the onset of puberty, only 400,000 remain. THIS CONSTITUTES THE ENTIRE SUPPLY OF POTENTIAL OVA FOR THE WOMAN'S REPRODUCTIVE LIFE BECAUSE NO NEW OOGONIA CAN BE FORMED. With continuing attrition, very few oocytes are left when menopause begins and reproductive capacity ends. This contrasts sharply with the male, in whom the supply of spermatogonia is continually being renewed (see Chapter 49).

Development of the ovarian follicle

Oocytes induce a surrounding supportive and protective follicle

The follicle develops in distinct stages (Figure 50-1). The first stage parallels the prophase of the oocyte and occurs very slowly. It begins in utero and ends at any time during reproductive life. As an oocyte enters meiosis, it induces a single layer of spindle-shaped cells from the stroma to surround it completely. They form cytoplasmic processes that attach to the plasma membrane of the oocyte. Simultaneously a membrane called the

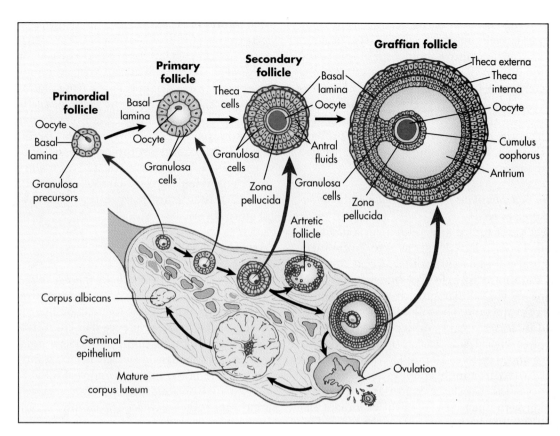

Figure 50-1 Schematic representation (not to scale) of the structure of the ovary, showing the various stages in the development of the follicle and its successor structure, the corpus luteum. The oocyte is shielded from indiscriminate exposure to plasma and interstitial fluid contents by the basal lamina and the cytoplasm of the surrounding granulosa cells. *(Redrawn from Ham AW, Leeson TS:* Histology, *ed 4, Philadelphia, 1968, JB Lippincott.)*

basal lamina forms outside the spindle cells. This delimits the **primordial follicle,** which has a diameter of 25 μm, from the surrounding stroma (Figure 50-1).

At 5 to 6 months of gestation, the spindle-shaped cells in some of the primordial follicles are transformed into cuboidal **granulosa cells,** thereby forming a **primary follicle.** As these granulosa cells divide and create several layers around the oocyte, the complex becomes a **secondary follicle.** The granulosa cells secrete mucopolysaccharides, which form a protective halo, the **zona pellucida,** around the oocyte (Figure 50-1). However, the cytoplasmic processes of the granulosa cells continue to penetrate the zona pellucida and provide nutrients and hormonal signals to the enclosed maturing primary oocytes. The cytoplasm of the granulosa cells also forms a filter through which plasma substances must pass before reaching the germ cell (compare to Sertoli cells and spermatocytes in Figure 49-1).

The secondary follicle grows to a diameter of about 150 μm. At this point, the oocyte has reached its maximum diameter of 80 μm. Concurrently, a new layer of cells from the stroma is "recruited" outside the basal lamina and forms the **theca interna.** The granulosa cells then begin to extrude small collections of fluid around and among them. This completes the first, or preantral, stage and is the maximal degree of follicular development ordinarily found in the prepubertal ovary.

A small number of follicles enlarge and develop further functional capability after menarche

The second stage of follicular development ordinarily begins only after the onset of menstrual cycling. This stage may require up to 70 to 85 days, and it spans parts of three menstrual cycles until completion. Past the midpoint of each cycle, a small number of secondary follicles are recruited for further development. The small collections of follicular fluid coalesce into a single area called the **antrum** (Figure 50-1). The fluid of the antral follicle contains a complex of substances, some secreted by the granulosa and theca cells and some transferred from the plasma through the granulosa cell cytoplasm. Included are mucopolysaccharides, plasma proteins, electrolytes, enzymes of steroid synthesis, steroid hormones, follicle-stimulating hormone (FSH), luteinizing hormone (LH), inhibin, oxytocin, arginine vasopressin, proopiomelanocortin derivatives, and other granulosa cell products. The steroid hormones reach the antrum via secretion from granulosa cells and via diffusion from theca cells. A nonsteroidal substance capable of inhibiting oocyte meiosis (possibly antimüllerian hormone) is also secreted into the antrum.

As the granulosa cells proliferate, they form a syncytium with electrical and chemical intercommunication. The oocyte is displaced into an eccentric position on a stalk, where it is surrounded by a distinctive layer, the

cumulus oophorus, which is two to three cells thick (Figure 50-1). The cells of the theca interna also proliferate and are transformed into cuboidal steroid-secreting cells. Additional layers of spindle cells from the stroma form an outer vascularized layer called the **theca externa.** The new blood vessels carry blood-borne substances such as LH and FSH to the follicle. At the end of this stage the entire complex, which is called a **preovulatory,** or **graafian, follicle** (Figure 50-1), has reached an average diameter of 2 to 5 mm.

The selection of a dominant follicle precedes and is essential for ovulation to occur

In the final stage of follicular development, one of the graafian follicles is "selected" by day 5 to 7 of a menstrual cycle, and it dominates the other second-stage follicles. This **dominant follicle** now undergoes further rapid expansion via cellular growth and augmented production of antral fluid. The colloid osmotic pressure of this fluid increases because of depolymerization of the mucopolysaccharides. However, the total pressure remains unchanged at 16 to 20 mm Hg. The granulosa cells spread apart, the cumulus oophorus loosens, and the vascularity of the theca layers increases greatly. With exponential growth, the total size of the dominant follicle reaches 10 to 20 mm during the last 48 hours before the midpoint of the cycle, when **ovulation** (release of the ovum) occurs. At a critical point, the basal lamina adjacent to the surface of the ovary undergoes proteolysis. The follicle gently ruptures, releasing the oocyte with its adherent cumulus oophorus into the peritoneal cavity. At this time, the initial meiotic division of the oocyte is completed. The resulting **secondary oocyte** is drawn into the closely approximated fallopian tube. The other daughter cell receives very little cytoplasm. It is called the first **polar body** and is discarded. In the fallopian tube, sperm penetration completes the second meiotic division, resulting in a haploid (23-chromosome) **ovum** and a second polar body. The remaining nondominant and unsuccessful follicles from that cycle undergo **atresia** (see later section) within the ovary (Figure 50-1).

Corpus luteum formation

After fertilization, the zygote is supported by a new structure formed from the ruptured follicle

The residual elements of the ruptured dominant follicle next form a new endocrine unit, the **corpus luteum** (Figure 50-1). THE CORPUS LUTEUM PROVIDES THE NECESSARY STEROID HORMONE BALANCE THAT OPTIMIZES CONDITIONS FOR IMPLANTATION OF A FERTILIZED OVUM AND FOR SUBSEQUENT MAINTENANCE OF THE ZYGOTE UNTIL THE PLACENTA IS ABLE TO DO SO. The corpus luteum is made up mainly of granulosa cells. These hypertrophy and form rows, and numerous lipid droplets appear within their cytoplasm. This process, which is called **luteinization,** begins just before ovulation and is greatly accelerated by the exit of the oocyte from the follicle. The rest of the corpus luteum consists of somewhat luteinized theca cells arranged in folds along its outer surface. In the next important step, the basal lamina disappears, allowing ingrowth of more blood vessels that supply the granulosa cells directly.

The corpus luteum regresses after a 14-day life span if conception does not follow ovulation. In this process of regression, known as **luteolysis,** the granulosa and theca cells undergo necrosis, and after the structure is invaded by leukocytes, macrophages, and fibroblasts, the corpus luteum degenerates to an avascular scar (Figure 50-1).

Atresia of follicles

The fate of unsuccessful follicles is programmed cell death

During an average woman's reproductive life span, only 400 to 500 oocytes (usually one per month) undergo the complete sequence that culminates in ovulation. The remaining millions of oocytes disappear in a process called **atresia,** which begins almost with the appearance of the initial primordial follicles. Atresia is caused by **apoptosis,** or programmed cell death. In first-stage follicles, the oocyte simply becomes necrotic, and the granulosa cells degenerate. This accounts for almost all of the oocytes. In second-stage follicles (Figure 50-1), necrosis of the granulosa cells farthest from the oocyte may precipitate a resumption of meiosis in the oocyte to the point of extrusion of the first polar body. However, the granulosa cells in the cumulus oophorus also eventually die, the unsupported oocyte degenerates, and everything inside the basal lamina collapses into a scar. The theca cells dedifferentiate and return to the stroma.

Hormonal patterns during the menstrual cycle

The menstrual cycle is divided physiologically into three phases (Figure 50-2) that correspond with the dominant events in the monthly development of each ovum. The **follicular phase** begins with the onset of menstrual bleeding and averages 15 days (range, 9 to 23 days). The succeeding **ovulatory phase** lasts only 1 to 3 days. The final **luteal phase** lasts 13 to 14 days and ends with the onset of menstrual bleeding. A normal menstrual cycle may range from 21 to 35 days, depending mainly on the length of the follicular phase.

Levels of pituitary gonadotropins and ovarian steroids fluctuate in a regular, interrelated pattern throughout the cycle

Normal reproductive function is characterized by cyclic changes in ovarian steroid hormone and inhibin production that are consequent to cyclic changes in pituitary LH and FSH secretion and hypothalamic gonadotropin-releasing hormone (GnRH) pulses. Both

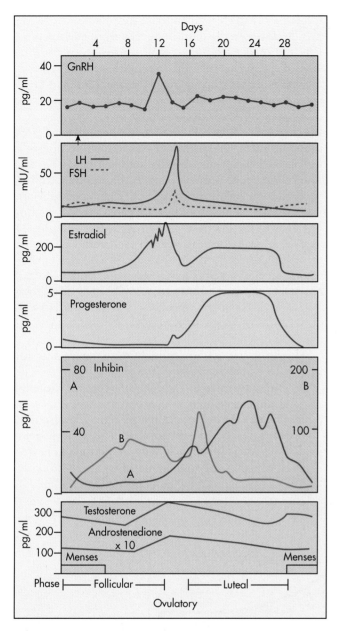

Figure 50-2 Profile of plasma hormone levels throughout the menstrual cycle. The dominant follicle is the source of the rising estradiol level in the later part of the follicular phase. The ovulatory surges of LH and FSH are preceded by increases in the levels of estradiol and gonadotropin-releasing hormone *(GnRH)*. The broad peaks of progesterone and estradiol in the luteal phase result from secretion by the corpus luteum. The earlier inhibin B peak results from follicle production; the later inhibin A peak originates from corpus luteum production.

negative- and positive-feedback loops are involved in creating this complex pattern.

The critical regulators of the ovarian cycle are FSH and LH. Just before the start of the follicular phase, plasma FSH and LH concentrations are at their lowest (Figure 50-2), and the LH/FSH ratio is slightly greater than 1. The FSH level begins to rise gradually 1 day before menses begins, and it continues to do so through the first half of the follicular phase. The level of LH rises later.

During the second half of the follicular phase, the FSH level falls slightly, whereas the LH level continues to rise so that the LH/FSH ratio reaches about 2. Stimulated by the early rise in FSH levels, the plasma estradiol concentration also increases gradually during the critical first 6 to 8 days. Later in the follicular phase the plasma estradiol level increases much more sharply and reaches a peak just before the ovulatory phase (Figure 50-2). THIS ESTRADIOL IS SECRETED BY THE GRANULOSA CELLS OF THE DOMINANT FOLLICLE. The higher estradiol level, along with increased granulosa cell secretion of inhibin B, then feeds back to decrease the plasma FSH concentration during the second half of the follicular phase. LH levels continue to rise slowly, as do androgens produced by theca cells.

The succeeding ovulatory phase is uniquely characterized by a very large but transient spike in the plasma LH level, with a lesser spike in the FSH level. This surge in gonadotropin is preceded first by the "sawtooth" estradiol peak of the late follicular phase and then by an increase in GnRH pulses (Figure 50-2). At the same time, the plasma progesterone level rises slightly. Together these changes suggest that both the ovary and the hypothalamus contribute to the ovulatory surge of LH and FSH.

Corpus luteum function determines the hormone pattern in the postovulatory second half of the cycle

After ovulation, negative feedback from the corpus luteum causes LH and FSH levels to decline during the luteal phase and reach their nadirs toward its end (Figure 50-2). The pulse frequency of gonadotropin secretion is also diminished. The most distinctive feature of the luteal phase is a tenfold increase in plasma levels of progesterone from the corpus luteum. Levels of estradiol, which is also secreted by the corpus luteum, increase again, and there is a large rise in inhibin A concentrations. If pregnancy does not occur and the corpus luteum degenerates, progesterone, estradiol, and inhibin A levels decrease dramatically to their lowest at the end of the luteal phase, FSH secretion increases, and menstrual bleeding starts.

Hormonal Regulation of Oogenesis

The first stage of follicle formation is not absolutely hormonally dependent

The initial growth of the primordial follicle appears to be a local phenomenon that is independent of gonadotropins and one in which factors from the oocyte stimulate granulosa cell development. In turn, granulosa cell products initiate formation of the theca and then stop maturation of the oocyte once it reaches about 80 μm in diameter. This first stage, from primordial to primary follicle, continues to occur until menopause, apparently independent of the state of reproductive cycling. However, the transient surge of FSH and LH in midgestation and even the low levels of gonadotropins secreted during childhood appear to be necessary for an adequate rate of follicular growth throughout the rest of life. Females with inactivating mutations of the FSH β subunit gene or of the FSH receptor gene are infertile.

The exact mechanism by which a particular group of resting primordial follicles is recruited to descend from the cortex into the interstitium toward the medulla and to initiate development into primary follicles is unknown. However, the most "selectable" follicles are those whose theca interna begin to develop during the periovulatory phase of that cycle, when the surge of gonadotropin release increases the vascularity of the follicles and helps protect them from atresia.

Follicular development

A high level of estradiol production is essential to a follicle's "success"

The second stage of follicular development begins in the early luteal phase of one cycle and continues gradually until the late luteal phase two cycles later. A small number of follicles that have acquired FSH and LH receptors are recruited, and they grow slowly over this period. From each group of approximately 20 follicles of 2 to 4 mm, a single dominant follicle is "selected" by the fifth to seventh day of the ensuing follicular phase, usually in only one ovary each month. The early rise in FSH

levels during the follicular phase stimulates mitosis and proliferation of the granulosa cells in the selected follicle. FSH acts by inducing gene expression and production of cyclin D_2, one of the regulators of the cell cycle clock apparatus during the G_1 phase. FSH ALSO STIMULATES ACTIVITY OF THE KEY ENZYME AROMATASE, CAUSING ESTRADIOL SYNTHESIS FROM ANDROGENS TO BE MARKEDLY ENHANCED IN THE DOMINANT FOLLICLE (Figure 50-3). The high local estradiol concentration then increases its own receptors as well as FSH receptors. This further sensitizes the granulosa cells to both hormones, and even more estradiol is produced. In addition, granulosa cell hypertrophy and hyperplasia are enhanced by local generation of insulin-like growth factors (IGF-1 and IGF-2) (see Chapter 44) as well as transforming growth factor and epidermal growth factor. ONCE STARTED, SECOND-STAGE FOLLICULAR DEVELOPMENT THUS BECOMES A SELF-PROPELLING MECHANISM THAT COMBINES ENDOCRINE, AUTOCRINE, AND PARACRINE EFFECTS AND THAT REQUIRES FINE COORDINATION BETWEEN THE PITUITARY GLAND AND THE OVARY. THE OUTCOME IS EXPONENTIAL FOLLICULAR GROWTH.

Three further actions contribute to continuing follicular development (Figure 50-3):
1. FSH and estradiol induce LH receptors on the granulosa cells.
2. The slowly rising plasma estradiol level conditions the GnRH-gonadotropin axis to decrease FSH secretion slightly but still permits LH secretion to increase slightly. Pituitary stores of LH are

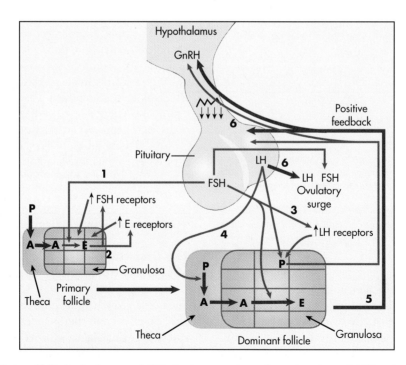

Figure 50-3 Hormonal regulation of follicular development. *1,* FSH stimulates granulosa cell growth and estradiol *(E)* synthesis in a small cohort of primary follicles. *2,* The local estradiol increases its own receptors and FSH receptors, amplifying both hormones' effects. Thus a self-propelling mechanism is set into motion. *3,* FSH later increases LH receptors, initiating granulosa responsiveness to LH. *4,* LH stimulates theca cell growth and androgen *(A)* production. Androgen is then converted to estradiol in the granulosa cells. LH also stimulates progesterone *(P)* production in the granulosa cells and adds to the effects of FSH by increasing cyclic AMP levels. *5,* As a result of theca and granulosa cell synergism, the dominant follicle emerges as a very efficient secretor of estradiol. *6,* Rising estradiol levels, with late potentiation by progesterone, feed back positively on the pituitary gland and hypothalamus to evoke the preovulatory surge of LH and FSH.

also built up, thereby creating a supply for the coming surge of LH in the ovulatory phase. This estradiol effect occurs partly within the gonadotroph cells and is mediated partly via interaction with dopaminergic and endorphinergic neurons inhibiting GnRH release

3. Estradiol increases LH receptors on theca cells.

Theca and granulosa cells cooperate to boost estradiol synthesis and to induce the ovulatory surge of luteinizing hormone

THE UNIQUE ROLE OF LH IN THE SECOND HALF OF THE FOLLICULAR PHASE IS TO STIMULATE THECA CELLS TO PRODUCE INCREASING AMOUNTS OF ANDROSTENEDIONE AND TESTOSTERONE. These androgens diffuse across the basal lamina into the granulosa cells, where they serve as essential precursors to estradiol (see Figures 48-1 and 50-1). In addition, LH stimulates more granulosa cell production of progesterone. The maturation of the dominant follicle depends on a complex set of interactions between its component theca and granulosa layers (Figure 50-3). These interactions underlie the critical goal: a high enough output of estradiol to trigger ovulation. The FSH-specific granulosa cells are greatly dependent on the LH-specific thecal cells for a sufficient supply of androgens to be converted to estrogens. This reaction is catalyzed by the action of aromatase, which is up-regulated by FSH-stimulated cyclic AMP levels. The FSH-induced recruitment of LH receptors on granulosa cells also allows LH to augment cyclic AMP levels and thus to directly contribute to estradiol production in those cells. Another granulosa cell product induced by FSH (namely inhibin B) stimulates androgen production by the theca cells. In turn, androgens stimulate inhibin production by granulosa cells. This local positive-feedback loop, as well as paracrine effects of locally produced IGF-1 and its binding proteins, contributes to the striking synthetic momentum of the dominant follicle and its production of estradiol.

FSH also stimulates enhanced granulosa cell production of trace metal and vitamin binding proteins, and substrates for energy generation in germ cells. Levels of molecules involved in the mechanism of ovulation (such as plasminogen activator and cytokines) are also increased by FSH during the preovulatory period.

Both ovaries presumably receive similar amounts of FSH and LH. Therefore THE EMERGENCE OF ONE DOMINANT FOLLICLE IN EACH CYCLE MAY RESULT FROM ITS POSSESSING MORE FSH RECEPTORS AND GREATER AROMATASE ACTIVITY AT THE OUTSET. Such characteristics would permit this particular follicle to exceed the others in early estradiol production. Conversely, the other second-stage follicles undergoing atresia have relatively low ratios of estradiol to androgen in the antral fluid. This likely reflects declining FSH availability as FSH secretion is reduced by estradiol and by inhibin B released from the dominant follicle.

Ovulation

The ovulatory surge of luteinizing hormone and follicle-stimulating hormone is triggered by a positive-feedback effect of estradiol

A critical plasma estradiol level of at least 200 pg/ml, sustained for at least 2 preceding days, is required to trigger ovulation (Figures 50-2 and 50-3). The proportionally smaller preovulatory increase in plasma progesterone synergizes with estradiol to amplify and prolong the gonadotropin surge. This positive-feedback effect takes place at both pituitary and hypothalamic levels. Estradiol and progesterone augment the flow of GnRH pulses from the hypothalamus to the pituitary gland. The pituitary gland, appropriately primed by the preceding pattern of ovarian steroid exposure, now responds to these repetitive GnRH pulses in exaggerated fashion. Furthermore, the secreted LH molecules are more biologically active.

A hormonally stimulated pseudoinflammatory response ruptures the follicle and releases the ovum

The hypothalamic-pituitary unit is conditioned by ovarian steroids to provide a sudden increase in gonadotropin (mainly LH) stimulation of the dominant follicle. This triggers ovulation 12 hours later via a multicomponent mechanism:

1. LH neutralizes the action of a peptide oocyte maturation inhibitor. A sterol (4,4 dimethyl zymosterol) in follicular fluid also activates meiosis. These effects allow the completion of meiosis. At the same time, further replication of granulosa cells is halted.
2. LH stimulates progesterone synthesis; the increased progesterone augments proteolytic enzyme activity, which loosens the wall and increases the distensibility of the follicle.
3. A pseudoinflammatory response ensues; this response is characterized by local synthesis of prostaglandins, leukotrienes, and thromboxanes, some of which are required for follicular rupture.
4. FSH stimulates the production of glycosaminoglycans, which mucify the environment and disperse the cumulus oophorus. FSH also induces proteolytic enzymes, which catalyze the final breakdown of the follicular wall.
5. Immediately after ovulation, there is a rapid fall in estradiol production, which also contributes to the loss of integrity of the follicle.

Corpus luteum function

The development and functioning of the corpus luteum are under hormonal control

The ovulatory LH surge stimulates the luteinization of granulosa cells. Subsequent lower-frequency, higher-amplitude luteal phase pulses of LH can then maintain a very high rate of progesterone production by the corpus luteum as well as a substantial rate of estradiol production (Figure 50-2). Exposure to proper amounts of FSH in the preceding follicular phase ensures the presence of sufficient corpus luteum receptors for LH action. Vascular ingrowth into the corpus luteum is also important for delivery of the LH and cholesterol necessary to sustain progesterone secretion. The lower levels of FSH and LH during the luteal phase withdraw support from the other follicles of this cohort and hasten their atresia.

When pregnancy occurs, an early placental hormone saves the corpus luteum from atresia

If pregnancy is initiated, the earliest placental cells rapidly begin secreting **human chorionic gonadotropin (HCG)** with LH bioactivity. If pregnancy does not ensue and the declining LH levels of the late luteal phase are not replaced by the equivalent HCG, the corpus luteum begins to regress after the eighth postovulatory day, and its secretion of progesterone and estradiol ceases completely by the fourteenth day. By then, corpus luteum secretion has fallen low enough to release the pituitary gland from feedback inhibition of FSH by estradiol and inhibin A and allow the FSH rise of the next cycle to begin. The process of luteolysis is partly mediated by prostaglandins.

Extraordinary coordination between the various elements of the female hypothalamic-pituitary-ovarian axis is required for ovulation and conception. This creates numerous possibilities for failure, and infertility arising from dysfunction of this system is common. Disease or conditions that disrupt GnRH release or impair the gonadotrophic responsiveness prevent the necessary initial FSH pattern to recruit a dominant follicle, and they may result in complete loss of menses **(amenorrhea).** A dominant follicle may produce enough estrogen for uterine bleeding to occur (see later section) but not enough to induce a midcycle peak of LH; this causes **anovulatory cycles.** On the other hand, an elevated ratio of LH to FSH in the follicular phase is associated with excessive theca cell production of androgens and the formation of numerous atretic and cystic follicles; this constitutes the **polycystic ovary syndrome.** Even if ovulation occurs, an **inadequate luteal phase,** either too short or substandard in progesterone production, may lead to poor preparation of the reproductive tract for either fertilization or implantation.

Various manipulative medical therapies are available for female infertility, in contrast to the situation in men. For example, the drug **clomiphene** is an estrogen antagonist that blocks the estrogen receptor in the hypothalamus. By simulating estrogen deficiency and producing negative feedback, clomiphene produces an increase in GnRH and gonadotropin secretion in women with a hypothalamic origin of infertility. Alternatively, endogenous pituitary

---

function can be suppressed with a long-acting GnRH superagonist, and ovulation can be induced by carefully timed doses of exogenous FSH and LH or by pulses of native GnRH.

The menstrual cycle originates in the ovary

Substantial evidence supports the thesis that in humans, THE MONTHLY CYCLE OF THE LH/FSH SURGE AND CONSEQUENT OVULATION IS MAINLY A RHYTHM INDUCED BY THE OVARY ITSELF RATHER THAN THE RESULT OF AN INHERENT RHYTHM GENERATED WITHIN THE CENTRAL NERVOUS SYSTEM. No cycle of LH/FSH release is observed in the absence of functional ovaries. The gonadotropin surge occurs only when the dominant follicle has reached the receptive preovulatory stage of development irrespective of the number of days required for this to occur. Estradiol itself, administered in a proper fashion, can induce an LH surge. Finally, in primates if the pituitary gland is experimentally severed from the hypothalamus and GnRH pulses of appropriate frequency and amplitude are provided externally to the pituitary gland in a proper but fixed pattern, then a preovulatory surge of LH and ovulation occur without abruptly altering the profile of the GnRH input.

The close coordination between the emergence of a single dominant follicle and the ovulatory signal it recruits makes multiple pregnancies unlikely in humans. For example, the natural rate of occurrence of **dizygotic twins** is less than 1% of live births. This is further emphasized by the much higher rate (15%) of multiple ova produced during cycles in which follicular development and ovulation are produced artificially "from above" by superimposed profiles of stimulation with exogenous FSH and LH. Multiple pregnancies are also more common (5%) when endogenous FSH and LH are released in response to clomiphene administered on the fifth day of the cycle to infertile women.

The ovarian signals that induce ovulation can be overridden by other influences. Loss of cyclic gonadotropin secretion can occur as a result of caloric deprivation, habitual strenuous exercise, stress, and emotional disturbances such as depression. The inhibitory influences on GnRH or LH and FSH secretion may be mediated by endorphins, dopamine, corticotropin-releasing hormone (CRH), or all three in concert and in some instances by changing the levels of cortisol, androgens, or thyroid hormone.

Well-known examples of anovulation or even complete loss of menses occur in women with **anorexia** nervosa, in ballet dancers, or in marathon runners.

The ovarian dysfunction can be so serious that it causes profound estrogen deficiency with consequent **osteoporosis.**

The Cyclic Changes in Ovarian Hormone Secretion Affect All the Reproductive Tract Tissues Involved in Conception

Fallopian tubes

Fertilization normally occurs in the fallopian tubes. Each tube ends in fingerlike projections called **fimbriae** that lie close to the adjacent ovary. The tubes consist of a muscular layer enclosing an epithelial lining containing secretory and ciliated cells that beat toward the uterus. During the follicular phase of the cycle, estradiol increases the number of cilia and their rate of beating. At ovulation the fimbriae undulate to draw the shed ovum into the tube, and tubal contractions move the ovum toward incoming sperm. During the luteal phase, progesterone maximizes this ciliary beat, thereby facilitating movement of any fertilized ovum toward the uterus. Estradiol and progesterone also regulate the tubal secretion of mucoid fluids, ions, and substrates that facilitate movement of the ovum and sperm and help sustain a zygote.

Uterus

The uterus houses and nurtures the developing conceptus and ultimately evacuates the mature fetus. This muscular organ encloses a cavity lined with a mucous membrane called the **endometrium.** At the start of each menstrual cycle, the endometrium is thin, and its glands are sparse and straight, with a narrow lumen (Figure 50-4); it exhibits few mitoses and is incapable of receiving a conceptus. After menstruation has ceased, the rise in plasma estradiol concentration during the follicular phase increases endometrial thickness threefold to fivefold. Mitoses appear in the glands and stroma, the glands become tortuous, and the spiral arteries that supply the endometrium elongate. This is the characteristic appearance of the **proliferative phase** of the endometrium. Estradiol also changes the mucus elaborated by the cervix (the opening to the uterus) from a scant, very viscous material to a copious, more watery but more elastic substance. This mucus can be stretched into a long, fine thread, and it produces a characteristic fernlike pattern when dried. Such cervical mucus creates channels that facilitate the entrance of the sperm into the uterine cavity.

Shortly after a woman ovulates, the rise in the plasma concentration of progesterone greatly alters the endometrium and produces the characteristic appearance of the **secretory phase** (Figure 50-4). The rapid growth and mitotic activity of the endometrium are inhibited. The glands become much more tortuous and accumulate glycogen. As the luteal phase of the cycle progresses, the glycogen vacuoles move from the base toward the lumen, and the glands

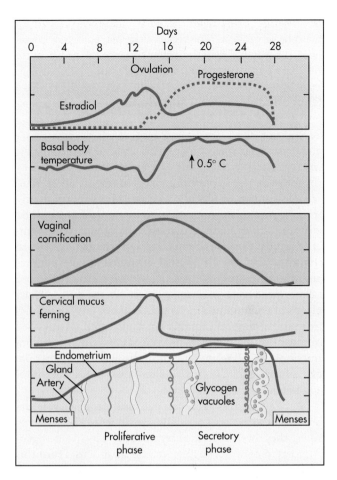

Figure 50-4 Correlation of changes in body temperature, vaginal cytology, and endometrial structure and function with the profiles of plasma estradiol and progesterone concentrations. *(Redrawn from Odell WD. In DeGroot LJ et al, eds:* Endocrinology, *vol 3, New York, 1989, Grune & Stratton.)*

greatly increase secretion. The stroma of the endometrium becomes edematous; the spiral arteries elongate further and coil. These changes enable the endometrium to accept, implant, and nourish a conceptus. At the same time, progesterone decreases the quantity of cervical mucus and returns it to its thick, nonelastic, and nonferning state.

If conception does not occur, the abrupt loss of progesterone and estradiol from the corpus luteum causes spasmodic contractions of the spiral arteries. These contractions are mediated by increased levels of prostaglandins and leukotrienes. The resultant loss of blood supply produces tissue death, and the superficial endometrial cells are shed along with clotted blood. This constitutes the **menstrual flow.**

Vagina

The vaginal canal is lined with a stratified squamous epithelium that is highly sensitive to estradiol. In its absence, only a layer of basal cells is present. As estradiol levels rise during the follicular phase, more layers of epithelium are added, and the maturing vaginal cells accumulate glycogen. They become large and **cornified,** and their nuclei shrink or disappear. The percentage of such cells is a quantitative index of estrogenic activity (Figure 50-4). In the luteal phase, progesterone reduces the percentage of cornified cells. Vaginal secretions that enhance the prospect for fertilization are also increased by estradiol.

Reproductive sexual functioning

Several processes combine to accomplish the acceptance and inward transmission of sperm. In some women the desire for sexual activity is increased just before ovulation by the midcycle rise in plasma androgens (Figure 50-2). With sexual stimulation, vascular erectile tissue beneath the clitoris is activated by parasympathetic impulses. During heterosexual intercourse, this causes the vagina to be tightened around the penis. Simultaneously the glands beneath the labia and in the vaginal entrance secrete copious amounts of mucus. The secretions lubricate the vagina and help it produce a massaging effect on the penis. These glands are maintained by estradiol action. Orgasm results from spinal cord reflexes that are similar to those involved in male ejaculation. Orgasm consists of involuntary contractions of the skeletal muscle of the perineum; musculature of the vagina, uterus, and fallopian tubes; and rectal sphincter.

Many spermatozoa are trapped and within a few hours are destroyed in the vagina. The remainder reach the cervix, where they dwell in storage crypts formed by the estrogen-stimulated convoluted mucosa and its mucus. From this reservoir, capacitated spermatozoa migrate into the uterine cavity and fallopian tubes over 24 to 48 hours. Of these, as few as 50 to 100 spermatozoa eventually reach an ovum, but they are sufficient for fertilization.

Breasts

The mammary glands consist of lobular ducts lined by an epithelium capable of secreting milk. These ducts empty into larger milk-conveying ducts that converge at the nipple. The glandular structures are embedded in supporting adipose and connective tissue. Before puberty, the breasts grow only in proportion to the rest of the body. The development of adult breasts depends on estradiol, but progesterone, insulin, growth hormone (GH), IGF-1, cortisol, epidermal growth factor, and prolactin have synergistic effects. After puberty, estradiol stimulates the growth of lobular ducts in the area around the nipple. Estradiol also selectively increases the adipose tissue, giving the breast its distinctive female shape. Progesterone stimulates outpouching of the lobular ducts to form numerous alveoli capable of milk secretion. Cyclic changes in the breast occur in conjunction with the fluctuations in estradiol and progesterone levels during the menstrual cycle.

Ovarian steroid effects on other tissue

During puberty, estradiol is to the female what testosterone is to the male. Estradiol causes almost all the somatic changes that result in the female adult appearance. In addition to stimulating growth of the internal reproductive organs and breasts, estrogens cause pubertal enlargement of the labia majora and labia minora. Linear body growth is accelerated by estradiol; however, because the epiphyseal growth centers are more sensitive to estradiol than to testosterone, they close sooner. For this reason, the average height of women is less than that of men. The hips enlarge, and the pelvic inlet widens, facilitating future accommodation of pregnancy. The predominance of estradiol over testosterone is responsible for women's total weight of adipose tissue being twice as great as that of men, whereas muscle and bone mass are only two thirds that of men.

The adult skeleton, the kidneys, and the liver are also target tissues of estrogens. Estradiol inhibits bone resorption; loss of this important action can contribute to a declining bone mass and an increased fracture rate. Estradiol stimulates the reabsorption of sodium from the renal tubules, and this may contribute to cyclic fluid retention before menses.

Estradiol increases hepatic synthesis of binding proteins for thyroid and steroid hormones, of the renin substrate angiotensinogen, of clotting factors, and of very-low-density lipoproteins. The latter actions can lead to hypertension, venous thrombosis, and hyperlipidemia in estrogen-treated women.

The effects of estradiol on the vasculature are vasodilatory and antivasoconstrictive. It increases the local release of vasodilators such as nitric oxide, prostaglandin E_2, and prostacyclin, and it decreases the production or activity of endothelin-1, a potent local vasoconstrictor. The marked fall in estradiol secretion at the end of the luteal phase alters the endometrial balance from vasodilator to vasoconstrictor and helps initiate the ischemic necrosis of the endometrium. The vasodilatory effect of estradiol may protect women from coronary thrombosis and myocardial infarction before menopause.

Progesterone produces the 0.5° C rise in body temperature that occurs shortly after ovulation (Figure 50-4). Central nervous system actions of progesterone include an increase in appetite, a decrease in wakefulness, and a heightened sensitivity of the respiratory center to CO_2.

Estrogens and Progesterone Modulate Gene Expression

Estrogens and progesterone enter cells freely and bind to cytoplasmic/nuclear receptors of the superfamily described in Chapter 40. There are several types of estrogen receptors. The estradiol-receptor complex undergoes an activation step that allows its translocation into the nucleus and enhances its binding to target DNA molecules. The receptors can also be phosphorylated by a protein kinase dependent on cyclic AMP. The estrogen receptors can dimerize, thereby increasing their binding efficiency to estrogen regulatory elements on target DNA molecules. By inducing or repressing transcription of the respective genes, estradiol increases or decreases the synthesis of numerous proteins that have reproductive functions. Some early and relatively rapid effects of estradiol are due to activation of the protooncogene transcription factors, C-jun and C-fos. Progesterone and its receptor interact in a manner similar to that of cortisol (see Chapter 46), and some cross-reaction occurs.

Because spare receptors generally are not present, the responsiveness of various tissues to ovarian steroids is proportional to receptor concentration. Estradiol and progesterone can fortify or inhibit each other's actions through receptor recruitment. Estradiol increases the number of its own receptors and the number of progesterone receptors in the uterus during the latter part of the proliferative phase. Conversely, progesterone decreases the number of estradiol receptors, and therefore estrogen action on the endometrium diminishes during the secretory phase.

Estradiol and Progesterone Circulate Bound to Protein

Estradiol and estrone bind to sex steroid–binding globulin, but their affinities are lower than that of testosterone. They also circulate largely bound to albumin, and this fraction, along with the free steroids, is biologically active. In women who menstruate, most of the circulating estrogen is estradiol from the ovaries. Estrogens are excreted in the urine as sulfate and glucuronate conjugates, and hydroxylation of the aromatic ring produces **catechol estrogens** that may have antiestrogen effects in the brain. Progesterone circulates bound largely to albumin. It is reduced to pregnanediol, which is then secreted in the urine.

Female Puberty

The general process of the initiation of puberty is described in Chapter 48. Reproductive function begins after gonadotropin secretion increases from the low levels of childhood (Figure 50-5). Budding of the breasts is the first physical sign of puberty, and it coincides with the initial increase in plasma estradiol concentration. The onset of menses occurs approximately 2 years later, at 11 to 15 years of age, after LH levels have risen more sharply.

The positive-feedback effect of estradiol on gonadotropin secretion is the last step in the maturation of the hypothalamic-pituitary-ovarian axis; thus ovulation usually does not occur in the first few menstrual cycles. These cycles are irregular in length because the bleeding is induced by the withdrawal of estrogen secretion from graafian follicles undergoing atresia.

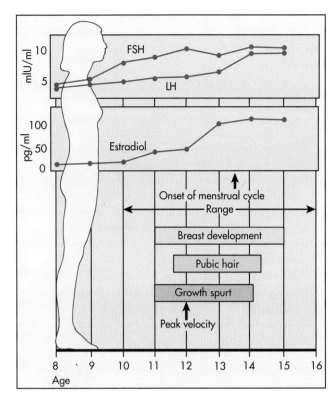

Figure 50-5 Average chronological sequence of hormonal and biological events in female puberty. The growth spurt starts earlier and is shorter than it is in males. *(Redrawn from Lee PA et al: J Clin Endocrinol Metab 43:775, 1976; and Marshall WA, Tanner JM: Arch Dis Child 45:13, 1970.)*

The growth spurt and peak velocity of growth are characteristically attained earlier in girls than in boys. Height increase usually stops 1 to 2 years after the onset of menses. The development of pubic hair precedes menses and correlates best with rising levels of adrenal dehydroepiandrosterone sulfate (DHEA-S). The time of onset of female puberty is influenced by race, individual heredity, and degree of obesity, and it occurs earlier in tropical zones.

Estrogen Deficiency Characterizes Menopause

The reproductive capacity of women usually wanes in the fifth decade of life, and menses terminate at an average age of 50. For several years before, the frequency of ovulation decreases. Menses occur at variable intervals, and the decreased menstrual flow is caused by irregular peaks of estradiol secretion and inadequate secretion of progesterone in the luteal phase. With the disappearance of almost all follicles, ovarian secretion of estradiol virtually ceases, and estrone produced from theca cell and adrenal androgens becomes the predominant estrogen.

As menopause approaches, follicular sensitivity to gonadotropin stimulation diminishes, and plasma FSH and LH levels gradually increase. Once menopause occurs, loss of negative feedback from estradiol and inhibin increase plasma gonadotropins to levels four to ten times those characteristic of the follicular phase, and FSH levels exceed LH levels (see Figure 48-3). Although the cycle of gonadotropin secretion is lost, pulsatility persists.

The manifestations of ovarian insufficiency, most particularly estradiol deficiency, depend on the stage of female life. **Intrauterine estradiol deficiency**—even caused by complete absence of the ovaries—does not prevent expression of the basic feminine phenotype (see Chapter 48), although the external genitalia may appear somewhat undersized. During puberty, estrogen deficiency causes a lack of breast development and menses. The uterus and ovaries remain infantile in size. In an **XX individual,** instead of a growth spurt, there is slow but prolonged growth until the epiphyses close late.

In women whose reproductive function is terminated early by disease and in postmenopausal women, estrogen deficiency causes thinning of the vaginal epithelium, loss of its secretions, and discomfort during intercourse. A decrease in breast mass and thinning of the skin also occur. Vascular flushing and emotional lability are disturbing symptoms. Of great importance is a sharp increase in the incidence of **coronary artery disease.** In women with relatively low bone mass caused by other factors such as poor calcium intake in earlier life, accelerated further bone loss from estrogen deficiency causes **osteoporosis,** with fractures of the wrist, spine, and hips. Hip fractures become a common and major source of morbidity after age 80.

Endocrine Aspects of Pregnancy

Fertilization of an ovum by a single sperm depends on a complex set of interactions

After the ovum enters the widened proximal end of the fallopian tube (ampulla), it is transported down to the junction with the isthmus. There, the ovum must encounter sperm within 12 to 24 hours for fertilization to occur. The sperm in turn must reach the ovum within 48 hours after entering the vagina. Contact between the sperm and ovum is facilitated by a mixing motion of the fallopian tube. When sperm come very close to an ovum, they undergo the **acrosomal reaction.** Access of the sperm to the ovum then begins with dispersal of the granulosa cells of the cumulus oophorus (Figure 50-1). Dispersal is achieved through the action of **hyaluronidase** and a **corona-dispersing enzyme,** both of which are contained in the acrosomal cap of the sperm (see Figure 49-2). The underlying zona pellucida of the ovum (Figure 50-1) contains species-specific receptors for sperm. The single fertilizing sperm penetrates this barrier by releasing **acrosin,** a proteolytic enzyme. Penetration is followed by Ca^{++} uptake into the ovum, which then releases ovum materials contained in granules. These substances block the entrance of other sperm. This prevents **polyploidy,** which is the production of an individual with more than two sets of homologous chromosomes. The polar body resulting from the second reduction division is then ejected from the ovum, leaving a haploid female pronucleus with 23 chromosomes. After fusion of their respective membranes, the DNA of the sperm head is engulfed by the ovum and forms the male pronucleus with 23 chromosomes. The two pronuclei then generate a spindle on which the chromosomes are arranged, and a zygote with 46 chromosomes is created.

Implantation of a zygote within the uterine endometrium requires complex interactions

The zygote develops by mitosis into a **blastocyst,** which traverses the fallopian tube in about 3 days. Within another 2 or 3 days, implantation in the uterus begins. IMPLANTATION CONSISTS OF THREE CONSECUTIVE PROCESSES: ADHESION, PENETRATION, AND INVASION. The requisite dissolution of the zona pellucida is initiated by alternate contraction and expansion of the blastocyst, as well as by the action of lytic substances in the uterine secretions. These and other maternal factors necessary for implantation depend on adequate maternal levels of progesterone and early paracrine signals from the zygote. From the initial solid mass of cells, a layer of **trophoblasts** separates. Microvilli of these cells interdigitate with those of endometrial cells, and junctional complexes form between the cell membranes. Adhesion is aided by a variety of endometrially produced molecules such as **laminin** and **fibronectin.** Once firmly attached, trophoblasts penetrate between and beneath endometrial cells by lysing the intercellular matrix with a variety of enzymes and by phagocytizing and digesting dead endometrial cells.

The depth of penetration by the trophoblasts is limited by changes in the endometrium. Late in the luteal phase, uterine stromal cells, stimulated by progesterone, enlarge and accumulate glycogen and lipid. Now called **decidual cells,** they disappear unless pregnancy supervenes and the corpus luteum is maintained. In that case, continuing progesterone and estrogen stimulation rapidly changes the entire stroma into a sheet of decidual cells. This **decidua** functions initially as a source of nutrients for the embryo, until trophoblastic invasion establishes vascular connections between the fetus and the mother. Thereafter, the decidua provides a mechanical and an immunological barrier to further invasion of the uterine wall. The decidua also secretes prolactin, relaxin, prostaglandins, and other molecules with paracrine effects on the uterine muscle and on the fetal membranes **(chorion** and **amnion).**

Implantation is even more susceptible to mishap than conception. Approximately 70% of all conceptions result in **miscarriage.** The majority occur within 14 days and are unrecognized by the woman, who may only have a slightly delayed menstrual period. Miscarriages later in the first trimester may still reflect suboptimal maternal-fetal attachment but are also caused by fetal anomalies.

The placenta is an endocrine organ whose products affect both the mother and the fetus

Pregnancy is marked by the development of a unique organ, the **placenta,** which has a limited life span. This organ serves (1) as the fetal gut, supplying nutrients; (2) as the fetal lung, exchanging O_2 and CO_2; and (3) as the fetal kidney, regulating fluid volumes and disposing of waste metabolites. In addition, the placenta is an extraordinarily versatile endocrine gland capable of synthesizing and secreting numerous protein and steroid hormones that affect maternal and fetal metabolism. These hormones can be found in fetal plasma and amniotic fluid, and they exhibit characteristic concentration profiles in maternal plasma (Figure 50-6).

Trophoblasts differentiate into an inner layer of **cytotrophoblasts** and an outer layer of **syncytiocytotro-**

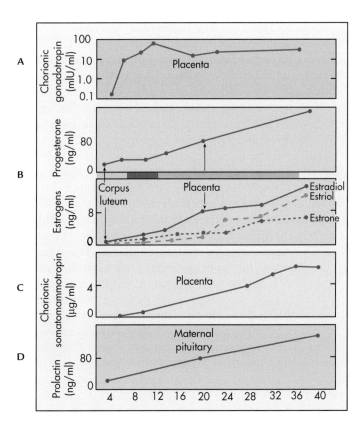

Figure 50-6 Profile of maternal plasma hormone changes in human pregnancy. **A,** Note the logarithmic scale for HCG. **B,** Between 6 and 12 weeks, the source of estrogens and progesterone shifts from the corpus luteum to the placenta. **C,** The placenta also secretes large amounts of chorionic somatomammotropin. **D,** The maternal pituitary contributes the excess prolactin. *(Redrawn from Goldstein DP et al: Am J Obstet Gynecol 102:110, 1968; Rigg LA et al: Am J Obstet Gynecol 129:454, 1977; Selenkow HA et al. In Pecile A, Frinzi C: The foetoplacental unit, Amsterdam, 1969, Excepta Medical; Tulchinski D et al: Am J Obstet Gynecol 112:1095, 1972.)*

phoblasts, which are fused. The inner cytotrophoblasts secrete hypothalamic-like stimulatory and inhibitory peptides, such as CRH, that may regulate in paracrine manner the secretion of pituitary-like peptides, such as adrenocorticotrophic hormone (ACTH), by the outer syncytiocytotrophoblasts. The latter also secrete increasingly large amounts of sex steroid hormones as pregnancy progresses.

Human chorionic gonadotropin replaces luteinizing hormone as the hormone that sustains corpus luteum function

HCG is the first key hormone of pregnancy. PLACENTAL SYNCYTIOCYTOTROPHOBLAST CELLS STIMULATED BY GNRH FROM ADJACENT CYTOTROPHOBLASTS SECRETE HCG. THIS GONADOTROPIN CAN BE DETECTED IN MATERNAL PLASMA AND URINE WITHIN 9 DAYS OF CONCEPTION, AND IT SERVES AS A RELIABLE PREGNANCY TEST. HCG is a glycoprotein with two subunits. The α subunit is identical to that of thyroid-stimulating hormone (TSH), FSH, and LH. The β subunit is closely homologous to that of LH, and the two hormones have indistinguishable biological actions. Maternal plasma HCG concentrations increase at an exponential rate, reach a peak at 9 to 12 weeks of gestation, and then decline to a stable plateau for the remainder of pregnancy (Figure 50-6).

HCG maintains the function of the corpus luteum, which would otherwise degenerate in the absence of pregnancy. It stimulates the corpus luteum to secrete progesterone and estradiol via mechanisms identical to those of LH. Later, when the placenta itself synthesizes these steroids in adequate amounts, HCG secretion declines, and the corpus luteum regresses. HCG also stimulates essential DHEA-S production by the fetal zone of the adrenal gland (see later section). In males, HCG stimulates the early secretion of testosterone by the Leydig cells, an action that is critical to masculine genital tract differentiation (see Chapter 48). The very high HCG levels have enough structural overlap with TSH to stimulate increased maternal thyroid activity early in pregnancy.

Progesterone is essential for successful implantation, initial sustenance, and long-term maintenance of the fetus

Progesterone stimulates the endometrial glands to secrete nutrients on which the early zygote depends. Thereafter, progesterone maintains the decidual lining of the uterus, where it induces prolactin synthesis. The latter helps inhibit maternal immune responses to fetal antigens of male parent origin, and thus it helps prevent rejection of the fetus. Progesterone transferred to the fetus is the substrate for the synthesis of cortisol and aldosterone by the fetal adrenal cortex (Figure 50-7). The latter cannot itself synthesize progesterone from pregnenolone because it lacks 3β-ol-dehydrogenase, $\Delta^{4,5}$-isomerase activity (see Figures 46-3 and 48-1).

Progesterone quiets uterine muscle activity by inhibiting prostaglandin production and responsivity to oxyto-

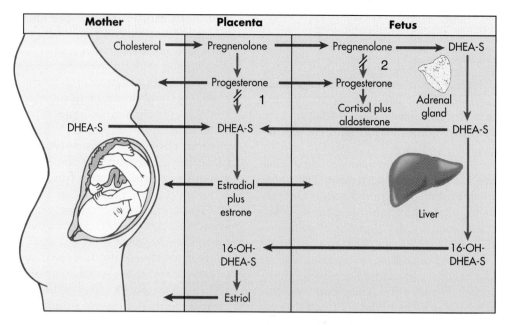

Figure 50-7 Maternal-fetal-placental unit in steroid hormone synthesis. Progesterone is synthesized in the placenta from maternal cholesterol. In turn, this progesterone acts on the mother and serves as the precursor to fetal adrenal cortisol and aldosterone synthesis. Estradiol and estrone are synthesized in the placenta from maternal and fetal adrenal DHEA-S and estriol from 16-α-hydroxydehydroepiandrosterone sulfate *(16-OH-DHEA-S)*, which is synthesized in the fetal liver. *1*, 17-hydroxylase/17,20-desmolase; *2*, 3β-ol-dehydrogenase, $\Delta^{4,5}$-isomerase.

cin (see Chapter 44). This prevents premature expulsion of the fetus. Also, it stimulates mammary gland development and greatly enhances the eventual capacity to secrete milk. Finally, progesterone increases the rate of maternal ventilation, which is needed for removal of the increased load of CO_2 created by metabolism in the pregnant state.

The placenta begins to synthesize progesterone at about 6 weeks, and by 12 weeks, it produces enough to replace the corpus luteum source (Figure 50-6). Cholesterol extracted from maternal plasma serves as the major precursor for placental progesterone. The synthetic pathway is identical to that of the adrenal gland and ovary. By the end of pregnancy, placental progesterone production reaches a level that is tenfold greater than peak production by the corpus luteum.

Estrogens prepare maternal tissues for labor, delivery, lactation, and nursing

Progressive increases in **estradiol, estrone,** and **estriol** occur throughout pregnancy. These estrogens stimulate continuous growth of the uterine muscles necessary for labor. They foster relaxation and softening of the pelvic ligaments and junction of the pelvic bones; this allows better accommodation of the expanding uterus. In addition, estrogens augment growth of the ductal system of the breast to prepare it for lactation.

Estrogens are initially produced by the corpus luteum. The placenta subsequently assumes this role, but because it lacks 17-hydroxylase/17,20-desmolase activity, it cannot produce the necessary androgen precursors (see Figure 48-1). Therefore the placenta requires androgen substrates

from the maternal and fetal compartments (Figure 50-7). This exemplifies coordinated maternal-placental-fetal function. Thus the placenta extracts DHEA-S derived from the maternal and fetal adrenal glands, removes the sulfate, and aromatizes the androgen to estradiol and estrone (Figure 50-7). In the case of **estriol,** the fetal liver must first 16-hydroxylate DHEA-S before the placenta can act on this precursor androgen (Figure 50-7).

Human chorionic somatomammotropin

A protein hormone unique to pregnancy is **human chorionic somatomammotropin (HCS),** also called **human placental lactogen.** Its structure is determined by a gene in the GH family.

HCS synthesis by placental trophoblasts is regulated by GH-releasing hormone and somatostatin from other trophoblasts and occurs within 4 weeks; maternal plasma HCS concentration rises steadily throughout pregnancy. The peak HCS production rate far exceeds that of any other human protein hormone. Although its growth-promoting activity is only a fraction of that of GH, the high maternal plasma concentration of HCS makes it capable of contributing to anabolism in the mother. HCS stimulates lipolysis and is an insulin antagonist. Thus HCS raises maternal free fatty acid and glucose levels. As discussed later, a major function of HCS is to direct maternal metabolism to shunt these substrates to the fetus.

Other placental hormones

The placenta produces hypothalamic- or pituitary-like peptides, including GnRH, thyrotropin-releasing hormone, CRH, GH-releasing hormone, somatostatin, ACTH, and TSH. CRH levels, in particular, become very high in maternal plasma, and peak during labor. In addition, a unique placental GH variant is synthesized and becomes the dominant GH in maternal plasma. Placental ACTH and TSH may augment maternal adrenal and thyroid gland activity, and placental GH acts on maternal target tissues. The placenta also synthesizes 1,25-hydroxyvitamin D, which helps regulate calcium homeostasis and skeletal formation in the fetus (see Chapter 43). Inhibin A from the placenta replaces that from the corpus luteum, and it suppresses maternal FSH secretion and more follicle development in the mother during pregnancy.

Hormones of maternal origin

Prolactin maintains breast milk production and suppresses ovulation in the nursing mother

Prolactin secretion from the maternal pituitary gland increases greatly (Figure 50-6) in response to high maternal estrogen levels. The prolactin is in the nonglycosylated active form, and it specifically stimulates the lactogenic apparatus of the breast (see Chapter 44). During pregnancy, however, lactation itself is inhibited by the great excess of estrogen and progesterone. After delivery of the fetus, true milk synthesis is initiated by the precipitous drop in steroid hormone levels. Thereafter, milk synthesis is maintained in a nursing mother by prolactin and is facilitated by insulin and cortisol. Although basal prolactin concentrations gradually decline by 8 weeks after delivery, they are transiently elevated during each period of suckling. This helps sustain milk secretion.

Prolactin also suppresses reproductive function in the nursing mother. During the first 7 to 10 days after delivery, plasma FSH and LH levels remain low. FSH levels then rise, but LH levels do not; this pattern simulates that in early puberty. In the nursing mother, this pattern persists because of the inhibitory effects of prolactin on GnRH secretion. A decrease in circulating prolactin that follows the cessation of nursing triggers LH release and initiates a resumption of menstrual cycling.

Relaxin is a peptide hormone that is structurally similar to proinsulin

Relaxin is produced by the corpus luteum, decidua, and placenta under HCG stimulation. Maternal plasma relaxin levels rise to a peak in the first trimester and then decline somewhat. This hormone relaxes the mother's pelvic outlet and softens the cervix by increasing collagenase activity and decreasing tissue collagen content. Relaxin also decreases uterine muscle contractility by reducing the activity of myosin kinase. Thus relaxin acts initially to maintain uterine quiescence and prevent early abortion, but later it facilitates easier passage of the fetus into the birth canal once labor has begun.

The pregnant state induces changes in the function of all maternal endocrine glands

After the third month of pregnancy, maternal insulin secretion increases in response to glucose challenge or meals. It peaks during the last trimester and acts to compensate for the insulin resistance caused by HCS, placental GH, and cortisol.

Aldosterone secretion increases throughout pregnancy because of estrogen-induced augmentation of renin and angiotensinogen levels. The higher levels of angiotensin II stimulate the adrenal zona glomerulosa to increase aldosterone secretion (see Chapter 46). This induces a positive sodium balance, which is needed to support a high maternal plasma volume and to build the extracellular fluid of the fetus. Another mineralocorticoid, deoxycorticosterone (see Chapter 46), is synthesized by maternal kidneys during pregnancy, and it also contributes to sodium retention.

Total plasma thyroxine and cortisol levels are elevated because of estrogen-induced increases in their respective binding globulins. Levels of free thyroxine and triiodothyronine may be increased in the first trimester, and these hormones may be transferred to the fetus. The level of plasma free cortisol also rises modestly, and this may contribute to maternal adipose tissue gain and to mammary gland development.

Parathyroid hormone secretion also increases. This hormone augments maternal plasma levels of 1,25-hydroxyvitamin D, which in turn increases dietary calcium absorption. This action enhances the maternal supply of calcium for the growing fetal skeleton (see Chapter 43).

Maternal FSH and LH secretion is suppressed by high concentrations of estrogen, progesterone, and prolactin and by inhibin A from the corpus luteum and placenta. Similarly, maternal pituitary GH secretion is decreased through negative feedback resulting from the actions of HCS and placental variant GH actions.

Maternal-Fetal Metabolism

Maternal metabolism is adapted to the changing needs of the mother and fetus

During pregnancy, the average gain in maternal weight is 11 kg. Approximately half of this can be attributed to changes in maternal tissues and half to the fetus and placenta. The mother must ingest approximately 300 extra kilocalories and 30 extra grams of protein daily to support fetal development, enlarge maternal energy stores, and sustain growth of certain maternal tissues.

DURING THE FIRST HALF OF PREGNANCY, THE MOTHER IS IN AN ANABOLIC STATE, and the conceptus represents an insignificant nutritional drain. This phase is characterized by normal or even increased maternal sensitivity to insulin. Maternal plasma levels of glucose, free fatty acids, glycerol, and amino acids are normal or slightly decreased. Dietary carbohydrate and protein loads are rapidly used. Maternal lipogenesis is favored, glycogen stores are expanded, and protein synthesis is enhanced. These actions support the early growth of the breasts and uterus and prepare the mother to withstand the later metabolic demands of the enlarging fetus during maternal fasting periods.

DURING THE SECOND HALF OF PREGNANCY THE MOTHER SHIFTS INTO A CATABOLIC STATE APTLY DESCRIBED AS "ACCELERATED STARVATION" (SEE CHAPTER 41). INSULIN SENSITIVITY IS REPLACED BY INSULIN RESISTANCE. This resistance causes elevation of postprandial plasma levels of glucose and amino acids as the uptake of dietary carbohydrate, protein, and fat by maternal tissues is reduced. Consequently, the diffusion of glucose and the facilitated transport of amino acids across the placenta into the fetus are accelerated. During maternal fasting intervals, plasma glucose and amino acid levels fall more rapidly than in nonpregnant women because the fetus continues to siphon off these substances. Maternal lipolysis is excessively stimulated, ensuring alternate oxidative fuels for the mother and even for the fetus, to whom ketoacids and free fatty acids can be transferred across the placenta. HCS is a key hormone responsible for maternal insulin resistance and for lipid mobilization during fasting in this later stage of pregnancy. Elevated estrogen, progesterone, and cortisol levels also antagonize insulin action in the mother. Estrogens also stimulate hepatic production of very-low-density lipoproteins (see Chapter 41). The extra triglycerides are stored in breast tissue to be used later for milk production.

The insulin resistance of pregnancy, when added to an underlying vulnerability to diabetes, produces **gestational diabetes** in 4% of pregnancies. Hyperglycemia appears around week 24 to 28 of gestation, and this occurrence may have serious consequences for the fetus. Maternal hyperglycemia is transmitted to the fetus and stimulates fetal hyperinsulinemia; the latter causes heavier babies that are harder to deliver and a tendency toward hypoglycemia in the newborn infant. Immature lungs that lack surfactant can cause respiratory distress, and sudden death caused by heart muscle abnormalities may occur in utero. even near term.

Parturition

Just as the maintenance of the pregnant state depends on a unique hormonal milieu, its termination probably also depends on specific hormonal changes

In humans, the exact mechanism by which parturition, or the process of giving birth, is initiated remains uncertain. Cortisol, estrogen, progesterone, CRH, prostaglandins, oxytocin, catecholamines and inflammatory cytokines may all participate in complex interrelationships that result in the initiation and maintenance of labor and in the

final uterine evacuation. Because species variations exist, it is difficult to extrapolate data from animal studies directly to humans. Figure 50-8 illustrates current concepts of the endocrine regulation of parturition.

Throughout pregnancy, the uterine myometrium exhibits long episodes of low-amplitude contractions referred to as **contractures.** These are perceived by the mother beginning at least one month before the end of gestation and are called **Braxton Hicks** contractions. They are uncoordinated and ineffective. Progesterone helps maintain this myometrial state of functional quiescence.

The onset of true labor has a circadian rhythm, with a peak between midnight and 5 AM, during which period the sensitivity of the myometrium to stimulation by prostaglandins and oxytocin is heightened and the secretion of maternal oxytocin peaks. Some signal from the fetus probably initiates labor contractions. In sheep, fetal cortisol has been strongly implicated as the signal. Although gestation is prolonged in women when the fetus lacks an intact hypothalamic pituitary adrenal unit, the evidence for a surge of fetal cortisol secretion immediately preceding human parturition is weak. However, a marked late gestational increase in fetal cortisol secretion is important to survival of the newborn (Figure 50-8).

CRH produced by the placenta stimulates the fetal pituitary to secrete ACTH which in turn increases fetal cortisol and dehydroepiandrosterone (DHEA) production. The extra DHEA substrate fuels placental estradiol production (Figure 50-7), which is also increased by cortisol stimulation. In an unusual positive-feedback effect, the fetal cortisol also amplifies (rather than inhibits, as expected) placental CRH synthesis (see Chapter 46). This phenomenon generates a powerful momentum to increase both factors exponentially. The late rapid rise in CRH production is reflected by escalating levels of maternal plasma CRH.

A central role for CRH is supported by several other observations. CRH receptors are present in the myometrium, and CRH potentiates the contractile responses to both oxytocin and prostaglandins. In another positive-feedback loop, CRH and prostaglandins stimulate each other's production. Finally, an inverse correlation exists between maternal plasma CRH levels early in pregnancy and the absolute length of the gestational period. Higher CRH levels predict shorter gestational periods. Thus a placental clock based on the inherent ability of the placenta to produce CRH may be set early in pregnancy; cortisol from the fetus may trigger a CRH alarm to start labor once the hormone reaches a high enough level in the uterus. Increased fetal cortisol levels also stimulate lung maturation, increase stores of liver glycogen, induce intestinal transport systems and digestive enzymes, and promote closure of the ductus arteriosus, all of which prepare the fetus for the abrupt transition to extrauterine life (Figure 50-8).

Late in pregnancy, increases in the secretion of estradiol by the placenta prepare the myometrium to contract in a forceful and coordinated manner by increasing the concentrations of contractile proteins, myosin and actin, as

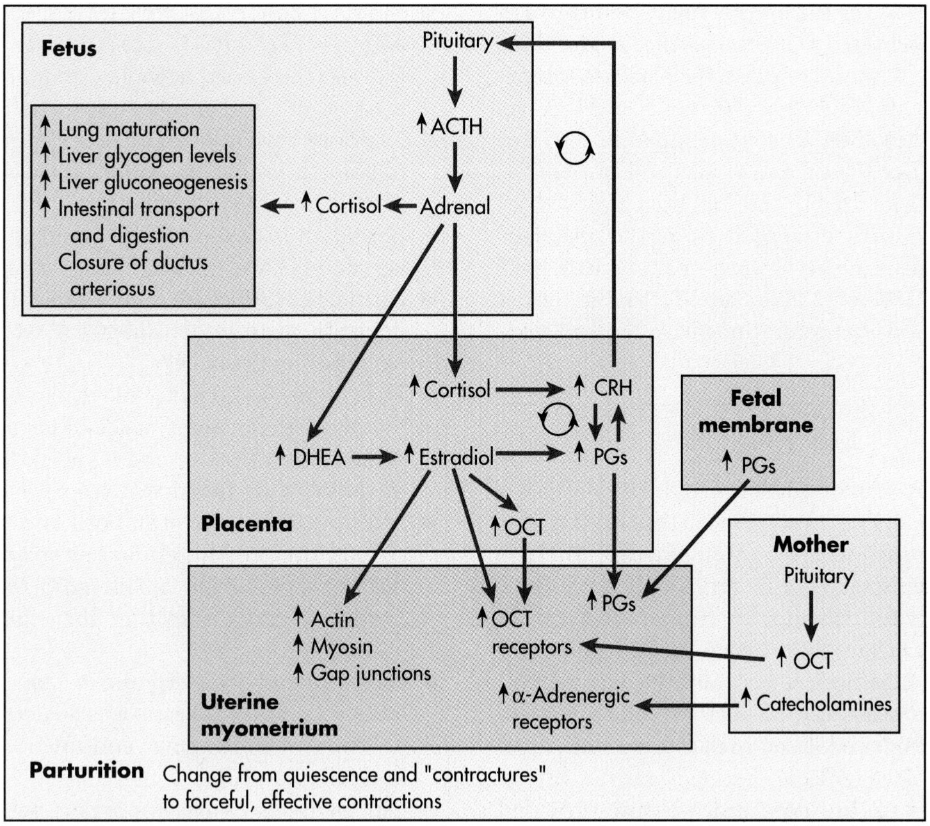

Figure 50-8 Endocrine regulation of parturition. A positive-feedback loop between cortisol and placental CRH production appears to initiate parturition. A rising fetal adrenal supply of dehydroepiandrosterone *(DHEA)* augments estradiol production. This leads to increased prostaglandin *(PGs)* levels, which are the main stimuli of uterine labor contractions. Oxytocin *(OCT)* produced locally in the placenta and decidua and a small maternal component coupled with increased myometrial oxytocin receptors may contribute to labor but is not essential. However, oxytocin sustains uterine contractions after expulsion of the fetus to minimize maternal loss of blood. Maternal catecholamines may add to the hormonal cascade stimulating contractions. Cortisol also prepares the fetus to maintain its own supply of O_2 and substrates after birth.

well as the gap junctions between fibers. Oxytocin receptors and prostaglandins are also increased by estradiol. It is still moot whether a decrease in local effective free progesterone levels in the uterus is an essential component to the overall process. However, mechanisms whereby this can occur have been described, and progesterone withdrawal would augment the effects of increased estradiol and would favor CRH production. The progesterone antagonist **mifepristone** (RU-486) is a potent abortifacient.

A LARGE INCREASE IN THE LOCAL CONCENTRATION OF PROSTAGLANDINS INCREASES MYOMETRIAL CELL Ca^{++} LEVELS AND TRIGGERS UTERINE CONTRACTIONS. The prostaglandins are produced by the maternal uterine tissues (decidua) and the fetal chorion and amnion as evidenced by an increase in amniotic fluid prostaglandins before the onset of labor. Certain prostaglandins are also abortifacients.

Another major stimulator of myometrial contractions is **oxytocin.** Although the concentration of oxytocin in maternal plasma does not increase consistently just before labor, the frequency of oxytocin pulses does increase. Furthermore, myometrial oxytocin receptor content rises dramatically at term, as does the local synthesis of oxytocin by the decidua and the fetal membranes. Thus maternal, placental, and even fetal oxytocin may reinforce labor contrac-

tions, and immediately after delivery, oxytocin probably maximizes the contractions that minimize maternal blood loss. Uterine contractions can also be modulated by catecholamines; α-adrenergy is stimulatory, and β-adrenergy is inhibitory. Both estradiol and prostaglandins increase myometrial α-adrenergic receptors.

In addition to uterine contractions, the rapid changes that occur in placental and cervical tissue are also important components of labor. At term, the concentrations of inflammatory cytokines, such as interleukin-6 and interleukin-8, rise sharply in amniotic fluid. These cytokines are produced by maternal decidua and fetal membranes, probably under hormonal paracrine stimulation. They attract neutrophils, which then release collagenase. This enzyme loosens the attachments between the maternal and fetal tissue planes and decreases the cervical resistance to pressure from the fetal head.

Once labor has begun, it proceeds in three clinically recognized stages. In the first stage, which lasts several hours, the uterine contractions, which originate at the fundus and sweep downward, force the head of the fetus against the cervix. Under this pressure, the cervix progressively widens and thins the opening to the vaginal canal. In the second stage, which lasts less than 1 hour, the fetus is forced out of the uterine cavity and through the cervix and is delivered from the vagina. In the third stage, which lasts 10 minutes or less, the placenta is separated from the decidual tissue of the uterus and is forcefully evacuated. Myometrial contractions during this stage act to constrict the uterine vessels and prevent excessive bleeding. Once the placenta has been removed, all its hormonal products disappear from the maternal plasma at a rate determined by their characteristic half-lives. In general, by 48 to 72 hours after birth, the steroid and protein hormone concentrations have reached non-pregnancy levels.

Lactation

The maternal provision of nutrients to the newborn begins within 48 hours of delivery. First, a thin fluid that is known as **colostrum** and that contains lactose and proteins but little fat is secreted in very small quantities. True milk delivery follows shortly. Human breast milk contains 1% protein, largely as casein, lactalbumin, and lactoglobulin. In addition, it contains 7% lactose and 3.5% fat, equivalent to about 70 kcal/l00 ml. By 1 week, 550 ml/day are produced; later, maximum amounts of up to 2000 ml/day may occur. Large quantities of calcium and phosphorus are also needed by and provided to the infant. Milk also contains immunoglobulins, which protect against infection. There are over 160 other constituents, including many peptide hormones and growth factors, that are synthesized in the breast or actively transported from maternal plasma into the milk. These may act directly on the infant's gastrointestinal tract or even be absorbed to act systemically. Typically, infants nurse for 6 to 12 months.

Mammary cells package proteins, lactose, calcium, and phosphate in secretory vesicles and fat in droplets. Prolactin is essential to these processes (see Chapter 44). Immunoglobulins, combined with membrane receptors in vesicles, enter the cells. All these products are then secreted into the alveoli. Suckling and even anticipatory signals, such as the infant's cry, stimulate oxytocin release via neural sensory pathways and the central **nucleus tractus solitarius.** Oxytocin causes contraction of myoepithelial cells around the alveoli and smooth muscle cells in the duct walls. This "lets the milk down" into the areolar area, where the infant obtains it through holes in the nipple.

Summary

- In the ovary, oocytes that are suspended in the prophase of meiosis are secluded in primordial follicles. These follicles undergo slow, hormonally independent development to primary follicles, which are composed of nurturing, surrounding granulosa cells.

- Monthly cohorts of follicles are stimulated sequentially by FSH and LH to progress in development. From each cohort, a single dominant follicle emerges each month and grows exponentially.
- The dominant follicle produces enough estradiol and inhibin to inhibit its cohort follicles, prepare reproductive organs for fertilization, and condition the hypothalamus and pituitary gland to provide a timed surge of LH and FSH to cause ovulation.
- Estradiol production by the follicular granulosa cells depends on androgen substrate, which is provided by neighboring theca cells.
- The monthly cyclicity of ovulation is determined mainly by the ovary. A surge of LH and FSH secretion occurs when the dominant follicle secretes sufficient estradiol in an appropriate temporal pattern.
- After ovulation, the granulosa and theca cells form a corpus luteum. This endocrine structure secretes sufficient progesterone and estradiol to condition the reproductive organs so that they can receive and implant a zygote.
- Estradiol and progesterone in sequence and together induce cyclic changes in the structure and secretory function of the vagina, endometrium of the uterus, and fallopian tubes.
- Estrogens also have important actions on bone remodeling, the hepatic synthesis of proteins, and other systemic target tissues.
- After implantation of a conceptus, the placenta is formed from fetal trophoblasts, which initially secrete HCG that sustains the corpus luteum. Eventually the placenta itself produces the important hormones of pregnancy, such as estrogens, progesterone, and a variety of proteins and peptides that resemble hypothalamic and pituitary hormones.
- Early in pregnancy, the mother is in a metabolic state that facilitates the growth of reproductive tissues and energy stores. Later, she becomes insulin resistant, which allows her to shunt substrates to the growing fetus.
- The endocrine mechanism of parturition is not yet completely defined. An increased ratio of estradiol to progesterone in uterine tissue augments the production of prostaglandins, which are the main stimulators of uterine contractions.

BIBLIOGRAPHY

Apter D et al: Gonadotropin-releasing hormone pulse generator activity during pubertal transition in girls: pulsatile and diurnal patterns of circulating gonadotropins, *J Clin Endocrinol Metab* 76:940, 1993.

Crisp TH: Organization of the ovarian follicle and events in its biology: oogenesis, ovulation or atresia, *Mutat Res* 296:89, 1992.

Gougeon A: Regulation of ovarian follicular development in primates: facts and hypotheses, *Endocr Rev* 17:121, 1996.

Hillier SG: Current concepts of the roles of follicle stimulating hormone and luteinizing hormone in folliculogenesis, *Human Reprod* 9:188, 1994.

Hillier SG, Whitelaw PF, Smyth CD: Follicular oestrogen synthesis: the "two-cell, two-gonadotrophin" model revisited, *Mol Cell Endocrinol* 100:51, 1994.

Hsueh AJW, Billig H, Tsafriri A: Ovarian follicle atresia: a hormonally controlled apoptotic process, *Endocr Rev* 15:707, 1994.

Kelly RW: Pregnancy maintenance and parturition: the role of prostaglandin in manipulating the immune and inflammatory response, *Endocr Rev* 15:684, 1994.

McLean M et al: A placental clock controlling the length of human pregnancy, *Nat Med* 1:460, 1995.

Olson DM, Mijovic JE, Sadowsky DW: Control of human parturition, *Semin Perinatol* 19:52, 1995.

Rories C, Spelsberg TG: Ovarian steroid action on gene expression: mechanisms and models, *Annu Rev Physiol* 51:653, 1989.

Rossmanith WG: Contemporary insights into the control of the corpus luteum function, *Horm Metab Res* 15:192, 1993.

Turner RT, Riggs BL, Spelsberg TC: Skeletal effects of estrogen, *Endocr Rev* 15:275, 1994.

White MM et al: Estrogen, progesterone, and vascular reactivity: potential cellular mechanisms, *Endocr Rev* 16:739, 1995.

Yeh J, Adashi EY: The ovarian cycle. In Yen SSC, Jaffe RB, eds: *Reproductive endocrinology*, Philadelphia, 1999, WB Saunders.

Yen SSC: The human menstrual cycle: neuroendocrine regulation. In Yen SSC, Jaffe RB, eds: *Reproductive endocrinology*, Philadelphia, 1999, WB Saunders.

▷ CASE STUDIES

Case 50-1

A 28-year-old healthy woman with regular menstrual cycles since age 12 was a passenger on a bus that overturned and submerged in a lake. She was uninjured, but was one of only four passengers who escaped death by drowning. Her menses ceased completely in the ensuing year, during which she had frequent recurring nightmares about the accident.

1. Which of the following most likely mediates her amenorrhea?

- **A.** Increased CRH secretion
- **B.** Decreased prolactin secretion
- **C.** Decreased dopamine secretion
- **D.** Decreased endorphin secretion
- **E.** Increased norepinephrine levels

2. Which of the following findings would be expected in this estrogen deficient patient?

- **A.** Hyperplasia of the endometrium
- **B.** Cornification of the vaginal epithelium
- **C.** Profuse secretion of an elastic cervical mucus
- **D.** Decreased libido
- **E.** Decreased breast mass

Case 50-2

A 30-year-old married woman consults her physician for infertility. She has regular menstrual cycles. Daily home urine LH measurement shows a midcycle surge in LH secretion, and intercourse has been appropriately timed thereby. Her husband's sperm count and analysis are normal. Her physical examination is entirely normal.

1. Which of the following is the most likely cause of her infertility?

- **A.** Progesterone excess
- **B.** Inhibin A excess
- **C.** Failure to form an adequately functioning corpus luteum
- **D.** Failure to develop a dominant follicle
- **E.** Estradiol deficiency

2. Which of the following findings would confirm the diagnosis?

- **A.** Low plasma estradiol on day 28 of her cycle
- **B.** Low plasma estrone on day 1 of her cycle
- **C.** High plasma prolactin on day 14 of her cycle
- **D.** Low plasma progesterone on day 21 of her cycle
- **E.** Low plasma progesterone on day 7 of her cycle

Answers to Case Studies

Case 1-1

1. **A** is incorrect because the level of cholesterol synthesis by hepatocytes is also elevated, since their intracellular levels of cholesterol are low and the normal suppression of cholesterol synthesis by intracellular cholesterol is not as effective as normal.
   B is correct because elevated cholesterol synthesis contributes as explained in the answer to **A**.
   C is incorrect because xanthomas are due primarily to cholesterol deposition.
   D is incorrect because only 1 in 500 individuals is heterozygous for this disorder.
   E is incorrect because the high levels of LDL cholesterol are conducive to atherosclerosis and to significantly increased rates of heart attack and stroke.

2. **A** is correct because the cells of a patient with one normal copy and one mutant copy of the LDL receptor might have about 50% of the normal capacity to bind LDL with high affinity.
   B is correct because the cells of a homozygous individual might have essentially no high-affinity binding of LDL.
   C is correct because in some causes of familial hypercholesterolemia, mutant LDL receptors bind LDL normally but cannot be internalized by receptor-mediated endocytosis.
   D is correct because in all the forms of the disease the uptake of LDL by cells is deficient, and thus LDL catabolism is reduced.
   E is correct because **A** through **D** are all correct.

3. **A** is incorrect because dietary restriction of fat intake can decrease plasma cholesterol levels 10% to 15% at the most.
   B is incorrect because dietary restriction alone does not reduce the patient's cholesterol level enough to markedly reduce the risk for heart attack.
   C is incorrect because increased hepatic synthesis of cholesterol contributes to the patient's elevated serum cholesterol level, so inhibition of cholesterol synthesis would be a helpful intervention in this patient and would help reduce serum cholesterol levels.
   D is incorrect because the transplanted liver would have normal LDL receptors but the patient would still have elevated LDL as a result of deficient uptake of LDL in other tissues.
   E is correct because the combination of a diet very low in lipids and a drug that suppresses hepatic synthesis produces a much greater decrease in plasma cholesterol than either of these interventions alone and is a recommended treatment for this patient.

Case 1-2

1. **A** is incorrect because maltose is a disaccharide of glucose monomers and if this were the deficit, then feeding glucose should not have caused diarrhea.
   B is incorrect because plant starch is a polymer of glucose units and if this were the deficit, the feeding glucose should not have caused diarrhea.
   C is incorrect because lactose is a disaccharide of glucose and galactose and if this were the deficit, then feeding glucose should not have caused diarrhea.
   D is incorrect because glucoamylase hydrolyzes glucose from linear polymers of glucose and if this were the deficit, feeding glucose should not have caused diarrhea.
   E is correct because **A** through **D** are incorrect. Feeding glucose caused the diarrhea. All of the sugars that were fed contain glucose, and they all caused diarrhea. The most likely problem is that the small intestine of this infant cannot absorb glucose and probably is deficient in the Na^+-powered facilitated transporter that transports glucose and galactose across the brush border membrane. This disorder is very rare and is called **familial glucose/galactose malabsorption syndrome.**

2. **A** is incorrect because if the baby cannot absorb glucose from the small intestine, it is almost certain that she cannot absorb galactose either, since glucose and galactose are handled by the same transport proteins.
   B is incorrect because if this were the problem, then feeding glucose should not have caused diarrhea.
   C is incorrect because feeding a formula with fructose as its carbohydrate source would cause diarrhea to abate.
   D is correct because since glucose and galactose are handled by the same transport proteins, the baby is probably deficient in the glucose-galactose transport protein SGLT1.
   E is incorrect because **D** is a correct answer.

3. **A** is incorrect because the small intestine contains NaCl at concentrations similar to those in plasma. Feeding NaCl would not substantially alter the NaCl concentration in the small intestine.
   B is incorrect because feeding hypertonic NaCl would cause osmotic flow of water into the small intestine until the contents reached isotonicity. This increased volume of fluid would likely increase the baby's diarrhea.
   C is incorrect because as explained in the answer to Question 2, the baby most likely has a deficit in the protein responsible for absorption of glucose and galactose across the brush border membrane, so galactose would be malabsorbed and if fed, would cause diarrhea.
   D is correct because SGLT1 is probably deficient in this infant's small intestine.
   E is incorrect because **D** is the correct answer.

Case 2-1

1.   **A** is incorrect because the reduced size would, if anything, contribute to increased resistance to osmotic hemolysis.
     B is correct because when a normal erythrocyte hemolyzes, it first swells to an approximately spherical shape. Any attempt to increase its volume beyond this point causes hemolysis.
     C is incorrect because the elevation in Na^+ permeability does contribute to the destruction of the patient's erythrocytes in the spleen (see answer to Question 2, **D**, below) but is not responsible for increased osmotic fragility in hypotonic solutions.
     D is incorrect because the elevated Na^+,K^+-ATPase level helps the erythrocyte resist osmotic swelling resulting from Na^+ entry and does not play a role in the increased osmotic fragility.
     E is incorrect because the levels of Na^+ and K^+ in fresh erythrocytes are normal.

2.   **A** is incorrect because the patient's rate of erythropoiesis is normal or elevated.
     B is incorrect because the patient's spleen is normal. This is demonstrated by the observation that erythrocytes from a normal donor have a normal life span in the patient's circulation.
     C is incorrect because the elevated Na^+,K^+-ATPase helps resist hemolysis of the erythrocytes in the patient's spleen.
     D is correct because when the patient's erythrocytes are in the spleen and are subject to low levels of ATP and glucose, Na^+ entry contributes to hemolysis.
     E is incorrect because the increased anemia after a fever results from suppression of erythropoiesis by the fever.

3.   **A** is incorrect because levels of Na^+ and K^+ in the patient's erythrocytes are normal.
     B is correct because diminished deformability of the patient's spherical erythrocytes is conducive to their destruction in the spleen as a result of the erythrocytes being trapped in the splenic cords.
     C is incorrect because the patient's erythrocytes were stated to have a diminished life span in the circulation of a normal individual.
     D is incorrect because the therapeutic benefit of splenectomy is that it reduces the rate of destruction of the patient's erythrocytes.
     E is incorrect because K^+ tends to diffuse out of the erythrocyte (see Chapter 2) and thus does not contribute to osmotic hemolysis.

Case 2-2

1.   **A** is incorrect because increased conductance to Cl^- would be expected to stabilize the resting membrane potential near its normal value (-90 mV).
     B is incorrect because Cl^- is expected to be in equilibrium across the plasma membrane of the muscle cell. A decreased electrical force for Cl^- to leave the cell should raise intracellular $[Cl^-]$.
     C is incorrect because the sum of $[K^+]$ and $[Na^+]$ in the cytosol is expected to be roughly constant. The decrease in cellular $[K^+]$ should be accompanied by an increased intracellular $[Na^+]$.
     D is correct because an increased resting conductance to Na^+ would tend to diminish the resting membrane potential (see Equation 2-8). An increased resting inflow rate of Na^+ should elevate intracellular $[Na^+]$, which would

stimulate the activity of Na^+,K^+-ATPase so that the rate of extrusion of K^+ would be increased, leading to the diminished intracellular $[K^+]$ and the increased extracellular $[K^+]$.
     E is incorrect because the decreased intracellular $[K^+]$ would lead to hyperpolarization.

2.   **A** is incorrect because the function of the neuromuscular junction was not impaired.
     B is incorrect because insulin improves the patient's condition by stimulating the uptake of K^+ by muscle cells and the efflux of Na^+ from them (see Chapter 42).
     C is incorrect because salbutamol improves the situation by producing a long-term increase in the number of active Na^+,K^+-ATPases present in the muscle cells.
     D is incorrect because although diminishing the K^+ conductance alone would lead to depolarization of the cell, it would not explain the diminished intracellular $[K^+]$ in the muscle cells.
     E is correct because statements **A** through **D** are all incorrect.

3.   **A** is correct because if inactivation of the Na^+ channel were impaired, a prolonged influx of Na^+ might occur after a train of action potentials. This might lead to an elevated intracellular $[Na^+]$, thereby stimulating Na^+,K^+-ATPase to extrude K^+ at a greater rate, leading to a decreased intracellular $[K^+]$ and an increased extracellular $[K^+]$ as described in the answer to **D** of the previous question.
     B is incorrect because the increased inflow of Na^+ should be associated with increased intracellular $[Na^+]$.
     C is incorrect because the increased intracellular Na^+ would be expected to stimulate the activity of Na^+,K^+-ATPase in the patient's muscle cells.
     D is incorrect because the mutation is consistent with depolarization of the cell by increasing the conductance to Na^+ (see Equation 2-8).
     E is incorrect because paralysis might, in theory, result from either an increased or a decreased resting membrane potential. Hyperpolarization takes the muscle cell farther from threshold and makes it more difficult to stimulate. Depolarization may diminish the number of Na^+ channels that can participate in an action potential (see Chapter 3).

Case 3-1

1.   **A** is incorrect because if the resting K^+ conductance had been reduced, the resting membrane potential would have been smaller (less negative) than normal.
     B is incorrect because the duration of the action potential was normal.
     C is correct because saxitoxin (like tetrodotoxin) binds to Na^+ channels and prevents them from opening in response to depolarization.
     D is incorrect because the time course of the action potential was normal.
     E is incorrect because the time course of the action potential was normal.

2.   **A** is incorrect because the patient ultimately had trouble walking, which indicates that the motor system is involved too.
     B is incorrect because the patient had tingling and numbness, which indicates malfunction of the cutaneous sensory system.
     C is correct.

D is incorrect because the symptoms and tests point to deficits in the nervous system. Whether the muscle cells can fire normal action potentials is unknown.

E is incorrect because **C** is the correct answer.

3. **A** is incorrect because saxitoxin should affect all normal individuals.

    B is incorrect because this patient might go into respiratory failure and need ventilatory support.

    C is correct.

    D is incorrect because this patient is no more susceptible to shellfish poisoning than any other individual.

    E is incorrect because the excretion of saxitoxin requires about 24 hours, and after most of the saxitoxin is excreted, the patient should suffer no more symptoms.

Case 3-2

1. **A** is incorrect because the conductance to Na^+ is a small fraction of the total conductance, so decreasing the Na^+ conductance would not result in a large decrease in the total conductance. Also, a decrease in the Na^+ conductance would be expected to increase the resting membrane potential.

    B is incorrect because if g_K were reduced, there should have been a reduction in the resting membrane potential.

    C is correct because Cl^- is the most conductive ion in muscle, so a decrease in g_{Cl} should lead to an increase in the membrane resistance. Because Cl^- is at equilibrium at the resting potential, a decreasing g_{Cl} should not influence the resting membrane potential.

    D is incorrect because the resting g_{Ca} is so low that decreasing it further would have no influence on membrane resistance.

    E is incorrect because **C** is the right answer.

2. **A** is incorrect because during the action potential, Cl^- is not at equilibrium and Cl^- should flow to help bring the membrane potential back toward -90 mV. If g_{Cl} is reduced, the Cl^- currents will be smaller, and repolarization will take longer.

    B is incorrect because with a larger membrane resistance a smaller stimulating current will be required to bring the membrane to threshold ($\Delta V = IR$).

    C is incorrect because the repetitive action potentials are explicable in terms of the lower g_{Cl}. Some of the K^+ that flows out of the muscle cell during the action potential accumulates in the transverse tubules (see Chapter 13) and causes depolarization there. In a normal individual, the high g_{Cl} helps clamp the surface plasma membrane to -90 mV in spite of the depolarization existing in the T tubules. In myotonia congenita, because of the lowered g_{Cl}, the depolarization in the T tubules causes depolarization of the surface membrane, leading to spontaneous action potentials in the surface membrane.

    D is incorrect because as explained in **B**, with a larger membrane resistance a smaller membrane current is required to reach threshold.

    E is correct because **A** through **D** are all incorrect.

3. We assume, for simplicity, that in the dominant disorder, the individual has three times as much normal Cl^- channel polypeptide as mutant polypeptide and that in the recessive disease, the individual has equal amounts of normal and mutant channel peptides.

    A is correct because if only one mutant polypeptide in a tetramer is required to dramatically diminish Cl^- conductance, only 6% of the tetramers formed will have no mutant polypeptide and will therefore be normal. This is consistent with the 90% (approximately) reduction in g_{Cl} in the disorder.

    B is incorrect because if only one mutant polypeptide in a tetramer is sufficient to dramatically reduce Cl^- conductance, the individual should not require two mutant alleles to manifest the disease; one mutant allele should suffice, and the disorder should show dominant inheritance.

    C is incorrect because if only tetramers with three or more mutant polypeptides have reduced conductance (assume zero conductance for simplicity), then since a majority of the tetramers will have two or fewer mutant peptides/tetramer, it should not be possible to have the 90% reduction of g_{Cl} that occurs in the disease.

    D is incorrect because there will be more tetramers with one or two mutant polypeptides than with three or four mutants/tetramer; if three or more mutants/tetramer are required to greatly reduce conductance, it should not be possible to reduce the g_{Cl} to about 10% of normal as is observed in the disorder.

    E is incorrect because **A** is the correct answer.

Case 4-1

1. **A** is incorrect because salivation depends on cholinergic nerves too (see Chapter 33), so a defect in acetylcholine release by presynaptic nerve terminals would diminish salivation.

    B is incorrect because facilitation only persists for a fraction of a second. The improvement might result from post-tetanic potentiation, however.

    C is incorrect because there was no defect in nerve conduction velocities.

    D is correct because smaller endplate potentials would be expected to increase the failure rate at the neuromuscular junction.

    E is incorrect because **D** is the correct answer.

2. **A** is incorrect because MEPPs do not depend on voltage-gated Ca^{++} channels. Consequently the frequency of the patient's MEPPs should not differ much from normal.

    B is incorrect because ionophore treatment will raise the level of Ca^{++} in motor nerve terminals and increase the frequency of MEPPs.

    C is correct because the patient's nerve terminals will have fewer functional voltage-gated Ca^{++} channels.

    D is incorrect because increasing extracellular K^+ will cause a smaller increase in MEPP frequency in the patient than in a normal individual.

    E is not correct because **C** is the correct answer.

3. **A** is correct because this would diminish the level of circulating antibodies.

    B is correct because this will prolong the action potential and allow more Ca^{++} to enter the nerve terminal.

    C is correct because this would diminish the level of circulating antibodies.

    D is correct because this will prolong the action potential and allow more Ca^{++} to enter the nerve terminal.

    E is correct because **A** through **D** are correct.

Case 4-2

1. **A** is incorrect because the nicotinic AChR is very highly conserved among species, especially the α subunit. Most

patients with myasthenia gravis have antibodies against the α subunit.

B is incorrect because even though most anti-AChR antibodies are directed against the α subunit, there is a large number of different epitopes.

C is incorrect because the absolute titer of anti-AChR does not correlate well with the severity of the disease; changes in the titer in a given patient are useful indicators.

D is incorrect because a few patients with myasthenia gravis have no detectable anti-AChR in their sera.

E is correct because none of the other options is correct.

2. **A** is incorrect because the compound muscle action potential is likely to decrease during sustained effort.

B is incorrect because nerve conduction time should be unaffected.

C is incorrect because the level of AChR is very likely to be decreased.

D is correct because the failure rate of neuromuscular transmission increases with time during sustained effort.

E is incorrect because D is the correct response.

3. **A** is incorrect because the patient is likely to have thymic hyperplasia.

B is incorrect because removal of the thymus is likely to improve the symptoms of patients in whom the onset of disease occurs before age 40.

C is incorrect because immunosuppression with doses of prednisone given on alternate days is likely to improve the patient's symptoms.

D is correct because treatment with azathioprine is highly likely to be effective.

E is incorrect because **D** is correct.

Case 5-1

1. **A** is incorrect because cholera toxin is produced by *Vibrio cholerae*.

B is incorrect because adenylyl cyclase is not activated by having ADP-ribose transferred to it.

C is correct because elevated cyclic AMP levels increase the open time of the Cl^- channel in the luminal membranes of the crypt cells, thereby causing the secretion of NaCl and water.

D is incorrect because the increased levels of cyclic AMP cause diminished absorption of salts and water by the villous epithelial cells, but they are still net absorbers of salts and water (see Chapter 40).

E is incorrect because α_i is not affected by cholera toxin.

2. **A** is incorrect because dehydration is the major cause of weakness.

B is incorrect because the diarrhea itself does an adequate job of clearing *Vibrio cholerae* from the intestine.

C is correct because the loss of water from the body is the primary cause of all the symptoms of cholera.

D is incorrect because if the patient is kept adequately hydrated and in electrolyte balance, the disease will abate with no additional therapy.

E is incorrect because loss of K^+ and HCO_3^- in the diarrheal fluid may lead to acidosis and to hypokalemia (see Chapter 38).

3. **A** is correct because Na^+ and glucose in the oral rehydration fluid stimulate the absorption of salts and water (see Chapter 34).

B is incorrect because it will take only 3 or 4 days for the diarrhea to abate, since the entire epithelial cell population turns over every 3 or 4 days.

C is incorrect because G_i administered by mouth would be digested, and if it were not, it could not enter the intestinal epithelial cells in its intact form (see Chapter 34).

D is incorrect because the diarrheal flow is sufficient to clear *Vibrio cholerae* from the intestine.

E is incorrect because drugs that suppress motility may prolong the disease by decreasing the rate of clearance of *Vibrio cholerae* by the diarrheal flow.

Case 5-2

1. **A** is incorrect because only the hyperpigmentation is due to elevated ACTH.

B is incorrect because elevated levels of ACTH would not be present if levels of CRH were inadequate.

C is incorrect because the administration of cortisol diminishes levels of ACTH.

D is incorrect because the patient already has elevated levels of ACTH and it was found that administration of ACTH did not elevate serum cortisol levels.

E is correct because these symptoms are all associated with cortisol deficiency (see Chapter 46).

2. **A** is incorrect because a decreased number of ACTH receptors might cause this disorder.

B is correct because ACTH receptors with very low affinities for ACTH could account for the low cortisol levels in the presence of elevated levels of ACTH.

C is incorrect because an inability of liganded ACTH receptors to activate α_s, which would then fail to activate adenylyl cyclase, might be the cause of the disorder.

D is incorrect because a defect in the biosynthetic pathway for cortisol could cause this disorder.

E is incorrect because if the receptor's affinity for ACTH were sufficiently reduced, there might be no response to elevated levels of ACTH.

3. **A** is incorrect because if the patient had one normal form of the ACTH receptor gene, then about half of his ACTH receptors should be normal, and thus administration of ACTH should cause some elevation of serum cortisol levels.

B is incorrect because the presence of two normal ACTH receptor genes does not completely rule out some problem with the receptor; however, it makes other causes of the disorder more likely.

C is correct because the presence of two mutant, unresponsive forms of the ACTH receptor could account for the failure of cortisol levels to increase in response to elevated levels of ACTH.

D is incorrect because if the disease is recessive and both parents are heterozygous for this defect, then they might be asymptomatic or have milder symptoms.

E is incorrect because a person with one normal and one mutant ACTH receptor gene might require elevated ACTH levels to produce normal serum cortisol levels.

Case 6-1

1. **A** is incorrect because the motor deficit is uncharacteristic for this disease.

B is incorrect because a brain tumor was not revealed in the magnetic resonance scan and microorganisms were found in the CSF.

C is incorrect because encephalitis would not generally be associated with markedly dilated ventricles, and it would have a more acute course.

D is correct because hydrocephalus is due to obstruction of the ventricles as a result of cryptococcal meningitis.

E is incorrect because the findings of blood chemistry tests were normal.

2. **A** is incorrect because the MRI would show distention of the subarachnoid space and cryptococcal meningitis is more likely to affect the base of the brain.

B is incorrect because if the cerebral aqueduct were occluded, only the lateral and third ventricles would be dilated.

C is incorrect because if one interventricular foramen were blocked, only one lateral ventricle would be distended.

D is correct because the roof of the fourth ventricle can be occluded by meningitis at the base of the brain.

E is incorrect because obstruction of the third ventricle would result in distention of the lateral ventricles and interventricular foramina.

Case 6-2

1. **A** is incorrect because astrocytes affect nerve impulse activity only indirectly.

B is incorrect because the patient had disruption of sensation (vision, hearing) as well as motor difficulties, and the motor disorders included interruption of the voluntary motor pathways; the stretch reflexes were increased on one side, whereas diseases of motor neurons result in reduced stretch reflexes.

C is correct because oligodendroglia provide myelin sheaths for CNS axons and demyelinating diseases that affect these cells disrupt function by slowing or interrupting nerve impulse conduction.

D is incorrect because the function of these neurons on one side was temporarily affected secondarily to the disorder of oligodendroglial cells that provided the myelin sheaths for pyramidal cell axons.

E is incorrect because Schwann cells myelinate axons in the PNS, whereas the disorder in this patient affected the CNS.

2. **A** is incorrect because there are no known disorders that cause localized and changeable disorders of axonal transport.

B is correct because the disorder, multiple sclerosis, affects localized groups of oligodendroglial cells, resulting in demyelination of axons of neurons in a particular location and therefore having a particular function; remissions often occur as the oligodendroglial cells recover and remyelinate the axons.

C is incorrect because chromatolysis results from transection of axons, which could not occur in a disease in which symptoms recover in as short a time as a few weeks; the interruption of axons in the CNS usually results in a permanent impairment because of the very limited capability of CNS neurons to regenerate.

D is incorrect because no disorders are known that result in localized and migratory failures of synaptic transmission in different neural systems.

E is incorrect for the same reasons that are discussed under answer **C**.

Case 7-1

1. **A** is incorrect because such a lesion might interrupt the medial lemniscus and pyramid (see Chapter 9), causing some of the symptoms, but the spinothalamic tract would be unaffected, and chronic pain would not be expected.

B is incorrect because it would be unlikely that a cortical lesion would involve both the arm and face, since these are supplied by different cerebral arteries.

C is incorrect because peripheral polyneuropathies are symmetrical and would not be restricted to one side.

D is correct because somatosensory loss can result from a lesion affecting the VPL nucleus. The motor deficit could be caused by extension of the lesion into the internal capsule (see Chapter 9). A thalamic pain syndrome can result from a lesion of the VPL nucleus.

E is incorrect because a hemisection of the spinal cord above C5 on the right would result in a loss of fine tactile discrimination on the right and of pain and temperature sensation on the left.

2. **A** is incorrect because if these ascending projections of the reticular formation were interrupted, the patient would be comatose (see Chapter 11).

B is incorrect because the pain in patients who have the thalamic syndrome is very real and can lead to suicide.

C is correct because spinothalamic input to the VPL nucleus is largely interrupted, but there are plastic changes in denervated cortical circuits.

D is incorrect because mechanoreceptors do not convert to nociceptors, although their activation can trigger discharges in wide-dynamic-range nociceptive neurons in the central nervous system.

E is incorrect because nociceptive neurons would not stop responding to pinprick, although they might well develop more spontaneous activity and discharge more vigorously to tactile stimuli after injury to the nervous system.

Case 7-2

1. **A** is incorrect because morphine is unlikely to reach the periaqueductal gray.

B is correct because there are opiate receptors in the spinal cord dorsal horn, and their activation will reduce nociceptive transmission.

C is incorrect because there is no evidence that morphine would act on cancer cells in the pelvic region, preventing these cells from inducing pain.

D is incorrect because nociceptors in the meninges are unlikely to be responsible for the pain, unless metastases have reached the spinal cord; in this case, morphine would not act like a local anesthetic to block their activity.

E is incorrect because when morphine reaches the spinal cord, it will diminish the release of substance P from the terminals of nociceptors in the dorsal horn.

2. **A** is incorrect because morphine could cause respiratory depression if it reached the medulla.

B is incorrect because the local infusion of morphine may cause itching sensations.

C is incorrect because tolerance to morphine may develop.

D is incorrect because morphine will block only some types of pain.

E is correct because morphine will only block pain, whereas the local anesthetic will block all somatovisceral sensations.

Case 8-1

1. **A** is incorrect because this visual field defect involves a loss of vision in the temporal half of the visual field in each eye.
B is incorrect because a scotoma implies an area of visual loss that corresponds to an area within the visual field of one eye.
C is correct because homonymous means that the visual loss is in the corresponding region in both eyes (e.g., on the left or on the right in both eyes). Hemianopsia means "half-blindness," so the loss is in half of each visual field. Macular sparing means that vision in the central parts of the visual fields is relatively spared.
D is incorrect because this visual field defect is a loss of vision in the lower quadrants in the two eyes. Homonymous means that the loss is in the corresponding quadrants (e.g., both left or both right quadrants).
E is incorrect because the loss is in the upper right or upper left quadrants in both eyes.

2. **A** is incorrect because this artery supplies the medial parts of the frontal and parietal lobes and has nothing to do with vision.
B is incorrect because although it does supply the optic tract, a lesion of the optic tract would produce homonymous hemianopsia without macular sparing. In addition, it supplies structures belonging to the motor system that are not impaired in this patient.
C is incorrect because one of the branches of the internal carotid is the ophthalmic artery, which supplies the retina. Occlusion of the blood flow in the ophthalmic artery would cause blindness in one eye.
D is incorrect because interruption of the middle cerebral artery on the left side might produce a homonymous hemianopsia without macular sparing by interrupting the optic radiation, but it would also cause motor and somatosensory impairments and a language disorder.
E is correct because it supplies the striate cortex. Macular sparing can result if there is enough collateral circulation.

3. **A** is incorrect because destruction of a lateral geniculate nucleus would produce a homonymous hemianopsia without macular sparing.
B is correct because macular sparing can occur because of the large representation of the macula in the cortex near the occipital pole and the possibility of collateral circulation from branches of the middle cerebral artery.
C is incorrect because a lesion there would produce a bitemporal hemianopsia if only the crossing fibers from the nasal hemiretinas were interrupted. This is unlikely with a vascular lesion but can occur in cases of pituitary tumor.
D is incorrect because a lesion of the optic tract is likely to result in homonymous hemianopsia without macular sparing.
E is incorrect because a lesion within the retina would cause a scotoma.

Case 8-2

1. **A** is incorrect because with a conduction deficit, the Rinne tests would be expected to show that bone conduction is better than air conduction.
B is incorrect because the boy can hear, although his hearing is impaired.
C is incorrect because in this case, the sound should have been localized to the impaired side in Weber's test and bone conduction should have been better than air conduction on that side.
D is correct because Weber's test is inconclusive, and therefore the hearing loss is symmetrical. The Rinne tests show the normal relationship of air to bone conduction. Audiometry shows a severe hearing loss that includes part of the region important in understanding spoken language.
E is incorrect because in this case, sound should have been localized to the left side in Weber's test.

2. **A** is incorrect because deafness is generally not associated with a cortical lesion, although problems with language are.
B is incorrect because although damage to both cochlear nerves would result in a similar pattern of sensorineural deafness, the history of listening to loud music suggests another cause.
C is correct because the loud music has evidently resulted in damage to hair cells as a result of excessive deflections of the basilar membrane in the region corresponding to the range of hearing loss detected by audiometry.
D is incorrect because such a disruption would result in a conduction deficit.
E is incorrect because a problem with the tympanic membranes would also cause conduction deafness.

Case 9-1

1. **A** is incorrect because disorders of the basal ganglia do not produce weakness or hyperactive stretch reflexes.
B is incorrect because cerebellar disorders are likely to reduce muscle tone and stretch reflexes.
C is correct because the corticospinal, corticobulbar, and corticoreticulospinal pathways, as well as the thalamocortical projections from the somatosensory thalamus, are interrupted.
D is incorrect because the face, arm, and leg areas of the precentral and postcentral gyri would probably not all be damaged in a stroke that left the patient able to function relatively well because the cerebral arteries that supply the leg differ from those that supply the arm and face.
E is incorrect because although a high cervical lesion could cause spastic paralysis of the arm and leg and interrupt transmission of somatic sensations in the dorsal column, no paralysis or sensory loss would occur in the head.

2. **A** is incorrect because Babinski's sign indicates that the lateral corticospinal tract has been interrupted; however, this sign can be elicited whether or not the paralysis is of the spastic type.
B is correct because spasticity is characterized by hyperactive stretch reflexes.
C is incorrect because sensory loss is independent of the presence or absence of spasticity.
D is incorrect because the tongue can be weak either because of interruption of the corticobulbar tract or because of a lesion of the hypoglossal nucleus or nerve.
E is incorrect because weakness can be present without spasticity.

Case 9-2

1. **A** is correct because individuals with Parkinson's disease have lost many of the dopaminergic neurons of the substantia nigra, so dopamine levels in the striatum are reduced.

B is incorrect because damage to the corticoreticulospinal inhibitory pathway contributes to spasticity.

C is incorrect because a lesion of these nuclei will result in cerebellar signs such as ataxia.

D is incorrect because a lesion in the primary motor cortex will cause weakness and perhaps also Babinski's sign.

E is incorrect because a lesion in the supplementary motor cortex may interfere with motor performance, but it will not produce Parkinson's disease.

2. **A** is correct because the main problem is the reduction in the number of dopaminergic neurons in the substantia nigra. Replacement of the dopamine by L-DOPA can be an effective therapy, at least in the early stages of Parkinson's disease, because it can cross the blood-brain barrier.

B is incorrect because epinephrine will not cross the blood-brain barrier.

C is incorrect because this inhibitory neurotransmitter used in the basal ganglia circuits will not cross the blood-brain barrier.

D is incorrect because glutamate is used in many excitatory synapses in the brain, including in the basal ganglia circuits, so even if it crossed the blood-brain barrier, it would have generalized effects.

E is incorrect because substance P would be broken down in the blood and would not cross the blood-brain barrier.

Case 10-1

1. **A** is incorrect because the ascending pathways from the spinal cord are interrupted, as is the hypothalamospinal tract.

B is incorrect because the bladder may become excessively distended in the spinal shock phase of spinal cord injury, but it becomes spastic in the chronic phase. No pain can be felt in either phase.

C is incorrect because the main concern with bacterial infection is hypotension and shock if bacterial products reach the systemic circulation.

D is incorrect because the target organs of sympathetic postganglionic neurons have not been denervated, so there should be no change in postsynaptic receptors in the target organs.

E is correct because both autonomic and somatic reflexes become exaggerated after spinal cord transection.

2. **A** is correct because the hypothalamus is disconnected from the spinal cord autonomic centers.

B is incorrect; although relatively vasodilated because of loss of central autonomic drive, the patient will not be able to lose heat via increased vasodilation and sweating in response to a hot environment.

C is incorrect because the patient would not be able to shiver effectively.

D is incorrect because the thermoreceptors would presumably react to thermal stimuli in a normal fashion, but in any event the hypothalamic signals that mediate thermoregulation are impaired.

E is incorrect because hypothalamic regulation in either direction is prevented by the spinal cord transection.

Case 11-1

1. **A** is incorrect because interruption of the corpus callosum will produce problems other than a language disorder.

B is correct because Broca's area has been damaged, which leads to an expressive aphasia.

C is incorrect because in most people, Broca's area is in the left hemisphere.

D is incorrect because this region of the superior temporal gyrus is part of Wernicke's area, and damage here would result in a receptive aphasia.

E is incorrect because this region does not have a language function.

2. **A** is correct because language functions of all types, not just speech, would be impaired.

B is incorrect because this type of tremor would be expected from a cerebellar lesion.

C is incorrect because this would involve the right hemisphere.

D is incorrect because unilateral deafness is usually due to a conduction deficit or to a sensorineural deficit involving the cochlea, cochlear nerve, or cochlear nuclei, not a brainstem or cortical lesion.

E is incorrect because the motor deficit would be on the right; the patient could have Babinski's sign on the right if projections from the leg representation are interrupted in the internal capsule.

Case 12-1

1. **A** is incorrect because the muscle can generate about 3×10^5 N/m^2 at its optimum length in an isometric contraction, but this is not the maximum force possible.

B is incorrect because the only forces in a relaxed muscle are those caused by extension of connective tissue or cytoskeletal elements.

C is incorrect because forces decrease when muscles shorten below their optimum length.

D is correct because a contracting muscle can withstand an externally imposed force about 60% greater than the maximum force it will develop.

E is incorrect because the forces on rapidly shortening cells are low.

2. **A** is correct because the muscles are not rigid and hence this is not a reasonable explanation.

B is correct because metabolic factors are unlikely to be a direct contributor to soreness.

C is correct because it is unlikely that structural damage occurred in cells with the highest rates of ATP consumption.

D is correct because in the absence of sustained contractions a reduction in blood flow would not occur.

E is correct and is the best answer as it is the most complete.

3. **A** is incorrect because not all of the leg muscles are involved in the fitness test.

B is incorrect because there were differences in muscle use between the legs.

C is correct because muscles in the left leg were used to decelerate the body and gravity imposed high loads on contracting motor units that caused injury and soreness.

D is incorrect because these motor units were shortening and insufficiently loaded to cause injury.

E is incorrect because unstimulated muscle cells provide little resistance to stretch.

Case 13-1

1. **A** is incorrect because injuries and other diseases can elevate serum myoplasmic protein concentrations.

B is correct because the sarcolemma barrier must be broken to allow proteins to escape.

C is incorrect because the proteins of interest are expressed only in skeletal muscle and are not secreted.

D is incorrect because any increase in myoplasmic proteins in the serum caused by a rare exercise-related injury would be small and of short duration.

E is incorrect because atrophy results from decreased synthesis of muscle proteins.

2. **A** is correct because girls will have an X chromosome from both their father and their mother. The dystrophin gene from the father must be normal, or he would have died before adolescence.

    B is incorrect because testosterone increases the synthesis of muscle proteins but dystrophin is normally expressed in both sexes.

    C is incorrect because dystrophin is essential for the structural integrity of all skeletal muscle. Girls must inherit one normal dystrophin gene from their fathers, so they cannot be homozygous for the recessive defective allele.

    D is incorrect because there is a pattern of expression of muscle protein isoforms during fetal and neonatal development that differs somewhat from that in adults. These isoforms are associated with some protection from the defective dystrophin gene because muscular dystrophy develops only later in childhood.

    E is incorrect because most girls will have the normal dystrophin gene in both X chromosomes and their sons will not be at risk for Duchenne's muscular dystrophy.

3. **A** is incorrect because ingested proteins are broken down to small peptides and amino acids before entering the bloodstream.

    B is incorrect because gene therapy is not practical now.

    C is incorrect because replication is not the problem. Regeneration is important in delaying the progression of muscular dystrophy.

    D is correct because an exercise program is key to minimizing the progression of muscular dystrophy. There is no cure. Activity stimulates regenerative processes and also induces adaptive hypertrophic responses in synergistic muscles that may not be affected by the disease.

    E is incorrect because injected proteins would not leave the muscle vascular system, nor be taken up by the muscle cells.

Case 13-2

1. **A** is incorrect because the muscle relaxant would block neuromuscular transmission even if the motor systems became hyperexcitable.

    B is incorrect because contractures arising from the persistence of acetylcholine would be blocked by the muscle relaxant.

    C is incorrect because an influx of Ca^{++} through the sarcolemma would only be prevented by Ca^{++} channel blockers.

    D is correct because it is the most reasonable explanation of the symptoms, given the success of the treatment with a drug that blocks Ca^{++} release from the sarcoplasmic reticulum.

    E is incorrect because the muscle relaxant would block neuromuscular transmission.

2. **A** is incorrect because although a contributing factor, cycling rates would be at their slowest in rigid, isometrically contracting muscle cells.

    B is correct because the defective Ca^{++} channels in the pa-

tient's sarcoplasmic reticulum were locked open by the anesthetic, creating a short circuit for Ca^{++} to be pumped inside only to diffuse out again.

C is incorrect because heat is dissipated by evaporation of sweat, increased respiratory rate, and increased blood flow from skeletal muscle to tissues where heat transfer takes place, and most or all of these dissipative factors were increased.

D is incorrect because the increased metabolism is a consequence of ATP hydrolysis and is not the cause of the temperature rise.

E is incorrect because the presence of a mutant gene is not the cause of the hyperthermia, although the defective gene made it possible to trigger the episode.

Case 13-3

1. **A** is correct because most tasks are effortless in microgravity.

    B is incorrect because deceleration can impose greater than normal loads on the body.

    C is incorrect because reentry would impose gravitational and deceleration loading of muscle, leading to weakness with rapid fatigue characteristic of fast, glycolytic motor units.

    D is incorrect because recovery requires the remineralization of bone and protein synthesis in muscle and tendons in the normal adaptive response to increased muscular activity. Also involved are the heart and respiratory muscles that are fundamental to sustained muscular activity.

    E is incorrect because normal gravitational loads will stress the weakened bones and muscles.

2. **A** is incorrect because the loss of muscle mass reflects disuse.

    B is incorrect because the weakness is due to a lack of exercise.

    C is incorrect because microgravity and reinnervation by an inexcitable motor neuron both involve conversion to fast motor units as the result of infrequent recruitment.

    D is incorrect because a reduction in muscle mass follows a decrease in exercise.

    E is correct because the absence of the cytoskeletal protein dystrophin is responsible for this genetic disease.

3. **A** is incorrect because appropriate exercise has positive effects.

    B is incorrect because information can be obtained that is not possible with astronauts. In addition, the effects of microgravity occur several times faster in small mammals with high metabolic rates and rapid protein turnover, effectively modeling the effects of much longer periods in space for humans.

    C is incorrect because autopilots would minimize the physical stress on shuttle pilots.

    D is correct because skeletal muscle is voluntary and can be recruited in an effective exercise program. This strategy has no apparent merit.

    E is incorrect because this is the only way to avoid all risk to crews.

Case 14-1

1. **A** is incorrect because fatigue of the diaphragm and other respiratory muscles caused by impaired O_2 delivery was a consequence of the episode rather than the cause.

B is incorrect because edema would not be alleviated by the treatment.

C is correct as shown by the response to epinephrine, which relaxes airway smooth muscle.

D is incorrect because airway O_2 content would not fall.

E is incorrect as shown by the response to epinephrine.

2. **A** is correct because the diaphragm and other respiratory skeletal muscles, the heart, and the airway and other smooth muscles were active.

B is incorrect because airway smooth muscle constriction caused the difficulty in breathing.

C is incorrect because respiratory muscles are skeletal and their activity to increase air flow was largely responsible for the fatigue.

D is incorrect because the airway smooth muscle is involuntary.

E is incorrect because the skeletal muscles involved are voluntary.

3. **A** is incorrect because relaxation is a physiological response to enhanced pulmonary ventilation during exercise.

B is incorrect because phasic contraction is a physiological response to increased air flow velocity during a cough reflex.

C is incorrect because maintenance of airway dimensions is an important physiological role.

D is correct because skeletal muscle generates the pressure gradients responsible for airflow.

E is incorrect because adjustments in regional airflow are important.

Case 14-2

1. **A** is incorrect because the cyanosis induced by anoxia was due to abnormally high O_2 extraction rather than delivery of poorly oxygenated blood, which would affect all tissues.

B is incorrect because the symptoms were triggered by cold rather than work by the hands.

C is correct because peripheral vasoconstriction would reduce blood flow and produce all of the symptoms.

D is incorrect because both hands would not be affected by vascular blockade, nor would they be triggered by cold.

E is incorrect because anything that decreased O_2 binding by hemoglobin in the periphery would increase O_2 delivery.

2. **A** is incorrect because the restoration of normal flow would restore only normal color.

B is correct because the accumulation of metabolites and other vasodilators is followed by a period of increased flow (termed reactive hyperemia).

C is incorrect because the bluish color, or cyanosis, observed initially was due to deoxygenation of these pigments.

D is incorrect because sympathetic activity constricts vascular smooth muscle.

E is incorrect because this would not significantly affect O_2 delivery to the hands.

3. **A** is incorrect because the severe reduction in blood flow was responsible for the pain.

B is correct although the mechanisms triggering the vasospasm are unknown.

C is incorrect because there was no drop in core temperature in the absence of flow from the hands.

D is incorrect because blood flow is regulated, in part to maintain normal temperatures.

E is incorrect because cooling would not be expected to increase metabolite production and many metabolites are vasodilators.

Case 15-1

1. **A** is incorrect because the wide pulse pressure produces a pulsatile flow in the nail bed.

B is correct because the circulation time will be shortened because some blood passes through the shunt (short circuit).

C is incorrect because the pulse pressure is increased secondary to reduced peripheral resistance.

D is incorrect because the velocity of blood flow is still greatest in the aorta, where the cross-sectional area of the vasculature is smallest.

E is incorrect because the right atrial pressure is less than vena caval pressure; otherwise blood would not be able to return to the heart.

Case 16-1

1. **A** is incorrect because chronic blood loss results in red cells with considerable size variation, typical of microcytic anemia.

B is incorrect because the hematocrit would be greatly reduced below a normal of 45%.

C is incorrect because the red cell count would be below the normal level of 5 million cells/μL.

D is correct because the normal blood hemoglobin level is 15 g/dl. A value of 6 g/dl indicates severe anemia.

E is incorrect because the hemoglobin/red cell ratio would be reduced. Each red cell would contain less than the normal amount of hemoglobin.

Case 16-2

1. **A** is incorrect because she would get a severe reaction to type A blood. Because she is Rh positive, she can receive either Rh-negative or Rh-positive blood.

B is incorrect because she would get a severe reaction to type AB blood. Because she is Rh positive, she can receive either Rh-negative or Rh-positive blood.

C is incorrect because she would get a severe reaction to type AB blood. Because she is Rh positive, she can receive either Rh-negative or Rh-positive blood.

D is correct because the patient can receive only group O blood.

E is incorrect because she would get a severe reaction to type B blood. Because she is Rh positive, she can receive either Rh-negative or Rh-positive blood.

Case 17-1

1. **A** is incorrect because a less negative transmembrane potential (V_m) inactivates fast Na^+ channels, and this decreases propagation velocity.

B is incorrect because ventricular myocardial cells are fast-response fibers, and such fibers do not display postrepolarization refractoriness.

C is correct because when the extracellular K^+ concentration increases, the Nernst equation indicates that the transmembrane potential will become less negative.

D is incorrect because ordinary myocardial cells do not possess the property of automaticity.

E is incorrect because reentry is more likely to occur when propagation is retarded.

2. **A** is incorrect because the slope of the automatic cell upstroke does not appreciably affect the firing frequency.
    B is correct because when the slope of the slow diastolic depolarization is increased, the firing threshold of the automatic cells is reached more quickly.
    C is incorrect because increasing the firing threshold per se would actually decrease the firing frequency of the automatic cells.
    D is incorrect because increasing the maximum negativity would prolong the time required for V_m to reach threshold.
    E is incorrect because changes in the amplitude of the action potential upstroke of an automatic cell do not appreciably affect the firing frequency of that cell.

3. **A** is incorrect because if a bypass tract had been present, the ventricle would contract at the same frequency (90 beats/min) as did the atria.
    B is incorrect because ordinary ventricular myocytes can become automatic only under very unusual conditions.
    C is incorrect because if such ventricular cells did exist, they would fire at the prevailing frequency (90 firings/min) of the SA node cells.
    D is correct because the Purkinje fibers are automatic fibers, and they generate action potentials at a low frequency when they are not depolarized by action potentials originating in higher-frequency pacemaker sites.
    E is incorrect because myoneural junctions (between nerve and muscle cells), such as those in skeletal muscle, do not exist in cardiac muscle.

4. **A** is correct because pacing cardiac tissue at a frequency substantially greater than the natural firing frequency of the intrinsic ventricular pacemakers (Purkinje cells) causes an excessive influx of Na^+ into the cardiac cells, including the automatic cells, and this leads to overdrive suppression.
    B is incorrect because overdrive suppression is readily induced in isolated cardiac tissues that have been completely denervated.
    C is incorrect, also because overdrive suppression is readily induced in isolated cardiac tissues that have been completely denervated.
    D is incorrect because overdrive suppression is a characteristic of automatic, not of ordinary, myocardial cells.
    E is incorrect because overdrive suppression is readily induced in isolated cardiac tissues that have been completely denervated.

Case 18-1

1. **A** is incorrect because the patient's murmur is diastolic, not systolic.
    B is incorrect for the same reason as for **A**.
    C is incorrect because the characterizations of this murmur (soft, high pitched) and its location are compatible with aortic regurgitation, not mitral stenosis.
    D is correct because the murmur is characteristic of mitral stenosis.
    E is incorrect because for the same reason as for **A**.

2. **A** is incorrect because cardiac rhythm is irregular in atrial fibrillation.
    B is incorrect because some weak beats are not palpable at the wrist but are heard over the precordium.
    C is correct because the pulse is totally irregular.

D is incorrect because beats after inadequate ventricular filling are felt as weaker than those after adequate ventricular filling.
E is incorrect because P waves are replaced by F waves in the electrocardiogram.

3. **A** is incorrect because a pacemaker cannot take over the rhythm in atrial fibrillation.
    B is correct because a phlebotomy would relieve the excessive preload and allow the ventricles to contract more efficiently.
    C is incorrect because a saline infusion would add to the high preload and aggravate the congestive failure.
    D is incorrect because adenosine will have no effect on atrial fibrillation.
    E is incorrect because the heart needs more intracellular Ca^{++}, not less.

4. **A** is incorrect because the serum albumin level would not be elevated. It might even be reduced.
    B is correct because the elevated left atrial pressure would be transmitted back to the wedged catheter (wedge pressure).
    C is incorrect because Na^+ excretion would be reduced in a patient in congestive heart failure.
    D is incorrect because peripheral resistance would be increased in a patient with heart failure and a low cardiac output.
    E is incorrect because the pulse pressure would be either normal or reduced in a patient with a low cardiac output.

5. **A** is incorrect because dicumarol would prevent clot formation in the fibrillating atria and thereby prevent the release of emboli from the atria.
    B is incorrect because digoxin strengthens the cardiac contractions by raising intracellular Ca^{++} levels.
    C is incorrect because procainamide can sometimes stop atrial fibrillation.
    D is incorrect because the diuretic, hydrochlorothiazide enhances the renal excretion of NaCl and water, thereby reducing blood volume and cardiac preload.
    E is correct because nitroglycerin is prescribed for angina pectoris caused by myocardial ischemia and is not prescribed for congestive heart failure.

6. **A** is incorrect.
    B is incorrect.
    C is correct because:

    $$\frac{300}{0.18-0.08} = \frac{300}{0.10} = 300 \text{ ml/min} = 3 \text{ L/min}$$

    D is incorrect.
    E is incorrect.

Case 19-1

1. **A** is incorrect because a decrease in the arterial pressure would reflexly increase sympathetic activity and decrease vagal activity, both of which would increase myocardial contractility.
    B is incorrect because a decrease in the arterial pressure would reflexly increase sympathetic activity and decrease vagal activity, both of which would shorten the cardiac cycle.
    C is incorrect because a decrease in the arterial pressure would reflexly increase sympathetic activity and decrease

vagal activity, both of which would enhance AV conduction.

D is correct because a decrease in the arterial pressure would reflexly increase sympathetic activity and thereby increase the neuronal release of norepinephrine.

E is incorrect because a decrease in the arterial pressure would increase the neuronal release of norepinephrine and thereby increase calcium conductance.

2. **A** is incorrect because the acetylcholine (ACh) released by the vagal fibers markedly shortens the atrial action potentials, which curtails the influx of Ca^{++} into the myocytes and thus weakens their contractions.

   B is incorrect because the ACh released from vagal endings inhibits the release of norepinephrine from nearby sympathetic nerve endings.

   C is incorrect because the distribution of vagal nerve fibers and of muscarinic cholinergic receptors is sparse in these tissues.

   D is correct because the ACh released from vagal fibers acts on muscarinic receptors on SA node automatic cells, and these receptors interact very quickly with specific K^+ channels because no second messenger intervenes.

   E is incorrect because the neurally released ACh hyperpolarizes the conduction fibers and thereby retards conduction.

3. **A** is correct because the cardiac responses to vagal stimulation develop and decay rapidly, but the responses to sympathetic stimulation develop and decay very slowly. Hence respiratory arrhythmia is mediated almost entirely by the vagus nerves, and this arrhythmia would be abolished by a potent muscarinic antagonist.

   B is incorrect because vagally released ACh weakens the contractions of atrial myocytes; a muscarinic antagonist would prevent this effect.

   C is incorrect because vagally released ACh retards AV conduction; a muscarinic antagonist would prevent this effect.

   D is incorrect because vagally released ACh decreases the action potential duration of atrial myocytes; a muscarinic antagonist would prevent this effect.

   E is incorrect because vagally released ACh hyperpolarizes the atrial myocytes during phase 4; a muscarinic antagonist would prevent this effect.

4. **A** is correct because the heart rate increases during inspiration in this arrhythmia; this increase is mediated mainly by a reduction in vagal activity.

   B is incorrect because decreased sympathetic activity would tend to decrease the heart rate during inspiration.

   C is incorrect because a decreased rate of slow diastolic depolarization would decrease the heart rate during inspiration.

   D is incorrect because hemorrhage decreases vagal activity and would thereby attenuate the arrhythmia.

   E is incorrect because propranolol attenuates the sympathetic effects on the heart; such effects have little influence on the respiratory arrhythmia.

5. **A** is incorrect because if the cardiac automatic cells became more responsive, the heart rate response would decay less rapidly.

   B is incorrect because ACh is removed from the cardiac interstitium by hydrolysis, not by uptake by the vagus nerve endings.

   C is incorrect because ACh is removed from the cardiac interstitium by hydrolysis, not by uptake by the cardiac myocytes.

D is incorrect because the synthetic mechanisms in the nerve endings can usually produce new ACh at a rate equal to its release rate.

E is correct because acetylcholinesterase is abundant in atrial tissues, especially the SA and AV nodes.

Case 20-1

1. **A** is incorrect.
   B is correct because:

   $$\frac{Pa - Pa}{Q} = \frac{100 - 10}{300} = 0.3 \text{ mm Hg/ml/min}$$

   C is incorrect.
   D is incorrect.
   E is incorrect.

2. **A** is incorrect.
   B is incorrect.
   C is incorrect.
   D is correct because the left [(100 − 10)/500] and right [(100 − 10)/300] vascular resistances were 0.18 and 0.30 mm Hg/ml/min, respectively, and the reciprocals of those resistances were 5.56 and 3.33 ml/min/mm Hg, respectively. Hence the reciprocal of the sum (8.89 ml/min/mm Hg) of these reciprocals equals 0.11 mm Hg/ml/min.
   E is incorrect.

3. **A** is correct because:

   Resistance to flow =

   $$\frac{\text{Pressure diference across the plaque}}{\text{Flow past the plaque}} =$$

   $$\frac{100 - 80 \text{ mm Hg}}{300 \text{ ml/min}} = 0.066 \text{ mm Hg/ml/min}$$

   B is incorrect.
   C is incorrect.
   D is incorrect.
   E is incorrect.

Case 21-1

1. **A** is correct because the mean arterial pressure in the systemic and pulmonary vascular beds depends on the outputs of the left and right ventricles and the systemic vascular resistances. Over any substantial time interval, the outputs of the two ventricles are equal, but the systemic vascular resistance far exceeds the pulmonary vascular resistance.

   B is incorrect because the mean arterial pressure is not affected by the arterial compliance.

   C is incorrect because over any substantial time interval, the outputs of the right and left ventricles must equal each other.

   D is incorrect because the total cross-sectional area of the systemic capillary bed is much greater than the total cross-sectional area of the pulmonary capillary bed.

   E is incorrect because the durations of the rapid ejection phases of the right and left ventricles are virtually equal.

2. **A** is incorrect because the systemic vascular resistance increases considerably in patients with essential hypertension.

   B is incorrect because the duration of the reduced ejection phase of the left ventricle has only a negligible effect on the arterial pulse pressure.

C is correct because when the arterial pressure rises, the arteries become less compliant (as does a balloon); also, the arterial compliance decreases with age.

D is incorrect because the total cross-sectional area of the systemic capillary bed does not change substantially in hypertensive subjects.

E is incorrect because if the aortic compliance increased, the arterial pulse pressure would tend to decrease.

Case 22-1

1.   **A** is incorrect.
     B is incorrect.
     C is incorrect.
     D is correct because $(44 + 2) - (23 + 8) = 15$.
     E is incorrect.

2.   **A** is incorrect because dialysis would be of no value. It is used in cases of kidney failure to remove waste products normally eliminated by the kidneys.

     B is incorrect because a high-fat diet is contraindicated because it would put an added burden on the cirrhotic liver.

     C is correct because portal-caval shunt (portal vein to inferior vena cava) could reduce the high venous pressure in the mesentery by allowing mesenteric blood to bypass the high vascular resistance in the liver. This would aid in eliminating the ascites.

     D is incorrect because cholecystectomy would be of no value.

     E is incorrect because erythromycin is an antibiotic and would not be indicated because alcoholic cirrhosis is not an infectious disease.

3.   **A** is incorrect because sodium, chloride, and potassium are equally distributed across the capillary membrane and hence do not exert an osmotic force between intravascular and extracellular spaces.

     B is correct because albumin is small enough (low molecular weight) to exert the main osmotic force of plasma and large enough to remain within the vascular compartment.

     C is incorrect because sodium, chloride, and potassium are equally distributed across the capillary membrane and hence do not exert an osmotic force between intravascular and extracellular spaces.

     D is incorrect because globulin is a large protein (high molecular weight) and hence exerts only a small osmotic force.

     E is incorrect because sodium, chloride, and potassium are equally distributed across the capillary membrane and hence do not exert an osmotic force between intravascular and extracellular spaces.

Case 22-2

1.   **A** is incorrect because although saline can help restore blood volume, it would be rapidly lost from the burned surfaces.

     B is incorrect because although whole blood can restore blood volume, it would not be the most effective treatment. The patient has a high hematocrit, which indicates a concentration of red cells in his circulation. Therefore red cells are not needed, and whole blood would not correct the hemoconcentration.

     C is incorrect because isotonic glucose would only temporarily restore blood volume, and as with saline, the water would be lost from the burned surfaces.

     D is incorrect because although dextran can help restore blood volume and the oncotic pressure, it would not restore albumin levels to normal.

     E is correct because the albumin concentration in the patient's blood is low because of loss of albumin from the burned tissues. This results in a decreased plasma oncotic pressure; this plus the loss of fluid from the damaged microvessels leads to a decreased blood volume and an increased red cell concentration. Therefore a plasma transfusion, which supplies albumin plus saline without red cells, is the most effective treatment.

2.   **A** is incorrect because a reflex constriction of arterioles in the feet would not occur as a consequence of standing erect.

     B is incorrect because tissue pressure is normally close to atmospheric pressure and it could only reach high levels if severe subcutaneous edema occurred. Even then, the pressure would not equal intracapillary pressure in the feet in the standing position.

     C is incorrect because the total capillary cross-sectional area is not involved. The pressure would be high and equal in all of the capillaries of the feet.

     D is correct because the small diameter (or radius) of the capillaries is responsible for the low wall tension, according to the law of Laplace: T (wall tension) = P (pressure) × r (radius of capillary). The low wall tension protects against capillary rupture.

     E is incorrect because capillaries do not constrict. They are passive in response to intravascular pressure changes.

Case 23-1

1.   **A** is incorrect because the intravascular pressure in the arterioles is decreased, not increased, and because the arterioles are maximally dilated by the local release of metabolites.

     B is correct because the arterioles are maximally dilated secondary to the inadequate blood flow that causes the local release of vasodilation metabolites.

     C is incorrect because maximally dilated vessels do not autoregulate.

     D is incorrect because local metabolites override a myogenic response.

     E is incorrect because this would occur only with the washout of metabolites, not with their presence.

2.   **A** is correct because use of tobacco is believed to be a contributing factor to the cause and exacerbation of thromboangiitis obliterans.

     B is incorrect because a vasodilator drug would be valueless. The resistance vessels are already maximally dilated.

     C is incorrect because the arterioles cannot be dilated further by interrupting their nerve supply.

     D is incorrect because heat would increase the metabolic rate of the ischemic tissue and would thereby aggravate the problem.

     E is incorrect because a vasoconstrictor drug would reduce blood flow to the lower leg and exacerbate his symptoms.

Case 23-2

1.   **A** is incorrect because a hypersensitive carotid sinus can produce fainting, especially with tight collars.

B is incorrect because episodes of heart block can produce fainting (Stokes-Adams syndrome) when the ventricular rate falls to very low levels and blood pressure falls.

C is incorrect because some individuals experience severe hypotension when they change from the horizontal to the vertical position, a condition usually observed in astronauts when they return to earth.

D is incorrect because severe tachycardia can interfere with ventricular filling, which can result in low blood pressure and syncope.

E is correct because diabetic coma is not characterized by repeated brief bouts of unconsciousness.

2. **A** is incorrect because adenosine as a bolus injection is the drug of choice in the treatment of supraventricular tachycardia (SVT).

B is incorrect because the Valsalva maneuver can terminate SVT by depressing atrial ventricular conduction via enhanced cardiac vagal activity.

C is correct because digitalis is not prescribed for SVT unless there is also impaired myocardial function.

D is incorrect because carotid sinus massage can terminate SVT by the same mechanism as with Valsalva's maneuver.

E is incorrect because in severe and prolonged cases of SVT the ectopic focus is located with a cardiac catheter tip and is ablated with an electric current.

Case 24-1

1. **A** is incorrect because the blood loss would decrease the central venous pressure, but this reduction in cardiac preload would decrease the cardiac output.

B is incorrect because the blood loss would decrease the central venous pressure.

C is correct because the blood loss would decrease the central venous pressure; this reduction in cardiac preload would decrease the cardiac output.

D is incorrect because the reduced cardiac preload would decrease the cardiac output and thus would decrease the mean arterial pressure.

E is incorrect because the decrease in the central venous pressure (preload) would decrease the stroke volume and thus the aortic pulse pressure.

2. **A** is correct because a drug that improves cardiac contractility would increase cardiac output, which would tend to increase the arterial blood volume. Hence if the total blood volume remains constant, the venous blood volume would decrease. Consequently, the central venous pressure would decline.

B is incorrect because a drug that improves cardiac contractility would increase cardiac output. Consequently, mean arterial pressure would increase.

C is incorrect because a drug that improves cardiac contractility would increase cardiac output. Consequently, the increased cardiac output would redistribute the blood volume such that the arterial volume would increase and the venous volume would decrease. Hence central venous pressure would decrease.

D is incorrect because a drug that improves cardiac contractility would, by definition, enhance the efficacy of the cardiac contractile proteins and thereby increase cardiac output.

E is incorrect because a drug that improves cardiac contractility would increase cardiac output, and would therefore decrease central venous pressure.

3. **A** is incorrect because gravity acts to pool blood in the compliant, dependent veins. Hence, the volume of blood in the central veins diminishes, and central venous pressure falls.

B is incorrect because gravity acts to pool blood in the compliant, dependent veins, and hence pressure increases in the foot veins.

C is incorrect because gravity acts to pool blood in the compliant, dependent veins; hence the central venous volume and pressure diminish. The consequent reduction in preload reduces the cardiac output and therefore the mean arterial pressure.

D is incorrect because gravity acts to pool blood in the compliant, dependent veins, and hence the pressure in the foot veins will increase.

E is correct because gravity acts to pool blood in the compliant, dependent veins; hence the pressure in the foot veins will increase. The redistribution of the venous blood volume will cause the central venous volume and pressure to diminish. The consequent reduction in preload decreases the cardiac output.

4. **A** is incorrect because when the heart rate is abnormally high (250 beats/min), the cardiac output declines substantially, and hence mean arterial pressure is diminished.

B is correct because when the heart rate is abnormally high, cardiac filling is inadequate; therefore stroke volume and cardiac output are decreased.

C is incorrect because cardiac filling is inadequate; therefore stroke volume is decreased.

D is incorrect because cardiac filling is inadequate; therefore cardiac output is decreased.

E is incorrect because cardiac filling is inadequate; therefore stroke volume is decreased. The reduction in stroke volume causes the arterial pulse pressure to decrease.

Case 25-1

1. **A** is incorrect because in severe bradycardia, blood pressure and hence coronary perfusion pressure are low, and the reduced transmural pressure might elicit a myogenic dilation but not a constriction.

B is incorrect because myocardial metabolic activity is reduced and would produce vasoconstriction.

C is incorrect because local factors predominate over neural factors. Also, there is no reason to invoke a reflex response.

D is correct because two factors operate in bradycardia. At the slower rate, more time is spent in diastole, which decreases coronary resistance (less extravascular compression). However, at the slower rate the heart uses less O_2, and fewer vasodilator metabolites are present, which permits greater expression of basal tone (coronary constriction). The result is the algebraic sum of these two opposing factors.

E is incorrect because the epicardial/endocardial blood flow rate is not significantly affected in bradycardia.

2. **A** is correct because the coronary vessels are maximally dilated as a result of the accumulation of vasodilator metabolites consequent to an inadequate O_2 supply to the myocardial cells. If any vasoconstriction occurred it would be transient.

B is incorrect because both the atrial and ventricular rate would increase.

C is incorrect because both the atrial and ventricular rate would increase.

D is incorrect because the coronary resistance vessels are already maximally dilated.

E is incorrect because the accumulated vasodilator metabolites would override a neural vasoconstrictor response.

3. **A** is incorrect because nitroglycerin is a vasodilator.
   B is correct because endothelin is a powerful vasoconstrictor.
   C is incorrect because prostacyclin is a vasodilator.
   D is incorrect because adenosine is a vasodilator.
   E is incorrect because acetylcholine is a vasodilator.

4. **A** is incorrect because a transplanted heart is denervated.
   B is incorrect because a transplanted heart is denervated.
   C is incorrect because a transplanted heart is denervated and the respiratory effect on heart rate is mediated by the cardiac nerves.
   D is incorrect because a transplanted heart is denervated and the respiratory effect on heart rate is mediated by the cardiac nerves.
   E is correct because with exercise a denervated heart increases the stroke volume more than the heart rate to meet the required cardiac output. Any increase in heart rate must come from release of epinephrine and norepinephrine from the adrenal medulla.

Case 25-2

1. **A** is correct because hepatic fibrosis increases the hepatic vascular resistance; therefore the pressure in the vessels downstream to the liver is elevated. Consequently, the balance of Starling forces in the splanchnic capillaries favors the movement of fluid out of the capillaries and into the abdominal cavity.
   B is incorrect because the hepatic artery pressure would be equal to the aortic pressure, which is not appreciably affected by cirrhosis.
   C is incorrect because the resistance vessels between the portal and hepatic vessels cause a pressure drop as blood flows from the portal to the hepatic veins.
   D is incorrect because the pressure in the splenic vein virtually equals that in the portal vein, since the splenic vein is a tributary of the portal vein. Hence the resistance vessels between the splenic and hepatic veins cause a pressure drop, as explained in **C**.
   E is incorrect because the hepatic vascular resistance was increased.

Case 26-1

1. **A** is incorrect because the active muscles were capable of using more O_2 if it were provided by the circulation.
   B is incorrect because the arterial blood was fully saturated with O_2 even at a high rate of blood flow through the lungs.
   C is incorrect because there is no reason to suspect that the splanchnic vessels and those in the inactive muscle were not constricted.
   D is correct because his heart became unable to pump enough blood per unit time as a result of a decrease in stroke volume and hence in cardiac output.
   E is incorrect because the arteriovenous O_2 difference was at maximum.

   A is correct because his body temperature reached an alarmingly high level as a result of inadequate heat loss via the skin (vasoconstriction secondary to decrease in blood

pressure) in the face of the great heat production in the active muscles.
   B is incorrect because the heart rate reached a maximum level before his collapse.
   C is incorrect because his skin blood vessels constricted in response to a fall in blood pressure.
   D is incorrect because his blood pH decreased caused by the release of lactic acid from the active muscles.
   E is incorrect because his blood pressure fell as a result of the reduction of stroke volume.

Case 26-2

1. **A** is incorrect because there are very few parasympathetic nerves to the skin and because the released acetylcholine would dilate, not constrict, the cutaneous vessels.
   B is incorrect because there are very few parasympathetic nerves to the skin; the released vasoactive intestinal peptide would dilate, not constrict, the cutaneous vessels.
   C is incorrect because there are very few parasympathetic nerves to the skin; they do not release neuropeptide Y.
   D is incorrect because the sympathetic nerves to the skin do not release much nitric oxide; the nitric oxide would dilate, not constrict, the cutaneous vessels.
   E is correct because the hypotension would act via the arterial baroreceptors to activate the sympathetic nerves to the skin. The consequent release of norepinephrine would constrict the cutaneous arterioles, and the skin temperature would drop.

2. **A** is correct because the abnormally low mean arterial pressure ($\approx$72 mm Hg) would signify an abnormally small cardiac output. The low mean arterial pressure could not have been caused by arteriolar vasodilation because the baroreceptor reflex response to such a low pressure would be vasoconstriction, not vasodilation. The low pulse pressure (20 mm Hg) would signify an abnormally small stroke volume.
   B is incorrect because over any substantial time the outputs of the two ventricles must be equal.
   C is incorrect because the small pulse pressure (20 mm Hg) denotes a small stroke volume (and there is no reason to believe that the arterial compliance is abnormally great).
   D is incorrect because blood loss would lead to reflex vasoconstriction. A normal cardiac output would lead to a higher-than-normal mean arterial pressure if generalized vasoconstriction prevailed.
   E is incorrect because over any substantial time, the output of the two ventricles must be equal.

3. **A** is incorrect because any acute change in red cell volume would most likely be produced by a change in the osmolarity of the plasma; blood loss does not acutely alter the osmolarity of the extracellular fluid (or blood plasma) substantially.
   B is correct because the decrease in capillary hydrostatic pressure draws interstitial fluid into the plasma compartment and thereby dilutes the red cell component of whole blood.
   C is incorrect because hemorrhage would have no direct effect on the leukocytes, but the dilution effect of the influx of interstitial fluid into the plasma compartment would tend to dilute the leukocyte component of whole blood.
   D is incorrect because the dilution effect of the influx of interstitial fluid into the plasma compartment would tend to diminish the concentration of albumin in the plasma.

E is incorrect because the dilution effect of the influx of interstitial fluid into the plasma compartment would tend to diminish the concentration of globulin in the plasma.

Case 27-1

1. **A** is incorrect because this patient likely has severe obstructive lung disease, probably emphysema, based on the reduced expiratory flows. Emphysema may lead to ventilation/perfusion mismatching, causing a low Pa_{O_2}. Unfortunately, this is unpredictable based on the severity of lung disease.
   B is incorrect because patients with severe emphysema may have difficulty with Pa_{CO_2} retention. In some emphysema patients, the anatomical dead space increases to the point that minute ventilation is impaired, resulting in a high Pa_{CO_2} (see Chapter 28). This is unpredictable based on the severity of lung disease.
   C is incorrect because the Pa_{CO_2} could be decreased or increased (as in **B**).
   D is incorrect because the arterial pH may be decreased when the Pa_{CO_2} levels rise acutely, as in **B**; however, this is unpredictable.
   E is correct because the effect of this patient's severe obstructive lung disease on gas exchange is unpredictable.

2. **A** is incorrect because as the lungs become hyperinflated in a patient with emphysema, the diaphragm often becomes flattened—a finding evident on chest x-ray films (see Chapter 28).
   B is correct because it is false. The maximal inspiratory pressure is a measurement of the amount of pressure a person can generate when inspiring forcefully. Because the diaphragm is the primary inspiratory muscle, the maximal inspiratory pressure reflects diaphragmatic function. In this patient, the maximal inspiratory pressure would be normal or reduced because of the disadvantageous flattening of the diaphragm that occurs with emphysema.
   C is incorrect because the flattening diaphragm muscles will not be at the optimal length-force relationship; therefore diaphragmatic movement or contractility is impaired.
   D is incorrect because the principal inspiratory muscle, even in emphysema patients, is the diaphragm.
   E is incorrect because the sternocleidomastoid and scalenus muscles can aid inspiration in the setting of respiratory failure.

Case 27-2

1. **A** is incorrect because ventilation/perfusion mismatching is a common cause of hypoxemia. In this patient, aspiration pneumonia leads to inadequate ventilation to portions of the lung, which are still being perfused (low $\dot{V}/\dot{Q}$).
   B is correct because it is unlikely that this patient had a ventricular septal defect that was unrecognized since birth. Furthermore, the lack of a cardiac murmur makes this possibility even more remote.
   C is incorrect because a diffusion abnormality in the setting of pneumonia is common as a result of alveolar filling and disruption of the alveolar-capillary interface.
   D is incorrect because hypoventilation caused by central respiratory drive depression from drugs (e.g., narcotics, alcohol) can cause hypoxemia.
   E is incorrect because the aspirated stomach contents could block a bronchus.

2. **A** is incorrect because CO_2 freely diffuses across the alveolar-capillary interface, and therefore there is no gradient.
   B is incorrect because the alveolar-arterial O_2 difference is usually between 5 and 15 mm Hg. A large difference between PA_{O_2} and Pa_{O_2} indicates a significant defect in getting O_2 from the alveoli to the pulmonary circulation.
   C is incorrect because using the alveolar gas equation for O_2 (see Equation 28-3), one can determine the alveolar-arterial O_2 gradient. If the gradient is normal, hypoventilation is the most likely cause because there is no defect in getting O_2 across the alveoli to the capillaries, such as would occur with aspiration pneumonia.
   D is correct because carbon monoxide freely diffuses across the alveolar-capillary interface, and therefore there is no gradient.
   E is incorrect because the alveolar gas equation (see Equation 28-3) requires that the clinician know the barometric pressure to determine the PA_{O_2}.

Case 28-1

1. **A** is incorrect.
   B is incorrect.
   C is incorrect.
   D is incorrect.
   E is correct because alveolar ventilation is determined by the difference between tidal volume and anatomical dead space multiplied by breathing frequency. Therefore:

   $$(600 \text{ ml} - 200 \text{ ml}) \times 30 \text{ breaths/min} =$$
   $$12{,}000 \text{ ml/min} = 12 \text{ L/min}$$

2. **A** is incorrect.
   B is correct because by the alveolar ventilation equation:

   $$\dot{V}_A \text{ (L/min)} \times Pa_{CO_2}\text{(mm Hg)} = \dot{V}_{CO_2} \text{ (ml/min)} \times K$$

   Therefore:

   $$12 \text{ L/min} \times 30 \text{ mm Hg} =$$
   $$360 \text{ ml/min} \times 0.863 = 310 \text{ ml/min.}$$

   C is incorrect.
   D is incorrect.
   E is incorrect.

3. **A** is correct because of the alveolar gas equation:

   $$PA_{O_2} = PI_{O_2} - Pa_{CO_2}\left(\frac{1 - FI_{O_2}}{R}\right)$$

   Therefore:

   $$PI_{O_2} = (PB - 47)FI_{O_2} = (760 - 47)0.21 = 149.7 \text{ mm Hg}$$

   The second half of the equation is:

   $$Pa_{CO_2}\left[FI_{O_2} + \left(\frac{1 - FI_{O_2}}{R}\right)\right] = 30\left[0.21\left(\frac{1 - 0.21}{0.8}\right)\right] = 35.9$$

   So the $PA_{O_2} = 149.7 - 35.9 = 113.8$. The A − a gradient for O_2 would then be $Pa_{O_2} - PA_{O_2} = 114 - 60 = 54$.
   B is incorrect.
   C is incorrect.
   D is incorrect.
   E is incorrect.

Case 28-2

1. **A** is incorrect.
    B is incorrect.
    C is incorrect.
    D is correct because compliance is the measurement of how much pressure is required to overcome the elastic forces of a structure (in this case, the lungs and chest wall together). It is important that this measurement be made in a patient who is not exerting effort and at the point of no airflow so that airway resistance will not affect the pressure being measured. So the compliance of the respiratory system in this patient is:

    $$\frac{100 \text{ ml}}{100 \text{ cm H}_2\text{O} - 0 \text{ cm H}_2\text{O}} = 40 \text{ ml/cm H}_2\text{O}$$

    E is incorrect.

2. **A** is incorrect.
    B is incorrect.
    C is incorrect.
    D is correct because airway resistance is equal to the change in pressure divided by airflow. The pressure difference in this situation is the difference between the pressure at the mouth (P_{ao}) and the alveolar pressure (P_{alv}). In an intubated patient the peak airway pressure during airflow is P_{ao}, and pressure during occlusion (i.e., air is not flowing) is equal to P_{alv}. Therefore:

    $$\text{Airway resistance (RAW)} = \frac{P_{ao} - P_{alv}}{\text{Flow}}$$
    $$= \frac{35 \text{ cm H}_2\text{O} - 15 \text{ cm H}_2\text{O}}{1 \text{ L/sec}}$$
    $$= 20 \text{ cm H}_2\text{O/L/sec}$$

    E is incorrect.

Case 29-1

1. **A** is incorrect because the rise in pulmonary artery pressure is transient.
    B is incorrect because the rise in pulmonary artery pressure and pulmonary vascular resistance is transient.
    C is correct because after a pneumonectomy, the pulmonary artery pressure and pulmonary vascular resistance rise in the immediate postoperative period until the remaining lung is able to recruit more pulmonary capillaries. Once the additional capillaries open, the pulmonary pressure and pulmonary vascular resistance return to normal. In the immediate postoperative period after a pneumonectomy, surgeons often use inhaled nitric oxide to selectively decrease the pulmonary artery pressure.
    D is incorrect because the patient may not be hypoxemic. This depends on the lung reserve remaining in the right lung and whether there is ventilation/perfusion mismatching, shunting, or a diffusion abnormality.
    E is incorrect because the patient may not be hypoxemic (as discussed in D) and may not be hypercarbic. The latter is determined by the adequacy of ventilation in the remaining right lung.

2. **A** is incorrect because there would be no circulation to the left side after a pneumonectomy; the pulmonary arterial circulation is removed with the lung.
    B is correct because after a pneumonectomy the remaining lung will receive twice the ventilation and perfusion, but

the V̇/Q̇ ratio will not be appreciably altered. Exercise tolerance is decreased because the remaining lung has no or little reserve for increasing alveolar ventilation with exercise.
C is incorrect because the P_{aO_2} and P_{aCO_2} levels should remain the same, given that the V̇/Q̇ ratio will not significantly change.
D is incorrect because the right lung can recruit additional capillaries; therefore the V̇/Q̇ ratio should not change.
E is incorrect because ventilation and perfusion should rise equally in the right lung.

Case 29-2

1. **A** is correct because the pulmonary vascular resistance (PVR) is calculated by dividing the transpulmonary pressure by the flow. The standard formula is:

    PVR =
    $$\frac{\text{Mean pulmonary pressure } (\overline{P}pa) - \text{Mean left atrial pressure } (\overline{P}la)}{\text{Flow } (\dot{Q})} =$$
    $$\frac{45 - 15}{3} = 10 \text{ mm Hg/L·min}$$

    because in this example, cardiac output is used in the denominator (i.e., equals flow), and the pulmonary artery occlusion pressure (PAOP) reflects the mean left atrial pressure. Clinically, the pulmonary vascular resistance is reported as dyne·sec/cm^{-5}. The numerator is multiplied by 80 to convert to dyne·sec/cm^{-5}; therefore the PVR in this case would be reported as 800 dyne·sec/cm^{-5}.
    B is incorrect.
    C is incorrect.
    D is incorrect.
    E is incorrect.

2. **A** is incorrect because nitric oxide (NO), previously known as endothelium-dependent relaxation factor, when delivered as an inhaled gas selectively vasodilates the pulmonary vasculature in acute and chronic pulmonary hypertension patients. NO binds to the heme iron in hemoglobin in the pulmonary capillary blood, which reduces its systemic vasodilator activity.
    B is incorrect because inhalation of 100% O_2 may reverse any potential hypoxia-induced vasoconstriction component of pulmonary hypertension.
    C is incorrect because Ca^{++} channel blockers, such as nifedipine, are used in large doses to dilate the pulmonary vasculature. They may lower the cardiac output because of their vasodilator effect on the peripheral circulation.
    D is incorrect because prostacyclin (available as epoprostenol) is a potent pulmonary vasodilator, although unfortunately, it must be given as a continuous intravenous infusion, since it has a short half-life in the circulation.
    E is correct because leukotriene D_4 is not a known vasodilator of the pulmonary circulation; furthermore, it is thought to cause bronchoconstriction when inhaled.

Case 30-1

1. **A** is incorrect because O_2 delivery would be affected by the binding of carbon monoxide to hemoglobin.
    B is correct because the hemoglobin-O_2 equilibrium curve would be shifted downward and to the left. Carbon monoxide displaces O_2 from hemoglobin at the alveolar-capillary level because the affinity of carbon monoxide for

hemoglobin is 200 times that of O_2. This causes a downward shift in the curve, resulting in a lower O_2 saturation for a given PaO_2. The curve is shifted to the left because of the effect of carbon monoxide and the increased pH. A leftward shift indicates more O_2 taken up by hemoglobin in the pulmonary capillaries; however, at this level, the downward shift has much more effect than the left shift. Therefore the SaO_2 is always reduced in carbon monoxide poisoning. The leftward shift is detrimental because it inhibits O_2 unloading in the systemic capillaries.

C is incorrect because O_2 unloading in the tissue is inhibited.

D is incorrect because an increase in pH would cause a leftward shift in the curve.

E is incorrect because O_2 delivery depends primarily on the O_2 bound to hemoglobin and not the PaO_2.

2. **A** is correct because the alveolar gas equation states:

$$P_{AO_2} = F_{IO_2}(P_B - P_{H_2O}) - P_{aCO_2}\left[F_{IO_2} + \frac{1 - F_{IO_2}}{R}\right]$$

The barometric pressure (P_B) minus the partial pressure of water (47) is multiplied by the inspired fraction of O_2 (in this problem = 100%). Therefore:

$$P_{AO_2} = 100\%(738 - 47) - 36\left[1 + \left(\frac{1 - 1.0}{8}\right)\right] = 691 - 36 = 655$$

The PaO_2 is 155, so the A − a gradient, or difference between alveolar and arterial O_2 pressure, is 500. This patient's PaO_2, while seemingly high at 155 mm Hg, is actually much less than expected for a high F_{IO_2}. The widened A − a gradient in this case is probably due to a parenchymal lung problem such as pulmonary edema from the smoke inhalation. Such damage results in ventilation/perfusion mismatching and diffusion abnormality.

B is incorrect as proved by the alveolar gas equation.

C is incorrect as proved by the alveolar gas equation.

D is incorrect as proved by the alveolar gas equation.

E is incorrect as proved by the alveolar gas equation.

Case 30-2

1. **A** through **C** and **E** are incorrect according to the arterial content equation.
D is correct because the arterial blood O_2 content (CaO_2) is markedly reduced in this patient as a result of the chronic anemia. The arterial O_2 content is equal to the amount of O_2 bound to Hb plus the dissolved O_2:

$$CaO_2 = (SaO_2 \times Hb\ [g/dl] \times 1.34\ ml\ O_2/g\ Hb) +$$
$$(0.003\ mg\ O_2/mm\ Hg\ PaO_2/dl \times PaO_2)$$

Therefore:

$$CaO_2 = (92\% \times 7.0\ g/dl \times 1.34) + (0.003 \times 60)$$
$$= 8.6\ ml\ O_2/dl + 0.18\ ml\ O_2$$
$$= 8.8\ ml\ O_2/dl\ or\ 88\ ml/L$$

2. **A** is correct based on the Fick equation. O_2 consumption can be directly measured by analyzing inspired and expired gases or by using the Fick equation:

$$\dot{V}O_2 = \dot{Q}(CaO_2 - C\bar{v}O_2)$$

where $\dot{Q}$ is the cardiac output (L/min) and CaO_2 and $C\bar{v}O_2$ are the O_2 content of arterial and mixed venous blood, respectively. Because CaO_2 was calculated previously, only the $C\bar{v}O_2$ must be calculated:

$$C\bar{v}O_2 = (S\bar{v}O_2 \times Hb\ [g/dL] \times 1.34\ ml\ O_2/g\ Hb) +$$
$$(0.003\ ml\ O_2/mm\ Hg\ P\bar{v}O_2/dl \times P\bar{v}O_2)$$

Therefore:

$$C\bar{v}O_2 = (73\% \times 7.0\ mg/dl \times 1.34) + (0.003 \times 40) =$$
$$6.85\ ml\ O_2/dl + 0.12\ ml\ O_2 = 6.97\ ml\ O_2/dl = 70\ ml/L$$

Thus $\dot{V}O_2 = 8(88 - 70) = 144\ ml/min$.

B is incorrect according to the equation in **A**.

C is incorrect according to the equation in **A**.

D is incorrect according to the equation in **A**.

E is incorrect according to the equation in **A**.

3. **A** is correct because an increase in the hemoglobin level from 7 to 10 g/dl provides a 43% increase in hemoglobin-bound O_2 content, thereby directly increasing O_2 delivery.

B is incorrect because an increase in the cardiac output will have no effect on arterial O_2 content but will increase O_2 delivery by only 20%.

C is incorrect because an increase in O_2 concentration by 20% will increase the PaO_2 and SaO_2 by only a small amount.

D is incorrect because increasing venous return to the heart will not appreciably affect oxygenation.

E is incorrect because the use of antibiotics will not affect O_2 delivery.

Case 31-1

1. **A** is incorrect because this transection level is below the brainstem. Therefore the only innervation that would be interrupted would be the phrenic nerve. Transection at the level of the middle pons with the vagus nerves intact would only moderately slow the breathing frequency.

B is incorrect because the transection level is below the brainstem.

C is incorrect because the transection level is below the brainstem; also, one would expect the reticular activating system to be intact.

D is correct because the phrenic nerve arises from C3-5— below the level of the lesion in this case.

E is incorrect because the dorsal respiratory group is in the medulla, above the lesion at C2.

2. **A** is correct because apneic episodes would occur only with damage or destruction of the reticular activating system in the brainstem.

B is incorrect because a decreased tidal volume would occur with a C2 lesion and cause loss of innervation to the diaphragm via the phrenic nerve.

C is incorrect because mild hypercapnia and hypoxemia could occur with loss of diaphragmatic function. Mild hypercapnia would result from decreased alveolar ventilation. Mild hypoxemia could occur with atelectasis (collapse of alveoli) in parts of the lung that are not adequately ventilated, and result in ventilation/perfusion mismatching (see Chapter 30).

D is incorrect because diaphragmatic movement would be decreased with loss of innervation via the phrenic nerve.

E is incorrect because a decreased maximal inspiratory pressure is a test of inspiratory muscle strength. Because the diaphragm is paralyzed, one would expect reduced inspiratory pressures (usually more negative than −20 cm H_2O).

Case 31-2

1. **A** is incorrect because the clinician would suspect that this patient has obstructive sleep apnea and therefore would expect that periods of absent airflow could occur and be associated with O_2 desaturation.

    B is incorrect because the clinician would expect the presence of abdominal and chest wall movement in the setting of obstructive apnea as the body attempts to overcome the obstruction of the upper airway.

    C is correct because the clinician would *not* expect abdominal and chest wall movement to be absent. This finding is characteristic of central sleep apnea and can be associated with arousals.

    D is incorrect because the clinician would expect airflow to be decreased with obstructive sleep apnea, which could result in O_2 desaturation.

    E is incorrect because the clinician would expect airflow and movement of the abdominal and chest wall to be decreased with obstructive sleep apnea.

2. **A** is incorrect because there is evidence of worsening dead space gas exchange (see Chapter 28), given that the Pa_{CO_2} increased (decreased alveolar ventilation).

    B is incorrect because increased levels of CO_2 are reflected by an upward shift of the O_2 ventilatory response curve (see Figure 31-7).

    C is incorrect because increased levels of O_2 will not stimulate the peripheral chemoreceptors.

    D is incorrect because the development of an acidosis would be reflected by a leftward shift of the CO_2 ventilatory response curve and an increase in sensitivity to CO_2.

    E is correct because the increased levels of O_2 administered would be reflected by a rightward shift of the CO_2 ventilatory response curve and a decreased sensitivity to CO_2. This explains the worsening hypercapnia and the sleepiness in this patient (CO_2 narcosis).

Case 32-1

1. **A** is incorrect because the normal resting pressure in the LES is about 25 mm Hg.

    B is correct because the pressure in the relaxed normal LES is close to zero.

    C is incorrect because the LES fails to relax on swallowing; therefore the pressure increase caused by contraction of the upper esophagus is immediately transmitted along the entire length of the esophagus.

    D is incorrect because the failure of the LES to relax appropriately while the patient swallows can explain the failure to clear barium at a normal rate.

    E is incorrect because **B** is the correct answer.

2. **A** is incorrect because the response to amyl nitrate does not rule out hypertrophy of the LES.

    B is incorrect because the innervation of the LES is not properly signaling the LES to relax.

    C is correct because achalasia is the most likely cause of her disorder.

    D is incorrect because diffuse esophageal spasm would not be characterized by elevated pressures in the LES.

    E is incorrect because **C** is the correct answer.

    A is incorrect because dilation tears smooth muscle cells in the LES; once they heal, the problems with swallowing are ~ly to occur.

B is incorrect because a Ca^{++} channel blocker ingested just before a meal may alleviate the symptoms.

C is correct because a common treatment for this disorder is to incise the full depth of the LES musculature, thereby permanently weakening the LES.

D is incorrect because another dilation would likely have an effect similar to the first one.

E is incorrect because **C** is the correct answer.

Case 32-2

1. **A** is incorrect because the normal reflex relaxation is absent in a significant number of normal infants.

    B is incorrect because the next step should be a suction mucosal biopsy, since it does not require anesthesia.

    C is incorrect because the absence of ganglion cells in the submucous plexus and the presence of enlarged nerve trunks in the mucosa would help confirm the diagnosis.

    D is correct because this would reveal a lack of ganglion cells in the submucosal plexus and the presence of enlarged nerve fibers in the submucosa of the affected segment of colon.

    E is incorrect because **D** is the correct answer.

2. **A** is incorrect because although the disease is clearly familial, the risk among siblings is only 5% to 10% and is independent of gender.

    B is incorrect because the disorder will not improve with age.

    C is incorrect because there is currently no effective pharmacological therapy.

    D is correct because removal of the affected segment of colon is the only effective therapy.

    E is incorrect because **D** is the correct answer.

3. **A** is incorrect because this would possibly cause subsequent rupture of this segment.

    B is incorrect because only the aganglionic portion of the colon should be removed.

    C is incorrect because in almost all cases an anastomosis of unaffected colon to the rectum just proximal to the anal sphincter is effective.

    D is correct because there is no reason to remove normal colon.

    E is incorrect because **D** is the correct answer.

Case 33-1

1. **A** is correct because HCl and gastrin are both effective secretagogues for pepsinogens.

    B is correct because the duodenal mucosa is poorly protected against acid and pepsin.

    C is correct because pancreatic lipase is inactivated at a low pH, leading to steatorrhea.

    D is correct because the actions of gastrin, both on parietal cells and on ECL cells, are potentiated by acetylcholine.

    E is correct because **A** through **D** are all correct.

2. **A** is incorrect because hyposecretors of HCl also have elevated gastrin levels because of lack of feedback inhibition of H^+ on gastrin secretion.

    B is incorrect because if the diagnosis is correct, the patient has an ectopic gastrin-secreting tumor that will not respond to amino acids and peptides in the stomach and duodenum.

C is correct because gastrin is trophic and increases the number of oxyntic glands and the number of parietal cells in the glands.

D is incorrect because high rates of HCl secretion are very rarely associated with gastric ulcers.

E is incorrect because **C** is the correct answer.

3. **A** is incorrect because many ectopic gastrinomas are malignant; therefore it is important to find the tumor and excise it.

B is incorrect because H$_2$-receptor blockers will reduce HCl secretion but not to the same extent as in a normal individual.

C is incorrect because sectioning these vagal branches would substantially diminish HCl secretion.

D is correct because omeprazole directly inhibits H$^+$,K$^+$-ATPase; it will strongly suppress HCl secretion, even in the presence of elevated gastrin levels.

E is incorrect because **D** is the correct answer.

Case 33-2

1. **A** is correct because 70% of gallstones in the United States are cholesterol stones.

B is correct because when gallstones contain calcium salts, they are radiopaque.

C is correct because ultrasonography is effective at detecting gallstones.

D is correct because calcified stones are not very effectively disrupted by lithotripsy.

E is correct because **A** through **D** are all correct.

2. **A** is correct because when cholesterol secretion into bile is high, relative to the amounts of bile acids and phospholipids in bile, cholesterol gallstones tend to form.

B is incorrect because hypomotility of the gallbladder frequently contributes to gallstone formation.

C is incorrect because mucus secretion enhances gallstone formation.

D is incorrect because nonsteroidal antiinflammatory drugs depress mucus secretion by the gallbladder and thereby decrease the likelihood of gallstone formation.

E is incorrect because **A** is correct.

3. **A** is incorrect because treatment with these bile acids would tend to dissolve cholesterol gallstones but would take many months or years of treatment to dissolve stones 5 to 10 mm in diameter.

B is incorrect because this patient is a good candidate for lithotripsy based on the size of the gallstones and their lack of calcification.

C is incorrect because treatment with an inhibitor of HMG-CoA reductase would diminish the rate of cholesterol secretion into bile; in combination with other therapies, this would be useful.

D is incorrect because gallstones recur in about 50% of patients who have previously been cleared of them.

E is correct because **A** through **D** are incorrect.

Case 34-1

1. **A** is incorrect because the absorption of neutral amino acids from dipeptides and tripeptides is usually adequate to maintain good nutrition.

B is correct because even though dietary niacin is over the minimum daily requirement, the patient is missing some of the large fraction of niacin synthesized from tryptophan. Because 60 mg of tryptophan are required to produce 1 mg of niacin, the patient requires doses of niacin much greater than the minimum daily requirement.

C is incorrect because as a result of the absorption of neutral amino acids in dipeptides and tripeptides, plasma levels of the neutral amino acids will not be markedly reduced.

D is incorrect because high urinary levels of most neutral amino acids are the hallmark of Hartnup's disease.

E is incorrect because **B** is the correct response.

2. **A** is correct because a diet richer in protein would improve the patient's protein nutrition and by providing more tryptophan, help remedy the niacin deficit.

B is correct because the renal and intestinal transporter responsible for absorbing most of the neutral amino acids in the jejunum is defective in Hartnup's disease.

C is correct because the disorder is recessive, so both parents are most likely carriers.

D is correct because pellagra is, strictly speaking, a disease caused by a dietary deficiency of niacin. The patient is deficient in niacin but has a niacin intake in excess of the minimum daily requirement.

E is correct because **A** through **D** are all correct.

3. **A** is incorrect because the amino acid transporter that transports these amino acids across the brush border membrane of the jejunum and proximal renal tubule is deficient.

B is incorrect because glycine, methionine, and cysteine are reabsorbed from the renal proximal tubule by other transporters that are not defective in Hartnup's disease (see Chapter 35).

C is correct because Hartnup's disease is quite rare. It is most likely that both parents are carriers.

D is incorrect because the patient's ability to absorb dipeptides and tripeptides is not deficient.

E is incorrect because **C** is the correct response.

Case 34-2

1. **A** is incorrect because pancreatic insufficiency is quite common in cystic fibrosis.

B is incorrect because cystic fibrosis is the most common autosomal recessive disorder, occurring in about 1 in 2000 live births.

C is incorrect because the baby is as likely to be deficient in pancreatic proteases as lipases.

D is incorrect because a low-fat diet would exacerbate the baby's malnutrition.

E is correct because **A** through **D** are all incorrect.

2. **A** is correct because this will improve the digestion of fats, carbohydrates, and proteins.

B is correct because decreased gastric acid secretion will decrease acid inactivation of pancreatic enzymes, since the baby will have decreased bicarbonate from pancreatic juice.

C is correct because the absorption of fat-soluble vitamins is likely to be deficient.

D is correct because medium-chain triglycerides will be more completely digested and absorbed than long-chain triglycerides.

E is correct because **A** through **D** are all correct.

3.   **A** is incorrect because as a result of the destruction and fibrosis of pancreatic tissue, as the child develops, there is an increased likelihood that islets of Langerhans will be destroyed and diabetes mellitus will ensue.

B is incorrect because there is no deficiency of brush border enzymes associated with cystic fibrosis.

C is correct because ongoing destruction of acinar cells will release trypsinogen. In later life, when the exocrine pancreas is essentially gone, serum trypsinogen levels may be below normal.

D is incorrect because as a result of protein malnutrition, the baby may have decreased levels of plasma proteins.

E is incorrect because **C** is the correct response.

Case 35-1

1.   **A** is incorrect because the serum creatinine concentration does not depend on changes in the RBF.

B is incorrect because the serum creatinine concentration does not depend on urine output.

C is incorrect because creatinine metabolism rarely changes except in exceptional circumstances.

D is correct because the serum creatinine concentration is inversely related to GFR.

E is incorrect because the serum creatinine concentration is not related to blood volume.

2.   **A** is incorrect because nonsteroid antiinflammatory drugs such as prostaglandin cause vasodilation and thereby increase RBF. Thus reduced renal prostaglandin levels would allow sympathetic nerves to go unopposed, induce renal vasoconstriction, and decrease the RBF.

B is correct because decreased prostaglandin levels would cause constriction of the afferent and efferent arterioles, which would reduce the GFR.

C is incorrect because decreased prostaglandin levels would reduce the GFR and urine output.

D is incorrect because a decrease in prostaglandin levels would not affect protein excretion, since prostaglandins do not have any effect on the amount of protein in the ultrafiltrate or on protein absorption by the proximal tubule.

E is incorrect because prostaglandins have no effect on creatinine excretion in the steady state.

Case 35-2

1.   **A** is incorrect because the filtration rate of Na^+ is not affected by the integrity of the filtration barrier (i.e., it is filtered freely) and the amount of Na^+ in the urine is determined by its rates of reabsorption along the nephron.

B is incorrect because the filtration rate of K^+ is not affected by the integrity of the filtration barrier (i.e., Na^+ is filtered freely) and the amount of K^+ in the urine is determined by the rates of K^+ secretion and reabsorption along the nephron.

C is correct because serum albumin is not normally found in the urine. However, when the glomerular filtration barrier is damaged, the amount of albumin filtered increases and overwhelms the ability of the proximal tubule to resorb albumin. Thus albumin appears in the urine.

D is incorrect because the filtration rate of creatinine is not affected by the integrity of the filtration barrier (i.e., creatinine is filtered freely) and the amount of creatinine in the urine is determined by the rate of creatinine reabsorption along the nephron.

E is incorrect because the filtration rate of urea is not affected by the integrity of the filtration barrier (i.e., urea is filtered freely) and the amount of urea in the urine is determined by the rate of urea reabsorption and secretion along the nephron.

Case 36-1

1.   **A** is incorrect because damage to the glomerulus would not increase the excretion of organic molecules (except protein). Glucose and amino acids are normally filtered freely across the glomerulus and reabsorbed by the nephron.

B is correct because the proximal tubule is the portion of the nephron responsible for reabsorbing the organic molecules entering the tubular fluid via glomerular filtration.

C is incorrect because damage to the thick ascending limb of the loop of Henle would not result in the increased excretion of organic molecules, since they are reabsorbed by the proximal tubule.

D is incorrect because damage to the distal tubule would not result in the increased excretion of organic molecules. They are reabsorbed by the proximal tubule.

E is incorrect because damage to the collecting duct would not result in the increased excretion of organic molecules. They are reabsorbed by the proximal tubule.

2.   **A** is correct because a decrease in the ECF volume will activate the renin-angiotensin-aldosterone system (see Chapter 37). Aldosterone will act on the collecting duct to increase the reabsorption of Na^+, the appropriate adaptive response (i.e., increase renal Na^+ reabsorption).

B is incorrect because ANP is secreted in response to an increase in the ECF. Also, ANP inhibits Na^+ reabsorption by the collecting duct.

C is incorrect because urodilatin is produced by the kidneys in response to an increase in ECF volume. Also, urodilatin inhibits Na^+ reabsorption by the collecting duct.

D is incorrect because dopamine is released in response to an increase in the ECF. Also, dopamine inhibits Na^+ reabsorption by the proximal tubule.

E is incorrect because hydrostatic pressure in the peritubular capillaries will be decreased in the setting of reduced ECF volume.

Case 36-2

1.   **A** is incorrect because the glomerulus is not a site of action of diuretics. Diuretics inhibit the specific membrane transport proteins along the nephron.

B is incorrect because the large increase in fractional excretion of Na^+ seen in this case is not typical for diuretic agents acting on the proximal tubule. In addition, increased excretion of organic molecules would also be seen if the diuretic acted on the proximal tubule.

C is correct because the pattern of excretion, especially the large increase in fractional excretion of Na^+, is exactly what is expected for a diuretic acting on the thick ascending limb of the loop of Henle.

D is incorrect because diuretics that act on the distal tubule will not cause the large increase in the fractional excretion of Na^+ seen with this agent. The distal tubule reabsorbs only about 7% of the filtered load of Na^+.

E is incorrect because diuretics that act on the collecting duct will not cause the large increase in the fractional excretion of Na^+ seen with this agent. The collecting duct reabsorbs a low percentage of the filtered load of Na^+.

2. **A** is incorrect because the Na$^+$-glucose symporter is found in the proximal tubule and because no glucose was found in the urine.

B is incorrect because inhibition of the Na$^+$-H$^+$ antiporter would likely be seen with diuretics affecting the proximal tubule. Also, inhibition of this transporter would result in the excretion of large amounts of HCO$_3^-$.

C is correct because the 1Na$^+$-1K$^+$-2Cl$^-$ symporter is responsible for NaCl reabsorption in the thick ascending limb of the loop of Henle, this diuretic's site of action.

D is incorrect because the Na$^+$-Cl$^-$ symporter is localized to the distal tubule.

E is incorrect because the Na$^+$ channel is localized to the collecting duct.

Case 37-1

1. **A** is incorrect because changes in Na$^+$ balance usually result in changes in the volume of the ECF, not the [Na$^+$]. Hyponatremia indicates a problem with water balance, not Na$^+$ balance.

B is incorrect because as noted, this man has a problem with water balance, not Na$^+$ balance.

C is correct because hyponatremia indicates a problem in water balance. In this case the amount of water excreted by the kidneys is less than the amount of water ingested. Also, this man's kidneys are producing concentrated urine, a finding that indicates that ADH levels are elevated. This in turn prevents the kidneys from excreting water. The elevated level of ADH is unexpected because his body fluid osmolality is reduced (2 × [Na$^+$] = 260 mOsm/kg H$_2$O), and his ECF volume appears to be normal. Therefore he must have inappropriate secretion of ADH, probably caused by the infection in his lungs.

D is incorrect because a shift of water from the ICF to the ECF could cause the [Na$^+$] to decrease. However, this man has developed hyponatremia as a result of a positive water balance. Therefore the ECF becomes diluted, which causes water to move from the ECF into the ICF.

E is incorrect because the distribution of Na$^+$ between the ICF and ECF is maintained by Na$^+$,K$^+$-ATPase. Because the activity of this enzyme is not altered in this case, a shift of Na$^+$ from the ECF to ICF is not expected.

2. **A** is incorrect because this man's ADH level is already elevated, causing the reduced excretion of water. The administration of ADH would only make this situation worse.

B is correct because this is a case of positive water balance, in which the ability of the kidneys to excrete water is impaired as a result of inappropriately elevated levels of ADH. To reestablish water balance, this patient's water intake must be reduced.

C is incorrect because as noted, water intake needs to be restricted. Increased water intake would make the hyponatremia worse.

D is incorrect because the man is in Na$^+$ balance. Therefore altering his NaCl intake would be inappropriate.

E is incorrect because as noted, this man is in Na$^+$ balance, and altering NaCl intake would be inappropriate.

Case 37-2

1. **A** is correct because this woman is in positive Na$^+$ balance (presence of edema) and positive water balance (presence of hyponatremia). As a result of her heart failure, her volume sensors are sending signals to the kidneys to reduce both NaCl and water excretion. Therefore her intake of NaCl and water must be restricted to match the reduced excretory capacity of the kidneys.

B is incorrect because while restriction of NaCl intake would be beneficial in treating her ECF volume expansion, increasing her water intake will intensify the hyponatremia.

C is incorrect because although restriction of water intake would be beneficial in treating the hyponatremia, increasing her NaCl intake would further increase the volume of the ECF and make the edema worse.

D is incorrect because as noted, NaCl and water intake must be restricted, not increased.

E is incorrect because this woman is in positive Na$^+$ and water balance as a result of reduced excretion of NaCl and water by her kidneys. Reestablishing balance would require that her current levels of NaCl and water ingestion be reduced.

2. **A** is incorrect.

B is incorrect.

C is incorrect.

D is correct because the ACE inhibitor blocks the conversion of angiotensin I to angiotensin II. As a result, angiotensin II levels drop. Because angiotensin II inhibits renin secretion (negative feedback), renin levels increase after the administration of the ACE inhibitor. Also, ACE breaks down bradykinin, a potent vasodilator. After administration of ACE inhibitor, bradykinin levels increase.

E is incorrect.

Case 38-1

1. **A** is incorrect because frequent urination (i.e., an increase in urine flow rate) would tend to increase urinary K$^+$ excretion and cause hypokalemia.

B is incorrect because ketoacidosis would have no effect on plasma K$^+$. Ketoacids do not cause K$^+$ to shift into cells.

C is correct because increased plasma glucose levels would increase plasma osmolality. An increase in plasma osmolality causes K$^+$ to leave cells and thereby increase the plasma [K$^+$].

D is incorrect because the presence of glucose and ketones in the urine has no effect on the plasma [K$^+$].

E is incorrect because the patient does not have metabolic alkalosis.

2. **A** is correct because insulin promotes K$^+$ uptake into cells.

B is incorrect because although insulin corrects the ketoacidosis, K$^+$ will not enter cells in exchange for H$^+$ as the ketoacidosis is corrected. Ketoacids are organic acids, and they do not cause K$^+$ to be exchanged for H$^+$ across cell membranes.

C is incorrect because although insulin reduces the polyuria, a reduction in urine flow in this setting has little effect on the amount of K$^+$ excreted in the urine or the plasma [K$^+$].

D is incorrect because insulin stimulates glucose uptake by cells, lowers plasma osmolality, and thereby causes K$^+$ to enter cells.

E is incorrect because insulin stimulates Na$^+$,K$^+$-ATPase and thereby stimulates K$^+$ uptake into cells.

Case 38-2

1. **A** is correct because you would expect to see an increase in the serum $[Ca^{++}]$ and a decrease in the serum [Pi] as a result of an elevation of PTH.
    B is incorrect.
    C is incorrect.
    D is incorrect.
    E is incorrect.

2. **A** is incorrect.
    B is incorrect.
    C is incorrect.
    D is correct because PTH stimulates Ca^{++} reabsorption only in the distal tubule.
    E is incorrect.

3. **A** is incorrect.
    B is correct because PTH decreases Pi reabsorption only in the proximal tubule.
    C is incorrect.
    D is incorrect.
    E is incorrect.

Case 39-1

1. **A** is correct because this is a case of diabetic ketoacidosis as a result of the lack of insulin. The blood gases show that the patient has metabolic acidosis with appropriate respiratory compensation secondary to the generation and accumulation of ketoacids that occur when insulin levels are not adequate.
    B is incorrect because the patient is acidotic not alkalotic.
    C is incorrect because with respiratory acidosis the PCO_2 is increased. The laboratory data show a decreased PCO_2 consistent with respiratory compensation for metabolic acidosis.
    D is incorrect because the patient is acidotic not alkalotic.
    E is incorrect because although a mixed disorder consisting of metabolic acidosis and respiratory alkalosis would have decreased the $[HCO_3^-]$ and PCO_2, the history and laboratory values are more consistent with simple metabolic acidosis with appropriate respiratory compensation (see Figure 39-5).

2. **A** is incorrect because although an increase in the PCO_2 will also increase the ventilation rate, this man's PCO_2 is reduced.
    B is incorrect because hypoxemia also stimulates ventilation; however, the man has a normal PO_2.
    C is correct because the normal respiratory response to metabolic acidosis is an increase in the ventilation rate (i.e., rapid and deep breathing) to reduce the PCO_2. This respiratory compensation is mediated by the respiratory center's response to the acidosis.
    D is incorrect because although this man reports having the "flu," there is no evidence that he has a lung infection. If he did have an infection that impaired gas exchange, he would probably have hypoxemia.
    E is incorrect because aspirin can stimulate the respiratory centers, but only at doses exceeding the two tablets that he reported he took for the headache. Moreover, an aspirin overdose would more likely present as a mixed acid-base disorder.

3. **A** is incorrect because the decrease in plasma $[HCO_3^-]$ caused by the ketoacidosis decreases the filtered load of HCO_3^- in this case.
    B is incorrect because the secretion of H^+ by the proximal tubule is increased, not decreased, in this situation because of the systemic acidosis.
    C is correct because the renal system compensates for metabolic acidosis by increasing the excretion of net acid. This occurs primarily through the production and excretion of NH_4^+. Moreover, the expression and activity of the proximal tubule enzymes responsible for glutamine metabolism are increased by acidosis.
    D is incorrect because H^+ secretion by the collecting duct is increased in this situation because of the systemic acidosis.
    E is incorrect because the secretion of HCO_3^- by the collecting duct is stimulated in alkalosis but not acidosis.

Case 39-2

1. **A** is incorrect because the patient is alkalotic not acidotic.
    B is correct because the loss of gastric contents from vomiting and nasogastric suction has resulted in the development of metabolic alkalosis. The results of tests of arterial blood gases also confirm the presence of metabolic alkalosis.
    C is incorrect because the patient is alkalotic, not acidotic.
    D is incorrect because with respiratory alkalosis the PCO_2 is decreased. The laboratory data show an increased PCO_2 consistent with respiratory compensation for metabolic alkalosis.
    E is incorrect because a mixed disorder consisting of metabolic alkalosis and respiratory acidosis would have increased the $[HCO_3^-]$ and PCO_2. The history and laboratory values are more consistent with a simple metabolic alkalosis with appropriate respiratory compensation (see Figure 39-5).

2. **A** is correct because the loss of gastric fluid has resulted in volume depletion. As a result, the kidneys are conserving Na^+. An important mediator for this response is the renin-angiotensin-aldosterone system (see Chapter 37). Because Na^+ reabsorption in the proximal tubule is coupled to the secretion of H^+ and because Na^+ reabsorption is enhanced, all of the filtered load of HCO_3^- is reabsorbed. The elevated levels of aldosterone stimulate not only collecting duct Na^+ reabsorption but also intercalated cell H^+ secretion. As a result, HCO_3^- excretion is reduced, collecting duct H^+ secretion is stimulated, and the urine pH is acidic. This occurs despite the presence of metabolic alkalosis.
    B is incorrect because as just described, H^+ secretion by the proximal tubule is enhanced as a result of this nephron segment's need to increase its reabsorption of Na^+.
    C is incorrect because although the plasma $[HCO_3^-]$ is increased, the glomerular filtration rate is reduced because of the volume depletion. Therefore the filtered load of HCO_3^- is probably decreased, not increased. Moreover, an increase in the filtered load of HCO_3^- would result in a more alkaline urine, not the acidic urine seen in this woman.
    D is incorrect because NH_4^+ production and excretion would be reduced secondary to the metabolic alkalosis.
    E is incorrect because the most abundant urinary buffer is phosphate. Because phosphate is reabsorbed in the proximal tubule with Na^+ (see Chapter 38), less will be excreted in the setting of volume depletion.

Case 40-1

1. **A** is incorrect because a mutant receptor with a reduced affinity for hormone X or a decreased concentration of receptors for the hormone could be overcome by increasing the concentration of the hormone, as was the case in this patient. [XR], which initially determines the biological effect, can be increased by increasing [X] to overcome a decrease either in K or in [R] (see Equation 39-5).

    B is incorrect because of the same reasons as **A**.

    C is incorrect because an excess of a competitive antagonist (A) (e.g., another hormone that cross-reacts with the same receptor to bind to the receptor but not generate a signal) can be overcome by increasing the concentration of hormone X. This would lead to more [HR] and less inactive [AR].

    D is correct because if the patient's problem was inability to transduce the primary signal of hormone X because its second messenger could not be generated as a result of a severe lack of the necessary enzyme, then no amount of hormone X could be expected to elicit a normal response. The patient would be resistant to the hormone with a decrease in maximal responsiveness.

    E is incorrect because if a mutant hormone X were altered in structure so that it could bind to the receptor but not generate a signal, then it would act like a competitive antagonist as in **C**.

    NOTE: In **A** through **C** and **E**, the patient would be insulin resistant because of decreased sensitivity to hormone X. In all the answers, the lack of normal hormone effect would generate negative feedback on the gland of origin and thus increase the secretion of and plasma levels of hormone X (as measured by immunoassay).

2. **A** is incorrect because the patient would need all the hormone X that he or she could possibly secrete to bind to a mutant receptor with decreased affinity for the hormone, so an inhibitor of secretion would be counterproductive.

    B is incorrect because when there is a deficiency of the receptor, a higher hormone concentration would increase the concentration of the hormone-receptor complex.

    C is incorrect because the effect of a competitive antagonist could be overcome by more hormone.

    D is incorrect because less hormone would only magnify the problem of generating too little second messenger.

    E is correct because reduction of the level of mutant hormone X would allow greater access of genuine hormone X to its receptor binding sites and thus decrease the dose of hormone X that would be needed for therapy.

Case 41-1

1. **A** is correct because the avid hepatic uptake and conversion to glucose of this important gluconeogenic amino acid would exceed its release from protein stores.

    B is incorrect because urine nitrogen levels would increase in the first 2 or 3 days, reflecting an increased protein breakdown. However, after a further 10 to 12 days, metabolic adaptation to prolonged fasting would decrease protein breakdown to conserve body structure and function, and urine nitrogen would decline to a constant low level.

    C is incorrect because markedly increased lipolysis of stored triglycerides would raise plasma FFA levels.

    D is incorrect because markedly increased β-oxidation of FFAs would raise plasma ketoacid levels.

    E is incorrect because plasma glucose level would be decreased. This would occur because the brain continues to use glucose despite the lack of exogenous carbohydrate and because the increase in hepatic production of glucose does not initially quite keep up with the substrate's use.

2. **A** is incorrect because 2550 g would require that he had expended a normal total of 2300 calories/day; however, he cannot move, so this is highly unlikely.

    B is incorrect because 1550 g would require that his basal metabolic rate had remained at a constant 1400 calories/day for the whole time.

    C is correct because in a resting state, the metabolic rate would be about 20 cal/kg body weight, or 1400 calories/day. After about 3 days of fasting and a lower body temperature, the BMR would decline. Assuming a decrease in the BMR of about 10% to 1260 calories, (3 × 1400) + (7 × 1260) = 13,020 calories expended in the 10 days of fasting. At 9 calories/g, this would be provided by 1450 g of fat.

    D is incorrect because this caloric value of 4 calories/g for carbohydrate was used in the final step of the calculation performed in **C**.

    E is incorrect both because the caloric value of 4 calories/g was used in the final step in the calculation and the value of 2300 calories/day was used as in **A**.

Case 41-2

1. **A** is incorrect because neuropeptide Y stimulates eating. An inactive mutant would cause decreased appetite, not obesity.

    B is correct because an inactive mutant β-adrenergic receptor would prevent normal sympathetic nervous stimulation of obligatory thermogenesis in adipose tissue, thus preventing increased energy expenditure when even occasional ingestion of excess calories occurred. This could lead to obesity.

    C is incorrect because an overactive leptin receptor would falsely report the presence of an excess of adipose tissue. This would stimulate downstream mechanisms to reduce adipose tissue, not increase it.

    D is incorrect because overactivity of UCP would increase thermogenesis and decrease adipose tissue mass.

    E is incorrect because lipoprotein lipase is required to transfer FFA from circulating triglycerides into adipose tissue for reesterification with glycerol and storage. An inactive form of the enzyme would decrease fat storage.

2. **A** is incorrect because theoretically a single abnormal set point for appetite would have made weight loss more difficult and such an abnormality could have been compensated for at least partially by an increase in energy expenditure for thermogenesis.

    B is incorrect because leptin secretion stimulated by a lower-than-normal adipose mass should cause lower-than-normal body weight, not obesity.

    C is incorrect because theoretically a single abnormal set point for energy expenditure could have been compensated for at least partially by a decrease in appetite.

    D is incorrect because if UCP production was stimulated at a lower-than-normal adipose mass, this should cause a lower-than-normal body weight, not obesity.

    E is correct because her return after weight loss to about her original weight suggests an abnormal set point for energy stores (i.e., adipose tissue mass).

Case 42-1

1.   **A** is incorrect because though her dietary protein intake is reduced, her endogenous protein breakdown is excessive as a result of the lack of insulin's inhibitory action on proteolysis. The carbon skeletons of the excess amino acids are used for accelerated gluconeogenesis, and the amino groups are incorporated into urea and excreted in urine.
     B is incorrect because plasma glucagon levels will be high in the absence of insulin's inhibitory action on glucagon secretion.
     C and **E** are incorrect because both FFA and acetoacetate levels will be high as a result of the loss of insulin's inhibitory action on lipolysis and ketogenesis and as a result of elevated glucagon levels.
     D is correct because the patient is almost certainly in diabetic ketoacidosis caused by insulin deficiency. To compensate for this metabolic acidosis, she is hyperventilating to excrete the extra CO_2 generated from $NaHCO_3$, which is used to buffer the large amounts of strong ketoacids produced by the liver. Therefore the P_{CO_2} will be reduced.

2.   **A** is incorrect because lipoprotein lipase activity will decrease, enhancing clearance of VLDL triglycerides from the plasma.
     B is incorrect because insulin will cause K^+ to move back into cells.
     C is correct because lipoprotein lipase activity is stimulated by insulin. Therefore plasma triglyceride levels will decrease, making **A** incorrect.
     D is incorrect because the restoration of insulin will decrease adipose tissue lipase activity, in part by decreasing cyclic AMP levels in that tissue.
     E is incorrect because insulin promotes phosphate uptake by cells. It also promotes glucose uptake.

Case 42-2

1.   **A** is incorrect because this insulin/glucagon state will not promote lipolysis in adipose tissue and gluconeogenesis in the liver as efficiently as the state in **D.**
     B is incorrect for the same reason as **A.**
     C is incorrect for the same reason as **A.**
     D is correct because to support prolonged aerobic exercise, this woman needed to mobilize endogenous substrates (i.e., free fatty acids, glucose) at maximum rates. This required a decrease in insulin levels and an increase in glucagon concentrations to promote lipolysis in adipose tissue and gluconeogenesis in the liver, respectively.
     E is incorrect for the same reason as **A.**

2.   **A** is incorrect because the formation of fructose-6-phosphate (gluconeogenesis) would be favored over that of fructose 1,6 biphosphate (glycolysis).
     B is incorrect because the activity of this key enzyme of gluconeogenesis would be increased.
     C is correct because when insulin levels are deficient and glucagon levels excessive, the formation of fructose 2,6-biphosphate is decreased. This favors the activity of fructose 1,6-biphosphatase over that of 6-phosphofructokinase so that gluconeogenesis predominates over glycolysis.
     D is incorrect because glucose-6-phosphatase activity would be high to catalyze release of glucose from the liver.
     E is incorrect because phosphorylase activity would be high to favor glycogenolysis over glycogen synthesis and

prevent storage of glucose when glucose needs to be exported to the exercising muscles.

Case 43-1

1.   **A** is incorrect because increased 1,25-$(OH)_2$-D would slightly increase plasma calcium levels. Both would then decrease PTH levels via negative feedback.
     B is incorrect because a decrease in PTH levels would lead to increased renal tubular phosphate reabsorption and hence decreased urine phosphate levels.
     C is incorrect because increased 1,25-$(OH)_2$-D and calcium levels would decrease 1,24-$(OH)_2$-D formation.
     D is correct because phosphate deficiency would decrease plasma and renal cortical phosphate levels. This would increase 1,25-$(OH)_2$-D synthesis.
     E is incorrect because bone formation would decrease as a result of lack of phosphate for mineralization.

2.   **A** is incorrect because the 1,25-$(OH)_2$-D increase would enhance the gastrointestinal absorption of calcium.
     B is correct because 1,25-$(OH)_2$-D levels would increase secondary to phosphate deficiency. This would tend to raise plasma calcium concentration, which with the rise in 1,25-$(OH)_2$-D values, would decrease PTH levels.
     C is incorrect because to the extent that the increased amount of 1,25-$(OH)_2$-D could increase bone resorption, this action would increase hydroxyproline excretion.
     D is incorrect because urine calcium excretion would increase, partly as a result of the decrease in PTH levels.
     E is incorrect because an increase in plasma calcium levels would increase calcitonin secretion.

Case 43-2

1.   **A** is incorrect because urine cyclic AMP levels would be increased by excess PTH action on renal tubular cells.
     B is incorrect because urine phosphate levels would be increased by excess PTH action on renal tubular cells.
     C is incorrect because excess PTH would increase the differentiation of osteoclast precursors into active osteoclasts and increase their number.
     D is incorrect because although excess PTH secretion stimulates bone resorption, the principle of coupling suggests that bone formation would secondarily increase.
     E is correct because excess PTH action on the kidney would decrease plasma phosphate levels.

2.   **A** is incorrect because the sudden cessation of excess PTH-stimulated bone resorption would shift the balance to the coupled excess of bone formation. This action would "pull" phosphate out of the plasma into bone and plasma phosphate levels would decrease.
     B is correct because nerve excitability had been previously suppressed by hypercalcemia and would increase rapidly. Plasma calcium levels might well drop below normal for reasons stated in **C** through **E,** and the patient might develop tetany.
     C is incorrect because unopposed bone formation would also "pull" calcium out of the plasma, plasma calcium levels would decrease, the renal filtered load of calcium would decrease, and urine calcium concentrations would decrease (despite a decrease in the tubular reabsorption of calcium).
     D is incorrect because neither PTH nor Ca^{++} primarily affects the heart rate.

E is incorrect because the loss of PTH would lower plasma calcium levels. Moreover, PTH does not directly affect the equilibrium between ionized and protein-bound calcium levels. However, withdrawal of the excess PTH would remove the hormone's inhibition of renal tubular bicarbonate reabsorption. This would tend to increase the pH of plasma, which in turn would decrease the ionized calcium fraction.

Case 44-1

1. **A** is incorrect because somatostatin inhibits GH secretion.
    B is incorrect because somatostatin inhibits GH secretion.
    C is incorrect because the combination of IGF-1 with its receptor mediates many of the actions on tissue growth of GH. **E** might also lead to a compensatory increase in IGF-1 levels, which would inhibit GH secretion via negative feedback.
    D is correct because increased GHRH receptor activity would generate excess cyclic AMP in the pituitary somatotroph, causing hyperplasia of somatotroph cells, excess GH secretion, and consequent tissue overgrowth.
    E is incorrect (see **C**).

2. **A** is incorrect because GHRH release would be decreased through negative feedback.
    B is incorrect because somatostatin release would be increased through negative feedback.
    C is correct because high levels of GH and its peripheral product IGF-1 would feed back negatively on GHRH neurons to decrease their activity and would feed back to increase the secretion of the GH inhibitor or somatostatin. Both actions would have the effect of trying to decrease the excess secretion of GH.
    D is incorrect (see **A** and **B**).
    E is incorrect because it does not take into account the regulatory pathways stimulated by GH.

3. **A** is incorrect because GH stimulates the production of some IGF-1 binding proteins.
    B is correct because high GH levels stimulate protein synthesis, putting the patient in positive nitrogen balance. Hence the amount of urea produced and excreted would be less than expected.
    C is incorrect because GH is an antagonist to insulin action. Therefore plasma glucose levels would be higher, not lower.
    D is incorrect because GH is an antagonist to insulin action. Therefore compensatory plasma insulin levels would be higher, not lower.
    E is incorrect because although glucose normally suppresses GH secretion, it would fail to do so when GH is secreted autonomously by a tumor. Plasma GH levels may even rise paradoxically after a glucose load.

Case 44-2

1. **A** is incorrect because the loss of water would increase the serum concentrations of sodium.
    B is incorrect because the loss of water would increase the serum concentrations of sodium and hence osmolality.
    C is incorrect because a water deficit of large magnitude would lead to a decrease in circulating blood volume and hence GFR, so blood urea concentrations would rise.
    D is incorrect because a low circulating blood volume would distend the cardiac atria less and decrease ANP production.
    E is correct because the sudden onset of such severe polyuria strongly suggests traumatic hypothalamic damage resulting in ADH deficiency. In the absence of ADH, the kidney cannot conserve water and the urine is very dilute (i.e., hypoosmolar).

2. **A** is incorrect because cyclic AMP is the second messenger for ADH action on the renal tubules and its levels would increase in the urine.
    B is correct because ADH has a vasoconstrictive effect through its V_1 receptor.
    C is incorrect because water retention caused by ADH would decrease serum osmolality.
    D is incorrect because ADH has no significant effect on the metabolism of potassium.
    E is incorrect because ADH stimulates adrenocorticotropin and hence cortisol secretion.

Case 45-1

1. **A** is incorrect because it is a product of T_4, which is present in excessive amounts. There may be relatively less excess T_3 than rT_3 to compensate for the decreased effects of the active T_3 metabolite on tissues.
    B is incorrect because it is a product of T_4, which is present in excessive amounts. There may be relatively less excess T_3 than rT_3 to compensate for the decreased effects of the active T_3 metabolite on tissues.
    C is correct because exogenous T_4 will feed back negatively on the hypothalamus-pituitary axis to decrease TRH and TSH secretion.
    D is incorrect because high levels of total T_4 will also increase levels of free T_4 unless thyroid binding globulin were also increased. If anything, this globulin may actually be slightly decreased.
    E is incorrect because high levels of total T_3 will also increase levels of free T_3 unless thyroid binding globulin were also increased. If anything, this globulin may actually be slightly decreased.

2. **A** is correct and largely accounts for the rapid heart rate.
    B is incorrect because hyperthyroidism causes defects in generating ATP and leads to reduced stores of creatine phosphate.
    C is incorrect because the activity of the sympathetic nervous system is diminished by excess thyroid hormone, and this is reflected in lower levels of plasma norepinephrine.
    D is incorrect because thyroid hormone increases tissue use of O_2 and production of CO_2, which causes vasodilation and lowers systemic vascular resistance.
    E is incorrect because the vasodilation noted in **D** decreases the diastolic blood pressure.

3. **A** is incorrect because a low TSH level (see previous question) would decrease iodide trap activity.
    B is correct because the low TSH stimulation (see previous question) would decrease the proteolysis of thyroglobulin and the release of T_4, so some colloid might initially accumulate.
    C is incorrect because it is dependent on the action of TSH, so peroxidase activity, the height of thyroid epithelial cells, and thyroglobulin synthesis would all decrease eventually, since TSH levels remain low.
    D is incorrect for the same reasons as **C**.
    E is incorrect for the same reasons as **C**.

Case 45-2

1. **A** is incorrect because it could cause hypothyroidism and thyroid enlargement secondary to the elevated TSH. The patient's thyroid gland uptake of a radioactive iodide isotope would be increased.

    B is incorrect because it could cause hypothyroidism and thyroid enlargement secondary to the elevated TSH. Thyroid uptake would be decreased because iodide could not be incorporated into tyrosine.

    C is correct because the patient's skeletal maturation would be retarded, not accelerated, by thyroxine deficiency.

    D is incorrect because water does accumulate in the tissues held by increased ground substance.

    E is incorrect because central nervous system development would be retarded in hypothyroidism.

2. **A** is incorrect because sensitivity to adrenergic stimulation would increase and so would heart rate, contractile force of cardiac muscle, and systolic blood pressure.

    B is incorrect for the same reasons as **A**.

    C is incorrect because linear growth at the epiphyseal centers of long bones and consequently height would increase.

    D is incorrect because diuresis of excess interstitial water would occur, and enhanced lipolysis would decrease adipose tissue; both effects would contribute to an initial weight loss.

    E is correct because O_2 use and CO_2 production would increase, necessitating increased ventilation.

Case 46-1

1. **A** is incorrect because the high cortisol levels will bind to the type 1 glucocorticoid (mineralocorticoid) receptor in the renal tubules and stimulate potassium excretion. As a result, serum potassium levels would be decreased.

    B is correct because ACTH is cosecreted with molecules that have melanocyte stimulating activity from a common precursor, proopiomelanocortin. Therefore high levels of expression of the ACTH gene cause increased skin pigmentation.

    C is incorrect because ACTH from the tumor is stimulating the adrenal cortex to secrete excessive amounts of cortisol. The cortisol suppresses both hypothalamic CRH and pituitary ACTH secretions via negative feedback.

    D is incorrect for the same reasons as **C**.

    E is incorrect because the mineralocorticoid effect of cortisol expands extracellular fluid volume, and this effect would suppress renin.

2. **A** is incorrect because the zona fasciculata will be hyperplastic, not atrophied, from stimulation by tumor ACTH.

    B is correct because excessive amounts of cortisol from tumor ACTH have blocked the effects of CRH on the pituitary adrenocorticotrophs, causing suppression of their ACTH release and loss of CRH's trophic effect on these cells; hence they atrophy and cannot immediately provide sufficient ACTH to meet the major stress of lung surgery. The patient's hypotension, fever, and anorexia reflect the resultant acute cortisol deficiency, as does the hyponatremia, which results from the retention of water given as intravenous infusions.

    C is incorrect because ADH deficiency would cause hypernatremia, not hyponatremia, and would not cause fever and anorexia.

    D is incorrect because the zona glomerulosa will be maintained via stimulation by tumor ACTH. However, renin and angiotensin levels will be decreased because of the expanded extracellular fluid volume.

    E is incorrect because the zona reticularis will also be hyperplastic from tumor ACTH stimulation. Dehydroepiandrosterone secretion may be excessive; because this steroid is largely an androgen precursor, it is likely the cause of the excessive hair growth.

Case 46-2

1. **A** is correct because this patient probably has hyperaldosteronism secondary to reduced blood flow in the right renal artery. This would increase renin secretion from the juxtaglomerular apparatus of the right kidney, in turn increasing angiotensin levels and aldosterone secretion.

    B is incorrect because it would be increased for the reasons stated in **A**. The elevated angiotensin level is causing the acute rise in blood pressure. The elevated aldosterone level would increase potassium excretion and cause hypokalemia.

    C is incorrect because it would be increased for the reasons stated in **A**. The elevated angiotensin level is causing the acute rise in blood pressure. The elevated aldosterone level would increase potassium excretion and cause hypokalemia.

    D is incorrect because it would be increased for the reasons stated in **A**. The elevated angiotensin level is causing the acute rise in blood pressure. The elevated aldosterone level would increase potassium excretion and cause hypokalemia.

    E is incorrect because high aldosterone levels would cause sodium retention and elevated extracellular fluid volume. The increased pressure on the atrial myocytes would increase the secretion of atrial natriuretic peptide.

2. **A** is incorrect because it is involved in generating the effects of the increased angiotensin level on the zona glomerulosa and causing hyperaldosteronism.

    B is incorrect for the same reasons as **A**.

    C is incorrect for the same reasons as **A**.

    D is incorrect for the same reasons as **A**.

    E is correct because angiotensin does not work through cyclic AMP as second messenger.

Case 47-1

1. **A** is incorrect because cortisol acts via gene transcription, and this mechanism is unlikely to cause abrupt hypertension.

    B is incorrect because the bradycardia would be an uncharacteristic effect of epinephrine, which typically causes tachycardia.

    C is correct because paroxysmal hypertensive episodes of such severity suggest sudden secretion of a catecholamine hormone. Norepinephrine causes extreme vasoconstriction, and the resultant hypertension activates baroreceptors and produces a reflex bradycardia. Stimulation of K^+ uptake into muscle cells would explain the slight hypokalemia.

    D is incorrect for the same reason as **A**.

    E is incorrect for the same reason as **A**.

    NOTE: All 3 of the steroid hormones (those in **A, D,** and **E**) could produce the hypokalemia by stimulating the excretion of renal potassium.

2. **A** is correct because it would rapidly relieve vasoconstriction in the renal, splanchnic, and cutaneous vascular beds and lower the blood pressure.

B is incorrect because reduced cardiac contractility would not decrease the diastolic blood pressure, which prevails during two thirds of the cardiac cycle.

C is incorrect because blocking the β_2 action could further decrease an already slow heart rate and might raise the blood pressure by leaving α_1 effects unopposed by the vasodilator action of the β_2-receptors.

D is incorrect because α_2-receptors are primarily located not in blood vessels but in platelets and gastrointestinal cells.

E is incorrect because the hypertension is not caused by an excessive amount of aldosterone; even if it were, the response to an aldosterone antagonist would be much too slow.

Case 47-2

1. **A** is incorrect because C peptide is released with insulin in response to hyperglycemia, not hypoglycemia. In addition, there would be no functioning β-cells left after 40 years of type 1 diabetes.

B is incorrect because although α-cells of the pancreatic islets are innervated by the sympathetic nervous system, these cells can also respond directly to a low ambient glucose level by releasing glucagon.

C is correct because epinephrine release by the adrenal medulla requires stimulation by the sympathetic splanchnic nerve with acetylcholine as the preganglionic mediator.

D is incorrect because cortisol release depends on ACTH, not sympathetic nerve stimulation.

E is incorrect because GH release is modulated both negatively (β-adrenergy) and positively (α-adrenergy) by the sympathetic nervous system at the hypothalamic, not the peripheral, level. Hypoglycemia triggers GH release by decreasing the release of somatostatin, an inhibitor of GH secretion.

2. **A** is incorrect because GH does not directly stimulate glycogenolysis.

B is correct because glucagon immediately stimulates glycogenolysis in the liver as well as the rapid release of glucose.

C is incorrect because cortisol does not directly stimulate glycogenolysis. Cortisol does increase gluconeogenesis, which would be necessary for a sustained increase in glucose.

D is incorrect because insulin lowers blood glucose levels.

E is incorrect because somatostatin would have counterproductive effects on the response to hypoglycemia by inhibiting glucagon and GH release.

Case 48-1

1. **A** is incorrect because the patient has excellent breast development, which requires estrogen.

B is correct because the external genitalia are not masculinized and there is no pubic or axillary hair—all effects that require androgen action.

C is incorrect because the patient lacks a uterus and upper vagina. That is, antimüllerian hormone has been present to suppress development of the müllerian ducts into female internal genitalia.

D is incorrect because FSH has no known direct effect on differentiation of the genitalia. In addition, the biological action of estrogen on the breast suggests FSH stimulation of either ovarian granulosa cells or analogous testicular cells.

E is incorrect because there is no known effect of IGF-1 on genital patterning. In addition, the patient is of normal height, implying normal growth hormone and IGF-1 action.

2. **A** is incorrect because the patient would be very unlikely to have a high testosterone level and evidence of antimüllerian hormone without a Y chromosome.

B is incorrect because a Y chromosome would direct formation of the testes, not the ovaries.

C is incorrect because LH levels would be elevated as a result of lack of negative feedback caused by inactive androgen receptors in the pituitary.

D is correct because this explains the absence of androgen effects despite a high testosterone level; the latter has resulted from the lack of negative feedback by testosterone on pituitary gonadotrophs that are also missing a competent androgen receptor.

E is incorrect because the patient's well-developed breasts show the presence of estrogen receptors.

Case 48-2

1. **A** is correct because although androgen stimulates the wolffian duct to develop into the vas deferens, it is local testosterone from the ipsilateral testis that is responsible. However, the patient has two X chromosomes, and no testes should be present. The patient likely has 21-hydroxylase deficiency (congenital adrenal hyperplasia), which was inadvertently treated for the first time with glucocorticoids at age 15. These suppressed the greatly elevated ACTH levels and reduced the high adrenal androgen levels; the latter had been suppressing LH and FSH secretion. Removal of these androgens permitted expression of her hypothalamic-pituitary-ovarian axis and menstrual bleeding.

B is incorrect because in an individual with two X chromosomes, ovaries will develop. Without testes, antimüllerian hormone will be lacking, and the müllerian duct will develop into a uterus and fallopian tubes.

C is incorrect for the same reasons as **B**.

D is incorrect for the same reasons as **B**.

E is incorrect because this individual with two X chromosomes has had enough masculinization of her external genitalia since birth to have led to assignment of the male gender and to rearing as a male. Because there are no testes, the requisite androgen derives from the adrenal zona reticularis (see **A**).

2. **A** is incorrect because no steroid hormone directly causes skin to darken.

B is incorrect for the same reasons as **A**.

C is incorrect for the same reasons as **A**.

D is incorrect because LH has no MSH activity.

E is correct because ACTH has MSH activity.

Case 49-1

1. **A** is incorrect because the lack of the pubertal increase in testosterone level, stimulated by GnRH and LH secretion, leads to failure of the epiphyses (growth centers) to close. Hence the long bones continue to grow slowly for years after the normal closure time of 15 to 18 years, leading to long arms and legs relative to height.

B is incorrect because sexual differentiation occurs before the Leydig cells of the testes become dependent on fetal pituitary LH secretion stimulated by fetal GnRH. The testosterone necessary for the male pattern of external genitalia is secreted by the fetal testis in response to chorionic gonadotropin secreted by fetal placental cells.

C is incorrect because the lack of pubertal testosterone and its product DHT would not allow the prostate to develop to even a normal size.

D is correct because lack of FSH to initiate spermatogenesis would lead to its absence and to small testes, since 80% of testicular volume is accounted for by the seminiferous (spermatogenic) tubules.

E is incorrect because without FSH, the spermatid stage of spermatogenesis is unlikely to be reached.

2. **A** is incorrect because testosterone produced in high concentrations by LH stimulation within the testis must synergize with FSH to initiate and maintain spermatogenesis.

B is incorrect because neither it nor LH alone can sustain spermatogenesis. However, some men with this problem produce sperm if both gonadotropins are injected in proper doses with proper timing.

C is incorrect because neither it nor FSH alone can sustain spermatogenesis. However, some men with this problem produce sperm if both gonadotropins are injected in proper doses with proper timing.

D is incorrect because constant GnRH stimulation of the pituitary gonadotrophs down-regulates GnRH receptors and leads to LH and FSH deficiency.

E is correct because pulsatile stimulation of the pituitary will generate pulses of gonadotropins to the testis, which will result in the optimum intratesticular hormonal environment to initiate and support spermatogenesis.

Case 49-2

1. **A** is incorrect because inhibin is a product of FSH action.

B is incorrect because there is presently no known relationship between FSH action and antimüllerian hormone secretion.

C is incorrect because inhibin has less of a negative-feedback effect on LH secretion than on FSH secretion.

D is correct because FSH action on Sertoli cells would be lacking. This would lead to low inhibin levels. The lack of negative feedback of inhibin on the pituitary gonadotrophs would then result in elevated FSH levels.

E is incorrect because FSH action on the testis has no direct effect on testosterone secretion.

2. **A** is incorrect because testosterone levels would remain normal with selective loss of FSH action but retention of LH action.

B is incorrect because LDL is increased by testosterone and would remain normal in testosterone deficiency.

C is correct because without FSH, spermatogenesis would be reduced; hence sperm count would decrease below normal.

D is incorrect because red blood cell production is increased by testosterone, which is not deficient in this case.

E is incorrect because testosterone increases bone density, but testosterone is not deficient here.

Case 50-1

1. **A** is correct because this is classic, stress-induced amenorrhea with increased CRH secretion suppressing GnRH release.

B is incorrect because prolactin inhibits GnRH release.

C is incorrect because dopamine inhibits GnRH release.

D is incorrect because endorphin inhibits GnRH release.

E is incorrect because α-adrenergic pathways stimulate GnRH release.

2. **A** is incorrect because estrogen increases endometrial hyperplasia.

B is incorrect because estrogen increases vaginal epithelial cornification.

C is incorrect because estrogen increases secretion of an elastic cervical mucus.

D is incorrect because insofar as is known, there is no direct effect of estrogens on libido. Androgens are stimulatory. However, prolonged CRH excess might decrease the patient's libido.

E is correct because the estrogen-sensitive ductal tissue of the breast would partly atrophy.

Case 50-2

1. **A** is incorrect because progesterone helps elicit the LH surge and is required to support a conceptus.

B is incorrect because inhibin A is a product of the corpus luteum and is probably deficient in this woman.

C is correct because the LH surge suggests that the patient probably ovulates, but after the ovum is fertilized, the zygote probably fails to implant. This suggests inadequate progesterone secretion from the corpus luteum. This causes poor preparation of the endometrium to support a conceptus adequately.

D is incorrect because without a well-functioning dominant follicle, no LH surge would occur.

E is incorrect because a late rise in estradiol during the follicular phase is essential for an LH surge to occur.

2. **A** is incorrect because this is a normal finding on day 28, when corpus luteum functioning has normally just ceased and no dominant follicle has yet formed.

B is incorrect because this is a normal finding on day 1, when corpus luteum functioning has normally just ceased and no dominant follicle has yet formed.

C is incorrect because there is no notable variation in prolactin secretion during the menstrual cycle. Moreover, prolactin helps increase LH receptors, which would enhance corpus luteum function.

D is correct because with a normally functioning corpus luteum, plasma progesterone levels would be greatly elevated on day 21.

E is incorrect because plasma progesterone levels are at a relatively low point normally on day 7.

Index